Research Anthology on Food Waste Reduction and Alternative Diets for Food and Nutrition Security

Information Resources Management Association
USA

Volume I

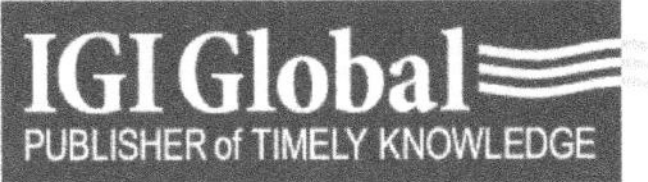

Published in the United States of America by
IGI Global
Engineering Science Reference (an imprint of IGI Global)
701 E. Chocolate Avenue
Hershey PA, USA 17033
Tel: 717-533-8845
Fax: 717-533-8661
E-mail: cust@igi-global.com
Web site: http://www.igi-global.com

Library of Congress Cataloging-in-Publication Data

Names: Information Resources Management Association, editor.
Title: Research anthology on food waste reduction and alternative diets for
  food and nutrition security / Information Resources Management
  Association, editor.
Description: Hershey, PA : Engineering Science Reference, an imprint of IGI
  Global, [2021] | Includes bibliographical references and index. |
  Summary: "This book explores methods for reducing waste and cutting food
  loss in order to help the environment and support local communities as
  well as solve issues including that of land space. It also provides
  vital research on the development of plant-based foods, meat-alternative
  diets, and nutritional outcomes"-- Provided by publisher.
Identifiers: LCCN 2020009128 (print) | LCCN 2020009129 (ebook) | ISBN
  9781799853541 (hardcover) | ISBN 9781799853558 (ebook)
Subjects: LCSH: Food industry and trade--Waste disposal.
Classification: LCC TD899.F585 R47 2020 (print) | LCC TD899.F585 (ebook)
  | DDC 363.72/88--dc23
LC record available at https://lccn.loc.gov/2020009128
LC ebook record available at https://lccn.loc.gov/2020009129

British Cataloguing in Publication Data
A Cataloguing in Publication record for this book is available from the British Library.

For electronic access to this publication, please contact: eresources@igi-global.com.

List of Contributors

Table of Contents

Section 2
Food Supply Chain Management

Section 3
Repurposing Wasted Food

Section 4
Sustainable Agricultural Production

Section 5
Sustainable Consumption and Alternative Diets

Preface

Of the utmost importance in every country are the accessibility, availability, and stability of food. As increasing populations, reduction in farmland, climate change, improper transportation of food, unbalanced dieting habits, increased cases of foodborne illness, and other factors have put a strain on resources, issues with food waste, food scarcity, and food safety have increased. It has become imperative for sustainable agriculture to be discussed and transformed through the use of technologies that can increase efficiency and crop output. Similarly, food supply chains and food preservation must be reexamined to procure solutions that mitigate the amount of food that is wasted due to such factors as improper refrigeration or handling methods that render the products unsafe for consumption.

Alternatively, this distinctive reference source also looks past the technological and sustainable methods that can be applied to the production and distribution of food and incorporates applications for repurposing food that is wasted. This innovative research examines the conversion of waste byproduct into livestock feed, value-added products, and more. Additionally, the content includes a unique perspective on eating habits and the ways in which society can transform to include more sustainable and environmentally-friendly food products into their diets. Such research includes the analysis of plant-based proteins, soybeans, insects, and new meat alternatives that present sustainable food consumption options without sacrificing nutrition security as well. The book serves to incorporate case studies and applications in these areas in order to assist in reducing food waste, increasing consumer awareness of their food choices, and improving the quality of the farming industry and agricultural technologies of the future.

Thus, the *Research Anthology on Food Waste Reduction and Alternative Diets* seeks to fill the void for an all-encompassing and comprehensive reference book covering the latest and emerging research, concepts, and theories for the better understanding of food waste reduction and management and the technologies being implemented for both. This two-volume reference collection of reprinted IGI Global book chapters and journal articles that have been handpicked by the editor and editorial team of this research anthology on this topic will empower farmers, experts in the agricultural industry, nutritionists, supply chain managers, food safety experts, technologists, policymakers, professionals, students, researchers, and academicians with a strong understanding of critical issues within food waste reduction by exploring preservation technologies, food safety, food supply chain management and improvement, along with the conversion of waste into useful byproducts and the ethical production and consumption of food.

The *Research Anthology on Food Waste Reduction and Alternative Diets* is organized into five sections that provide comprehensive coverage of important topics. The sections are:

1. Food Safety and Preservation Technologies;
2. Food Supply Chain Management;

3.   Repurposing Wasted Food;
4.   Sustainable Agricultural Production;
5.   Sustainable Consumption and Alternative Diets.

The following paragraphs provide a summary of what to expect from this invaluable reference tool.

Section 1, "Food Safety and Preservation Technologies," opens this comprehensive reference work with research on the latest tools and technologies being used to safely preserve various types of food products. Opening this book is "Food Quality and Safety Regulation Systems at a Glance," by Profs. Arvind Kumar Singh and Dixit V. Bhalani of Central Salt and Marine Chemicals Research Institute, India and Prof. Poonam Singh Thakur from Rashtrasant Tukadoji Maharaj Nagpur University, India, which explains the role of various assessment agencies and their rights and workflows in ensuring the quality and safety of food products. The next chapter, "Ecological Chemistry Aspects of Food Safety," written by Prof. Rodica Sturza of the Technical University of Moldova, Moldova, reflects on the studies carried out over the last decade, with the subject being soil, water, vegetal raw materials, and wines from the Republic of Moldova. Following this is the chapter "Food Safety and Climate Change: Case of Mycotoxins," by Prof. Abdellah Zinedine of Chouaib Doukkali University, Morocco and Prof. Samira El Akhdari from the Ministry of National Education, Morocco, which gives an overview about the major mycotoxins, masked mycotoxins, and emerging mycotoxins found on various grains and agricultural commodities and their negative impacts. The chapter "Investigation Into Fermentation: A Journey Into Cultural Relevance and Mindful Eating," by Prof. Kris Krautkremer of Kingsport City Schools, USA and Prof. Cerrone Renee Foster of East Tennessee State University, USA, focuses on fermentation, its role in cellular respiration, and practical uses of fermentation for food preservation and nutrient bioavailability. The next chapter, "Technologies for Monitoring the Safety of Perishable Food Products," authored by Prof. Pedro Dinis from Gaspar University of Beira Interior, Portugal; Prof. Pedro Dinho da Silva of the University of Beira Interior, Portugal; Profs. Luís Pinto Andrade and José Nunes from the Polytechnic Institute of Castelo Branco, Portugal; and Prof. Christophe Espírito Santo from the Agrofood Technological Center, Portugal, addresses food safety issues, namely factors related to microbial growth responsible for food deterioration, and modern monitoring technologies. The chapter "Closed Refrigerated Display Cabinets: Is It Worth It for Food Quality?" by Prof. Onrawee Laguerre of the National Research Institute of Science and Technology for Environment and Agriculture IRSTEA, France and Prof. Nattawut Chaomuang from King Mongkut's Institute of Technology Ladkrabang, Thailand, presents state-of-the-art studies on refrigerated display cabinets with further information on the airflow and temperature profile in the closed display cabinet, the influence of the presence of doors, and the frequency of door openings and the room temperature. The following chapter, "Nanocomposites in the Food Packaging Industry: Recent Trends and Applications," by Prof. Dheeraj Kumar of the National Institute of Technology, Durgapur, India and Prof. Md. Farrukh from the Echelon Institute of Technology, India, focuses on nano-composite materials that enhance the antimicrobial, mechanical, thermal, as well as barrier properties against the migrating element in the food packaging system. "Non-Thermal Food Preservation Methods in the Meat Industry," by Prof. Basak Gokce Col of Istanbul Gelisim University, Turkey and Profs. Sergen Tuggum and Seydi Yıkmış of Tekirdağ Namık Kemal University, Turkey, focuses on two novel approaches to meat preservation: non-thermal Pulsed Electric Field and Atmospheric Pressure Cold Plasma APCP Technologies. Next is "Non-Thermal Preservation of Dairy Products: Principles, Recent Advances, and Future Prospects," written by Profs. Alperen Koker and İlhami Okur from Middle East Technical University, Turkey; Prof. Sebnem Ozturkoglu-Budak of Ankara University, Turkey; and Prof. Hami

Alpas from Middle East Technical University, Turkey, which gives general principles of non-thermal techniques, current applications with dairy products, and recent advances in the dairy industry. The following chapter, "Novel Packaging Technologies in Dairy Products: Principles and Recent Advances," by Profs. Sebnem Ozturkoglu-Budak and Nazli Turkmen from Ankara University, Turkey informs about the general principles of the novel packaging techniques, such as nanotechnology, active packaging, and intelligent/smart packaging, and their current applications in dairy technology. "Biopreservatives for Improved Shelf-Life and Safety of Dairy Products: Biopreservatives for Dairy Products," by Profs. Sarang Dilip Pophaly, Tejinder Pal Singh, and Ruby Siwach of the College of Dairy Science and Food Technology, India provides a scientific background on bio preservation, a detailed look at its functionality, as well as giving food applications and further commercial aspects of bio preservatives derived from microbial sources. Concluding this section is the chapter "Resource-Saving Technology of Dehydration of Fruit and Vegetable Raw Materials: Scientific Rationale and Cost Efficiency," by Profs. Inna Simakova, Victoria Strizhevskaya, and Igor Vorotnikov of Saratov State Vavilov Agrarian University, Russia and Prof. Fedor Pertsevyi of Sumy National Agrarian University, Ukraine. It presents a solution to the insufficient consumption of fruits and vegetables in the diet of modern people with the development of technology for the dehydration of fruit and vegetables applicable directly at the harvesting site.

Section 2, "Food Supply Chain Management," presents extensive coverage on the latest findings in identifying and managing risks in food supply chain management as well as providing coverage on the technological advancements for managing food loss and waste. Starting off this section is the chapter "Managing Risk in Global Food Supply Chains: Improving Food Security and Sustainability" by Prof. Marco A. Miranda-Ackerman from the Universidad Autónoma de Baja Callifornia, Mexico; Profs. Betzabé Ruiz-Morales and Irma Cristina Espitia-Moreno from the Universidad Michoacana de San Nicolás de Hidalgo, Mexico; Prof. Citlali Colin-Chávez of CONACYT, Centro de Investigación en Alimentación y Desarrollo, Mexico & Centro de Innovación y Desarrollo Agroalimentario de Michoacán, Mexico; and Prof. Karina Cecilia Arredondo-Soto from the Universidad Autónoma de Baja Callifornia, Mexico, which presents an overview of the main risks involved in global food supply chains, as well as some techniques for risk management. The next chapter, "Risks in Sustainable Food Supply Chain Management," written by Prof. Yogesh Kumar Sharma of Graphic Era University, India; Prof. Sachin Kumar Mangla from the University of Plymouth, UK; and Prof. Pravin P. Patil of Graphic Era University, India, discusses the risks in the adoption of sustainable food supply chain management SFSCM and ranks the risks by using the Fuzzy Analytic Hierarchy Process FAHP technique. "Building a Sustainable Food Supply Chain and Managing Food Losses," by Profs. A D Nuwan Gunarathne, D. G. Navaratne, M. L. S. Gunaratne, Amanda Erasha, and Yasasi Tharindra Perera of the University of Sri Jayewardenepura, Sri Lanka, provides a conceptual model, incorporating stakeholder management and other behavioral aspects, to build a sustainable food supply chain while minimizing the food waste that occurs at different stages. The following chapter, "Logistic Strategies to Minimize Losses and Waste in Food Supply Chains," authored by Prof. Betzabé Ruiz-Morales from the Universidad Michoacana de San Nicolás de Hidalgo, Mexico; Prof. Marco A. Miranda-Ackerman of Universidad Autónoma de Baja Callifornia, Mexico; and Prof. Irma Cristina Espitia-Moreno from Universidad Michoacana de San Nicolás de Hidalgo, Mexico, proposes sustainable supply chains in agrifoods, achieved through logistical strategies to minimize food waste and losses. "From Information Sharing to Information Utilization in Food Supply Chains," by Prof. Kasper Kiil from Norwegian University of Science and Technology, Trondheim, Norway & Aalborg University, Aalborg, Denmark; Prof. Hans-Henrik Hvolby from Aalborg University, Aalborg, Denmark & Norwegian University of Science and Technology, Trondheim, Norway; Profs. Jacques

Trienekens and Behzad Behdani from Wageningen University, Wageningen, The Netherlands; and Prof. Jan Ola Strandhagen of Norwegian University of Science and Technology, Trondheim, Norway, uses a case study methodology and literature review to identify the characteristics of information sharing, and conceptualize how to move from information sharing to information utilization in food supply chains. The next chapter, "IoT-Based Cold Chain Logistics Monitoring," written by Profs. Afreen Mohsin and Siva S. Yellampalli of UTL Technologies, India aims to reduce the extent of human presence along the cold chain and fill existing gaps through the use a powerful tool in the form of the IoT. "An Exploratory Study on Blockchain Application in a Food Processing Supply Chain to Reduce Waste," by Ms. Emily Anne Carey from Samsung Electronics, UK and Dr. Nachiappan Subramanian an Independent Researcher, UK, uses a case study approach to explore the feasibility of using blockchain in the beef supply chain to reduce waste. Next is "Performance Evaluation of Food Cold Chain Logistics Enterprise Based on the AHP and Entropy," by Profs. Yazhou Xiong, Jie Zhao, and Jie Lan from Hubei Polytechnic University, Huangshi, China, evaluates the system of food cold chain logistics from four aspects, including the financial management, cold chain logistics process, development ability and customer service, based on the analytic hierarchy process. The chapter "A Circular Economy Perspective for Dairy Supply Chains," by Profs. Dimitrios Vlachos and Christina Paraskevopoulou of Aristotle University of Thessaloniki, Greece, provides a CE perspective for the dairy supply chain by identifying and analyzing the associated technologies and strategies through a literature review taxonomy based on the related stage of the supply chain. The following chapter, "Consumer Purchase Preference for the Perception of Quality of Perishable Products in a Smart City," by Profs. Iván Alonso Rebollar-Xochicale and Fernando Maldonado-Azpeitia from the Universidad Autónoma de Querétaro, Mexico, discusses the consumers role in determining food waste along the supply chain and how companies can correctly implement supply chains in smart cities for perishable products. "Methodology for the Design of Traceability System in Food Assistance Supply Chains: Case Bienestarina, Colombia," by Prof. Feizar Javier Rueda-Velasco of Universidad Distrital "Francisco José de Caldas", Colombia; Prof. Angie Monsalve-Salamanca from Universidad Nacional de Colombia, Colombia; and Prof. Wilson Adarme-Jaimes from Universidad Nacional de Colombia, Colombia, proposes a methodology for the design of traceability systems in FAP which allows increasing supply chain visibility, coordination between deliveries and social conditions, and therefore, possible impacts on public policy implications. Next is "Analyzing Sustainable Food Supply Chain Management Challenges in India," written by Profs. Pravin P. Patil, Sachin Kumar Mangla, Yogesh Kumar Sharma, and Surbhi Uniyal from Graphic Era University, India. It identifies 11 challenges in sustainable food supply chain management and uses the integration of fuzzy with DEMATEL to analyze the challenges in SFSCM. "Wastage and Cold Chain Infrastructure Relationship in Indian Food Supply Chain: A Study From Farm to Retail," by Profs. Saurav Negi and Neeraj Anand from the University of Petroleum and Energy Studies, India, outlines the extent of fruits and vegetables waste in India (at various stages from farm to retail) and its ramifications on food production and safety in the cold chain sector. The chapter "Perishable Goods Supply Cold Chain Management in India," authored by Prof. Anju Bharti from Maharaja Agrasen Institute of Management Studies, India and Prof. Arun Mittal of Birla Institute of Technology, India, explores the cold chain potential in India that still remains untapped and the challenges the country faces in becoming a part of the global trade in perishable products and quality produce. This section ends with the chapter "Factors That impact Quality during the Transportation of Tomatoes: Evidence From India," by Profs. Saurav Negi, Neeraj Anand, and Shantanu Trivedi from the University of Petroleum and Energy Studies, Dehradun, India. It provides information on the current status of tomato transportation and related issues and challenges in India and the ways in which stakeholders can improve efficiency in the transportation stage of the supply chain.

Section 3, "Repurposing Wasted Food," reveals the latest research on the history, process, technologies, and conversion of food waste into value added byproducts. The opening chapter, "Food Waste Reduction Towards Food Sector Sustainability," by Profs. Giovanni Lagioia, Vera Amicarelli,, Teodoro Gallucci, and Christian Bux from the University of Bari Aldo Moro, Italy, reviews the magnitude of FLW at a global and European level and its environmental, social, and economic implications as well as using Material Flow Analysis to support and improve FLW management and application. The following chapter, "Utilization and Management of Food Waste," by Prof. Shriram M. Naikare of SNDT College of Home Science, India, explores how the different types of food industrial waste can be converted into byproducts for livestock feed, bioenergy production, artificial fertilizer and more. Next is "Various Approaches for Food Waste Processing and Its Management," by Prof. Priyanka Harishchandra Tripathi from National Institute of Pathology ICMR, India and Profs. Anupam Pandey, Ashutosh Paliwal, Ankita Harishchandra Tripathi, Satish Chandra Pandey, Tushar Joshi, and Veena Pande from Kumaun University Nainital, India, looks into global food wastage and the approaches to manage and reduce the high environmental, social, and economic impacts associated with this type of waste. "Value-Added Products From Food Waste," written by Dr. Baban Baburao Gunjal of Sunrise Biotech Organisation, India, explains how the management of food waste can be done by conversion to different value-added products. The chapter "Microbe Mediated Bioconversion of Fruit Waste Into Value Added Products: Microbes in Fruit Waste Management," by Profs. and Thazeem Basheer from Bharathiar University, India, summarizes microbe mediated fermentative utilization of fruit waste for the production of value-added products like organic acid, single cell protein, bioplastics, enzymes, and biogas. The next chapter, "Industrially Important Enzymes Production From Food Waste: An Alternative Approach to Land Filling," by Prof. Madhuri Santosh Bhandwalkar of S. B. B. Alias Appasaheb Jedhe College, India, focuses on the production of industrially important enzymes from food waste such as pectinase, peroxidase, lipase, glucoamylase, and protease. "Recent Advances in Waste Cooking Oil Management and Applications for Sustainable Environment," by Prof. Ching Thian Tye from Universiti Sains Malaysia, Malaysia, discusses the management of waste cooking oil WCO in a sustainable manner and provides an overview of the most recent approaches in WCO recycling and applications. "Impacts of Food Industrial Wastes on Soil and Its Utilization as Novel Approach for Value Addition," by Prof. Ifra Ashraf from SKUAST-K, India; Prof. Shazia Ramzan of University of Kashmir, India; and Prof. Nowsheeba Rashid from Amity University, India, describes the new, innate, and monetary sources of colorants, protein, dietary fiber, flavoring, antimicrobials, and antioxidants, which can be utilized in the food industry as a basis of natural food additives. The next chapter, "Allocation Optimization Problem for Peruvian Food Bank," by Prof. Ricardo Campos-Caycho, Renzo A. Benavente-Sotelo, Yasser A. Hidalgo-Gómez, Christian A. Blas-Bazán, Pamela Ivonne Borja-Ramos, Stephanie M. Dueñas-Calderón, Patricia Elkfury-Cominges, Pamela Arista-Yampi, and Jorge Luis Yupanqui-Chacón from Pontificia Universidad Católica del Perú, Peru, uses the tools of operations research to determine a solution to the problem of maximizing the combination of food orders to be distributed based on their total nutritional value to the beneficiaries, seeking maximum coverage and minimum logistic costs. The final chapter in this section, "Economic and Environmental Costs of Meat Waste in the US," by Profs. Nicholas Hardersen and Jadwiga R. Ziolkowska of University of Oklahoma, USA, monetizes the annual costs of natural resources including water, land, and energy, as well as emissions of methane and nitrous oxide embedded in wasted meat in the United States.

Section 4, "Sustainable Agricultural Production," discusses leading research on the issues, challenges, and benefits in smart farming and the tools, techniques, and technologies that have been studied in a variety of regions to improve agricultural production. Opening this chapter is "Tropospheric Ozone Pollution, Agriculture, and Food Security," by Prof. Pooja Singh from Banaras Hindu University, India; Prof. Abhijit Sarkar of the University of Gour Banga, India; and Prof. Sambit Datta from the University of Calcutta, India, reviews the available literature and discusses the impact of tropospheric ozone 03 gas on modern day agricultural production worldwide. The next chapter, "Technical Equipment of Agricultural Production: The Effects for Food Security," written by Prof. Mikail Khudzhatov from Peoples' Friendship University of Russia RUDN University, Russia and Prof. Alexander Arskiy of Russian Academy of Personnel Support for the Agroindustrial Complex, Russia, analyzes the current state of the world market of agricultural machinery, develops the methodology of assessment of the competitiveness of agricultural machinery in the domestic market, and elaborates the definition of effective methods of management of logistics costs at the operation of agricultural machinery. The chapter "Issues and Challenges in Smart Farming for Sustainable Agriculture," by Profs. Immanuel Zion Ramdinthara and Shanthi Bala P. of Pondicherry University, India, focuses on sustainable agriculture and covers the benefits, where it can be used, and common practices. Next is "Disrupting Agriculture: The Status and Prospects for AI and Big Data in Smart Agriculture," by Profs. Omar F. El-Gayar and Martinson Q. Ofori from Dakota State University, USA. It conducts a systematic review focusing on big data and artificial intelligence in agriculture and emphasis the potential, key drivers, and challenges of its use. "Agbiotech, Sustainability, and Food Security Connection to Public Health," by Prof. Ike Valentine Iyioke from Michigan State University, USA, includes an integrative model of food security linking sociocultural, public policy, and ecological aspects to public health and analyzes both sides of the argument for and against agricultural biotechnology. The following chapter, "Agricultural Cooperatives for Sustainable Development of Rural Territories and Food Security: Morocco's Experience," by Prof. Maria Fedorova from Omsk State Technical University, Russia and Prof. Ismail Taaricht of Cadi Ayyad University, Morocco, uses the Moroccan agriculture cooperatives as a case of cooperative longevity and survival in order to observe the evolution and processes of adaptation to the distinct economic, social, and environmental demands of a broad range of member-owners. The next chapter, "Towards the Development of Salt-Tolerant Potato," written by Prof. John Okoth Omondi from Ben Gurion University of the Negev, Israel, explores the salinity management of potatoes and breeding and genetic engineering towards the development of salt-tolerant potatoes. "Local Production-Based Dietary Supplement Distribution in Emerging Countries: Bienestarina Distribution in Colombia," by Prof. Jesus Gonzalez-Feliu from Mines Saint-Etienne, France; Prof. Carlos Osorio-Ramírez of National University of Colombia, Colombia; Prof. Laura Palacios-Arguello from Mines Saint-Etienne, France; and Prof. Carlos Alberto Talamantes from Autonomous University of Ciudad Juarez, Mexico, presents an analysis of the Bienestarina supply chain based on the four elements: steering, organization, development, and financial issues. The chapter "State Support of Agricultural Production in Emerging Countries as a Tool to Ensure Food Security," by Profs. Anna Ivolga and Marina Lescheva from Stavropol State Agrarian University, Russian Federation and Prof. Oleksandr Labenko from National University of Life and Environmental Sciences of Ukraine, Ukraine, explores how agricultural protectionism and support of domestic farmers affect the level of food security on the emerging markets in the conditions of expanding globalization and liberalization of trade in food. The following chapter, "New Approaches to Agricultural Production Management in the Arctic: Organic Farming and Food Security," by Prof. Mykhailo Guz from the National University of Life and Environmental Sciences of Ukraine, Ukraine, discusses the potential of organic farming as a solution to the food insecurity problem and sustainable development in the rural northern areas in the Arctic. Next is "Produce Internationally, Consume Locally: Changing Paradigm of China's Food Security Policy," by Prof. Vasilii Erokhin of Harbin Engineering University, China. It discusses how China's Belt and Road Initiative may serve improving food security of the country by establishing of a predictable system of agricultural production and trade across Eurasia, particularly with the involvement of land-abundant Russia and the countries of Central Asia. The chapter "Financing and Training Imperatives for Resilient Agriculture in Nigeria," by Augustine Odinakachukwu Ejiogu from Imo State University, Nigeria, focuses on the financing and training imperatives for resilient agriculture in Nigeria and proposes a twin-track approach to addressing the challenge of agriculture as a development issue by both encouraging agri-business and supporting the large population of smallholders. The next chapter, "Determinants of Agricultural Production in Romania: A Panel Data Approach," by Profs. Alina Zaharia and Simona Roxana Pătărlăgeanu of The Bucharest University of Economic Studies, Romania, examines a panel data approach to determine the contribution of several factors on the agricultural output in terms of value and of yield in Romania. Closing this section is "Farm Security for Food Security: Dealing With Farm Theft in the Caribbean Region," by Profs. Wendy-Ann Isaac, Wayne Ganpat, and Michael Joseph, The University of Trinidad and Tobago, Trinidad and Tobago, examines the current status of farm theft in the Caribbean region, explores some of the main factors influencing farm theft, reviews some of the strategies attempted in the Caribbean and other places around the world, and makes several suggestions to create a more secure food region.

Section 5, "Sustainable Consumption and Alternative Diets," concludes this reference work with research on the way consumers choose their food and diets, the alternative diet types and foods that can be consumed to increase sustainability and the effects of consumption choices in climate change and possible solutions for the future. Opening the last section of this reference book is "A Review on Impact of Changing Climate on Sustainable Food Consumption," by Prof. Tosin Kolajo Gbadegesin from the University of Ibadan, Nigeria. It examines the impact of the changing climate on sustainable food consumption by identifying the effects of this changing climate on nutrition, food production, and food consumption, and also provides recommendations on sustainable food consumption measures. The next chapter, "Comparing the Effects of Unsustainable Production and Consumption of Food on Health and Policy Across Developed and Less Developed Countries," by Prof. Josue Mbonigaba of the University of KwaZulu-Natal, South Africa, aims to document the evidence of the difference in nature and extent of unsustainable food consumption across high-income countries HICs and low-income countries LICs. Following this chapter is "Sustainable Food Consumption in the Neoliberal Order: Challenges and Policy Implications," by Profs. Luke A. Amadi and Henry E. Alapiki from the University of Port Harcourt, Nigeria, which turns to the original impetus of sustainable food consumption and the question of how neoliberal order can be reconciled with the need to save the ecology. Next is "Food and Environment: A Review on the Sustainability of Six Different Dietary Patterns," by Prof. Pedro Pinheiro Gomes of National Statistics Institute, Portugal. It assesses the impacts of six dietary patterns while emphasizing protein overconsumption and sustainability of food systems and the nutritional disparities existent within these different patterns and the potential to make changes. "Re-Thinking Meat: How Climate Change Is Disrupting the Food Industry," by Dr. Jeff Anhang from The World Bank Group, USA, describes the ideal that sacrificing meat will benefit the climate; however, these efforts have not been linked to reduced meat consumption and instead this chapter offers alternative modes to disrupting meat production and consumption. The chapter "Normality, Naturalness, Necessity, and Nutritiousness of the New Meat Alternatives," by Prof. Diana Bogueva from Curtin University, Australia and Prof. Kurt Schmidinger of

Vienna University, Austria, examines the social readiness and acceptability of new meat alternatives as normal, natural, necessary, and nutritious amongst Gen Y and Gen Z consumers. The following chapter, "New Meat Without Livestock," by Profs. Dora Marinova and Diana Bogueva of Curtin University, Australia and Prof. Kurt Schmidinger from the University of Vienna, Austria, summarizes the global problems associated with livestock production and meat consumption and shows solution strategies through replacing animal products with plant-based alternatives. "Application of the Dietary Processed Sulfur Supplementation for Enhancing Nutritional and Functional Properties of Meat Products," by Prof. Chi-Ho Lee from Konkuk University, South Korea, focuses on strategies to investigate the changes in physical, physicochemical, and microbial properties of meat and meat products in dietary processed sulfur fed animals. Another chapter, "Nutritional Benefits of Selected Plant-Based Proteins as Meat Alternatives," written by Prof. Seydi Yıkmış from Tekirdağ Namık Kemal University, Turkey; Prof. Ramazan Mert Atan of Bandırma Onyedi Eylül University, Turkey; Prof. Nursena Kağan from Tekirdağ Namık Kemal University, Turkey; Prof. Levent Gülüm of Abant İzzet Baysal University, Turkey; Prof. Harun Aksu from Istanbul University – Cerrahpaşa, Turkey; and Prof. Mehmet Alpaslan from Tekirdağ Namık Kemal University, Turkey, describes the nutritional benefits and current uses of nine non-animal protein sources and the health benefits arising from replacing animal protein. The chapter "Understanding Gender Identities and Food Preferences to Increase the Consumption of a Plant-Based Diet With Heuristics," by Prof. Estela Seabra from The New School, USA, discerns existent food preferences and their correlation with women and men, and gender biases, in America and accounts for gender norms, cultural roles, and subconscious behavior in these decisions. The following chapter, "Lifelong Consumption of Plant-Based GM Foods: Is It Safe?" authored by Prof. Matthew Chidozie Ogwu of Seoul National University, South Korea, seeks to highlight general concerns and potential lifelong effects of consuming GM plant-based food including socioeconomic effects, development of new diseases, and potential effects on the environment and biodiversity. The chapter "Nutritional Properties of Edible Insects," by Prof. Anna K. Żołnierczyk from Wrocław University of Environmental and Life Sciences, Poland, explores how the consumption of edible insects can build a well-balanced diet, the nutrients within insects, and the benefits of insect production as compared to livestock production. Another chapter, "The Nutritional and Health Potential of Blackjack Bidens pilosa l.: A Review – Promoting the Use of Blackjack for Food," by Dr. Rose Mujila Mboya an Independent Researcher, Pietermaritzburg, South Africa, reviews the advantages and disadvantages of blackjack and argues for the deliberation of promoting its use for food. "Special Legume-Based Food as a Solution to Food and Nutrition Insecurity Problem in the Arctic," by Prof. Liudmila Nadtochii of ITMO University, Russia; Prof. Anna Veber from Omsk State Agrarian University, Russia; Prof. Svetlana Leonova of Bashkir State Agrarian University, Russia; Prof. Nina Kazydub from Omsk State Agrarian University, Russia; and Prof. Inna Simakova from Saratov State Agrarian University, Russia, discusses the potential of legume-based food products to contribute to the improvement of food and nutrition security in northern communities. Another chapter, "Soybeans Consumption and Production in China: Sustainability Perspective," by Profs. Dora Marinova and Xiumei Guo from Curtin University, Australia; Prof. Amzad Hossain of Curtin University, Australia & Rajshahi University, Bangladesh; Prof. Xiaoling Shao from Nanjing Audit University, China; and Prof. Shagufta M. Trishna from Curtin University, Australia, examines the trends in soy consumption and production in China and explores people's dietary preferences for soybeans, including concerns about the import of genetically modified soybeans. The next chapter, "The Potential of Traditional Leafy Vegetables for Improving Food Security in Africa," by Profs. Praxedis Dube, Wim J. M. Heijman, and Rico Ihle from Wageningen University, The Netherlands and Prof. Justus Ochieng from World Vegetable Center, Eastern and Southern Africa, Tanzania, assesses the potential of traditional leafy vegetables in improving food security in Africa by proposing research on the seeds, seed systems, processing methods, and increasing of consumption. Concluding this reference book is "Veganism in the Bhagwad Gita," by Prof. Pratyush Ranjan of G. M. University, India, which seeks directions from the Gita (the Song of the Spirit) on the appropriate principled responses to the animal agriculture industry, including that of changing dietary habits towards plant-based sources, before finally exploring whether the Gita would promote veganism.

Although the primary organization of the contents in this work is based on its five sections, offering a progression of coverage of the important concepts, methodologies, technologies, applications, social issues, and emerging trends, the reader can also identify specific contents by utilizing the extensive indexing system listed at the end. As a comprehensive collection of research on the latest findings related to reducing food waste and managing food waste, the *Research Anthology on Food Waste Reduction and Alternative Diets* provides farmers, experts in the agricultural industry, nutritionists, policymakers, researchers, academicians, students, and all audiences with a complete understanding of sustainable agriculture, food waste, food consumption, and food security through the lens of upcoming technologies, case studies, current methodologies, and theories. Given the vast number of issues concerning food waste and agricultural sustainability throughout countries around the world, this extensive book addresses the demand for a resource that encompasses the most pertinent research in methods being employed to globally bolster sustainability when it comes to food and agriculture.

Section 1
Food Safety and Preservation Technologies

Chapter 1
Food Quality and Safety Regulation Systems at a Glance

Dixit V. Bhalani
Central Salt and Marine Chemicals Research Institute, India

Arvind Kumar Singh Chandel
Central Salt and Marine Chemicals Research Institute, India

Poonam Singh Thakur
Rashtrasant Tukadoji Maharaj Nagpur University, India

ABSTRACT

The quality and safety of all food products are the essential parameter for both ends manufactures and end consumers. This parameter of the food products we cannot overlook or liberalize in any situation. More than two-thirds of diseases are spread through the contaminated or spoiled food source. Looking at the importance of quality and safety management issue, the various governments made a series of rules and regulations for the assessment of food products. This chapter explains the role of various assessment agencies and their rights and workflows.

INTRODUCTION

With the correct ventures and assets, agribusiness can give satisfactory, moderate, protected and nutritious nourishment to everybody, all over the place, each day. However, notwithstanding critical advance, the world keeps on bearing a triple weight of lack of healthy sustenance. As indicated by 2016 information, around 800 million individuals around the world one of every four individuals in Sub-Saharan Africa and one out of six individuals in South Asia - still did not expend their base dietary vitality needs. Less advance has been accomplished in handling different types of ailing health. More than 2 billion individuals do not have the micronutrients required for development, improvement and malady anticipation. More than 2 billion individuals experience the ill effects of the antagonistic wellbeing impacts of being overweight or fat. Tainted sustenance is likewise a broad issue, affecting the wellbeing of 1 out of 10

DOI: 10.4018/978-1-7998-5354-1.ch001

individuals internationally every year and contrarily influencing the livelihoods of agriculturists, nourishment organizations and exchange. Hunger and nourishment borne ailments force huge present and future human, financial, social and monetary expenses on nations. Lessening these expenses requires multi-sectoral approaches: There is extraordinary potential for powerful mediations through horticulture and the sustenance framework generally speaking.

Regardless of the enormous endeavours paid by the nourishment security experts, masters and industry, sustenance wellbeing still stays basic and frequently is coming into spotlights pulling in media's consideration with flare-ups that can bring a pile of different negative outcomes. Such real occasions like BSE in 2000, dioxin or PCB (polychlorinated biphenyls) emergency in 1999 and others doubted the viability of the sustenance quality confirmation frameworks and nourishment security administration connected and exhibited that new device is expected to supplement the genuine frameworks set up. While assessing the negative outcomes one need to consider the restorative expenses brought about, the practical misfortunes that can gravely shake nearby little enterprises, and minimum yet not last consumers` trust. The worldview food security is that in spite of the fact that nourishment is more secure, consumers` demeanour is commanded by elevated amounts of vulnerability. In this changing atmosphere, we are that as it may, require perceiving the exertion EU experts make to re-establish consumers` trust and authorize new directions and better impart nourishment wellbeing related issues. An imperative highlight of sustenance industry is that makers, to adapt to showcase needs and lawful prerequisites, need to fulfil both wellbeing and quality criteria for their items. Having various choices as various quality as well as administration frameworks, nourishment makers ought to choose the most proper one for its particular movement and should build up, archive and execute powerful frameworks for overseeing quality also, security (van der Speigel et al., 2003).

Among the accessible Quality Assurance (QA) frameworks there are within reach today frameworks, for example, GMPs (Good Manufacturing Practices), GHPs (Good Cleanliness Practices), GAPs (Good Agricultural Practices) or other essential frameworks and HACCP (Hazard Analysis. Basic Control Points) (van der Speigel et al., 2003; Rotaru et al., 2015). This chapter also covers the following point mainly:

- Recommended international code of practice - general principles of food hygiene.
- Good Manufacturing Practices (GMPs)
- Good Hygiene Practices GHPs
- The hazard analysis and critical control point (HACCP) System.
- International Organization for Standardization

RECOMMENDED INTERNATIONAL CODE OF PRACTICE: GENERAL PRINCIPLES OF FOOD HYGIENE

Codes of Practice

Codes of practice are a group of guidelines, or one can be described as process specifications. These guidelines and specifications are generally helpful in providing constructive advice to manufacturers who have the same production facilities and manufacturing similar kind of products. These guidelines involve endorsements for the operational method, the design of construction facility, plant cleaning procedures, personal hygiene, quality and type of equipment, standard packaging procedures, and the handling of various raw materials at various stage of production. Codes of practice were prepared by the Codex Alimentarius Commission. For example, the international codes for various fish products were also prepared by the commission, it contains numerous commendations for each product, and starting from its raw material, vessel design and ends up to goods retail practices. It details the codes of practice includes regulations for the processing facility, sanitation procedures, growing areas and harvesting techniques. Some the codes of practice are made compulsory by governments. Such as, the Code of Federal Regulations concerning to human food production in the United States of America, which is imposed by the USFDA (Royce et al., 1996; Rosentrater et al., 2017).

Codes of practice and government authorities are in interference with free trade, and it is needed some practical attitude to the questions, such as what can be done and how costly it will be. Consumers can only be protected by eliminating the doubtful products from the market via strong rules and regulations. There are numbers of products in the market, so it was very difficult to command it uniformly. Codes and standards should full proof, fair, widely acceptable, easy to understand, and can be easily managed. It can be effectively applied by the good collaboration between government authorities and industry (Royce et al., 1996).

Codex Alimentarius

The Codex Alimentarius Commission was formed by the Food and Agriculture Organization (FAO) of UN (United Nations) in November 1961, and in June 1962 it was further joined by WHO (World health organization). In October 1963, the first meeting of Codex Alimentarius Commission was held in Rome. The contents are established and maintained by commission (Ottaway et al., 2003).

The commission had narrated Codex Alimentarius. It is mainly providing information regarding the HACCP system and also defines its lacking. FAO/WHO commission had accepted the HACCP system in early 1990 and comprises it into the Codex Alimentarius. It provides the details about the need for hygiene rules in the supply chain, regarding the HACCP, phases of implementation and also discuss the definitions. In general, the Codex Alimentarius is a set of internationally accepted guidelines, standards, codes of practice, and some other recommendations concerning to food safety, foods, and food production (Sorreaux et al., 2015; Sikora et al., 2005).

The Codex Alimentarius includes every food products, raw, processed, or semi-processed. It includes specific standards for specific foods as well as some general standards for other. General standards provide details about additives, labelling, hygiene, pesticide residue, and methods for evaluating food quality. The Codex Alimentarius also provides guidelines about the official management, such as import and export examination by government and food certification systems. The Codex Alimentarius is available in the six certified languages of the United Nations (UN): French, Arabic, Russian Chinese, Spanish, and English (CODEX Alimentarius: Understanding Codex". FAO and WHO. 1999. Retrieved 6 September 2012).

The aim of the commission was shielding the public health by implementing standard practices in manufacturing and international trading of products. The World Trade Organization renowned the Codex Alimentarius as an international reference for resolving clashes related to consumer protection and food safety (Winickoff et al., 2010; Agreement on the Application of Sanitary and Phytosanitary Measures. World Trade Organization. Accessed 3 September 2008).

The Codex Organizations

In Codex organization the detailed work is alienated within several committees. Numbers of committees were structured separately for focusing on 'horizontal' concerns like food labelling, whereas some others were focusing on 'vertical' concerns like specific needs for foods for its particular dietary uses. In the developing stage of the standards, it will be accepted by both kinds of the committee. In addition these committees, there are other five regional committees including Europe, Africa, Latin America, Asia, Caribbean, South-West Pacific and North America. The Codex Alimentarius Commission and their committees can take guidance from WHO and FAO expert Committees. Three other intergovernmental bodies are also there which deals with some particular commodities groups. They are also reporting to the commission. These are united committee of WHO and FAO of Government Experts officials on the Code of Principles regarding to the Milk and related products, a united Codex group of experts/ UNECE (United Nations Economic Commission for Europe) on fruit juices, and a combined UNECE and Codex Group of Experts on quick frozen foods (Ottaway et al., 2003).

As we mentioned earlier, the Codex committees are differentiated in two parts: specific and general subject committees. There are nine committees currently working on horizontal subjects (Labelling, pesticide residue and food additives). The rest of 15 Codex Commodity Committees are dealing with specific commodity groups (vegetable proteins, oils, and fats).

As per the Codex policy, every Codex committee has a host country. The host countries and their governments are responsible for their allotted committee's meeting arrangement and the administrative infrastructural facilities for meetings should also be provided by those countries. The country is also liable for the financial support for meeting arrangements, most of the currently hosting countries are in Western Europe and North America. The Meat Hygiene Committee was hosted by New Zealand from 1972 until its suspension 1983, and in 1972, the Methods of Analysis and Sampling Committee was taken by Hungary from Germany, and Mexico hosting the Committee on Tropical Fresh Fruits and Vegetables, which was made in 1988. Codex has prepared a task force on biotechnology, because of the fast growth in biotechnology, specifically genetic engineering. In March 2000 in their first meeting, they were agreed for the development principles regarding the risk assessment of foods prepared from modern biotechnology and also agreed for preparing guidelines for the safety analysis of food products made by those types of processes. The Codex Alimentarius Commission has 186 members of 186 member countries and one additional, the European Union as a member organization in 2012. It had 16 United Nations (UN) organizations, 215 codex observers, 150 non-governmental organizations and 49 intergovernmental groups (Randell et al., 1997; Sikes et al., 1998; Codex Alimentarius Commission: procedural manual. Food & Agriculture Org. 2007).

The Codex General Principles of Food Hygiene

1. Primary production
2. Establishment: Design and Facilities
3. Control of operation
4. Establishment: Maintenance and sanitation
5. Transportation
6. Product information and consumer awareness
7. Training

Table 1. General standards and specific standards of the Codex Alimentarius Commission (Joint FAO/ WHO Codex Alimentarius Commission, Codex Alimentarius Commission, & Joint FAO/WHO Food Standards Programme. (2001). Codex alimentarius: fats, oils and related products (Vol. 8). Food & Agriculture Org; Joint FAO/WHO Codex Alimentarius Commission, Joint FAO/WHO Food Standards Programme, & World Health Organization. (2003). Codex Alimentarius: Food hygiene, basic texts. Food & Agriculture Org; Joint FAO/WHO Codex Alimentarius Commission, Joint FAO/WHO Food Standards Programme, & World Health Organization. (2001). Codex Alimentarius: General requirements (food hygiene) (Vol. 1). Food & Agriculture Org; Masson-Matthee et al., 2007)

General Standards	
Food Hygiene	It includes codes and general principle of hygienic practice in particular industries or guidelines for the implementation of the HACCP system, and food handling establishments. These guidelines were represented in broad spectrum. Its primary objective is to ensure that whether the food products are safe for the intended purpose or not.
Food Labelling	It includes guidelines regarding labelling claims and some general guidelines and standards on nutrition (Cheftel et al., 2005).
Risk Assessment	Methods for evaluating safety of food which were prepared through biotechnology such as DNA-modified micro-organisms, DNA-modified plants, and allergens (Poli et al., 2004).
Food Additives	It includes general standard regarding quality specification of food grade chemicals, and its approved utilization (Alimentarius, C., 2009).
Methods	Process and techniques for sampling and analysis.
Food Contaminants	It includes standards and tolerance limits for particular contaminants such as aflatoxins, mycotoxins and radionuclides (Henry et al., 1999; D'Mello et al., 2003; WHO., 1999).
Specific Standards for Specific Products	
Special Dietary Foods	It includes baby formula foods, infant formula and specially manufactured foods for particular purposes (Joint FAO/WHO Codex Alimentarius Commission. 1994).
Meat	It provides guidelines about frozen meat, fresh meat, processed meat and also about poultry (Mead et al., 2006).
Oils and Fats	It includes information about the oil-fats products and their derivatives (Alimentarius, C., 1999; Alimentarius, C., 2012).
Fish and Fishery	It involves fish and fishery products from aquaculture, marine water, and fresh water (Ababouch et al., 2006; Tacon and Metian et al., 2008).
Dairy Products	It includes guidelines related to milk processing and other dairy product (Koletzko et al., 2005; Rastogi et al., 2004; Wiles et al., 1998).
Miscellaneous Food Products	It includes standards for sugar, mineral water, chocolate, and honey products (Kugonza et al., 2008; Rizelio et al., 2012; Baba et al., 2008; Semerjian et al., 2011; Man et al., 2015; Copetti et al., 2014; Chopra et al., 2002).

(Joint FAO/WHO Codex Alimentarius Commission, Joint FAO/WHO Food Standards Programme, & World Health Organization. (2003). Codex Alimentarius: Food hygiene, basic texts. Food & Agriculture Org)

Principle 1: Primary Production

The primary food production should be managed in such a way that, it can ensure the food safety and can also confirm its suitability for intended utilization (Cerf et al., 2011). Primary production involves:

- The plants and animals should be kept in proper atmosphere so that they are free from diseases and contaminants. This ultimately eliminates threats to food safety.
- The use environmental threaten areas is evaded.
- For the hygienic atmosphere and conditions, the standard practices and measures should be considered and this will ensure food safety (Joint FAO/WHO Codex Alimentarius Commission, Joint FAO/WHO Food Standards Programme, & World Health Organization. (2003). Codex Alimentarius: Food hygiene, basic texts. Food & Agriculture Org).

Figure 1. Important factors involved in primary production

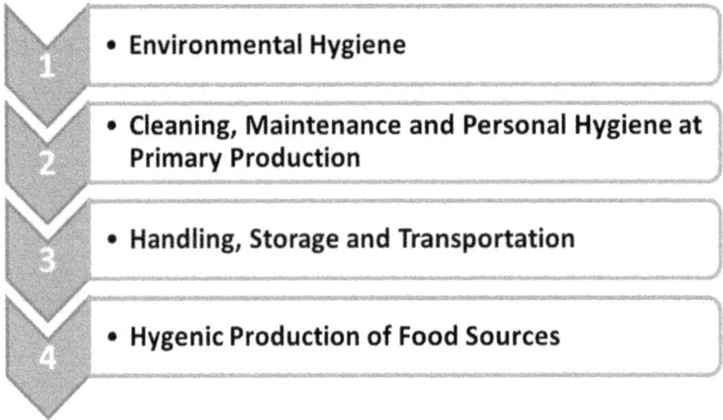

Principle 2: Establishment: Design and Facilities

Construction and designing of equipment, premises, and facilities should be done with consideration of associated risks and the nature of the operation. The appropriate hygienic construction and design, suitable location, availability of facilities are required for controlling hazards effectively. The design and facilities should such that:

- Contamination is diminished;
- Layout and designing are suitable to easy cleaning, sanitation, disinfections, maintenance, and reduce air-borne contamination (Cramer et al., 2013).
- Materials and surfaces which come in contact with food should be inert, non-toxic, durable, and should be easy to clean and maintain.
- Required facilities should be available for controlled conditions such as humidity, temperature, and other necessary controls.

Principle 3: Control of Operation

The food products consumed by human should be suitable and safe. This can be only achieved by operational control. So the food safety can be achieved by designing appropriate control and monitoring systems for raw materials, raw material composition, processing practices, distribution and handling. Proper designing, implementation, process monitoring and documents reviewing and verification are

Figure 2. Schematic representation shows the parameters involved in design and facility establishment (Joint FAO/WHO Codex Alimentarius Commission, Joint FAO/WHO Food Standards Programme, & World Health Organization. (2003). Codex Alimentarius: Food hygiene, basic texts. Food & Agriculture Org; Cramer et al., 2013)

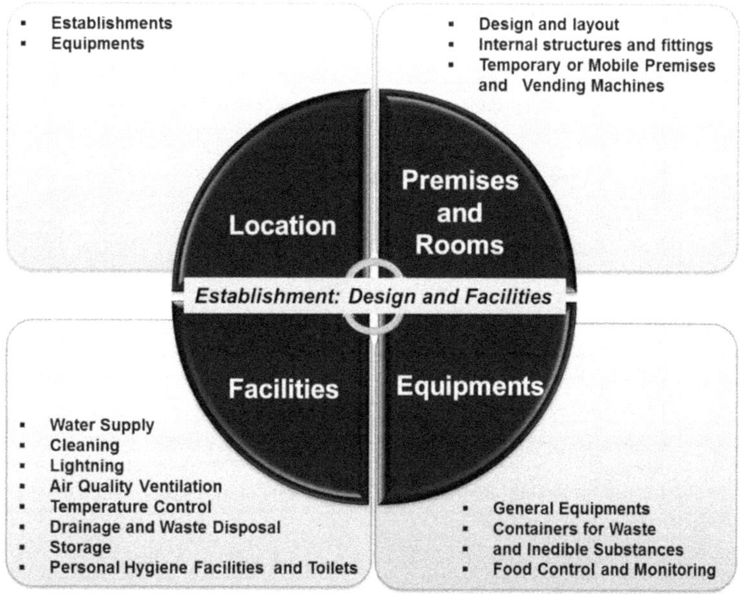

the effective control systems. The corrective and preventive actions should be taken at every stage of operation; this will be helpful in minimizing the food hazards. The business operators should implement HACCP type of systems. It should be implemented in whole food chain to control hygiene. The shelf-life of food can be protected by appropriate designing of process and product. Proper monitoring methods and analytical techniques for analysing physical, chemical, and microbial contamination. For prevention of contamination and cross-contamination, the personal entry in the controlled area is monitored by implementing area wise accessing protocols. Portable water should be used food processing. In case of threat to any food product, the product recall channel should be very effective.

Principle 4: Establishment - Maintenance and Sanitation

For the development of efficient food processing system, the following steps are the most necessary.

- The periodically pest control in the facility (Troller et al., 2012).
- Corrective and preventive maintenance after some fixed time intervals.
- Cleaning and cleaning records.
- Waste management systems should be implemented.
- Sanitation and maintenance should be effectively observed and maintained (Troller et al., 2012).

Table 2. Important measures and steps for the control of operation (Joint FAO/WHO Codex Alimentarius Commission, Joint FAO/WHO Food Standards Programme, & World Health Organization. (2003). Codex Alimentarius: Food hygiene, basic texts. Food & Agriculture Org).

Control of Food Hazards	• Identification of critical steps. • Implementation of control procedures. • Monitoring for ensurement of effectiveness. • Reviewing.
Incoming Material Requirements	• Specifications for the raw materials should be prepared and employed. And incoming material should be properly inspected.
Important Aspects of Hygiene Control Systems	• Controlling time and temperature. • Specific Process Steps. • Physical and chemical contamination. • Microbiological and other specifications. • Microbiological cross contamination (Van Schothorst et al., 1998).
Management and supervision	• Supervisors and managers should be highly knowledgeable, effective and able to take proper corrective and preventive actions.
Packaging	• It should provide satisfactory protection. • Packaging material should be inert and non-toxic.
Documentations and Records	• Proper record keeping of manufacturing, processing and distribution up to the shelf life of the food product. • It will increase the effectiveness and credibility of food safety control system.
Water	• In processing and handling of food only portable water should be used. • Water is used as ingredient, steam and in ice from in food processing.
Recall	• For the prevention of food safety hazard, the recall procedure should be rapid. • The recall products are kept in supervision and then destroyed.

Table 3. Steps involved in establishment of maintenance and sanitation (Lelieveld et al., 2014; Marriott et al., 2018; Joint FAO/WHO Codex Alimentarius Commission, Joint FAO/WHO Food Standards Programme, & World Health Organization. (2003). Codex Alimentarius: Food hygiene, basic texts. Food & Agriculture Org)

Maintenance and Cleaning
• General maintenance. • Cleaning procedures and techniques.
Pest Control Systems
• General pest control. • Harbourage and infestation. • Preventing access. • Eradication. • Monitoring and detection.
Cleaning Programmes
• Disinfection and cleaning should guarantee that each parts of facility are clean. • These programmes should be continuously monitored and documented. • The cleaning and sanitation programme should be designed by consulting with relevant experts.
Monitoring Effectiveness
• Verification for the effectiveness of sanitation systems. • Microbiological assessment of working environment, and contact surfaces should be inspected and reviewed regularly.
Waste Management
• The waste accumulation in working and storage areas must be prevented. • Some regulatory protocols should be followed for the storage and elimination of waste.

Principle 5: Establishment - Personal Hygiene

The establishment of personal hygiene is necessary because those who are in direct contact of food may be contaminating the food. By maintaining appropriate personal cleanliness and hygiene, the contamination can be minimized. And also by following the standard operating and working procedures, the chances of contaminations can be reduced. Personal hygiene is helpful in preventing the food contamination due to the personal illness (Lelieveld et al., 2014).

Table 4. Factors to be considered for the establishment of personal hygiene (Joint FAO/WHO Codex Alimentarius Commission, Joint FAO/WHO Food Standards Programme, & World Health Organization. (2003). Codex Alimentarius: Food hygiene, basic texts. Food & Agriculture Org)

Health Status
• If any personal is suffering illness or disease, then he should not be allowed to enter in food processing area. • Any kind of illness or symptoms of personal should be informed to the management.
Personal Cleanliness
• The food handling personal should maintain personal hygiene and cleanliness by using personal protective equipments such as apron, shoe cover, head cap, and hand gloves. • The workers should always wash their hand before and after food handling activities.
Illness and Injuries
• If any working personal is suffering from jaundice, fever, vomiting, diarrhoea and sore throat with fever. Then the situations should be informed to management, so that further medical examination can be done.
Visitors
• The visitors coming to the manufacturing facilities should were personal protective cloths for avoiding threat to food contamination.
Personal Behaviour
• During food handling activities spitting, smoking, eating, chewing, sneezing, and coughing will contaminate foods. So that it should be avoided. • Watches, jewellery, pins and other items should avoid to worn during food handling.

Principle 6: Transportation

Food transportation should be done under control measures. Transportation is comes under food supply chain and distribution. The food should be provided to end user in suitable form without any contamination. During food transportation following measures should be taken:

- The food products should be protected from damaging, so that its not became unsuitable for the end user.
- The food must be protected from its effective source of contamination.
- The transportation environment must be suitable to the quality sustenance of the product. Appropriate environmental conditions will protect the food from micro-organism and pathogenic growth.

The type food containers and packaging form will depends on the nature of foods. The food products should be transported in their suitable conditions. The designing and construction of bulky food containers should be according to following requirements:

- The food containers should not contaminate foods.
  - There should be an appropriate separation of foods and food from non-food materials.
  - They should be easy to clean and easy to be disinfected.
  - The containers have to maintain humidity, temperature, atmosphere and other required conditions to protect food from deterioration and microbial growth.
  - The container should design in such a way that the food products are free from fumes and dust.
  - The design should be such that the humidity, temperature and other conditions can be easily checked and operated.

(Joint FAO/WHO Codex Alimentarius Commission, Joint FAO/WHO Food Standards Programme, & World Health Organization. (2003). Codex Alimentarius: Food hygiene, basic texts. Food & Agriculture Org)

Principle 7: Product Information and Consumer Awareness

The food products should contain proper details. The sufficient and manageable should be available to the food chain personal so that they can be easily stored, handle, prepare and display products correctly and safely. With the help of product information, it can be rapidly identified and recalled. The consumers should be aware of food hygiene so that they can easily understand the significance of product information. The end user should have appropriate information and awareness so that they can eliminate contamination and microbiological and pathogens growth. The end user information and trade information can be easily distinguishable (Ababio et al., 2012; Gendel., 2012; Caswell et al., 1996).

Principle 8: Training

Personals who are working in food processing or who are in direct or indirect contact of food should be well instructed and trained for food hygiene and safety. They should be trained for following standard codes of practice so that the level of food hygiene can be maintained in the processing facility (Ehiri et al., 1996; da Cunha et al., 2014). The Components of training are mentioned below:

Awareness and Responsibilities: The training is one of the most necessary thing to maintain food hygiene. All the workers should be aware of their working responsibility for personnel should be aware of their role and responsibility in guarding foods against deterioration and contamination.

Instruction and Supervision: There should be regular supervision of instruction and training programmes. The efficiency of training should also monitor. Supervisors should be knowledgeable about food hygiene safety principles and practices. And they should be able to identify the risk and take corrective actions.

Training Programmes: Workers should be frequently trained for the procedures to be followed during the handling, packaging, and storing.

Figure 3. Schematic representation shows the important factors involved in product information and consumer awareness (Ababio et al., 2012; Gendel., 2012; Caswell et al., 1996; Joint FAO/WHO Codex Alimentarius Commission, Joint FAO/WHO Food Standards Programme, & World Health Organization. (2003). Codex Alimentarius: Food hygiene, basic texts. Food & Agriculture Org)

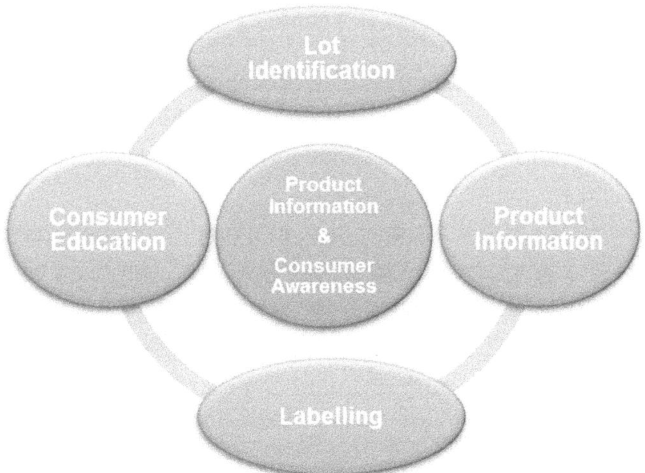

Refresher Training: The personal training should be frequently observed, modified and updated as per the norms and necessity.

(Mayes et al., 1994; Moy et al., 1994; Khandke et al., 1998; Joint FAO/WHO Codex Alimentarius Commission, Joint FAO/WHO Food Standards Programme, & World Health Organization. (2003). Codex Alimentarius: Food hygiene, basic texts. Food & Agriculture Org)

GOOD MANUFACTURING PRACTICE (GMPs)

Good Manufacturing Practices (GMP) is a collection of detailed information and guidelines for the act and standard operating procedures to be followed, and their requirements should be fulfilled. GMP is implemented for the ensurement of food safety. GMP covers the basic activity of the facility. The activities should be as per the standard procedures and norms so that the quality food products can be prepared (Sikora and Strada, 2003; Rotaru et al., 2005; Sikora 2005).

GOOD HYGIENE PRACTICE (GHPs)

Good Hygienic Practices (GHP) contains a collection of guidelines focusing on the hygienic conditions which should be at a satisfactory level and monitored at every stage of the food chain for the assurance of safety of food. Following the GHP rules and regulations is generally making all the activities in the preparation process and in the profit of foods with ensuring appropriate conditions to foods and their decent health quality. In the case of the Health Conditions of Foods and Nutrition, the GMP and GHP are explained differently, both are intimately connected, and both are implemented for hygienic requirements in the facility. Both the GMP and GHP are employed and properly maintained and documented (Sikora and Strada, 2003; Rotaru et al., 2005; Sikora 2005).

HAZARD ANALYSIS AND CRITICAL CONTROL POINT (HACCP)

The HACCP was constructed for the assurance of food health and safety. It is composed of two main stakes: Health hazard analysis and critical control points which were settled after the completion of hazard analysis. An improper following of guidelines and conditions leads to health hazards. The health hazards cannot be controlled by conventional tools.

In accordance with the HACCP system, each deviation and potential hazards in the manufacturing method will be identified at a time of production or before that. The main objective of the HACCP is to eliminate any hazards before its establishment. In the early time of system establishment, primarily it was just designed to prevent every microbiological hazard. Secondly, it was employed to physical, chemical and biological hazards.

Basic steps of implementation of HACCP system: the 1st is hazard analysis for identifying the possible danger related to food processing at each stage up to the consumption. In the next step, monitoring methods should be developed, and observations should be mentioned in registers.

The proper employment of HACCP system needs:

- Appropriate designing of the documentation process.
- Carrying out detailed hazard analysis.
- Designing of control points and critical control points.
- Structuring of monitoring methods.

Figure 4. The schematic representation shows the characteristics of HACCP systems

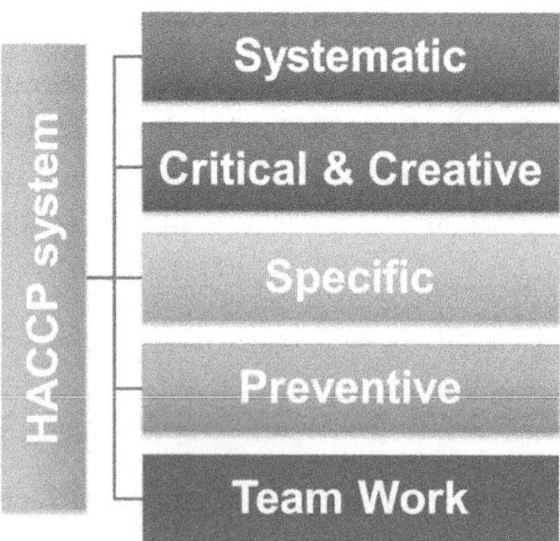

The HACCP system should be systematic. The manufacturing processes and practices should be performed according to the seven basic rules. The HACCP system should be specifically designed according to every enterprise. The system should be capable of the prevention of all possible hazards. For defeating the problems and issues, the system should be creative and innovative in the finding of new solutions. Teamwork is most necessary for proper implementation of the system because personals with diverse specialization are involved.

Advantages of the HACCP system:

- By the implementation running the HACCP system, there is no needs of permanent control on the end product.
- Preventive and corrective features of system will defeat the problem before tis arising.
- Working according to the HACCP system will ensures the quality food production without any health hazards.
  (Sikora, 2005; Kijowski et al., 2003; Sun and Ockerman, 2005; Motarjemi et al., 1996)

INTERNATIONAL ORGANIZATION FOR STANDARDIZATION

On 23 February 1947, the International Organization for Standardization (ISO) is an international standard-setting body was created that's representatives from various national standards organizations. The ISO 22000 addresses the food safety standard management issue, the significances of unhygienic and unsafe food can be harmful to the health, The ISO's food safety management standards service organizations categorise and regulator the food safety standard and hazards (Arvanitoyannis, 2009).

Nowadays many food products frequently cross national boundaries, so the international standards are required to certify the safety of the worldwide food supply chain. The ISO 22000:2018 fixed the necessities for a food safety management system and can be certified the food products. It recognizes which organization needs to do validate its ability to regulate food safety and standards and hazards to certify that food is safe or not. More than two hundred diseases are speeds only because of contaminated or spoiled food stuff so that it is very clear the hygienic, safe, sustainable food production is one of our extreme challenges. The food trade globalization is further complicated because of maintaining the food safety standards. The food safety is about the elimination, avoidance, and regulates the food products from the foodborne hazards factors, from the production site to the utilization site.

Meanwhile, food safety standards and hazards may be introduced at any stage of the food processing. Each food supply chain company must implement adequate hazard controls. Food safety can be secured only by the united efforts of all parties: producers, governments, retailers and end customers.

The new edition of ISO 22000 improved the clarity of understanding for the many of companies globally that already used this standard. Its latest following improvements comprise:

- Implementation of the High-Level Structure common to all ISO management system standards, creating it easier for organizations to combine ISO 22000 with other management systems (such as ISO 14001 or ISO 9001) at any given time
- A different approach to risk as an important concept in the food product business – which differentiates between risk at the working level and the corporate level of the management system
- Strong links to the Codex Alimentarius, a United Nations food group that develops food safety guidelines for government authorities.

The new ISO 22000 standard offers a forceful control of food safety hazards coalescing the following generally recognized key elements: systems management, interactive communication, Prerequisite Programmes (PRPs), and Critical Control Points (HACCP), and the principles of Hazard Analysis (Arvanitoyannis, 2009; Surak, 2005)

FOOD SAFETY LEGISLATION

Legislative regulations which people need to be aware of are:

- Food Safety Act 1990
- Food Hygiene Regulations (Northern Ireland) 2006
- Food Hygiene (Scotland) Regulations 2006
- Food Safety and Hygiene (England) Regulations 2013
- Food Hygiene (Wales) Regulations 2006

These regulations make compulsory implementation of HACCP based food safety management procedures for all food businesses.

- **Food Safety Acts in Europe and the United Kingdom:** The European Union established the European Food Safety Authority in the year 2002 which is an independent source of scientific advice. The independent Food Standards Agency (FSA) was established in 2001 by the government of UK. FSA was made by merging various prevailing agencies under one body. The aim behind FSA is to promote standards and to advise the government.
- **India's Food Safety Act:** India implemented the Food Safety and Standards Act in 2006, which merged various existing organisations to establish the Food Safety and Standards Authority of India (FSSAI).
- **Food Safety Modernization Act (FSMA):** On 4 Jan 2011, the FSMA was signed into law by US President Obama. FSMA gives major importance on food safety and public health assurance by using preventive action, rather than countering after cases of contamination. It will modify the role of the USFDA. FSMA gives the FDA legal authority.

CONCLUSION

The quality and safety assessment of all food products are the very essential step for the entire food chain from the manufacturer to end consumers. Because of the causes of the maximum disease are reported from the contaminated or unhygienic food source so that the food safety and quality standard assessment is very crucial before selling or consuming the food products. This chapter summarises, in brief, the analysis of the specific and integrated/advanced food quality and safety management system, along with the identification and analysis of the factors that can influence the employment process. The various investigating and assessment agencies and their role in the hole process of quality and safety assessment for the food products. The efficiency of the ISO systems is based on the association between external and internal organizational factors. In addition to that, these factors act into the food industry have to balance the food quality and safety assurance management systems, select the appropriate ones permitting to its resources and requirements and implement tolerable outfits for continuously evaluating and measuring the quality safety and performance of the individual or advanced/integrated management systems.

ACKNOWLEDGMENT

Dr P S Thakur thanks to Department of Zoology S. A. Sci. College, RTM University Nagpur, for providing research facility, and Dixit V. Bhalani thanks DST for providing DST-INSPIRE Fellowship. And Arvind K. Singh Chandel thank CSIR, India for providing a research fellowship (CSIR-JRF). DV and AKSC also thanks to CSIR-CSMCRI for providing research facility

REFERENCES

Ababio, P. F., Adi, D. D., & Amoah, M. (2012). Evaluating the awareness and importance of food labelling information among consumers in the Kumasi metropolis of Ghana. *Food Control, 26*(2), 571–574. doi:10.1016/j.foodcont.2012.02.015

Ababouch, L. (2006). Assuring fish safety and quality in international fish trade. *Marine Pollution Bulletin, 53*(10-12), 561–568. doi:10.1016/j.marpolbul.2006.08.011 PMID:17052733

Agreement on the Application of Sanitary and Phytosanitary Measures. (2008, September 3). World Trade Organization.

Alimentarius, C. (1999). Codex standard for edible fats and oils not covered by individual standards. *Codex stan, 19*, 1981.

Alimentarius, C. (1999). Codex standard for named vegetable oils. *Codex Stan, 210*, 1–13.

Alimentarius, C. (2009). General standard for food additives. *Codex stan*, 192-1995.

Alimentarius, C. (2012). International food standards. Standard for Foods for Special Dietary Use for Persons Intolerant to Gluten. *Codex Stan*, 118-1979.

Arvanitoyannis, I. S. (2009). *HACCP and ISO 22000: Application to foods of animal origin.* John Wiley & Sons. doi:10.1002/9781444320923

Baba, A., Ereeş, F. S., Hıçsönmez, Ü., Cam, S., & Özdılek, H. G. (2008). An assessment of the quality of various bottled mineral water marketed in Turkey. *Environmental Monitoring and Assessment, 139*(1-3), 277–285. doi:10.100710661-007-9833-9 PMID:17577674

Caswell, J. A., & Hooker, N. H. (1996). HACCP as an international trade standard. *American Journal of Agricultural Economics, 78*(3), 775–779. doi:10.2307/1243303

Cerf, O., & Donnat, E.Farm HACCP Working Group. (2011). Application of hazard analysis–Critical control point (HACCP) principles to primary production: What is feasible and desirable? *Food Control, 22*(12), 1839–1843. doi:10.1016/j.foodcont.2011.04.023

Cheftel, J. C. (2005). Food and nutrition labelling in the European Union. *Food Chemistry*, *93*(3), 531–550. doi:10.1016/j.foodchem.2004.11.041

Chopra, M., Galbraith, S., & Darnton-Hill, I. (2002). A global response to a global problem: The epidemic of overnutrition. *Bulletin of the World Health Organization*, *80*, 952–958. PMID:12571723

Codex Alimentarius Commission, Joint FAO/WHO Food Standards Programme, & World Health Organization. (2007). *Codex alimentarius commission: procedural manual*. Food & Agriculture Org.

Copetti, M. V., Iamanaka, B. T., Pitt, J. I., & Taniwaki, M. H. (2014). Fungi and mycotoxins in cocoa: From farm to chocolate. *International Journal of Food Microbiology*, *178*, 13–20. doi:10.1016/j.ijfoodmicro.2014.02.023 PMID:24667314

Cramer, M. M. (2013). *Food plant sanitation: design, maintenance, and good manufacturing practices*. CRC Press. doi:10.1201/b14902

D'Mello, J. F. (Ed.). (2003). *Food safety: contaminants and toxins*. CABI. doi:10.1079/9780851996073.0000

da Cunha, D. T., Stedefeldt, E., & de Rosso, V. V. (2014). The role of theoretical food safety training on Brazilian food handlers' knowledge, attitude and practice. *Food Control*, *43*, 167–174. doi:10.1016/j.foodcont.2014.03.012

Ehiri, J. E., & Morris, G. P. (1996). Hygiene training and education of food handlers: Does it work? *Ecology of Food and Nutrition*, *35*(4), 243–251. doi:10.1080/03670244.1996.9991494

FAO. (1999). *CODEX Alimentarius: Understanding Codex*. FAO and WHO.

Gendel, S. M. (2012). Comparison of international food allergen labeling regulations. *Regulatory Toxicology and Pharmacology*, *63*(2), 279–285. doi:10.1016/j.yrtph.2012.04.007 PMID:22565206

Henry, S. H., Bosch, F. X., Troxell, T. C., & Bolger, P. M. (1999). Reducing liver cancer--global control of aflatoxin. *Science*, *286*(5449), 2453–2454. doi:10.1126cience.286.5449.2453 PMID:10636808

Joint FAO/WHO Codex Alimentarius Commission. (1994). *Codex Alimentarius: Foods for Special Dietary Uses Including Food for Infants and Children*. Food & Agriculture Org.

Joint FAO/WHO Codex Alimentarius Commission, Codex Alimentarius Commission, & Joint FAO/WHO Food Standards Programme. (2001). *Codex alimentarius: fats, oils and related products* (Vol. 8). Food & Agriculture Org.

Joint FAO/WHO Codex Alimentarius Commission, Joint FAO/WHO Food Standards Programme, & World Health Organization. (2001). *Codex Alimentarius: General requirements (food hygiene)* (Vol. 1). Food & Agriculture Org.

Joint FAO/WHO Codex Alimentarius Commission, Joint FAO/WHO Food Standards Programme, & World Health Organization. (2003). *Codex Alimentarius: Food hygiene, basic texts*. Food & Agriculture Org.

Khandke, S. S., & Mayes, T. (1998). HACCP implementation: A practical guide to the implementation of the HACCP plan. *Food Control*, *9*(2-3), 103–109. doi:10.1016/S0956-7135(97)00065-0

Kijowski, J., & Sikora, T. (2003). *Food quality and safety management. Integration and computerization of systems*. Warsaw: WNT.

Koletzko, B., Baker, S., Cleghorn, G., Neto, U. F., Gopalan, S., Hernell, O., ... Pzyrembel, H. (2005). Global standard for the composition of infant formula: Recommendations of an ESPGHAN coordinated international expert group. *Journal of Pediatric Gastroenterology and Nutrition, 41*(5), 584–599. doi:10.1097/01.mpg.0000187817.38836.42 PMID:16254515

Kugonza, D. R., & Nabakabya, D. (2008). *Honey quality as affected by handling, processing and marketing channels in Uganda*. Academic Press.

Lelieveld, H. L., Holah, J., & Napper, D. (Eds.). (2014). *Hygiene in food processing: principles and practice*. Elsevier.

Man, Y. C., Syahariza, Z. A., Mirghani, M. E. S., Jinap, S., & Bakar, J. (2005). Analysis of potential lard adulteration in chocolate and chocolate products using Fourier transform infrared spectroscopy. *Food Chemistry, 90*(4), 815–819. doi:10.1016/j.foodchem.2004.05.029

Marriott, N. G., Schilling, M. W., & Gravani, R. B. (2018). *Principles of food sanitation*. Springer. doi:10.1007/978-3-319-67166-6

Masson-Matthee, M. D. (2007). *The codex alimentarius commission and its standards*. Academic Press.

Mayes, T. (1994). HACCP training. *Food Control, 5*(3), 190–195. doi:10.1016/0956-7135(94)90082-5

Mead, G. (Ed.). (2006). *Microbiological analysis of red meat, poultry and eggs*. Woodhead Publishing. doi:10.1201/9781439823880

Motarjemi, Y., Käferstein, F., Moy, G., Miyagawa, S., & Miyagishima, K. (1996). Importance of HACCP for public health and development the role of the world health organization. *Food Control, 7*(2), 77–85. doi:10.1016/0956-7135(96)00003-5

Moy, G., Käferstein, F., & Motarjemi, Y. (1994). Application of HACCP to food manufacturing: Some considerations on harmonization through training. *Food Control, 5*(3), 131–139. doi:10.1016/0956-7135(94)90072-8

Ottaway, P. B. (2003). *Legislation Codex*.

Poli, S. (2004). The European Community and the adoption of international food standards within the Codex Alimentarius Commission. *European Law Journal, 10*(5), 613–630. doi:10.1111/j.1468-0386.2004.00234.x

Randell, A. W., & Whitehead, A. J. (1997). Codex Alimentarius: Food quality and safety standards for international trade. *Revue Scientifique et Technique (International Office of Epizootics), 16*(2), 313–318. doi:10.20506/rst.16.2.1019 PMID:9501343

Rastogi, S., Dwivedi, P. D., Khanna, S. K., & Das, M. (2004). Detection of aflatoxin M1 contamination in milk and infant milk products from Indian markets by ELISA. *Food Control, 15*(4), 287–290. doi:10.1016/S0956-7135(03)00078-1

Rizelio, V. M., Gonzaga, L. V., Borges, G. D. S. C., Micke, G. A., Fett, R., & Costa, A. C. O. (2012). Development of a fast MECK method for determination of 5-HMF in honey samples. *Food Chemistry, 133*(4), 1640–1645. doi:10.1016/j.foodchem.2011.11.058

Rosentrater, K. A., & Evers, A. D. (2017). *Kent's Technology of Cereals: An introduction for Students of Food Science and Agriculture*. Woodhead Publishing.

Rotaru, G., Sava, N., Borda, D., & Stanciu, S. (2005). Food quality and safety management systems: A brief analysis of the individual and integrated approaches. *Scientifical Researches Agroalimentary Processes and Technologies, 11*(1), 229–336.

Royce, W. F. (1996). Introduction to the Practice of Fishery Science (rev. ed.). Elsevier.

Semerjian, L. A. (2011). Quality assessment of various bottled waters marketed in Lebanon. *Environmental Monitoring and Assessment, 172*(1-4), 275–285. doi:10.100710661-010-1333-7 PMID:20148363

Sikes, L. (1998). FDA's consideration of Codex Alimentarius Standards in light of international trade agreements. *Food and Drug Law Journal, 53*, 327. PMID:10346688

Sikora, T. (2005). Methods and systems of food quality and safety assurance. *Polish Journal of Food and Nutrition Sciences, 14*(1), 41.

Sikora, T., & Strada, A. (2003). *Safety and Quality Assurance and Management Systems in Food Industry: An Overview*. Academic Press.

Sorreaux, G., & Thiry, C. (2015). *Food Regulation and Enforcement in Belgium*. Academic Press.

Sun, Y. M., & Ockerman, H. W. (2005). A review of the needs and current applications of hazard analysis and critical control point (HACCP) system in foodservice areas. *Food Control, 16*(4), 325–332. doi:10.1016/j.foodcont.2004.03.012

Surak, J. G. (2005). ISO 22000: Requirements for food safety management systems. In *ASQ World Conference on Quality and Improvement Proceedings* (Vol. 59, p. 211). American Society for Quality.

Tacon, A. G., & Metian, M. (2008). Aquaculture feed and food safety: The role of the food and agriculture organization and the codex alimentarius. *Annals of the New York Academy of Sciences, 1140*(1), 50–59. doi:10.1196/annals.1454.003 PMID:18991902

Troller, J. A. (2012). *Sanitation in food processing*. Academic Press.

Van der Spiegel, M., Luning, P. A., Ziggers, G. W., & Jongen, W. M. F. (2003). Towards a conceptual model to measure effectiveness of food quality systems. *Trends in Food Science & Technology, 14*(10), 424–431. doi:10.1016/S0924-2244(03)00058-X

Van Schothorst, M. (1998). Principles for the establishment of microbiological food safety objectives and related control measures. *Food Control, 9*(6), 379–384. doi:10.1016/S0956-7135(98)00129-7

Wiles, P. G., Gray, I. K., & Kissling, R. C. (1998). Routine analysis of proteins by Kjeldahl and Dumas methods: Review and interlaboratory study using dairy products. *Journal of AOAC International, 81*(3), 620–632. PMID:9606925

Winickoff, D. E., & Bushey, D. M. (2010). Science and power in global food regulation: The rise of the codex alimentarius. *Science, Technology & Human Values, 35*(3), 356–381. doi:10.1177/0162243909334242

World Health Organization. (1999). *Food safety* (No. EM/RC46/6). WHO.

This research was previously published in Novel Technologies and Systems for Food Preservation edited by Pedro Dinis Gaspar and Pedro Dinho da Silva; pages 275-293, copyright year 2019 by Engineering Science Reference (an imprint of IGI Global).

Chapter 2
Ecological Chemistry Aspects of Food Safety

Rodica Sturza

https://orcid.org/0000-0002-2412-5874

Technical University of Moldova, Moldova

ABSTRACT

The presented results reflect the researches carried out over the last decade, having as their object the soil, water, vegetal raw materials, and wines from the Republic of Moldova. The analysis of the possible anthropogenic contamination (NAA method) demonstrated the absence of systematic soil pollution. A total of 30 elements were determined in soil samples and the soil-leaves-fruit transfer factors were calculated. Approximately 3000 samples of local wines have been analysed to determine the residual quantities of pesticides. POPs were not found in any of the wine samples. In most of the examined cases (> 60% of samples), the lack of organic pesticide residues was observed. The migration of phthalates into different solutions from polymeric materials (PVC, rubber) and the influence of the temperature on the extraction rate were investigated. It has been shown that the contamination with phthalate residues occurs predominantly at the stage of grape processing, technological treatment, and storage.

INTRODUCTION

Food is a system that is closely related to the individual and it is the fundamental biological link of man to the environment (Weiss, 2016). Thus, any environmental disturbance finds the ideal way to reach man via food. A characteristic of food products is the wide variety of factors that can influence safety and hygienic quality (Mylona, 2016). In a brief classification, they can be distributed as follows: biological pollution agents, pollution and chemical contamination agents, natural toxic substances and toxic compounds formed by food processing.

The main agents that can reduce or even annihilate food safety, with varying degrees of harmfulness and extremely random penetration, can be synthesized in the following groups (Sturza, 2017):

DOI: 10.4018/978-1-7998-5354-1.ch002

– Toxic compounds can be found naturally in foods, including toxic aminoacids in seeds, unripe fruits and vegetables. Biogenic amines, alkaloids, glycosides releasing hydrogen cyanide, toxins from fungi fall also into this category. Their effects on the body are manifested by growth retardation and renal tissue damage (produced by amino acids), cardiac lesions, effects on the adrenal gland, increased blood pressure (caused by amines), gastrointestinal disorders, vomiting, diarrhea, haemolytic lesions by alkaloids), nerve disorders and even death caused by toxins from poisonous fungi.

– Toxic compounds that are formed in foodstuffs within technological and preservation processes: nitrosamines from plants grown on nitrogen-treated lands, condensed polycyclic hydrocarbons (3 – 4 benzo[a]pyrene), azotates and nitrites from plants, meat, milk. These chemicals have irritating action on the digestive tract, causing congestion and haemorrhage, increased blood pressure, severe hepatotoxic effects, liver damage.

– Pesticides and fertilizers representing the chemicals used in agriculture and veterinary medicine to combat various pest categories: fungicides, insecticides, rodenticides; act primarily on the liver which increases its volume and intensifies enzymatic action, causing disturbances in human metabolism and leading to tumor formation.

– Industrial chemicals: organics, packaging materials, plastics, synthetic rubber, lacquers, industrial solvents, aerosols, nitrates and nitrites, polycyclic aromatic hydrocarbons, metals with toxic potential, antibiotics, hormones, detergents, radionuclides, etc.

The large number of exogenous aggression factors on food requires food control throughout the food chain. As the chemicals diffuse into the food chain, the chemicals and their metabolites accumulate at all levels of the food chain. Effects on living organisms can range from mild discomfort to serious illness, such as cancer or physical deformities. Experts recognize that the effects of pollution are quite often underestimated and that more research is needed to understand the connections between pollution and its effects on all forms of life. Conditions related to water polluted by chemicals (such as pesticides, hydrocarbons, persistent organic pollutants, phthalates, heavy metals, nitrates) can induce cancer, hormonal problems that can disrupt reproduction and development processes, damage to the nervous system, liver and kidneys, DNA damage. Soil pollution also has many effects, including cancer and leukemia. Lead from the soil can be transfer in food via fruits and vegetables; it is particularly dangerous for children, causing damage to brain development. Mercury increases the risk of kidney damage; pesticide residues can cause liver toxicity. Other effects may include neuromuscular blockage, central nervous system depression, headaches, nausea, fatigue, eye irritation and rash. The random nature and impact of different types of toxins implies the knowledge of the sources of pollution.

The purpose of this study was to elucidate the impact of same exogenous factors (environmental contamination) on food harmlessness. These aspects will be examined, such as the heavy metal accumulation in plant foods depending on the soil composition, the mineral transfer factor in the soil-leaf-fruit systems; accumulation of pesticide residues in horticultural products; the causes of contamination of the food chain with phthalate residues.

CIRCUIT OF MINERAL ELEMENTS IN THE SOIL-PLANT-FRUIT-PRODUCTS SYSTEM BACKGROUND

Analysis of published data indicates that heavy metals, such as cadmium, arsenic, chromium, lead and mercury, naturally occur. However, anthropogenic activities contribute significantly to environmental contamination. The heavy metal contamination of food products by vegetal origin comes from soil and atmosphere, especially when the crops are approximately enterprises, urban wastewaters, and intensely circulated streets. These metals are systemic toxins known to induce adverse effects on human health. Toxic elements induce cardiovascular disease, developmental abnormalities, neurological disorders, diabetes, hearing loss, hematological and immunological disorders and cancer. The severity of adverse effects on health is related to the type of heavy metals and their chemical form; it is dependent on the exposure time and the dose. An essential role in the toxic kinetics of metals have valence, solubility, bioavailability and chemical form. Their bioavailability is influenced by physical factors, such as temperature, phase association, adsorption and sequestration. It is also affected by chemical factors that influence thermodynamic balance, complexation kinetics, lipid solubility and partition coefficients. Biological factors such as species characteristics, trophic interactions and biochemical / physiological adaptation also play an important role.

All metals are toxic at higher concentrations. Excessive levels can be damaging to the organism (Reena Singh, 2011). If the acute and chronic effects are known for some elements, little is known about the impact of mixtures of toxic elements. It have pointed that toxic elements may interfere metabolically with nutritionally essential metals such as iron, calcium, copper, and zinc (López Alonso M, 2004). The literature is low regarding the combined toxicity of heavy metals. Simultaneous exposure to several heavy metals can produce a toxic effect that is additive, antagonistic or synergistic (Paul B Tchounwou, 2012). There is a potential synergism between Cu and Zn, Cu and As, Zn and As, but an antagonism between these elements and Pb. The synergistic or antagonistic effect depends on the dose and duration of application of the substances (Sturza, 2016).

Lead is used in the form of lead tetraethyl on the gasoline additive. By removing it from the exhaust gases, the air and the adjacent land of the road are polluted over a distance of 200 – 250 m. Plants such as cabbage, celery, beet, corn, peach collect a lot of lead (Botnari, 2016).

Mercury comes from the use of pesticides, from gas or industrial emissions. It can to precipitate cytoplasmic proteins and block some enzymes. Cadmium is used in stainless steel alloys, dental technology, dye enameling, etc. The use of fertilizers (with Cd residue) leads to its accumulation in the soil, where it is taken up by the plants, rapidly migrating into their organs. Rice, wheat accumulate large amounts of cadmium. Zinc has an important biological role, but in the case of high amounts, it produces toxic effects. It is used in the form of compounds (oxide, sulfide, sulfate, chloride) for various industrial uses. The use of insecticides and fungicides based on organic zinc compounds leads to contamination of agro-food products and feed. It is accumulated in beans, corn, sorghum (Veliksar, 2016).

Copper is used in phytosanitary treatments (control of green algae in ponds, vine diseases) as well as in industry. It originates from the soil, absorbed by plants, but also as a result of the antifungal treatments with copper-based preparations, copper oxychloride (Stasiev, 2016). It is accumulated mainly in root vegetables. Although copper is part of the category of essential elements, being present in excessive amount (> 1 mg / kg) can cause intoxication of the body?

Tin (Sn) is used both in industry (metal packaging for cans, cutlery) and in agriculture. Products are contaminated by the use of various fungicides and through contact with processing equipment or storage packaging. Arsenic is an element being present in organisms, having an incompletely elucidated role. It is used in therapeutics, food industry and agriculture, its residues being active for years (Balan, 2008).

At the same time, the elements are an important component of food. Sources that contribute to the elemental composition of food products can be distinguished into two groups: natural and anthropic, allowing the definition of a representative "fingerprint", which is particularly important for foods manufactured in specific regions, such as Protected Designation of Origin (Galani-Nikolakaki S. M., 2007). The natural factors that influence the endogenous metallic content are the metabolic specificity of the plants, the degree of maturity, the climatic conditions, the nature of the soil, the quality of the water. The technological factors that influence the metal content include fertilizers, inorganic pesticides, processing equipment, steel containers and pollution of the surrounding environmental industries.

The elemental analysis of food products is of great interest to consumers and producers, as it can offer guarantees of quality and harmlessness, identify the geographical origin of the product, determining criteria for their price (Frontasyeva M.V., 2011).

Issues, Controversies, Problems

Are there soil pollution with mineral elements? What is the transfer rate of soil minerals in plants, fruits and food? Can the transfer of heavy metals from soil to food affect health? Can the content of mineral elements provide information on the origin of food?

Study carried out by Epithermal Neuron Activation Analysis (NAA) was focused on the distribution of microelements in the soils of the Republic of Moldova (Zinicovscaia, 2018). The comparison of two analytical techniques – inductively coupled plasma atomic emission spectroscopy (ICP-AES) and NAA using as example eight matrix and trace elements: Al, Ba, Ca, Fe, K, Mg, Na, and Zn was previously performed (Sturza, 2015). All data, interpreted within the Upper Continental Crust model, showed first of all that within experimental uncertainties, the soils of both vineyards are identical and close to the average composition of the UCC. A more detailed analysis of the distribution of Rb, Sr, and Zr revealed a significant degree of chemical weathering as well as a prolonged process of sorting and recycling of minerals.

At the same time, the soil content of Cr, Mn, Co, Zn and As proved, exception for As, the absence of any systematic heavy element pollution. In this regard, although the As content exceeds the UCC value of 1.5 mg/kg, almost reaching the alarm threshold according to some national regulations, its increased content can be regarded, according to literature data, as a characteristic of Moldavian soils, without any traces of anthropogenic contamination (Stasiev, 2016).

In a recent study, metals Transfer Factor (TF) was analyzed from soil to plant (Zinicovscaia, 2018). The transfer factor (TF) is defined in the following equation: $TF = \dfrac{C_{plant}}{C_{soil}}$, where C_{plant} is the concentration of an element in the plant material (dry weight basis) and C_{soil} is the total concentration of the same element in the soil (dry weight basis) where the plant was grown. The higher the value of the TF, the more mobile/available the metal is.

The values of TF were calculated to reveal accumulation of elements the following systems: $TF_{L/S}=C_{leaves}/C_{soil}$, $TF_{F/S}=C_{fruits}/C_{soil}$, $TF_{F/L}=C_{fruits}/C_{leaves}$, $TF_{F/St}=C_{fruits}/C_{stone}$, and $TF_{St/S}=C_{stone}/C_{soil}$. The content of major and trace elements in selected varieties of fruits (apple, plum and grape) as well as in leaves and soils samples were determined using neutron activation analysis. A total of 30 elements were determined in soil samples and 25 elements in fruit samples, originals from the Republic of Moldova.

It has been found that in leaves from soils mostly there have been accumulated K ($TF_{L/S}=3.1$), Zn ($TF_{L/S}=2.1$), Sr ($TF_{L/S}=1.9$), and Mo ($TF_{L/S}=1.1$) and Ca ($TF_{L/S}=0.96$). In a smaller extent there have been accumulated Ca ($TF_{L/S}=0.96$) and Br ($TF_{L/S}=0.73$). For other elements $TF_{L/S}$ values were found to be lower than 1.0, for most of them in the order of 0.1. Concerning the elements transfer from soil in fruits the highest TF values were obtained for Ca ($TF_{L/S} = 3.3$), Sr ($TF_{L/S} = 2.8$) and K ($TF_{F/S}= 1.6$).

In system leaf- fruit (apple) TF> 1.0 was obtained for Na, Cl, and Cr. For all studied systems, the accumulation of elements (both rare earth and pollutants) was very low. It is known that plants act as a barrier to accumulation of pollutants in the food chain. The low level of uptake and the accumulation of some elements in fruits can also be explained by the low level of available forms of these elements in the soil, as well as to the slightly acid to neutral soil pH, which is unfavorable in terms of their uptake (Murtić, 2014).

It is known that the macro-and microelement composition of plants and living organisms depends on the elemental composition of the habitat (Balasubramanian, 2008). European researchers found that even 10 years after bottling, the wine still carries the "chemical signature" of the vineyard and the forest from which the barrel was made, in which the wine was aged (Amorós, 2013). Naturally, this fact can be used to confirm the origin of wines with a geographical name, as well as to detect falsification of wine.

Identification of a product by its place of origin means that it has some special characteristics associated with this territory due to the unique natural and climatic conditions and existing traditions. Also, the geographical name carries the information that there is a specific control over such production. In essence, this is recognition of the product's valorization due to its place of origin.

A large number of natural and anthropogenic factors such as soil characteristics, grape type, production area, environment conditions, fertilizers, inorganic pesticides, winemaking practices, application of additives, transport and storage could significantly influence the concentration of the major and trace elements in wine (Geana, 2012).

From a toxicological point of view, the determination of the content of some mineral elements – possible contaminants (Pb, Cd, Cu, Zn, As, Hg) is mandatory for all food products. At the same time, some countries include in the list of requested characteristics of wine and other macronutrients – potassium (normally its content in wine varies in the range of 0.5–0.8 g/l), sodium (0.02 – 0.35 g/l), calcium (0.1 – 0.5 g/l), magnesium (0.05 – 0.4 g/l). Some micro and oligoelements like F, Al, B, Mn, Se, Br differ in a larger range in which concentrations can vary – fluorine: 0.6 – 2.8 mg/l; aluminum: 1 – 5 mg/l; bromine: 0.1 – 0.7 mg/l; selenium: 0.02 – 0.8 mg/l; manganese: 0.4 – 2.0 mg/l), etc. Therefore, if in the first case the content of macronutrients is of interest mainly from a technological point of view, in the case of trace elements their content / ratio is a carrier of information on the geographical origin of the product (Gonzálvez, 2009).

The ICP-AES and NAA techniques was used to determine 35 elements in vineyard chernozem soil and 18 elements in wines from Republic of Moldova and expand our understanding of the elemental transfer from soil to wine (Zinicovscaia, 2017). Soil elemental content allowed evidencing more similarities between considered soils and the Upper Continental Crust and the World Average Soil as well as to calculate the soil-to-wine transfer factor for 18 of investigated elements. From all 28 trace elements evidenced in soil, only 13, the soluble ones, were found in all wine samples, which finally allowed determining the corresponding transfer factors whose values varied between 0.02 mg/l (U) and 38 mg/l (K). In this regard, all sorts of wines showed a significant concentration of potassium, varying from 370 to 700 mg/l. Comparison of the results obtained for Na, K, Ca, Fe, Zn, and Ba (figure 1) show a good agreement between ICP-AES and NAA techniques. In case of Mg and Al the correlation between methods was better than wines were divided by producers. Mg and Al can be defined as a representative "fingerprint" for grouping wines into distinct classes, depending on their origin (figure 1).

In conclusion, the activation analysis enabled to evidence the presence of all seven major elements, which are present in soil, i.e., Na, Mg, Al, K, Ca, Mn, and Fe, and only 10 soluble trace elements, i.e., Co, Ni, Zn, As, Br, Rb, Sr, Sb, Cs, Ba, and U, whose concentrations were above the detection limits.

Figure 1. Comparison of ICP-AES and NAA data for K and Al

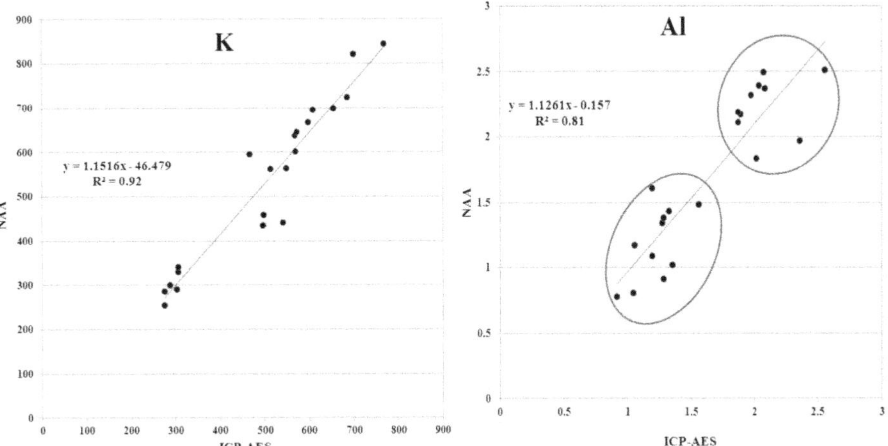

All types of wine presented a high content of K, whose average values varied between 383 mg/l (white wine) and 693 mg/l (red wine), results which are in good concordance with literature data which also point toward a significantly increased content of K in all sorts of wine.

The content of 18 elements detected in all 24 wine samples examined allowed, through discriminatory analyzes, the classification of wines into distinct categories according to sort, type (red and white) and vineyard, which proves that multielement analysis represents a valid tool for the determination of the origin of wines.

ANALYSIS OF CONTAMINATION OF FOODSTUFFS WITH RESIDUES OF PLANT PROTECTION PRODUCTS – BACKGROUND

The presence of pesticide residues in food is a major concern for consumers. A Eurobarometer about EU citizens' general fears and fears about food shows that 63%are worried about the presence of pesticide residues in food (EURACTIV, 2019).

A recent report provides an overview of the 2016 the results of control program (EUCP) and the results of national control programs (NP) about the situation of pesticide residues in food products that are the most widely consumed in the EU, carried out in the European Union (EU) Member States, Iceland and Norway. Overall, 98.3% of the samples analyzed in the 2016 EUCP fell within the legal limits (11,965 samples); 6,367 samples (52.3%) were free of quantifiable residues (residues below the limit of quantification (LOQ). The number of samples with quantified residues, but within the legally permitted level (at or above the LOQ but below the maximum residue level (MRL) was 5,598 (46.0%). In 1.7% of the samples analyzed the MRL was exceeded (203 samples). In total, 0.9% of the samples (107 samples) were considered to be not compliant with the legal limits taking into account the measurement uncertainty (EU Report, 2018). Compared with 2013, when the same commodities were analyzed, the MRL exceedance rate in 2016 is higher (1.7% in 2016 compared to 0.9% in 2013). This significant increase was mainly driven by the high number of exceedances regarding residues of chlorpyrifos, an active substance for which the MRLs were lowered for many crops during 2016 (59 exceedances were reported out of the 10,212 samples analyzed for this pesticide).

The presence of considerable levels of pesticide residues in the European food chain is the direct result of pesticide dependence on conventional agriculture. Each year, over 220 000 tons of pesticides are used in the European Union environment. The European Union annual results on the use of pesticides show that 108 000 tons of fungicides, 84 000 tons of herbicides, 21 000 tons of insecticide and 7 000 tons of plant growth regulators – representing approximately one kilo of the active substance per capita (Eurostat, 2010).

The study *"Message in a Bottle", 2008* on the presence of pesticide residues in wine present in the European consumer network was coordinated by Pan-Europa and supported by MDRGF for France, Global 2000 for Greenpeace Austria and Germany. 40 bottles of red wine from France, Austria, Germany, Italy, Portugal, South Africa, Australia and Chile were analyzed, of which 34 were from intensive agriculture and 6 from organic farming. Wines have been selected from the least-priced brands as well as the world's most famous brands. 100% of the conventional wines tested were contaminated. It has been established that each sample from traditional agriculture contains more than 4 different pesticide residues in the environment, the most contaminated among them containing up to 10 pesticides. In some of the wines tested, the residual content of plant protection products exceeded 5800 times the maximum allowable concentrations authorized for drinking water.

These numerous residues characterize a very intensive use of pesticides in viticulture. Many of these are carcinogenic or potentially toxic for reproduction or development. Altogether, 15 different pesticide residues were detected in conventional-grape wines. Among the most dangerous substances there was procymidone, classified as a carcinogen and endocrine substance. The study shows that the intensive use of pesticides in viticulture leads to the systematic presence of many phytosanitary residues in wine. It has been established that about 1/3 of the pesticides present in grapes are systematically transferred to the finished product („Message in a Bottle", 2008).

The amount of pesticide (active substance) used in viticulture is 21.4 kg of active ingredients (AI) per hectare. Much of this refers to the application of sulfur – relatively less dangerous than the chemicals used to protect against oidium (Cabras, 2000). However, in addition to sulfur-based fungicides, grapes receive doses of synthetic fungicides averaging 4.7 kg/ha – and higher than any other crop, except for potatoes. Of the 2163 grape samples, 57% of the tests were positive for at least one pesticide, 5% of the samples contained more pesticides than the legal limits. Among the most frequently, detected residues there were many synthetic fungicides: procymidone, dicarboximide (present in 22.41% of grape samples evaluated), iprodione, imidazole present in 16.26% of evaluated grape samples (Čuš, 2010).

The results obtained in these studies are by no means able to alleviate public opinion – procymidone, incriminated as a substance with potential carcinogenic, toxic for reproduction / development and deregulator of the endocrine system, which is the leader in this chapter, was detected in 22.41% of contaminated grape seed samples. Chlorpyrifos – a substance with neurotoxic effect present in 17.33% of cases, carcinogenic iprodione – in 16.26%, and for maneb (substance with carcinogenic potential and endocrine deregulator), the incidence is 14.33%. Numerous researches have shown that people with frequent activities requiring contact with pesticides (field spraying, chemical plants, etc.) show a higher incidence of respiratory problems, chronic rhinitis, cancer and chromosomal abnormalities, alterations in neurological capacity associated with the risk of occurrence of neurodegenerative diseases.

The results of these studies show that only the issue of contact with pesticides either directly (people involved in agricultural works, for example) or indirectly – contamination with residues present in food can significantly affect the health of the population. A major issue – the cumulative effect of pesticide residues remains on the agenda and requires extensive research (Grinbaum, 2010).

Issues, Controversies, Problems

What is the rate of accumulation of organic pesticide residues in horticultural products? In wines? Transfer of pesticide residues into wine can affect health?

In the Republic of Moldova, the area of the vineyard plantations is about 150 thousand hectares. For phytosanitary protection of the vineyards, 1000 tons of pesticides (per active substance) are used annually, which is an average of 6.5 kg per hectare. The State Register includes 158 pesticides, approved for the protection of vineyards, including 112 fungicides. In 2007, it was decided to include in the State Register and to admit only plant and plant products of grade III and IV of toxicity (with a medium and low toxicity level) for plant protection (State Register of Pesticides, 2016).

Approximately 3000 samples of wine have been analyzed to determine the residual quantities of pesticides in wines produced in the Republic of Moldova. Persistent organic pollutants, POPs (DDT and its isomers / metabolites DDE, DDD), alpha-, beta-, gamma-HCH, Aldrin and Heptaclor were not found in any of the wine samples. Chlorinated organic pesticides have been banned for use in the Republic of Moldova since 1970, including DDT and its metabolites: hexachlorocyclohexane, heptachlor, aldrin, etc. banned after 1980. The lack of POPs in wine products is an extremely important thing, which proves that there is no systemic pollution of the vineyards (Gh. Duca, 2012).

In wine samples there were identified insignificant quantities of metalaxyl and mefenoxam or its isomer (metalaxyl-M). Mefenoxam and metalaxyl are active ingredients of some modern systemic fungicides, such as Ridomil Gold, Protexyl, Acedan, Metaxyl, applied on vineyards with the purpose to control diseases caused by air- and soil-borne Peronosporales.

Detected residues of metalaxyl and mefenoxam in wine were generally lower than MAL (Maximal Admitted Level) for grapes – 0.03 mg/kg and EU MAL – 0.2 mg/kg. The results obtained during 2008 – 2009 are presented in Table 1.

After the return of Moldovan wine from Russia under the pretext of containing pesticide residues, 384 raw material wine and bottled wine samples were analyzed in order to determine the organic pesticide residue content. This category does not include the lots, which according to phytosanitary certificate, there were not treated with organic pesticides, but with sulfur-based fungicides.

The distribution median for metalaxyl in the examined wines can serve as a statistical index. At the same time it must be noted that wine production originating from the same enterprises presents, in most cases, similar data about metalaxyl residual content or the lack of this (for the same crop year). The generalized data regarding the distribution of wine samples tested for pesticide residues is presented in Table 2.

The monitoring of pesticide residues content in grapes and wine has a short history in Republic of Moldova. Before 2006, when the embargo for Moldovan wines in Russian Federation was imposed, the content of pesticide residues in wines was not analyzed, and this one was not regulated (moreover, this has not changed at present). In addition, there persists the opinion that pesticide residues cannot be accumulated, because during technological treatment these are eliminated. In grapes only the residual content of persistent pesticides (chlorinated organic) - DDT and metabolites, hexachlorocyclohexane, heptachlor, aldrin was analyzed. The methods used for residual analysis of pesticides in grapes were very simple – thin layer chromatography, which had not allowed a veridical analysis.

Table 1. Pesticide residues in wines produced in Republic of Moldova

Found active ingredient	Corresponding pesticide	Concentration, µg/l	MAL µg/kg, grapes	Wines
metalaxyl	Profexyl 350 FS Ridomil Gold MZ 68 WG Valsalaxil720 WP Pyrenomil720WP	6 7 9 30-35	30	Cabernet[1] Merlot[1] Muscat[1] wine raw material[3]
vinclozolin	Ronilan 50 WG	13	300	Kahor[2]
metalaxyl	Profexyl 350 FS, Ridomil Gold MZ 68 WG	16 2 3-13 11 16 6	30	Muscat[4] Cabernet[5] Chardonnay[5] Feteasca[6] Portwein[7] Zemfira[8]
metalaxyl, procymidone	Sumilex, WG	13 49	30 500	Sauvignon[9] Chardonnay[9]
tebuconazole azoxystrobin metalaxyl	Falcon 460 EC, Quadris 250 EC	11 9 22	25* 50 30	Wine raw material[10] Riesling[6] Aligote[6]
kresoxim-methyl azoxystrobin metalaxyl	Stroby, Quadris 250 EC	2 9 23	50 50 30	Sauvignon[6]
azoxystrobin mefenoxam	Quadris 250 EC, Ridomil Gold MZ 68 WG	7 6	50 30	Rkatsiteli[6]

*for grains, not allowed in grapes; [1-10] –wine samples originating from different regions

Table 2. Distribution of pesticide active ingredients found in wine samples

Wine category	Metalaxyl[1] residues µg/l				
	<5	5-10	10-20	20-30	[3]30
Raw material wine: white	10	17	18	7	3
red	16	19	23	9	2
Bottled white wines (including sparkling wines)	6	2	3	-	-
Bottled red wines	5	7	3	3	-
Total	37	45	47	19	5
Median of distribution	3.77±0.89	7.98±1.02	13.66±1.56	24.21±2.07	35.2±6.28

[1]MAL for metalaxyl – 30 µg/l

Almost in all cases, for which traces of pesticides' active ingredients were found, their residual content in wine was not exceeding MAL (for grapes). However, if the fact that some pesticides contain 2 – 3 active ingredients is considered and every active ingredient presents a different degree of toxicity, it is obvious that the cumulative effect of these must be taken into account.

Based on the results obtained in 2008 the Interagency Council approved a decision on increasing the waiting period (time between last treatment and grape harvest) from 20 to 60 days, no later than two weeks after the flowering of vine. The Council decision had a beneficial effect – not only the range of active ingredients' residues of detected pesticides was significantly reduced, but also the contamination level of wine products.

By July 2010 the analysis of pesticide residues in wines bears a random character, dictated by the demands of importers (Belarus, Russian Federation). After the return of Moldovan wines from Russian Federation on the grounds of metalaxyl residues detection (in two cases the concentrations of 0.037 and 0.032 mg/l metalaxyl were reported) the Ministry of Agriculture and Food Industry has ordered compulsory testing of the pesticide residue content for each batch of exported wine. For organic pesticide testing, the phytosanitary certificate, which indicates the used pesticide and date of last treatment, must be taken into account.

According to the obtained results of 384 analyzed samples, in 231 cases traces of organic pesticides were not found, although according to the phytosanitary certificate, they have been used for vine treatment. Thus, if the pesticide application doses and the waiting period are met, they can be used without causing damage to the products. The lack of organic pesticide traces in 60% of examined cases evidence that most growers comply with the rules of use of organic pesticides.

With regard to wine samples in which organic pesticide residues were detected, it should be noted that in most cases metalaxyl was found, which indicates that the pesticides mainly used to treat vines were Profexyl 350 FS, Ridomil Gold MZ 68 WG, Pyrenomil 720 WP, Valsalaxil 20 WP. In terms of quantity, the distribution of samples is shown in Figure 1 (white wine) and 1b (red wine).

The data analysis from Table 2 attests that most manufacturers test raw materials before bottling, allowing them to reduce the cost of analysis and product losses related to the refusal by the importer. It appears, that in 24% of the cases, the content of metalaxyl in raw material and wine samples did not exceed 5 µg/l. In 30% of the cases it was situated within 5 to 10 µg / l; in 30.5% of the cases the residue content of metalaxyl was varying within the range 10 – 20 µg/l, which is well below the MAL established in Russian Federation for wines at 30 µg/l. In 12% of samples positively attested to the presence of metalaxyl, its concentration was located near the MAC and varied within 20 to 30 µg/l. In 3% of the cases excesses of the MAL were discovered. It is noted that excesses of the MAL were not observed in finished products (bottled wines). In addition, values close to the MAL, located within 20 to 30 µg/l were only found in a very small number of examined samples.

In red wines, the percentage of samples without organic pesticide residues was 56%. For white wines, pesticide residues were not detected in 64% of examined samples. Decreased rate of contamination of white wines compared to red wines suggests the idea that there might be a correlation between applied winemaking technology, red or white – the skin maceration could contribute to a higher degree of pesticide residues' transfer in wine.

In addition to wine samples, at the demand of importers from Russian Federation some manufacturers have tested spirits category – divin, wine and brandy distillates (a total of 42 samples). Divin is a spirit drink obtained from wine distillates, aged at least 3 years, with the addition of softened water, sugar syrup and, where appropriate, with caramel sugar and alcoholic water, up to the organoleptic and physico-chemical characteristics established in the respective regulations. Divin (from Latin *divinus*) is a product with a geographical indication from the Republic of Moldova, synonymous with the well-known Cognac.

Traces of pesticides were not found in any of the examined samples confirming the lack of pesticide residues transfer in the process of wine distillation. Obviously, this conclusion cannot be generalized, because previous data on the content of organic pesticide residues in raw materials subjected to wine distillation are lacking.

The following conclusions can be made from the generalization of the data presented:

The problem of organic pesticide residues in wines is significant for countries with intensive viticulture. In the Republic of Moldova it is noted a low level of organic pesticide residues in wines, taken in relation to the major wine-producing countries. Persistent organic pesticides (chlorinated organic) were not detected in any of the samples examined in the last three years (over 3000 samples) using advanced methods with high-resolution, GC/MS. The presence of multi residues is rarely detected. The active ingredient most commonly found in wine production is metalaxyl.

The lack of organic pesticide residues is attested in most of the examined cases (60% of samples). This is due firstly to the relatively low number of applied phytosanitary treatments, but also the prevalence of sulfur-based fungicides. The increase of the waiting period at vineyards treatment with organic pesticides also had an important role. The share of MAL (for grapes) excess cases is very low – <3%, and refers only to raw material wines. In bottled wines, MAL surpluses were not registered.

In order to reduce the contamination risks of wine production with organic pesticide residues, it is necessary to revise the list of pesticides approved for the treatment of vineyards in the State Register, taking into account the degree of toxicity, and to inform the grape producers about the effectuated changes.

FOOD CHAIN CONTAMINATION WITH PHTHALATE RESIDUES

BACKGROUND

Phthalates (esters of phthalic acid) are included in the compositions of almost all types of plastics, rubber, paints and varnishes, giving them elasticity and strength. The annual production of phthalates was estimated by the World Health Organization (WHO) to approach 8 million tons (by data on 1992) and 5 million tons by data on 2011 (Phthalates, 2011). Most phthalates produced (90%) are used as plasticizers (Wei Wang, 2018). Since February 2017, 4 phthalates (DEHP, DIBP, DBP and BBzP) are recognized by European regulations REACH on the list of substances of very high concern to humans. DEHP is classified as a carcinogen (category 2B) by the International Agency for Research on Cancer (IARC). DEHP and DBP are classified as Category 1B reproductive toxic (likely effect in human). Standards are defined based on the individual data of each phthalate, but they can act according to a cocktail effect, including with other currently unregulated phthalates (eg DEP).

The main source of contamination is food, due to the ingestion of food contaminated by phthalate migration from plastic packaging (Arnold Schecter, 2013). When DEHP, a semi-volatile organic compound, is used in floor coverings, it constitutes 20 to 40% of the weight. As it is not chemically related to materials, it is slowly emitted in the indoor environment. An American study has calculated that the estimated exposures from this source range from 5µg / kg / day to 180µg/kg/day with a median at 38µg/kg/day, twice the toxic value of reference of the US EPA (Marianne Balck, 2015).

The authors (van Gelder, 2010) provided that phthalates be accumulated in the human body. Phtalates negatively affect hormones, liver and kidneys and can also cause allergies, asthma, neurodeveloped disorders and abnormalities in the development of children (Lacey Robinson, 2015). A mixture of plastic derived compounds, phthalates can promote epigenetic transgenerational inheritance of adult onset disease. The sperm provide potential epigenetic biomarkers for transgenerational disease and/or ancestral environmental exposures (Mohan Manikkam, 2013).

Most researchers from different organizations suggest that in most cases, the influence of phthalates is less than tolerable daily doses (Jung-Wei Chang, (2017). However, it is difficult to accurately determine the exposure dose as the spread of phthalates is everywhere (Xu-Liang Cao, 2010). Determination of the sources and causes of food contamination with phthalates is the key moments in the issue of product safety. A number of European laboratories investigated the migration of harmful substances from the polymer by acting on them with solutions simulating saliva, blood, milk, soft drinks, etc. Most of the procedures of the study of migration are described of existing publications and directives (Chatonnet, 2014, Yukihiro Ouchi, 2019).

Issues, Controversies, Problems

What are the factors that influence the migration of phthalates in wines and other beverages?

Migration of phthalates has been studied in samples of rubber and plasticized PVC. For each series of experiments, samples of polymers were taken with the same mass (5.0g of rubber, 1.0g of PVC) and surface area S=32,98см² and S=15,57см² respectively. The volumes of extractants are also the same for every series – 100 ml. As the solvents, there were investigated: water – as a basic component of alcoholic beverages (T=25,0°C), solution of water/alcohol (1:1) for modeling strong alcoholic beverages (T=25,0°C), wine simulant (T=25,0°C), alcohol ethylic – as an essential component (T=0,0°C, 25,0°C, 50,0°C, 75,0°C), chloroform as alternative organic solvent (T=25,0°C), alcohol ethylic (T=25,0°C under the ultrasonic influence). All samples of polymers, completely immersed in the extractants, were kept for 7 hours at static conditions, except the case of ultrasonic extraction. Samples were taken for analysis every hour (all extractions were performed in two parallels). DBP and DEHP were detected in the investigated samples of polymers.

Figure 2 shows the kinetic curves reflecting the migration of DBP (fig. 2a) and DEHP (fig. 2b) from PVC in different solvents, at different temperatures.

Figure 2. Migration of DBP (a) and DEHP (b) in various solvents from PVC.

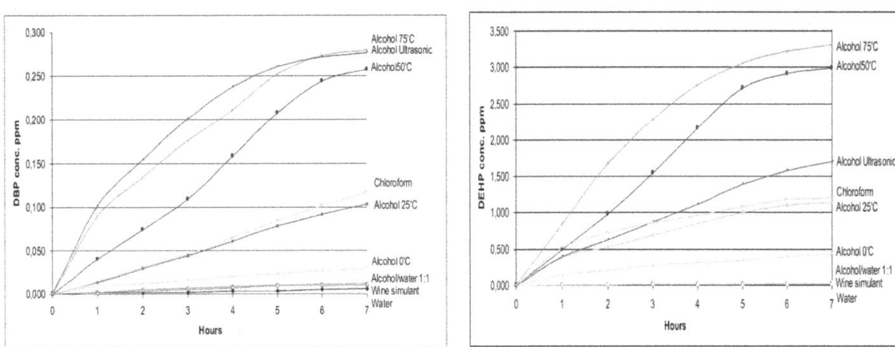

The migration of DBP and DEHP in water, wine simulant (12% vol. ethanol) and water/ethanol solution (1: 1) runs slowly during the examined time (25°C). The migration rate of phthalates in chloroform and ethanol (25°C) is considerably higher. The temperature and the action of the ultrasound accelerate exponentially the migration process of phthalates into alcohol.

The study of phthalates migration from the rubber was carried out similar to the same experiment with PVC (figure 3). Although the allure of the curves is similar to that attested for PVC, the migration of phthalates in similar time intervals is considerably higher, a fact most likely caused by the texture of the material.

Figure 3. Migration of DBP (a) and DEHP (b) in various solvents from rubber

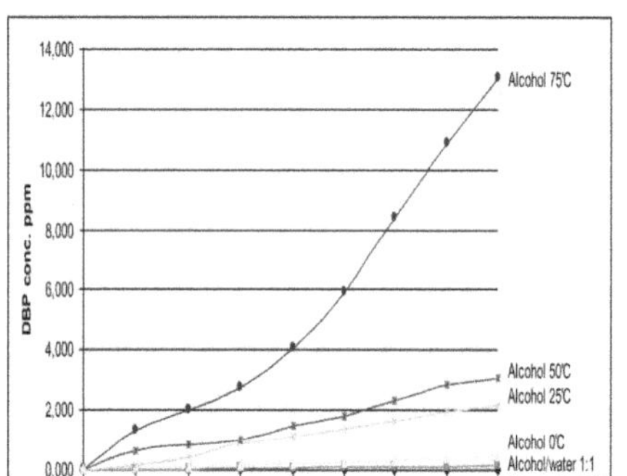

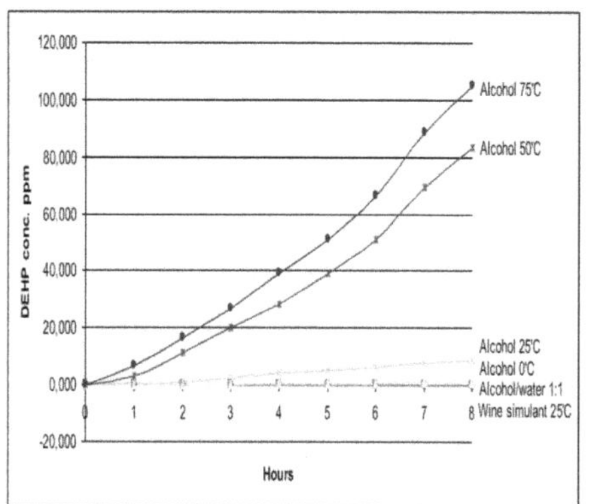

The migration of phthalates from polymeric materials proceeds extremely fast, depending on the nature and texture of the polymer, but also on the nature of the solution. In solutions with a low degree of polarity, the intensity of the transfer is considerably higher than in water and low alcohol solutions. Extraction at high temperatures increase the migration of phthalates .For every 10°C in water, there is an increase of 1.5 – 2.5 times, and for alcohol - an increase of 2.5 – 15 times. The use of the ultrasonic bath (45 kHz, 100 W) for the study of migration initially increases the migration rate up to 6 – 10 times.

The samples of polymeric materials in contact with wine /wine raw material at different stages of production were investigated. The samples for study, such as lining for containers, hoses, rubber and PVC pipe have been provided by some manufacturers, to determine the availability for use in the winery. Results of the phthalates migration in alcohol are given in tab.3. The data are expressed as mg phthalate per kg of investigated material (25°C, 1 hour).

Also 36 different samples of cork stoppers (for wine and brandy), 6 samples of polymer stoppers for sealing wines and more than 20 samples of caps, seals, dispensers bottle and other polymer elements, which can contact with bottled alcoholic beverages have been studied as a potential source of contamination. All the samples were crushed to accelerate the potential migration of phthalates in the model solution and better quantify the amount of phthalates present.

In some cases, migration of phthalates was determined from the surface of the products. As the model solutions there was used water-alcohol solution and acidic water-alcohol mixture simulating wine. As a result, it should be noted that DBP was detected in trace amounts only in four of the investigated samples. In these cases, the observed DBP was on the surface of cork, that is probably due to a violation of the

Table 3. Migration of phthalates in alcohol from polymeric materials for 1 hour, mg/L

Polymeric material	DMP	DEP	DBP	DEHP
Paints	<LD	<LD	0 – 867.4	0 – 55.7
Lining for containers	<LD	<LD	0 – 94.6	0 – 34.44
Enamels	<LD	<LD	0 – 29.5	0 – 11.589
Varnish	<LD	<LD	63.7	13.15
Hardenger	<LD	<LD	33.2	<LD
Hoses	<LD	<LD	0 – 170.0	0 – 2478.5
Filter paper	<LD	<LD	0.052	0.042
Filter sheets	<LD	0 – 0.020	0.068 – 0.406	0.025 – 0.241
Perlite	<LD	<LD	0.000	0.000
Nutrient additions	<LD	<LD	0 – 0.019	0 – 1.016
Bentonite	<LD	<LD	0.023	0.000
Gelatin	<LD	<LD	0.000	0.000
Kieselguhr	0 – 0.082	0 – 0.104	0.05 – 4.204	0 – 0.067

conditions of capping material storage. No significant amounts of phthalates were found in any of the samples studied by coating materials (Duca, 2014).

Although the costs of replacing DBP and DEHP include both the higher cost of alternative materials, exposure risks can not be ruled out as a contributing factor to multiple health hazards (Sturza, 2017).

CONCLUSION

The environment influences food along the raw material-finished product pathway, at different times the food-environment relationship causes changes that concern the composition and harmlessness of the product intended for human consumption. The raw materials make the first impact with the environment. The study of the ways and dimensions in which the environment interacts with the raw materials involves assessing the transfer mechanisms, the persistence and the accumulation of various xenobiotics. The research allows us to draw the following conclusions:

- The analysis of the possible anthropogenic contamination content, made by the Neutron Activation Analysis (NAA) has demonstrated, with the exception for the As, the absence of any systematic soil pollution in the Republic of Moldova. In this respect, although the As content exceeds a few times the UCC value of 1.5 mg / kg, reaching the alarm threshold according to some national regulations, its increased content can be considered, according to the literature, as a characteristic of soils Moldovans, without traces of anthropogenic contamination.
- The TF values were calculated to show the accumulation of elements in the following systems: $TF_{L/S}=C_{leaves}/C_{soil}$, $TF_{F/S}=C_{fruits}/C_{soil}$, $TF_{F/L}=C_{fruits}/C_{leaves}$, $TF_{F/St}=C_{fruits}/C_{stone}$, and $TF_{St/S}=C_{stone}/C_{soil}$. A total amount of 30 elements were determined in soil samples and 25 elements in the samples of leaves and fruits (apples, plums and grapes), originating from the Republic of Moldova. For all

studied systems, the accumulation of rare earth elements and elements, which can be considered as environmental pollutants, was very low.

- The NAA was used to determine 35 elements in vineyard chernozem soil and 18 elements in wines from Republic of Moldova. From all 28 trace elements evidenced in soil, only 13, the soluble ones, were found in all wine samples. Using discriminant analysis, the content of each element and wine sample could be classified into categories according to sort, type (red and white) and vineyard. The method can be applied to guarantee origin and quality of wines of controlled origin from the Republic of Moldova, as well as to prevent fraud.

- In the Republic of Moldova it is noted a low level of organic pesticide residues in wines, taken in relation to the major wine producing countries. Persistent organic pesticides (chlorinated organic) were not detected in any of the samples examined in the last three years (over 3000 samples) using advanced methods with high-resolution, GC/MS. The presence of multi residues is rarely detected. The active ingredient most commonly found in wine production is metalaxyl. The share of MAC (for grapes) excess cases is very low – <3%, and refers only to raw material wines. In finished products, MAC surpluses were not registered.

- Migration of phthalates in various solutions from polymeric materials was investigated. A number of materials that might be potential sources of phthalates and influence of temperature on the rate and extent of extraction was carried out. It has been shown that the contamination with phthalate residues of beverages occurs predominantly at the stage of grape processing, technological treatments and storage.

FUTURE RESEARCH DIRECTIONS

Research has shown that environmental pollution, agrobiological and technological processes applied to the industrial processing of raw materials can be the cause of food contamination. It is necessary to monitor the content of pesticide residues in plant raw materials, as the active principles used are very varied. One concern is the contamination of foodstuffs with phthalates residues, both from environmental pollution, from packaging and utensils used to produce them. Thus, a rigorous and continuous control of the degree of environmental pollution and contaminants transfer factors in raw materials and food is necessary.

ACKNOWLEDGMENT

The author expresses his gratitude to all colleagues involved in the research mentioned in this chapter: ASM, JINR-Dubna, CNVCPA.

REFERENCES

Amorós, J. A., Pérez-de-los Reyes, C., Francisco, J. G. N., Bravo, S., Chacón, J. L., Martínez, J., & Ballesta, R. J. (2013). Bioaccumulation of mineral elements in grapevine varieties cultivated in "La Mancha". *Journal of Plant Nutrition and Soil Science, 176*(6), 843–850. doi:10.1002/jpln.201300015

Balan, V. (2008). Development of Fruit Growing In the Republic Of Moldova. *Bulletin UASVM. Horticulture*, *65*(1), 252–256.

Balasubramanian, A. (2008). *Ecosystem and its Components*. Technical Report. Retrieved from: https://www.researchgate.net/publication/314213426_ECOSYSTEM_AND_ITS_COMPONENTS

Balck, M. (2015). *Phthalates in preschool dust the relation between phthalates and parameters in the preschool environment*. Degree project in biology, Master of Science. Retrieved from https://www.diva-portal.org/smash/get/diva2:852215/FULLTEXT01.pdf

Botnari, V. (2016). Use of microelements in vegetable growing. In *Microelements in the composition of the biosphere and their application in agriculture and medicine* (pp. 164–167). Chisinau: ASM Publishing House.

Cabras, P., & Angioni, A. (2000). Pesticide Residues in Grapes, Wine, and Their Processing Products. *Journal of Agricultural and Food Chemistry*, *48*(4), 967–973. doi:10.1021/jf990727a PMID:10775335

Cao, X.-L. (2010). Phthalate Esters in Foods: Sources, Occurrence, and Analytical Methods. *Comprehensive Reviews in Food Science and Food Safety*, *9*(1), 21–43. doi:10.1111/j.1541-4337.2009.00093.x

Chang, J.-W., Lee, C.-C., Pan, W.-H., Chou, W.-C., Huang, H.-B., Chiang, H.-C., & Huang, P.-C. (2017). Estimated Daily Intake and Cumulative Risk Assessment of Phthalates in the General Taiwanese after the 2011 DEHP Food Scandal. *Scientific Reports*, *7*(1), 45009. doi:10.1038rep45009 PMID:28327585

Chatonnet, P., Boutou, S., & Plana, A. (2014). Contamination of wines and spirits by phthalates: Types of contaminants present, contamination sources and means of prevention. *Food Additives & Contaminants. Part A, Chemistry, Analysis, Control, Exposure & Risk Assessment*, *31*(9), 1–11. doi:10.1080/19440049.2014.941947 PMID:25099435

Čuš, F., Česnik, H. B., Bolta, Š. V., & Gregorčič, A. (2010). Pesticide residues in grapes and during vinification process. *Food Control*, *21*(11), 1512–1518. doi:10.1016/j.foodcont.2010.04.024

Determination of Migration Rates for Certain Phthalates. (2016). *Survey of chemical substances in consumer products No. 149*. Retrieved from https://www2.mst.dk/Udgiv/publications/2016/08/978-87-93529-01-4.pdf

Duca, G., Sturza, R., & Lazacovici, D. (2014, Dec.). Comparative study of the analysis techniques of phthalates in wine products. *Revue Roumaine de Chimie*, 11–15.

Duca, Gh., Sturza, R., & Siretanu, L. (2012). Estimation of organic pesticide residue content in wines. *CLEAN - Soil, Air, Water*, *40*(6), 661–666. doi:10.1002/clen.201100081

EURACTIV. (2012). *Pesticides are EU citizens' top food-related health concern*. Retrieved from: https://www.euractiv.com/section/health-consumers/news/pesticides-are-eu-citizens-top-food-related-health-concern/

European Union report on pesticide residues in food. Scientific Report. (2018). EFSA Journal, 16(7). doi:10.2903/j.efsa.2018.5348

Eurostat. (2010). *The use of plant protection products in the European Union.* Retrieved from: https://ec.europa.eu/eurostat/web/products-statistical-books/-/KS-76-06-669

Frontasyeva, M. V. (2011). Neutron activation analysis for the Life Sciences. A review. *Physics of Particles and Nuclei, 42*(2), 332–378. doi:10.1134/S1063779611020043

Galani-Nikolakaki, S. M., & Kallithrakas-Kontos, N. G. (2007). Elemental Content of Wines. In P. Szefer & J. O. Nriagu (Eds.), Mineral components in foods (pp. 323–338). Academic Press.

Geana, I., Iordache, A., Ionete, R., Marinescu, A., Ranca, A., & Culeac, M. (2013). Geographical origin identification of Romanian wines by ICP-MS elemental analysis. *Food Chemistry, 138*(2-3), 1125–1134. doi:10.1016/j.foodchem.2012.11.104 PMID:23411223

Gonzálvez, A., Llorens, A., Cervera, M. L., Armenta, S., & Guardia, M. (2009). Elemental fingerprint of wines from the protected designation of origin Valencia. *Food Chemistry, 112*(1), 26–34. doi:10.1016/j.foodchem.2008.05.043

Grinbaum. (2014). *Le point sur les résidus des produits phytosanitaires dans les vins. Œnologies Bordeaux.* Retrieved from: https://www.canal.tv/video/universite_de_bordeaux/

Kalliopi, Petros-Achillefs, Anne-Katrin, Jan, Sandra, & Franz (2016). *Delivering on EU Food Safety and Nutrition in 2050 – Future challenges and policy preparedness.* Publications Office of the European Union.

López Alonso, M., Prieto Montaña, F., Miranda, M., Castillo, C., Hernández, J., & Luis Benedito, J. (2004). Interactions between toxic (As, Cd, Hg and Pb) and nutritional essential (Ca, Co, Cr, Cu, Fe, Mn, Mo, Ni, Se, Zn) elements in the tissues of cattle from NW Spain. *Biometals, 17*(4), 389–397. doi:10.1023/B:BIOM.0000029434.89679.a2 PMID:15259359

Manikkam, M., Tracey, R., Guerrero-Bosagna, C., & Skinner, M. K. (2013). Plastics Derived Endocrine Disruptors (BPA, DEHP and DBP) Induce Epigenetic Transgenerational Inheritance of Obesity, Reproductive Disease and Sperm Epimutations. *PLoS One, 8*(1), e55387. doi:10.1371/journal.pone.0055387 PMID:23359474

Message in a Bottle. (2008). *Supporting Information.* Retrieved from: https://www.pan-europe.info/old/Resources/Briefings/Message_in_a_bottle_Background.pdf

Meyts, E. R.-D. (2006). Developmental model for the pathogenesis of testicular carcinoma in situ: Genetic and environmental aspects. *Human Reproduction Update, 12*(3), 303–323. doi:10.1093/humupd/dmk006 PMID:16540528

Murtić, S., Brkovic, D., Djuric, M., & Vujinovic, I. (2014). Heavy metal dynamics in the soil–leaf–fruit system under intensive apple cultivation. *Acta Agriculturae Serbica, 19*(38), 123–132. doi:10.5937/AASer1438123M

Ouchi, Y., Yanagisawa, H., & Fujimaki, S. (2019). Evaluating Phthalate Contaminant Migration Using Thermal Desorption–Gas Chromatography–Mass Spectrometry (TD–GC–MS). *Polymers, 11*(4), 683. doi:10.3390/polym11040683 PMID:30991697

Paul, B. (2012). Heavy Metals Toxicity and the Environment. *EXS, 101*, 133–164. doi:10.1007/978-3-7643-8340-4_6 PMID:22945569

Phthalates and their alternatives health and environmental concerns. (2011). University of Massachusetts Lowell.

Robinson, L., & Miller, R. (2015). The Impact of Bisphenol A and Phthalates on Allergy, Asthma, and Immune Function: A Review of Latest Findings. *Current Environmental Health Reports, 2*(4), 379–387. doi:10.100740572-015-0066-8 PMID:26337065

Rodica, S. (2016). Microelements in food. In Microelements in the composition of the biosphere and their application in agriculture and medicine, (pp.174-194). Chisinau: ASM Publishing House.

Rodica, S., Boris, G., Roxana, I. E., & Diana, C. (2017). The authenticity and harmlessness of uvological products. Chişinău, "MS Logo" Publishing House.

Schecter, A., Lorber, M., Guo, Y., Wu, Q., Yun, S. H., Kannan, K., ... Birnbaum, L. S. (2013). Phthalate Concentrations and Dietary Exposure from Food Purchased in New York State. *Environmental Health Perspectives, 121*(4), 473–479. doi:10.1289/ehp.1206367 PMID:23461894

Serrano, S. E. (2014, June 2). Phthalates and diet: A review of the food monitoring and epidemiology data. *Environmental Health,* 13. PMID:24894065

Singh, R., Gautam, N., Mishra, A., & Gupta, R. (2011). Heavy metals and living systems: An overview. *Indian Journal of Pharmacology, 43*(3), 246–253. doi:10.4103/0253-7613.81505 PMID:21713085

Stasiev, G., & Toma, S. (2016). Ecological content and evaluation of microelements in soil (2016). In *Microelements in the composition of the biosphere and their application in agriculture and medicine* (pp. 27–56). Chisinau: ASM Publishing House.

State Register of Pesticides Approved in the Republic of Moldova. (2016). Retrieved from http://www.pesticide.md/registrul-de-stat/

Sturza & Lazacovich. (2017). *Monitoring the overall phthalate burden – a public health problem.* RIVEmed no.2, "Grigore T. Popa" Publishing House Iasi.

Sturza, R., Bilici, C., Zinicovscaia, I., Culicov, O. A., Gundorina, S., & Duca, G. (2015). Moldavian wine analysis by ICP-AES and NAA techniques: Comparison study. *Revue Roumaine de Chimie, 60*(11-12), 1065–1071.

van Gelder, M. M. H. J., van Rooij, I. A. L. M., Miller, R. K., Zielhuis, G. A., de Jong-van den Berg, L. T. W., & Roeleveld, N. (2010). Teratogenic mechanisms of medical drugs. *Human Reproduction Update, 16*(4), 378–394. doi:10.1093/humupd/dmp052 PMID:20061329

Veliksar, S. (2016). Microelements in achieving the adaptive productivity potential and resistance in horticulture. In *Microelements in the composition of the biosphere and their application in agriculture and medicine* (pp. 142–163). Chisinau: ASM Publishing House.

Wang, W., Leung, A. O. W., Chu, L. H., & Wong, M. H. (2018). Phthalates Contamination in China: Status, Trends and Human Exposure-with an Emphasis on Oral Intake. *Environmental Pollution, 238,* 771–782. doi:10.1016/j.envpol.2018.02.088 PMID:29625301

Weiss, J. M., Lignell, S., Darnerud, P. O., & Kotova, N. (2016). Human Biomonitoring of Environmental Contaminants - Examples Offering Tools Towards Safe Food in Sweden. *European Journal of Nutrition & Food Safety*, 6(3), 132–147. doi:10.9734/EJNFS/2016/20212

Zinicovscaia, Duliu, Culicov, Frontasyeva, & Sturza. (2018). Major and trace elements distribution in Moldavian soils. Rom. Rep. Phys., 70(2).

Zinicovscaia, I., Duliu, O. G., Culicov, O. A., Sturza, R., Bilici, C., & Gundorina, S. (2017). Geographical Origin Identification of Moldavian Wines by Neutron Activation Analysis. *Food Analytical Methods*, 10(11), 3523–3530. doi:10.100712161-017-0913-3

Zinicovscaia, I., Sturza, R., Gurmeza, I., Vergel, K., Gundorina, S., & Duca, G. (2018). Metal bioaccumulation in the soil-leaf-fruit system determined by neutron activation analysis. *Journal of Food Measurement and Characterization*. doi:10.100711694-018-9972-4

This research was previously published in theHandbook of Research on Emerging Developments and Environmental Impacts of Ecological Chemistry edited by Gheorghe Duca and Ashok Vaseashta; pages 472-490, copyright year 2020 by Engineering Science Reference (an imprint of IGI Global).

Chapter 3
Food Safety and Climate Change:
Case of Mycotoxins

Abdellah Zinedine
Chouaib Doukkali University, Morocco

Samira El Akhdari
Ministry of National Education, Morocco

ABSTRACT

Mycotoxins are chemical compounds produced mainly by mounds of genera Aspergillus, Penicillium, and Fusarium on various grains and agricultural commodities at different stages in the field, before harvest, post-harvest, during processing, packaging, distribution, and storage. The production of mycotoxins depends on several environmental factors such as temperature and moisture. This chapter gives an overview about the major mycotoxins (e.g., aflatoxins, ochratoxin A, and Fusarium toxins), masked mycotoxins, and emerging mycotoxins. The toxicity of these mycotoxins and their negative economic impact was also discussed together with the effect of climate change on their production. A section on mycotoxins regulations by international agencies and organisms (WHO, FAO, EU, etc.) was discussed. Finally, the different strategies to reduce or eliminate the toxic effects of mycotoxins in contaminated foods and feeds by using chemical, physical, and biological/biotechnological methods or innovative approaches were explained.

INTRODUCTION

Fungi are considered ubiquitous microorganisms found in nature, their spores are able to travel across countries and continents on our planet (De Ruyck *et al*, 2015). They are known to produce active chemical compounds called mycotoxins, which are secondary metabolites that exert adverse negative effects both on human and animal health and may contaminate agricultural food products of vegetal and animal origin (Tantaoui-Elaraki *et al.*, *in press*).

DOI: 10.4018/978-1-7998-5354-1.ch003

Strains of the genera *Aspergillus*, *Penicillium*, *Fusarium* and *Alternaria* are the most mycotoxins producing fungi. Mycotoxins synthesis by toxigenic species depend widely on internal parameters of fungal strains (physiological, genetic and biochemical, etc.) but also on external factors (climatic factors) such as humidity and temperature.

The genus *Aspergillus* was described by Pier Antonio Micheli in 1729. It was reported that *Aspergillus* species that produce mycotoxins are more common in the warmer, subtropical and tropical areas than in the temperate areas of the world (Wilson *et al.*, 2002). *Aspergilli* species are soil fungi or saprophytes, and several are able to produce active compounds especially aflatoxins, ochratoxins, citrinin, penicillic acid, sterigmatocystin, cyclopiazonic acid, gliotoxin, citreoviridin and other important metabolites. All these compounds are produced by a high number of fungal mycotoxin species producers belonging to the genus *Aspergillus* including *A. flavus, A. niger, A. nomius, A. ochraceus, A. parasiticus, A. candidus, A. clavatus, A. restrictus, A. tamarii, A. terreus, A. versicolor*, etc. (Frisvad & Samson, 1991).

Mycotoxins are known as low molecular weight (below 700 Da) chemical substances and are produced on various grains and agricultural commodities at different stages in the field, before harvest, post-harvest, during processing, packaging, distribution and storage (Creppy *et al.*, 2002). Modified mycotoxins called also "masked mycotoxins" can be produced by fungi or generated as part of the defense mechanism of the infected plant. They can be produced during the processing of contaminated food processing (e.g. cooking), then can be converted to the original mycotoxin by the metabolism of animals and humans (Berthiller *et al.*, 2013). The conversions of these modified mycotoxins to their free form possibly increased the bioavailability of the parent mycotoxin and induce potential risk to human health (Paris *et al.*, 2014). Some species belonging to the *Fusarium* genus are responsible for the production of another group of bioactive compounds called *emerging* or *minor* mycotoxins. This group includes enniatins (A, A1, B and B1), fusaproliferin, beauvericin, and moniliformin (Jestoi, 2008).

Some mycotoxins are known of their acute toxic properties on humans (ergot alkaloids) and animals (aflatoxins, OTA, *Fusarium* toxins), but the majority of them are of chronic toxicological effects (Zinedine & Mañes, 2009).

Several mycotoxins are correlated with toxicological effects including hepatotoxicity, teratogenicity, carcinogenicity, neurotoxicity, immunosuppressive effects as well as reproductive and developmental toxicity in humans and animals. Among these substances, aflatoxins, ochratoxin A, fumonisins, zearalenone, trichothecens, T-2, HT-2 toxins are of a great concern because of their negative impact on human and animal health (Bennett & Klich, 2003). Mycotoxins are also known with their negative economic impacts. Indeed, according to FAO, one third of all foodstuffs produced for world's population are lost from field to consumer, reaching nearly 1.3 billion metric tons each year; and that 25% of the crops in the world are damaged by mould or fungal growth (FAO, 2012).

The mycotoxin problem in public health is longstanding and all humans and animals are at risk for mycotoxin exposure. People are mainly exposed via the ingestion of contaminated foods; however, alternate routes include dermal absorption and inhalation of toxinogenic molds containing mycotoxins. The major regulated mycotoxins and the most associated producing fungi are summarized in Table 1.

The climate change is likely to alter the degree of human exposure to pollutants and the response of human populations to these exposures. The contamination of food and feed by mycotoxins, and the production of these compounds by fungi can be very sensitive to environmental factors such as temperature and humidity. Paterson and Lima (2010) showed that indirect effects of climate change may also be important; for example, changes in the distribution and activity of insect vectors may increase the exposure and vulnerability of plants to mycotoxins. It was reported that climate change could have a

Table 1. Major mycotoxins and associated fungi (AFSSA, 2009 with modifications)

	Mycotoxins	Associated Fungi
Major Legislated mycotoxins	Aflatoxins: B1, B2, G1 and G2	*Aspergillus flavus, A. parasiticus, A. nomius*
	Ochratoxin A	*Penicillium verrucosum, A. ochraceus, A. carbonarius*
	Patulin	*P. expansum, A. clavatus, Byssochlamys nivea*
	Fumonisins B1, B2 and B3	*Fusarium verticillioides, F. proliferatum*
	Trichothecens (types A and B)	*F. langsethiae, F. sporotrichioides, F. poae, F. graminearum, F. culmorumF. crookwellense, F. tricinctum, F. acuminatum*
	Zearalenone	*Fusarium graminearum, F. culmorum F. crookwellense.*
Others mycotoxins	Citrinin	*A. terreus, A. carneus, A. niveus P. verrucosum, P. citrinum, P. expansum*
	Alternaria toxins	*Alternaria alternata, Alternaria solani*
	Cyclopiazonic acid	*A. flavus, A. versicolor, A. tamari, P. camemberti*
	Sterigmatocystin	*A. nidulans, A. versicolor, A. flavus*
	Stachybotryotoxin	*Strachybotrys chartarum*

positive effect on exposure, but in most instances an adverse effect is anticipated in certain regions and it is possible that this will result in adverse health outcomes (Tirado *et al.*, 2010). In regions of some developing countries, the increase in the extent and magnitude of episodes of fungal infestations is likely to correspond to increasing mycotoxin exposures, with attendant increasing occurrence of target organ toxicity and cancer, especially in areas where fungal infestations are endemic and populations are vulnerable (Balbus *et al,* 2013).

MAJOR MYCOTOXINS

Aflatoxins

Aflatoxins (AFs) are widely distributed toxins produced by *Aspergillus* species including *A. flavus, A. parasiticus, A. nomius, A. pseudotamarii, A. bombycis, A. ochraceoroseus,* and *A. australis* (IARC, 2002). According to Creppy (2002), *A. flavus* strains produce only type B aflatoxins (B1 and B2), while the other strains produce both B and G aflatoxins (B1, B2, G1 and G2). *A. flavus* and *A. parasiticus* are responsible for the largest proportion of aflatoxins found in foodstuffs throughout the world. Of the other species, it was reported that only *A. australis*, which appears to be widespread in the southern hemisphere and is common in Australian peanut soils, may also be an important source of aflatoxins in some countries (IARC, 2002).

AFs (Figure 1) were the first mycotoxins isolated in the 1960th after hard investigations following the "Turkey-X-disease" outbreaks in the UK. AFs are well known with their heat-stability and their resistance to several food processes such as cooking, baking and extrusion (Marin *et al.*, 2013). AFs are able to contaminate a wide range of food commodities including grains (wheat, maize, barley, rice, and sorghum, etc.), nuts (almonds, peanuts, walnuts, and pistachios, etc.), spices (red paprika, ginger, chili powder, etc.) and animal feeds (Dragacci *et al.*, 2011). Nowadays, AFs are recognized as the most relevant mycotoxins worldwide because of their confirmed toxicity to humans and animals, their widespread occurrence and their economic losses. In term of biological activity, AFs are of great concern because of their detrimental effects on the health of humans and animals, including carcinogenic, mutagenic, teratogenic and immunosuppressive effects (Eaton & Gallagher, 1994).

Figure 1. Chemical structure of aflatoxins (B1, B2, G1, G2, M1 and M2)

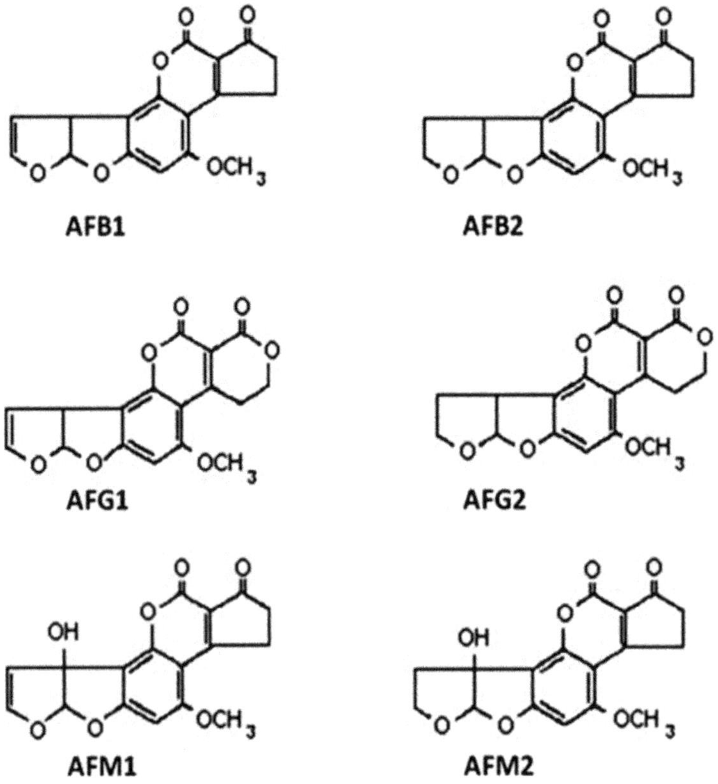

Recently, AFs acute poisoning outbreaks affecting a large geographical area and causing over 123 deaths were reported in Kenya in 2004 and 2005. Epidemiological studies from this case showed a relationship between the outbreak and the local methods of harvesting, storing and preparing maize. Contamination of maize with AFs was found up to 1000 µg/Kg (Centers for Disease Control, 2004). The early symptoms of AFB1-induced hepatotoxicity in human are anorexia, malaise and low-grade fever and it can progress with vomiting abdominal pain and even may be associated to diarrhea (Sherif *et al.*, 2009).

Until now, twenty molecules of AFs are chemically known and identified in the world; however, only six aflatoxin compounds (B1, B2, G1, G2, M1 and M2) are the most significant and interesting. AFM1 and AFM2 are the main monohydroxylated derivatives respectively of AFB1 and AFB2 forming in liver of lactating mammals by means of cytochrome P450-associated enzymes (Bennett & Klich, 2003).

AFs were evaluated several times in IARC Monographs, and were confirmed as a Group 1 like carcinogenic to humans. IRAC monographs states that there is sufficient evidence in humans for the carcinogenicity of AFs. Indeed, AFs cause cancer of the liver (hepatocellular carcinoma) and there is sufficient evidence in experimental animals for the carcinogenicity of naturally occurring mixtures of AFs, and of AFB1, AFG1 and AFM1. However, there is limited evidence in experimental animals for the carcinogenicity of AFB2 and there is inadequate evidence in experimental animals for the carcinogenicity of AFG2 (IARC, 2018).

The weight of evidence for the classification of the aflatoxins as group-1 carcinogens was driven by statistically significantly increased risks for hepatocellular carcinoma (HCC) in individuals exposed to aflatoxins, as measured by aflatoxin-specific biomarkers in cohort studies in Shanghai and Taiwan provinces in China. On one hand, these studies reported statistically significant effects of exposure to AFs on the development of HCC and also confirmed that in the presence of HBV exposure, as judged by HBsAg status, there is a greater than multiplicative interaction between aflatoxin and HBV, increasing the risk for HCC. On the other, it was demonstrated that aflatoxins are able to induce a specific mutation in codon 249 of the TP53 tumor-suppressor gene (IARC, 2018).

Since milk is a major commodity for introducing AFs in the human diet, evidence of hazardous human exposure to AFM1 through dairy products has been shown by several studies. Compared to its parent molecule, AFM1 has a carcinogenicity of 2–10%. It is secreted into milk in the mammary glands of dairy cows that have consumed feeds containing AFB1. AFM1 could be detected in milk 12–24 h after the first AFB1 ingestion, reaching a high level after a few days (Zinedine *et al.* 2007a). When the intake of AFB1 has finished, AFM1 amounts decreases to undetectable levels after 72 h (Van Egmond, 1989). The amount of AFB1 present in contaminated feed is usually 1–3% but values as high as 6% were reported (Pittet, 1998). According to Yousef and Marth (1985), the residues of AFM1 remain stable when milk is heat-treated, and the level of AFM1 did not change with concentrating, drying, freezing or cold storage of contaminated milk.

Ochratoxin A

Ochratoxin A (OTA) is a mycotoxin isolated and characterized after the discovery of AFs. It was described for the first time by Van der Merwe *et al.* (1965). Chemically, OTA is known as: N-{[(3R)-5-chloro-8-hydroxy-3-methyl-1-oxo-7-isochromanyl]-carbonyl}-3-phenyl-L alanine (Figure 2). According to Abarca *et al.* (2003), OTA is a ubiquitous secondary fungal metabolite produced by wide varieties of species of the genus *Aspergillus* (e.g., *A. ochraceus, A. niger, A. carbonarius,* etc.) in temperate, tropical or warm climates (Africa, Asia), and by *Penicillium verrucosum* in cold climates (Northern Europe, Canada). OTA has been widely detected in several food commodities of plant origin (cereals, coffee beans, raisins,

Figure 2. Chemical structure of ochratoxin A

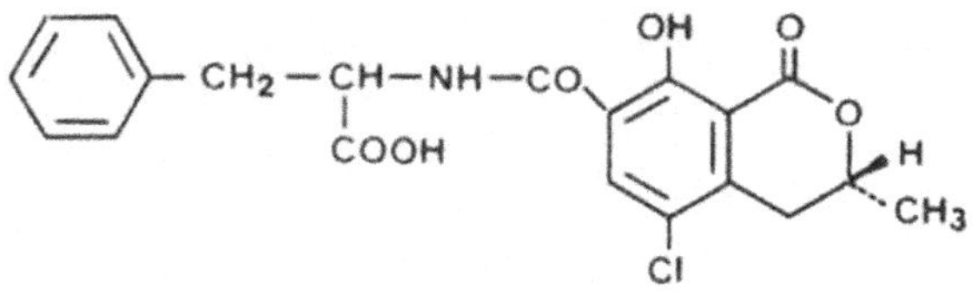

wine, beer, and grape juice) and commodities of animal origin such as pork and poultry meats, eggs, milk, and dairy products due to the carryover effect (Peraica *et al.*, 2014).

OTA has been implicated in a human disease of kidney referred to as Balkan endemic nephropathy, characterized by tubule interstitial nephritis and associated with high incidence of kidney, pelvis, ureter and urinary bladder tumors in some Eastern European countries (Pfohl-Leszkowicz *et al.*, 2002). In experimental and domestic animals the main target organs of OTA toxicity are the kidney and liver, but it also affects other targets as the heart, blood, lymphoid tissue, and bone marrow. Several mechanisms are involved in OTA toxicity such as the production of reactive oxygen species, the mitochondrial respiration inhibition, the protein synthesis inhibition; and particularly OTA is known to cause DNA damage (Creppy, 2002). It was described that OTA is reabsorbed by the upper gastro-intestinal tract and persists in the circulation for a long time due to binding to plasma proteins; OTA plasma half-life in humans was estimated to 35.5 days, which is extremely long and makes OTA of plasma a good biomarker of exposure (Zepnik *et al.*, 2003).

OTA has been classified as a possible human carcinogen (group 2B) by the International Agency for Research on Cancer (IARC, 1993). The Joint Committee FAO/WHO of Experts on Food Additives (JECFA) has established the provisional tolerable weekly intake (PTWI) of OTA at 100 ng/Kg of body weight (bw) corresponding to approximately 14 ng/Kg bw/day (JECFA, 2001). The European Food Safety Authority (EFSA) has proposed a new safety value of 120 ng OTA/Kg bw as a Tolerable Weekly Intake, which corresponds to a TDI of 17.1 ng/Kg bw (EFSA, 2006).

Fumonisins

Fumonisins (FUM) are a group of 15 mycotoxins produced by *Fusarium* species (e.g. *F. verticilloides*, *F. moniliforme*, etc.). FUM were isolated for the first time in 1988 (Gelderblom *et al.*, 1988). They contaminate various cereal grains, but are common in maize and sorghum which are the main sources of the exposure to FUM in humans. In naturally contaminated grains, the most frequent is fumonisin B1 (FB1), often accompanied by small amounts of fumonisin B2 (FB2) and fumonisin B3 (FB3). FUM are chemically similar to sphinganine which is the backbone of sphingolipids (Figure 3).

Figure 3. Chemical structure of fumonsin B1

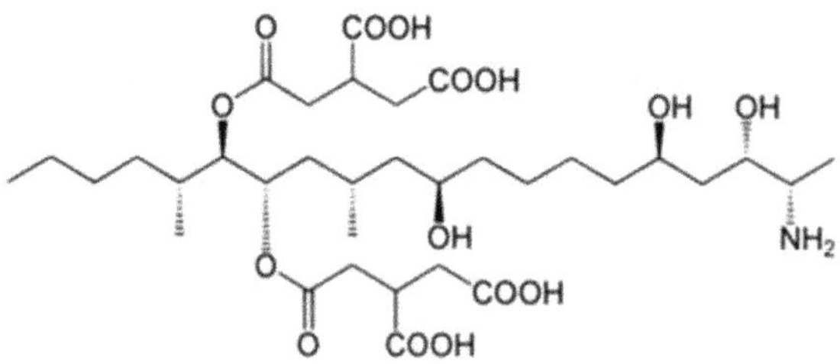

FUM are poorly absorbed by the gastro-intestinal tract and quickly eliminated from plasma with low accumulation in the kidney and liver (Soriano *et al.*, 2005). Bhat *et al.* (1997) reported a possible case of acute exposure to FB1 involved 27 villages in India, where consumption of unleavened bread made from moldy sorghum or corn, containing up to 64 mg/Kg FB1, was associated with an outbreak of human disease involving gastrointestinal symptoms (transient abdominal pain, borborygmus, and diarrhea).

Fumonisins target different organs in domestic and experimental animals: in horses they cause leukoencephalomalacia, in pig pulmonary oedema, in rats they are predominantly nephrotoxic, and in mice they are hepatotoxic and teratogenic, causing neural tube defects (Soriano *et al.*, 2005). In some world areas where maize is considered as staple food (Southern Africa, China, and Northern Italy), the high frequency of the incidence of esophageal cancer is believed to be related to exposure to FUM or their producers (Marasas *et al.*, 1988). In the early of the 1990th, a higher prevalence of neural tube defects was observed in children born along the Texan and Mexican border by Mexican-American women, and it was suggested that this was caused by fumonisin exposure in the first trimester of pregnancy (Hendricks *et al.* 1999). High prevalence of these defects was also found in the Transkei region in Southern Africa, northern Iran, and several regions of China (Peraica *et al.*, 2014). FB1 was reported to be the most widespread toxin in the group of FUM and was classified by the International Agency for Research on Cancer in 2B group as a possible carcinogenic to humans (IARC, 1993). A provisional maximum for tolerable daily intake (PMTDI) is fixed for fumonisins B1, B2 and B3 alone or in combination, of 2 µg/Kg bw/day on the basis of the NOEL of 0.2 mg/Kg bw/day and a safety factor of 100 (Creppy, 2002).

Zearalenone

Zearalenone (ZEA) is a mycotoxin produced by *Fusarium* fungi in temperate and warm countries (Bennett & Klich, 2003). ZEA is chemically known as 6-[10-hydroxy-6-oxo-trans-1-undecenyl]-B-resorcyclic acid lactone (Figure 4). ZEA producing fungi contaminate cereals and derivatives, especially wheat, oats, corn, barley, millet, sorghum and rice (Zinedine *et al*, 2007b). Furthermore, the toxin has been detected in cereal products such as flour, malt, soybeans and beer. It was reported that species of the genus *Fusarium* infect cereals in the field. The ZEA derivatives (α-zearalenol, β-zearalenol, α-zearalanol, β-zearalanol and zearalanone) can also be detected in food commodities, especially in corn and derivatives. ZEA and its metabolites represent a serious hazard to animals and human health. They have been shown to bind competitively to estrogen receptors (ER-α and ER-β) because of their structural similarity to the sex hormone, 17β-estradiol, they activate the estrogen gene and cause reproductive disorders (Zinedine *et al*, 2007b). Several authors reported that ZEA is of a relatively low acute toxicity after oral administration in mice, rats and guinea pigs (SCF, 2000). ZEA produces hematologic, cytotoxic, genotoxic, immunotoxic and hepatotoxic effects. Concerning long-term toxicity, ZEA has shown adverse liver lesions with subsequent development of hepatocarcinoma. ZEA also affected some enzymatic parameters of the hepatic function in rats and in rabbits. Conková *et al.* (2001) reported the effects of ZEA on the changes in enzymatic activities of aspartate aminotransferase, alanine aminotransferase, alkaline phosphatase, γ-glutamyl transferase and total lactate dehydrogenase in rabbits, indicating the possible liver toxicity due to the chronic effects of the toxin.

ZEA was found to to induce DNA-adduct formation in vitro cultures of bovine lymphocytes (Lioi *et al.*, 2004), DNA fragmentation and micronuclei production in cultured DOK, Vero and Caco-2 cells, in Vero monkey kidney cells and in bone marrow cells of mice (Ouanes *et al.*, 2003). However, previous studies showed the potential for ZEA to stimulate growth of human breast cancer cells containing estrogen response receptors (Yu *et al.*, 2005).

Figure 4. Chemical structure of zearalenone

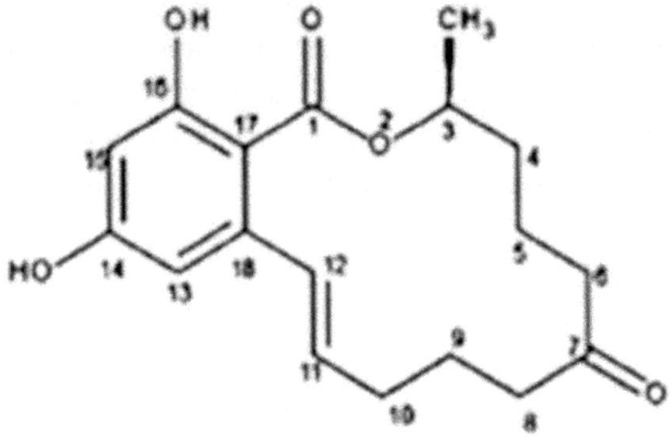

For the ZEA risk assessment, JECFA (2000) established a Provisional Maximum Tolerable Daily Intake of 0.5 µg/kg b.w. This decision was based on the NOEL of 40 µg/Kg b.w. per day obtained in a 15-day study in pigs and the lowest observed effect level of 200 µg/Kg b.w. per day in this study.

Trichothecens

Trichothecens is a heterogeneous family of mycotoxins all produced by toxingenic fungi on foods and feeds. The term trichothecene is derived from trichothecin, which was the one of the first members of the family identified (Zinedine & Mañes, 2009). All trichothecenes contain a common 12,13-epoxy-trichothene skeleton and an olefinic bond with various side chain substitutions (Bennett and klich, 2003). The trichothecenes constitute a family of more than sixty sesquiterpenoid metabolites produced by a number of fungal genera, including *Fusarium, Myrothecium, Phomopsis, Stachybotrys, Trichoderma and Trichothecium*. The most serious and regulated mycotoxins in this family are Deoxynivalenol (DON), T-2 and HT-2 toxins.

Deoxynivalenol

Deoxynivalenol (DON) is a mycotoxin of the type-B trichothecenes, which are epoxy-sesquiterpenoids. The toxin DON (Figure 5) often contaminates cereal grains such as wheat, barley and maize, but less found on oats, rice, rye and sorghum. According to several toxicological studies, the toxin DON shows adverse health effects after acute, short-term, or long-term administration to animals. Indeed, two characteristic toxicological effects appear after acute administration of the toxin: anorexia (decrease in feed consumption) and vomiting. For this, DON is also known under its synonym "vomitoxin" and its presence in foods can cause clinical or subclinical manifestations to humans and animals (Pestka, 2010). The toxin DON is the most prevalent in its group and was commonly described as a serious mycotoxin several cereals such as wheat, corn, barley, rye, safflower seeds, and animal mixed feeds.

Figure 5. Chemical structure of deoxynivalenol

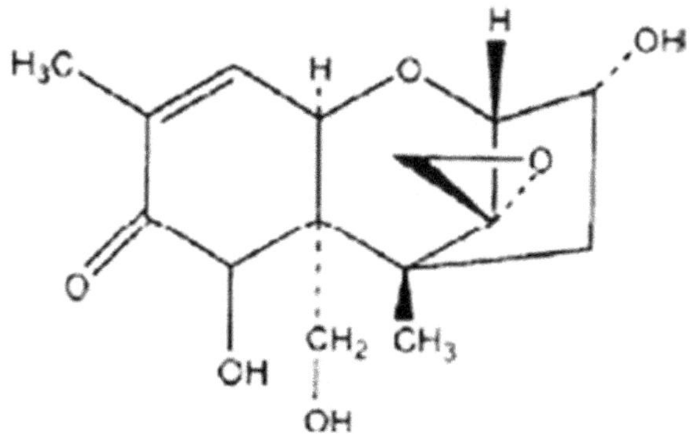

T-2 and HT-2 Toxins

The toxin T-2 (Figure 6) and its derivative (HT-2) are type A trichothecenes. Chemically, they are closely related epoxy, sesquiterpenoids. Previous reports showed the occurrence of both T-2 and HT-2 toxins in cereal grains especially in wheat, maize, oats, barley, rice, beans, and soya beans and in processed cereals. According to Creppy (2002), T-2 and HT-2 toxins are produced by several *Fusarium* species such as *F. sporotrichioides, Fusarium poae, Fusarium equiseti* and *Fusarium acuminatum*. T-2 and HT-2 toxins were implicated in acute poisoning outbreaks with several symptoms that included nausea, vomiting, pharyngeal irritation, abdominal pain, diarrhea, bloody stools, dizziness and chills. According to Bennett and Klich, (2003), T-2 toxin was associated with *Alimentary Toxic Aleukia (ATA)*, a human disease that affected a large population of the former USSR during the 1940th. The symptoms include inflammation of the skin, vomiting, and damage to hematopoietic tissues.

Figure 6. Chemical structure of T-2

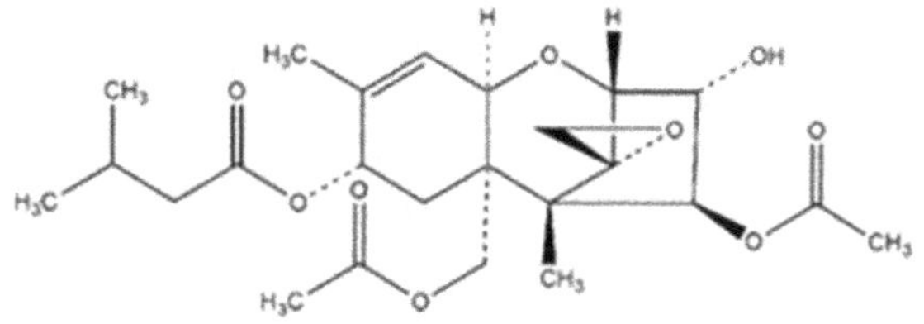

Ergot Alkaloids

The genus *Claviceps* is composed of about 36 species of fungi responsible for the production of more than 40 known ergot alkaloids (Arroyo-Manzanares et al., 2014). Although some *Aspergilli* species also produce ergot alkaloids, the most popular producer is *Claviceps purpurea*. Common growth substrates for these species include cereal grains and feeds ingredients, such as corn, barley, oats, rice, rye and sorghum. Some plants of the family of *convolvulaceae* covering the soil are also known to produce ergot alkaloids, although the consumption of these plants by humans or livestock is minimal. The most known acute effects of ergot poisoning, called "ergotism," imply powerful and very painful vasoconstrictor effects on the peripheral circulation, often leading to gangrene, to loss of limbs or even death (Schiff, 2006). Different ergot alkaloids may also produce another group of acute poisoning symptoms, including abdominal pain, seizures, vomiting, insomnia, burning skin and other hallucinations (Tudzynski & Neubauer 2014). Figure 9 below illustrates the chemical structure of ergotamine, the main mycotoxin produced by *Claviceps purpurea* and responsible for ergotism or "burning pain".

MODIFIED AND MASKED MYCOTOXINS

In addition to the known mycotoxins, scientists started to use the terms "modified mycotoxins" and "masked mycotoxin" in the mid of the 1980th. Indeed, it was reported that some cases of mycotoxicosis did not correlated with the mycotoxins detected in the suspected foods. Thus, the high toxicity could be due to the presence of unknown mycotoxins forms (Freire & Sant'Ana, 2018). The term "modified mycotoxins" was launched on the metabolites which cannot be detected during the analysis of the parent mycotoxins by official analytical methods. Nowadays, different forms of mycotoxin are still confusing, the term "masked mycotoxins" has been indicated to be used exclusively for compounds derived from mycotoxins that were formed by plants' defense mechanisms. According to Berthiller *et al.* (2013), mycotoxin-derived compounds can also be formed by other pathways, such as food processing and animal metabolism. Moreover, the term "modified mycotoxin" was commonly used for all derived-mycotoxins compounds that could be formed by food processing, produced by microorganisms, or obtained from the plants metabolism.

The first modified mycotoxin reported was AFM1, a substance formed from the hydroxylation of AFB1 and eliminated in the milk of animals that consumed AFB1 feed contaminated. The degradation of OTA after the high thermal treatment (roasting coffee) resulted in the formation of its modified forms including ochratoxin α amide, 14-(R)-ochratoxin A and 14-decarboxyochratoxin A (Bittner *et al.*, 2015). Deoxynivalenol-3-glucoside (D3G), one of the most common modified forms of DON, is formed through the plant defense mechanism, in which glycosyltransferase enzymes bind an endogenous glucose molecule to the hydroxyl group of carbon 3 of the DON molecule (Freire & Sant'Ana, 2018). In ZEA-treated barley seedlings, the metabolites ZEA-16-glucoside (ZEA-16G) and ZEA-14G were detected in the roots, although in small amounts (Paris *et al.*, 2014).

Little information is now available on the toxicity of the modified or masked mycotoxins to humans and animals. However, according to Rychlik *et al.*, (2014), there is a potential risk of release of the parent mycotoxins by hydrolysis during food processing and by the digestion and/or metabolism in humans and animals. Indeed, it was suggested that the conversions of these modified or masked mycotoxins to their free form possibly may increase the bioavailability of the parent mycotoxins and may enhance the potential risk to human health. Due to this risk, The Panel on Contaminants in the Food Chain of the European Food Safety Authority decided that during risk assessment, the modified mycotoxins must be considered with the same toxicity of the parent mycotoxins (EFSA, 2014).

EMERGING MYCOTOXINS

In addition to the production of trichothecenes, ZEA and FUM, toxigenic fungi species of *Fusarium* are also able to produce a second group of bioactive compounds already called "minor" mycotoxins but now are known as "emerging mycotoxins" because of their widespread in cereal grain and the phenomenal levels usually detected (Jestoi, 2008). This group includes enniatins (A, A1, B and B1), beauvericin and fusaproliferin, etc. First investigations on this mycotoxin group started on the 2000th, and now several papers are worldwide published on the occurrence of these toxins in cereal grains and processed cereals in the USA, in European Nordic countries, in Italy (Uhlig, 2006; Jestoi, 2008), in Spain (Meca *et al.*, 2010) and in Morocco (Zinedine *et al.*, 2011; Mahnine *et al.*, 2011). However little information is still available in the literature about their toxicity and to assess their risk for humans.

Enniatins

The enniatines (ENs, Figure 7) were first isolated from cultures of *F. orthoceras Appl.* and *F. oxysporum.* Nowadays, more than 23 different ENs compounds (and analogues) were identified and described in the literature (Meca *et al.*, 2010). Until now, several papers reported that four ENs occurs naturally in cereal grains, these are ENA, ENA1, ENB and ENB1 (Figurc7). Enniatins arc produccd mainly by strains of some species of *Fusarium*. But, other fungal genera including *Alternaria*, *Halosarpheia* and *Verticillium* were also described to produce ENs. These mycotoxins are of high interest because of their wide range of biological activity. This bioactivity has long been assumed to be associated with their ionophoric properties (Uhlig *et al.*, 2009). ENs inhibit the enzyme acyl-CoA:cholesterol acyl transferase (ACAT) (Tomoda *et al.*, 1992). They are also known as phytotoxins and are associated with plant diseases characterized by wilt and necrosis (Burmeister and Plattner, 1987). Other studies reported the bioactivity of ENs against Mycobacterium sp. and Plasmodium falciparum (Nilanonta *et al.*, 2000; Supothina *et al.*, 2004). Hiraga *et al.* (2005) showed that ENs have been identified as inhibitors of major drug efflux pumps in *Saccharomyces cerevisiae*.

Bauvericin

The mycotoxin beauvericin (BEA, Figure 7) is a cyclic lactone trimer containing an alternating sequence of three N-methyl L-phenylalanyl and three D-α-hydroxyisovaleryl residues. BEA was isolated for the first time from the culture of the insect-pathogenic fungus *Beauverina bassiana*. More recently, it was reported that several fungal species such as *F. bulbicola, F. denticulatum, F. lactis, F. phyllophilum, F. pseudocircinatum and F. succisae* are able to produce this mycotoxin (Moretti *et al.*, 2007).

BEA affected the electromechanical and physiological properties of isolated smooth and heart muscle preparations (Lemmens-Gruber *et al.*, 2000). BEA is a specific cholesterol acyltransferase inhibitor (Tomoda *et al.*, 1992). BEA is toxic to several human cell lines (Logrieco *et al.*, 2002) and can induce apoptosis and DNA fragmentation (Ojcius *et al.*, 1991). This mycotoxin inhibited the Ltype Ca2+ current in the NG108-15 neuronal cell line and increased the intracellular calcium by increasing the formation of cation selective channels in lipid membrane (Wu *et al.*, 2002; Kouri *et al.*, 2003). Previous studies have shown that BEA induced cell death can be prevented by administration of intracellular calcium chelator-BAPTA/AM (Jow *et al.*, 2004) in human lymphoblastic leukemia CCRF-CEM cells, indicating that the intracellular Ca2+ plays an important role in cell death signaling.

Figure 7. Chemical structure of enniatins (A, A1, B, B1) and beauvericin

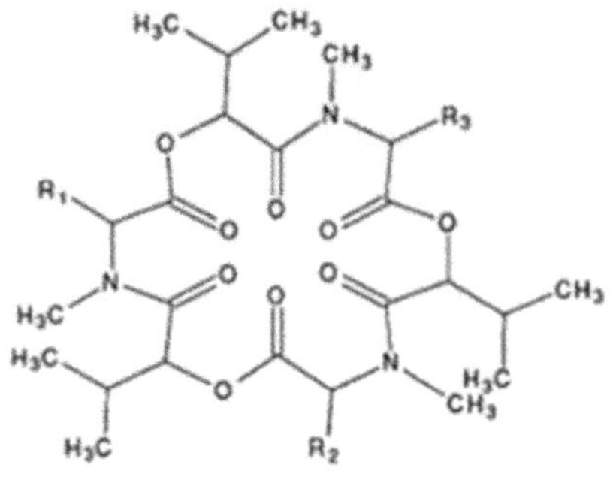

	R$_1$	R$_2$	R$_3$
BEA	phenylmethyl	phenylmethyl	phenylmethyl
A	*sec*-butyl	*sec*-butyl	*sec*-butyl
A$_1$	*sec*-butyl	*sec*-butyl	isopropyl
B	isopropyl	isopropyl	isopropyl
B$_1$	isopropyl	isopropyl	*sec*-butyl

Fusaproliferin

Fusaproliferin (FUS) is a bicyclic sesterterpene (Figure 8) consisting of five isoprenic units, which was originally isolated from a pure culture of *Fusarium proliferatum* (Randazzo *et al.*, 1993). Moretti *et al.* (2007) reported that FUS could be produced by F. *antophilum, F. begoniae, F. bulbicola, F. circinatum, F. concentricum, F. succisae and F. udum*. FUS is also produced by *F. subglutinans* (Ritieni *et al.*, 1995; Meca *et al.*, 2009). FUS is produced through the isoprenoid pathway via common terpene intermediates originating from acetyl-CoA subunits. Preliminary studies indicated that FUS has been found to be toxic in the brine shrimp (*Artemia salina*) larve bioassay (Ritieni *et al.*, 1995) and mammalian cells (Logrieco *et al.*, 1996) and causes teratogenic effects on chicken embryos (Ritieni *et al.*, 1997).

MYCOTOXINS AND ECONOMIC IMPACTS

Economic losses due to the presence of mycotoxins in food and feed are diverse and can be associated with the decrease of their quality. The food production industry is most commonly affected by mycotoxins. Major financial losses of mycotoxins are attributable to AFs because of their strict regulations and confirmed carcinogenic effects. The estimated losses in wheat and barley attributable to the *Fusarium* mycotoxins in US alone were estimated to about $ 2.9 billion a year (Windels, 2000). In a study by Robens and Cardwell in 2003, loss due to AF contaminated corn and peanuts, as well as FB contaminated corn and DON contaminated wheat resulted in estimated loss ranging from $ 0.5 million to over $ 1.5 billion for the U.S. (Robens & Cardwell, 2003).

Figure 8. Chemical structure of fusaproliferin

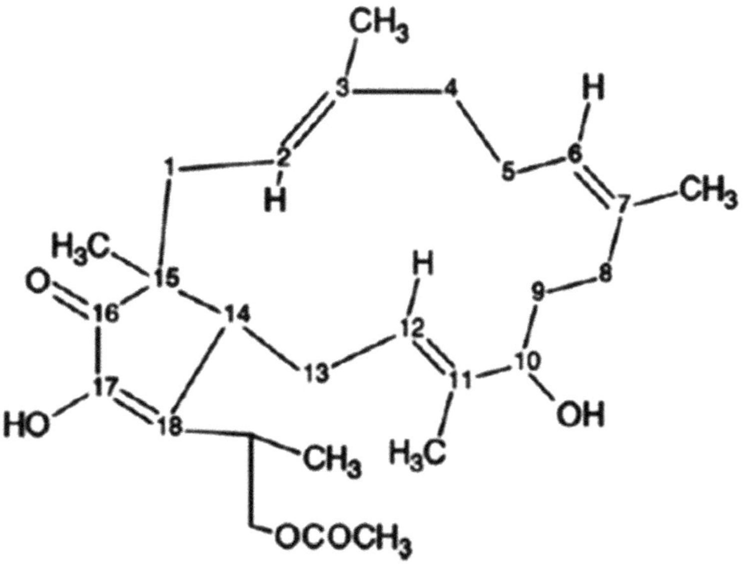

Animal Productivity Losses

Overall, most mycotoxins cause immunosuppression which can make animals more prone to disease by weakening their immune system or making them less responsive to vaccinations. In acute cases, losses are related to animal mortality. Other subclinical effects may cause many productivity losses such the decrease in the quantity and/or quality of animal by-products (milk, eggs and meat), and reduced weight gains and feed efficiency. The reduction in animal production could be due to feed refusal or diseases, increasing medical cost for toxicosis treatments, to find alternative foods, to design adequate management of contaminated supplies, to improve detection and quantification methods and to develop strategies to reduce toxin exposure. More specific reproductive effects are frequently associated with the negative effects of the estrogenic mycotoxin ZEA, these effects may cause infertility and abortion predominantly in swine. In animals, trichothecenes can cause weight loss by inhibition of protein synthesis, nutritional impairment as well as immunosuppression. In the case of dairy industry, losses involve the times farmers have to wait in order to allow animals to excrete all AFM1 form before milk collecting.

Food Unavailability

Economic loss related to unavailability of foods can be more dramatic if the affected foods are the most important ones. For example, cereals (wheat, maize and corn) are the most consumed staple food worldwide and are estimated to feed near 4 billion people all together. They are commonly reported with mycotoxin contamination; especially aflatoxins, OTA, citrinin, DON, fumonisins, fusarenon-X, nivalenol, sterigmatocystin and ZEA (Tanaka *et al.*, 2007). It is evident that loss due to mycotoxins in this widely consumed cereal may have disastrous monetary impacts not just for the producers but for all of the world population. Moreover, food recalls or food detentions due to mycotoxins are familiar to all countries that enforce regulations. Besides loss of production, food recalls of already produced cereals and grains constitute important losses. Indeed, many countries have records of recalls but not many of them make this information available.

MYCOTOXINS AND CLIMATE CHANGE

Climate change is predicted to have significant impacts on the quality and availability of staple food commodities. According to FAO guidelines, food security is determined by three key components: (a) sufficient food availability, (b) access to this food and (c) quality and use of the food in terms of both nutritional and cultural perspectives (FAO, 1996).

Several environmental factors contribute to the presence of mycotoxins in foods. Some factors are related to susceptibility of crops, plant stress, harvesting practices, and storage of grains. Intrinsic factors from the fungi are strain specific and vary according to the availability of substrates in which the mold grows. Broad environmental conditioners include climate changes that directly influence fungal contamination of foods.

The change in climate is a widely acknowledged fact and a trend of warming around the globe has been documented based on evidence taken from increased global average air and ocean temperatures, melting of snow and ice, and rising of global average sea levels (IPCC, 2007). Previous literature revisions describe how the plausible changes in temperature, rain precipitation, drought occurrence, and CO_2 increase pose a significant risk to the food supply.

Based on present available data, atmospheric concentrations of CO_2 are expected to double or triple (from 350-400 to 800-1200 ppb) in the next 25 to 50 years. Thus, different regions in Europe will be impacted by the increases in temperature of 2-5 °C coupled with elevated CO_2 and drought episodes. This will have profound impacts on pests and diseases. Similar impacts have been predicted in other areas of the world, especially parts of Asia, and Central and South America which are important producers of wheat, maize and soya beans for food and feed uses on a global basis. Miraglia *et al.* (2009) reported that recent outbreaks of aflatoxins in foods have been reported in some regions of Europe as a result of prolonged dry weather.

Temperature

Temperature is a primary determining factor that modulates fungal growth and mycotoxin production. *Fusarium* growth is more common in temperate weathers at temperatures ranging from 26–28 °C and water activity (A_w) > 0.88, while *Aspergillus* (i.e. *A. flavus*) grows better under warm temperatures. According to the strain and substrate specificities, the optimal temperature for AFs production can vary from 24 to 30 °C (Klich, 2007). Water activity is another important factor that modulates fungal growth and mycotoxin production. Recent studies evaluating the effect of A_w and temperature on AF production by *A. flavus* show that the highest AF concentrations were found in inoculated brown and polished rice under A_w ranges of 0.9-0.92 at 21 °C after 21 days of incubation.

Drought

Drought is another modulator of mycotoxin contamination that is expected to be more frequent depending on geography. For the current century, longer and more severe droughts are projected for West Africa and southern Europe, while for central Europe, central North America, Central America, northeast Brazil and southern Africa the projections of intense drought are moderated (IPCC, 2012).

Pluvial Precipitation

Pluvial precipitation is another environmental factor that plays an important role in mycotoxin food contamination. In India, sorghum grown in the rainy season (Kharif or monsoon crops) during 2006–2007 resulted with higher levels of AF compared to other years (Ratnavathi *et al.*, 2012). Severe rains, while plants are in anthesis (flowering), are associated with increase dispersion of *Fusarium* to corn ears (Parry *et al.*, 1995) which may lead to higher mycotoxin production. Similarly, the production of fumonisins has been associated with dry weather and late season rains (Munkvold & Desjardins, 1997). Unseasonable rains can also affect mycotoxin production by forcing people to harvest earlier when grains are not completely dry hence favoring mold contamination. This was the case of the maize implicated in the Kenyan outbreak of 2004, where 317 clinical cases and 125 deaths for aflatoxicosis were reported (CDC, 2004). Tantaoui-Elaraki *et al.* (*in press*) reported that stachybotryotoxicosis caused in November of 1991 the death of 216 equines in Morocco that had been fed straw moulded with *Stachybotrys atra* and that 8 strains of *S. atra* strains were isolated from the mouldy straw incriminated in this poisoning. This poisoning was explicated by the changes of the climate during autumn after unseasonable rainfall followed by a hot-climate that accelerated mould growth and mycotoxins production. Other outbreaks of aflatoxins occurred under similar conditions of unseasonable rainfall during 1981 in the Makueni District of Kenya (Ngindu *et al.*, 1982) and in western India in 1975 (Krishnamachari *et al.*, 1975). On the other hand, lack of rainfall brings other problem to consider, since it causes stress to the plants.

Due to intensifications of hydrological cycle in the planet, it's been predicted that pluvial precipitations will be reduced in subtropical regions (Solomon *et al.*, 2007) which may lead to stressed crops. The European Food Safety Authority (EFSA) has examined the potential impact of climate change in Europe and has suggested that effects will be (a) regional and (b) detrimental or advantageous depending on geographical region (Battilani et al., 2012). This suggests that in northern Europe the effects may be positive, while the Mediterranean basin may be a hot spot where many effects will be negative, with extreme changes in rainfall/drought, elevated temperatures and CO_2 impacting on food production. Effects of climate change on cereals will be significant and detrimental as ripening in southern and central Europe will occur much earlier than at present. This will influence pests and diseases with decreasing yields and increasing mycotoxins contamination. Indeed it has been suggested that climate change may be responsible for up to a 1/3 of yield variability in key staple commodities on a global basis (Ray *et al.*, 2015). This will have profound impacts on food security in different continents. Recently, several mathematical models have been elaborated to predict the potential impacts of climate change scenarios on mycotoxins and fungi. In northern Europe, Van Der Fels-Klerx *et al.*, (2012) focused a mathematical model on DON. While, another model focused on aflatoxins contamination of maize, wheat and rice grown in Europe (Battilani *et al.*, 2016).

MYCOTOXINS REGULATION

Mycotoxin-producing mold species are extremely common, and they can grow on a wide range of substrates under a wide range of environmental conditions. Mycotoxins can enter the food chain in the field, during storage, or at later points. Mycotoxin problems are exacerbated whenever shipping, handling, and storage practices are conducive to mold growth. The end result is that mycotoxins are commonly found in foods. Several authors classified mycotoxins as the most important chronic dietary risk factor, higher than synthetic contaminants, plant toxins, food additives, or pesticide residues. The economic consequences of mycotoxin contamination were well demonstrated.

Since the discovery of the AFs in 1960, regulations have been established in many countries to protect consumers from the harmful effects of mycotoxins that may contaminate foodstuffs, as well as to ensure fair practices in food trade. Various factors play a role in decision-making processes focused on setting limits for mycotoxins. These include scientific factors to assess risk (such as the availability of toxicological data), food consumption data, detailed knowledge about possibilities for sampling and analysis, the distribution of the mycotoxins over commodities and socio-economic issues. Each process for mycotoxins legislation should take into account also the situation in the other countries with which trade contacts exist.

Food security, as defined by the WHO at the World Food Summit of 1996, only exists when people have continuous access to safe and nutritious food in order to maintain a healthy and active life. Despite the efforts made by different agencies and organizations like the Food and Agriculture Organization (FAO), the World Health Organization (WHO) and country specific agencies in setting regulations to limit the amounts of mycotoxins in foods, up to day, mycotoxin regulation is not global and many countries still lack appropriate guidelines to manage these toxins (particularly in Africa and Latin America). Because of their significant toxicological impacts on both human and animal health, the focus on mycotoxins has been a high priority by the FAO and WHO and other international organisms. This has resulted in strict legislative limits for mycotoxins in many parts of the world in a wide range of foodstuffs with the strictest limits in the EU countries, USA and other countries. For example, in EU countries, several regulatory limits were adopted and revised (European Commission, 2006, 2007, 2010 and 2012), a summary of EU legislation on the aflatoxins, the most serious mycotoxins, is given in Table 2.

In contrast, if mycotoxins hazards are seriously considered and these substances strictly regulated in food and feed in developed countries, mycotoxin legislation is almost absent in some countries of the world, particularly in Africa and Latin America; and if it does exist, it serves only to control food products exported to developed countries, or it remains without any real application by official control laboratories for the determination of levels of mycotoxins in contaminated food. In these cases consumption of mycotoxins contaminated staple foods is a significant risk, especially in rural populations and sub-groups such as children and immunocompromised people.

Zinedine and Mañes (2009) reported that fifteen countries in Africa were known to have specific mycotoxins regulations. These countries cover approximately 59% of the inhabitants of the continent. For the majority of the African countries, specific mycotoxin regulations (probably) do not exist. The fact that some countries have no specific regulatory limit for mycotoxins does not mean that the problem is ignored. Several of these countries recognize that they have problems due to mycotoxins and that regulations should be adopted as soon as possible.

STRATEGIES TO REDUCE MYCOTOXINS

Nowadays, it is well known that the good manufacturing (GMP) and good agricultural (GAP) practices are the most effective worldwide strategies recommended for the prevention of the growth of mycotoxigenic

Table 2. Maximum limits for aflatoxins set by European countries

Mycotoxins	Food Commodities	European Limits * (µg/Kg)
AFB1	Groundnuts (peanuts) and other oilseeds and processed products thereof, intended for direct human consumption	2
	Almonds, pistachios and apricot kernels, intended for direct human consumption	8
	Hazelnuts and Brazil nuts, intended for direct human consumption	5
	Dried fruit and processed products thereof, intended for direct human consumption	2
	Cereals and cereal products	2
	Spices	5
	Processed cereal-based foods and baby foods for infants and young children	0.1
	Dried figs	6
Total AFs B1+B2+G1+G2	Groundnuts (peanuts) and other oilseeds and processed products thereof, intended for direct human consumption	4
	Almonds, pistachios and apricot kernels, intended for direct human consumption	10
	Hazelnuts and Brazil nuts, intended for direct human consumption	10
	Dried fruit and processed products thereof, intended for direct human consumption	4
	Cereals and cereal products	4
	Spices	10
	Dried figs	10
Aflatoxin M1	Liquid milk	0.05
	Baby milk	0.025
	Dietary foods for special medical purposes intended specifically for infants	0.025

* European Regulations (EC, 2006, 2010 and 2012)

fungi and the production of mycotoxin. In developed countries, people are less exposed to mycotoxins hazards compared to those in developing countries. Indeed, the European Commission and the Codex Alimentarius Commission established several practices for the controlling of mycotoxin contamination in food and feed. The first step of each strategy is based on the control of mold growth and mycotoxins production of the prevention strategies. Common strategies for contaminated foods and feeds to reduce or eliminate the toxic effects of mycotoxins by chemical, physical, and biological/biotechnological methods are crucial to improve food safety, prevent economic losses, and reclaim contaminated products. The use of biotechnology to develop host resistance plant and to manage fungal growth and mycotoxins accumulation is the most promise approach for the prevention of mycotoxins contamination in the future. Moreover, the storage conditions are very important to control for the prevention of fungal growth and the reduction of mycotoxins biosynthesis. Biological detoxification using microorganisms (lactic acid bacteria, yeast, etc.) as biological adsorbents was widely described. Several mycotoxins, including ZEA, OTA, AFs and DON can be bind to lactic acid bacteria adsorbed by the bacterial surface (Tantaoui-Elaraki *et al.* in press). On the other, physical methods were also applied for the decontamination of mycotoxins including immersing and washing, sorting and separation, filtering and adsorption as well as irradiation. The immersing and washing is considered an effective method for the reduction of mycotoxins contamination in grains. Finally, chemical agents were also applied for their efficiency to decontaminate mycotoxin including the organic acids, bases and oxidizing agents. Although ammonia was effective to inhibit fungal growth and reduce AFs, FUM and OTA to undetectable levels in animal feeds, this process was not permitted for decontaminating food destined to human consumption (Peraica *et al.*, 2002). Some innovative strategies were also proposed to reduce mycotoxins such as the use of essential oils extracted from aromatic herbs and the use of some anti-oxidants compounds (flavonoides and polyphenols) for their inhibitory effect on fungi growth. More attention is nowadays given to the use of nanoparticles and magnetic materials, these materials appear more effective in the removal of mycotoxins and are considered promising tools for adsorption in the food industry (Sun *et al.*, 2016).

REFERENCES

Abarca, M. L., Accensi, F., Bragulat, M. R., Castella, G., & Cabañes, F. J. (2003). Aspergillus carbonarius as the main source of ochratoxin a contamination in dried vine fruits from the Spanish market. *Journal of Food Protection*, *66*(3), 504–506. doi:10.4315/0362-028X-66.3.504

AFSSA. (2009). Agence Française de Sécurité Sanitaire des Aliments. Évaluation des risques liés à la présence de mycotoxins dans les chaînes alimentaires humaine et animale. Rapport final.

Arroyo-Manzanares, N., Malysheva, S. V., Vanden Bussche, J., Vanhaecke, L., Diana Di Mavungu, J., & De Saeger, S. (2014). Holistic approach based on high resolution and multiple stage mass spectrometry to investigate ergot alkaloids in cereals. *Talanta*, *118*, 359–367. doi:10.1016/j.talanta.2013.10.002

Balbus, J. M., Boxall, A. B. A., Fenske, R. A., Mckone, T. E., & Zeisel, L. (2013). Implications of global climate change for the assessment and management of human health risks of chemicals in the natural environment. *Environmental Toxicology and Chemistry*, *32*(1), 62–78. doi:10.1002/etc.2046

Bennett, J. W., & Klich, M. (2003). Mycotoxins. *Clinical Microbiology Reviews*, *16*(3), 497–516. doi:10.1128/CMR.16.3.497-516.2003

Berthiller, F., Crews, C., Dall'Asta, C., De Saeger, S., Haesaert, G., Karlovsky, P., ... Stroka, J. (2013). Masked mycotoxins: A review. *Molecular Nutrition & Food Research*, *57*(1), 165–186. doi:10.1002/mnfr.201100764

Bhat, R. V., Shetty, P. H., Amruth, R. P., & Sudershan, R. V. (1997). A foodborne disease outbreak due to the consumption of moldy sorghum and maize containing fumonisin mycotoxins. *Journal of Toxicology. Clinical Toxicology*, *35*(3), 249–255. doi:10.3109/15563659709001208

Bittner, A., Cramer, B., Harrer, H., & Humpf, H. (2015). Structure elucidation and in vitro cytotoxicity of ochratoxin α amide, a new degradation product of ochratoxin A. *Mycotoxin Research*, *31*(2), 83–90. doi:10.100712550-014-0218-y

Bottalico, A., Visconti, A., Logrieco, A., Solfrizzo, M., & Mirocha, C. J. (1985). Occurrence of zearalenols (diastereomeric mixture) in corn stalk rot and their production by associated Fusarium species. *Applied and Environmental Microbiology*, *49*, 547–551.

Burmeister, H. R., & Plattner, R. D. (1987). Enniatin production by Fusarium tricinctum and its effects on germinating wheat seeds. *Phytopathology*, *77*(10), 1483–1487. doi:10.1094/Phyto-77-1483

Centers for Disease Control and Prevention-CDC. (2004). Outbreak of aflatoxin poisoning eastern and central provinces, Kenya, January–July 2004. *MMWR. Morbidity and Mortality Weekly Report*, *3*, 790–793.

Čonková, E., Laciaková, A., Pástorová, B., Seidel, H., & Kováč, G. (2001). The effect of zearalenone on some enzymatic parameters in rabbits. *Toxicology Letters*, *121*(3), 145–149. doi:10.1016/S0378-4274(01)00312-5

Creppy, E. E. (2002). Update of survey, regulation and toxic effects of mycotoxins in Europe. *Toxicology Letters*, *127*(1-3), 19–28. doi:10.1016/S0378-4274(01)00479-9

De Ruyck, K., De Boevre, M., Huybrechts, I., & De Saeger, S. (2015). Dietary mycotoxins, co-exposure, and carcinogenesis in humans: Short review. *Mutation Research/Reviews in Mutation Research*, *766*, 32–41. doi:10.1016/j.mrrev.2015.07.003

Eaton, D. L., & Gallagher, E. P. (1994). Mechanisms of aflatoxins carcinogenesis. *Annual Review of Pharmacology and Toxicology*, *34*(1), 135–172. doi:10.1146/annurev.pa.34.040194.001031

European Commission. (2006). *Commission Regulation No. 1881/2006 of December 19th setting maximum levels of certain contaminants in foodstuffs*. Official Journal of the European Union No. L364/5.

European Commission. (2010). Commission Regulation (EC) No 165/2010 of 26 February 2010 amending Regulation (EC) No 1881/2006 setting maximum levels for certain contaminants in foodstuffs as regards aflatoxins. *Official Journal of the European Union, L*, *50*(8).

European Commission. (2012). Commission Regulation (EC) No 1058/2012 of 12 November 2012 amending Regulation (EC) No 1881/2006 setting maximum levels for certain contaminants in foodstuffs as regards maximum levels for aflatoxins in dried figs. *Official Journal of the European Union, L*, *313*(14).

European Food Safety Authority (EFSA). (2006). Opinion of the scientific panel on contaminants in the food chain on a request from the commission related to ochratoxin A in food (Question No. EFSA-Q-2005-154). The EFSA Journal, 365.

FAO. (2012). *Statistical year book 2012*. Retrieved from http://www.fao.org /docrep/015 /i2490e/ i2490e00.htm

Freire, L., & Sant'Ana, A. S. (2018). Modified mycotoxins: An updated review on their formation, detection, occurrence, and toxic effects. *Food and Chemical Toxicology*, *111*, 189–205. doi:10.1016/j.fct.2017.11.021

Frisvad, J. C., & Samson, R. A. (1991). Mycotoxins produced by species of Penicillium and Aspergillus occurring in cereals. In J. Chelkowski (Ed.), *Cereal Grain Mycotoxins, Fungi and Quality in Drying and Storage*. Amsterdam: Elsevier.

Gelderblom, W. C. A., Jaskiewicz, K., Marasas, W. F. O., Thiel, P. G., Horak, R. M., Vleggaar, R., & ... . (1988). Fumonisins-Novel mycotoxins with cancerpromoting activity produced by Fusarium moniliforme. *Applied and Environmental Microbiology*, *54*, 1806–1811.

Gelderblom, W. C. A., Jaskiewicz, K., Marasas, W. F. O., Thiel, P. G., Horak, R. M., Vleggaar, R., & ... . (1988). Fumonisins – Novel mycotoxins with cancerpromoting activity produced by Fusarium moniliforme. *Applied and Environmental Microbiology, 54*, 1806–1811.

Hendricks, K. A., Simpson, J. S., & Larsen, R. D. (1999). Neural tube defect along the Texas-Mexico border, 1993-1995. *American Journal of Epidemiology, 149*(12), 119–127. doi:10.1093/oxfordjournals.aje.a009766

Hendrickse, R. G. (1997). Of sick Turkeys, Kwashiorkor, malaria, perinatal mortality, Herion addicts and food poisoning: Research on influence of aflatoxins on child health in the tropics. *Journal of Tropical Medicine and Parasitology, 91*, 87–93.

Hiraga, K., Yamamoto, S., Fukuda, H., Hamanaka, N., & Oda, K. (2005). Enniatin has a new function as an inhibitor of Pdr5p, one of the ABC transporters in Saccharomyces cerevisiae. *Biochemical and Biophysical Research Communications, 328*(4), 1119–1125. doi:10.1016/j.bbrc.2005.01.075

IARC. (2002). *Some traditional herbal medicines, some mycotoxins, naphthalene and styrene.* IARC..

IARC. (2018). *Aflatoxins.* Available at https://monographs.iarc.fr/wp-content/uploads/2018/06/mono100F-23.pdf

International Agency for Research on Cancer (IARC). (1993). Evaluation of carcinogenic risks of chemical to humans. In Some naturally-occurring substances: Food Items and Constituent. IARC.

JECFA-Joint FAO/WHO Expert Committee on Food Additives. (2000). Zearalenone. In: JECFA (Ed.), Safety evaluation of certain food additives and contaminants. WHO.

JECFA-Joint FAO/WHO Expert Committee on Food Additives. (2001). *Safety evaluation of certain mycotoxins in food.* Prepared by the 56th Meeting of the Food Additives Series No. 47. Geneva.

Jestoi, M. (2008). Emerging *Fusarium*-mycotoxins fusaproliferin, beauvericin, enniatins, and moniliformin-a review. *Critical Reviews in Food Science and Nutrition, 48*(1), 21–49. doi:10.1080/10408390601062021

Jow, G. M., Chou, C. J., Chen, B. F., & Tsai, J. H. (2004). Beauvericin induces cytotoxic effects in human acute lymphoblastic leukemia cells through cytochrome c release, caspase 3 activation: The causative role of calcium. *Cancer Letters, 216*(2), 165–173. doi:10.1016/j.canlet.2004.06.005

Kouri, K., Lemmens, M., & Lemmens-Gruber, R. (2003). Beauvericin-induced channels in ventricular myocytes and liposomes. *Biochimica et Biophysica Acta, 1609*(2), 203–210. doi:10.1016/S0005-2736(02)00689-2

Lemmens-Gruber, R., Rachoy, B., Steininger, E., Kouri, K., Saleh, P., Krska, R., ... Lemmens, M. (2000). The effect of the *Fusarium* metabolite beauvericin on electromechanical and physiological properties in isolated smooth and heart muscle preparations of guinea pigs. *Mycopathologia, 149*(1), 5–12. doi:10.1023/A:1007293812007

Lioi, M. B., Santoro, A., Barbieri, R., Salzano, S., & Ursini, M. V. (2004). Ochratoxin and zearalenone: A comparative study on genotoxic effects and cell death induced in bovine lymphocytes. *Mutation Research, 557*(1), 19–24. doi:10.1016/j.mrgentox.2003.09.009

Logrieco, A., Rizzo, A., Ferracane, R., & Ritieni, A. (2002). Occurrence of beauvericin and enniatins in wheat affected by Fusarium avenaceum head blight. *Applied and Environmental Microbiology, 68*(1), 82–85. doi:10.1128/AEM.68.1.82-85.2002

Marasas, W. F., Kellerman, T. S., Gelderblom, W. C., Coetzer, J. A., Thiel, P. G., & van der Lugt, J. J. (1988). Leukoencephalomalacia in a horse induced by fumonisin B1 isolated from Fusarium moniliforme. *The Onderstepoort Journal of Veterinary Research, 55*, 197–203.

Marasas, W. F. O., Jaskiewicz, K., Venter, F. S., & Van Schalkwyk, D. J. (1988). Fusarium moniliforme contamination of maize in esophageal cancer aereas in Transkei. *South African Medical Journal, 74*, 110–114.

Marin, S., Ramos, A. J., Cano-Sancho, G., & Sanchis, V. (2013). Mycotoxins: Occurrence, toxicology, and exposure assessment. *Food and Chemical Toxicology, 60*, 218–237. doi:10.1016/j.fct.2013.07.047

Meca, G., Sospedra, I., Soriano, J. M., Ritieni, A., Valero, M. A., & Mañes, J. (2009). Isolation, purification and antibacterial effects of fusaproliferin produced by Fusarium subglutinans in submerged culture. *Food and Chemical Toxicology, 47*(10), 2539–2543. doi:10.1016/j.fct.2009.07.014

Meca, G., Zinedine, A., Blesa, J., Font, G., & Mañes, J. (2010). Further data on the presence of Fusarium emerging mycotoxins enniatins, fusaproliferin and beauvericin in cereals available on the Spanish markets. *Food and Chemical Toxicology, 48*(5), 1412–1416. doi:10.1016/j.fct.2010.03.010

Moretti, A., Mulè, G., Ritieni, A., & Logrieco, A. (2007). Further data on the production of beauvericin, enniatins and fusaproliferin and toxicity to Artemia salina by Fusarium species of Gibberella fujikuroi species complex. *International Journal of Food Microbiology, 18*(2), 158–163. doi:10.1016/j.ijfoodmicro.2007.07.004

Nilanonta, C., Isaka, M., Kittakoop, P., Palittapongarnpim, P., Kamchonwongpaisan, S., Pittayakhajonwut, D., ... Thebtaranonth, Y. (2000). Antimycobacterial and antiplasmodial cyclodepsipeptides from the insect pathogenic fungus Paecilomyces tenuipes BCC 1614. *Planta Medica, 66*(8), 756–758. doi:10.1055-2000-9776

Ojcius, D. M., Zychlinsky, A., Zheng, L. M., & Young, J. D. E. (1991). Ionophore-induced apoptosis: Role of DNA fragmentation and calcium fluxes. *Experimental Cell Research, 197*(1), 43–49. doi:10.1016/0014-4827(91)90477-C

Ouanes, Z., Abid, S., Ayed, I., Anane, R., Mobio, T., Creppy, E., & Bacha, H. (2003). Induction of micronuclei by zearalenone in Vero monkey kidney cells and in bone marrow cells of mice: Protective effect of vitamin E. *Mutation Research, 538*(1-2), 63–70. doi:10.1016/S1383-5718(03)00093-7

Paris, M. P. K., Schweiger, W., Hametner, C., Stückler, R., Muehlbauer, G. J., Varga, E., & ... . (2014). Zearalenone-16-O-glucoside: A new masked mycotoxin. *Journal of Agricultural and Food Chemistry, 62*(5), 1181–1189. doi:10.1021/jf405627d

Paterson, R. R., & Lima, N. (2010). Toxicology of mycotoxins. *EXS, 100*, 31–63. doi:10.1007/978-3-7643-8338-1_2

Peraica, M., Richter, D., & Rasi, C. D. (2014). Mycotoxicoses in children. *Arhiv za Higijenu Rada i Toksikologiju, 65*(4), 347–363. doi:10.2478/10004-1254-65-2014-2557

Peraica, M., Richter, D., & Rašić, D. (2014). Mycotoxicoses in children. *Arhiv za Higijenu Rada i Toksikologiju, 65*(4), 347–363. doi:10.2478/10004-1254-65-2014-2557

Pestka, J. (2010). Deoxynivalenol: Mechanisms of action, human exposure, and toxicological relevance. *Archives of Toxicology, 84*(9), 663–679. doi:10.100700204-010-0579-8

Pestka, J. J. (2010). Deoxynivalenol: Mechanism of toxicological relevance. *Archives of Toxicology, 84*, 663–679. doi:10.100700204-010-0579-8

Pfohl-Leszkowicz, A., Petkova-Bocharova, T., Chernozemsky, I. N., & Castegnaro, M. (2002). Balkan endemic nephropathy and associated urinary tract tumors: A review on etiological causes and the potential role of mycotoxins. *Food Additives and Contaminants, 19*(3), 282–302. doi:10.1080/02652030110079815

Pittet, A. (1998). Natural occurrence of mycotoxins in foods and feeds—an updated review. *Revue de Medecine Veterinaire, 6*, 479–492.

Randazzo, G., Fogliano, V., Ritieni, A., Mannina, L., Rossi, E., Scarallo, A., & Segre, A. L. (1993). Proliferin, a new sesterterpene from Fusarium proliferatum. *Tetrahedron, 49*(47), 10883–10896. doi:10.1016/S0040-4020(01)80241-6

Ritieni, A., Fogliano, V., Randazzo, G., Scarallo, A., Logrieco, A., Moretti, A., ... Bottalico, A. (1995). Isolation and characterization of fusaproliferin, a new toxic metabolite from Fusarium proliferatum. *Natural Toxins, 3*(1), 17–20. doi:10.1002/nt.2620030105

Ritieni, A., Monti, S. M., Randazzo, G., Logrieco, A., Moretti, A., Peluso, G., ... Fogliano, V. (1997). Teratogenic effects of fusaproliferin on chicken embryos. *Journal of Agricultural and Food Chemistry, 45*(8), 3039–3043. doi:10.1021/jf960890v

Robens, J., & Cardwell, K. (2003). The costs of mycotoxin management to the USA:management of aflatoxins in the United States. *Journal of Toxicology, 22*, 139–152.

Rychlik, M., Humpf, H. U., Marko, D., Danicke, S., Mally, A., Berthiller, F., ... Lorenz, N. (2014). Proposal of a comprehensive definition of modified and other forms of mycotoxins including "masked" mycotoxins. *Mycotoxin Research, 30*(4), 197–205. doi:10.100712550-014-0203-5

SCF. (2000). *Opinion on Fusarium Toxins – Part 2: zearalenone (ZEA)*. Retrieved from http://ec.europa.eu/food/fs/sc/scf/out65_en.pdf

Schiff, P. L. Jr. (2006). Ergot and its alkaloids. *American Journal of Pharmaceutical Education, 70*(5), 98. doi:10.5688/aj700598

Sherif, S. O., Salama, E. E., & Abdel-Wahhab, M. A. (2009). Mycotoxins and child health: The need for health risk assessment. *International Journal of Hygiene and Environmental Health, 212*(4), 347–368. doi:10.1016/j.ijheh.2008.08.002

Soriano, J. M., González, L., & Catalá, A. I. (2005). Mechanism of action of sphingolipids and their metabolites in the toxicity of fumonisin B1. *Progress in Lipid Research, 44*(6), 345–356. doi:10.1016/j.plipres.2005.09.001

Sun, X. D., Su, P., & Shan, H. (2017). Mycotoxin contamination of rice in China. *Journal of Food Science, 82*(3), 573–584. doi:10.1111/1750-3841.13631

Supothina, S., Isaka, M., Kirtikara, K., Tanticharoen, M., & Thebtaranonth, Y. (2004). Enniatin production by the entomopathogenic fungus Verticillium hemipterigenum BCC 1449. *J. Antibiot., 57*(11), 732–738. doi:10.7164/antibiotics.57.732

Tantaoui-Elaraki, A., Riba, A., Oueslati, S., & Zinedine, A. (2018). Toxigenic fungi and mycotoxin occurrence and prevention in food and feed in northern Africa – a review. Special issue: "Mycotoxins in Africa. *World Mycotoxin Journal, 11*(3), 385–400. doi:10.3920/WMJ2017.2290

Tirado, M. C., Clarke, R., Jaykus, L. A., McQuatters-Gollop, A., & Frank, J. M. (2010). Climate change and food safety: A review. *Food Research International, 43*(7), 1745–1765. doi:10.1016/j.foodres.2010.07.003

Tomoda, H., Huang, X.-H., Cao, J., Nishida, H., Nagao, R., Okuda, S., ... Inoue, K. (1992). Inhibition of acyl-CoA: Cholesterol acyltransferase activity by cyclodepsipeptide antibiotics. *J. Antibiot., 45*(10), 1626–1632. doi:10.7164/antibiotics.45.1626

Tudzynski, P., & Neubauer, L. (2014). Biosynthesis and Molecular Genetics of Fungal Secondary Metabolites. Academic Press. doi:10.1007/978-1-4939-1191-2_14

Uhlig, S., Ivanova, L., Petersen, D., & Kristensen, R. (2009). Structural studies on minor enniatins from Fusarium sp. VI 03441: Novel N-methyl-threonine containing enniatins. *Toxicon, 53*(7-8), 734–742. doi:10.1016/j.toxicon.2009.02.014

Uhlig, S., Torp, M., & Heier, B. T. (2006). Beauvericin and enniatin A, A1, B and B1 in Norwegian grain: A survey. *Food Chemistry, 94*(2), 193–201. doi:10.1016/j.foodchem.2004.11.004

Van der Merwe, K. J., Steyne, P. S., Fourie, L. F., Scott, D. B., & Theron, J. J. (1965). Ochratoxin A, a toxic metabolite produced by Aspergillus ochraceus Wilh. *Nature, 205*(4976), 1112–1113. doi:10.1038/2051112a0

Van Egmond, H. P. (1989). *Mycotoxins in dairy products*. London: Elsevier Applied Science.

Wilson, D. M., Mubatanhema, W., & Jurjevic, Z. (2002). Biology and ecology of mycotoxigenic aspergillus species as related to economic and health concerns. In J. W. De Vries, M. W. Trucksess, & L. S. Jackson (Eds.), *Mycotoxins and Food Safety*. New York: Kluwer Academic / Plenum Publishers. doi:10.1007/978-1-4615-0629-4_2

Wu, S. N., Chen, H., Liu, Y. C., & Chiang, H. T. (2002). Block of L-type Ca2+ current by beauvericin, a toxic cyclopeptide in the NG108-15 neuronal cell line. *Chemical Research in Toxicology, 15*(6), 854–860. doi:10.1021/tx020003k

Yousef, A. E., & Marth, E. H. (1985). Degradation of aflatoxin M1 in milk by ultraviolet energy. *Journal of Food Protection, 48*(8), 697–698. doi:10.4315/0362-028X-48.8.697

Yu, Z., Zhang, L., Wu, D., & Liu, F. (2005). Anti-apoptotic action of zearalenone in MCF-7 cells. *Ecotoxicology and Environmental Safety*, *62*(3), 441–446. doi:10.1016/j.ecoenv.2004.10.003

Zepnik, H., Völkel, W., & Dekant, W. (2003). Toxicokinetics of the mycotoxin ochratoxin A in F 344 rats after oral administration. *Toxicology and Applied Pharmacology*, *192*(1), 36–44. doi:10.1016/S0041-008X(03)00261-8

Zinedine, A., Gonzales-Osnaya, L., Soriano, J. M., Moltó, J. C., Idrissi, L., & Mañes, J. (2007a). Presence of aflatoxin M1 in pasteurized milk from Morocco. *International Journal of Food Microbiology*, *114*(1), 25–29. doi:10.1016/j.ijfoodmicro.2006.11.001

Zinedine, A., & Mañes, J. (2009). Occurrence and legislation of mycotoxins in food and feed from Morocco. *Food Control*, *20*(4), 334–344. doi:10.1016/j.foodcont.2008.07.002

Zinedine, A., Meca, G., Mañes, J., & Font, G. (2011). Further data on the occurrence of Fusarium emerging mycotoxins enniatins (A, A1, B, B1), fusaproliferin and beauvericin in raw cereals commercialized in Morocco. *Food Control*, *22*(1), 1–5. doi:10.1016/j.foodcont.2010.05.002

Zinedine, A., & Ruiz, M. J. (2014). Zearalenone. In *Mycotoxins and their implications in food safety*. Future Science Ltd. Retrieved from www.future-science.com

Zinedine, A., Soriano, J. M., Moltó, J. C., & Mañes, J. (2007b). Review on the toxicity, occurrence, metabolism, detoxification, regulations and intake of zearalenone: An oestrogenic mycotoxin. *Food and Chemical Toxicology*, *45*(1), 1–18. doi:10.1016/j.fct.2006.07.030

This research was previously published in the Handbook of Research on Global Environmental Changes and Human Health edited by Kholoud Kahime, Moulay Abdelmonaim El Hidan, Omar El Hiba, Denis Sereno, and Lahouari Bounoua; pages 74-97, copyright year 2019 by Engineering Science Reference (an imprint of IGI Global).

Chapter 4
Technologies for Monitoring the Safety of Perishable Food Products

Pedro Dinis Gaspar
University of Beira Interior, Portugal

Pedro Dinho da Silva
 https://orcid.org/0000-0003-2204-3397
University of Beira Interior, Portugal

Luís Pinto Andrade
Polytechnic Institute of Castelo Branco, Portugal

José Nunes
Polytechnic Institute of Castelo Branco, Portugal

Christophe Espírito Santo
 https://orcid.org/0000-0002-9800-4186
Agrofood Technological Center, Portugal

ABSTRACT

Food safety and eradication of food waste are current concerns of society and governments due to health, ethics, and sustainable economics. There are multiple technologies for monitoring food safety at different chain stages, among them, time-temperature integrators (TTI). Temperature is a major factor affecting food quality and safety during its life cycle. This parameter can be monitored using TTI devices on food packages, allowing users to know the thermal exposure. This chapter addresses food safety issues, namely factors related to microbial growth responsible for food deterioration. Moreover, TTI monitoring technologies are also described, focusing on features, advantages, disadvantages, applicability, and product examples. Analysis of the current state of TTI and technological evolution, a prediction is provided for future TTI devices designed for more assertive, traceable, safe, and quality food products.

DOI: 10.4018/978-1-7998-5354-1.ch004

INTRODUCTION

Food waste is a persistent reality in the actual society. This is an upmost issue with substantial relevance, not only by the intrinsic ethical questions, but also to the relation between food consumer and producer (APIC, 2006). Food shortage in the world are due to lack of socio-economic conditions of parts of the population, this causes an immorality that condemns the existence of food waste, specially that 925 million people suffer of malnutrition in the world (APIC, 2006). Additionally, food waste is translated into costs to final consumers, distributors and producers. Lastly, food waste leads to degradation of natural resources such as water, soil, or energy consumption, affecting biodiversity preservation and air quality (ANCIPA, 2005). In recent years, a major priority for distributors is to provide high quality food (in a good state of conservation) to consumers, which became more aware and concerned with food quality standards (ANCIPA, 2005).

The Food and Agriculture Organization of the United Nations (FAO) estimates that one-third of the total food produced for human consumption is lost or wasted, approximately 1.3 billion of tons. This corresponds to annual costs of 750 billion dollars (FAO, 2011). The economical impact is significant due to loss of product value, nevertheless the environmental impact has to be accounted too, food waste leads also to waste of natural resources, such as water, land, energy, and unnecessary green gas emissions leading to global warming and climate change. This, in turn, affects agriculture and food production. Moreover, the FAO CEO, Graziano da Silva, reported during the Global Green Grout Forum (3GF) realized in Copenhagen (Denmark) in October of 2013, that food waste reduction to zero could provide sufficient food for 2 billion people. Thus, the FAO appeals for innovative ways to control and reduce this global food waste problem. FAO indicates that the major food waste happens in post-production phase, as well as during the harvest, transportation and storage. In developing countries, food waste is related with inadequate infrastructures, while in developed countries is a problem between commercialization and consumption phases (Gogou *et al.*, 2013).

In the 27-member states of the European Union (EU), annual food waste is about 89 million tons, with a prediction of a rise to 126 million tons in 2020. In the case of perishable food products, such as the horticultural products, 30% of the European production is wasted after harvest (FAO, 2013). According to 2012 data, only in Portugal, about 1 million tons of food is wasted, i.e., about 17% of the total production (O'Connor, 2014).

The European Parliament declared 2014 as the European Year against the Food Waste, in order to take measures to solve this problem.

This is a worldwide problem, from agricultural field to consumers. Significant part of the problem is due to consumer behaviour, i.e. avoiding to buy "imperfect" horticultural products or with "small dimension" or products with closer expiry date.

To overcome this problem with serious ethical, social, environment and economic consequences, the European Parliament called a collective and urgent action to reduce food waste in half until 2025. Nonetheless, European Commission hopes to reach this target by 2020, since the "Roadmap to a Resource Efficient Europe" has been given a priority (Baptista *et al.*, 2012) This ambition involves an assertive effort between all food chain parties. Additionally, many initiatives and campaigns have started to sensitize producers, sellers and consumers for the food waste problem.

Alternatively, ensuring food safety will reduce waste in the production, transportation and food display, and will help consumers to change their behaviour (APIC, 2006).

The time span, under storage conditions, which food remains acceptable for human consumption (in terms of safety, nutritional attributes, and sensory characteristics) is known as shelf life (Bell & Labuza, 1992; Corradini & Peleg, 2006; van Boekel, 2009; Jedermann *et al.*, 2014). Food progressively deteriorates leading to loss of quality and safety, this is accelerated by inadequate storage and distribution conditions, such exposure to high temperatures or humidity (Taoukis *et al.*, 1997; Labuza, 2001; van Boekel, 2008).

Perishable food products have high quantity of water and nutrients, essential elements for microorganisms to develop. This type of products requires special conditions to its conservation, storage and transportation (EU, 2015). Low temperature conservation is constantly required to extend lifespan and avoid deterioration. Examples of perishable products are all the fresh products of meat, fish, fruits and vegetables as well milk and its derivatives. Non-perishable foods, on the other hand, have low water content. Most of these products are vegetables, which can be stored in a dry environment at room temperature (for example: rice, beans, etc.). This type of food is a concern for production and distribution companies because they do not need specific conditions of preservation to be maintained. Fundamentally, conditions are harsh for microbial development (ANCIPA, 2005). Thus, the lifespan is longer and conservation requirements are lower.

Researchers focus towards creating new tools and improving the tracking capability/food safety in situ monitorization, in particular, the refrigerated chain, where quality and contamination risk is higher (FAO, 2011). At the retail stores around 15% of perishable foods are wasted as a consequence of damage and spoilage (Ferguson & Ketzenberg, 2006). This increases to approximately 35% when proper temperature conditions are not applied (Zoller *et al.*, 2013). Therefore, monitoring food distribution and storage is critical to avoid food deterioration and waste, and ensuring the costumer on the product freshness (Annese *et al.*, 2015). Hence, developing technologies to monitor quality of food products during all stages, from production to consumer, is crucial to reduce food safety outbreaks and lower food waste (ANCIPA, 2005).

HYGIENE AND FOOD SECURITY

The Role of Food Hygiene in Ensuring the Viability/Food Security

Food hygiene is the upmost important method to maintain product safety. Consisting on a set of measures that ensures safety and healthiness during food production: processing, manufacturing, packaging, storage, distribution, handling and sale (ANCIPA, 2005). Food contamination during preparation can lead to quicker food deterioration or worse, by jeopardizing safety causing diseases to consumers. The most infamous food contamination case was Typhoid Mary. In the 19th century Typhoid fever was identified and *Salmonella enterica* serovar Typhi was isolated. At that time, no antibiotics were available and mortality rate was at least 10%. Mary Mallon, named Typhoid Mary, carried the disease but never had any symptoms. In multiple occasions she was forbidden to practice cooking with enforced isolation, but anyway she constantly found a way to handle food for other people. Only Mallon infected 51 people, 3 of whom died. This stubbornness made society aware and started to protect itself (Brooks, 1996).

The Regulation (EC) No 852/2004 of the European Parliament and of the Council of 29 April 2004 on the hygiene of food, as well as the Portuguese Law by Decree-Law n ° 67/98, establishes general rules that for food safety (Venâncio & Batista, 2003; ANCIPA, 2005). This was recently changed by Regulation (EC) no. ° 219/2009 of the European Parliament and of the Council of 11 March 2009. In addition, the traceability and consequent contact between foods within packing is governed by the EC Regulation n.º 178/2002 and it should be rigorously followed.

Food Hazards

Besides physical (harmful materials, such as sharp metals) and chemical hazards (harmful toxic chemicals, such as cleaning agents), biological hazards are the source most concerns. Avoiding biological hazards is difficult and complicated due to the dependence of several factors. The food processing and the development of pathogenic bacteria rely heavily on the exposure. This can be caused by a macro-biologic agent (presence of flies or other insects) or microbiological agent (pathogenic bacteria, viruses and parasites).

Hazard severity and frequency classification is achieved by implementing a Hazard Analysis and Critical Control Point (HACCP) certification (Venâncio & Batista, 2003). This determines which hazards are more significant (Ellouze & Augustin, 2010).

Microbial Growth Factors

Microbial development is dependent of favourable conditions. The rate of microbial growth becomes exponential after cell adaptation to the environment. When nutrients are depleted or inhibitory metabolites are accumulated, growth reaches the stagnation phase or stationary phase.

Regarding the factors that affect the rate of microbial growth in food, these have the ability to determine the nature of the damage and thus have some risks to health. Some of these factors affecting the rate of microbial growth in food product are shown in Table 1 (Venâncio & Batista, 2003).

Table 1. Factors affecting the rate of microbial growth in food products (Venâncio & Batista, 2003)

Microbial Growth Factors	Example
Intrinsic	Physicochemical food properties
Extrinsic	Storage environment conditions
Processing factors	Disregard for proper food manufacture (time and temperature)

Extrinsic Microbial Growth Factors

Extrinsic factors are environmental conditions for storing food products that affect microbial growth. These factors are relative humidity, temperature and atmospheric composition (Venâncio & Batista, 2003).

Relative Humidity

Humidity is the moisture content of air, being the mass ration of water vapor to dry air. Relative humidity is the ratio as a percentage of the partial pressure of water vapor in air to the vapor pressure of liquid water at a given temperature. This is an essential measure of water activity of the gas phase. In regions where the water activity is low and the food is stored in atmospheres with high relative humidity.

Water can be transferred to the gas phase in foods and promote the growth (germinate and grow) of microorganisms that remained viable until the point, but unable to develop themselves.

Temperature

Microbial growth can occur at a wide temperature range depending on the microbe. Growth can be explained as simple as by the cell enzymatic activity. Enzymes are designed by biological organisms to have an optimum activity to allow the best adaptation to the environment temperature, pressure, pH, aw, etc. Temperature affects activity and can even lead to enzymatic denaturation (microbial inactivation). Low temperatures, slow down enzymatic reactions, growth rate is low (this is what happens in freezing or refrigerating temperatures). High temperatures, also inhibit enzyme activity, but it can lead to denaturation, growth is inhibited and microbes are inactivated (i.e. cooking food, pasteurization, sterilization). Higher temperature and longer exposure time will determine the amount of microbial inactivation. Microbial growth occurs when optimum temperature range is met, at lower temperatures growth rate is lower, at high temperature growth is also lower but if temperature is too high growth can be completely inhibited. An important requirement is the presence of liquid water as a basis that supports the growth.

Atmosphere Composition

Oxygen presence in the atmospheric composition and its potential influence on the oxidation/reduction allows the development of microbes. The common methods to reduce the microbial growth based in modified atmosphere packaging consist in: inhibitory effect of atmosphere enrichment with carbon dioxide CO_2 (with the consequent reduction of oxygen, O_2, and pH change on the food surface); oxygen impoverishment in the atmosphere (reducing respiratory intensity and consequent delay in maturation); and atmosphere modification with an inert gas such as the nitrogen, N_2. Though, lowering or removing completely oxygen from the atmospheric composition can lead to anaerobic microbial growth. Pathogenic bacteria such as *Clostridium* species are anaerobic and can lead to serious infections, for example, the ingestion of botulinum toxin produced by *Clostridium botulinum*. Increasing CO_2 can help inhibiting bacterial growth by lowering the pH.

Intrinsic Factors of Microbial Growth

Microbial growth also depends on factors related with the food itself.

Nutrients

For microbial growth to occurs the right carbon and nitrogen source need to be present. If the right nutrient is present in the food composition, growth will occur, i.e., key nutrients concentration, in some cases, can determine the rate of microbial growth. Examples of nutrients that promote microbial growth are: carbohydrates, proteins, fats, minerals and vitamins.

pH

Depending on the food type, pH can be optimum for microbial growth. Food pH has an important effect on growth and viability of microorganisms. This is also explained by stability of biomolecules, cells need to maintain an intracellular pH above a critical limit, otherwise denaturation of proteins occurs. Therefore, each microbe has a specific pH range which they can grow. In general, most microbes grow best around neutral pH values (6.5 - 7.0). However, different microorganisms resist to different pH's, some can resist in extreme pH conditions (pH as low as 1 and high as 9), yet these microbes are found in extreme conditions in the nature. In food environments, Yeasts and Moulds and some bacteria are more resistant to lower pH (low as 3.0), due to the production of acidic compounds from their metabolism, such as lactic acid (lactic acid bacteria) and acetic acid (yeasts and others). Generally bacterial pathogen growth is inhibited at pH lower than 4, that is the case of some preserves and fermentation processes.

Naturally acidic type of foods are fruits, been the reason why yeasts and mould are more susceptible to develop and cause spoilage. Neutral pH, such as meat, are more prone for pathogenic bacteria to grow.

Carbohydrate rich food tend to deteriorate by acid hydrolysis, reducing pH (reducing the risk of pathogens), protein-rich food, the pH increases, when spoiled, meaning its less safe with a higher risk of a pathogen to grow.

Oxidation/Reduction Potential

Chemical composition of foods influences the oxidation/reduction potential (Eh), thus affecting microbial growth. Positive redox potential is required for aerobic microorganisms, whereas anaerobes need a negative potential. Oxygen plays an important part in the redox potential due to our oxidizing atmosphere, however, oxygen presence is not an utter prerequisite for redox reactions since other compounds can accept electrons.

Plant origin foods have a typical Eh of +300 to 400 mV, aerobic growth is favoured. On the other hand, anaerobic growth is favoured on meat products due to the redox potential of -200 mV

Water Activity (a_w)

Free water in the food is required for microbial growth, in other words, for all cellular biochemical reactions to occur: transport nutrients, remove released products of enzymatic reactions for the synthesis of cellular materials and participate in other biochemical reactions. Each microbial species (or group) has an optimum level, maximum and minimum of water activity for growth. When a_w is reduced until a minimum level for microbial growth, the cells remain viable temporarily. However, if the water activity is dramatically reduced, the microbial cells lose their viability, usually more quickly at first and then slowly. Most enzymatic reactions require aw levels higher than 0.85, bacterial growth does not occur at aw levels lower that 0.9, and for moulds and yeasts the aw limit of growth is between 0.8 to 0.9. However, food cannot be all converted to low aw levels to ensure microbial inhibition, for example, fresh fruits need to be stored with other means because high air moisture will preserve the texture and the a_w will remain higher than 0.95.

Antimicrobials

Natural antimicrobial substances are present in food, these substances are able to inhibit microbial growth. Some examples are lysozyme in eggs, essential oils, lactoferrin from cows' milk, among others.

Common Bacteria Responsible for Food Contamination

In a review about food hazards, microorganisms are those that provide greater danger (Surak, 2003; Ellouze & Augustin, 2010).

The attention given by the producers to food hazards focus primarily on microbiological hazards that represent a significantly higher number of cases than the other types of contamination.

Among the microorganism variables that are possible to identify are:

- The variability expression of the many pathogenic mechanisms;
- The microorganism potential to cause disease;
- The sensitivity of the microorganism to the food substrate characteristics and with the surrounding environmental conditions;
- The nature of the interactions with other organisms.

Table 2 includes examples of common bacteria in food contamination and the main conditions to the occurrence of some of the biological dangers (Venâncio & Batista, 2003).

Table 2. Examples of common bacteria in food contamination and the main conditions to the occurrence of some of the biological dangers (Venâncio & Batista, 2003)

Bacteria	Parameters					
	T_{min} (°C)	T_{max} (°C)	pH_{min}	pH_{max}	$a_{w\,min}$	$NaCl_{max}$ (%)
Bacillus cereus	5	55	4.9	8.8	0.93	10
Campylobacter jejuni	32	45	4.9	9.0	0.98	2
Clostridium perfringens	12	50	5.5	9.0	0.943	7
Escherichia coli	7	46	4.4	9.0	0.95	6.5
Listeria monocytogenes	0	45	4.39	9.4	0.92	10
Salmonella spp.	5	47	4.2	9.5	0.94	8
Shigella spp.	7	47	4.9	9.3	0.97	5.2
Vibrio parahaemolyticus	5	43	4.8	11	0.94	10
Yersinia enterocolitica	-1	42	4.2	9.6	0.97	7

Bacteria in a certain concentration can be considered as having an infective dose, because has the minimum number of microorganisms necessary to cause a disease. This can change from individual to individual due to the fact that is necessary to have in consideration that there is a set of physiological nature factors that influence the level of minimum infective dose (degree of gastric acidity, intestinal flora, immunity, nutritional status and individual stress, ...).

Preventive Measures

To prevent the contamination of food is essential to implement some good practices that support this goal. In the food industry, the food products mixing and heat supply is made simultaneously to ensure safety and to avoid physiological damage to the consumer.

Processes Used in Minimizing Food Contamination

The mixture of certain levels of nutrients, oxygen and favourable pH are necessary conditions to provide the microorganism growth. Perishable foods are the foods most susceptible to deterioration by microbial growth (Mehauden, 2009; Li & Wang, 2012).

By microorganisms' growth, there is a consumption of nutrients and the production of enzymes that contribute for the loss/contamination of flavours or synthesis of compounds, which will cause the food to become unsuitable to consumption, ultimately could cause disease. However, not all microorganisms are pathogenic, this parameter depends on its concentration in the food product (infective dose).

Effectiveness of Thermal Treatments (Production of Food Safe)

Due to consumer pressure, regulations have been created and applied on food safety and quality to ensure consumer protection. The food producers are responsible for the safety of their products. To ensure this security, the food products are submitted to different techniques that allow the reduction of the number of microorganisms or eliminate pathogenic microorganisms in food (Mehauden *et al.*, 2007). Table 3 describes several food preservation techniques.

Heat Treatments

The quality requirements on food manufacturing became increasingly demanding over the last 20 years. Fundamentally, the product may not cause damage to the consumer. To ensure food safety, manufacturers have been using different techniques for preservation (Mehauden *et al.*, 2007).

The food treatment by heat consists in an operation that aims cooking/food producing and simultaneously reduce/prevent the microbial growth responsible for the "poisoning". The impact of these preservation techniques in food safety and quality is quantified by its effectiveness. Table 4 describes thermal treatments ranked according to their temperatures (Mehauden, 2009).

Theoretically, the duration of treatment by heating depends on several parameters (Surak, 2003):

- Thermal resistance of the microorganisms and spores hypothetically present in the food;
- Thermal characteristics;
- The food pH and characteristics of its nutrients;
- Shape and size of the package;
- Physical conditions of food (liquid, solid or mixture).

The thermal processes used can be determined from mathematical modelling. Mathematical models depend on the product time-temperature profile and the elimination kinetics of the desired microorganism. The thermal process calculation is based on the amount of destruction of the heat-resistant bacterium, *Clostridium botulinum* (Mehauden, 2009).

Table 3. Food preservation techniques

Preservation Technique	Description
Hygiene	- The microorganisms' growth can be delayed or prevented by the fulfilment of hygiene rules for food production.
HACCP	- The food security methodology can be applied to reduce contamination; - Depends on the identification of Critical Control Points (CCP) in the food production and preparation process; - The food products are strictly monitored in order to ensure the food safety for consumption.
Chemistry preservation	- Chemicals such as salt or acid can be added on foods to reduce its pH or reduce the water activity (a_w), thus limiting the growth of microorganisms.
Biological fermentation	- The fermentation purpose is to allow the growth of unwanted microorganisms. These are added on food in order to compete with the unwanted and harmful microorganisms causing its annulation; - It is the oldest method of food preservation.
"Smart packing"	- Used in order to extend the food product shelf life, through oxygen removal, capturing of carbon dioxide and mixing with control agents or antimicrobial agents inside of the product packaging.
Microorganisms removal by microfiltration	- Considered a "cold" pasteurization; - Used for liquid products such as milk and beer.
Thermal treatment	- Unlike the heat treatment, the cold preservation does not eliminate the microorganisms present, but slows their growth; - Low temperature methods include refrigeration and freezing.
Irradiation	- In this technique, electromagnetic waves or electrons are applied in food; - Ionization and UV radiation causes damages on microorganism DNA and lethal injuries; - This application is limited due to the damages that they may cause to the consumer.
High pressure (Pascalization)	- The pressures in the range of 200 MPa to 800 MPa are applied to food causing the damage in cell membrane of the microorganism and denaturation of its proteins; - This technique (recent) is very appealing in the food production industry.
Pulse electric field	- The application of an electric field in food usually causing damage on the membrane of microorganism during the voltage application; - Can only be applied to liquid food such as orange juice.

Table 4. Thermal treatments ranked according to their applied temperatures (Mehauden, 2009)

Treatment	Description
Pasteurization	- Heating food process in order to eliminate the microorganisms endowed with the capacity to cause damage to the consumer (example: bacteria, virus); - Does not eliminate all microorganisms present. Only reduces the number of sensitive microorganisms to heat for safe levels and stops the activity of most enzymes; - Is a soft treatment and temperature applied does not exceed the 100 °C; - Pasteurized products are constantly refrigerated and should be consumed before its expiry date.
Sterilization (Ultra High Temperature - UHT)	- Temperatures range between the 135 ° C and 150 ° C during 2 to 4 seconds; - Treatment goal is to extinguish all pathogenic organisms and their toxins; - Based on the destruction of the bacterium *Clostridium botulinum*, which can be lethal if swallowed.

Note: Clostridium botulinum - produces a botulinum exotoxin highly resistant to temperature. Its growth occurs in anaerobic environments and in conditions of pH > 4.5 allowing their growth after packaging of food products.

MONITORING TECHNOLOGY OF FOOD SAFETY OF PERISHABLES FOOD PRODUCTS

Food monitoring allows, to some point, to improve the distribution and supply of these products to the sales centres and to evaluate quality at different phases/stages of the food chain (Gogou *et al.*, 2014).

To this end, electronic devices named Time-Temperature data logger are used to evaluate food quality. There are several types of these devices, depending on their operating principle (Taoukis *et al.*, 2010).

Monitoring of Food Products

Perform the tracking of a product along all the food chain is the best way to evaluate the various steps or critical points (Taoukis *et al.*, 2010). This is also the best way to reduce food waste and maximize the producer profits (Mehauden *et al.*, 2007).

The consumer is aware that perishable foods products suffer quality and safety alteration when badly preserved (in not recommended environments). Thus, the consumer always chooses the product with longer expiry date (presuming to be fresher) or the one that presents most appealing organoleptic conditions. Therefore, producers become aware of the importance dynamics of the quality parameters after production of the food type, from preservation to transportation. This conscience improves the transportation, storage and sale quality standards, and clearly identifies the critical points of each key phase (Li & Wang, 2012).

Note that the lifespan or shelf-life of food products is a parameter that depends mostly on the temperature to which it is subjected. Consequently, producers consider this parameter to be crucial factor and aim to extend it to the maximum. Based on studies conducted in the food chain of Greece and France, the critical points where the food product is more subject/susceptible to thermal variations are in the transition phases along the distribution chain (small temperature oscillation) and, especially in the last stage of the chain, when consumer purchases the food product. Transition phase from supermarket to the domestic fridge/freezer and maintenance of food in this environment are the most critical points for food quality conservation (Gogou *et al.*, 2013).

Electronic devices, such as miniNOMAD, OM-84-TMP (Omega Engineering Inc., Stamford, USA) can be incorporated in the packaging monitoring effectively from food production line to consumers' homes (Gogou *et al.*, 2013).

As shown in Figure 1, we are able to through the analysis of results of this study it is possible understand where are the critical points on the chilled food chain. We can also conclude that food is maintained at a higher temperature and higher temperature variations during storage in domestic refrigerators (Figure 1). These thermal levels remain practically constant since the final phase of the step in which the food is placed in the supermarket display cabinets (at this stage food may be located closer to the display cabinet door that can be opened several times a day, leading to higher temperature variations). Table 5 shows the average temperature/duration of food at each recorded stage in the study carried out on the chilled French supermarkets chain (Gogou et al., 2013).

Results presented in Table 5 show that although consumer food transportation phase (supermarket/domestic refrigerator) exposed food to higher temperatures, this is performed in a short period of time. However, this can be harmful to food integrity, such as the temperature relation of domestic refrigerator/duration (time before consumption).

Figure 1. Historical time-temperature that the perishable foods cross through a chilled chain (Gogou et al., 2013)

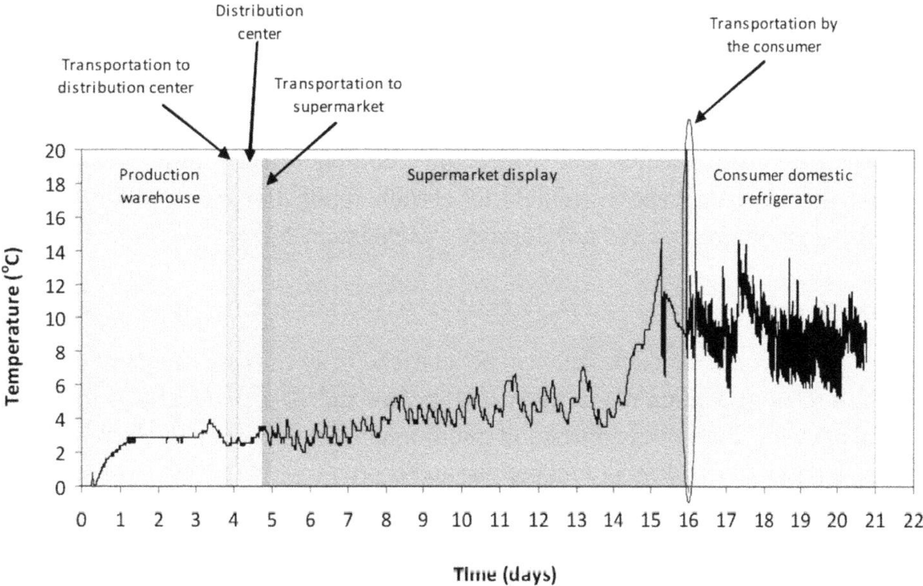

Table 5. Average temperature/duration of food at each recorded stage in the study carried out on the chilled French supermarkets chain (Gogou et al., 2013)

Phase of the chilled chain	Average temperature (°C)	Duration (days)
Production / Warehouse	3.4	2.7
Transportation / Distribution centre	3.9	0.4
Distribution centre / Transportation / Market	3.8	1.9
Supermarket	4.0	22.4
Transportation by the consumer	9.8	0.02 (48 min.)
Domestic refrigerator	6.8	16

Traditional Monitoring

Traditional monitoring consists in the verification of the thermal treatment effectiveness during food production phase. These treatments are used to eliminate any pathogenic agent during the production phase and the monitoring is realized in order to evaluate treatment effectiveness (Mehauden, 2009).

Thermocouples and Dataloggers

These electronic devices are incorporated on food products and used to check the thermal treatments validation/effectiveness (Mehauden, 2009).

They can be inserted into the food packaging and its objective is record the temperature inside the package during a period of time. Temperature records collected can be visualized using a graphical chart of temperature in function to time. This way of evaluating the effectiveness of thermal treatment is widely used and data analysis easier and fast (Gogou *et al.*, 2013).

However, these electronic systems present some drawbacks in some thermal processes. For example, analysing fluid food, the electronic equipment may interfere with the proper motion of the fluid in the container, leading to an incorrect temperature recording. In many cases, it is impracticable to put it in the right place, preferably in the coolest zone of the package.

The equipment size is also a barrier that affects the recording effectiveness. A wireless datalogger, due to its big size (battery), may not be suitable for certain application cases, although this restriction has been a priority area of research and development (Mehauden, 2009).

Count of Microorganisms

The effectiveness of thermal treatments can also be analysed from the assessment of changes in quality and attributes of the food (counting microorganisms) before and after treatment. A food sample is collected before and after the thermal treatment and microorganisms are counted. However, this technique can be laborious, lengthy (takes days of incubation) and costly.

Due to the disadvantages of these two presented techniques led to the development of a new monitoring technique, the use of Time-Temperature Integrators (TTI) (Mehauden, 2009).

Monitoring for Time-Temperature Integrators (TTI)

TTI devices are shelf-life indicators, alternative to conventional temperature control systems and as potential replacement for conventional open labelling (Farquhar, 1977; Taoukis & Labuza, 1989; Fu *et al.*, 1991; Shimoni *et al.*, 2001; Taoukis *et al.*, 2010; Taoukis, 2010). These devices have the purpose to measure the direct impact of storage conditions on the food product, allowing to quantify the impact of a certain temperature condition on a product attribute (Taoukis *et al.*, 2010). Thus, the real freshness of the product is reported instead of a static label. Producers, retailers, and consumers can, institutively, visually verify the cumulative time-temperature history of a product (Sherlock et al., 1991; Giannakourou & Taoukis, 2002; Giannoglou *et al.*, 2014). These simple devices are normally characterized of a label/sticker that changes coloration irreversibly, indicating the real food storage history. Degradation kinetics are temperature dependent, under an incorrect storage temperature, a chromatic change is triggered. This change can be quantified with a value of P (statistical value that refers the probability of rejecting the null hypothesis when it is true, i.e., considers two different groups that are not) (Mehauden, 2009).

Features

The fundamental characteristics of any of these types of temperature monitoring devices are (Kim *et al.*, 2012; Brizio & Prentice, 2015; Tsironi *et al.*, 2017):

- Small;
- Resistant;
- The time-temperature history is not necessary to determine the impact of the thermal treatments on foods.

Types

TTI devices are classified depending on two parameters. These can be classified according to their origin/application in food or in accordance with the substance containing (Mehauden *et al.*, 2007).

- **Classification according to the origin/application:**
  - **Intrinsic TTI:** Used in natural form in foods. The thermal treatments efficiency is evaluated through the specified quantification before and after the process. The most important advantage, is the homogeneously dispersed intrinsic TTI in the foods (Mehauden, 2009).
  - **Extrinsic TTI:** Used in artificial form in foods, and it can be subdivided into three groups:
    - TTI added directly to food, blended together with food;
    - Permeable TTI, which are placed in separate units that contain a permeable barrier which allows exchanges between food and TTI;
    - Isolated TTI, placed in a separate unit and the barrier is not permeable. Thus, no exchanges between device and food is made.
- **Classification according to the contained substance:**
  - Depending on the substance contained in the TTI, these can be subdivided into the types (Taoukis *et al.*, 2010):
    - Enzymatic TTI;
    - Microbiological TTI;
    - Chemical TTI;
    - Physical TTI.

Types of TTI Devices Depending on the Contained Substance

This section describes the basic principle, applications, advantages and disadvantages of different types of TTI classified according to type of contained substance.

Enzymatic TTI

The principle of operation is based on the quantification of the enzyme activity (Giannoglou *et al.*, 2014; Brizio & Prentice, 2015; Tsironi *et al.*, 2017). Accumulation of the substrate hydrolysis shows the impact of temperature variation suffered by the product. Having a high thermal stability allows its usage in a wide range of temperatures. These devices are best suited for pasteurization and sterilization (Mehauden, 2009).

The enzyme choice must satisfy certain conditions (Kim *et al.*, 2012):

- The isothermal enzyme inactivation has to follow a known kinetic order;
- The enzyme needs to be thermally resistant;
- The enzyme needs to have a Z value (the value of the accumulated probability) until a point that corresponds with the study of microorganisms rather than only be used as a security tool.

The most commonly used enzyme is *α-amylase* whose characteristics and properties that makes it suitable are:

- Belongs to microorganism *Bacillus spp*;
- Good thermal resistance;
- *Z* value roughly equivalent to the recipient organism (*Clostridium botulinum*);
- Denaturation follows a kinetic reaction of 1st order[1];
- Industrial application in the production of beer, processes of making paper and detergent;
- Produced to industrial scale by the microorganism *Bacillus spp*;
- Stable at pH values in the range of 5.5 to 8;
- The stability can be modulated by calcium addition. Hence, the enzyme can withstand high temperatures (up to 90 °C) during a specific time interval.

The most usual applications of these types of devices are on pasteurization and sterilization processes. In the pasteurization process its application are related with (Mehauden, 2009):

- The existence of enzymes thermally stable, common in pasteurization temperatures;
- Specific systems are not necessary to protect the enzyme.

The applicability in the case of sterilization processes results on:

- To find thermally stable enzymes in higher temperatures (sterilization temperatures) is more difficult.

The device response is characterized by:

- Quantifying enzyme denaturation due to the thermal treatment (enzyme activity decrease);
- The quantification of change between before and after treatment demonstrates the impact of enzymatic activity in the TTI device.

The utilization advantages of this type of devices are (Pavelkova, 2013):

- Small size;
- Low cost;
- Wireless;
- Shock resistant (available for processes where thermocouples and dataloggers cannot be used);
- Rapid analysis when compared with microbiological devices.

The application disadvantages of this type of device are (Mehauden *et al.*, 2007):

- Inability to allow online monitoring;
- Its small dimensions can difficult their recovery between foods;
- Need to know the value of Dt^2 and Z value (value of the cumulative probability to data processing) - helps determine the monitoring effectiveness and comparing the data. Necessary to have some preliminary experiments and enzyme calibration before the device is ready to use (Maesmans *et al.*, 1994).

Microbiological TTI

This is the mostly used type of TTI devices in the food industry, and it relies on the growth of microorganisms, such as yeast or lactic acid bacteria, which in turn release metabolites that change the environment pH leading to a colour change of a pH indicator (Kim *et al.*, 2013; Choi *et al.*, 2014; Zhang *et al.*, 2016). It can be divided in two types of analytical principles. The first, analyses the process impact based on the quantification of the number of surviving microorganisms. The second one, only detects if there are or not the microorganisms growth (Sun, 2012).

The operation basic principle consists in a carrier system, inoculated with a determined microorganism concentration and a thermal resistance. The cutting level of activity of the microbiological integrators in the sterilization provides the magnitude/effect of the process (Sun, 2012).

The characteristics of the microbiological integrator can be summarized in:

- The organism must be stable in respect to its quantity and thermal resistance. The results must be reproducible with low variability;
- The microbiological system (microorganisms, carrier system and procedure used) need to be calibrated for specific sterilization conditions;
- The relationships between the microbiological integrator and the load of pathogenic microorganisms in food products must be known so that the validity of the sterilization process can be ensured.

Depending on the intended application, the microorganism that will serve as a biological indicator has to be chosen. The most resistant species are generally the most used in the process, however, under certain conditions, less resistant microorganisms, quite similar to natural microflora or easily detectable can be used. Examples are (Sun, 2012):

- *Bacillus stearothermophilus* spores are the more used as biological indicators in sterilization process in humid heat conditions;
- *Bacillus subtilis* spores are used to the dry heat treatment and in processes where the ethylene oxide is used;
- *Bacillus pumilus* spores are used to sterilization processes by pathways of ionic radiation.

To determine the impact of thermal treatment, it is necessary to use spores previously calibrated and valid in relation to physical parameters known.

The utilization advantage of this type of device is that the microorganisms are easily disseminated in the food product, while that the main disadvantage is the difficulty to provide high accuracy results (Mehauden, 2009).

Chemical TTI

These are employed as a label on the product packaging with a very simple and intuitive reading so that the end consumer is able to gather the information and decide by himself about his purchase (Sun, 2012).

This type of indicator is based on chemical reactions, such as polymerization, photochromic, or oxidation reactions (Mai *et al.*, 2011; Brizio & Prentice, 2014). The specific molecule has no colour in its basic state, becoming dark blue when is activated when exposed to ultraviolet radiation (UV). The molecule reverts to colourless depending on the temperature (based in the Arrhenius equation[3]).

The label should be hidden under an anti UV filter after its activation avoiding another colour change. Consequently, if in the package label there is a change from dark blue to blue standard, the indicator show that the product remains in conditions to be consumed, because the extrinsic conditions of the food safety are within limits. If the label has grey or white, the product should not be consumed.

The labels may be stored in a room with any temperature, but without light until its utilization. The support paper must be specified, whereas the printing on a plastic substrate is possible (Hightech Europe, 2014).

The thickness of the ink is not easy to measure, but this parameter is read indirectly through the activation and colour measurement. The distance between the product and the packaging is the minimum recommended. This should be reduced for that food temperature history and the TTI device are as identical as possible (Hightech Europe, 2014).

As limitation of this type of TTI devices, it can be noted that the reference colours used are not very appealing/instinctive to the consumer. Reference colours used: blue (good condition) and grey (poor condition). Additionally, may be subject to product adulteration activities, such as re-packaging in cases that the expiration date of foods has been exceeded and can be placed a new label of fresh reference (dark blue).

Nanoparticle TTI

Nanoparticles can change shape, size or surface morphology depending on the temperature exposure. This leads to alteration of the light absorption spectra by the particle (different wavelength absorption), characterized by visual chromatic shift (Wang *et al.*, 2017).

Physical TTI

The operation basic principle of this type of TTI device is based on the phenomenon of diffusion. The system consists of a chemical coloured substance that can melt and be absorbed by an absorbent paper under the effect of moist heat (steam). Usually used as an indicator of thermal processes (Sun, 2012).

The response of this type of device is calculated by measuring the distance reached by the compound that is submitted to the diffusion process.

Its major disadvantage is the impossibility to use with dry heat thermal processes. Additionally, it cannot be included in the product because this device is only activated by steam.

TTI: INTEGRATORS TIME-TEMPERATURE

This section describes various TTI devices available on the market. Their specifications are described, as well as their advantages and disadvantages. Note that only some examples are shown. In the market, other TTI brands making use of the same concept are available.

TTI 3M MonitorMark™

Concept

Physical TTI device capable of indicating food products temperature over time, expressing this cumulative distribution by diffusion (3M, 2018). Consisting on accelerated diffusion of colored fatty acids at high temperatures (Jafry *et al.*, 2017), this is an irreversible thermal exposure record.

This type of equipment is used for a wide range of temperatures and is typically applied near the food products sensitive to temperature variations (usually applied in the packaging).

As a disadvantage this device does not provide specific information about the product quality, but only the food thermal exposure is reported (parameter that is related to the quality). The equipment dimensions are approximately 95x19x2 mm^3 (Figure 2).

Figure 2. TTI 3M MonitorMark (3M, 2018)

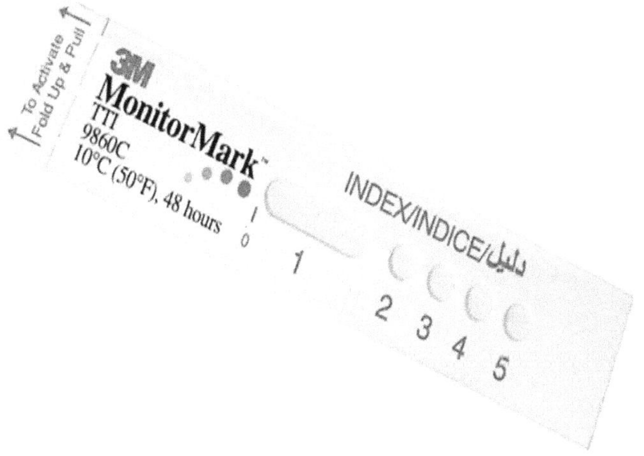

Features

The main features are:

- Rectangular shape, with a pellicle or adhesive slick/laminate;
- The dispersion of the blue compound allows to quantify temporally the threshold temperature at which the product was subject;
- The pressure sensitive adhesive allows their aggregation (the dispersion of blue compound) in any clean and dry surfaces.

Advantages

The main advantages offered are:

- Low cost;
- Works as accessory (label) on the outside of product packaging;
- The results are visual, easy and intuitive to interpret, indicating immediately the occurrence of thermal mishandling.

Equipment Models

The 3M MonitorMar device presents several specific models (see Table 6) designed to function on different temperature ranges and several time intervals that the cumulative records.

Table 6. Available models by the brand of the equipment (3M, 2018)

Model	Activation temperature range $A_{ctivation}$ (°C)- *Registration time*	Typical temperature °C to not *accumulate*	Conditional temperature °C *(minimum 2 hours)*
9860[a]	*-15°C – 48 hours*	*-20°C*	*≤ -25°C*
9860B	*5°C -48 hours*	*0°C*	*≤ -4°C*
9860C	*10°C – 48 hours*	*7°C*	*≤ 5°C*
9860D	*10°C - 1 weeks*	*7°C*	*≤ 5°C*
9860E	*26°C – 48 hours*	*24°C*	*≤ 21°C*
9860H	*31°C - 1 weeks*	*29°C*	*≤ 26°C*
9861[a]	*10°C - 2 weeks (End point 34°C)*	*7°C*	*≤ 5°C*
9864C	*10°C – 24 hours (End point 17°C)*	*7°C*	*≤ 5°C*

As can be seen by analysing the data presented in Table 6, the most suitable models to record temperature mishandling of perishable foods are the 9860B, 9860C (see Figure 3) and 9860D models, due to its activation and typical temperature characteristics described in Table 6.

These devices provide a general reference on exposure to a constant temperature and must be used with a combination of general knowledge about the terms of product display, in order to estimate the time-temperature exposure. The indicator verifies the exposure of temperature and not product quality. Its purpose is to visually indicate when the product quality should be checked (3M, 2018).

Figure 3. The Model 9860C of 3M MonitorMark (3M, 2018)

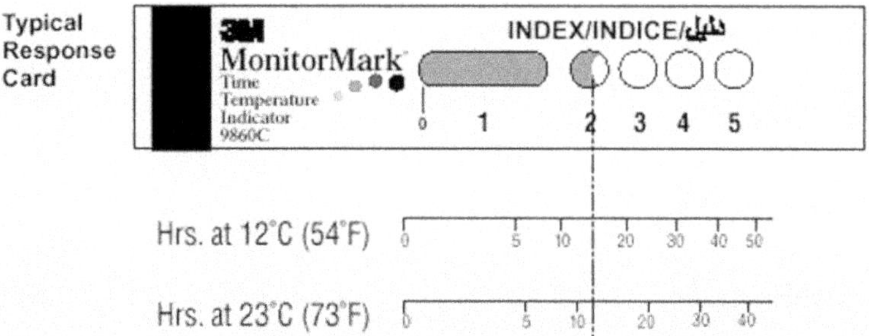

TTI Timestrips

Concept

The Timestrips is a unitary chemical indicator manually activated by the consumer in order to verify the elapsed time since the food package opening or since its first use (Timestrip, 2018).

In terms of dimensions, the standard size of this equipment is 19x40 mm^2.

This is designed to allow consumers to track down the time elapsed since label activation. This feature is particularly suitable for packaging, labelling of perishable foods or products that require maintenance and regular place relocation (chilled and frozen products).

The thermal monitoring tagged Timestrips is always available to be activated in the right time, because they are completely inert at the temperature at this stage and may be stored to the environment temperature, unlike other temperature recorders that need to be stored in controlled environments to ensure its functionalities.

Advantages

The main advantages offered by this indicator are:

- High accuracy and advantage cost/benefit;
- Easy handling and reading, being directly applied to the product or packaging.

This brand has two different types of devices with the same functionalities, but with different purposes. One type is used to monitor thermal mishandling in the ascending threshold recommended, and the other in descending threshold (Timestrip, 2018).

Timestrips Plus

This equipment works as indicator of the thermal exposures occurring in the ascending thresholds to the recommended or to its temperature range (Timestrip, 2018).

The specific features of this model are:

- "Button" which confirms the indicator activation to know when the device is in the cumulative record mode;
- Extensive validity;
- Water resistant.

Timestrips Plus type has several models that cover several temperature ranges (-20 °C to 38 °C). See sone examples on Table 7. Once again, this diversity exists so that it is possible to cover a wider range of foods in which it can be included because the foods do not have the same range of conservation values recommended (Timestrip, 2018).

As showed in the Table 7, the choice of device to be applied depends on the range of recommended food temperature and the time intended to be measured.

These models have a unique serial number on the label to improve its traceability.

Table 7. Description of the Timestrips Plus models (Timestrip, 2018)

Model:	Timestrip Plus 058	Timestrip Plus 077	Timestrip Plus 076
Application	Frozen foods	Frozen foods	Chilled foods
Temperature range	*-14°C*	*0°C*	*5°C*
Time scale	24 hours	12 hours	8 hours
Figure	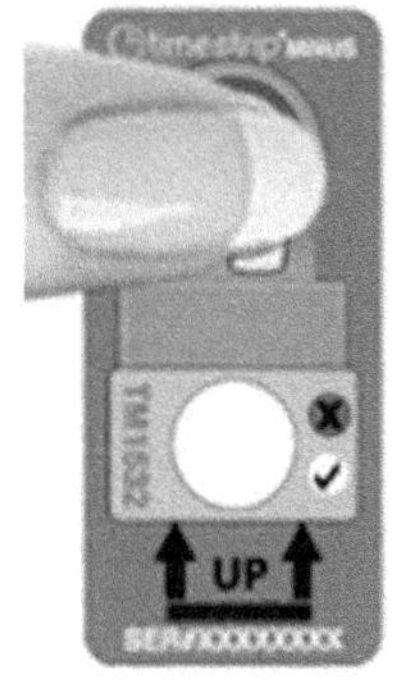	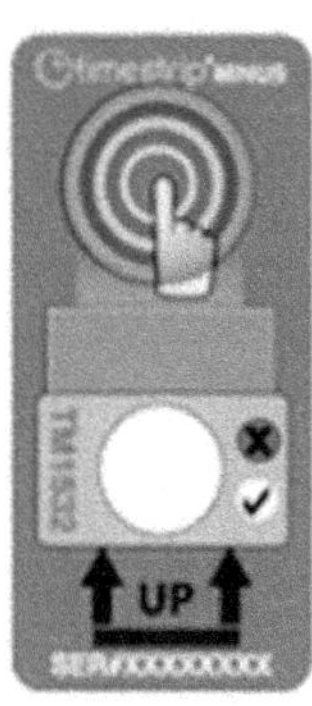	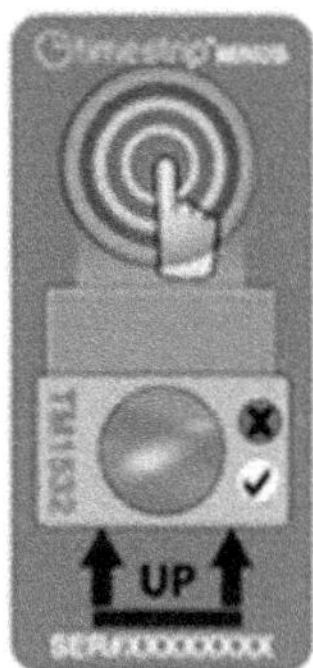

The models also include an activation button, which once pressed, measures the temperature violations. If the temperature falls below the threshold, a white circle changes to red colour irreversibly. This can be seen in the sequential process of images in Figure 4. The colour change is recognizable/appealing (from white to red) in order to be more effective to catch user attention (Timestrip, 2018).

Figure 4. Activation process of the temperature measurer equipment (Timestrip, 2018)

These devices type, when following the food products, have the task to show if the perishable food was exposed to temperatures in its limit descending threshold. Low temperature values also impair the quality and freshness of perishable foods, if the freezing point is reached. Table 8 shows some of these models.
These models have each one its serial number (unique) on each label in order to improve its traceability.

Table 8. Description of the Timestrips Minus models (Timestrip, 2018)

Model:	Timestrip Minus 0°C	Timestrip Minus 2°C
Application	*0°C*	*2°C*
Temperature range	Manual	Manual
Time scale	*Sole*	*Sole*
Figure		

Timestrips Complete

Timestrip Complete provides an active monitoring of the boundaries above and below of environment temperature. The combination of Timestrip Plus (ascending temperature threshold) with the Timestrip Minus (descending temperature threshold), provides a viable alternative for monitoring food safety in the range of 2°C-8°C. Thus, this device prevents the two risk sources interfering in the food quality, i.e., high temperatures and low temperatures (Timestrip, 2018).

The normally used package contains:

- **Timestrip Minus:** Limit to 2 °C
- **Timestrip Plus**: Limit to 8 °C (other temperatures available).

TTI Fresh-Check®

The food exhibition at temperatures above the recommended is reflected in its freshness. Then these abuses have effects on taste, smell, texture, quality and bacteria proliferation in the food product. The Fresh-Check® indicators are used to prevent these effects by providing an indication of when the food products are subject to some mishandlings (Pavelkova, 2013).

Concept

Its principle relies on a polymerization reaction in the solid state, resulting in a coloured polymer regarded as a temperature-sensitive ink that is invisible in its initial state, but in case of temperature excess, it darkens. The indicator consists on a polymer in a small circle surrounded by a printed ring of reference.

Features

The main features are:

- The chromic indicators is sensitive to temperatures since the -25 ºC;
- Accuracy of +/- 1 ºC;
- They exist on several sizes;
- The storage must be done at low temperatures;
- Its visual sensor is irreversible.

Figure 5. Timestrips complete (Timestrip, 2018)

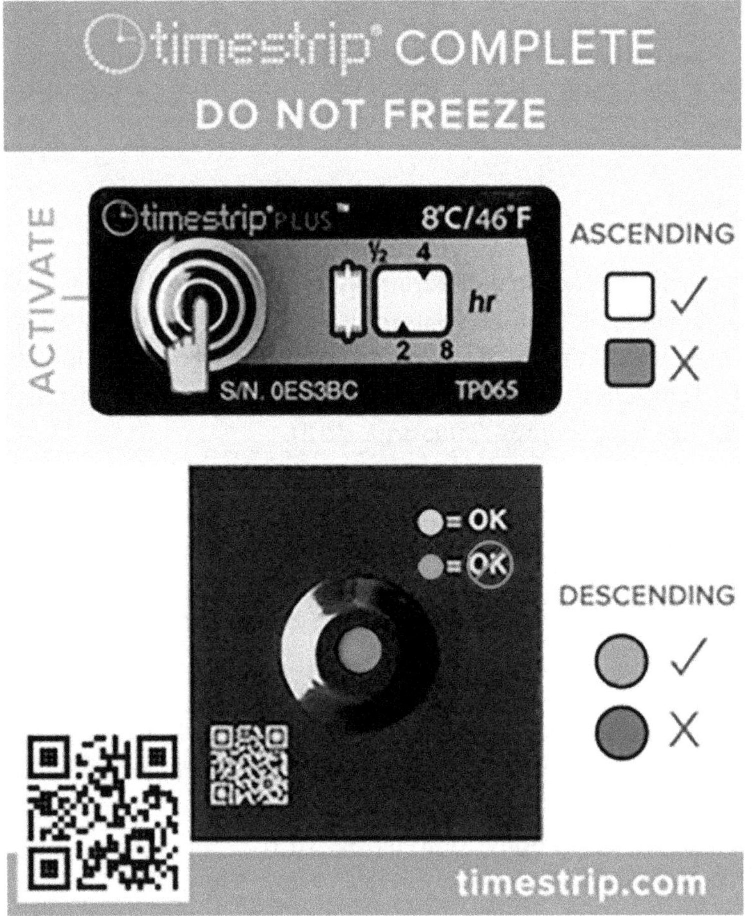

Operating Mode

The polymeric circle darkens if the product packaging was subjected to a thermal exposure outside of its range. The colour intensity is measured and compared to the reference colour on the label - on the reference ring (see Figure 6). Colour change of the polymer follows the temperature gradient, i.e., as higher the temperature variation, faster is the colour transition (Taoukis *et al.*, 2010).

Figure 6. Label Fresh-Check (Taoukis et al., 2010)

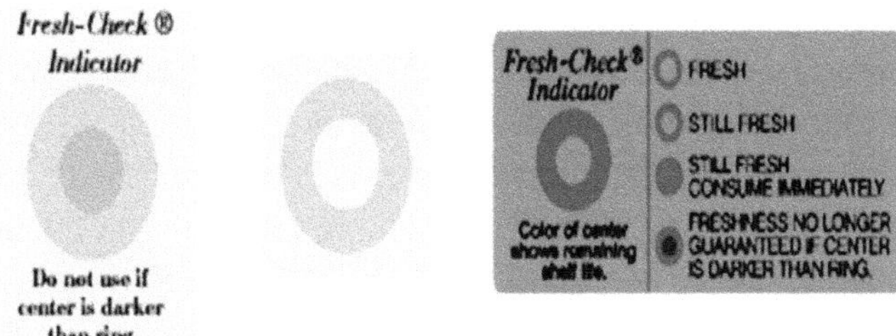

The indicator response is measured by decrease in reflectance quantification. This is due to the ratio between the electromagnetic flow radiation incident on a surface and the reflected flow. This indicator is used in different designs by different supermarkets. The principle is the same, the colour and display features are different depending on the supermarkets.

TTI CheckPoint (Vitsab L5-8 Smart TTI Seafood Label)

Concept

This enzymatic indicator allows a complete record of Time-Temperature (see Figure 7), i.e., responds continuously (accumulates) regardless of the temperature, unlike the partial history indicators, which accumulate when the temperature reaches the limit. Their cumulative is continuous *(Kaur & Puri, 2017)*.

Figure 7. Representative graphs of the temperature as a function of time, of the two types of historical that indicators can provide (Kaur & Puri, 2017)

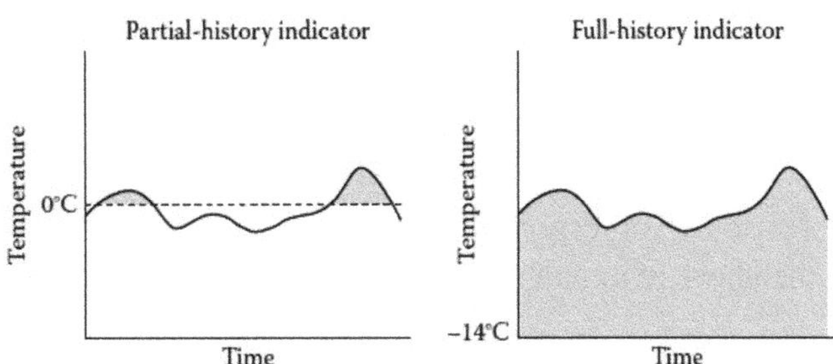

As indicated in Figure 7 b), the response of a full-history indicator does not alert, only when it reaches the temperature limit.

Operating Mode

This simple adhesive sticker has a basic enzymatic system principle: colour change caused by the pH decrease. After activation, the capsule is broken, substrate and enzyme are mixed, leading to an enzymatic hydrolysis of a lipid substrate by a lipase enzyme.

The substrate hydrolysis causes the acid release and the pH decreases, leading to a colorimetric change from dark green to bright yellow and then to red.

The combination of several types of enzymatic substrates at different concentrations can be used to provide a variety of responses depending on the temperature.

This indicator provides essentially the forecast percentage of load based on all temperatures that the equipment was subject over time, i.e., provides the remaining validity of the equipment or products where is inserted. As shown in the sequence of images displayed in Figure 8, initially, before being activated, the label has a background of neutral colour that is changing to green in its first phase of monitoring. Over time, the label changes shades of orange/red, indicating that the product is no longer in conditions to be consumed (see Figure 9) (Taoukis *et al.*, 2010).

Figure 8. Cumulative percentage relation/ring colour during the first phase after label activation, while still is viable (Taoukis et al., 2010)

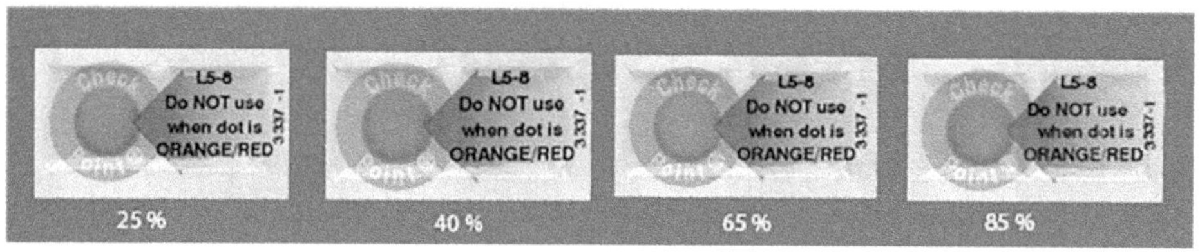

Figure 9. Cumulative percentage relation/ring colour during the last phase of monitoring (the label is no longer viable) (Taoukis et al., 2010)

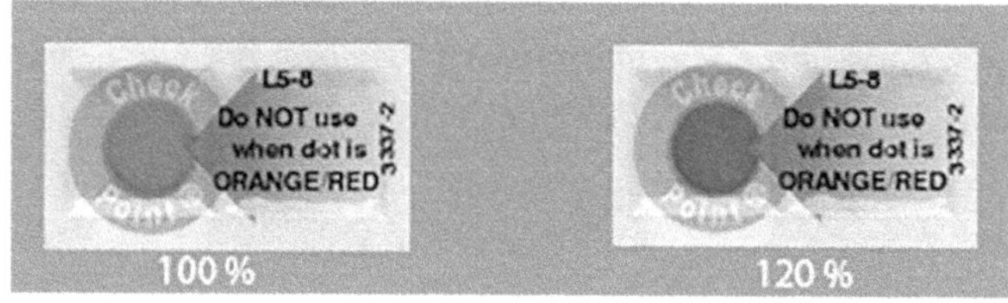

This device provides a progressive response of the product life instead of the final breaking point, after this be subjected to the above recommended temperatures.

TTI OnVu

Concept

This indicator is based in photosensitive chemical compounds and organic pigments. Example: Benzylpyridines - changes its colour depending on the subjected temperature over time. The indicator substance is activated by UV radiation, which can be visualized by a dark blue coloration. After application on the package, this indicator has a UV filter to protect the substance to be reactivated to dark blue (Figure 10). Over time and temperature exposures the colour fades away, indicative of wrong temperature conservation or food product lifespan expiration (Figure 11). The indicator can be calibrated according to the temperature range and product lifespan (Pavelkova, 2013).

Figure 10. Standard OnVu indicator (Taoukis et al., 2010)

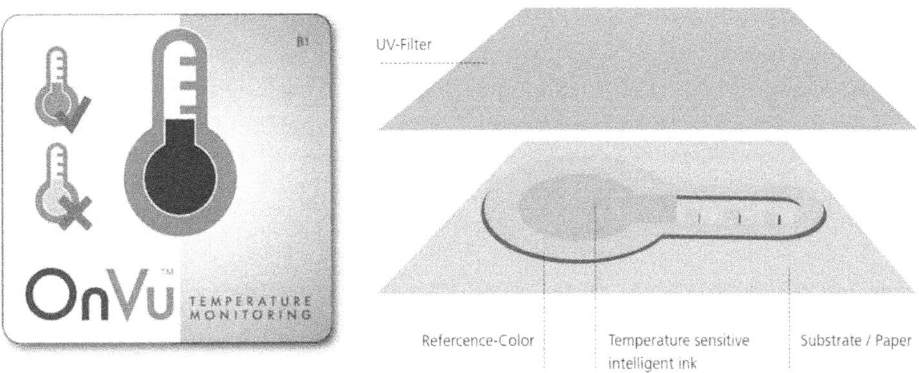

Figure 11. Registration and tendency of discoloration in the relation exposure time elapsed/temperature (Taoukis et al., 2010)

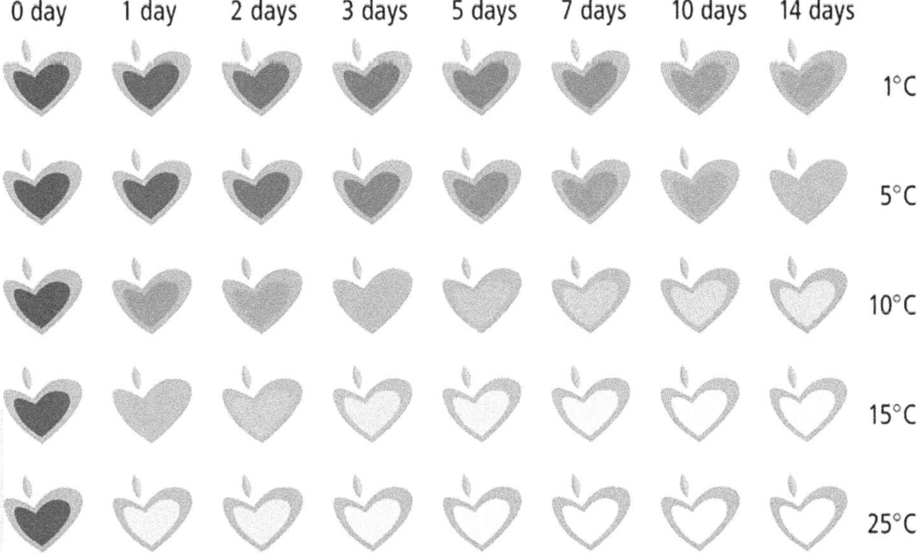

Response Analysis

The indicator is dependent of UV radiation to be activated, after that the indicator needs to be protected by a UV filter to prevent reactivation. Reference colour fades away due to two parameters, temperature and time, consequence of three different situations (Figure 11):

- Exposure to high temperature for a short time period;
- Exceeding the product life span by exposing to the recommended temperature during a long time period;
- Exposure to different temperatures and time (usual conservation experience).

In conclusion, this device has a unique property to relate time and temperature, giving a more detailed information of the food product conservation state.

Additionally, other models of the OnVu device are offered based on the same principle, but with different applications (see Figure 12) (Freshpoint, 2018). Since the reference colour can be calibrated to different temperature ranges, the different models can have applications to refrigerated products as well as frozen products. This TTI demonstrates to be very versatile and takes in consideration time and temperature, leaving consumers more informed on the food product conservation state.

Figure 12. Detailed description of the OnVu models (Freshpoint, 2018)

Model (logo)	Description	Application	Advantages/benefits	Design
ONVU Logistic active ink technology	The marker is dark blue colour after activation, colour fades away when product is subjected to temperature excess, the reference scale (by letters) helps determine if the refrigeration temperatures were respected during food logistics and distribution.	· Refrigerated food products.	· Easy to apply; · Immediate visual indicator; · Flexible design and size; · Activated by UV radiation; · Low cost.	
ONVU Ice active ink technology	· Indicator that shows if the product suffered a thawing event after production; · The used marker offers the consumer a warranty seal certifying that the product was maintained frozen since its production.	· Suitable for a wide range of frozen products (including ice cream, meat, fish, vegetables, ...);	· Can be calibrated to match with the recommended range of freeze/thaw temperatures; · Flexible design and size; · Low cost.	
ONVU active ink technology	· Product freshness indicator, after UV activation the marker is dark blue, over time and temperature differences colour fades; · Reference scale for comparison is below the marker.	· Available for food with short expiration date that require refrigeration (meats, fresh produce, juices).	· High accuracy; · Size and flexible design; · Can easily be incorporated in the food package; · Can be calibrated according to the food lifespan.	

CoolVu™ and BestBy™ TTi

OnVu new generation TTI, has similar performance changes colour from green or grey to red or white, respectively. These kinds of labels are used to follow conservation in the food chain (CoolVu™) and also as time from opening indicators (BestBy™), helping the costumer decide until when the product is safe to consume after opening (Freshpoint, 2018). The unique aspect of this label is to be very intuitive and simple to use, helping customer on the product freshness (Figure 13). Additionally, a mobile app was developed to help read these labels, enabling customers to have more information on the product.

TTI (eO)

This microbiological TTI is based on pH variations. Colour gradually changes when pH is lowered (from green to red, Figure 14) by a controlled microbial growth contained in the TTI marker gel (Chiellini, 2008; Pavelkova, 2013). Depending on the application, this device can be adjusted by selecting the right microorganism and gel composition (Chiellini, 2008). Before application, labels are stored frozen (-18 °C) to prevent the bacterial growth.

Figure 13. Different customisable models of the Freshpoint labels (Freshpoint, 2018)

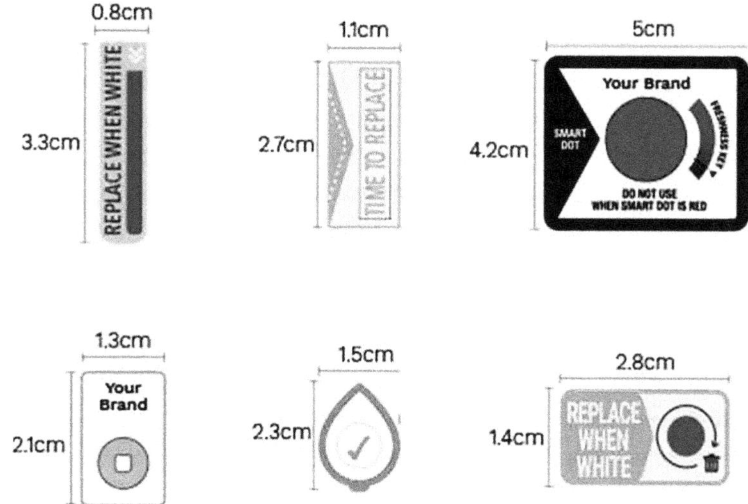

Figure 14. eO indicator (Pavelkova, 2013)

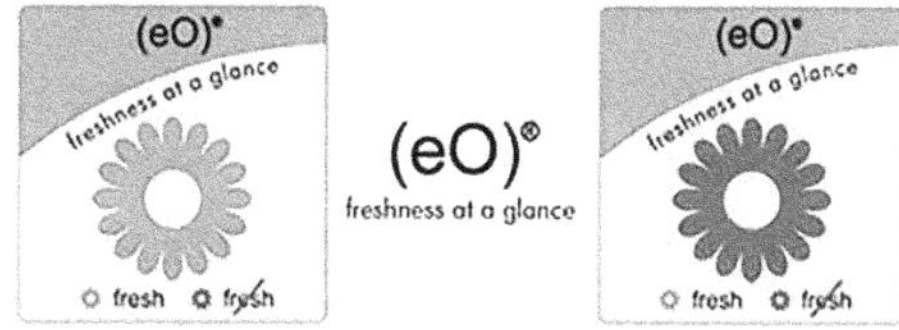

Activation is very simple, since the device is very thin, the label can be thawed at room temperature for a few minutes (Pavelkova, 2013).

Once placed on the food package, by exceeding the temperature or the expiry date, the microbial growth occurs and causes a decrease in pH and an irreversible colour change (Taoukis *et al.*, 2010).

FUTURE TRENDS/PROPOSED MODEL

There is no doubt that time temperature integrators are able to inform consumers and improves the whole food chain quality from production, distribution, sale and consumers, just by a simple, intuitive, clear and easy indication on the food product.

Consequently, consumers will purchase items with better quality, by a real-time result of good conservation conditions, instead of only focusing on the expiry date, which does not guarantee good conservation practices of the product.

Despite the extensive work that has been performed to advance this field and the valuable contribution that TTIs can bring in terms of eliminating consumer confusion and reducing food waste, there are still several limitations that hinder their extensive use in food products. Additionally, although the clear TTI application advantages, there are still improvements and limitations to overcome on future devices. Here we some issues that can be improved:

Price Dynamics

The consumer becomes increasingly aware of product life changes by indicators present in package, consequently this is a high priority to invest in a pricing strategy. Product prices become a dynamic parameter which decreases as the quality characteristics decreases. Therefore, food waste (before expiry date) will be reduced and producers' profits will increase. By creating a price dynamic and having a quality assurance indicator will increase changes of consumers buying the product. Consumer decisions are based on quality but also on pricing. Thus, consumers will fell more confident and will rely on the conservation quality of food products under the expiry date (regardless if the product is the freshest).

To follow this dynamic strategy, a strategy has to be defined by pricing policies, i.e., one justification for the prices assignment and discounts, based on a detailed identification of the real time food product qualities.

This change would not only improve the management of food safety, but also become an innovation in areas as marketing strategies, quality food management, consumers purchasing habits and refrigerated chain operations.

Reference Colours

As described before, consumer purchase intention is a variable parameter, very unpredictable and dynamic, this depends on the confidence that perishable food product package gives him. With the introduction of these monitoring technologies, reflecting the temperature history, consumer will have access to a detailed food conditions analysis, helping making the decision of a purchase.

However, in a general way and having as base the technological equipment studied, most of those that are applied in the product package follows a trend in their reference colours that describes the product characteristics or its condition. For example, the green colour reflects the good food conservation state and provides an idea of trust and safety to the consumer. By the other way, orange (middle term) and red (food safety limit) are appellative colours, which inform the consumer not to choose these foods items. When a food item contains a TTI with red indication, the commercial establishment has the responsibility of removing these products from the shelves. The problem arises when the TTI shows medium colours such as the smooth and dark orange. It must be highlighted that the consumer purchasing decisions, beyond being based in the price, are also based in the food quality. When the consumer faces a refrigerated display cabinet full of product packages with indicators reflecting a dark green colour or medium orange, he will manage his choice based on the product with better conservation state.

The food quality is in its maximum potential when arrives to the commercial establishment coming from the distributor, which does not mean that any foods indicator with a colour besides the green one is in bad conservation condition. However, knowing the consumer about the presence of indicators in food packages, his tendency will always search the entire display cabinet for a package with a green indicator. The consequences of these actions are the larger resident time of food items with less safety on display cabinet and the consequent accumulation of products which indicator will turn red. Thus, the food waste will not be successfully controlled. Thus, a new strategy for the aesthetics of the label is needed, specifically on the indicator reference. As example, the TTI OnVu has a reference scale not in colours but in letters (OnVu Logistic) or with several classification levels (OnVu active ink technology).

"Moment of Consumption" Scale

An alternative proposal only results if the consumer requires the food chain to comply strictly with the - uncontrolled parameter.

The products whose indicators are between the term of excellent conservation (green) and unacceptable food quality (red) are products that are still advisable to consumption. However, these suffer some unfair discrimination by the consumer. Depending on how purchase management is done, which varies from person to person, but always with the same principles ("last minute shopping" and "shopping to store in the storeroom"). Often, the consumer goes to a store knowing the food products what he needs to buy. Usually, he also knows when he will consume the products (in that day or in the next one or if he will store during some time). So, the reference scale of a label can be based in this idea.

Thus, a change in the reference scales used to identify the product state from a colours scale ("food preservation scale") to a "consumption time scale" would help choosing the products that are in the middle term. Probably, this condition will help to eliminate the existing discrimination with the orange indicator. Exchanging the orange indicator by a reference "Fast Consumption" and a green one by "Consumption in the forthcoming days" combined with price dynamics, above mentioned, could somehow eliminate the permanence of middle term products in the display cabinets until their food quality become unacceptable.

Combination of Features and Evaluation Parameters

Due to the extensive research, several TTI equipments were developed and are now available commercially with different functionalities and product organoleptic parameters evaluation.

Relatively to TTI functionalities, there are devices capable of indicating the consumer the product conservation status before its purchase, and others capable of evaluating the product state after package opening in a domestic environmental (or its remaining life time).

Thus, achieving the combination of these capabilities in a single equipment will increase slightly the average label size and its occupied space on the product package. However, on the other hand, this will become a lot more useful and versatile, since it includes two functions, one that evaluates the conservation state along the cold chain or in refrigerated location (either supermarket or domestic fridge) while the package is sealed, and other that starts operating when the package is opened.

Relative to evaluation parameters, several equipments have the capacity to evaluate, through microbiological, physical or chemical, organoleptic characteristics of foods. Nevertheless, other parameters can also be evaluated, such as, oxygen or humidity percentage present in the package. The development of an equipment with the ability to perform these three evaluations on the product, allows a better understanding of its conservation status.

Another perspective could pass through the inclusion of an antenna on the TTI device, making this device in a passive Radio Frequency Identification (RFID) tag. Based in an electrochemical process, the tag can provide the indication of conservation status when passing by an RFID antenna/reader. If these elements are located along all the cold chain, i.e., in the inputs/outputs of warehouses/stores, of transport/distribution vehicles, of commercial establishments (cash registers), it would be possible to obtain the real time data of each product (namely the temperature history along the cold chain), allowing to analyse the weaker links and act to promote the food security. Some studies demonstrate the efficiency of this kind of combined technology (Bibi *et al.*, 2017; Lorite *et al.*, 2017). This kind of device permits intelligent packaging which give more information on the product itself and its quality throughout the food chain. This device enables the package to be tracked down by GPS or mobile network, providing real time information. Depending on the type of RFID tag, the cost can vary between 40 to 50-euro cent per tag. This price can seem to be high, nevertheless when compared with temperature loggers, it is cheaper. With commercially available devices, this will lead the price to become lower and lower.

Potential Toxicity

Among some TTIs, there is a potential of migration of noxious reactants and the presence potential and actual toxic components. Some chemical TTIs use anthraquinone derivatives, which are structurally related to anthracene, which are potential carcinogenic and toxic (Wang *et al.*, 2015; Zhang *et al.*, 2016). Additionally, the usage of silver and gold nanoparticles, can lead to toxic effects to pulmonary cells (Ávalos *et al.*, 2015).

New TTIs need to take this into consideration, and replace toxic compounds with natural or generally recognized as safe (GRAS) indicators, subsequently diminishing user risk.

For example, Wei et al., reported the usage of the natural polyphenol anthocyanin (Wei *et al.*, 2017) as an indicator for food freshness. Another study demonstrated the usage of the combination of laccase, guaiacol, and cysteine as O_2 concentration indicators (Won *et al.*, 2016).

CONCLUSION

This chapter describes the literature of several technologies used for food safety monitoring of perishable products, which due to their susceptibility in losing nutritional qualities or organoleptic characteristics, deserve a special care by the producers/distributors and world organizations devoted to eradicate the world food waste.

The time-temperature indicators are used to optimize the product distribution and increase its lifespan, allowing a considerable waste reduction. The low cost, the trust that the consumer puts on the indicator and the record efficiency are the appointed criteria for the success of this type of equipment.

Currently, these systems provide a reproducible and assertive/precise answer according to their specifications. The TTI devices provide a visual summary of the product accumulated temperature.

This is a modern safety system of evaluation the food quality, preventing contamination through the monitoring, registration and control of the critical parameters during the entire food life cycle. There are devices commercially available to perform this evaluation, but for sure, the research and technological evolution will provide in the future new devices with extended functionalities that will develop this area, promoting its generalized use in the food chain.

REFERENCES

3M. (2006). *MonitorMark™ Time Temperature Indicators*. Ref: 78-6901-2024-7.

ANCIPA, FORVISÃO, IDEC, FUNDACION LAVORA, & SINTESISF. (2004-2005). *HYGIREST - Programa de Formação sobre Higiene e Segurança Alimentar para Restaurantes e Estabelecimentos Similares*. Leonardo da Vinci transational project, PA: ANCIPA.

Annese, V. F., Cipriani, S., Biccario, G., Di Marzio, D., & de Venuto, D. (2015). Wireless shelf life monitoring and real time prediction in a supply-chain of perishable goods. In *Proc. AASRI Int. Conf. Circuits Syst.* (pp. 322–26). Paris: Atlantis Press. 10.2991/cas-15.2015.77

APIC – Associação Portuguesa dos Industriais de Carnes. (2006). *Legislação alimentar - carnes e produtos cárneos*. Lisbon: APIC.

Ávalos, A., Haza, A. I., Mateo, D., & Morales, P. (2015). Effects of Silver and Gold Nanoparticles of Different Sizes in Human Pulmonary Fibroblasts. *Toxicology Mechanisms and Methods*, *25*(4), 287–295. doi:10.3109/15376516.2015.1025347 PMID:25798650

Baptista, P., Campos, I., Pires, I., & Vaz, S. (2012). *Do Campo ao Garfo. Desperdício Alimentar em Portugal*. Lisbon: CESTRAS - Centro de Estudos e Estratégias para a Sustentabilidade.

Bell, L. N., Fu, B., & Labuza, T. P. (1992). *Criteria for Experimental Kinetic Design and Prediction of Food Shelf-Life*. Boca Raton, FL: CRC Press.

Bibi, F., Guillaume, C., Gontard, N., & Sorli, B. (2017). A review: RFID technology having sensing aptitudes for food industry and their contribution to tracking and monitoring of food products. *Trends in Food Science & Technology*, *62*, 91-103. doi:10.1016/j.tifs.2017.01.013

Brizio, A., & Prentice, C. (2014). Use of smart photochromic indicator for dynamic monitoring of the shelf life of chilled chicken based products. *Meat Science*, *96*(3), 1219–1226. doi:10.1016/j.meatsci.2013.11.006 PMID:24334043

Brizio, A., & Prentice, C. (2015). Development of an intelligent enzyme indicator for dynamic monitoring of the shelf-life of food products. *Innovative Food Science & Emerging Technologies*, *30*, 208–217. doi:10.1016/j.ifset.2015.04.001

Brooks, J. (1996). The sad and tragic life of Typhoid Mary. *CMAJ: Canadian Medical Association Journal*, *154*(6), 915–916. PMID:8634973

Chiellini, E. (2008). *Environmentally compatible food packaging*. Woodhead Publishing Limited.

Choi, D. Y., Jung, S. W., Lee, D. S., & Lee, S. J. (2014). Fabrication and characteristics of microbial time temperature indicators from bio-paste using screen printing method. *Packaging Technology & Science*, *27*(4), 303–312. doi:10.1002/pts.2039

Corradini, M. G., & Peleg, M. (2006). Shelf-life estimation from accelerated storage data. *Trends in Food Science & Technology*, *18*(1), 37–47. doi:10.1016/j.tifs.2006.07.011

Ellouze, M., & Augustin, J.-C. (2010). Applicability of biological time temperature integrators as quality and safety indicators for meat products. *International Journal of Food Microbiology*, *138*(1-2), 119–129. doi:10.1016/j.ijfoodmicro.2009.12.012 PMID:20074826

European Commission (EU). (2011). A resource-efficient Europe - Flagship initiative under the Europe 2020 Strategy. Communication from the commission to the European parliament, the council, the European Economic and Social Committee and the Committee of the Regions. Brussels: European Union.

FAO - Food and Agriculture Organization of the United Nations. (2013, October 21). Monitoring food loss and waste essential to hunger fight. *FAO News*.

Farquhar, J. (1977). Time-temperature indicators in monitoring the distribution of frozen foods. *Journal of Food Quality, 1*(2), 119–123. doi:10.1111/j.1745-4557.1977.tb00934.x

Ferguson, M. E., & Ketzenberg, M. E. (2006). Information sharing to improve retail product freshness of perishables. *Production and Operations Management, 15*, 57–73.

Food and Agriculture Organization (FAO) of the United Nations. (2011). *Global Food Losses and Food Waste*. FAO.

Freshpoint™. OnVu™ Technology. (n.d.). Retrieved May 26, 2014, from http://www.freshpoint-tti.com/technology/default.aspx

Fu, B., Taoukis, P. S., & Labuza, T. P. (1991). Predictive microbiology for monitoring spoilage of dairy-products with time-temperature integrators. *Journal of Food Science, 56*(5), 1209–1215. doi:10.1111/j.1365-2621.1991.tb04736.x

Giannakourou, M. C., & Taoukis, P. S. (2002). Systematic application of time temperature integrators as tools for control of frozen vegetable quality. *Journal of Food Science, 67*(6), 2221–2228. doi:10.1111/j.1365-2621.2002.tb09531.x

Giannoglou, M., Touli, A., Platakou, E., Tsironi, T., & Taoukis, P. S. (2014). Predictive modeling and selection of TTI smart labels for monitoring the quality and shelf-life of frozen seafood. *Innovative Food Science & Emerging Technologies, 26*, 294–301. doi:10.1016/j.ifset.2014.10.008

Gogou, E., Derens, E., Alvarez, G., & Taoukis, P. (2014). *Field Test Monitoring of the Food Cold Chain in European Markets. 3rd IIR International Conference on Sustainability and the Cold Chain*, London, UK.

Hightech Europe. (n.d.). *Time temperature integrator/indicator (TTI): photochromic/photochemical TTI*. Hightech Europe.

Jafry, A. T., Lim, H., Sung, W. K., & Lee, J. (2017). Flexible time-temperature indicator: A versatile platform for laminated paper-based analytical devices. *Microfluidics and Nanofluidics, 21*(3), 57. doi:10.100710404-017-1883-x

Jedermann, R., Nicometo, M., Uysal, I., & Lang, W. (2014). Reducing food losses by intelligent food logistics. *Philos. Trans. A, 372*(2017), 20130302. doi:10.1098/rsta.2013.0302 PMID:24797131

Kaur, S., & Puri, D. (2017). Active and intelligent packaging: A boon to food packaging. *International Journal of Food Sciences and Nutrition, 2*(4), 15–18.

Kim, E., Choi, D. Y., Kim, H. C., Kim, K., & Lee, S. J. (2013). Calibrations between the variables of microbial TTI response and ground pork qualities. *Meat Science, 95*(2), 362–367. doi:10.1016/j.meatsci.2013.04.050 PMID:23747630

Kim, K., Kim, E., & Lee, J. S. (2012). New enzymatic time-temperature integrator (TTI) that uses lactase. *Journal of Food Engineering, 113*(1), 118–123. doi:10.1016/j.jfoodeng.2012.05.009

Labuza, T. (2001). Shelf life testing of foods. *Am. Chem. Soc., 222*, U26.

Laidler, K. J. (1987). *Chemical Kinetics* (3rd ed.). New York, PA: Harper & Row.

Li, D., & Wang, X. (2012). A dynamic product quality evaluation based pricing model for perishable food supply chains. *Omega, 40*(6), 906–917. doi:10.1016/j.omega.2012.02.001

Lorite, G. S., Selkälä, T., Sipola, T., Palenzuela, J., Jubete, E., Viñuales, A., … Toth, G. (2017). Novel, smart and RFID assisted critical temperature indicator for supply chain monitoring. *Journal of Food Engineering, 193*, 20-28. doi:10.1016/j.jfoodeng.2016.06.016

Maesmans, G. J., Hendrickx, M. E., De Cordt, S. V., & Tobback, P. (1994). Feasibility of the use of a time temperature integrator and a mathematical model to determine fluid to particle heat transfer coefficients. *Food Research International, 27*(1), 39–51. doi:10.1016/0963-9969(94)90176-7

Mai, N. T. T., Gudjonsdottir, M., Lauzon, H. L., Sveinsdottir, K., Martinsdottir, E., Audorff, H., … Arason, S. (2011). Continuous quality and shelf life monitoring of retail-packed fresh cod loins in comparison with conventional methods. *Food Control, 22*(6), 1000–1007. doi:10.1016/j.foodcont.2010.12.010

Mehauden, K. (2009). *Evaluation of the Thermal and Mixing Performance of an Agited Vessel for Processing of Complex Liquid Foodstufs*. University of Birmingham.

Mchauden, K., Cox, P. W., Bakalis, S., Simmons, M. J. H., Tucker, G. S., & Fryer, P. J. (2007). A novel method to evaluate the applicability of time temperature integrators to different temperature profiles. *Innovative Food Science & Emerging Technologies, 8*(4), 507–514. doi:10.1016/j.ifset.2007.03.001

Mendoza, T. F., Welt, B. A., Otwell, S., Teixeira, A. A., Kristonsson, H., & Balaban, M. O. (2006). Kinetic parameter estimation of time-temperature integrators intended for use with packaged fresh seafood. *Journal of Food Science, 69*(3).

O'Connor. (2014, October). *Quantification of Food Waste in the EU*. Food Chain Analysis Network Meeting, Paris, France.

Pavelkova, A. (2013). Time temperature indicators as devices intelligent packaging. *ACTA Univ. Agric. Silvic. Mendelianae Brun, 61*(1), 245–251. doi:10.11118/actaun201361010245

Sherlock, M., Fu, B., Taoukis, P. S., & Labuza, T. P. (1991). A systematic evaluation of time-temperature indicators for use as consumer tags. *Journal of Food Protection, 54*(11), 885–889. doi:10.4315/0362-028X-54.11.885

Shimoni, E., Anderson, E. M., & Labuza, T. P. (2001). Reliability of time temperature indicators under temperature abuse. *Journal of Food Science, 66*(9), 1337–1340. doi:10.1111/j.1365-2621.2001.tb15211.x

Sun, D.-W. (2012). *Thermal Food Processing: New technologies and Quality Issues* (2nd ed.). CRC Press. doi:10.1201/b12112

Surak, J. G. (2003). HACCP and ISO development of a food safety management standard. Department of Food Science and Human Nutrition, Clemson University.

Taoukis, P., Labuza, T., & Saguy, I. (1997). Kinetic of food deterioration and shelf-life prediction. In K. Valentas, E. Rotstein, & R. Singh (Eds.), *Handbook of Food Engineering Practice* (pp. 361–403). Boca Raton, FL: CRC Press.

Taoukis, P., Tsironi, T., Giannoglou, M., Metaxa, I., & Gogou, E. (2010). *Historical review and state of the art in Time Temperature Integrator (TTI) technology for the management of the cold chain of refrigerated and frozen food.* Paper presented at the 4th International Workshop - Cold chain management, Bonn, Germany.

Taoukis, P. S. (2010). Commercialization of time-temperature integrators for foods. In C. J. Doona, K. Kustin, & F. E. Feeherry (Eds.), *Case Studies in Novel Food Processing Technologies: Innovations in Processing, Packaging, and Predictive Modelling* (pp. 351–366). Cambridge, UK: Woodhead Publ. doi:10.1533/9780857090713.3.351

Taoukis, P. S., & Labuza, T. P. (1989). Applicability of time-temperature indicators as shelf-life monitors of foodproducts. *Journal of Food Science, 54*(4), 783–788. doi:10.1111/j.1365-2621.1989.tb07882.x

Timestrip. (2008). *Timestrip® Product&Company Overview.* ISO 9001:2008.

Timestrip. (n.d.). *Timestrip® Cold Chain Products for Food.* Retrieved from http://www.timestrip.com/coldchain_food.php

Tsironi, T., Ronnow, P., Giannoglou, M., & Taoukis, P. (2017). Developing suitable smart TTI labels to match specific monitoring requirements: The case of Vibrio spp. growth during transportation of oysters. *Food Control, 73,* 51–56. doi:10.1016/j.foodcont.2016.06.041

Tucker, G. S., Lambourne, T., Adams, J. B., & Lach, A. (2002). Application of a biochemical time temperature integrator to estimate pasteurisation values in continuous food processes. *Innovative Food Science & Emerging Technologies, 3*(2), 165–174. doi:10.1016/S1466-8564(02)00006-1

van Boekel, M. A. J. S. (2008). Kinetic modeling of food quality: A critical review. *Comprehensive Reviews in Food Science and Food Safety, 7*(1), 144–158. doi:10.1111/j.1541-4337.2007.00036.x

van Boekel, M. A. J. S. (2009). *Kinetic Modeling of Reactions in Foods.* Boca Raton, FL: CRC Press.

Venâncio, A., & Batista, P. (2003). *Os perigos para a segurança alimentar no processamento de alimentos* (1st ed.). Guimarães, PA: FORVISÃO – Consultoria em Formação Integrada.

Wang, S. D., Liu, X. H., Yang, M., Zhang, Y., Xiang, K. Y., & Tang, R. (2015). Review of time temperature indicators as quality monitors in food packaging. *Packaging Technology & Science, 28*(10), 839–867. doi:10.1002/pts.2148

Wang, Y. C., Lu, L., & Gunasekaran, S. (2017). Biopolymer/gold nanoparticles composite plasmonic thermal history indicator to monitor quality and safety of perishable bioproducts. *Biosensors & Bioelectronics, 92,* 109–116. doi:10.1016/j.bios.2017.01.047 PMID:28199952

Wei, Y. C., Cheng, C. H., Ho, Y. C., Tsai, M. L., & Mi, F. L. (2017). Active gellan gum/purple sweet potato composite films capable of monitoring pH variations. *Food Hydrocolloids, 69,* 491–502. doi:10.1016/j.foodhyd.2017.03.010

Won, K., Jang, N. Y., & Jeon, J. (2016). A natural component-based oxygen indicator with in-pack activation for intelligent food packaging. *Journal of Agricultural and Food Chemistry, 64*(51), 9675–9679. doi:10.1021/acs.jafc.6b04172 PMID:27976882

Zhang, X. S., Sun, G. G., Xiao, X. Q., Liu, Y. R., & Zheng, X. P. (2016). Application of microbial TTIs as smart label for food quality: Response mechanism, application and research trends. *Trends in Food Science & Technology*, *51*, 12–23. doi:10.1016/j.tifs.2016.02.006

Zoller, S., Wachtel, M., Knapp, F., & Steinmetz, R. (2013). Going all the way: detecting and transmitting events with ¨ wireless sensor networks in logistics. *Proc. IEEE Workshop Practical Issues Build. Sens. Netw. Appl.*, 39–47. 10.1109/LCNW.2013.6758496

ENDNOTES

[1]   *Kinetic reaction of 1ˢᵗ order* – Is one that occurs with speed directly proportional to the concentration of the reagent. For a reaction of this type to a constant volume (*mono-molecular, irreversible and of 1ˢᵗ order* – because the reagent concentration is elevated to the exponent 1) obtains the form: Reagent → Product.

[2]   *Dt* - Decimal value of the reduction time that corresponds to the amount of time required to reduce 1/10 the population of a microorganism subjected to a particular thermal treatment

[3]   *Arrhenius equation:* In many cases, the observed speed of a chemical reaction increases as the temperature increases, but the extent of this increase varies a lot of from reaction to reaction. In terms of the rate equation, the cause of variation of the reaction rate with temperature is in the constant k when this varies with the temperature changes.

According to Arrhenius equation, the value of the constant of speed k increases with temperature. This means that an increase in temperature would produce an increase in the reaction speed, which is usually observed (Laidler, 1987).

The Arrhenius equation is useful because it expresses the quantitative relationship between temperature, activation energy and rate constant. Its greatest usefulness lies in determining the energy of a reaction, from the velocity measurements at different temperatures (Laidler, 1987).

Note: ACTIVATION ENERGY: Energy from the collision between molecules to form the activated complex, an unstable set of atoms weakly bound to each other and that can decompose into molecules of reactants or products.

APPENDIX

Nomenclature

a_w: Water activity;
CO_2: Chemical symbol of carbon dioxide;
Dt: Decimal time reduction corresponding to the amount of time needed to reduce 1/10 of microorganisms' population subject to a certain thermal treatment;
Ea: Activation energy;
K: Constant;
N_2: Chemical symbol of nitrogen;
$NaCl_{max}$: Maximum amount of saline concentration admitted;
pH: Physical-chemical quantity of the hydrogen potential that indicates the acidity, neutrality or alkalinity of an aqueous solution;
$T_{Activation}$: Activation temperature;
T_{max}: Maximum temperature;
T_{min}: Minimum temperature;
P: Statistical value of the probability to obtain a statistic test equal or more extreme than the observed in a sample, under the null hypothesis;
Z: Statistical value of the accumulated probability.

Abbreviation List

3GF: Global Green Growth Forum;
AND: Deoxyribonucleic acid;
CE: European Community;
CCP: Critical Control Points;
EU: European Union;
FAO: Food and Agriculture Organization of the United;
HACCP: Hazard Analysis and Critical Control Points;
MAP: Modified Atmosphere Packaging;
Redox: Chemical reaction of oxidation-reduction;
TTI: Time-Temperature Integrator;
UV: Ultra-Violet.

Chapter 5
Closed Refrigerated Display Cabinets:
Is It Worth It for Food Quality?

Onrawee Laguerre
National Research Institute of Science and Technology for Environment and Agriculture (IRSTEA), France

Nattawut Chaomuang
 https://orcid.org/0000-0001-6231-4759
King Mongkut's Institute of Technology Ladkrabang, Thailand

ABSTRACT

The use of closed refrigerated display cabinets in supermarkets is in progression because of the potential energy saving compared to the open ones with an air infiltration at the front. However, the influence of the presence of doors on product temperatures (determining factor of product quality) is much less studied. For better understanding the interest of the use of closed display cabinets, this chapter presents the state of the art of field studies, the airflow and temperature profile in the closed display cabinet, the influence of the presence of doors/the frequency of door openings and the room temperature. Finally, a literature review of studies on food quality in the closed display cabinet is presented.

INTRODUCTION

Numerous studies on retail refrigerated display cabinets have been carried out over the past two decades, awareness of food product quality and energy efficiency is rising continuously. Open display cabinets are a refrigeration equipment typical used for food display in retail stores. In this cabinet type, there is no physical barrier between customers and products, except an air curtain which allows infiltration of warm and humid air from surroundings. This issue still poses problems in many research and development contexts even through plenty of research studies were undertaken by means of both experimental and numerical approaches. The application of closed doors is becoming an alternative solution and

DOI: 10.4018/978-1-7998-5354-1.ch005

several studies have demonstrated that fitting cabinets with doors can provide several benefits. Since there is no clear observation on the loss of sales of products due to the use of doors, many researchers are conducting investigations on the influence of the presence of doors. Nevertheless, most of these studies focused on the energy efficiency perspective. Its impact on internal temperature variations, which directly affect food quality and safety, requires further elucidation. The objective of this book chapter is therefore to highlight the new trend for the use of closed display cabinets in supermarkets and its associated implications on food quality.

BACKGROUND

About 66-77% of heat input in an open refrigerated display cabinet come from the infiltration of warm and humid ambient air in a supermarket (Gaspar, Carrilho Gonçalves, & Pitarma, 2011; Tassou, Ge, Hadawey, & Marriott, 2011) which is one of the main causes of internal temperature heterogeneity. Temperature differences of more than 5°C can be found on cabinet shelves (Willocx, Hendrick, & Tobback, 1994) where the highest temperature is regularly located at the front of the cases (Evans, Scarcelli, & Swain, 2007; Laguerre, Hoang, Osswald, & Flick, 2012). To overcome this major drawback, installation of doors becomes an alternative and attracts more and more attention, and it will account for 75% of all display cabinets in retail stores by the end of 2020 in France (RPF, 2016). Closed refrigerated display cabinets have been increasingly used because of their potential energy savings of between 20-70% (Fricke & Becker, 2010; Lindberg, Axell, & Fahlén, 2010; Rhiemeier, Harnisch, Ters, Kauffeld, & Leisewitz, 2009; Rolfsman & Borgqvist, 2014). Such savings were mainly achieved through a reduction in the entrainment of ambient warm and moist air into the shelves-space storage, thus, less frost is deposited on cooling coils and compressor energy demand becomes less (Faramarzi, Coburn, & Sarhadian, 2002). The difference in the energy consumption from these studies depends on a number of factors, for example, the number of door openings, the door itself, the door seals/gaskets and the level of air infiltration during door openings (Evans, 2014). Among these influencing factors, the frequency, duration of door openings and air gaps between the doors are important which can result in higher energy consumption (Li, Zhu, Wang, & Zeng, 2007). The refrigeration energy consumption of closed display cabinets during stable night condition was approximately 10% lower than that of the display cabinet operated under periodically door openings (Vallée, 2015). Despite these findings, the energy consumption between these two cabinet types may not significantly different when the estimation of the mean total energy consumption is based on a unit display area because of the difference of cabinet design (Evans & Swain, 2010). Further research is required to access additional data.

Temperature performance of closed refrigerated display cabinets was investigated particularly in regard to spatial and temporal temperature variations. A decrease in the overall air temperature of at least 2°C in display cabinets was achieved when retrofitted with doors (Lindberg et al., 2010). Chaomuang, Flick, Denis, and Laguerre (2019) reported that the studied cabinet with doors provided less temperature heterogeneity (ΔT_{max}=2.1°C) compared to the case without doors (ΔT_{max}=4.9°C). About 124 closed display cabinets were tested by Evans and Swain (2010) and the comparative results obtained with open and closed display cabinets revealed that the temperature variation within the closed cabinets was lower than that within the open ones. About 94% of the products with the highest temperature were located at the front of the chilled display cabinet, and nearly half of them (49%) were located on the bottom shelf. Most often, the products with the lowest temperatures were located at the rear of the cabinet and about 70% were on the top shelf. Another study of Atilio de Frias, Luo, Kou, Zhou, and Wang (2015) also affirmed that the temperature heterogeneity in the closed cabinet was less compared to the open one because of the decrease of spatial temperature differences almost by 6°C. As the quality of chilled/frozen food products is directly affected by storage temperature, the improvement in temperature homogeneity in display cabinets would be expected to provide better food quality during storage. The same authors reported that higher visual quality and lower decay rate of minimally processed vegetables could be achieved by the installation of doors on display cabinets. Details of the research studies with a view to improve the performance of the display cabinets, through both experimental and numerical approaches are highlighted by Chaomuang, Flick, and Laguerre (2017).

MAIN FOCUS OF THE CHAPTER

The aim of this book chapter is to highlight the new trend for closed display cabinet use in supermarkets. The chapter is composed of 7 sections:

1. Field studies of product temperature in display cabinets,
2. Experimental air temperatures in a closed display cabinet,
3. Influence of the presence of doors,
4. Influence of the frequency and the duration of door openings,
5. Influence of room temperature on the temperature performance of the cabinet,
6. Modelling of heat transfer and airflow in closed display cabinets
7. Product quality in closed display cabinet

The presented information can enable design improvements to align with user requirements.

Field Studies of Product Temperature in Display Cabinets

This section presents the field studies for both open and closed display cabinets. Derens, Palagos, and Guilpart (2006) conducted a survey of temperature in French cold chain for three chilled products (yoghurt, prepared meals and meat). A further study was later performed for sliced cooked ham (Derens-Bertheau, Osswald, Laguerre, & Alvarez, 2015). Regarding their survey method, temperature recorders were put in the product packages after fabrication in plants. These products were transferred in the cold chain until the consumption point, and the consumers returned temperature recorders to the laboratory for analysis by the experts. The analysis of the measured temperatures of these four chilled products showed that 30% of products during retail displays were 2°C above their recommended storage temperatures (6°C for yoghurt and 4°C for prepared meals, meat and sliced cooked ham) as shown Figure 1. Mean temperatures (standard deviation) of 4.2°C (±2.4°C), 3.1°C (±2.6 °C), 3.4°C (±1.8°C) and 2.8 (±1.2°C) were observed for yoghurt, prepared meals, meat and sliced cooked ham, respectively. This obtained product temperature profile made possible the interpretation of the moment where the product stayed in display cabinets.

Figure 1. Product temperatures in retail display cabinets measured in France (a) in 307 supermarkets for yoghurt, prepared meals and meat (Derens et al., 2006) (b) in 83 supermarkets for sliced cooked ham (Derens-Bertheau et al., 2015)

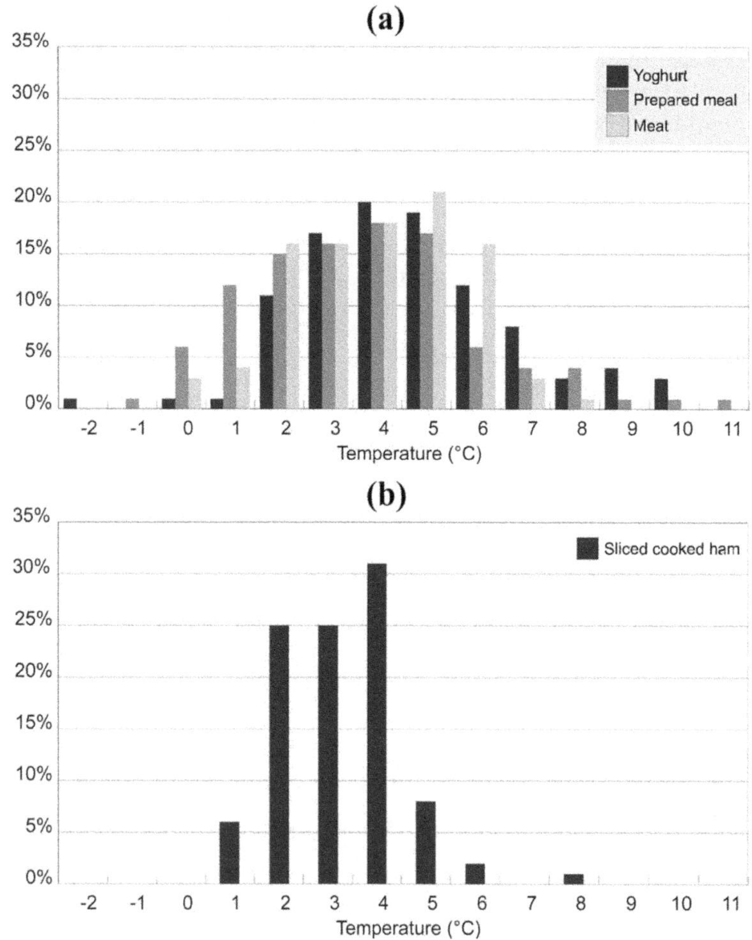

Willocx et al. (1994) measured the air temperature in open display cabinets with three decks over which minimally processed vegetables were displayed in Belgian supermarkets. They showed that the differences of more than 5°C were detected on the decks. The temperature also increased towards the end of the day in certain locations by 4°C and towards the end of the week by almost 7°C.

In Ireland, the Food Safety Authority of Ireland (FSAI) found that the temperatures of pre-packed sandwiches were above 5°C in 57% of cases (FSAI, 2002). In a similar study in 2003, the FSAI found that 14% of pre-cooked sliced ham was stored above 5°C (FSAI, 2003).

Studies in the USA have shown the temperature of foods in chilled food distribution channels were frequently in the range of 7.2°C to 12.8°C (Food Spectrum, 2002). Jol, Kassianenko, Wszol, and Oggel (2006) claimed that 20% of domestic and commercial refrigerators operated at a temperature of more than 10°C. Audits International (1999) found that 48% of product temperatures in retail refrigerators were above 5.0°C and 17% were above 8.3°C. Table 1 summarizes the field studies carried out in several countries.

Table 1. Field studies conducted on display cabinets in various countries

Country	Sample	Temperature (°C)			% of samples at specified temperature	Reference
		Min.	Mean	Max.		
Canada	Beef	-2.0	2.6	10.6	18% > 4 °C	Gill et al. (2003)
	Fresh-cut lettuce		4.1			McKellar, LeBlanc, Rodríguez, and Delaquis (2014)
Denmark	Chilled product			14.0	50% > 5°C	Bøgh-Sorensen (1980)
France	Yogurt	-2.1	4.2	9.8	18% > 6°C	Derens et al. (2006)
	Processed meat	-1.1	3.3	10.2	36% > 4°C	
	Ham	0.2	2.8	7.0	12% > 4°C	Derens-Bertheau et al. (2015)
	Bakery, pock and dairy products			16.0	70% > 7°C	Morelli, Noel, Rosset, and Poumeyrol (2012)
Finland	Fish	0.3	3.5	8.6	53% > 5°C	Lundén et al. (2014)
	Minced meat	0.1	3.1	6.9	10% > 7°C	
Germany	Chilled products			11	87.9% > 4°C 39.4% > 7°C	Murmann and Häger Kuhlung (1987)
Greece	Pasteurized milk	0	4.9	11.7	35% > 6°C	Koutsoumanis, Pavlis, Nychas, and Xanthiakos (2010)
	Smoked sliced turkey		4.0			Gogou, Katsaros, Derens, Alvarez, and Taoukis (2015)
Ireland	Cooked sliced ham	1.5	5.7	12.7	14% > 5°C	FSAI (2003)
Slovenia	Meat products Dairy products	0 0	3.8 5.6	10.5 16.0		Likar and Jevšnik (2006)
Spain	Meat products	-1.8	4.3	9.9	43% > 4°C	Baldera Zubeldia, Nieto Jiménez, Valenzuela Claros, Mariscal Andrés, and Martin-Olmedo (2016)
	Fish	2.9	6.2	10.0	75% > 4°C	
	Dairy products	1.2	6.4	15.3	57% > 8°C	
Sweden	Chilled product	-1.0	4.9	16.0	36% > 5 °C	Bøgh-Sørensen and Olsson (1990)
UK	Cooked meat				28% > 5 °C	Sagoo, Little, Allen, Williamson, and Grant (2007)
	Chilled products				55% > 5 °C	Evans (2010)
USA	Leafy green salad				40% > 7.2°C	Brown, Ryser, Gorman, Steinmaus, and Vorst (2016)
	Meat, Fish and dairy products	-10.0	5.4	21.1	47% > 5°C 22% > 7°C	Audits International (1999)
	Meat products			20.0	38% > 4°C	Rogers and Althen (1980)

Source: (Chaomuang et al., 2017)

Experimental Air Temperatures in a Closed Display Cabinet

Like other refrigerating equipment, the cooling system of display cabinets is composed of an evaporator, compressor, condenser and expansion valve. The operation of this system is presented in several books (ASHRAE, 2002; Evans & Foster, 2015; Meunier, Rivet, & Terrier, 2010). The airflow in closed and open display cabinets is illustrated in Figure 2. In both cases, air flows downward from the Discharge

Air Grille (DAG, front top) to the Return Air Grille (RAG, front bottom). This airflow, termed as the cold air curtain, provides not only cooling capacity but also insulation from ambient air. Air also flows horizontally from the rear to the front through a Perforated Back Panel (PBP). The air flows through the evaporator where it is cooled and then is circulated upward. This air circulation is provided by fans allowing uniformity of air temperature and effective food protection. It is to be emphasized that this airflow directions are available for vertical multi-deck display cabinets with an evaporator at the bottom; the airflow can be different for other display cabinet types. The air velocity can be adjusted with respect to the product characteristics to reduce the product weight loss due to water evaporation particularly in un-wrapped food. The air velocity in the air curtain may vary from 0.1 m/s at the edge to 1.0 m/s at the middle of air curtain (Laguerre, Hoang, Osswald, et al., 2012). For the open display cabinet (Figure 2b), there is an additional air infiltration from outside.

Figure 2. Airflow schematic in (a) closed and (b) open refrigerated display cabinets

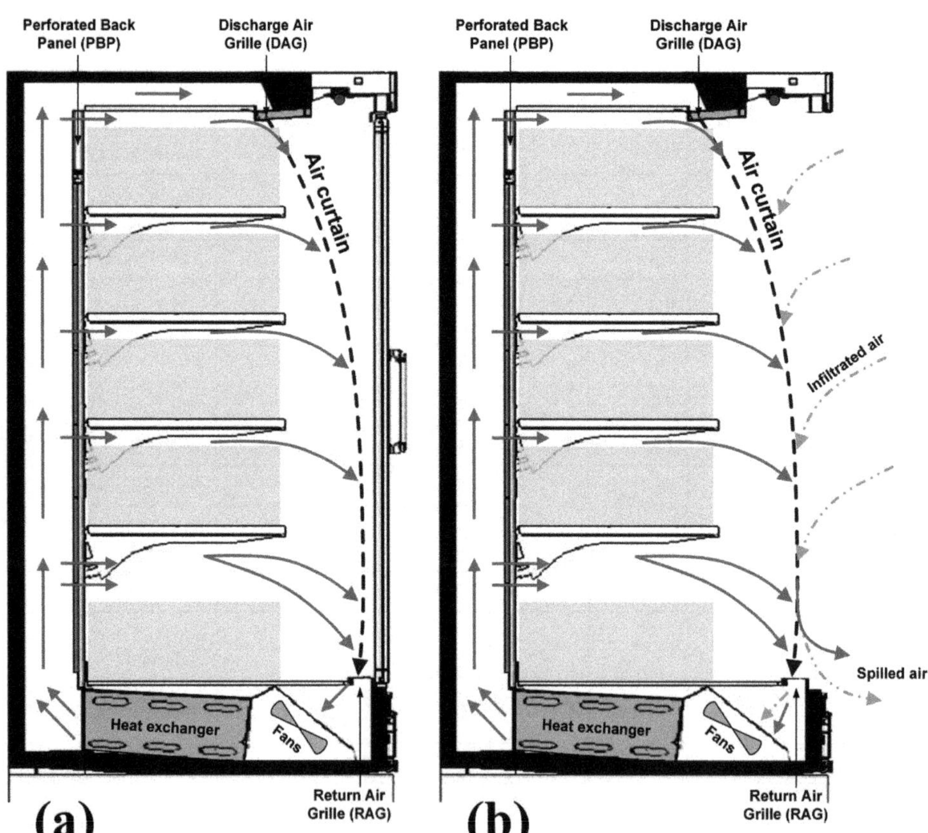

An experimental investigation of air temperature and airflow in an empty and loaded closed refrigerated display cabinet was presented in Chaomuang et al. (2019). In this study, the measurements of air temperature (with thermocouples) and of air velocity (with a hot-wire anemometer) were presented at various positions in the shelves-space storage and in the air curtain. In order to gain the knowledge of spatial and temporal temperature variations in the closed display cabinet, only the part of temperature measurement was addressed in this chapter. Figure 3 shows the air temperature evolution at different positions on the center plane of the display cabinet together with time-averaged temperatures and standard deviations during the quasi-steady state. It can be noticed that the min/max temperature variations changed from one position to another with the same frequencies due to the on/off compressor regulation. Because of negligible thermal inertia of air, there was not time lag of air temperature change at different positions. The air temperature variation curve at the bottom of the vertical rear duct (Figure 3a), near the thermostat sensor, provided information on the compressor working cycles.

Temperature fluctuations of the air in the vertical rear duct (positions a, b and c in Figure 3) had relatively greater amplitudes, compared to the air at the other positions. At these positions, an increase in the minimum temperature was observed while the maximum temperature was relatively similar at all positions. The heat loss through the cabinet walls explains a slight increase in the average temperature. The standard deviation, however, became slightly lower because of stabilization due to the thermal inertia of the wall of the rear duct. The same phenomena were observed in the upper horizontal duct from "c" to "d": an increase in the average temperature due to heat losses and a lower standard deviation due to exchanges with duct walls and the honeycomb of the DAG.

In the area in which food products are stored (positions e, f, g, h, i and j in Figure 3), the average air temperature was below 2°C, which is the recommended temperature for perishable foods (for example meat and fish). As the temperature was slightly negative at the bottom (position "i" and "j"), it could cause freezing damage to foods stored at these positions.

The average temperatures at the front of the shelves (positions f, h and j in Figure 3) were higher than at the DAG. This is because the air curtain exchanges heat with doors, through which heat is transferred from the external ambient, as well as the infiltration of external air through the gaps. The average temperatures at the back of the shelves (positions e, g and i in Figure 3) were lower than those at the front, especially on the bottom shelf. This is because of the higher percentage of holes at the bottom of the PBP of the studied display cabinet which allows higher air flow rate from the rear duct.

Air temperature is generally displayed on a monitoring screen to ensure that food products are stored at appropriate temperature in the display cabinet (Baldera Zubeldia et al., 2016). As this displayed value corresponds to an instantaneous air temperature at a given position, it should be preferable to display the temperature at the warmest and coldest positions, which may vary due to cabinet types.

Influence of the Presence of Doors

A comparative study of cabinet performance in terms of temperature distribution was performed between an empty and loaded display cabinet with doors and without doors.

Doors on the studied display cabinet were removed to investigate the influence of the presence of doors on the temperature performance. Figure 4a and 4b shows the time-averaged air temperature (and standard deviation) of the empty cabinet. These temperatures were calculated from the measurement at the center plane. Thus, the edge effect can be considered as negligible. The temperature profile in the empty cabinet with and without doors had the same trend: the highest temperature at the front of the top shelf (position "f") and the lowest temperature at the back of the bottom shelf (position "i"). Without doors, the average air temperatures in the storage zone increased in all positions, compared to the case with doors. The comparison of the air temperature at 4 cm from the shelf edges (positions "k" and "ℓ")

Figure 3. Air temperature fluctuations during quasi-steady state in various positions (on the center plane) in the closed display cabinet for a room temperature of 19°C
Source: Chaomuang et al. (2019)

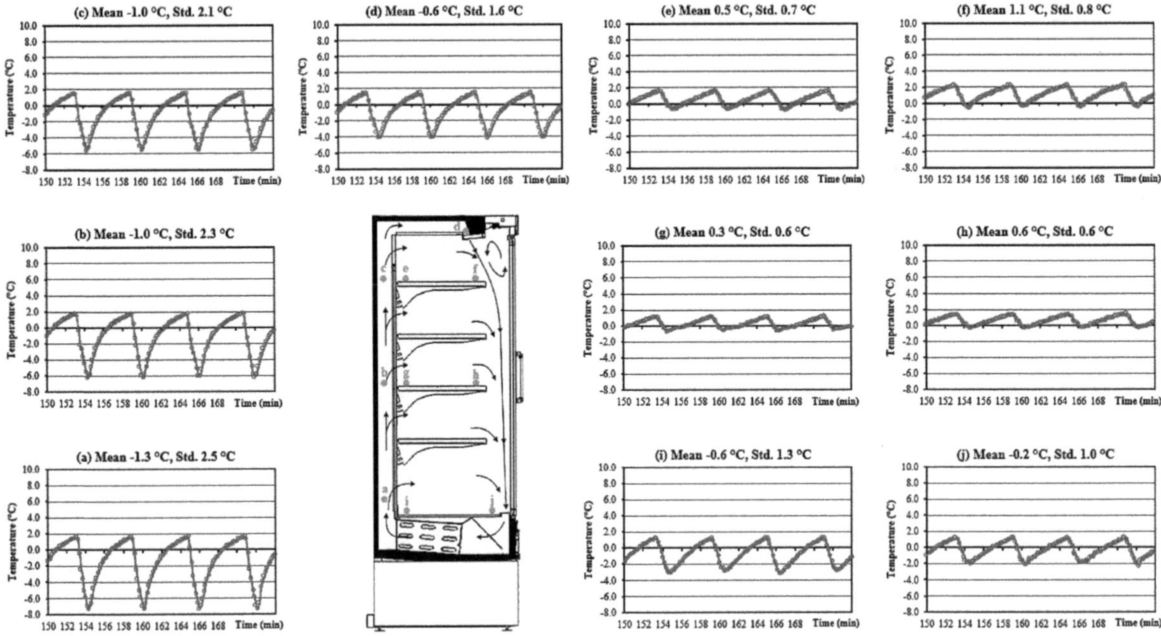

shows a large increase at the top and at the mid-height. This can be explained by the measurement positions which located at the outside of the air curtain. It is to be emphasized that the airflow underneath the DAG (position "k") is complex because of the mixing of the cold air from the DAG with the horizontal air flow from the PBP and the warm air (from outside). The higher temperature at the RAG in the case without doors leads to higher heat loads on the evaporator.

Test product packages made of methylcellulose (dimensions of 20 cm × 10 cm × 5 cm) were placed in the cabinet with an occupied volume of about 60% of total storage volume. The averages and standard deviations of product (core and surface) and air temperatures on the center plane are depicted in Figure 4c (with doors) and Figure 4d (without doors). The highest product temperature at the front of the top shelf can be explained by interdependencies among various influencing factors. At this position, the products were mainly subjected to heat exchanges with the air curtain, heat diffusion through the glass doors, and heat generation due to (visible) light absorption in the products. It can be noticed (Figure 4c) that product surface temperature was slightly higher than that of the surrounding air and that of its core temperature.

The products located at the back of the bottom shelf had the lowest temperature because of more cooled air from the back delivers to the storage. This low temperature position was already observed in the empty case (Figure 4a).

Product temperature difference between the front and the back was also observed, of which the highest difference was on the top shelf. This results from a combination of convection between product and cold air coming from the PBP and conduction within and between the products.

Figure 4. Average air and product temperatures and standard deviation (°C) during quasi-steady state (average of the measurements on the center plane) of the display cabinet exposed to a room temperature of 19°C (a) empty cabinet with doors and (b) empty cabinet without doors (c) loaded cabinet with doors and (b) loaded cabinet without doors Source: Chaomuang et al. (2019).

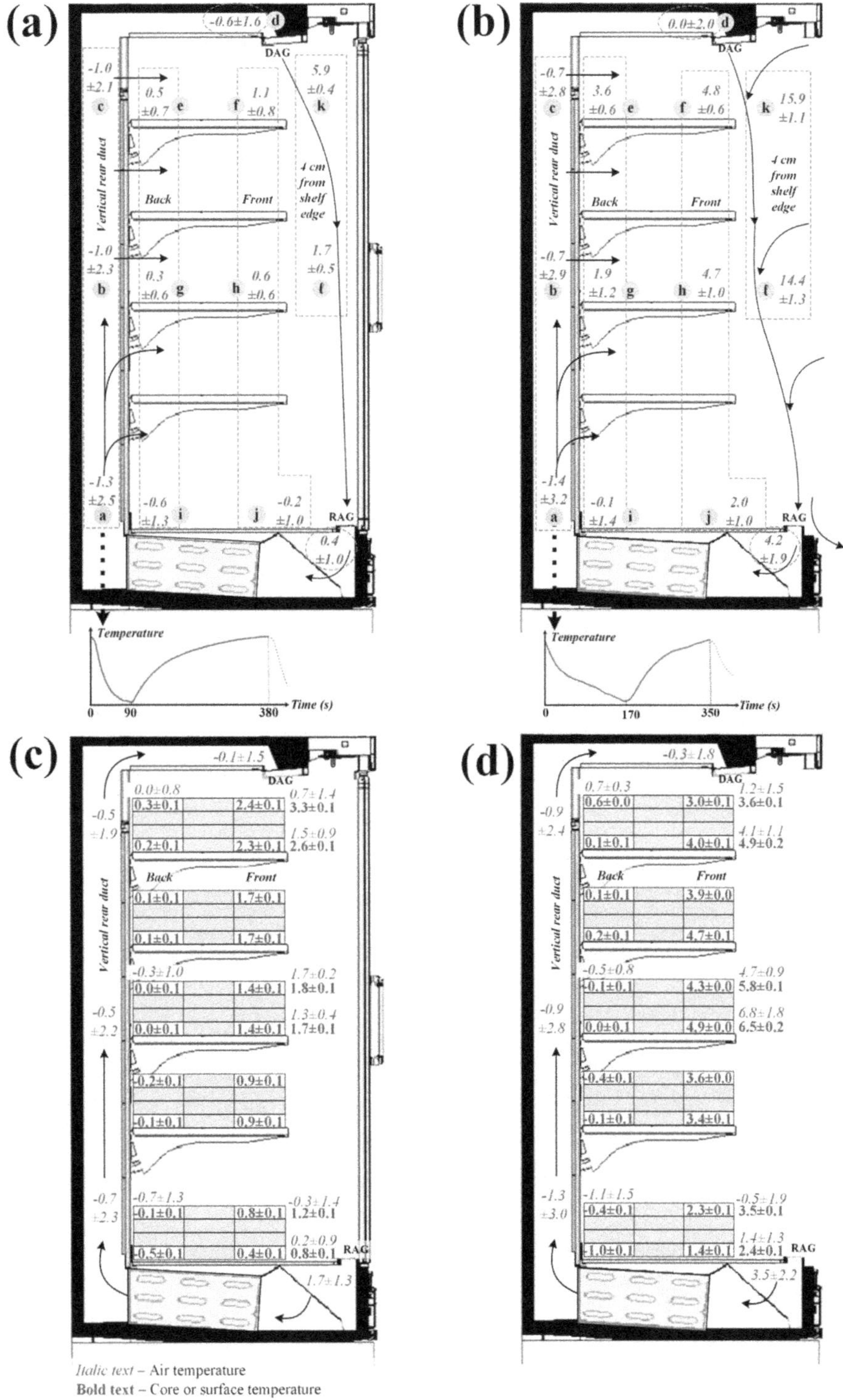

The results of the cabinet without doors (Figure 4d) show that product and air temperatures at the front areas remarkably increased at all positions. This can be explained by the external warm air infiltration mixing with the air curtain. Product and air temperatures at the back of the cabinet without doors was slightly lower than that of the cabinet with doors because higher refrigeration capacity is required to compensate additional heat loads due to warn air infiltration. As observed in the case of loaded and closed display cabinet, product surface temperature was slightly higher than that of the surrounding air and that of its core temperature.

Globally, lower (air and product) temperatures and less temperatures heterogeneity was observed in the storage of the closed display cabinet, thus, better temperature performance compared to the open one.

Figure 5. Comparison of energy consumption between open and closed refrigerated display cabinets

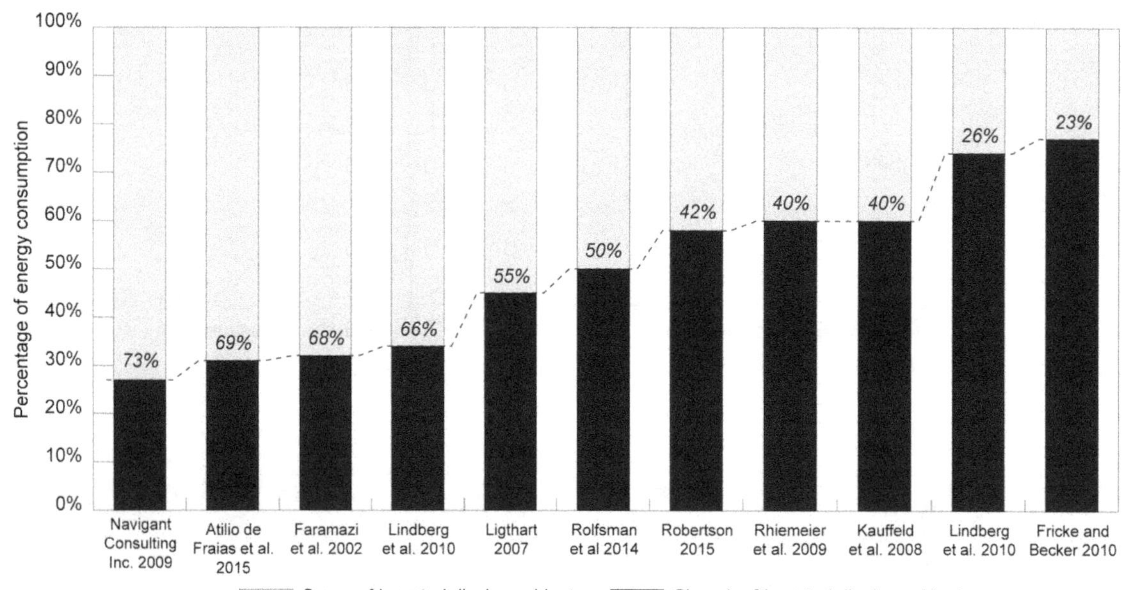

Influence of the Frequency and the Duration of Door Openings

Numerous works were carried out to study the influence of the presence of doors on the energy consumption, compared to the absence of doors (Atilio de Frias et al., 2015; Faramarzi et al., 2002; Fricke & Becker, 2010; Ligthart, 2007; Lindberg et al., 2010; Navigant Consulting Inc., 2009; Rhiemeier et al., 2009; Robertson, 2015; Rolfsman & Borgqvist, 2014). The comparison of energy consumption of open and closed display cabinets is shown in Figure 5. It can be seen that the percentage of energy savings varied from 23% to 73% when doors were fitted. The variations of these results can be explained by the difference of display cabinet configurations and the operating conditions used in the certain studies as summarized in Table 2.

The door opening frequency certainly affects the cabinet performance in terms of both temperature homogeneity and energy consumption. In spite of many tests of the impact of door openings, less published information is available on its influence on product temperature.

Table 2. Studies of the influence of open and closed display cabinets on the energy saving

Reference	Cabinet configuration	Operating condition	Door openings (OPH[a]/duration)	Night cover	Anti-sweat heaters
Atilio de Frias et al. (2015)	Two display cabinets: open and closed; both with LED lightings	• Thermostat setting at 0.6°C with a 12 h off-cycle defrost interval of 30 min (open) and a 24 h defrost interval of 30 min (closed). • Test room conditions of 21°C and 60–70% RH	6 OPH/12 s	n/a[b]	none
Faramarzi et al. (2002)	Open display cabinet retrofitted with doors	• Evaporator temperature at -5°C (23°F) with a 6 h off-cycle defrost. • Test room conditions of 24°C (75°F) and 55% RH.	5 OPH/16 s	n/a	YES
Fricke and Becker (2010)	Two display cabinets: open and closed	• Field measurement during 42-day test period in two supermarkets (20-45%RH, not mentioned store temperature)	6.3 OPH/5 s (mean value over the test period)	n/a	YES
Ligthart (2007)	Review from the literature	• n/a	n/a	n/a	n/a
Lindberg et al. (2010)	Open display cabinet retrofitted with doors	• Field measurement where the store conditions in front of the display cabinets were 15.9-17.3°C (38-43%RH) and 18.2-19.4°C (41%RH) for open and closed cases, respectively.	n/a	YES	n/a
Lindberg et al. (2010)	Open display cabinet fitted with doors	• Heat exchanger inlet temperature at -8°C for open cabinet and 2°C for closed cabinet • Test room conditions of 22°C and 65% RH.	10 and 30 OPH/ 6 s	YES	n/a
Navigant Consulting Inc. (2009)	Review from the literature	• n/a	n/a	NO	YES
Rhiemeier et al. (2009)	Review from the literature	• n/a	n/a	n/a	n/a
Robertson (2015)	Open display cabinet retrofitted with doors	• Test in the supermarket	n/a	YES	n/a
Rolfsman and Borgqvist (2014)	Open display cabinet retrofitted with doors	• Heat exchanger inlet temperature at -8°C for open cabinet and -1°C for closed cabinet • One-month test period in a supermarket.	n/a	n/a	n/a

[a]OPH: Number of door opening per hour per door;[b]n/a: Data not available

The cold loss was numerically quantified during a door opening procedure (opening, holding and closing) of close display cabinets with 1.8 m in height and 6 decks (Orlandi, Visconti, & Zampini, 2013). In this study, two three-door cabinets for chilled product were considered: one was equipped with sliding doors and the other one was equipped with hinged doors; only the central door opening was considered for the analysis. It was supposed in this study that the radiation and the thermal inertia of the cabinet solid parts were negligible. The comparative results showed that the internal temperatures were relatively the same for both door types when the doors remained closed. However, when doors were cyclically opened (10 openings/hour/door as prescribed in EN 23953:2005 for chilled cabinets and 60 openings/ hour/door for 15 s duration of each opening including 1 s opening, 13 s holding and 1 s closing), the air temperature at the return air duct in the cabinet with sliding doors was lower than that in the cabinet with hinged doors. This explained the display cabinet with sliding doors to consume 17% less energy than the cabinet with hinged doors. The same authors reported that the cold loss due to door openings was responsible for 12% of total heat extraction rate, while the contribution of lights was 25% (Figure 6). Nevertheless, when higher door opening frequency were applied (60 openings per hour for each door), the contribution to heat load due to door openings became significant. It accounted for 44% of the total. This very high frequency may not realistic. Fricke and Becker (2010) carried out measurements in supermarkets and found that in real-life situations, the most frequent door opening duration was 5 seconds and the daily average door opening frequency was about 6.3 openings per hour, which means one door being opened every 9.5 minutes.

Figure 6. Percentage of cold loss from the closed display cabinets due to different sources (Orlandi et al., 2013)

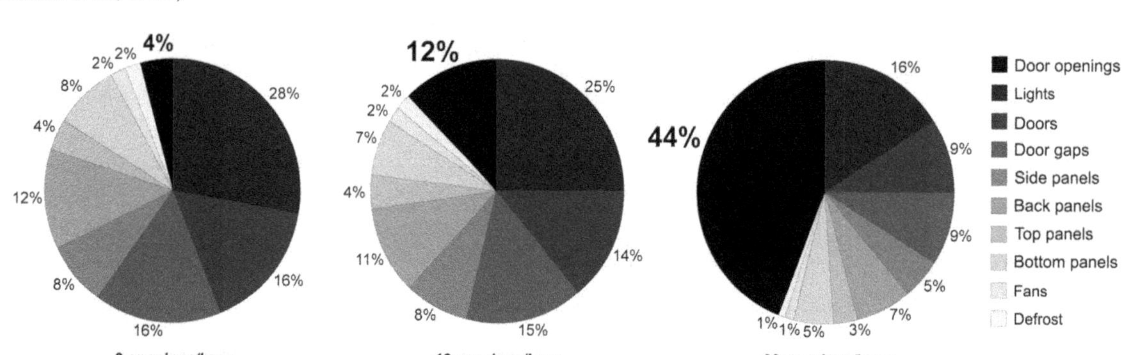

Influence of Room Temperature on the Temperature Performance of the Cabinet

As proven by many studies, ambient temperature in supermarkets has an impact on temperature distribution in open-front refrigerated display cabinets (Axell & Lindberg, 2005; Chen & Yuan, 2005; Heidinger, Nascimento, Gaspar, & Silva, 2013). To complement this knowledge the influence of ambient temperature on the temperature distribution in a closed display cabinet was carried out by Chaomuang et al. (2019) for three ambient temperatures.

Table 3 shows the influence of external ambient temperature (15°C, 19°C and 24°C) on the air temperature in the food storage zone (average value and standard deviation over 5 h of quasi steady state periods) of the studied closed display cabinet. The average temperature after the heat exchanger where the thermostat position was located (T_{th}) was slightly different for these three ambient temperatures. To be able to compare the results obtained under several ambient temperatures, temperature difference ($T–T_{th}$) is shown. Average for all positions $T–T_{th}$ increased from 1.1°C to 2.0°C when $\bar{T}_e - T_{th}$ rose from 15.2°C to 25.4°C. A dimensionless temperature defined as $T^* = \dfrac{T - T_{th}}{\bar{T}_e - T_{th}}$ was also calculated. It appeared that T^* was almost independent of $\overline{T}_e - T_{th}$. This is due to the linearity (between $\overline{T}_e$ and T_i) since the force convection and conduction are predominant heat transfer modes. In the closed configuration, free convection is negligible because of the rather high velocities at the DAG and PBP. Radiation is also limited because the glass doors shield the radiation from the external walls in opposite to the open configuration. The highest value of T^* was at the position f (the front of the top shelf) where $T–T_{th}$ is about 12% of $\overline{T}_e - T_{th}$. The lowest value of T^* is at the position i (the back of the bottom shelf) where the temperature is slightly higher than at the position after the heat exchanger.

Table 3. Effect of ambient temperature on the internal air temperature of the closed refrigerated display cabinet

Average ambient temperature $\pm$ standard deviation	Temperature difference	Number of compressor "on" cycles/5h		Temperature difference and time-averaged dimensionless temperature at a given position						All positions
T_e(°C)	$T_e–T_{th}$(°C)			e	f	g	h	i	j	
15 ± 0.5	15.2	36	$T–T_{th}$	1.1	1.7	1.0	1.4	0.3	0.8	1.1
			T^*	0.07	0.11	0.06	0.09	0.02	0.06	0.07
19 ± 0.4	20.3	44	$T–T_{th}$	1.5	2.4	1.2	1.8	0.4	1.1	1.4
			T^*	0.08	0.12	0.06	0.09	0.02	0.06	0.07
24 ± 0.3	25.4	52	$T–T_{th}$	2.3	3.7	1.6	2.4	0.6	1.5	2.0
			T^*	0.09	0.14	0.06	0.09	0.02	0.06	0.08
T* for all ambient temperatures				0.08	0.12	0.06	0.09	0.02	0.06	0.07

Source: (Chaomuang et al., 2019)

A comparison of the percentage of time "on" compared to the total time "on and off" of the compressor operation shows the significant influence of ambient temperature (Table 4). In fact, to maintain the desired supply air temperature, an increase in ambient temperature causes an increase in the frequency of compressor working cycles (shorter "off" period). This implies an increase in the energy consumption of the display cabinets installed in stores without air-conditioning systems in summer. Table 4 also shows that the percentage of time "on" compared to the total time "on and off" is not significantly different for the empty and loaded display cabinets.

Table 4. Percentage of time "on" compared to the total time "on and off" of the compressor under different conditions

Ambient temperature (°C)		Closed display cabinet		Open display cabinet	
		Empty	Loaded	Empty	Loaded
15	18				
19	21	21	49	47	
24	31				

Source: (Chaomuang et al., 2019)

Modelling of Heat Transfer, Airflow and Energy Consumption of Close Display Cabinet

In order to understand the mechanism of thermal transport phenomena occurring in a closed display cabinet experimental and numerical investigations are complementary. Several numerical studies were carried out on heat transfer and airflow in open refrigerated display cabinets (Alzuwaid, Ge, Tassou, & Sun, 2016; Gaspar, Gonçalves, & Pitarma, 2012; Ge, Tassou, & Hadawey, 2010; Hoang, Raoult, & Leducq, 2016; Laguerre, Hoang, & Flick, 2012; Moureh & Yataghene, 2016; Wu et al., 2014; Yu, Ding, & Chen, 2009; Zhijuan, Xuehong, Yanli, Qiuyang, & Wenhui, 2013).

Because of the lack of numerical study of closed display cabinets for chilled products, the one for frozen products with an air curtain flowing along the internal side of the door is presented (D'Agaro, Cortella, & Croce, 2006). In this study, a model of the misting and demisting process in the glass doors was developed. The main objective of this study was only to gain insight into the physical mechanism of the thermo-fluid phenomena of fogging and defogging taking place during the door openings as it is a very important issue for this cabinet type. The high fogging level leads to the poor transparency of the glass, thus influencing product visibility. Defogging with a heater is then required, which comes with higher energy demand and cooling load. However, no case study has shown to manifest the influence of these phenomena on the cabinet performance in terms of both energy efficiency and temperature distribution.

Product Quality in Closed Display Cabinet

Kou, Luo, Ingram, Yan, and Jurick (2015) studied the influences of thermostat settings (at -0.5°C and -2.2°C with the same defrosting interval of 12 h and duration of 30 min) on the product temperature and the quality of packaged baby spinach products at various locations in the open display cabinet. With the -2.2 °C thermostat temperature, the products located on the top shelf at the front of the display cabinet had the highest temperature (mean 6.5°C) and the temperature decreased towards the back of the cabinet. The lowest mean temperature was below zero (-0.6°C), thus, product located in this zone was subjected to freezing damage. To overcome this thermal problem, the temperature of thermostat was set at -0.5°C. However, the products in the front rows then underwent temperature abuse. This represents the situation in supermarkets and the major challenge is to control these temperature abuses so that all products are preserved at an adequate temperature without freezing problems. These results were in agreement with the results obtained by Laguerre, Hoang, Osswald, et al. (2012): warmer product temperature at the front and cooler product temperature at the rear for the same shelf.

Product temperatures in display cabinets can rise during the defrost operation (Lawrence & Evans, 2008). Temperature sensitive food products under fluctuating temperature condition can deteriorate at different rates than the ones under less fluctuating condition (Wells & Singh, 1989). The application of heat pipe and phase change materials (PCM) in the cabinet shelf was introduced to deal with this issue by Lu et al. (2010). Two cabinet prototypes, a shelf retrofitted with heat pipe and combined heat pipe with PCM, were experimentally tested in their study. Based on their results, the authors claimed that the use of heat pipe and PCM provides several advantages: the reduction of core product temperatures (3.0°C to 5.5°C lower with heat pipe alone), the improvement of temperature distribution homogeneity (small range of max-min temperatures during normal operation) and the reduction in temperature rise during defrost process (0.3°C rise with combined structure) with less energy consumption. The similar results were obtained by Alzuwaid, Ge, Tassou, Raeisi, and Gowreesunker (2015), they concluded that the use of PCM lowered cabinet temperatures and saved up to 5% of energy consumption. In spite of several studies on the influence of ambient temperature and humidity on the product quality (Paull, 1999; Ketsa & Pangkool, 1994; Sharkey & Peggie, 1984; Grierson & Wardowski, 1978.; Berg & Lentz., 1977), these influences on food quality displayed in closed display cabinets and door openings are less studied and still needed to fulfil.

FUTURE RESEARCH DIRECTIONS

Refrigerated display cabinets retrofitted with doors is an alternative to improve the cabinet performance since it is simple to implement. Many world's leading retailers have already fitted their display cabinet with doors and some extend the policy of putting doors as a standard for their new and/or renovated stores (EIA, 2014, 2017). This transition implies a more important role of closed refrigerated display cabinets in the future, and consequently generates research opportunities associated with this cabinet type.

The use of doors on chilled display cabinets reaps potential energy savings. However, attention must be paid since door installation can modify airflow pattern and temperature distribution within the cabinets (Faramarzi et al., 2002) which may result in a negative impact on food temperatures.

Door openings can also disrupt the air curtain of the closed display cabinet and induce the entrainment of warm and humid air from outside, thereby increasing temperature variation and energy consumption. An investigation into the effect of door opening frequency and duration on the cabinet performance is necessary. Determining the air infiltration rate during the door openings at different opening frequency and duration would bring more confidence in establishing if the closed display cabinet is worthwhile.

A change in the transport phenomena can be characterized using advanced air velocity field measurement such as Particle Image Velocimetry (PIV) and Laser Doppler Velocimetry (LDV). Additionally, Computational Fluid Dynamic (CFD) can be used to study the 3D airflow and heat transfer in display cabinets. The application of these methods on the closed refrigerated display cabinet is still rear.

As a complementary to the CFD model, a simplified heat transfer model based on a zonal approach should be developed to gain an insight into the mechanism of heat/mass transfer in a closed display cabinet. This model is rare while the ones for other refrigeration equipment were largely developed: processing plant (Lecoq, Flick, Derens, Hoang, & Laguerre, 2016), refrigerated vehicle (Hoang, Laguerre, Moureh, & Flick, 2012, cold room (Laguerre, Duret, Hoang, Guillier, & Flick, 2015) and household refrigerator (Laguerre & Flick, 2004). Such a model allows the prediction of product temperature at various positions in the equipment with a short calculation time. The closed display cabinet cabinets will be soon a new component of the series of refrigeration equipment in food cold chain. The simplified model of this cabinet type can be linked with the other models allows the knowledge of time-temperature history of food products from a production plant to a household refrigerator. Furthermore, predictive microbiological and/or quality models can also be established to evaluate the consumer risk (Duret et al., 2015).

CONCLUSION

Plenty of works on retail refrigerated display cabinets have been carried out for the last two decades particularly since there has been a greater awareness of food product quality and energy efficiency. Many researchers have tried to investigate and identify the key factors which influence the cabinet performance by the means of both experimental (field-based and laboratory-based) and numerical (in-house code and commercial code) approaches. The obtained knowledge will provide the opportunity to optimize this equipment in terms of both temperature homogeneity and energy consumption. The application of doors is an alternative solution and several studies have shown that doors can provide several advantages. Two studies (Carrington, 2012; Fricke & Becker, 2010) reported insignificant impact of the presence of doors on display cabinets on the product sale loss, thus, more studies should be carried out to confirm this observation. Most of studies tend to only focus on energy consumption.

Nomenclature

T: Temperature [°C or K]
$\bar{T}$: Mean temperature [°C or K]

T^*: Dimensionless temperature defined as $T^* = \dfrac{T - T_{th}}{\bar{T_e} - T_{th}}$

Subscripts

Th: thermostat
E: external ambient

Abbreviations

DAG: Discharge Air Grille
PBP: Perforated Back Panel
RAG: Return Air Grille
PCM: Phase Change Material

ACKNOWLEDGMENT

The work was supported by King Mongkut's Institute of Technology Ladkrabang (Thailand), the National Research Institute of Science and Technology for Environment and Agriculture (France) and the French Embassy in Thailand. The authors would like to thank EPTA (France), display cabinet manufacturer, for the industrial information.

REFERENCES

Alzuwaid, F., Ge, Y. T., Tassou, S. A., Raeisi, A., & Gowreesunker, L. (2015). The novel use of phase change materials in a refrigerated display cabinet: An experimental investigation. *Applied Thermal Engineering, 75,* 770–778. doi:10.1016/j.applthermaleng.2014.10.028

Alzuwaid, F. A., Ge, Y. T., Tassou, S. A., & Sun, J. (2016). The novel use of phase change materials in an open type refrigerated display cabinet: A theoretical investigation. *Applied Energy*, *180*, 76–85. doi:10.1016/j.apenergy.2016.07.088

ASHRAE. (2002). Household refrigerators and freezers. In M. S. Owen & H. E. Kennedy (Eds.), *ASHRAE Handbook: Refrigeration*. Atlanta, GA: American Society of Heating, Refrigerating and Air-Conditioning Engineers.

Atilio de Frias, J., Luo, Y., Kou, L., Zhou, B., & Wang, Q. (2015). Improving spinach quality and reducing energy costs by retrofitting retail open refrigerated cases with doors. *Postharvest Biology and Technology*, *110*, 114–120. doi:10.1016/j.postharvbio.2015.06.016

Audits International. (1999). *U.S. Cold temperature evaluation design and study summary*. Retrieved from foodrisk.org/default/assets/File/Audits-FDA_temp_study.pdf

Axell, M., & Lindberg, U. (2005). *Field measurements in supermarkets.* Paper presented at the Proceedings of the IIF-IIR Meeting Commercial Refrigeration, Vicenza, Italy.

Baldera Zubeldia, B., Nieto Jiménez, M., Valenzuela Claros, M. T., Mariscal Andrés, J. L., & Martin-Olmedo, P. (2016). Effectiveness of the cold chain control procedure in the retail sector in Southern Spain. *Food Control*, *59*, 614–618. doi:10.1016/j.foodcont.2015.06.046

Bøgh-Sorensen, L. (1980). *Product temperatures in chilled cabinets*. Paper presented at the 26th European Meeting of Meat Research Workers, Colorado Springs, CO.

Bøgh-Sørensen, L., & Olsson, P. (1990). The chill chain. In T. R. Gormley (Ed.), *Chilled foods: the state of the art* (pp. 245–267). London: Elsevier Applied Science.

Brown, W., Ryser, E., Gorman, L., Steinmaus, S., & Vorst, K. (2016). Temperatures experienced by fresh-cut leafy greens during retail storage and display. *Acta Horticulturae*, (1141), 103–108. doi:10.17660/ActaHortic.2016.1141.10

Carrington, D. (2012). Co-op supermarkets extend fridge door scheme. *The Guardian*. Retrieved from https://www.theguardian.com/environment/2012/dec/25/co-op-supermarkets-extend-fridge-door-scheme

Cemagref & ANIA. (2004). La chaine du froid du fabricant au consommateur: Résultats de l'audit ANIA/Cemagref. *Revue Générale du Froid*, *1042*, 29–36.

Chaomuang, N., Flick, D., Denis, A., & Laguerre, O. (2019). Experimental analysis of heat transfer and airflow in a closed refrigerated display cabinet. *Journal of Food Engineering*, *244*, 101–104. doi:10.1016/j.jfoodeng.2018.09.009

Chaomuang, N., Flick, D., & Laguerre, O. (2017). Experimental and numerical investigation of the performance of retail refrigerated display cabinets. *Trends in Food Science & Technology*, *70*(Supplement C), 95–104. doi:10.1016/j.tifs.2017.10.007

Chen, Y.-G., & Yuan, X.-L. (2005). Experimental study of the performance of single-band air curtains for a multi-deck refrigerated display cabinet. *Journal of Food Engineering*, *69*(3), 261–267. doi:10.1016/j.jfoodeng.2004.08.016

D'Agaro, P., Croce, G., & Cortella, G. (2006). Numerical simulation of glass doors fogging and defogging in refrigerated display cabinets. *Applied Thermal Engineering*, *26*(16), 1927–1934. doi:10.1016/j.applthermaleng.2006.01.014

Derens, E., Palagos, B., & Guilpart, J. (2006). *The cold chain of chilled products under supervision in France*. Paper presented at the 13th World Congress of Food Science & Technology, Nantes, France. 10.1051/IUFoST:20060823

Derens-Bertheau, E., Osswald, V., Laguerre, O., & Alvarez, G. (2015). Cold chain of chilled food in France. *International Journal of Refrigeration*, *52*, 161–167. doi:10.1016/j.ijrefrig.2014.06.012

Duret, S., Gwanpua, S. G., Hoang, H.-M., Guillier, L., Flick, D., Laguerre, O., ... Geeraerd, A. (2015). Identification of the significant factors in food quality using global sensitivity analysis and the accept-and-reject algorithm. Part II: Application to the cold chain of cooked ham. *Journal of Food Engineering*, *148*, 58–65. doi:10.1016/j.jfoodeng.2014.09.038

EIA. (2014). *Chilling Facts VI: Closing the door on HFCs*. Retrieved from https://eia-international. org/report/the-chilling-facts-vi-closing-the-door-on-hfcs

EIA. (2017). *Chilling Facts VII: Are Europe's supermarkets ready to quit HFCs?* Retrieved from https://eia-international.org/report/chilling-facts-vii

Evans, J. A. (2010). *Retail display*. Paper presented at 1st IIR Conference on Sustainability and the Cold Chain, Cambridge, UK.

Evans, J. A. (2014). *Are Doors on Fridges the Best Environmental Solution for the Retail Sector*. Paper presented at the London Chamber of Commerce and Industry, London, UK.

Evans, J. A., & Foster, A. M. (2015). *Sustainable retail refrigeration*. Oxford, UK: Wiley Blackwell. doi:10.1002/9781118927410

Evans, J. A., Scarcelli, S., & Swain, M. V. L. (2007). Temperature and energy performance of refrigerated retail display and commercial catering cabinets under test conditions. *International Journal of Refrigeration*, *30*(3), 398–408. doi:10.1016/j.ijrefrig.2006.10.006

Evans, J. A., & Swain, M. V. L. (2010). *Performance of retail and commercial refrigeration systems*. Paper presented at the IIR International Cold Chain Conference, Cambridge, UK.

Faramarzi, R. T., Coburn, B. A., & Sarhadian, R. (2002). Performance and energy impact of installing glass doors on an open vertical deli/dairy display case. *ASHRAE Transactions*, *108*, 673.

Food Spectrum, L. (2002). *Retail Prepared Refrigerated Foods: The Market and Technologies*. Retrieved from https://www.foodspectrum.com/pdf/1-RefrigeratedFoodsPublishedStudy-2002.pdf

Fricke, B., & Becker, B. (2010). *Energy use of doored and open vertical refrigerated display cases*. Paper presented at the International Refrigeration and Air Conditioning Conference, Purdue University.

FSAI. (2002). *3rd Quarter National Microbiology Survey 2002 (NS3): Microbiological safety of pre-packed sandwiches*. Retrieved from https://www.fsai.ie/uploadedFiles/3rdQuarter_prepacked_sandwiches .pdf

FSAI. (2003). *1st Quarter National Microbiological Survey 2003 (NS1): Microbiological quality/ safety of pre-packed cooked sliced ham*. Retrieved from https://www.fsai.ie/uploadedFiles/prepacked_ cooked_sliced_ham.pdf

Gaspar, P. D., Carrilho Gonçalves, L. C., & Pitarma, R. A. (2011). Experimental analysis of the thermal entrainment factor of air curtains in vertical open display cabinets for different ambient air conditions. *Applied Thermal Engineering, 31*(5), 961–969. doi:10.1016/j.applthermaleng.2010.11.020

Gaspar, P. D., Gonçalves, L., & Pitarma, R. (2012). Detailed CFD modelling of open refrigerated display cabinets. *Modelling and Simulation in Engineering, 2012*, 1–17. doi:10.1155/2012/867820

Ge, Y. T., Tassou, S. A., & Hadawey, A. (2010). Simulation of multi-deck medium temperature display cabinets with the integration of CFD and cooling coil models. *Applied Energy, 87*(10), 3178–3188. doi:10.1016/j.apenergy.2010.02.028

Gill, C. O., Jones, T., Houde, A., LeBlanc, D. I., Rahn, K., Holley, R. A., & Starke, R. (2003). The temperatures and ages of packs of beef displayed in multi-shelf retail cabinets. *Food Control, 14*(3), 145–151. doi:10.1016/S0956-7135(02)00058-0

Gogou, E., Katsaros, G., Derens, E., Alvarez, G., & Taoukis, P. S. (2015). Cold chain database development and application as a tool for the cold chain management and food quality evaluation. *International Journal of Refrigeration, 52*, 109–121. doi:10.1016/j.ijrefrig.2015.01.019

Grierson, W., & Wardowski, W. F. (1978). Relative humidity effects on the postharvest life of fruits and vegetables. *HortScience, 13*, 570–574.

Heidinger, G., Nascimento, S., Gaspar, P., & Silva, P. (2013). *Impact of environmental conditions on the performance of open multideck display case evaporators*. Paper presented at the 2nd IIR International Conference on Sustainability and the Cold Chain, Paris, France.

Hoang, H. M., Raoult, F., & Leducq, D. (2016). *Potential use of phase change materials in a display cabinet: development of a dynamic modelling approach*. Paper presented at the 11th IIR Conference on Phase Change Materials and Slurries for Refrigeration and Air Conditioning, Karlsruhe, Germany.

Hoang, M. H., Laguerre, O., Moureh, J., & Flick, D. (2012). Heat transfer modelling in a ventilated cavity loaded with food product: Application to a refrigerated vehicle. *Journal of Food Engineering, 113*(3), 389–398. doi:10.1016/j.jfoodeng.2012.06.020

Jol, S., Kassianenko, A., Wszol, K., & Oggel, J. (2005). Issues in time and temperature abuse of refrigerated foods. *Food Safety Magazine, 11*.

Ketsa, S., & Pangkool, S. (1994). The effect of humidity on ripening of durians. *Postharvest Biology and Technology, 4*(1-2), 159–165. doi:10.1016/0925-5214(94)90017-5

Kou, L., Luo, Y., Ingram, D. T., Yan, S., & Jurick, W. M. II. (2015). Open-refrigerated retail display case temperature profile and its impact on product quality and microbiota of stored baby spinach. *Food Control, 47*, 686–692. doi:10.1016/j.foodcont.2014.07.054

Koutsoumanis, K., Pavlis, A., Nychas, G.-J. E., & Xanthiakos, K. (2010). Probabilistic model for Listeria monocytogenes growth during distribution, retail storage, and domestic storage of pasteurized milk. *Applied and Environmental Microbiology, 76*(7), 2181–2191. doi:10.1128/AEM.02430-09 PMID:20139308

Laguerre, O., Duret, S., Hoang, H. M., Guillier, L., & Flick, D. (2015). Simplified heat transfer modeling in a cold room filled with food products. *Journal of Food Engineering, 149*, 78–86. doi:10.1016/j.jfoodeng.2014.09.023

Laguerre, O., & Flick, D. (2004). Heat transfer by natural convection in domestic refrigerators. *Journal of Food Engineering, 62*(1), 79–88. doi:10.1016/S0260-8774(03)00173-0

Laguerre, O., Hoang, M. H., & Flick, D. (2012). Heat transfer modelling in a refrigerated display cabinet: The influence of operating conditions. *Journal of Food Engineering, 108*(2), 353–364. doi:10.1016/j.jfoodeng.2011.07.027

Laguerre, O., Hoang, M. H., Osswald, V., & Flick, D. (2012). Experimental study of heat transfer and air flow in a refrigerated display cabinet. *Journal of Food Engineering, 113*(2), 310–321. doi:10.1016/j.jfoodeng.2012.05.027

Lawrence, J. M. W., & Evans, J. A. (2008). Refrigerant flow instability as a means to predict the need for defrosting the evaporator in a retail display freezer cabinet. *International Journal of Refrigeration, 31*(1), 107–112. doi:10.1016/j.ijrefrig.2007.05.015

Lecoq, L., Flick, D., Derens, E., Hoang, H. M., & Laguerre, O. (2016). Simplified heat and mass transfer modeling in a food processing plant. *Journal of Food Engineering, 171*, 1–13. doi:10.1016/j.jfoodeng.2015.09.026

Li, X., Zhu, D., Wang, N., & Zeng, X. (2007). *Influence of door opening on temperature fluctuation and energy consumption of refrigerated display cabinet.* Paper presented at the International Congress of Refrigeration, Beijing, China.

Ligthart, F. A. T. M. (2007). *Closed supermarket refrigerator and freezer cabinets: a feasibility study* (ECN-E-07-098). Retrieved from https://www.ecn.nl/publications/PdfFetch.aspx?nr=ECN-E--07-098

Likar, K., & Jevšnik, M. (2006). Cold chain maintaining in food trade. *Food Control, 17*(2), 108–113. doi:10.1016/j.foodcont.2004.09.009

Lindberg, U., Axell, M., & Fahlén, P. (2010). *Vertical display cabinets without and with doors–a comparison of measurements in a laboratory and in a supermarket.* Paper presented at the 1st IIR International Conference on Sustainability and the Cold Chain, Cambridge, UK.

Lu, Y. L., Zhang, W. H., Yuan, P., Xue, M. D., Qu, Z. G., & Tao, W. Q. (2010). Experimental study of heat transfer intensification by using a novel combined shelf in food refrigerated display cabinets (Experimental study of a novel cabinets). *Applied Thermal Engineering, 30*(2–3), 85–91. doi:10.1016/j.applthermaleng.2008.10.003

Lundén, J., Vanhanen, V., Myllymäki, T., Laamanen, E., Kotilainen, K., & Hemminki, K. (2014). Temperature control efficacy of retail refrigeration equipment. *Food Control, 45*, 109–114. doi:10.1016/j.foodcont.2014.04.041

McKellar, R. C., LeBlanc, D. I., Rodríguez, F. P., & Delaquis, P. (2014). Comparative simulation of *Escherichia coli* O157:H7 behaviour in packaged fresh-cut lettuce distributed in a typical Canadian supply chain in the summer and winter. *Food Control, 35*(1), 192–199. doi:10.1016/j.foodcont.2013.06.002

Meunier, F., Rivet, P., & Terrier, M. F. (2010). *Froid Industriel* (2nd ed.). Paris: Dunod.

Morelli, E., Noel, V., Rosset, P., & Poumeyrol, G. (2012). Performance and conditions of use of refrigerated display cabinets among producer/vendors of foodstuffs. *Food Control, 26*(2), 363–368. doi:10.1016/j.foodcont.2012.02.002

Moureh, J., & Yataghene, M. (2016). Numerical and experimental investigations on jet characteristics and airflow patterns related to an air curtain subjected to external lateral flow. *International Journal of Refrigeration, 67,* 355–372. doi:10.1016/j.ijrefrig.2016.03.002

Murmann, D., & Häger Kuhlung, O. (1987). von Hackfleisch im SB-Angebot. *Die Fleischwirtschaft (Frankfurt),* 245–248.

Navigant Consulting Inc. (2009). *Energy Savings Potential and R&D Opportunities for Commercial Refrigeration Final Report.* Retrieved from https://www1.eere.energy.gov/buildings/pdfs/commercial_re frigeration_equipment_research_opportunities.pdf

Olsson, P. (1990). *Chilled cabinet surveys* (Vol. 3). London: Elsevier Applied Science Publishers.

Orlandi, M., Visconti, F., & Zampini, S. (2013). *CFD assisted design of closed display cabinets.* Paper presented at the 2nd IIR International Sustainability and the Cold Chain Conference, Paris, France.

Paull, R. E. (1999). Effect of temperature and relative humidity on fresh commodity quality. *Postharvest Biology and Technology, 15*(3), 263–277. doi:10.1016/S0925-5214(98)00090-8

Rhiemeier, J., Harnisch, J., Ters, C., Kauffeld, M., & Leisewitz, A. (2009). Comparative assessment of the climate relevance of supermarket refrigeration systems and equipment. *Environmental Research of the Federal Ministry of the Environment, Nature Conservation and Nuclear Safety Research Report, 206*(44), 300.

Robertson, G. (2015). *Trial retrofit of doors on open refrigerated display cabinets.* Retrieved from https://www.airah.org.au/Content_Files/Resources/Trial-Retrofit-of-Doors-on-Open-Refrigerated-Display-Cabinets.pdf

Rogers, R. W., & Althen, T. G. (1980). Results of processed meat display case and storage cooler temperature survey. *Amer. Soc. Animal Sci. Southern Section, 45.*

Rolfsman, L., & Borgqvist, M. (2014). *Changes of the refrigeration system in the dairy section of a Supermarket-Field measurements.* Paper presented at the 3rd IIR International Conference on Sustainability and the Cold Chain, London, UK.

RPF. (2016). Fermeture des meubles réfrigérés: du positif pour les clients. *La Revue Pratique du Froid et du Conditionnement d'Air,* 26-28.

Sagoo, S., Little, C., Allen, G., Williamson, K., & Grant, K. (2007). Microbiological safety of retail vacuum-packed and modified-atmosphere-packed cooked meats at end of shelf life. *Journal of Food Protection, 70*(4), 943–951. doi:10.4315/0362-028X-70.4.943 PMID:17477265

Sharkey, P. J., & Peggie, I. D. (1984). Effects of high-humidity storage on quality, decay and storage life of cherry, lemon and peach fruits. *Scientia Horticulturae, 23*(2), 181–190. doi:10.1016/0304-4238(84)90022-0

Stoecker, W. F. (1998). *Industrial refrigeration handbook* (Vol. 10). New York, NY: McGraw-Hill.

Tassou, S. A., Ge, Y., Hadawey, A., & Marriott, D. (2011). Energy consumption and conservation in food retailing. *Applied Thermal Engineering, 31*(2–3), 147–156. doi:10.1016/j.applthermaleng.2010.08.023

Vallée, C. (2015). *Energy saving potential at partial load for vertical glass door refrigerated display cabinets.* Paper presented at the 24th IIR International Congress of Refrigeration, Yokohama, Japan.

Van Den Berg, L., & Lentz, C. P. (1977). Effects of relative humidity on storage life of vegetable. *Acta Horticulturae,* (62): 197–208. doi:10.17660/ActaHortic.1977.62.20

Wells, J. H., & Singh, R. (1989). A quality-based inventory issue policy for perishable foods. *Journal of Food Processing and Preservation, 12*(4), 271–292. doi:10.1111/j.1745-4549.1989.tb00086.x

Willocx, F., Hendrick, M., & Tobback, P. (1994). A preliminary survey into the temperature conditions and residence time distribution of minimally processed MAP vegetables in Belgian retail display cabinets. *International Journal of Refrigeration, 17*(7), 436–444. doi:10.1016/0140-7007(94)90003-5

Wu, X., Chang, Z., Yuan, P., Lu, Y., Ma, Q., & Yin, X. (2014). The optimization and effect of back panel structure on the performance of refrigerated display cabinet. *Food Control, 40*, 278–285. doi:10.1016/j.foodcont.2013.12.009

Yu, K. Z., Ding, G. L., & Chen, T. J. (2009). A correlation model of thermal entrainment factor for air curtain in a vertical open display cabinet. *Applied Thermal Engineering, 29*(14–15), 2904–2913. doi:10.1016/j.applthermaleng.2009.02.016

Zhijuan, C., Xuehong, W., Yanli, L., Qiuyang, M., & Wenhui, Z. (2013). Numerical simulation on the food package temperature in refrigerated display cabinet influenced by indoor environment. *Advances in Mechanical Engineering, 5*, 708–785. doi:10.1155/2013/708785

ADDITIONAL READING

Amin, M., Dabiri, D., & Navaz, H. K. (2011). Comprehensive study on the effects of fluid dynamics of air curtain and geometry, on infiltration rate of open refrigerated cavities. *Applied Thermal Engineering, 31*(14-15), 3055–3065. doi:10.1016/j.applthermaleng.2011.05.039

ASHRAE. (2010). *ASHRAE Handbook: Refrigeration.* Atlanta, GA: American Society of Heating, Refrigerating and Air-Conditioning Engineers.

D'Agaro, P., Cortella, G., & Croce, G. (2006). Two-and three-dimensional CFD applied to vertical display cabinets simulation. *International Journal of Refrigeration, 29*(2), 178–190. doi:10.1016/j.ijrefrig.2005.06.007

Hadawey, A. F., Jaber, T. J., Ghaffar, W. A., & Hasan, A. H. A. M. (2012). Air curtain design optimization of refrigerated vertical display cabinet using CFD. *International Journal of Scientific Engineering and Technology, 1*(4), 76–88.

Hale, E. T., Macumber, D. L., Long, N. L., Griffith, B. T., Benne, K. S., Pless, S. D., & Torcellini, P. A. (2008). *Technical Support Document: Development of the Advanced Energy Design Guide for Grocery Stores--50% Energy Savings*. Golden, CO: National Renewable Energy Laboratory. doi:10.2172/939005

Laguerre, O., Hoang, H. M., & Flick, D. (2013). Experimental investigation and modelling in the food cold chain: Thermal and quality evolution. *Trends in Food Science & Technology, 29*(2), 87–97. doi:10.1016/j.tifs.2012.08.001

Mercier, S., Villeneuve, S., Mondor, M., & Uysal, I. (2017). Time–Temperature Management Along the Food Cold Chain: A Review of Recent Developments. *Comprehensive Reviews in Food Science and Food Safety, 16*(4), 647–667. doi:10.1111/1541-4337.12269

Smale, N. J., Moureh, J., & Cortella, G. (2006). A review of numerical models of airflow in refrigerated food applications. *International Journal of Refrigeration, 29*(6), 911–930. doi:10.1016/j.ijrefrig.2006.03.019

KEY TERMS AND DEFINITIONS

Air Curtain: An air jet used to protect products stored in a refrigerated display cabinet from infiltration of warmer and humid external ambient air. For a vertical multi-deck display cabinet, which is widely used, the jet flows from discharge air grille at the top to return air grille at the bottom.

Air Infiltration: An entrainment of external air into a system.

Chilling Damage: An injury of fresh/chilled food produce that exposes to too low temperatures.

Closed Refrigerated Display Cabinet: A refrigerated display cabinet equipped with (glass/solid) doors used to display (chilled/frozen) food products for sale in a retail store/supermarkets.

Cold Chain: A supply chain in which perishable products (food, vaccines, etc.) are preserved under temperature-controlled environment from production to consumption.

Defrosting: A process to remove frost which deposits on surfaces of heat exchanger/evaporator/cooling coil of refrigeration equipment.

Heat Extraction Rate: A rate of heat or thermal loads removed by heat exchanger/evaporator/cooling coil per unit time.

Open Refrigerated Display Cabinet: A refrigerated display cabinet with air curtain and without another physical barrier between the product and the customer.

This research was previously published in Novel Technologies and Systems for Food Preservation edited by Pedro Dinis Gaspar and Pedro Dinho da Silva; pages 1-23, copyright year 2019 by Engineering Science Reference (an imprint of IGI Global).

Chapter 6

Nanocomposites in the Food Packaging Industry:
Recent Trends and Applications

Dheeraj Kumar
National Institute of Technology, Durgapur, India

Md. Farrukh
Echelon Institute of Technology, India

Nadeem Faisal
ITM University, Gwalior, India

ABSTRACT

The recent innovations in nanomaterials for the food packaging industry over the conventional food packaging material have made for a better quality of food product. The use of biodegradable materials is environmentally friendly and suitable for maintaining the quality of food. The chapter focuses on nano-composite materials that enhance the antimicrobial, mechanical, thermal, as well as barrier properties against the migrating element in the food packaging system. Bio-composite derivatives such as PLA, PCL, starch and cellulose, protein derivatives of nanocomposite materials have also been discussed in the chapter along with nano-sensors. Aspects of safety for human and environments and need for regulations of hazard assessment for safety purpose for the food packaging have also been discussed in this chapter. The chapter concludes by discussing the use of nanomaterials applications in food packaging for developing countries, forming some conclusions and leaving readers with thoughts for future research directions.

INTRODUCTION TO FOOD PACKAGING

Packing has been an essential aspect for the human being for a thousand years. When people started going from one place to another place, they felt the need for packing of the food products. The packaging concept lacked almost a hundred years ago, and food packaging industries were quick to realize this and

DOI: 10.4018/978-1-7998-5354-1.ch006

took the opportunity to fill the gap. Nowadays, the packaging is an essential need of the society, because it encompasses, and protects the goods. The importance of the packaging concept does not need to be justified, or it can be said that its values hardly needs stressing. The reason behind it is that no one can think of selling a product of food items without its packaging. However, knowing all about the importance of packaging and its role, it is quite common to observe, that people still have the mindset that the cost of the packing material is unnecessary and often the price of a product which is high just because of its packaging is taken as a negative aspect by the society. This is only due to the gap or lack of information about what a packaging performs. The people are not known for this information, or maybe because of misunderstanding and lack of information, consumers mostly concentrate on the end-product rather than the packaging of materials. At an earlier time, people were using skins, leaves, and bark materials for the packaging purpose of the food products (Driscoll rh et al., 1999).

The packaging concept holds a significant position in the food processing unit. Now in the present time, much progress, developments have been made in the food packaging industry. It can also be said that in the last three decades, the concept of packaging has been increased in a large volume and is also quite diversified (Coles R et al., 2003). For extending the life of the food product, i.e., Shelf-life, too much innovative idea has been applied in the packaging materials. The packaging is a socio, logical, and scientific discipline of thought which guarantees delivery of products to a consumer who needs those merchandise in the best condition suitable for their utilization. This concept of packing includes a package of food products in the form of pouches, bags, cups, trays, cans, tubes, bottles, or it may contain any container to perform some specific task function to protect the food products. From a survey, which was conducted in the United States, it has been shown that approximately 72% peoples are there in the United States of America who can pay extra money for the freshness of the food products, which have the assured certification of healthy food products and will not harm anymore. So, the concept of food packaging is growing hugely, and a lot of research work is going on for its development and providing better shelf-life of food products for the satisfaction of consumers.

PACKAGING AND PRESERVATION

It is a well-known fact that drying and freezing are the direct approaching techniques for the preservation of foods. Some other methods are there, which are quite necessary to be implemented for the packaging and preservation of food products. The indirect methods are also crucial factors to avoid the phenomenon of contamination or recontamination. These indirect tools are packaging concept and quality management which needs implementation.

Nevertheless, these techniques do not come in the category of food preservation techniques (Rahman et al., 1999). They are giving important consideration for maintaining the quality of the foods most securely and are also quite healthy. There are mainly five functions of the packaging concept. They are also known as (5Ps): and collectively called product containment, preservation, and quality, presentation and convenience, protection, and provide storage history (Figure 1).

Product Containment

The capability of containment and its protection is the first and most important function of the packaging concept. It can be easily explained the reason why the liquids, semiliquid, and powders, etc. like products

Figure 1. 5Ps of Food Packaging

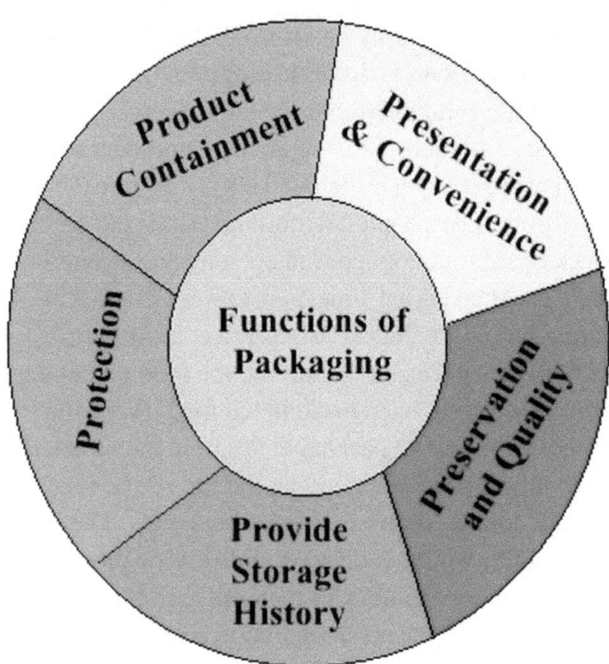

cannot be marketed without any packaged products. So, for packaging, it needs some containers of some desired quality according to the product kept within the package. So, it results that all the food products must be contained before storing and moving from one place to some other place. Containment talks only about the concept of holding product items compatible with transport also, and protection refers to the prevention against the deterioration of food products (Miltz et al., 1992).

Preservation by Maintaining Quality

The second most important function of the packaging is all about the maintenance of the food product and the local surroundings of its environment. The main objective is to provide enhanced storage life and safety issues. Three factors govern the products shelf-life; they are characteristics of the foods, their properties, and storage with the conditions of distribution for any individual packaging. The reactions which are going inside the packaging system deteriorate the quality of the food products inside the package. Moreover, these reactions include the following: chemical, physical, enzymatic, micro-biological changes occurred. Some other reasons may be due to the presence of insects, pesticides, and rodents also.

Presentation and Convenience

The third one conceptual function is about the presentation and its convenience. The labels which are available on the food items must have to follow the rules of the organizations of the food industry. These labels give essential information about the products so that the customers who are willing to buy that product can make it. However, customers need some attractiveness as well as the assurance of that product regarding health. A food package can be turned into a compelling package as it needs the presence of well-conditioned and its publicity of the product materials.

Convenience

For a food product, it should fulfill the need of the current, as well as that of future meeting style, and is demanding as per the society. Moreover, some other parameters decide the conveniences of the product. Those are opening, closing, enclosable, tamper-proof, smaller portions. The important thing is about the adaptation of the package size as per the needs of the consumer (size of the family, individuals, special sizes for the food delivery service) are important steps taken by the industries to enhance the conveniences of the food product with the help of packaging. Self-heating containers have already been developed only to provide convenience to the customers. There is no need to heat that food product before consumption again, so it provides convenience in this manner.

Protection during Processing and Distribution

The fourth important function in the food packaging is about protecting at the time when the product is transiting to the customer. Packing is an essential part of the distribution process. So, when the product is going to be delivered to the concern customers, at that time its main objective is to provide the facilities like handling and transportation. It is only the packing which can accept the challenges like heating, humidity or dew, etc. So, there is a need to be aware of the challenges that occurred while distribution, and how to design a comfortable package that fits suitable for that food product. A particular type of frame is there, which provides a base for the carrying purpose of packets.

Provide Storage History

An important consideration for the prediction of microbial concentration and other related parameters responsible for the quality of food products known as Time-temperature indicator (TTI). TTI has been divided into three parts according to the responsive mechanism. They are as follows: (i) Biological (ii) chemical (iii) physical systems. Two key issues are considered during the distribution chain. The first one is economics, and the second is about knowing food products. It should have a better understanding of the degradation kinetics of the products. It will elaborate on the things that how the quality characteristics of the product change and, accordingly the behavior related to time-temperature exposure.

IDEAL PACKAGING

There are no such conditions that exist which represent the ideal packaging. However, it can be tried to come closer to the conditions related to the ideal packaging. So, these are the criteria for an ideal packaging. They are as follows:

- Zero levels of toxicity behavior
- Higher visibility of the food product

- Marketing appeal should be powerful
- Ability to control the moisture and gas content
- Performance should be stable even at a high-temperature zone of working
- Readily available and having low-cost material
- Easy handling machines and low friction coefficient
- It should be properly labeled
- Migration resistant package
- Controlled transmission of the unwanted gases and particles
- It should be protected from the loss of flavor and odor also
- Having suitable mechanical strength properties
- Advanced closure characteristics like; opening, sealing, pouring, and resealing

TYPES OF PACKAGING MATERIAL USED FOR FOODS

At the earlier stage, the materials used for packaging were usually skins, leaves. And barks. However, nowadays, in the industry of food packaging, it has been observed that regarding the materials selections for the food packaging, a lot of developments and research work has been made in order to improve the quality of packing materials for foods. The main objective for materials selection is only to provide diversified materials and equipment, also having desired properties as per the requirement. For the classification of materials for packaging purposes, it has been divided into two parts; rigid and another of flexible type. There are some examples like plastic films, foil, textiles, papers come into the category of flexible nature and woods, glasses, metals, and plastic of hard materials are examples of rigid type packing. For the selection of proper material type as per the requirement, it is vital to consider the properties which needed as a barrier, mechanical, chemical, physical, optical, transport properties, and all.

METALS

For food packaging, the use of metal containers is considered as the most suitable materials. These materials provide almost all the desired properties which should be made available for food packaging. Those properties are mechanically strength behavior, barrier property, impermeable towards mass transfer and also to light, having good conductivity of heat, having the capability to resist high temperature, etc. Considering its opacity property, it is suitable for food products having light sensitivity, but on the other side, the contents inside the package are not visible. However, there are some more disadvantages to these metals can containers. It costs too much high as compared to other materials; mass is also dense, tending to react with the food products inside the metal container and also with an environmental condition resulting like corrosion in it is inside and outside surface.

Under the category of metals, mainly *Tinplate. Steel, Aluminum* is the most useful cans and canister used. The central concept of using metals as a packaging material is to ensure that the product which is kept inside the metal can is stable and seal given to it is complete. One thing significant for the manufacturing of the cans is coating or lacquering materials used. The lacquer is a type of resin material. Some of the examples of it are; acrylic materials having more resistive power towards to sustain in the high-temperature zones, phenolic, polybutadiene, oleo resinous, alkyd, and vinyl resins. In the present age of technologies used for coating materials, there are almost 200 different kinds of protective coatings available to use. If we talk about the thickness of the tin coatings, then its units are expressed in terms of pounds per base box (lb/bb). Food packaging book. The technique was used before 50 years back for the coating of steel plate surface with the tin material was "hot dip" method, and nowadays it has been changed with the technique of electrolytic deposition method. The main advantage of using this technique is that it provides a more uniform tin coating surface with less consumption per unit area. The disadvantage of using the tin coating technique is that if any small gaps are present there, then it will lead to the formation of the corrosion phenomenon.

Furthermore, after corrosion, it produces gases like hydrogen, which can make a possibility of a blow of can. The size of the can is being standardized specified by organizations. And criteria for the selection of cans are steel bae specification, a thin layer thickness of the tin coating, and type of channels, also the geometry of cans.

Now among metal packaging materials, the second priority comes to aluminum. The lightweight properties of the aluminum make this possibility. There are more desirable properties of aluminum, which enable it to be a good packing material of food products. They are optimum cost, resistive of corrosion, easy availability in nature, and most important is of recyclable property. Alumina does not have any need for protective coating material additionally to protect corrosion. This is because of the formation of the thin layer of aluminum oxide because this layer protects the parent materials for further corrosion when it comes into contact with oxygen.

Nevertheless, it is attacked by alkali metals. The disadvantage of using aluminum is that the cost is too high as compared to tinplate, but is lighter in weight. Aluminum is found in two categories in the packing materials. The first form is used as cans for packing of mainly beers and soft beverages. The second form is like aluminum foils. However, the purest form of aluminum is of ductile foil type, which is used for laminations of food products.

GLASS

A packaging material as glass containers is considered as the most renowned packaging means. It is mostly preferred for the packaging of wines, liqueurs, perfumes, and cosmetics items. The properties that make it enable to be favorable material for packaging. Those are its highly inert behavior, impermeable to vapors and gases also, and can behavior to any shape and size, i.e., easy to go for different shaping. There are so many benefits of glass as packing material. Those properties are mentioned below: transparent, but also can be given to any color as per the desire. Inert, impermeable nature, rigidness, thermal resistive, fits for the general consumer appeal, the most important thing is that it has selective light protection qualities. If it is focused on the compositions of the glass materials, then it is found that the bottle includes 68-73% of SiO_2. 12-15% of Na_2O, 10-13% CaO, and it has lesser proportions for the other oxides. Glass materials have better barrier properties for oxygen molecules, and it is entirely neutral when it comes to direct contact with the food particles. These days it can be a concluding remark about the glass materials is that it can be recycled again and again. However, it has also some disadvantages. They are brittleness, heavyweight, and it requires more energy to be manufactured. Glass can be recycled, but it has some difficulty in re-use. So, recycling is economically viable and technically also.

PAPER

For packaging purposes, paper products are used these days broadly. The use of paper bags for packaging materials is from the long term ago around the seventeenth century. Paper is defined in terms of its dimensional property, i.e., the sheet thickness is less than 0.23 mm, and following the weight, it is lighter than 220 g/m^2. The production of the paper and board materials are done from woods, rags, and other waste material. Firstly, it is treated so that it can be broken the lignin structure with the help of calcium bisulfite or using caustic soda. For a while, the paper material is decomposed first with the technique of bacterial action. As we can count this paper in the category of environment-friendly. But nowadays, due to the excessive use of plastic material for packaging application paper material is facing much competition in packing material in an open market.

The main advantages are low costing, readily anywhere available, lightweight, ability to print on itself, also having mechanical strength. However, due to some challenging problem of its property that the paper material is facing is turned into its disadvantage. Furthermore, those are low strength, resistive for water and gas (moisture). These disadvantages can be reduced up to more extent with some applications and treatments. Like, its nature towards moisture, i.e., its permeable nature for moisture and fat, can be minimized with a wax coating on its surface. The most markable thing is that now a day's paper is still used in the second priority for packaging, e.g., cardboard boxes or cartoon are the best examples of it.

PLASTICS

The most popular material used in these days in the food packaging industry is polymers. It was first in 1939 when the plastic material is entered into commercialized production. The reason behind its popularity for packaging purposes is its diverse nature and having broad-spectrum properties. Even more, plastics have unique qualities like, cheaper than other packing materials, can be easily shaped and processing is effortless, light in weight, very comfortable to seal, transparency or opaque. Plastics containers can be made of any shapes and sizes. The good thing is that their cost is too much lesser than the metals, glasses. If it is compared with the paper materials, then its density is higher than of it, but its density is lesser than half of the glass and aluminum density. The most relevant aspect of research work, which is going on currently is about the transport property in food packaging for the polymeric materials. Although metals and glasses do not show the behavior of permeability, polymers show their permeable nature for small particles. There are two limitations while using polymers as packing materials. They are permeability to gases and vapors, and another one is the migration of the packaged materials to the food products.

SHORTCOMINGS OF EXISTING PACKAGING MATERIALS: OPPORTUNITIES FOR NANOTECHNOLOGY

The concept of food packaging has been evolved its response towards the continuous development in the sector of materials science and technology. It is changing day per day according to the need of consumer's demand. In the present economy of the global world, the concept of packaging is not only to provide the effective distribution and food preservation assurance, but it is also concerned about communication and facilitation to their convenient end-use at all level of consumers who are using it.

The use of non-biodegradable based plastic materials for the food packaging application has brought a concerned issue of environmental problems of waste disposal. Day by day increasing demand for the quality improvement for the food products is the major key factor for the increasing rate of rapid development in the sector of biodegradable based nanomaterials for food packaging (Cutter, N.C. 2006)

The industries of food packaging are facing challenging problems in the sector of food technology. These problems are due to the lacking behavior of essential properties, and their absence made some opportunities for their innovations. If we try to enlist those needful properties that they are lacking can be listed as: (i) production materials are of non-sustainable type (ii) absence of the property like recycling (iii) not fulfilling the properties like such strength of mechanically and also barrier properties (Akbari, Z et al.,2007)

It is a well-known fact that about the plastics materials and metals that they have sufficient barrier properties to restrict the mass transfer of unwanted particles, which leads to the toxic behavior in food particles. However, their degradation is not possible in a biotic manner, and they are responsible for an unhealthy environment. Plastic materials are still accessible for the food packaging these days, also up to a percentage of 40% (Rhim, J.-W 2013). Because of their property of lightweight materials, formability, cost adequacy, and adaptable attributes. However, most of the food packaging materials come into the category of petroleum-based and which are non-sustainable if we consider the parameter of supply standpoint. The result is that the current scenario of North America is that out of the total amount of the municipal solid waste generated consists of 30% of the waste packaging materials, pressed the environmental issue. On the other side, if we talk about the barrier properties of water vapor and gases, then these packaging materials show weak behavior towards the barrier (Arvanitoyannis, I. S., & Bosnea, L. A., 2001). For example, packaging of live foods such as; green vegetables, fruits, and fresh products requires materials that permit O_2 through the package and behaves as permeable transmission materials having an optimal rate of transfer. However, processed products do not exhibit these types of mass transfer phenomena. Here, the most challenging thing is about barrier properties. The question arises here on how to ensure the availability of such thermoplastics, which have suitable matching barrier properties according to the specific kind of products? It is all about to increase the shelf life of the food products in contact with such thermoplastics. But to get rid of this problem, it has been developed the properties inside materials to expand their functional behavior like the thermoplastics, and for this polymer blends and multi-layered composite-like structure have been developed. The problem is remained unsolved due to the problem of costlier materials and also facing difficulty in recycling the material as mentioned above type properties. These days, manufacturers of the food products are facing trouble to set a balance between both the requirements of the society. It is about to get enough shelf-life for the product to be prepared with the best quality as well as a matter of the safety of the food products and consumers also. These problems are concerned about the countries which are now in the condition of the underdeveloped countries due to which they have no such technological development in regards to the distribution of foods and infrastructures for the preservation the food products.

There are some critical issues related to safety concerns and the quality of food products. Moreover, in the current scenario, there is an urgent need to overcome these lacking properties so that it should be clarified about their quality assurance of foods. They are listed below: (i) expansion of microorganism because of pollution and temperature abusement (ii) Due to the oxidation phenomenon, it has been noticed a decrement in the quality of nutritional amounts. (iii) Naturally, the interactions of the food particles with the solar light, oxygen content, and aqua particles used to change some of its intrinsic behavior and the resulting loss of organoleptic, i.e., qualities related to the nutrition system. So, the drawbacks, as mentioned earlier, are existing shortcomings that have to remove. So it can be assured 100% for the quality assurance of the food products as well as for human health. Over the previous decade, a lot of research work and development is being carried out for the use of nanocomposites in the sector of food packaging applications.

INNOVATIVE FOOD PACKAGING

During the storage and distribution of food products, food packaging technology provides us with protection and containment of the foods. This technology helps to keep away from the unwanted materials that may harm or can change the quality of the product. The unfavorable conditions may be in the category of the water vapor, released gases, orders, mechanical shocks, vibrations that may occur inside them, born microorganism, etc. (Duncan, T. V. 2011).

In modern society, due to complexity like human beings and their ongoing busy-life food manufacturers and industries are more concerned about the development process of the packaging concept system. They are continuously making an effort to add up more enhanced and convenience features according to the demand and also suitable for the safety issues of the food products, human beings, and environment. Orders, mechanical shocks, vibrations that may occur inside them, born microorganism, etc. (Lim, L. T. 2011).

There is great importance to innovations in the food packaging industry. These innovations in the packaging industries of food products have made a variety of new terms related to the aspects of safety, the shelf life of the food products, and the food product convenience. The surrounding climate of the sustenance inside the packaged product has a significant impact on the period of the product, i.e., shelf-life of the product. So, the principles needed to be followed while packaging products for maintaining the inside environment healthy for food products and better preservation are classified as; (i) passive, (ii) active, and (iii) intelligent packaging (also called sometimes smart packaging). The active system packaging itself consists of two types of packaging concepts; they are simple and advanced packing system. Moreover, the intelligent packing system itself includes two other types of packing concept. They are termed as simple and interactive packing system.

Passive Packing System

It is defined as a packaging system of the passive type, which provides a barrier physically in between the food product and the surrounding environment around it inside the package. They are supposed to protect the food in a possessive way.

If we consider the conventional type of packaging system for food products, then most of them come into the category of the passive packing system. Examples of the passive packing systems are metal cans, glass, bottles, many more of the packing materials, which shows its flexible nature provides the same physical barrier in between the food products and the environment around it inside the packaging. This passive packaging system ensures the migrations that usually happen with the food products when coming in contact with the packing materials. So, the passive system provides prevention of coming in contact with the environment properties and the agents which are contained in the same environment. In a general way, the expectations from this packing system are to get maximum protection of the food products, but the fact is that it is not more responsive to the properties of the container.

In these days, the development work has been going on for the generation of newer coating materials for the polymeric containers and films also. Here, the question arises that why only these coatings are focused on implementing in container body? The reason behind this is that they have full control over the permeability of the migrative agents, which raises safety issues of the food products and also shows a negative impact on the shelf-life of the food products stored inside the container.

Active Packaging

An active packaging system can get information about whatever changes are going inside the environment of packaging products. It sends the feedback regarding this change through its sensing device. This packaging system is supposed to provide full protection as well as the preservation of the foods with the help of some intrinsic/extrinsic mechanism factors. It is defined as the packing, which helps to modify or extend the life span of that food product and gives more safety concerns about the food product as well as human health.

Simple Active Packing

A food packing system that does not include the presence of a functioning ingredient or effectively functional polymer is termed as a simple active packing system. An active system shows its response to any changes that are going within the food packaging due to the transfer mechanism of the materials to the food particle.

There is a kind of active packing system which is called modified atmosphere packing (MAP). It has been defined as a packing technique in such a way that it provides a modified atmosphere in comparison to the surrounding air composition. A very quiet natural definition of it is that it includes both kinds of packing behavior like; vacuum packing and (controlled atmosphere packing (CAP). So the most accurate definition comes for the MAP is "providing and continuously improved the environment in which the proportion of air is as per the desired nature of food within the package. Initially, the product is kept in the desired mixture of gases, and its composition depends on the type of food product, the packaging material, its average life-span, and the storage atmosphere. So, it can be added a remarkable point that whatever is the atmospheric condition within the package is mostly the outcomes of the result of the respiratory result as formed by the food products, selectively permeable, and the presence of added modifiers.

An example of a MAP system is about packing films that help to fulfill the desired atmospheric condition in maintaining the concentration of O_2 and CO_2 for the vegetables and fruits packaging. For categorize, the product type which falls under this category is the products of dairy, bakery, meats, and muttons, poultry items, fishes, and fresh green vegetables and fruits.

Advance Active Packing

An advanced active system is a type of packing system which contains polymers having actively functional behavior or having some active ingredients. In this packaging system, advance principles are being used in the packaging material. Those principles are listed below: (i) atmosphere modifiers (ii) absorber particles of O_2 molecules (iii) CO_2 generators and the absorber particles (iv) moisture regulators and ethylene absorber particles. The advanced active system of packaging has divided into two categories of the packaging system. The oxygen scavenging action for the food packaging is an excellent example of a system, which can absorb the unwanted foreign particles generated within the packaging environment when it comes to the contact of the food particle.

MAP system is another excellent example of the advance active packing system. It provides a barrier property to maintain that level of steady-state condition of the inside atmosphere proportion of air properties together with released gas due to the presence of food particles.

For the removal of oxygen, iron oxidation is used. Similarly, it is imperative to remove ethylene from the packaged material for the prevention of accelerated ripening effects. This ethylene is being removed by adding some active carbon content, or it can also be done by the oxidation phenomenon by $KMnO_4$. Similarly, cyclodextrin is the most emerging material for the scavenger of unwanted particles present during the storage of food items. The development of antioxidant film properties of protecting the shelf-life of the food product can be a significant factor in improving the attributes related to sensing issues inside the packaging products.

Intelligent Packaging

A packing system which exhibits the properties sends the feedback or information of the changing environmental condition and take corrective action to protect the food products during storage is called an intelligent packaging system. The identification of the intelligent packing system is to continuously enhance the aspects of the communication, i.e. feedback response of a package. So that it can be known about the situations inside the package about food quality in real-time. This intelligent packing gives an investigation report regarding the dating approach of "Best Before" and "Use by."

The feedback response of the intelligent packing system not only gives the information regarding the safety and product quality but also can be useful for the manufacturers to make decisions for the support system to verify questions like when and what steps should be taken in order to make the distribution of the entire product channel and production process.

So, there are some primary objectives of the intelligent packing system which has been enlisted below:

1. More improvement in the quality-based and product value of food materials.
2. Increased convenience manner
3. To bring the changes in the permeability properties of the gas
4. It should be assurance regarding the protection against additional effects like; tampering, counterfeiting, and theft.

The intelligent packing has provided some additional properties for an effective packing system. It includes oxygen indicators, can detect the pathogenic micro-organism and spoilage phenomenon, indicators giving information of the time, temperature and humidity inside the package. It also gives information about freshness providing real-time data of storage and distribution. A temperature indicating labels has been attached to the packaged external surface. It also gives information about the limit of the maximum temperature that has been exposed to the outer surface. It also has a component of the internal indicator having information about the current level of gas inside the packaging. These indicators are for monitoring the level of oxygen (O_2) and carbon dioxide (CO_2). To get the information regarding the contents of the food product, weight, locations, and timing throughout the channel distribution, it has been attached a Radio Frequency Identification (RFID). In the future, it may be possible to attach RFID levels for every food product. A schematic figure is shown in figure 2.

Figure 2. Nanotechnology development and its implication in active and intelligent packaging

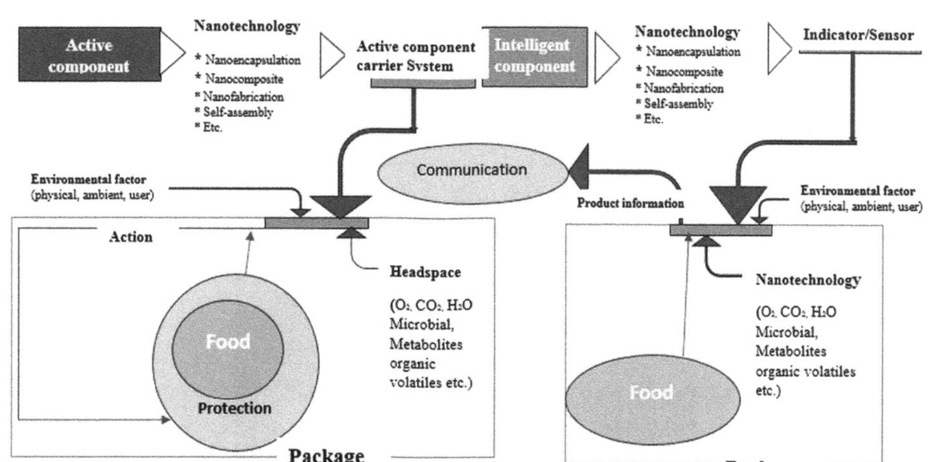

DEVELOPMENTS OF NANOCOMPOSITE FOR ENHANCED MECHANICAL AND BARRIER PROPERTIES FOR FOOD PACKAGING

Nanomaterials are known only due to their unique functional properties. It has a much larger surface to mass ratio as compared to larger-sized bulk materials. Nanocomposites are being incorporated with the polymer matrix to that substance due to their higher value of the surface area. Moreover, this increased surface area favors the filler-matrix, which is interacting in between and improving its performance. For the development of barrier properties introduction of nonreinforcement has been done, which provides a small barrier for the gases by complicating the path of that materials (Figure 3 & Figure 4).

Figure 3. Nanomaterials as building blocks for enhancing the mechanical strength

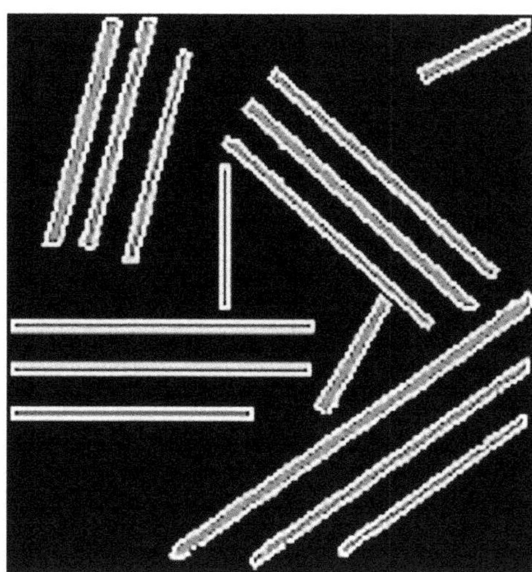

Figure 4. Nanomaterials providing plentiful surface area for filler matrix

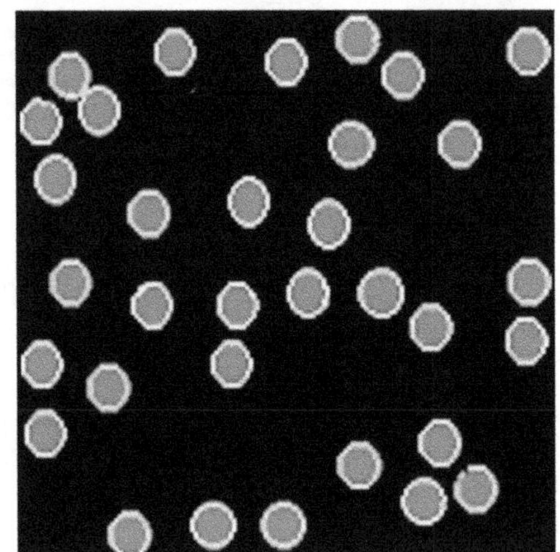

Barrier Protection

The protection of food products can be done by maintaining an inert and having a low oxygen content atmosphere within the packaging bags. This inert behavior of the inside environment provides a barrier to the exchange of gases. This barrier results accurately and provide a healthy environment and maintain the quality of food with the help of clays. The antimicrobial packaging concept terminates the formation of the bacterial growth and fungal organism or any pathogens and toxins inside the package. These antimicrobials are formed with the help of silver oxide, titanium oxide, and zinc oxide, or it may be other bio-nano particles or nano-composite material.

NANO-BASED SENSORS

Sensors are the devices that can be used to detect any changes that have been occurred in the system boundary of food packaging. These changes might be possibly related to the physical, mechanical, chemical one. So. The sensors detect that changes occurred within the environment of the food packaging system and convert these changes into some readable form of observable signals. In this way, sensors regulate all its internal environment of the foodstuffs and its properties are continuously sensed and indicated by sensors. These changes belong to temperature, humidity, levels of oxygen content, degradation of food products and contamination of microbial organisms.

When the nano-based sensors are being used in an integrated form with the food packaging, then it is quite easily possible to detect specific compounds, pathogens available, toxins, to eliminate the inaccuracy in expiration dates, to provide the real-time data for fresh products of foods.

There are some of the examples of sensors that are being used for food packaging. A most popular type of metal oxide gas sensor is used due to its high sensitiveness and stable nature. Conducting polymer nanocomposites (CPC) or metal oxides are one of the useful sensors used in food packaging for the identification of gas emissions due to micro-organism. TiO_2, SnO_2, are some examples of O_2 indicating sensors. The color response plays here an important role in sensing the O_2 exposed. So, it is bleached when it has not been exposed and blue when being exposed.

The current packaging concept is fulfilled with the oxygen scavengers, moisture absorbers, smart barrier packing. Moreover, for bakery and meat products, the pacing concepts are enabled with nano-enabled sensing elements continuously giving updates regarding the inside environment of packing. Not even this, nowadays nanosensors also gives the information related to the shelf life of the food products.

EXTENSION OF SHELF-LIFE OF FOOD PRODUCTS USING SILVER NANOPARTICLES AND NANOCOMPOSITES AS ANTI-MICROBIAL FOOD PACKAGING MATERIALS

After long-term research work, it has been observed and concluded that silver particles could perform itself as an antimicrobial agent in the food industry and also have applications like beverage storage. In ancient times silver made vessels have been used for the storage of wines and water. Russian MIR space stations were using silver as a sterilization agent for water. For the developing countries, silver's property of behaving like broad-spectrum antimicrobial and also relatively lower cost than others made it possible as an active disinfecting agent treated for water.

Silver particles dominate other anti-microbial agents. It is only due to its additional properties, and they are (i) self-stable (ii) having a broad spectrum (iii) effective at penetrating biofilms (iv) effective bactericides. Silver behaves like an anti-microbial agent, which prevents the growth of microbes. It has been found that silver nanoparticles (AgNPs) serve as potent agents against bacteria species. It has also been observed that AgNPs are very effective against the strains of an organism, which shows its resistive nature towards the potent chemical antimicrobials. It is a well-known fact that inorganic nanoparticles have some more advantages than the molecular antimicrobials. Furthermore, this is possible only due to the controlled release of the AgNPs. So, it can be concluded that AgNPs/polymer nanocomposites can be applicable in both the medical unit devices as well as for food packaging materials to increase the shelf-life in a preservative manner.

AgNPs nanocomposite material offers more stability and has some relaxed release of silver ions into the food products. Another polysaccharide named chitosan, if it is loaded with the AgNPs, then it has some more tensile strength and better gas barrier properties developed. Similarly, AgNPs proportions are there in the Chinese jujube fruits, which are stored in storage bags. On keeping the fresh melon cutting stored in the pads of AgNPs contains cellulose, then it has been lowered the counts of microbial growth.

Application Polymeric Nanocomposites as Anti-Microbial Properties

Polymer nanocomposite materials help a lot in controlling the growth of microorganisms inside the food packaged material. It becomes possible due to the desirable property of structural integrity and barrier properties, which is imparted by the polymeric matrix. It also enhances the antimicrobial properties due to the agents, which have already been embedded within it. Nanocomposites have a higher ratio of surface to volume, that is why they can attach themselves with more number of biological molecules. It leads to a higher value of efficiency when it is compared with its microscale counterparts. These materials are versatile so that it can be used in numerous means as antibiotic carriers, killing agents, or inhibitors, which helps in growing. (Shankar et al., 2016). Various research work has been enhanced its properties like; it has been noticed an increased efficacy against Escherichia coli when nanocomposite is with less silver as compared to micro composite with more silver content. (Shyam S. Sablani 2015)

Moreover, it is being concluded that when polyamide 6 is filled with a weight percentage of 2 of Ag-NPs shows a more useful nature against E. coli, even after immersing it into the water for 100 days. It has also been reported that it starts retarding the senescence of jujube, (a Chinese fruit) when PE nanocomposite film is mixed with Ag-NPs.(Emamifar A, 2011).

BIO-NANOCOMPOSITES FOR FOOD PACKAGING APPLICATIONS

Most of the materials used for food packaging comes in the category of non-biodegradable materials category. They are not fulfilling the increased demand of the society and also not so cared about the issues related to the sustainable development and safety of the environment. In order to reduce the dependency of the food packaging materials on fossil fuels, there are more innovative technologies are currently running so that it can be moved to a sustainable type of material. To enhance the quality of food and increase the shelf-life of the food products, a lot of efforts are going on to reduce the waste generations from the food packaging due to its non-biodegradable nature (Avella, M et al., 2005). The disadvantage of using non-biodegradable materials or plastics for packaging purposes is that these products have been derived from petroleum products. It creates a problem of waste disposal. Due to the weak mechanical strength and having not excellent barrier properties the application of biopolymers has been limited. Moreover, the scarcity of the desired property can be enhanced by the addition of reinforced nano-sized particles (Tang et al., 2012).

The establishment of the nanocomposite material has been done to improve the mechanical as well as barrier properties of the biopolymers for the food packaging. Bio-composites are multiphase-materials which have the continuous phase of the two or more constituent particles and having a discontinuity in nanofillers (<100 nm). The role of the nanofillers is more essential to improve the properties like mechanical and barrier. There are some examples of nanofillers (silicates, TiO_2, and clay) that not only improve the property mentioned above but; it offers some more critical functions. They are listed as an antimicrobial agent, bio-based sensor, and lastly, oxygen scavenger. At the earlier days, the application of biopolymers for packaging of food products were starch, cellulose, chitosan, and agar. The origin of the agar was from carbohydrates and gelatin, gluten, alginate, and collagen have been derived from protein. Recently, after a lot of research work, it became possible for bio-degradable polymeric nanocomposites to develop those properties which are more suitable for full applications in the packaging industries.

It can be concluded that for the packaging application, the most suitable biodegradable nanocomposite materials are polylactic acid (PLA), polybutylene succinate (PBS), polyhydroxy butyrate (PHB), aliphatic polyester (PCL) (Rhim, J.-W. et al., 2013).

Application of Bio Nanocomposites for Food Packaging

The extraction of the biodegradable packaging material is done from the resources of bio-based renewables. These materials are generally called as biopolymers having much good barrier and mechanical properties. They degrade biologically at the end of their life. These polymers have been evolved as an environmentally friendly substitute option for the non-biodegradable plastic materials for packaging purposes. (Pan et al., 2014).

Among most of the bio-polymers used for food packaging purposes are carbohydrates and their derivatives. Research shows that poor mechanical strength of starch can improved with mixing additives like; plasticizers, nanofillers. (Sorrentino et al., 2007).

Other biopolymer-based research work has been performed with cellulose acetate (Bruna et al., 2014), alginate (Shankar et al., 2016), pectin (Shankar et al., 2016c) synthetic biopolymer as PLA (Conte et al., 2013;), PHA (Bordes et al., 2009), PCL (Gorrasi et al., 2013, and microbial synthesized polymers such as; PBAT (Shankar and Rhim, 2016b)., agar (Orsuwan et al., 2016), chitosan. (Pereda et al., 2014).

PLA Nanocomposites

PLA is the most common bio-based nanocomposite material known for its bio-degradable nature in the environment. The production of the PLA is done from the lactic acid. It is a simple process that is produced through the fermentation process of the carbohydrates originated from plant resources. Some of the examples are sugar beet, molasses, wheat and corn (Sorrentino, A et al., 2007). The advantages are self-biodegradability and can be set as a personalized life span as per the requirements. There are mainly two forms of the lactic acid monomer (L form or D form). The properties of the L type PLA material are that it has a higher value of the melting point and also have higher crystalline behavior, whereas another form is a mixture of D and L- PLA has a lower value of transition temperature comes into the category of an amorphous polymer. So far, the production of the PLA type bio-degradable polyesters for the packaging material have some limitations regarding higher cost, and its performance is not so good.

PCL Nanocomposites

Polycaprolactone (PCL) is manufactured by the process of ring-opening polymerization of ε-caprolactone. This type of polyester has a linear shape and comes in the category of a semi-crystalline polymer. The level of crystallinity is around 50%. At the breaking point, it shows its mechanical behavior like high elongations at breaking point and low modulus value. Nowadays, PCL is getting popular only due to its excellent physical properties and its availability in a commercial manner for commodity application.

Starch Nanocomposites

After excellent research work, it has cleared that for the packaging of food products, Starch is the right choice for its utilization. The properties that enable starch for this capability is possible only due to its eco-considerate compliancy, a more extensive range of availability, cheaper rate. The resistance for the water has enhanced with the addition of matrices of the synthetic polymer and the use of inorganic materials.

Recently investigation has been performed on the blends of starch with the nanoclays. It has been reported from this investigation that it is compatible with food packaging due to its biodegradable nature and versatile applications. It has also been noticed an enhancement regarding its mechanical behavior. The most important thing is that consideration of MMT is responsible for enhanced tensile strength and modulus of elasticity. It has also minimized the chances of absorption of water molecules, and it becomes possible with the presence of MMT in starch. Recent data shows that as the concentration of the ZnO-CMC is increased from 0 to 5% by weight, then it leads an increment of 3.9 to 9.8 MPa in tensile strength, while there is a decrement in the elongation from 42.2% to 25.8%.

Cellulose Nanocomposites

Cellulose is an exceptionally strong natural polymer that exists in nature, and these are the building blocks of the long fibrous materials. The production of cellulose is done sustainably from the biomass and the places from the availability of natural polymers. The properties of the cellulose nanocomposites are so attractive that it makes them accessible in the application of food packaging. They are as follows: Lower cost, very high mechanical strength, the specific surface area is bigger, higher aspect ratio, lower value of density, lower thermal coefficient of expansion, tensile strength is good (Metzger, C. et al., 2018)

Cellulose nanofibrils (CNFs) are efficient nanomaterials because it acts as a barrier protection against the residue of mineral oil and oxygen content also. In a similar way methylcellulose (MC) is derived from the nanocomposites bio-film can minimize the challenging problem related to the environment.

Protein Nanocomposites

In recent years, the research has been focused on enhancing the properties of the protein on the film edible and coatings for the packaging material. These are the proteins that have been obtained from animals and can be utilized commercially. Most of the utilized zones are caseins, collagens, egg white, whey protein, and myofibrillar proteins (Jimenez. A et al., 2018), (Rocha. M et al.,2018)

Protein nanocomposites do not have good resistance ability for moisture content, but it has higher rigidity. Moreover, nowadays, whey protein isolate (WPI) has opted as an edible film as the best option for the food packaging materials (Sanyang M et al., 2018).

Recently, it has been derived from a hydrophobic protein from the corn kernels and named Zein. It has inherent characteristics of film formations. In the sector of food industries, Zein is used as coating substrate materials that have an inbuilt property of the biodegradable polymer. Soy protein is also a type of nanocomposite material when it is filled with nano-cellulose which is originated from a residue of licorice. This gives assurance for the sensitivity towards the water and also to increase mechanical strength (Orsuwan et al., 2018)

SAFETY ASSESSMENT OF NANOMATERIALS IN FOOD PACKAGING

The primary concern about the use of nanocomposite materials is how to ensure customers and environment also about its only global perspectives suitable for food packaging. To ensure its suitability and perfectness, it needs excellent evaluation for its properties and positive response. So, in that direction, research work needs to fulfill five markable questions to ensure that nanocomposite and nanotechnology is the better material technique for food packaging. Those cross-questions are enlisted below:

1. Firstly, how to determine or how to examine the presence of nanomaterials in the sector of food packaging sends potential hazards when they come into direct contact with the oral route? Because it is applicable for all nanoparticles used, so it is not a lack of knowledge issue, but any negative impact on the quality of food will raise the questions of hazards material. So, research needs to think over it seriously to overcome it (Simon. et al., 2008).
2. The second question is concerned about lacking the tools that tell us the exact exposure. That is, if the migration phenomenon is going on, then how much proportion is limited about it? Is it utterly

depending upon the concentration of the nanoparticles or on the number of particles present? Is it related to the size and shape of nanoparticles? So, how hazard type is being characterized? (Teide et al., 2008)

3. The third one is related to surface chemistry. It asks that is it the only reason for unwanted chemical reactions, which is due to the presence of nanomaterials. It is surface chemistry that gives elevation to the migration phenomenon which results in the formation of unwanted products during the fabrication and processing of the packaging materials (Teide et al.,2009).

4. The fourth question is all about what negative impact does nanomaterials shows towards the waste disposal streams. The concept of recycling and reuse, burning for recovery of energy, and lastly, a viable and straightforward arrangement for landfilling. Which option will be better whether the waste disposal system or recycling process? The matter is that when they are allowed for the transformation process, then they will able to retain their behavior like physical, chemical and toxic behavior or not? (Simon P et al.,2008)

5. Last but not least, the fifth point is about the real issues and worries on nanomaterials that they have cast a shadow on the conventional technologies for food packaging. A direct question arises about the differences between the already determined and has permission conventional technology and the novel one. In this manner, where and how the overlapping is happening in conventional technology?

Research only needs the answer to these above mentioned five critical questions to do the hazard assessment and its characterization successfully.

HAZARD ASSESSMENT OF ENGINEERED NANOPARTICLES IN FOOD: NANO-RISK CAT TOOL APPROACH

For the assessment of hazards and exposure potentials due to the presence of the nanomaterials in the food products, a systematic approach has been developed, which is named as a nano-risk Cat tool approach. It gives its analytical results in the form of dot indications. Moreover, all dots have different features related to potential hazards. The three consecutive dots representing for the professional users, for the consumers, and the third one is for the environment. The other two dots used for the denotation of the potential hazards for the human being and environment respectively. This technique can be used for understanding and distinguishing the exposure of known potential hazards, which will be caused due to the application of nanoparticles for food packaging. The essential features of this technique are that in case of where there is a lack of data that hampering the traditional risk assessment procedure. This analysis is only possible when there is the presence of the expert judgments opinion which can give their response based on the dots coming (EFSA., 2011)

The migration phenomenon of the nanocomposites packaging material in contact with the foods is one of the most critical worries for humans. Therefore, issues of health risks come. Furthermore, the effect of toxicity behavior present in the nanomaterials mainly depends upon the fact of how much concentration of food is consumed (Chen et al., 2013).

The researcher's considerations have been pulled towards the safety-related issues for nanocomposites due to their enormous use as a packaging material in the food industry. In the present age of commercialization, worldwide organizations are continuously giving their effort to gather information about the current health and safety risk associated with the use of nanocomposite materials for food packaging and production. These organizations are also concerned about the migration of materials when it comes in contact with the foods.

It can be easily seen from our daily life examples, that how these hazards quite naturally come, that we did not bother about it. Therefore, here are some enlisted examples who are responsible for all these things to happen, which are related to the health issues of human beings. Likewise, a person chewing the gum admitted into his body about 93% of TiO_2 of the nano-sized particle. Because it contains the same proportions into the chewing gum sugar-coated. Similarly, consuming foods that contain E551 allows inhalation of gut epithelium-like materials, which has very much tendency to be exposed towards SiO_2 nanomaterials (Margo et al.2014).

MIGRATION ASSESSMENT

Allergies

Two considerable critical issues show its adverse effects on exposure with nanomaterials are an allergy, and another one is massive metals release. As the food technology has been reached up to the right level of research work, still it cannot be ignored with the fact that the presence of nanoparticles can promote hypersensitive pneumonic inflammation in coming in contact with the food items. Moreover, from the previous research work, it can be revealed that due to their presence, the inflammatory response, and an increment in the ROS production, it has become a typical immune response with the exposure of nanomaterials. Even carbon contained nanomaterials are also responsible for the cause of allergic inflammable. It has also been found in the research work that carbon nanotubes of a single and multi-walled type tend to increase the lung type inflammation. A specific type of allergen level of IgE type of mice sensitized to the OVA-specific egg allergen.

Heavy Metal Release

It is a proven fact that the presence of metal-based nanomaterials not only encourage the mechanical strength, but it also provides barrier properties, and prevents the phenomenon of photo-degradation of plastics, and shows its properties like an effective antimicrobial in the form of bulkier ions of metals. However, on the other side, it has a contradictional argument about its toxic behavior. The release of heavy metals causes toxic outcomes due to the presence of nanomaterials. It is only due to long term contamination of the release of heavy metals into the food particle which shows an adverse effect. There are much more nanomaterials which are in the category of metal-based nanomaterials, but among them, three are of those type which is mostly recorded metal-leaching. They are ZnO, Ag, and CuO and their presence increase the level of intracellular ROS, which results in DNA damage and phenomenon like lipid peroxidation.

NEED FOR REGULATIONS

The safety issues of the nanocomposite materials in the food packaging are increasing rapidly; hence, attention has been attracted to the safety-related issues for both the human being as well as the environment. For the safety assessment, there needs to a granted market permission for the components like plastic materials for packaging purposes. As per the chemical and toxicity data submission through the manufacturer side, it is based on the guidelines of data requirement (Bradley., et al. 2011)

At present various world-wide agencies are working on getting the information regarding the health and risk related to the use of nanotechnology in the packaging of foods. An international organization WHO (World Health Organization) with FAO (Food and Agriculture Organization) (FAO, 2009) has given a recent report on the use of nanotechnology in the sector of food and agricultural growth in a meeting of a joint expert meeting which was held in 2009. It was totally about the potential food safety implications. Another establishment has been done by the organizational council for Economic Cooperation and Development (OECD) (OECD., 2009). The issues were related to the health of human beings and the safety aspects of the environment for nanomaterials in chemical sectors of food technology. Therefore, in the future, worldwide agencies are so much concerned about it. Continuously, they are raising the issues related to food safety, and their organizations are still working for the development of nanomaterials that are not harmful like the toxicity effect of nanomaterials.

The EFSA has been authorized to organize and give recommendations for the issues which govern the quality of the foods for the human being as well as the environment also. This regulation offers such recommendations only for European Commissions. These regulations provide us with information about the active components which are present in the nanomaterials used for the food packaging. It also gives realistic data about the maximized quantity that has been released from the active materials present in the nanoparticles (Schmidt et al., 2011). There is an urgent need for the overall safety of the environment from the disposal of packaging materials. Two paramount concern is there about global environment protection and second is saving the natural resources, need to develop environmentally-friendly packing concept. The concept is reusable, recyclable, and environmentally friendly disposal.

ASPECTS OF SAFETY TO HUMANS AND THE ENVIRONMENT

There are only two critical issues of significance related to the safety concerns of the use of nanocomposites materials for food packaging. The first and most preference goes to the safety and quality-based products of food and their impact on the consumer's health. The aspects of safety concern arise. The question is that the use of nanocomposites and technologies for food packaging and migration phenomenon puts negative questions impact the quality and assurance of the consumer's health.

Furthermore, if we talk about the second question related to the environment, if looked deeply into the environmental issues, then the first thing is about the manufacturing of the materials needed for packaging, but more important than this is how these materials are being disposed of when they have used up finished. This leads to the recycling concept of the nanomaterials. And another aspect is of compromising nature and performance quality of the product of nanomaterials after being recycled. What regulations and market uptake are obstructed by these uncertain natures belonging to the consumer as well as environmental safety issues.

The councils who defines some standard regulations keeping because of safety concern to protect human health and to prevent the adulteration of foodstuffs has set some limits of migration. It has been defined as two types of migration limits in case of the plastic materials used for packaging purposes for food (The Council of the European Communities.,1990). They are as follows:

1. The first one is about the Overall migration limit (OML) of the granted permission plastic materials when it comes in contact with the food materials is 60mg/kg of substances in any of the conditions.
2. Secondly, it is about the Specific migration limit (SML), which governs the migration level of materials that send hazardous toxic effects coming in contact with the food particles. These levels of migration are decided on the daily basis of tolerable daily intake (TDI), and another one is acceptable daily intake (ADI), which is highly recommended by the regulation of EFSA. These regulations also provide the procedures of testing like overall migration (The Council of the European Communities, 2007).

OPPORTUNITIES FOR DEVELOPING COUNTRIES

The advantages offered by the application of nanomaterials and nanotechnology are frequently realized in near-market applications. They include the following benefits: (i) innovations (ii) Light -weighing (iii) massive extent of protection and preservation of foods (iv) performance enhancement in the bio-based materials.

Nowadays, nanotechnology along with information communication technology (ICT), has emerged as a new technology for the developing country's markets. They are getting renovated or adapted with the new technology for storage and transport of agricultural products, animal products, and food products. For the developing countries, this real-life relevance is so much needful to the poor peoples.

CONCLUSION

The use of nanocomposites materials and nanotechnology offers new opportunities for the foods and agriculture-based industries. Nano-composite materials have greater surface area per unit mass and are more biological activity than the larger sized particles. Bio-nanocomposite materials have more improved mechanical, thermal, and barrier properties for gases within the food package. In place of conventional packaging materials, it is far better to use bio-degradable packaging materials. For packaging purposes, silver nanocomposites, protein, starch, cellulose, PLA, PCL based nanocomposites are being used these days as they are bio-degradable. So, they are environment-friendly and also satisfy the need for customer safety.

Nanotechnology has more significant potential to provide a better quality of food products by making the food items tastier, healthy, and safety for the consumers. This technology innovates some new food products and improves the way of packaging and storage. In addition to food packaging, nano-sensors holds a vital place for maintaining food preservation. They detect whatever changes are going on inside the packaged food product and regulate the internal environment of foods. They are responsible for the enhanced shelf-life of the food products. Nanotechnology provides the benefits not only within the food packaging but also around the packaging. The application of nanocomposites/ nanotechnology detects the presence of bacteria, shows healthy behavior and also shows color response as per the inside quality of foods. Nanomaterials provide secure barrier property for the safety of food products. So, it will be better to communicate the benefits of using nanocomposite materials in food packaging to increase the level of acceptance of consumers towards this technology.

FUTURE SCOPE & RESEARCH DIRECTIONS

For ideal packaging, most of the target is to satisfy the standards as well as the customers, which have been discussed in this chapter. However, still, there is a compromise between the choice of package and the desired objectives. In the development of food packaging, quality assurance, safety, freshness, and convenience are considered as future needs and targets. Future trends arise questions on the characteristics like; opening case, small portions, consumer safety, environmentally friendly packaging, methods compatible with tamper-proof, and reclosable packaging.

Oxygen scavenging, revolutionary advancements in all cases optimum condition should be fulfilled. In the future, the driving forces of more research work, more innovations will be generated from the following mentioned questions which are: Who and Whom should pay for the collections and sorting? Is packaging has been done excessively? What management should be done to reduce the condition of excessive packaging? So, for this, the consumer should be educated to understand all the needs/ aspects of edible food packaging. How to make the right partner in food packaging for future development? These concepts and thoughts can help to get safe packaging for the customers.

ACKNOWLEDGMENT

The authors sincerely acknowledge the suggestions and comments of the authors are heavily indebted to them in providing their valuable suggestions and insights.

REFERENCES

Akbari, Z., Ghomashchi, T., & Moghadam, S. (2007). Improvement in food packaging industry with biobased nanocomposites. *International Journal of Food Engineering*, *3*(4). doi:10.2202/1556-3758.1120

Arvanitoyannis, I. S., & Bosnea, L. A. (2001). Recycling of polymeric materials used for food packaging: Current status and perspectives. *Food Reviews International*, *17*(3), 291–346. doi:10.1081/FRI-100104703

Avella, M., De Vlieger, J. J., Errico, M. E., Fischer, S., Vacca, P., & Volpe, M. G. (2005). Biodegradable starch/clay nanocomposite films for food packaging applications. *Food Chemistry*, *93*(3), 467–474. doi:10.1016/j.foodchem.2004.10.024

Bordes, P., Pollet, E., & Avérous, L. (2009, February 1). Nano-biocomposites: Biodegradable polyester/ nanoclay systems. *Progress in Polymer Science*, *34*(2), 125–155. doi:10.1016/j.progpolymsci.2008.10.002

Bradley, E. L., Castle, L., & Chaudhry, Q. (2011). Applications of nanomaterials in food packaging with a consideration of opportunities for developing countries. *Trends in Food Science & Technology*, *22*(11), 604–610. doi:10.1016/j.tifs.2011.01.002

Bruna, J. E., Galotto, M. J., Guarda, A., & Rodríguez, F. (2014, February 15). A novel polymer-based on MtCu2+/cellulose acetate with antimicrobial activity. *Carbohydrate Polymers*, *102*, 317–323. doi:10.1016/j.carbpol.2013.11.038 PMID:24507287

Chen, X. X., Cheng, B., Yang, Y. X., Cao, A., Liu, J. H., Du, L. J., ... Wang, H. (2013). Characterization and preliminary toxicity assay of nano-titanium dioxide additive in sugar-coated chewing gum. *Small*, *9*(9–10), 1765–1774. doi:10.1002mll.201201506 PMID:23065899

Coles, R., McDowell, D., & Kirwan, M. J. (2003). *Food packaging technology*. CRC Press.

Conte, A., Longano, D., Costa, C., Ditaranto, N., Ancona, A., Cioffi, N., ... Del Nobile, M. A. (2013, July 1). A novel preservation technique applied to fiordilatte cheese. *Innovative Food Science & Emerging Technologies*, *19*, 158–165. doi:10.1016/j.ifset.2013.04.010

Cutter, C. N. (2006). Opportunities for bio-based packaging technologies to improve the quality and safety of fresh and further processed muscle foods. *Meat Science*, *74*(1), 131–142. doi:10.1016/j.meatsci.2006.04.023 PMID:22062722

Driscoll, R. H., & Paterson, J. L. (1999). Packaging and food preservation. In Food science and technology, (pp. 687-734). Marcel Dekker.

Duncan, T. V. (2011). Applications of nanotechnology in food packaging and food safety: Barrier materials, antimicrobials and sensors. *Journal of Colloid and Interface Science*, *363*(1), 1–24. doi:10.1016/j.jcis.2011.07.017 PMID:21824625

EFSA Scientific Committee. (2011). Guidance on the risk assessment of the application of nanoscience and nanotechnologies in the food and feed chain EFSA Scientific Committee. *EFSA Journal*. doi:10.2903/j.efsa.2011.2140

Emamifar A. (2011). *Applications of antimicrobial polymer nanocomposites in food packaging*. Academic Press.

FAO. (2009). *WHO Expert Meeting on the Application of Nanotechnologies in the Food and Agriculture Sectors: Potential Food Safety Implications*. Meeting Report 1-102OECD. Guidance Manual for the Testing of Manufactured Nanomaterials, ENV/JM/MONO 20/REV.

Gorrasi, G., & Pantani, R. (2013, May 1). Effect of PLA grades and morphologies on hydrolytic degradation at composting temperature: Assessment of structural modification and kinetic parameters. *Polymer Degradation & Stability*, *98*(5), 1006–1014. doi:10.1016/j.polymdegradstab.2013.02.005

Jiménez, A., Requena, R., Vargas, M., Atarés, L., & Chiralt, A. (2018). Food Hydrocolloids as Matrices for Edible Packaging Applications. In Role of Materials Science in Food Bioengineering (pp. 263–299). doi:10.1016/B978-0-12-811448-3.00008-5

Lim, L. T. (2011). Active and Intelligent Packaging Materials. In Comprehensive Biotechnology, Second Edition (Vol. 4, pp. 629–644). doi:10.1016/B978-0-08-088504-9.00308-1

Magro, M., Campos, R., Baratella, D., Lima, G., Holà, K., Divoky, C., ... Vianello, F. (2014). A magnetically drivable nanovehicle for curcumin with antioxidant capacity and MRI relaxation properties. *Chemistry (Weinheim an der Bergstrasse, Germany)*, *20*(37), 11913–11920. doi:10.1002/chem.201402820 PMID:25079005

Metzger, C., Sanahuja, S., Behrends, L., Sängerlaub, S., Lindner, M., & Briesen, H. (2018). *Efficiently Extracted Cellulose Nanocrystals and Starch Nanoparticles and Techno-Functional Properties of Films Made Thereof.* Coatings. doi:10.3390/coatings8040142

Mihindukulasuriya, S. D. F., & Lim, L. T. (2014). Nanotechnology development in food packaging: A review. *Trends in Food Science & Technology*, *40*(2), 149–167. doi:10.1016/j.tifs.2014.09.009

Miltz, J. (1992). Food packaging. In D. R. Heldman & D. B. Lund (Eds.), *Handbook of Food Engineering* (pp. 667–740). New York: Marcel Dekker.

OECD. (2010). *Guidance manual for the testing of manufactured nanomaterials: OECD's sponsorship program.* OECD.

Orsuwan, A., Shankar, S., Wang, L. F., Sothornvit, R., & Rhim, J. W. (2016, October 1). Preparation of antimicrobial agar/banana powder blend films reinforced with silver nanoparticles. *Food Hydrocolloids*, *60*, 476–485. doi:10.1016/j.foodhyd.2016.04.017

Orsuwan, A., & Sothornvit, R. (2018). Active Banana Flour Nanocomposite Films Incorporated with Garlic Essential Oil as Multifunctional Packaging Material for Food Application. *Food and Bioprocess Technology*, *11*(6), 1199–1210. doi:10.100711947-018-2089-2

Pan, H., Xu, D., Liu, Q., Ren, H. Q., & Zhou, M. (2014). Preparation and characterization of corn starch-nanodiamond composite films. In *Applied Mechanics and Materials* (Vol. 469, pp. 156–161). Trans Tech Publications; doi:10.4028/www.scientific.net/AMM.469.156

Pereda, M., Dufresne, A., Aranguren, M. I., & Marcovich, N. E. (2014, January 30). Polyelectrolyte films based on chitosan/olive oil and reinforced with cellulose nanocrystals. *Carbohydrate Polymers*, *101*, 1018–1026. doi:10.1016/j.carbpol.2013.10.046 PMID:24299870

Rahman, M. S. (1999). Purpose of food preservation and processing. In M. S. Rahman (Ed.), *Handbook of food preservation* (pp. 1–10). New York: Marcel Dekker.

Rhim, J. W., Park, H. M., & Ha, C. S. (2013). Bio-Nanocomposites for Food Packaging Applications. *Progress in Polymer Science*, *38*(10-11), 1629–1652. doi:10.1016/j.progpolymsci.2013.05.008

Rocha, M., Alemán, A., Romani, V. P., López-Caballero, M. E., Gómez-Guillén, M. C., Montero, P., & Prentice, C. (2018). Effects of agar films incorporated with fish protein hydrolysate or clove essential oil on flounder (Paralichthys orbignyanus) fillets shelf-life. *Food Hydrocolloids*. doi:10.1016/j.foodhyd.2018.03.017

Sanyang, M. L., Ilyas, R. A., Sapuan, S. M., & Jumaidin, R. (2017). Sugar palm starch-based composites for packaging applications. In Bionanocomposites for Packaging Applications (pp. 125–147). doi:10.1007/978-3-319-67319-6_7

Schmidt, B., Katiyar, V., Plackett, D., Larsen, E. H., Gerds, N., Koch, C. B., & Petersen, J. H. (2011). Migration of nanosized layered double hydroxide platelets from polylactide nanocomposite films. *Food Additives & Contaminants. Part A, Chemistry, Analysis, Control, Exposure & Risk Assessment, 28*(7), 956–966. doi:10.1080/19440049.2011.572927 PMID:21614708

Shankar, S., & Rhim, J. W. (2016, October 1). Tocopherol-mediated synthesis of silver nanoparticles and preparation of antimicrobial PBAT/silver nanoparticles composite films. *Lebensmittel-Wissenschaft + Technologie, 72*, 149–156. doi:10.1016/j.lwt.2016.04.054

Shankar, S., & Rhim, J.W. (2016). Polymer nanocomposites for food packaging applications. *Functional and Physical Properties of Polymer Nanocomposites*. Doi:10.1002/9781118542316.ch3

Shankar, S., Tanomrod, N., Rawdkuen, S., & Rhim, J. W. (2016, November 1). Preparation of pectin/silver nanoparticles composite films with UV-light barrier and properties. *International Journal of Biological Macromolecules, 92*, 842–849. doi:10.1016/j.ijbiomac.2016.07.107 PMID:27492557

Simon, P., Chaundry, Q., & Bakos, D. (2008). Migration of engineered nanoparticles from polymer packaging to food - A physicochemical view. *Journal of Food and Nutrition Research, 47*(3), 105–113.

Sorrentino, A., Gorrasi, G., & Vittoria, V. (2007). Potential perspectives of bio-nanocomposites for food packaging applications. *Trends in Food Science & Technology, 18*(2), 84–95. doi:10.1016/j.tifs.2006.09.004

Tang, X. Z., Kumar, P., Alavi, S., & Sandeep, K. P. (2012). Recent Advances in Biopolymers and Biopolymer-Based Nanocomposites for Food Packaging Materials. *Critical Reviews in Food Science and Nutrition, 52*(5), 426–442. doi:10.1080/10408398.2010.500508 PMID:22369261

The Council of the European Communities. (1990). Relating to plastics materials and articles intended to come into contact with foodstuffs. *Official Journal of the European Union, L, 349*, 26–47.

The Council of the European Communities. (2007). *Relating to plastic materials and articles intended to come into contact with food and Council directive,* 85/572/ EEC laying down the list of simulants to be used for testing migration of constituents of plastic materials and articles intended to come into contact with foodstuffs. *Official Journal of the European Union, L, 91*, 17–36.

Tiede, K., Boxall, A. B. A., Tear, S. P., Lewis, J., David, H., & Hasellöv, M. (2008). Detection and characterization of engineered nanoparticles in food and the environment. *Food Additives & Contaminants. Part A, Chemistry, Analysis, Control, Exposure & Risk Assessment, 25*(7), 795–821. doi:10.1080/02652030802007553 PMID:18569000

Tiede, K., Hasellöv, M., Breitbarth, E., Chaudhry, Q., & Boxall, A. B. A. (2009). Considerations for environmental fate and ecotoxicity testing to support environmental risk assessments for engineered nanoparticles. *Journal of Chromatography. A, 1216*(3), 503–509. doi:10.1016/j.chroma.2008.09.008 PMID:18805541

Chapter 7
Non–Thermal Food Preservation Methods in the Meat Industry

Basak Gokce Col
https://orcid.org/0000-0002-7627-9867
Istanbul Gelisim University, Turkey

Sergen Tuggum
https://orcid.org/0000-0002-0519-7039
Tekirdag Namik Kemal University, Turkey

Seydi Yıkmış
https://orcid.org/0000-0001-8694-0658
Tekirdağ Namık Kemal University, Turkey

ABSTRACT

The most commonly used meat preservation methods include cooling, freezing, drying, vacuum packing, and curing. Meat quality is impaired by a wide range of changes including physical, chemical, microbiological, and enzymatic reactions. Food manufacturers focus on processes that require fewer chemical additives to meet the increased demand of consumers and to obtain more natural, healthy, and nutritious meat products. Non-thermal food preservation methods are one of the new trends to minimise thermal effects on texture, nutritional value, and flavor losses of meats. The chapter focuses on two novel approaches; non-thermal (Pulsed Electric Field) and Atmospheric Pressure Cold Plasma (APCP) Technologies.

INTRODUCTION

Containers or cases made of special materials such as metal, glass, plastic, which protect the products against external factors and facilitate the marketing and consumption of foods are referred to as food packages. The main purpose of food packaging is to ensure food safety by preserving the overall quality during the production, shelf life and consumption of products (Cutter, 2006).

DOI: 10.4018/978-1-7998-5354-1.ch007

The UK Packaging Institute defines packaging in three different ways (Gawith & Robertson, 2000):

1. Preparation of products for transportation, distribution, storage, retailing and final use in a coordinated manner,
2. Safe and cost-efficient delivery way of products to the final consumers,
3. Technological and economic function of the goal of minimizing delivery costs while maximizing sales and profits.

Food packaging is being developed day by day, upon the demands of the consumers and the novel trends applied in food industry. Four important functions should be considered when developing a food package: storage, protection, convenience and communication. In other words, package should be able to protect the product against external factors such as water, gas, odor, microorganisms, dust and pressure. They also have to contain information about the product and should be constantly improved to adapt to varying living conditions (Gawith & Robertson, 2000). Since milk and dairy products are particularly prone to physical, chemical and biological changes in a short time, the packaging technologies have been being developed in order to extend the shelf life of them.

The novel methods used in packaging technology can be listed as follows (Patel, Prajapati, & Balakrishnan, 2015):

1. Nanotechnology
2. Modified Atmosphere Packaging
3. Active Packaging
4. Intelligent/Smart Packaging

Nanotechnology

Nanotechnology is an applied science that provides the control of occurrences at atomic or molecular level below 100 nm (Anonymous, 2019). It is implemented in many food fields such as increasing food safety, reducing agricultural inputs and preventing the nutritional factors (Schnettler et al., 2013). In food science, food packaging is known as the most common field where the nanotechnology is applied (Sürengil & Kılınç, 2011) and dairy products are not exception.

Nanotechnology in food/dairy packaging can be used in three different ways (Duncan, 2011):

1. Producing synthetic polymer and biopolymer based packaging materials with improved barrier and mechanical properties.
2. Developing active packaging materials having properties antimicrobial or oxygen absorption such as Ag, ZnO, TiO_2.
3. Monitoring the storage conditions in which food products are exposed by use of different nanoparticles such as Fe_2O_3, TiO_2 in intellegent packaging technology and to produce markers that inform the manufacturer, seller and consumer.

Nanotechnological applications, in food/dairy technology, have various advantages and disadvantages as indicated in Figure 1.

Figure 1. The advantages and disadvantages of nanotechnological applications (Chau, Wu, & Yen, 2007; Buzby, 2010; Gruere, Narrod, & Abbott, 2011; Momin, Jayakumar, & Prajapati, 2013)

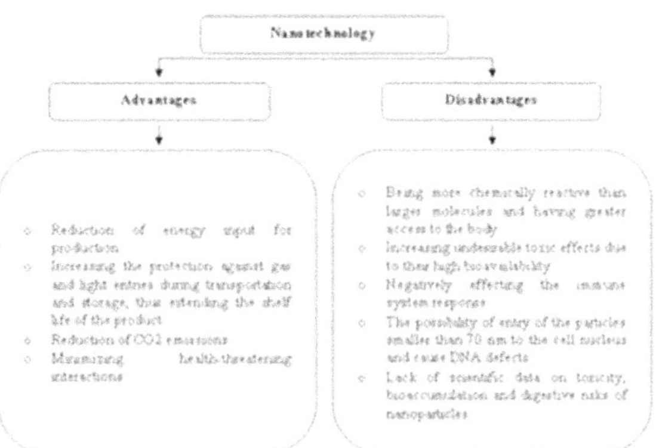

In addition to the disadvantages mentioned in Figure 1, major concerns with the nanotechnological applications in food/dairy products are the lack of scientific data. Therefore, nanotechnological applications in food/dairy packaging are considered to be more reliable than the applications in food products.

In a survey that examined the consumers' view about nanotechnological applications in the food industry, panelists stated that they would prefer to buy neither nanotechnological foods nor the products packaged with nanotechnological treatments (Siegrist, Cousin, Kastenholz, & Wiek, 2007). However, consumers also believe that the usage of nanotechnology in food packaging is more beneficial than the usage in foods. Siegrist, Stampfli, Kastenholz, & Keller (2008) also investigated the preference of 337 consumers in 19 nanotechnology products. Results showed that nanotechnological packaging materials were determined to be more reliable by consumers than the foods produced by nanotechnological approaches (Siegrist et al., 2008).

Modified Atmosphere Packaging

In 1930s, the great losses caused by the rapid deterioration of the products in the transportation especially of fruits and vegetables, led to new searches to increase the shelf life of food products. When CO_2 was supplied to the food stores, it was seen that the products could remain stable for a longer period and this has been the starting point for the development of Modified Atmosphere Packaging (MAP) technology (Demir, 1999).

MAP is based on the principle of replacing the air in the food package with a mixture of different gas or gases. This change can be implemented in two different ways: active MAP and passive MAP technology. In the Active MAP technology, the air in the package is directly replaced with the desired gas or gases. However, passive MAP technology is based on the occurrence of naturally desired composition in the atmosphere of package over time, depending on the respiration of the food and the permeability of the special packaging material used (Lee, Arul, Lencki, & Castaigne, 1996).

Oxygen (O_2), nitrogen (N_2) and carbon dioxide (CO_2) gases are the main gases used in MAP technology. In addition to these gases, carbon monoxide, ozone, ethylene oxide, nitrous oxide, sulfur dioxide, helium, neon, argon, propylene oxide, ethanol, hydrogen and chlorine are the gases that can be used in MAP technology. However, they are not preferred because they are costly and impair the sensory properties of the products (Farber, 1991; Sivertsvik et al., 2002).

During the storage of the product, O_2 is consumed and CO_2 is produced by food respiration. N_2 is an inert gas used to prevent shrinkage of packages due to CO_2 absorption (Sandhya, 2010). N_2 is a tasteless and a low solubility gas that is also insoluble in water and oil, which causes its not to be absorbed by foods, including dairy products. Although this gas alone does not have any antimicrobial effect, it is indirectly inhibits the development of aerobic microorganisms when used instead of O_2 to retard the oxidative rancidity in oxygen sensitive products (Farber, 1991; Sivertsvik et al., 2002).

It is stated that the development of aerobic bacteria will be supported by using high amounts of O_2 in MAP technology, on one hand the reactions of enzymatic discoloration and anaerobic fermentation can be prevented on the other hand (Van der Steen, Jacxsens, Devlieghere, & Debevere, 2002). In MAP technology, O_2 is mainly used for packaging fresh red meat products, by this way meat maintains its bright red color (Farber, 1991).

CO_2, one of the main gases used in MAP technology, is the only gas with a significant direct antimicrobial effect. Easy solubility of CO_2 in water and oil readily inhibits the microbial growth, and affects the lag phase (negatively or positively) leads to, maximum growth rate and maximum population density of microorganisms (Devlieghere & Debevere, 2000). Although the mechanism of action of CO_2 application is not known exactly, this gas penetrates into microbial cell and decrease the pH of stoplazm hence inhibiting the growth of microorganisms. It is reported that the use of CO_2 also prevents the bad odor that may occur during storage and transportation of the product (Mullan, 2002). CO_2 is also known as having a prevention effect on food respiration (Farber, 1991).

The degree of main gases effect used in MAP technology varies depending on the type of microorganism, temperature, water activity and characteristics of product (Oliveira et al., 2015). Therefore, combinations and usage rates of double or triple gas mixtures used in packaging change according to the characteristics of the food/dairy product (such as pH, water activity, type and amount of fat) to be maintained during storage. In this way, the product is effectively protected against microbiological, chemical and enzymatic changes (Devlieghere, Gil, & Debevere, 2002). As a result, the shelf life of a food product packaged by using MAP technology depends on the type and initial quality of the product, storage temperature, gas mixture used inside the package, gas / product volume ratio and the preservation properties of the packaging materials (Sivertsvik et al., 2002; Sivertsvik, Rosnes, & Jeksrud, 2004).

As mentioned above, within the scope of MAP technology, different concentrations of gas mixtures are used during the packaging of different types of foods. If the deterioration is mostly due to microbial spoilage, such as in milk and dairy products, the most important deterioration parameter is generally regarded as high water activity. In this case, the CO_2 value of the gas mixture used in MAP application recommended to be high. In foods where oxidative rancidity is observed, such as milk and dairy products, all atmosphere in the package must be replaced with nitrogen gas or CO_2/N_2 mixture, and O_2 should not be used in the packaging. In addition to the gas mixture applied in MAP technology, the packaging material also has a crucial effect on the shelf life of foods. Packaging materials such as polyester, polyethylene, nylon, polyvinyldichloride and polypropylene are frequently used in atmosphere modified packaging (Sivertsvik et al., 2002; Kılınç & Çaklı, 2004). When low permeability packaging material is used, the gas remains in the package for a longer period of time and if the permeability of the package increases, this gas escapes and lose its protective effectiveness (Batu, 1994).

Spoilage in milk and dairy products varies according to product properties. For example, it is usual to observe mould in products with low water activity such as hard cheeses. However, mainly yeast, bacterial spoilage, oxidative rancidity and physical separation are observed in products with higher water activity such as soft type cheeses and cream. It is possible to extend shelf life of products by applying the MAP technology on milk and dairy products (Sivertsvik et al., 2002; Velu et al., 2013). It is stated that the shelf life of cheeses which usually can be remain undeteriorated in refrigerator conditions for 3 weeks, can be extended as far as 8 weeks (Anonymous 1998: Batu et al., 2008). Since, especially some types of moulds can grow despite vacuum packaging, application of MAP technology is more effective on milk and dairy products in which mould development is observed. Similarly, the existence of gases used in MAP technology is effective in terms of preservation of integrity of products such as sliced cheese (Taniwaki, Hocking, Pitt, & Fleet, 2001). It is suggested to use the 30/70 proportion of CO_2/N_2 for the sliced cheeses (Farber, 1991). CO_2/N_2 composition is effective on the prevention of mould development, and it is usually used in packaging of hard cheeses. CO_2 proportion used in this stage is desired to be at least 30%, while this proportion can increase as far as 70%. On the other hand, N_2 proportion is suggested to be in the range of 30-100% (Farber, 1991; Fierheller, 1991). Since this gas composition is effective on the prevention of bacterial deterioration and oxidative rancidity, it is similarly used in soft cheeses. MAP technology can also be applied easily on crumbly cheeses which can be deformed when vacuum packaging is applied. It is inconvenient to apply MAP technology on mould-ripened cheeses since the gas composition prevents the mold growth which is desired to occur in the product (Fierheller, 1991). This packaging method is also used on headspace of fresh milk products such as pasteurized milk, yoghurt, ice cream, cream and sour cream by way of CO_2 application in different amounts for each product type (Hotchkiss & Chen, 1996; Batu et al., 2008).

Active Packaging

Active packaging is considered as an alternative method to chemical preservatives and MAP technology. With this method, it is made possible to protect the product characteristics and to extend the shelf life of product by adding specific substances into headspace, inner side between the different layers or surface of packaging material (Labuza & Breene, 1989; Dobrucka & Cierpiszewski, 2014). Active packaging is a packaging type which has an extra function providing a protective barrier for foods against external factors according to European Union Guidance to the Commission Regulation (EUGCR). The package used in this type of packaging absorbs the unwanted components from food and headspace surrounding the food or on the contrary it enables the release of components, preservatives and antioxidants which are intended to be supplied to food or the air surrounding the food (Anonymous, 2009). The fact that developed packaging machinery and packaging material of high barrier characteristics are the important advantages of this method over MAP technology (Gutiérrez et al., 2011).

Different systems are used in active packaging technology depending on the food/dairy product, which can be evaluated under two main headings: 1. Active absorber-scavenger systems, 2. Active release-emitter systems (Üçüncü, 2011). The most commonly used active absorber-scavenger systems are oxygen, carbon dioxide, ethylene, moisture scavenger systems, and the most commonly used active release-emitter systems are carbon dioxide, ethanol, antioxidant and antimicrobial emitter systems (Hurme, Sipilainen-Malm, & R. Ahvenainen, 2002). More than 15 active packaging products have been being used commercially, especially in Japan, Australia and the United States, with the majority of oxygen scavengers. Among these products, oxygen scavengers are followed by ethylene scavengers, antimicrobial emitters and moisture scavengers (Biji, Ravishankar, Mohan, & Gopal, 2015).

Oxygen Scavengers

O_2 present in the packages of foods such as dairy products can not be completely removed even with vacuum packaging and MAP technology, thus causes an increase in microbial load, aroma losses, unwanted odor, color changes and nutrition losses in time. The amount of O_2 in the package can be reduced to 0.01% in active packaging systems which O_2 scavengers are used. For this purpose, O_2 scavengers such as iron powder, ascorbic acid, enzymes and photosensitive dyes are used to absorb O_2 in the pack after packaging (Hurme et al. 2002; Göncü & Özkal, 2017). Another method used in this system is to absorb O_2 in the package by the use of sachets and pads placed inside the packaging material (Huff, 2008). Using oxygen scavengers, it is possible to prevent rancidity, discoloration and especially mould growth in cheese during storage of milk and dairy products (Kartal, 2010).

Among the O_2-scavenging components, iron-based ones are the most commonly used ones (Vermeiren et al., 1999). In these systems, the iron-based component reacts with O_2 and is oxidized to the iron oxide after packaging. Iron-based O_2 scavengers are effective in many food/dairy products with low, medium and high moisture content (Özdemir & Floros, 2004). When used for cheese-spreads, Gomes et al. (2009) showed that the active packaging using iron-based oxygen scavengers decreased the rancidity of samples and that all the product properties were preserved for a longer time period.

In addition to iron-based components, some enzymes such as glucose oxidase are also used as active O_2 scavengers during active packaging (Vermeiren et al., 1999). In these systems, the enzymes react with the O_2 capture substrate present in the package, thereby reducing the amount of O_2 in the package. However, due to the enzymes used, these systems are more expensive than iron based O_2 scavenging systems. In addition to being costly, these systems are highly sensitive to other factors such as temperature, pH, water activity and solvent/substrate balance in the package, and thus its use is very limited (Özdemir & Floros, 2004).

Carbon Dioxide Scavengers and Emitters

The amount of CO_2 required in the packaging material varies entirely depending on the type of product in the package. In some products, the amount of CO_2 in the package is desired to decrease while in some others to increase. Therefore, in the active packaging technology, it is possible to use CO_2 scavenger or CO_2 emitting components depending on the purpose.

CO_2 is produced as a result of spoilage or respiration by some foods, and may result in reduction in shelf life of the product, deformation or even the explosion of the package (Vermeiren et al., 1999). The use of CO_2 scavengers such as silica gel, calcium hydroxide, sodium hydroxide, potassium hydroxide, calcium oxide is effective in such products (Fang, Zhao, Warner, & Johnson, 2017).

In some cases, it is aimed to increase the CO_2 level in the package. It is because CO_2 has a direct inhibitory effect on many aerobic bacteria and fungi, and this effect varies according to the type of microorganism. For example, it is possible to inhibit *Pseudomonas* spp. with about 20% CO_2 while only a small proportion of pathogens such as *Clostridium perfringens*, *C. botulinum* and *Listeria monocytogenes* are inhibited with the presence of less than 50% CO_2 (Fang et al., 2017). CO_2 level in the package should be adjusted according to the type of microorganism which has a risk of occurrence in the product, by using various components in the packages. In such cases, it is aimed to spontaneously consume the O_2 present in the package and to produce CO_2, after packaging. Iron carbonate and ascorbic acid/sodium bicarbonate mixtures are generally used for this purpose. In addition to the above-mentioned effects on microorganisms, O_2 scavengers or CO_2 emitters are also used in active packaging technology to maintain a high volume in food packages and to preserve the appearance of bulk packages (Vermeiren et al., 1999).

Ethylene Scavengers

The use of ethylene scavengers in milk and dairy products where active packaging technology is applied is not very common. Ethylene scavengers are more important for fruits and vegetables as ethylene acts like a plant hormone accelerates the respiration rate and ripening. Furthermore, it causes softening in some fruit varieties and leads to yellowing of green vegetables. Therefore, the removal of ethylene from the package atmosphere is very important for fruits and vegetables, and for this purpose various ethylene scavengers are used in the active packaging technology. The most commonly used one is potassium permanganate and the minerals such as zeolite, silica gel and activated carbon are also used either alone or in combination to remove ethylene in the package (Vermeiren et al., 1999; Dainelli et al., 2008; Pereira de Abreu, Cruz, & Paseiro Losada, 2012) Ergun, 2016).

Moisture Absorbers

As in many foods, the water content is one of the most important causes for microbial spoilage in milk and dairy products. In the presence of high moisture, microbial growth is accelerated. In order to increase the shelf life of the product moisture content of the packages should be kept under control To do this, various moisture scavengers are used in the active packaging technology. Moisture absorbing pads and sheets are generally used where the moisture content is required to be kept under control., Active clay, silica gel and calcium oxide are commonly used components due to their high moisture-absorbing properties (Brody, Strupinsky, & Kline, 2001; Dobrucka, 2013; Biji et al., 2015).

Antimicrobial Emitters

Antimicrobial active packaging is a very important packaging method in the packaging of foods such as milk and dairy products containing many nutrients which are necessary for the development of microorganisms. The antimicrobial components used in this technique have an inhibitory effect on microorganisms by extending the lag phase and decreasing the expansion section of the microorganisms (Patel et al., 2015). The antimicrobial components are added to the packaging material or the product coating, and the mechanism of action of these components can be occur in two different ways. These components can migrate through food migration or prevent microbial growth that can be seen on the surface of the food without migration (Irkin & Esmer, 2015; Ergun, 2016). Examples of antimicrobial agents used in antimicrobial active packaging include alcohol, bacteriocin, nisin, natamycin and various metals such as silver, copper (Nicholson, 1998; Suppakul, Miltz, Sonneveld, & Bigger, 2003). In a study using antimicrobial active packaging in butter, it was determined that the product showed longer resistance to fungi and yeasts (Moraes et al., 2007).

Antioxidant Emitters

Lipid oxidation is one of the most important factors in shortening the shelf life of products such as milk and dairy products. The odor, aroma and color of the products change and also the nutritional value of food is lost with oxidation, due to the formation of toxic aldehydes and degradation of polyunsaturated fatty acid (PUFA) (Gomez-Estaca et al., 2014). To prevent the changes in the product occurred by oxidation and to prolong the shelf life of the foods, the antioxidants are usually incorporated into the packaging materials and these antioxidants pass into the food or air space around the food during storage. Waxed papers, butylated hydroxy toluene impregnated packaging materials and tocopherols, essential fatty acids and plant extracts obtained from plants such as rosemary, oregano and tea have been being used in antioxidant spreading systems. The effectiveness of α-tocopherol against lipid oxidation has already been shown in active packaged whole-fat milk Vitamins E and C appeared to be promising in these systems in recent years due to their antioxidative effects (Wessling, Nielsen, Leufvén, & Jägerstad, 1998; Tian, Decker, & Goddard, 2012; Yang, Lee, Won, & Song, 2016; Fang et al., 2017).

Ethanol Emitters

Ethanol emitters are especially used for active packaging of products with moderate moisture content against microbial spoilage and are particularly effective against mould growth. These components are also stated to be effective against yeasts and reduce staling and oxidative changes when used in high concentrations (Hurme et al. 2002; Suppakul et al., 2003; Dainelli et al., 2008). Ethanol emitters are reported to be particularly effective on bakery products (Dainelli et al., 2008).

The use of ethanol in active packaging technology can be applied in two ways: 1. Direct injection of ethanol into the package, 2. Use of packages with encapsulated ethanol that can release ethanol vapor (Hempel, O'Sullivan, Papkovsky, & Kerry, 2013).

Intelligent/Smart Packaging

Intelligent food packaging is defined as materials that can monitor the conditions of food and the surrounding environment. This technology, also known as smart labels, provides information to the producer, seller and consumer about changes in food during transport and storage (de Kruijf et al., 2002; Majid, Nayik, Dar, & Nanda, 2018). For this purpose, various sensors and indicators are integrated into the package or directly adhered to the package so that they provide information about some of the product characteristics such as freshness, shelf life and usage conditions. The working principle of these sensors and indicators is generally based on temperature-time measurements and the measurement of changes in chemical and microbiological properties (Yam, Takhistov, & Miltz, 2006; Dobrucka, 2013). Intelligent packaging technology provides useful information on the product in a short time, thus providing an alternative to time-consuming and costly analysis.

Sensors

Sensors are units that generally detect changes in the atmosphere of the product or packaging itself and transfer it to the manufacturer, seller and consumer. The sensors consist essentially of a receptor and a transducer. It is possible to examine the sensors used in smart packaging under different headings as biosensors, gas sensors, chemical sensors and pathogen sensors (Biji et al., 2015).

Biosensors

Devices that detect, record and transmit the biological reactions occur in food packages are called as biosensors. Biosensors, like other sensors, consist of a bioreceptor and energy converting devices (transducers). Bioreceptors are responsible for detecting the target parameter, usually organic materials such as various enzymes, antigens, hormones and nucleic acids. Transducers consist of electrochemical, optical or calorimetric systems that convert biological signals into measurable electrical messages (Smolander, 2003; Yam et al., 2006; Otles & Yalcin, 2008).

Gas Sensors

It is important that the gas mixture in the package does not change until it reaches to the consumer, particularly in products packaged using MAP systems, in order to maintain the quality of the product. Gas sensors are systems that detect and transmit the presence or absence of gases used in modified atmosphere packaging, packaging integrity and leaks (Otles & Yalcin, 2008; Robertson, 2012; Heising, Dekker, Bartels, & Van Boekel, 2014). O_2 and CO_2 sensors are the most commonly used gas sensors (Ergun, 2016).

Chemical Sensors

Chemical sensors detect the presence of a specific chemical or gas in the packaged product or in the headspace of the package. The substance detected by chemical sensors is converted into signals by transducers and enables the consumer to perceive the presence of the substance (Vanderroost, Ragaert, Devlieghere, & Meulenaer, 2014).

Pathogen Sensors

They are used for the detection of pathogenic microorganisms that infect the packaged products after production. Antibodies are generally used for this purpose and visual warning appears in the package as result of the reaction of these antibodies with the pathogens present in the product (Smolander, 2003).

Indicators

Indicators used in intelligent packaging technology indicate the presence, concentration or deficiency of a particular substance, particularly by color changes. They are generally classified as freshness indicators, time-temperature indicators (TTI), integrity indicators and Radio frequency information device (RFID) (Hogan & Kerry, 2008).

Freshness Indicators

The freshness indicators are generally used in products packaged with MAP technology, which informs the consumer on the change in gas composition in the package through the label printed on the package. If the necessary conditions are not met during the transportation and storage of foods, some microbiological spoilage may occur in the product and as a result of this deterioration, metabolites such as CO_2,

SO_2, NH_3 and ethanol are formed. Freshness indicators identify these metabolites and change the color of the label on the packaging, thus providing information about the quality of food (Smolander, 2003; Smolander, 2008). When classified according to working principles, it is possible to list the most frequently used freshness indicators as indicators; sensitive to pH change, volatile compounds, hydrogen sulfide (H_2S) and various microbial metabolites (Smolander, 2003; Gök, 2007).

Time-Temperature Indicators (TTI)

Time-temperature indicators (TTI) detect physical, chemical, enzymatic and microbial deteriorations in the product when food product is exposed to temperatures that they should not be exposed to during transport and storage. They are particularly effective in controlling temperature changes in refrigerated or frozen foods such as milk and dairy products. In case of temperature change, the barcode on the packaging turns into a dark color, thus it prevents the data transfer when the barcode is scanned and prevents the sale of the product. It is possible to classify the most commonly used time-temperature indicators as polymer, diffusion and enzymatic based ones (Riva, Piergiovanni, & Schiraldi, 2001; Taoukis & Labuza, 2003; Gök, 2007; Lee & Rahman, 2014; Taoukis & Tsironi, 2016). Time-temperature indicators can be used for all types of food products, including milk and dairy products (Ergun, 2016).

Integrity Indicators

The package may be punctured or torn particularly during transport of the products. Such situations can be detected and transferred to the seller and the consumer through integrity indicators. Among the integrity indicators, the most widely used ones are based on O_2 measurement. Integrity indicators detect O_2 entering the package when the package is punctured or torn and stain the active substance with redox effect (Mattila-Sandholm, Ahvenainen, Hurme, & Jarvi-Kaariainen, 1995; Davies & Gardner, 1996), indicating the integrity of the packaging material has been impaired.

Radio Frequency Information Device (RFID)

Radio frequency information device (RFID) is an advanced technology that make possible to read labels using radio waves without human intervention. In this system, unlike the other methods described above, various changes in food are not detected by physical interaction, but by radio waves through the microchips inserted into the product (Tajima, 2007; Lee & Rahman, 2014). RFID tags carry the information of all the changes in the food starting from the packaging of the product and allow remote monitoring of this information via radio waves thereafter (Karagöz & Demirdöven, 2017). RFID indicators can be found in many different forms such as disk, glass, capsule and label can also be combined with other indicators and can be used for all foods including milk and dairy products (Yuksel & Zaim, 2009; Ruiz-Garcia & Lunadei, 2011).

REFERENCES

Anonymous. (2009). *EU Guidance to the commission regulation (EC) No 450/2009 of 29 May 2009 on active and intelligent materials and articles intended to come into contact with food. Version 1.0. European Commission Health and Consumers Directorate-General Directorate E-Safety of the Food chain. E6- Innovation and sustainability.* Retrieved from https://ec.europa.eu/food/sites/food/files/safety/docs/cs_fcm_legis_active-intelligent_guidance.pdf

Anonymous. (2019). *Nanotechnology.* European Food Safety Authority. Retrieved from https://www.efsa.europa.eu/en/topics/topic/nanotechnology

Batu, A. (1994). Properties of modified atmosphere packaging films and application of fruits vegetables. *Gida, 19*(6), 397–403.

Batu, A., Caglar, A., & Kara, H. H. (2008). Afyon kaymagının raf ömrünün uzatılmasında modifiye atmosferde paketleme önerisi. *Gıda Teknolojileri Elektronik Dergisi, 2008*(2), 43-46.

Biji, K. B., Ravishankar, C. N., Mohan, C. O., & Gopal, T. S. (2015). Smart packaging systems for food applications: A review. *Journal of Food Science and Technology, 52*(10), 6125–6135. doi:10.100713197-015-1766-7 PMID:26396360

Brody, A. L., Strupinsky, E. R., & Kline, L. R. (2001). *Active packaging for food applications.* Boca Raton, FL: CRC Press. doi:10.1201/9781420031812

Buzby, J. C. (2010). Nanotechnology for food applications. More questions than answers. *The Journal of Consumer Affairs, 44*(3), 528–545. doi:10.1111/j.1745-6606.2010.01182.x

Chau, C. F., Wu, S. H., & Yen, G. C. (2007). The development of regulations for food nanotechnology. *Trends in Food Science & Technology, 18*(5), 169–280. doi:10.1016/j.tifs.2007.01.007

Cutter, C. N. (2006). Opportunities for bio-based packaging technologies to improve the quality and safety of fresh and further processed muscle foods. *Meat Science, 74*(1), 131–142. doi:10.1016/j.meatsci.2006.04.023 PMID:22062722

Dainelli, D., Gontard, N., Spyropoulos, D., Zondervan-van den Beuken, E., & Tobback, P. (2008). Active and intelligent food packaging: Legal aspects and safety concerns. *Trends in Food Science & Technology, 19*, 103–112. doi:10.1016/j.tifs.2008.09.011

Davies, E. S., & Gardner, C. D. (1996). *UK Patent No. GB-2298273.* Oxygen indicating composition, The Victoria University of Manchester.

de Kruijf, N. N., van Beest, M., Rijk, R., Sipilainen-Malm, T., Paseiro, L. P., & De Meulenaer, B. (2002). Active and intelligent packaging: Applications and regulatory aspects. *Food Additives and Contaminants, 19,* Suppl, 144-162.

Demir, M. (1999). *Modified atmosphere packaging.* Retrieved from http://www.apack.com.tr/images/userfiles/146705440090949918.pdf

Devlieghere, F., & Debevere, J. (2000). Influence of dissolved carbon dioxide on the growth of spoilage bacteria. *Lebensmittel-Wissenschaft + Technologie, 33*(8), 531–537. doi:10.1006/fstl.2000.0705

Devlieghere, F., Gil, M. I., & Debevere, J. (2002). Modified atmosphere packaging (MAP). In C. J. K. Henry, & C. Chapman (Eds.), *The nutrition handbook for food processors* (pp. 342–370). England: Woodhead Publishing. doi:10.1533/9781855736658.2.342

Dobrucka, R. (2013). The future of active and intelligent packaging industry. *LogForum, 9*(2), 103–110.

Dobrucka, R., & Cierpiszewski, R. (2014). Active and intelligent packaging food - Research and development - A review. *Polish Journal of Food and Nutrition Sciences, 64*(1), 7–15. doi:10.2478/v10222-012-0091-3

Duncan, T. V. (2011). Applications of nanotechnology in food packaging and food safety: Barrier materials, antimicrobials, and sensors. *Journal of Colloid and Interface Science, 363*(1), 1–24. doi:10.1016/j.jcis.2011.07.017 PMID:21824625

Ergun, M. (2016). Taze meyve ve sebzeler için aktif, zeki veya akıllı paketleme teknolojileri. *Alatarım, 15*(2), 51–60.

Fang, Z., Zhao, Y., Warner, R. D., & Johnson, S. K. (2017). Active and intelligent packaging in meat industry. *Trends in Food Science & Technology, 61*, 60–71. doi:10.1016/j.tifs.2017.01.002

Farber, J. M. (1991). Microbiological aspects of modified-atmosphere packaging technology - A review. *Journal of Food Protection, 54*(1), 58–70. doi:10.4315/0362-028X-54.1.58 PMID:31051584

Fierheller, M. G. (1991). Modified atmosphere packaging of miscellaneous products. In B. Ooraikul, & M. E. Stiles (Eds.), *Modified atmosphere packaging of food* (pp. 246–260). Boston, MA: Springer. doi:10.1007/978-1-4615-2117-4_8

Gawith, J. A., & Robertson, T. R. (2000). Wrapping up packaging technology. *Journal of the Home Economics Institute of Australia, 7*(2), 6–14.

Gök, V. (2007). Gıda paketleme sanayinde akıllı paketleme teknolojisi. *Gıda Teknolojileri Elektronik Dergisi, 2007*(1), 45-58.

Gomes, C., Elena Castell-Perez, M., Chimbombi, E., Barros, F., Sun, S., Liu, J. D., ... Wright, A. O. (2009). Effect of oxygen-absorbing packaging on the shelf life of a liquid-based component of military operational rations. *Journal of Food Science, 74*(4), 167–176. doi:10.1111/j.1750-3841.2009.01120.x PMID:19490321

Gomez-Estaca, J., Lopez-de-Dicastillo, C., Hernandez-Munoz, P., Catala, R., & Gavara, R. (2014). Advances in antioxidant active food packaging. *Trends in Food Science & Technology, 35*(1), 42–51. doi:10.1016/j.tifs.2013.10.008

Göncü, A., & Özkal, S. G. (2017). Ekmeklerde aktif paketleme uygulamaları. *Türk Tarım - Gıda Bilim ve Teknoloji Dergisi, 5*(11), 1264-1273.

Granda-Restrepo, D. M., Soto-Valdez, H., Peralta, E., Troncoso-Rojas, R., Vallejo-Córdoba, B., Gámez-Meza, N., & Graciano-Verdugo, A. Z. (2009). Migration of α-tocopherol from an active multilayer film into whole milk powder. *Food Research International, 42*(10), 1396–1402. doi:10.1016/j.foodres.2009.07.007

Gruere, G. P., Narrod, C. A., & Abbott, L. (2011). Agriculture, food, and water nanotechnologies for the poor: Opportunities and constraints, Policy briefs 19, International Food Policy Research Institute (IFPRI). Retrieved from http://cdm15738.contentdm.oclc.org/utils/getfile/collection/p15738coll2/id/124891/filename/124892.pdf

Gutiérrez, L., Batlle, R., Andújar, S., Sánchez, C., & Nerín, C. (2011). Evaluation of antimicrobial active packaging to increase shelf life of gluten-free sliced bread. *Packaging Technology & Science*, *24*(8), 485–494. doi:10.1002/pts.956

Heising, J. K., Dekker, M., Bartels, P. V., & Van Boekel, M. A. J. S. (2014). Monitoring the quality of perishable foods: Opportunities for intelligent packaging. *Critical Reviews in Food Science and Nutrition*, *54*(5), 645–654. doi:10.1080/10408398.2011.600477 PMID:24261537

Hempel, A. W., O'Sullivan, M. G., Papkovsky, D. B., & Kerry, J. P. (2013). Use of smart packaging technologies for monitoring and extending the shelf-life quality of modified atmosphere packaged (MAP) bread: Application of intelligent oxygen sensors and active ethanol emitters. *European Food Research and Technology*, *237*(2), 117–124. doi:10.100700217-013-1968-z

Hogan, S. A., & Kerry, J. P. (2008). Smart packaging of meat and poultry products. In J. Kerry & P. Butler (Eds.), *Smart packaging technologies for fast moving consumer goods* (pp. 33–59). West Sussex: John Wiley & Sons. doi:10.1002/9780470753699.ch3

Hotchkiss, J. H., & Chen, J. H. (1996). Microbiological effects of the direct addition of CO_2 to pasteurized milk. *Journal of Dairy Science*, *79*(Supplement 1), 87. PMID:8675787

Huff, K. (2008). *Active and intelligent packaging: Innovations for the future*. Retrieved from http://www.iopp.org/files/public/VirginiaTechKarleighHuff.pdf

Hurme, E., Sipilainen-Malm, T., & Ahvenainen, R. V. T. T. (2002). Active and intelligent packaging. In T. Ohlsson, & N. Bengtsson (Eds.), Minimal processing technologies in the food industry (pp. 87-123). Cambridge: CRC Press.

Irkin, R., & Esmer, O. K. (2015). Novel food packaging systems with natural antimicrobial agents. *Journal of Food Science and Technology*, *52*(10), 6095–6111. doi:10.100713197-015-1780-9 PMID:26396358

Karagöz, Ş., & Demirdöven, A. (2017). Gıda ambalajlamada güncel uygulamalar: Modifiye atmosfer, aktif, akıllı ve nanoteknolojik ambalajlama uygulamaları. *Gaziosmanpaşa Bilimsel Araştırma Dergisi*, *6*(1), 9–21.

Kartal, S. (2010). *Çileğin raf ömrünün mikroperfore filmler ve oksijen tutucular kullanılarak denge modifiye atmosfer ile arttırılması.* (Unpublished master's thesis). Çanakkale Onsekiz Mart University, Çanakkale, Turkey.

Kılınç, B., & Çaklı, Ş. (2004). Su ürünlerinin modifiye atmosferde paketlenmesi. *E.U. Su Ürünleri Dergisi*, *21*(3-4), 349–353.

Labuza, T. P., & Breene, W. M. (1989). Applications of "active packaging" for improvement of shelf-life and nutritional quality of fresh and extended shelf-life foods. *Journal of Food Processing and Preservation*, *13*(1), 1–69. doi:10.1111/j.1745-4549.1989.tb00090.x

Lee, L., Arul, J., Lencki, R., & Castaigne, F. (1996). A review on modified atmosphere packaging and preservation of fresh fruits and vegetables: Physiological basis and practical aspects-Part II. *Packaging Technology & Science, 9*(1), 1–17. doi:10.1002/(SICI)1099-1522(199601)9:1<1::AID-PTS349>3.0.CO;2-W

Lee, S. J., & Rahman, A. T. M. M. (2014). Intelligent packaging for food products. In J. H. Han (Ed.), *Innovations in food packaging* (pp. 171–209). Academic Press. doi:10.1016/B978-0-12-394601-0.00008-4

Majid, I., Nayik, G. A., Dar, S. M., & Nanda, V. (2018). Novel food packaging technologies: Innovations and future prospective. *Journal of the Saudi Society of Agricultural Sciences, 17*(4), 454–462. doi:10.1016/j.jssas.2016.11.003

Mattila-Sandholm, T., Ahvenainen, R., Hurme, E., & Jarvi-Kaariainen, T. (1995). *Finnish Patent No. FI-94802*. Leakage Indicator, VTT Biotechnology and Food Research.

Momin, J. K., Jayakumar, C., & Prajapati, J. B. (2013). Potential of nanotechnology in functional foods. *Emirates Journal of Food and Agriculture, 25*(1), 10–19. doi:10.9755/ejfa.v25i1.9368

Moraes, A. R. F., Gouveia, L. E. R., Soares, N. F. F., Santos, M. M. S., & Gonçalves, M. P. J. C. (2007). Development and evaluation of antimicrobial film on butter conservation. *Food Science and Technology (Campinas), 27*, 33–36. doi:10.1590/S0101-20612007000500006

Mullan, W. M. A. (2002). *Science and technology of modified atmosphere packaging*. Retrieved from https://www.dairyscience.info/index.php/packaging/117-modified-atmosphere-packaging.html

Nicholson, M. D. (1998). The role of natural antimicrobials in food/packaging biopreservation. *Journal of Plastic Film & Sheeting, 14*(3), 234–241. doi:10.1177/875608799801400306

Oliveira, M., Abadias, M., Usall, J., Torres, R., Teixido, N., & Vinas, I. (2015). Application of modified atmosphere packaging as a safety approach to fresh-cut fruits and vegetables - A review. *Trends in Food Science & Technology, 46*(1), 13–26. doi:10.1016/j.tifs.2015.07.017

Otles, S., & Yalcin, B. (2008). Intelligent food packaging. *LogForum, 4*(3), 1–9.

Özdemir, M., & Floros, J. D. (2004). Active food packaging technologies. *Critical Reviews in Food Science and Nutrition, 44*(3), 185–193. doi:10.1080/10408690490441578 PMID:15239372

Patel, R., Prajapati, J. P., & Balakrishnan, S. (2015). *Recent trends in packaging of dairy and food products*. Paper presented at the meeting National seminar on Indian Dairy Industry - Opportunities and Challenges. Gujarat, India.

Pereira de Abreu, D. A., Cruz, J. M., & Paseiro Losada, P. (2012). Active and intelligent packaging for the food industry. *Food Reviews International, 28*(2), 146–187. doi:10.1080/87559129.2011.595022

Riva, M., Piergiovanni, L., & Schiraldi, A. (2001). Performances of time–temperature indicators in the study of temperature exposure of packaged fresh food. *Packaging Technology & Science, 14*(1), 1–9. doi:10.1002/pts.521

Robertson, G. L. (2012). *Food packaging, principles and practice*. London, UK: CRC Press.

Ruiz-Garcia, L., & Lunadai, L. (2011). The role of RFID in agriculture: Applications, limitations, and challenges. *Computers and Electronics in Agriculture, 79*(1), 42–50. doi:10.1016/j.compag.2011.08.010

Sandhya. (2010). Modified atmosphere packaging of fresh produce: Current status and future needs. *Food Science and Technology, 43*, 381-392.

Schnettler, B., Crisostomo, G., Mora, M., Lobos, G., Miranda, H., & Grunert, K. G. (2013). Acceptance of nanotechnology applications and satisfaction with food-related life in southern Chile. *Food Science and Technology (Campinas), 34*(1), 157–163. doi:10.1590/S0101-20612014005000001

Siegrist, M., Cousin, M. E., Kastenholz, H., & Wiek, A. (2007). Public acceptance of nanotechnology foods and food packaging: The influence of affect and trust. *Appetite, 49*(2), 459–466. doi:10.1016/j.appet.2007.03.002 PMID:17442455

Siegrist, M., Stampfli, N., Kastenholz, H., & Keller, C. (2008). Perceived risks and perceived benefits of different nanotechnology foods and nanotechnology food packaging. *Appetite, 51*(2), 283–290. doi:10.1016/j.appet.2008.02.020 PMID:18406006

Sivertsvik, M., Rosnes, J. T., & Bergslien, H. (2002). Modified atmosphere packaging. In T. Ohlsson & N. Bengtsson (Eds.), *Minimal processing technologies in the food industry* (pp. 61–86). Cambridge: CRC Press. doi:10.1533/9781855736795.61

Sivertsvik, M., Rosnes, J. T., & Jeksrud, W. K. (2004). Solubility and absorption rate of carbon dioxide into non-respiring foods. Part 2: Raw fish fillets. *Journal of Food Engineering, 63*(4), 451–458. doi:10.1016/j.jfoodeng.2003.09.004

Smolander, M. (2003). The use of freshness indicators in packaging. In R. Ahvenainen (Ed.), *Novel food packaging techniques* (pp. 127–143). Cambridge: Woodhead Publishing. doi:10.1533/9781855737020.1.127

Smolander, M. (2008). Freshness indicators and food packaging. In J. Kerry, & P. Butler (Eds.), *Smart packaging technologies for fast moving consumer goods* (pp. 111–127). West Sussex: John Wiley & Sons. doi:10.1002/9780470753699.ch7

Suppakul, P., Miltz, J., Sonneveld, K., & Bigger, S. W. (2003). Active packaging technologies with an emphasis on antimicrobial packaging and its applications. *Journal of Food Science, 68*(2), 408–420. doi:10.1111/j.1365-2621.2003.tb05687.x

Sürengil, G., & Kılınç, B. (2011). Gıda - Ambalaj sektöründe nanoteknolojik uygulamalar ve su ürünleri açısından önemi. *Journal of Fisheries Sciences Com., 5*(4), 317–325.

Tajima, M. (2007). Strategic value of RFID in supply chain management. *Journal of Purchasing and Supply Management, 13*(4), 261–273. doi:10.1016/j.pursup.2007.11.001

Taniwaki, M. H., Hocking, A. D., Pitt, J. I., & Fleet, G. H. (2001). Growth of fungi and mycotoksin production on cheese under modified atmospheres. *International Journal of Food Microbiology, 68*(1-2), 125–133. doi:10.1016/S0168-1605(01)00487-1 PMID:11545212

Taoukis, P., & Tsironi, T. (2016). Smart packaging for monitoring and managing food and beverage shelf life. In P. Subramaniam, & P. Wareing (Eds.), *The stability and shelf life of food* (pp. 141–168). Woodhead Publishing. doi:10.1016/B978-0-08-100435-7.00005-8

Taoukis, P. S., & Labuza, T. P. (2003). Time-temperature indicators. In R. Ahvenainen (Ed.), *Novel food packaging techniques* (pp. 103–126). Cambridge: Woodhead Publishing. doi:10.1533/9781855737020.1.103

Tian, F., Decker, E. A., & Goddard, J. M. (2012). Development of an iron chelating polyethylene film for active packaging applications. *Journal of Agricultural and Food Chemistry, 60*(8), 2046–2052. doi:10.1021/jf204585f PMID:22288894

Üçüncü, M. (2011). *Gıda ambalajlanma teknolojisi.* İstanbul, Turkey: Ambalaj Sanayiciler Derneği.

Van der Steen, C., Jacxsens, L., Devlieghere, F., & Debevere, J. (2002). Combining high oxygen atmospheres with low oxygen modified atmosphere packaging to improve the keeping quality of strawberries and raspberries. *Postharvest Biology and Technology, 26*(1), 49–58. doi:10.1016/S0925-5214(02)00005-4

Vanderroost, M., Ragaert, P., Devlieghere, F., & Meulenaer, B. D. (2014). Intelligent food packaging: The next generation. *Trends in Food Science & Technology, 39*(1), 47–62. doi:10.1016/j.tifs.2014.06.009

Velu, S., Abu Bakar, F., Mahyudin, N. A., Saari, N., & Zaman, M. Z. (2013). Effect of modified atmosphere packaging on microbial flora changes in fishery products. *International Food Research Journal, 20*(1), 17–26.

Vermeiren, L., Devlieghere, F., Van Beest, M., De Kruijf, N., & Debevere, J. (1999). Developments in the active packaging of foods. *Trends in Food Science & Technology, 10*(3), 77–86. doi:10.1016/S0924-2244(99)00032-1

Wessling, C., Nielsen, T., Leufvén, A., & Jägerstad, M. (1998). Mobility of α-tocopherol and BHT in LDPE in contact with fatty food simulants. *Food Additives and Contaminants, 15*(6), 709–715. doi:10.1080/02652039809374701 PMID:10209582

Yam, K. L., Takhistov, P. T., & Miltz, J. (2006). Intelligent packaging: concepts and applications. *Journal of Food Science, 70*(1), 1–10. doi:10.1111/j.1365-2621.2005.tb09052.x

Yang, H. J., Lee, J. H., Won, M., & Song, K. B. (2016). Antioxidant activities of distiller dried grains with solubles as protein films containing tea extracts and their application in the packaging of pork meat. *Food Chemistry, 196,* 174–179. doi:10.1016/j.foodchem.2015.09.020 PMID:26593480

Yüksel, M. E., & Zaim, A. H. (2009). *Yeni nesil teknoloji olarak RFID, RFID sistem yapıları ve bir RFID sistem tasarımı yaklaşımı.* Paper presented at the meeting 5th International Advanced Technologies Symposium. Karabük, Turkey.

This research was previously published in Technological Developments in Food Preservation, Processing, and Storage edited by Seydi Yıkmış; pages 44-64, copyright year 2020 by Engineering Science Reference (an imprint of IGI Global).

Chapter 8
Non-Thermal Preservation of Dairy Products:
Principles, Recent Advances, and Future Prospects

Alperen Koker
Middle East Technical University, Turkey

İlhami Okur
https://orcid.org/0000-0002-2541-7123
Middle East Technical University, Turkey

Sebnem Ozturkoglu-Budak
Ankara University, Turkey

Hami Alpas
https://orcid.org/0000-0002-7683-8796
Middle East Technical University, Turkey

ABSTRACT

Dairy products include carbohydrates, protein, fatty acids, and different micronutrients, such as minerals and vitamins. Thermal treatment is generally used in dairy products to provide product safety and increase shelf life. But it can also lead to undesirable effects on dairy products such as protein denaturation, maillard reaction, and loss of vitamins. Non-thermal technology is an alternative method in the preservation of food products due to improving product safety and shelf life without any negative effects on food nutritional content. High hydrostatic pressure (HHP), pulsed electric field (PEF), ultrasound, cold plasma (CP), and pulsed light (PL) are the main non-thermal techniques that are used in the food industry. This chapter gives general principles of the non-thermal techniques, current applications in the dairy products, and recent advances in the dairy industry.

DOI: 10.4018/978-1-7998-5354-1.ch008

INTRODUCTION

Mammals secrete milk from their mammary glands and the primary function of milk is the nutrition of the mammalian neonates. Throughout history, milk and dairy products have been acknowledged as an important source of nutrition and humans domesticated variety of dairy animals such as cow, buffalo, goat, sheep, camel, and many other mammalian species. The major purpose was the production of an adequate amount of milk for the nutritional needs of a human i.e. higher amount of milk that is required for the nourishment of the dairy animal's offspring. Milk is available as a liquid form as pasteurized milk, sterilized milk, and milk of modified composition. Additionally, evaporated milk products, sweetened condensed milk products, and powdered milk products are available in the market. Another milk component, milk cream, is available in the market such as sterilized cream and whipping cream. Cheese, yogurt, butter, kefir, sour cream, fermented buttermilk, and many other fermented dairy products have been important for humans due to their longer shelf life compared with raw and heat-treated milk and nutritious properties developed during the fermentation process. In the class of dairy products, cheeses have the most number of varieties depending on milk type, starter culture, processing, and aging.

Non-thermal technologies are alternative methods in terms of preservation of food products to a certain shelf-life and providing both a healthy and quality product. These technologies have shown not to have any negative effects on the food nutritional content and other quality factors during the process stage (Putnik et al., 2019). Unlike heat treatment applications, non-thermal techniques are known as energy-efficient processes. For these reasons, in recent years non-thermal technologies have gained popularity in the food industry (Santhirasegaram et al., 2016) and there has been much research related to this subject. High hydrostatic pressure (HHP), pulsed electric field (PEF), ultrasound, cold plasma (CP), and pulsed UV-light are the main non-thermal techniques that are used in the industry. They have different microbial inactivation mechanisms and different effects on the physicochemical properties of foods. However, the effects of non-thermal techniques on foods and microorganisms are related to processing parameters, microorganism type and load, and properties of food. In recent years, there has been much research on non-thermal technology applications on milk and other dairy products such as cheese, yogurt, butter, kefir, ice-cream, sour cream, fermented buttermilk, and other fermented dairy products.

This chapter aims to give information about general principles of the non-thermal techniques, current applications in the milk and dairy products industry, recent advances, investigated novel approaches and future expectations from these technologies.

HIGH HYDROSTATIC PRESSURE (HHP)

High Hydrostatic Pressure (HHP), also known as a cold pasteurization technique or pascalization, is a non-thermal technique in which extremely high pressures (between 200 MPa and 800 MPa) are applied to foods that are submerged in a liquid -mostly water- for a desirable period of time (t) and at a desirable temperature (T) (Doona, Kustin, & Feeherry, 2010). It can be said that HHP is a 3-Dimensional process because of having three different parameters as pressure, time and temperature. HHP can destroy vegetative cells of microorganisms, and enzymes (Alpas et al., 1999; Alpas, Lee, Bozoglu, & Kaletunç, 2003). This technique can be applied to all solid and liquid foods except for porous and dry products (Morales-de la Peña, Welti-Chanes, & Martín-Belloso, 2019). Classic heat treatments usually cause the formation of undesirable compounds and caramelization of products due to Maillard reaction and affect color, texture, and flavor of processed foods. Contrary to heat treatment, HHP application retains the nutritional and functional ingredients in the food material (Khan et al., 2018; Misra et al., 2017). Besides, HHP treatment is independent of the mass and geometry of the products (Koutchma, 2014; Misra et al., 2017). Due to these reasons, HHP is one of the most popular non-thermal food processing methods and recently used for the preservation of a wide range of industrial food products like dairy, ready-to-eat, fruit juices and seafoods (Misra et al., 2017). Apart from these, HHP treated food market value is expected to be increased to $ 54.77 billion in 2025 (Huang et al., 2017).

Figure 1. HHP system

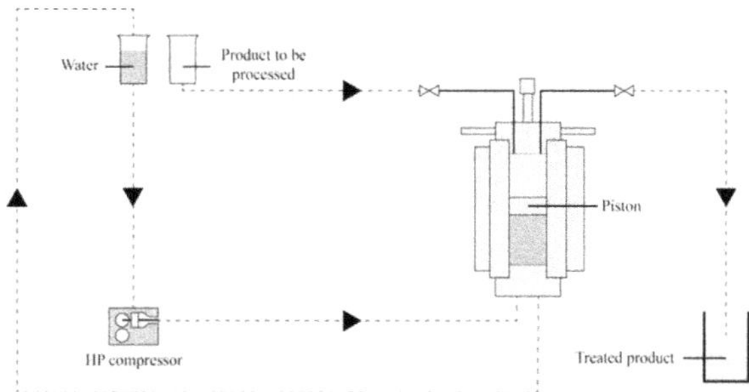

The typical HHP system consists of a high-pressure vessel and its closure, pressure generation device, temperature and pressure control device (Figure 1). Water is used mostly for pressure-transferring medium. Food is put into the pressure vessel with or without packaging. The closed pressure vessel is filled with a pressure transmitting medium and the liquid is compressed by a pump or pressure intensifier. The hydrostatic pressure distributes uniformly throughout the pressure vessel and equally in all directions of the food surfaces (Isostatic Pressure). The temperature of water raises roughly 3°C in each 100 MPa due to adiabatic heating during the pressure build-up (Bhattacharya, 2015; Durance, 2002; Doona et al., 2010; Morales-de la Peña et al., 2019).

EFFECT OF HHP ON MILK AND DAIRY PRODUCTS

In food science, application of HHP was first introduced by the study of Hite (1899) on raw milk, in which it was found that HHP treatment of milk at 600 MPa for 1 h at room temperature extended shelf life of raw milk. Subsequently, effect of HHP on spoilage and pathogenic microorganisms present in milk and on physicochemical properties of milk have been studied comprehensively.

In terms of extending shelf life, raw milk subjected to 350 MPa for 32 min was found to increase the shelf life of milk to 12, 18 and 25 days at 10, 5 and 0 °C, respectively (Mussa & Ramaswamy, 1997). High-pressure treatment of 300 MPa for 30 min at 20 °C and 500 MPa for 5 min at 20 °C was enough for obtaining shelf life of 10 days at 10 °C (Rademacher, Pfeiffer, & Kessler, 1998). Refrigeration storage (7 °C) of raw milk and application of pressure (400 MPa for 30 min at 25 °C) lead to lower amount of microbial count in pressurized milk after 45 days of storage comparing to microbial count of raw milk after 15 days of storage (García-Risco, Cortés, Carrascosa, & López-fandiño, 1998).

Effect of HHP on pathogenic microorganisms was investigated profoundly in pursuance of achieving food safety conditions for high-pressure treated milk. *Escherichia coli* is an indicator organism for fecal contamination and one of the most important foodborne pathogens for the food industry, particularly serotype *E. coli* O157: H7. Various studies were performed about the application of HHP on milk inoculated with *E.coli*. Patterson and Kilpatrick (1998) achieved 5 log CFU/ml reduction of *E. coli* O157: H7 NCTC 12079 with the high-pressure treatment of 400 MPa for 15 min at 50 °C. Application of high pressure within a range of 250 MPa and 400 MPa for 0 to 80 min as a holding time at two different temperatures of 3 °C and 21 °C on milk inoculated with *E. coli* ATCC-29055 demonstrated that higher reduction of *E. coli* was achieved at higher pressures, longer holding times and lower temperatures (Pandey, Ramaswamy, & Idziak, 2003). *Listeria monocytogenes* is another foodborne pathogen related to milk and dairy products, which cause listeriosis infection. Styles, Hoover, and Farkas (1991) achieved 6 log CFU/ml reduction in *L. monocytogenes* Scott A number when 345 MPa pressure was applied at 23 °C for 60 min and 80 min in raw and UHT milk, respectively. HHP application of 345 MPa for 5 min at 45 °C and 50 °C lead to 8 log CFU/ml reduction of *L. monocytogenes* CA and *L. monocytogenes* OH, respectively (Alpas, Kalchayanand, Bozoglu, & Ray, 2000). *Staphylococcus aureus* is the most pathogenic staphylococci, which are commonly related to food poisoning due to staphylococcal enterotoxins. *S. aureus* has very high-pressure resistance and pressure resistance of *S. aureus* increases in bovine milk (Patterson & Kilpatrick, 1998). Alpas et al. (2000) studied the reduction degree of *S. aureus, L. monocytogenes, E. coli*, and *Salmonella* spp. in case of HHP treatment and reported that HHP application of 345 MPa for 5 min at 50 °C destroyed *L. monocytogenes, E. coli*, and *Salmonella* spp. completely (8 log CFU/ml reduction), whereas *S. aureus* survived to a degree (5.33 log CFU/ml reduction).

The effect of HHP treatment on milk components, such as proteins and enzymes was also investigated. Casein is the major milk protein found in the cow's milk and due to its primary structure, casein micelles effected by HHP at higher pressure values than 300 MPa. Higher pressure values result in defragmentation of casein micelles as a result of interruption of casein micelle structure's electrostatic and hydrophobic interactions, and colloidal calcium phosphate solubilization (Schrader, Buchheim, & Morr, 1997). It was reported that micellar substructures of casein in HHP treated milk are similar to structures in untreated milk in the view of the electron microscope (Knudsen & Skibsted, 2010).

Main whey proteins present in bovine milk are α-lactoalbumin and β-lactoglobulin. The other whey proteins are found in smaller amounts such as immunoglobulins, bovine serum albumin, and lactoferrin. The effect of pressure treatment of 400 MPa for 15 min on β-lactoglobulin and α-lactoalbumin denaturation were investigated at different temperatures by García-Risco et al. (2000). The percentage loss of β-lactoglobulin was determined as 76 and 95% at the temperatures of 20 °C and 40 °C, respectively. They also found that α-lactoalbumin is more pressure resistant comparing to β-lactoglobulin, and the denaturation ratio was observed as only 3% at 40 °C and no denaturation was detected in α-lactalbumin at 20 °C at the pressure treatment of 400 MPa for 15 min. α-lactoalbumin and β-lactoglobulin denaturation was observed to increase with increasing temperature, treatment time and pH (Trujillo, Ferragut, Juan, Roig-Sagués, & Guamis, 2016).

Effect of HHP on milk enzymes is important considering their potential use of indicator for sufficient processing conditions and their effects on product quality. Rademacher et al. (1998) reported that enzyme activity loss of alkaline phosphatase, γ-glutamyltransferase, and phosphohexose isomerase starts at the HHP treatment of 600, 500 and 400 MPa for 8 min at 20 °C. Rademacher and Hinrichs (2006) proposed that γ-glutamyltransferase could be used as a process indicator for raw milk during HHP treatments as an alternative to alkaline phosphatase due to the efficient inactivation of foodborne pathogens in milk in case of the adequate (500 MPa) inactivation pressure is applied. Otherwise, HHP process indicator may lead to over processing due to the high-pressure inactivation value of alkaline phosphatase (600MPa).

HHP treatments were found to have effects on milk characteristics. It was reported that HHP application decreased the turbidity of milk up to 330 MPa. It was also determined that up to 220 MPa turbidity decreases with increasing processing time from 10 min to 20 min due to changes in casein micelle size (Altuner, Alpas, Erdem, & Bozoglu, 2006). Combination of temperature and high-pressure treatment increases phosphorus and calcium solubility slightly and decreases average particle diameter and lightness (Gaucheron et al., 1997). 40% reduction of level and rate of creaming occurs by the application of HHP higher than 400 MPa, and these creaming properties increases by 70% at pressure values lower than 250 MPa (Huppertz, Fox, & Kelly, 2003). Altuner et al. (2006) reported HHP application to milk leads to the repositioning of hydrophobic areas inside the micelles by the evidence of increasing binding strength and maximum surface allowable for binding. Water binding, gelling, foaming and emulsifying properties of milk is likely to change due to increased exposure of hydrophobic groups (Nakai & Li-chan, 1988). Production of low-fat yogurt from skim milk processed by a combination of heat treatment and HHP (400 MPa to 500 MPa) decreases syneresis and enhances yield stress and elastic modulus (Harte, Luedecke, Swanson, & Barbosa-Cánovas, 2010).

PULSED ELECTRIC FIELD (PEF)

PEF treatment is the application of high-voltage pulses (20–80 kV/cm) during a short time (1-10 µs) to food located between two electrodes. It is usually used for liquid foods (Doona et al., 2010; Shahbaz et al., 2018) and the food material must be homogenous for pasteurization process (Morales-de la Peña et al., 2019). Like HHP treatment, application of PEF also decreases the unacceptable changes in the food materials. The main food products treated with PEF technology are fruit juices, liquid egg, and milk for the purpose of their preservation.

Figure 2. PEF system

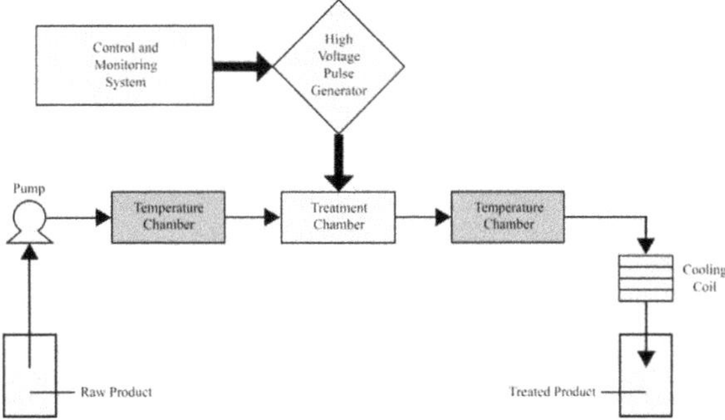

The typical PEF system includes voltage power supply and treatment chamber, which contains electrode, resistor and capacitor (Figure 2). When a voltage is applied to a cell, a sufficiently high transmembrane potential is induced across the cell membrane and this leads to rapture at the membrane (Doona et al., 2010). After damaging a cell, water starts to interrupt to cell and this leads to inactivation of the cell. Unlike HHP which temperature, pressure and time are critical parameters, PEF technology has so many critical parameters to the optimization of the processing system (Ahmed et al., 2010). These are treatment time, electric field strength (E), pulse shape, pulse-frequency, pulse-width, pulse polarity, and temperature. Although there are too many critical parameters to optimize the system, there have been too many researches to find the effects of PEF on food system (Misra et al., 2017).

EFFECT OF PEF ON MILK AND DAIRY PRODUCTS

In terms of extending shelf life, PEF application of 35.5 kV electric field strength for 1000 µs processing time with bipolar 7 µs pulses at 111 Hz on raw milk increased the shelf life of raw milk to 5 days, which is similar to high temperature short time pasteurization process (at 75 °C for 15 s) (Odriozola-Serrano, Bendicho-Porta, & Martín-Belloso, 2010). For the purpose of comparing the effects of conventional heat treatment and the combination of PEF and PEF with (or plus) heat treatment was investigated on the shelf life of skim milk. According to results the shelf life of milk increases to 14 days at 4 °C both for heat treatment at 65 °C for 21 s and PEF treatment of 28, 32 and 36 kV/cm for 30 pulses with a total processing time of 84 µs. Moreover, the combination of PEF and heat treatment increases the shelf life of skim milk to 30 days at the same storage conditions (Fernández-Molina et al., 2005).

In order to obtain milk without the presence of pathogenic microorganisms, the effects of PEF on foodborne pathogens are crucial. Treatment of milk containing *Escherichia coli* K-12 with preheating unit to increase the initial temperature to 60 °C and PEF application of 40 kVp with frequency of 100 Hz and post holding of milk for 20 s decreases *E. coli* count at least 7 log CFU/ml, and also reduces time required for low temperature long time pasteurization significantly (Ohshima, Tanino, Kameda, & Harashima, 2016). Combination of PEF and electrically induced heat application to pasteurized milk inoculated with *L. innocua* ATCC 51742 at 30 kV/cm, 10 pulses with a pulse width of 2.5 µs at initial temperature of 43 °C leads to 4.3 log CFU/ml reduction, and similar amount of *L. innocua* reductions occur by increasing pulse number and decreasing initial temperature of milk at the same electric field intensity (Guerrero-Beltrán, Sepulveda, Góngora-Nieto, Swanson, & Barbosa-Cánovas, 2010). PEF treatment of skim milk inoculated with *Staphylococcus aureus* ATCC 6538 with electric field strength of 35 kV/cm for 450 µs with bipolar square pulse waves of pulse width of 3.7 µs with 250 Hz pulse rate leads to 3.7 log CFU/ml reduction of *S. aureus* (Evrendilek, Zhang, & Richter, 2004). Heat treatment at 55 °C for 24 s prior to PEF treatment of 23 kV/cm electrical field strength with pulse width 20 µs for 70 µs processing time decreases *E. coli*, *L. innocua* and *S. aureus* below 2 log CFU/ml (Sharma, Bremer, Oey, & Everett, 2014). Comparing PEF resistance of *L. monocytogenes*, *E. coli* and *S. aureus*, with lethal and sublethal injury of these microorganisms, PEF treatment of 15, 20, 25 and 30 kV/cm electric field strength were applied for a treatment time between 0 to 600 µs with square waves of 2 µs width and 200 Hz rate. *L. monocytogenes* was found as the most resistant bacteria to PEF treatment, also inactivation kinetics of all these food-borne pathogens best fit with Hülsheger model (Zhao, Yang, Shen, Zhang, & Chen, 2013).

Application of PEF leads to protein modification and enzyme inactivation in milk as a result of changes in apparent charge of proteins following modification of ionic interactions of proteins (Jaeger, Meneses, & Knorr, 2014). Moreover, free radicals generated by energy absorption of proteins from PEF application can lead to disruption of interactions between proteins and unfolding due to cross-linking of free radicals with proteins (Han, Cai, Cheng, & Sun, 2018).

Loss of β-lactoglobulin, α-lactalbumin and serum albumin in milk after PEF application of 35.5 kV/cm with bipolar pulses of 7 µs pulse width for 1000 µs process time is 20.1%, 40% and 24.5%, respectively, which is similar to loss of whey proteins in milk with the application of traditional heat treatment (Odriozola-Serrano et al., 2010). PEF treatment of reconstituted skim milk (49 kV/cm, 19.36 µs, up to 70 °C) at pH values lower than 7.5 does not affect caseins and have a minor effect on whey protein denaturation. Besides, pH values higher than 7.5 cause dissociations of casein micelles, decrease milk protein sizes and increase casein amount in serum (Liu et al., 2015).

Application of PEF treatment to whey protein isolate at 30-35 kV/cm electric field intensity for a treatment time of 19.2-211 µs at 30-75 °C does not affect emulsification, surface hydrophobicity, and protein aggregation properties, however gel strength of whey protein isolate decreases and gelation time increases (Sui, Roginski, Williams, Versteeg, & Wan, 2011).

Considering milk-fat globule size distributions, the effect of PEF treatments with electric field intensities of 36 kV/cm for 24, 40, 60 pulses and 42 kV/cm for 8, 16, 24 pulses, respectively, gave similar results to thermal treatment at 63 °C for 30 min (Garcia-Amezquita, Primo-Mora, Barbosa-Cánovas, & Sepulveda, 2009). Yu, Ngadi, and Raghavan (2009) studied the effect of PEF on rennet coagulation and they found that increasing electric field intensity, pulse number, and treatment temperature effects coagulation properties of milk and they have concluded that combination of mild heat treatment (50 °C) with PEF (30 kV/cm, 120 pulse) of milk is suitable for cheese production due to increased coagulation activity (or coagulability) of PEF applied milk.

ULTRASOUND (US)

Ultrasound (US) is a novel food preservation technique, in which pressure waves are applied to food material (Morales-de la Peña et al., 2019). The main concept of this technology is to produce acoustic cavitation and this cavitation causes disruption of living cells by micro-mechanical shocks. According to frequency magnitude, US divides into three groups which are power ultrasound (with a frequency of 20-100 kHz), high frequency or extended range for sonochemistry (20 kHz–2 MHz) and diagnostic ultrasound (>1 MHz) (Figure 3) (Awad et al., 2012; Chemat et al., 2011). Furthermore, US types used in the food industry are divided into two groups according to frequency level; a high-frequency ultrasound (HFU) and a low-frequency ultrasound (LFU). A typical ultrasound system is shown in Figure 4.

HFU is used as a non-destructive, non-invasive analytical technique for quality assurance, process monitoring, and control in the food industry. At the low frequency, HFU is enough to lead acoustic cavitation so that minimal physicochemical changes occurred at food material during wave passes. On the other hand, LFU is used for process intensification. Even at the lower frequencies, LFU produces cavitation and it can cause physicochemical changes at food material (Ojha et al., 2017).

Figure 3. The frequency range of application of ultrasound technology reproduced from Ojha et al., (2017)

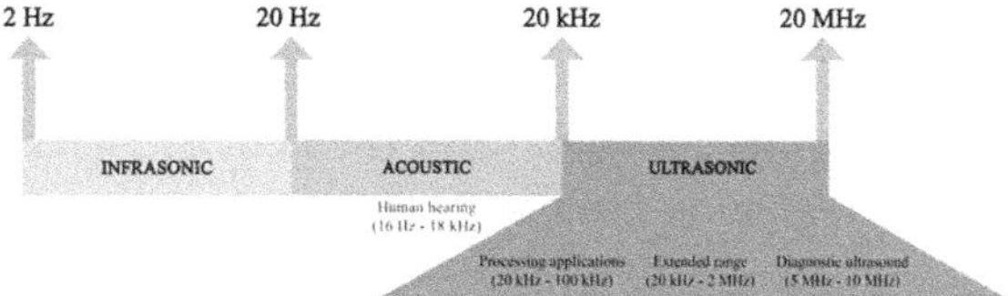

Figure 4. Ultrasound system reproduced from Moreno, (2017)

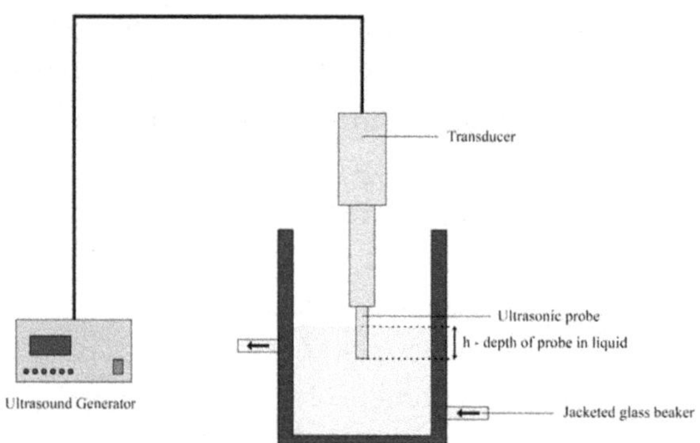

EFFECT OF US ON MILK AND DAIRY PRODUCTS

In terms of extending shelf life, UV treatment of raw milk initially containing 5.31 log CFU/ml coliform and 8.6 log CFU/ml total bacteria lead to 4.01 log CFU/ml and 1.31 log CFU/ml, respectively, in which the treatment conditions of 24 kHz frequency, 100% amplitude, and 15 min was applied (Şengül, Erkaya, Başlar, & Ertugay, 2011). Vijayakumar et al. (2015) studied the effect of thermosonication on coliform and total aerobic bacteria both in skim milk and cream, at 104 W power for 3 min and at 115 W power for 1 min. The authors reported a 2 log CFU/ml reduction in total aerobic bacteria and 3.65 log CFU/ml reduction in the coliform count.

Considering the health risks caused by foodborne pathogens, the effects of ultrasonication on pathogens, which may present in milk, are crucial. Cameron, McMaster, and Britz (2009) inoculated UHT milk with 10^6 CFU/ml *Escherichia coli* and *Listeria monocytogenes*, and obtained 5.34 log CFU/ml and 2.07 log CFU/ml reduction, respectively, after US treatment of 20 kHz for 10 min at 100% amplitude. US treatment (20 kHz, 100% amplitude, 6 min) of raw milk inoculated with 8 log CFU/ml decreased the *L. monocytogenes* ATCC 51414 number to 1.93 and 3.47 log CFU/ml at 20 °C and 57 ± 1 °C, respectively (D'Amico, Silk, Wu, & Guo, 2006). US treatment of 24 kHz, 100% amplitude and 300 s process time lead to 2.09 log CFU/ml reduction in *Escherichia coli* and 0.55 log CFU/ml reduction in *Staphylococcus aureus*. Sensorial deterioration was also observed during this stage (Marchesini et al., 2015). In an earlier study, Wrigley and Llorca (1992) applied US on skim milk inoculated with *Salmonella typhimurium* ATCC 14028 and observed a decrease of 2.5 and 3.0 log CFU/ml in cell numbers after the treatment of 30 min at 40 °C and 50 °C, respectively.

Effect of ultrasonication on milk proteins and enzymes also investigated by researchers because of their importance in milk and dairy products. Denaturation of whey proteins occurs at higher pH values and lower frequencies. In a research performed by Liu et al. (2014), an increase in protein solubilization, casein release and casein particle negative charge was observed in skim-milk within the US conditions of 20, 400 and 1600 kHz (energy provided for each system adjusted to 286 kJ/kg), at processing temperature lower than 30 °C between pH 6.7 and 8.0. Another study on the effect of US on surface hydrophobicity of reconstituted milk protein concentrate showed that surface hydrophobicity increased from 177.51 to 200.06 and 416.94 with 0.5 and 5 min, respectively. The authors concluded that unfolding of milk protein molecules occurs by US application (Sun et al., 2014). Application of thermo-sonication (115

W average power, 3 min) on skim milk and cream also decreased the total plasmin activity, a heat stable enzyme that can be found in milk, in a ratio of 94% (Vijayakumar et al., 2015).

US treatment of reconstituted milk protein concentrate at 20 kHz frequency and 50% amplitude decreased the particle size from 28.45 µm to 0.13 µm after 30 s of treatment and increased the solubility from 35.8% to 88.3% after 5 min of treatment (Sun et al., 2014). Chandrapala, Martin, Kentish, and Ashokkumar (2014) also examined the effect of US process (20 kHz, 50% amplitude, 10 min) both on solubilization of micellar casein powder and low solubility milk protein concentrate. Similar to the results of Sun et al. (2014), they obtained an increase in solubilization and decrease in average particle sizes. US also leads to a decrease in milk fat globule size due to the homogenization effect caused by the process (Cameron et al., 2009). Zhao et al. (2014) examined effect of US (20 kHz, 0-20 min) on coagulation aspects of goat milk and demonstrated that coagulation time increases 5 to 7 min, when US treatment applied. However, coagulation time again decreases to its original value in the subsequent 10 to 15 minutes, and increases slightly at 20 min. US also increased the coagulum strength, water holding capacity and gel firmness. Effect of US on the particle size of goat milk is similar to cow milk, with increasing processing time average particle size decreases and particle size distribution become more homogeneous.

COLD PLASMA (CP) TECHNOLOGY

Cold Plasma (CP) technology is one of the novel non-thermal technology for food processing that has gained attention from researchers on the world in recent years (Morales-de la Peña et al., 2019). This technology was used for rising surface energy of materials, ameliorating the printing and adhesion properties of polymers, and a variety of usage domains in electronics. However, it was shown that CP is a powerful method for the food industry (Chizoba Ekezie et al., 2017). Plasma is called the fourth state of matter which is an ionized gas including active species such as free radicals, ions, and electrons. Generally, plasma is divided into two groups that are thermal plasma and non-thermal plasma, which is also known as Cold Plasma (CP) (Coutinho et al., 2018; Misra et al., 2017; Misra, Oliver, Schlüter, 2016). In the simplest form, CP technology can be explained that plasma is generated by applying partially ionized state of a gas (usually O_2 and N_2) with free ions, electrons, molecules, atomic species, UV photons, and charged particles. These active species of plasma can react with food and inactivate target microorganism by releasing the stored energy (Misra et al., 2017). The process parameters of this technology are gas fed (type, flow, pressure, type, flow), electric field, time, and media.

EFFECT OF COLD PLASMA (CP) ON MILK AND DAIRY PRODUCTS

CP is an effective method to inactivate microorganisms present in milk (Coutinho et al., 2018; Segat et al., 2016). There are three basic mechanisms that cause inactivation of microorganisms. These mechanisms include;

1.   Etching of cell surfaces induced by reactive species formed during plasma generation,
2.   Volatilization of compounds and intrinsic photodesorption of ultraviolet (UV) photons,
3.   Destruction of genetic material (Laroussi, 2005).

Reactive species such as radicals and chemicals can cause lipid and protein oxidation and DNA damage (Coutinho et al., 2018). UV irradiation in cold plasma causes the breakdown of chemical bonds in bacteria. Then, by-products such as CO and CH_n from the intrinsic atoms of the bacteria occurs. Finally, replicate inhibition and activation of etching happens, which leads to inactivation of bacteria (Niemira, 2012). Changes in membrane integrity by charged particles action makes DNA breakdown interaction with a membrane protein. After this event, cell perforation occurs and DNA is released from the cell and genetic material is destructed (Moreau et al., 2008).

There is little information about the effects of cold plasma on dairy products (Coutinho et al., 2018). Low-Temperature Plasma for inactivation of *E. coli* in milk was examined by Gurol et al. (2012). At this study, three different milk having different fat contents were used. The time-dependent effect of atmospheric corona discharge produced with 9 kV of AC power supply and different exposure time (0, 3, 6, 9,12, 15 and 20 min) was applied. According to results, 4 log reduction occurred after 20 min application. Also, cold plasma treatment did not have any significant effect on the pH and color values of milk samples. Another study performed in terms of microbial inactivation by cold plasma processing is related to microbial safety and quality attributes of milk following treatment with atmospheric pressure encapsulated dielectric barrier discharge (DBD) plasma (Kim et al., 2015). Whole milk was inoculated with *E. coli*, *L. monocytogenes,* and *S. typhimurium*, and plasma were produced by using a plastic container (250 W, 15 kHz) for 10 min. It is stated that roughly 2.4 log reduction occurred after the treatment. Furthermore, pH value and a* of milk were decreased although L* and b* values were increased with respect to the color results. The study suggested that encapsulated DBD plasma treatment for less than 10 min should be done for improving the microbial quality without slight changes in physicochemical quality of milk. Yong et al. (2015) reported pathogen inactivation and quality changes in Cheddar cheese by using flexible thin-layer DBD plasma. *L. monocytogenes*, *E. coli* O157: H7 and *S. typhimurium* were used as pathogen bacteria and plasma was produced by conductive layer (100 W, 15 kHz) for 10 min. 2.1, 3.2, and 5.8 log CFU/g reductions were observed for *L. monocytogenes*, *E. coli* O157: H7, and *S. typhimurium,* respectively after cold plasma treatment. Although sensory attributes such as total color difference (ΔE), and color scores did not show significant changes. Whereas, a significant decrease was determined in flavor and overall acceptance of product after cold plasma treatment due to the increasing off-flavor.

Korachi et al. (2015) stated that there were no significant changes observed for the lipid composition of milk but the quantity of volatile compounds decreased significantly after 20 minCP treatment. Alkaline phosphatase activity has a similar Z-value to heat-resistant pathogens in milk therefore it is used as an indicator to evaluate the efficiency of heat- treatments. Segat et al. (2016) showed that CP technology having high voltages (40, 50 and 60 kV) could inactivate alkaline phosphatase within a few seconds of process time because of the fact that alkaline phosphatase has an α-helix structure and the structure was breakdown under cold plasma process, although the temperature did not change significantly. Moreover, the Weibull model is the best-described model for the inactivation of alkaline phosphatase.

PULSED LIGHT

Pulsed Light (PL) is an emerging technology that is based on the application of using intense and short pulses (100–400 µs) of white light (Li & Farid, 2016; Mahendran et al., 2019). The spectrum of PL consists of wavelengths ranging from ultraviolet to near-infrared region (Li & Farid, 2016). PL was approved by Food and Drug Administration (FDA) in 1996 during food applications up to a cumulative fluence of 12 J cm^{-2}, where emission spectra should be kept between 200 and 1100 nm and pulse duration at ≤ 2 ms (Rowan, 2019). At the beginning of the usage of this technology, it was used for surface and water decontamination. However, in recent years this technology is used for a wide range of food products such as liquid products, fruit, and vegetable surfaces (Morales-de la Peña et al., 2019). The main components of PL are shown in Figure 5, which includes power unit for generation of pulses in the treatment chamber.

Figure 5. Schematic diagram of PL technology system reproduced from Mahendran et al., (2019)

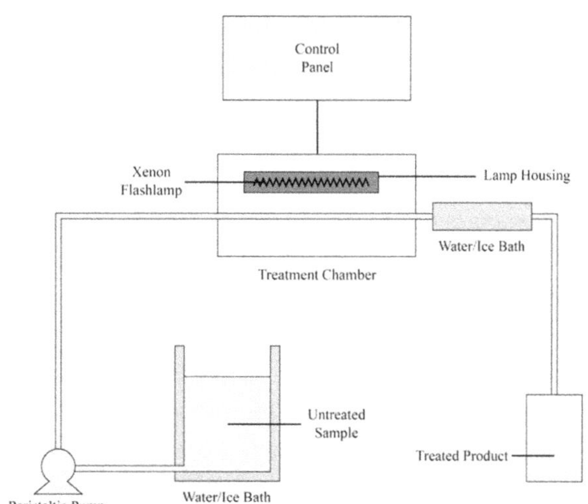

The principle of PL relies on the accumulation of high discharge voltage in a capacitor, where the stored energy is delivered in ultra-short pulses through a light source filled with xenon gas. The xenon-light source has a spectrum light flashes with the range of 200–1100 nm and this leads to photochemical modification of microorganism which means disinfection (Garvey & Rowan, 2019; Kramer et al., 2015; Rowan, 2019). The parameters of PL are the fluence (J cm^{-2}), pulse width (τ), number of the pulse (n), frequency (Hz), exposure time (s), and the peak power [W].

EFFECT OF PULSED LIGHT ON MILK AND DAIRY PRODUCTS

Little information is available on the application of PL to milk and dairy products. Effect of PL on pathogenic microorganisms was found profoundly in pursuance of achieving food safety conditions for PL-treated milk. The inactivation mechanism of PL is the impairment of the DNA of microorganism by forming thymine dimers that cause bacterial death. *Staphylococcus aureus* is one of the most important contagious mastitis foodborne pathogen in dairy products (Kümmel et al., 2016). In terms of inactivation of *S. aureus* in milk, different parameters (distance of the sample from the light strobe (5 to 11 cm), number of passes (1 to 3 passes), and flow rate (20 to 40 mL/min)) were applied into raw milk, which included roughly 8 to 9 log CFU/mL *S. aureus* (Krishnamurthy et al., 2007). Application of 11 cm distance with

2 passes, 11 run order and 30 mL/min flow rate or 8 cm distance with 1 pass, 4 run order and 20 mL/min flow rate showed the highest reduction in *S. aureus* count (roughly 7 $\log_{10}$ CFU/mL). In addition to this, the average bulk temperature of raw milk after PL treatment was found between 22-51°C. This temperature was derived from the distance of the sample to the light strobe (Krishnamurthy et al., 2007).

Inactivation of *E. coli* by using PL treatment was examined by Kasahara et al. (2015). According to the results, it was shown that 6 $\log_{10}$ CFU/mL reduction of *E. coli* was achieved when 10,000 mJ/cm^2 fluence was applied. Furthermore, the physical properties of goat milk such as viscosity, pH, and density were not changed significantly after PL treatment. Similar to physical properties, a chemical composition such as moisture, protein, lipid and ash content, and aroma profiles of the goat milk were not demonstrated any significant change after treatment (Kasahara et al., 2015). Innocente et al. (2014) investigated the effect of PL on the total microbial count and alkaline phosphatase activity of raw milk. In this study, different fluence (0.2626.25 J cm^2) was applied to raw milk. According to results, PL treatments inactivate alkaline phosphatase activity by photochemical and photothermal effects. Moreover, alkaline phosphatase activity was found more photo-resistant than microorganisms.

Effect of PL on pathogenic and spoilage microorganisms for PL-treated cheese surface was performed by Proulx et al., (2015). *Pseudomonas fluorescens* was used as spoilage bacteria, *E. coli* ATCC 25922 was used as a nonpathogenic form of *E. coli* O157: H7, and *L. innocua* was used as a nonpathogenic form of *L. monocytogenes* in this study. 5 or 7 log CFU/slice of bacteria was inoculated on the surface of the cheese and different fluences (1.02 to 12.29 J/cm ^{2}) were applied. Maximum inactivation was obtained at 3.07 J/cm^2 and the most sensitive microorganism to PL treatment was determined as *E. coli* with a nearly 5.4 log reduction. *P. fluorescens* (roughly 3.7 log reduction) and *L. innocua* (approximately 3.3 log reduction) followed *E. coli*, respectively. Proulx et al. (2017) also studied the reduction degree of *E. coli*, *P. fluorescens*, *L. innocua* in case of PL treatment in comparison to PL treatments combined with nisin and natamycin on Cheddar cheese. It was reported that nisin or natamycin before the application of PL treatment reduced the effectiveness of PL t for all bacteria due to decreasing the fluence received by the bacteria. However, the effectiveness of PL treatment increased for all bacteria, when these antimicrobials were applied after the treatment.

PL treatment was reported not to have any negative effects on the quality and sensory characteristics of dairy products. It was shown that no significant changes occurred in color and peroxide value of Cheddar cheese after the PL dose of 9.22 J/ cm^2. In addition to this, PL treatment has a significant effect to delay mold growth during 7 days of refrigeration storage treated with 9.22 J/ cm^2 fluence. It is also reported that PL treatment has an overall liking in terms of flavor, and appearance (Proulx et al., 2016). Protein oxidation in processed cheese slices treated with PL was also examined. Different fluences (0.7, 2.1, 4.2, 8.4 and 11.9 J/cm^2) were applied and it was found that PL treatments up to 4.2 J/cm^2 did not increase protein oxidation whereas higher fluences increased protein oxidation by absorption of light by amino acids or by the involvement of photosensitizers (Fernández et al., 2014).

CONCLUSION AND FUTURE PROSPECTS

Milk and dairy products are important nutrition sources for humans and to preserve the nutritional contents the novel processing method is thermal processing in this sector. Application of thermal treatment leads to the elimination of pathogenic and spoilage microorganisms, together with deterioration in the desirable as well as the undesirable changes of physicochemical properties products. It is possible to eliminate undesirable microorganisms in milk and dairy products without effecting fresh-like properties by application of non-thermal techniques. Microbiological and physicochemical effects of high hydrostatic pressure, pulsed electric field, ultrasound, cold plasma, and pulsed UV-light on milk and dairy products, and advantages of these non-thermal processing technologies comparing with thermal treatments reviewed in this chapter. Future applications of non-thermal processes with or without heat treatment for milk and dairy products will probably advance due to achievement of food safety without undesirable effects caused by thermal treatment, as well as the variety of physicochemical changes induced by non-thermal treatments.

REFERENCES

Ahmed, J., Ramaswamy, H. S., Kasapis, S., & Boye, I. (2010). *J.* Novel food processing effects on rheological and functional properties. CRC Group.

Alpas, H., & Bozoglu, F. (2000, June). The combined effect of high hydrostatic pressure, heat and bacteriocins on inactivation of foodborne pathogens in milk and orange juice. *World Journal of Microbiology & Biotechnology*, *16*(4), 387–392. doi:10.1023/A:1008936607413

Alpas, H., Kalchayanand, N., Bozoglu, F., & Ray, B. (2000). Interactions of high hydrostatic pressure, pressurization temperature and pH on death and injury of pressure-resistant and pressure-sensitive strains of foodborne pathogens. *International Journal of Food Microbiology*, *60*(1), 33–42. doi:10.1016/S0168-1605(00)00324-X PMID:11014520

Alpas, H., Kalchayanand, N., Bozoglu, F., Sikes, A., Dunne, C. P., & Ray, B. (1999). Variation in resistance to hydrostatic pressure among strains of food-borne pathogens. *Applied and Environmental Microbiology*, *65*(9), 4248–4251. PMID:10473446

Alpas, H., Lee, J., Bozoglu, F., & Kaletunç, G. (2003). Evaluation of high hydrostatic pressure sensitivity of Staphylococcus aureus and Escherichia coli O157:H7 by differential scanning calorimetry. *International Journal of Food Microbiology*, *87*(3), 229–237. doi:10.1016/S0168-1605(03)00066-7 PMID:14527795

Altuner, E. M., Alpas, H., Erdem, Y. K., & Bozoglu, F. (2006). Effect of high hydrostatic pressure on physicochemical and biochemical properties of milk. *European Food Research and Technology*, *222*(3–4), 392–396. doi:10.100700217-005-0072-4

Awad, T. S., Moharram, H. A., Shaltout, O. E., Asker, D., & Youssef, M. M. (2012). Applications of ultrasound in analysis, processing and quality control of food: A review. *Food Research International*, *48*(2), 410–427. doi:10.1016/j.foodres.2012.05.004

Bhattacharya, S. (2015). *Conventional and advanced food processing technologies*. Wiley Blackwell.

Cameron, M., McMaster, L. D., & Britz, T. J. (2009). Impact of ultrasound on dairy spoilage microbes and milk components. *Dairy Science & Technology*, *89*(1), 83–98. doi:10.1051/dst/2008037

Chandrapala, J., Martin, G. J. O., Kentish, S. E., & Ashokkumar, M. (2014). Dissolution and reconstitution of casein micelle containing dairy powders by high shear using ultrasonic and physical methods. *Ultrasonics Sonochemistry*, *21*(5), 1658–1665. doi:10.1016/j.ultsonch.2014.04.006 PMID:24798226

Chemat, F., Zill-e-Huma, & Khan, M. K. (2011). Applications of ultrasound in food technology: Processing, preservation, and extraction. *Ultrasonics Sonochemistry, 18*(4), 813–835. doi:10.1016/j.ultsonch.2010.11.023 PMID:21216174

Chizoba Ekezie, F. G., Sun, D. W., & Cheng, J. H. (2017). A review on recent advances in cold plasma technology for the food industry: Current applications and future trends. *Trends in Food Science & Technology, 69*, 46–58. doi:10.1016/j.tifs.2017.08.007

Coutinho, N. M., Silveira, M. R., Rocha, R. S., Moraes, J., Ferreira, M. V. S., Pimentel, T. C., ... Cruz, A. G. (2018). Cold plasma processing of milk and dairy products. *Trends in Food Science & Technology, 74*(February), 56–68. doi:10.1016/j.tifs.2018.02.008

D'Amico, D. J., Silk, T. M., Wu, J., & Guo, M. (2006). Inactivation of microorganisms in milk and apple cider treated with ultrasound. *Journal of Food Protection, 69*(3), 556–563. doi:10.4315/0362-028X-69.3.556 PMID:16541685

Doona, C. J., Kustin, K., & Feeherry, F. (2010). *Case studies in novel food processing technologies.* Woodhead Publishing; doi:10.1533/9780857090713

Durance, T. (2002). *Handbook of food preservation* (Vol. 35). Food Research International; doi:10.1016/S0963-9969(00)00143-5

Evrendilek, G. A., Zhang, Q. H., & Richter, E. R. (2004). Application of pulsed electric fields to skim milk inoculated with Staphylococcus aureus. *Biosystems Engineering, 87*(2), 137–144. doi:10.1016/j.biosystemseng.2003.11.005

Fernández, M., Ganan, M., Guerra, C., & Hierro, E. (2014). Protein oxidation in processed cheese slices treated with pulsed light technology. *Food Chemistry, 159*, 388–390. doi:10.1016/j.foodchem.2014.02.165 PMID:24767071

Fernández-Molina, J. J., Fernández-gutiérrez, S. A., Altunakar, B., Bermúdez-Aguirre, D., Swanson, B. G., & Barbosa-Cánovas, G. V. (2005). The combined effect of pulsed electric fields and conventional heating on the microbial quality and shelf life of skim milk. *Journal of Food Processing and Preservation, 29*(5–6), 390–406. doi:10.1111/j.1745-4549.2005.00036.x

Garcia-Amezquita, L. E., Primo-Mora, A. R., Barbosa-Cánovas, G. V., & Sepulveda, D. R. (2009). Effect of nonthermal technologies on the native size distribution of fat globules in bovine cheese-making milk. *Innovative Food Science & Emerging Technologies, 10*(4), 491–494. doi:10.1016/j.ifset.2009.03.002

García-Risco, M. R., Cortés, E., Carrascosa, A. V., & López-Fandiño, R. (1998). Microbiological and chemical changes in high-pressure-treated milk during refrigerated storage. *Journal of Food Protection, 61*(6), 735–737. doi:10.4315/0362-028X-61.6.735 PMID:9709260

García-Risco, M. R., Olano, A., Ramos, M., & López-Fandiño, R. (2000). Micelar changes induced by high pressure. influence in the proteolytic activity and organoleptic properties of milk. *Journal of Dairy Science, 83*(10), 2184–2189. doi:10.3168/jds.S0022-0302(00)75101-0 PMID:11049057

Garvey, M., & Rowan, N. J. (2019). Pulsed UV as a potential surface sanitizer in food production processes to ensure consumer safety. *Current Opinion in Food Science, 26*, 65–70. doi:10.1016/j.cofs.2019.03.003

Gaucheron, F., Famelart, M. H., Mariette, F., Raulot, K., Michel, F., & Le Graetf, Y. (1997). Combined effects of temperature and high-pressure treatments on physicochemical characteristics of skim milk. *Food Chemistry*, *59*(3), 439–447. doi:10.1016/S0308-8146(96)00301-9

Guerrero-Beltrán, J. Á., Sepulveda, D. R., Góngora-Nieto, M. M., Swanson, B., & Barbosa-Cánovas, G. V. (2010). Milk thermization by pulsed electric fields (PEF) and electrically induced heat. *Journal of Food Engineering*, *100*(1), 56–60. doi:10.1016/j.jfoodeng.2010.03.027

Gurol, C., Ekinci, F. Y., Aslan, N., & Korachi, M. (2012). Low temperature plasma for decontamination of E. coli in milk. *International Journal of Food Microbiology*, *157*(1), 1–5. doi:10.1016/j.ijfoodmicro.2012.02.016 PMID:22622128

Han, Z., Cai, M., Cheng, J., & Sun, D. (2018). Effects of electric fields and electromagnetic wave on food protein structure and functionality: A review. *Trends in Food Science & Technology*, *75*(March), 1–9. doi:10.1016/j.tifs.2018.02.017

Harte, F., Luedecke, L., Swanson, B., & Barbosa-Cánovas, G. V. (2010). Low-fat set yogurt made from milk subjected to combinations of high hydrostatic pressure and thermal processing. *Journal of Dairy Science*, *86*(4), 1074–1082. doi:10.3168/jds.S0022-0302(03)73690-X PMID:12741531

Hite, B. H. (1899). The effects of pressure in the preservation of milk. *Bulletin of the West Virginia University Agricultural Experimental Station Morgantown*, (58), 15–35.

Huang, H. W., Wu, S. J., Lu, J. K., Shyu, Y. T., & Wang, C. Y. (2017). Current status and future trends of high-pressure processing in food industry. *Food Control*, *72*(12), 1–8. doi:10.1016/j.foodcont.2016.07.019

Huppertz, T., Fox, P. F., & Kelly, A. L. (2003). High pressure-induced changes in the creaming properties of bovine milk, *4*(July), 349–359. doi:10.1016/S1466-8564

Innocente, N., Segat, A., Manzocco, L., Marino, M., Maifreni, M., Bortolomeoli, I., ... Nicoli, M. C. (2014). Effect of pulsed light on total microbial count and alkaline phosphatase activity of raw milk. *International Dairy Journal*, *39*(1), 108–112. doi:10.1016/j.idairyj.2014.05.009

Jaeger, H., Meneses, N., & Knorr, D. (2014). Pulsed electric field technology. In Y. Motarjemi, G. Moy, & E. Todd (Eds.), *Encyclopedia of food safety* (Vol. 3, pp. 239–244). Elsevier. doi:10.1016/B978-0-12-378612-8.00260-2

Kasahara, I., Carrasco, V., & Aguilar, L. (2015). Inactivation of Escherichia coli in goat milk using pulsed ultraviolet light. *Journal of Food Engineering*, *152*, 43–49. doi:10.1016/j.jfoodeng.2014.11.012

Khan, M. K., Ahmad, K., Hassan, S., Imran, M., Ahmad, N., & Xu, C. (2018). Effect of novel technologies on polyphenols during food processing. *Innovative Food Science and Emerging Technologies*, *45*(December 2017), 361–381. doi:10.1016/j.ifset.2017.12.006

Kim, H. J., Yong, H. I., Park, S., Kim, K., Choe, W., & Jo, C. (2015). Microbial safety and quality attributes of milk following treatment with atmospheric pressure encapsulated dielectric barrier discharge plasma. *Food Control*, *47*, 451–456. doi:10.1016/j.foodcont.2014.07.053

Knudsen, J. C., & Skibsted, L. H. (2010). High pressure effects on the structure of casein micelles in milk as studied by cryo-transmission electron microscopy. *Food Chemistry*, *119*(1), 202–208. doi:10.1016/j. foodchem.2009.06.017

Korachi, M., Ozen, F., Aslan, N., Vannini, L., Guerzoni, M. E., Gottardi, D., & Ekinci, F. Y. (2015). Biochemical changes to milk following treatment by a novel, cold atmospheric plasma system. *International Dairy Journal*, *42*, 64–69. doi:10.1016/j.idairyj.2014.10.006

Koutchma, T. (2014). *Adapting high hydrostatic pressure (HPP) for food processing operations. Adapting high hydrostatic pressure (HPP) for food processing operations.* doi:10.1016/C2013-0-12997-2

Kramer, B., Wunderlıch, J., & Muranyı, P. (2015). Pulsed light decontamination of endive salad and mung bean sprouts and impact on color and respiration activity. *Journal of Food Protection*, *78*(2), 340–348. doi:10.4315/0362-028X.JFP-14-262 PMID:25710149

Krishnamurthy, K., Demirci, A., & Irudayaraj, J. M. (2007). Inactivation of Staphylococcus aureus in milk using flow-through pulsed UV-light treatment system. *Journal of Food Science*, *72*(7), M233–M239. doi:10.1111/j.1750-3841.2007.00438.x PMID:17995646

Kümmel, J., Stessl, B., Gonano, M., Walcher, G., Bereuter, O., Fricker, M., ... Ehling-Schulz, M. (2016). Staphylococcus aureus entrance into the dairy chain: Tracking S. aureus from dairy cow to cheese. *Frontiers in Microbiology*, *7*(OCT), 1–11. doi:10.3389/fmicb.2016.01603 PMID:27790200

Laroussi, M. (2005). Low temperature plasma-based sterilization: Overview and state-of-the-art. *Plasma Processes and Polymers*, *2*(5), 391–400. doi:10.1002/ppap.200400078

Li, X., & Farid, M. (2016). A review on recent development in non-conventional food sterilization technologies. *Journal of Food Engineering*, *182*, 33–45. doi:10.1016/j.jfoodeng.2016.02.026

Liu, Z., Hemar, Y., Tan, S., Sanguansri, P., Niere, J., Buckow, R., & Augustin, M. A. (2015). Pulsed electric field treatment of reconstituted skim milks at alkaline pH or with added EDTA. *Journal of Food Engineering*, *144*, 112–118. doi:10.1016/j.jfoodeng.2014.06.033

Liu, Z., Juliano, P., Williams, R. P., Niere, J., & Augustin, M. A. (2014). Ultrasound effects on the assembly of casein micelles in reconstituted skim milk. *The Journal of Dairy Research*, *81*(2), 146–155. doi:10.1017/S0022029913000721 PMID:24351847

Mahendran, R., Ramanan, K. R., Barba, F. J., Lorenzo, J. M., López-Fernández, O., Munekata, P. E. S., ... Tiwari, B. K. (2018, December). Recent advances in the application of pulsed light processing for improving food safety and increasing shelf life. *Trends in Food Science & Technology*, *88*, 67–79. doi:10.1016/j.tifs.2019.03.010

Marchesini, G., Fasolato, L., Novelli, E., Balzan, S., Contiero, B., Montemurro, F., ... Segato, S. (2015). Ultrasonic inactivation of microorganisms: A compromise between lethal capacity and sensory quality of milk. *Innovative Food Science & Emerging Technologies*, *29*, 215–221. doi:10.1016/j.ifset.2015.03.015

Misra, N. N., Koubaa, M., Roohinejad, S., Juliano, P., Alpas, H., Inácio, R. S., ... Barba, F. J. (2017). Landmarks in the historical development of twenty first century food processing technologies. *Food Research International*, *97*(May), 318–339. doi:10.1016/j.foodres.2017.05.001 PMID:28578057

Misra, N. N., Oliver, K., & Schlüter, P. J. C. (2016). *Cold plasma in food and agriculture*. Academic Press; doi:10.1016/b978-0-12-801365-6.09991-1

Morales-de la Peña, M., Welti-Chanes, J., & Martín-Belloso, O. (2019). Novel technologies to improve food safety and quality. *Current Opinion in Food Science*, *30*, 1–7. doi:10.1016/j.cofs.2018.10.009

Moreau, M., Orange, N., & Feuilloley, M. G. J. (2008). Non-thermal plasma technologies: New tools for bio-decontamination. *Biotechnology Advances*, *26*(6), 610–617. doi:10.1016/j.biotechadv.2008.08.001 PMID:18775485

Moreno, S. E. H. (2017). Distribución de pesticidas en sistemas de abejas, polen, cera y miel. Análisis por LC-MS/MS. Retrieved from http://repositorio.ual.es/bitstream/handle/10835/6453/16628_Memoria_TFG FINAL2.pdf?sequence=1&isAllowed=y

Mussa, D. M., & Ramaswamy, H. S. (1997). Ultra high pressure pasteurization of milk: Kinetics of microbial destruction and changes in Physico-chemical characteristics. *Lebensmittel-Wissenschaft + Technologie*, *30*(6), 551–557. doi:10.1006/fstl.1996.0223

Nakai, S., & Li-chan, E. (1988). *Hydrophobic interactions in food systems authors*. Boca Raton, FL: CRC Press.

Niemira, B. A. (2012). Cold plasma decontamination of foods. *Annual Review of Food Science and Technology*, *3*(1), 125–142. doi:10.1146/annurev-food-022811-101132 PMID:22149075

Odriozola-Serrano, I., Bendicho-Porta, S., & Martín-Belloso, O. (2010). Comparative study on shelf life of whole milk processed by high-intensity pulsed electric field or heat treatment. *Journal of Dairy Science*, *89*(3), 905–911. doi:10.3168/jds.S0022-0302(06)72155-5 PMID:16507684

Ohshima, T., Tanino, T., Kameda, T., & Harashima, H. (2016). Engineering of operation condition in milk pasteurization with PEF treatment. *Food Control*, *68*, 297–302. doi:10.1016/j.foodcont.2016.03.047

Ojha, K. S., Mason, T. J., O'Donnell, C. P., Kerry, J. P., & Tiwari, B. K. (2017). Ultrasound technology for food fermentation applications. *Ultrasonics Sonochemistry*, *34*, 410–417. doi:10.1016/j.ultsonch.2016.06.001 PMID:27773263

Pandey, P. K., Ramaswamy, H. S., & Idziak, E. (2003). High pressure destruction kinetics of in raw milk at two temperatures. *Journal of Food Process Engineering*, *26*(3), 265–283. doi:10.1111/j.1745-4530.2003.tb00601.x

Patterson, M. F., & Kilpatrick, D. J. (1998). The combined effect of high hydrostatic pressure and mild heat on inactivation of pathogens in milk and poultry. *Journal of Food Protection*, *61*(4), 432–436. doi:10.4315/0362-028X-61.4.432 PMID:9709206

Proulx, J., Agustin, M., Sullivan, G., VanWees, S., Jian, J., Hilton, S. T., & Moraru, C. I. (2016). Short communication: Influence of pulsed light treatment on the quality and sensory characteristics of Cheddar cheese. *Journal of Dairy Science*, *100*(2), 1004–1008. doi:10.3168/jds.2016-11579 PMID:28012618

Proulx, J., Hsu, L. C., Miller, B. M., Sullivan, G., Paradis, K., & Moraru, C. I. (2015). Pulsed-light inactivation of pathogenic and spoilage bacteria on cheese surface. *Journal of Dairy Science*, *98*(9), 5890–5898. doi:10.3168/jds.2015-9410 PMID:26162787

Proulx, J., Sullivan, G., Marostegan, L. F., VanWees, S., Hsu, L. C., & Moraru, C. I. (2017). Pulsed light and antimicrobial combination treatments for surface decontamination of cheese: Favorable and antagonistic effects. *Journal of Dairy Science, 100*(3), 1664–1673. doi:10.3168/jds.2016-11582 PMID:28109595

Putnik, P., Kresoja, Ž., Bosiljkov, T., Režek Jambrak, A., Barba, F. J., Lorenzo, J. M., ... Bursać Kovačević, D. (2018, July). Comparing the effects of thermal and non-thermal technologies on pomegranate juice quality: A review. *Food Chemistry, 279*, 150–161. doi:10.1016/j.foodchem.2018.11.131 PMID:30611474

Rademacher, B., & Hinrichs, J. (2006). Effects of high-pressure treatment on indigenous enzymes in bovine milk: Reaction kinetics, inactivation and potential application. *International Dairy Journal, 16*(6), 655–661. doi:10.1016/j.idairyj.2005.10.021

Rademacher, B., Pfeiffer, B., & Kessler, H. G. (1998). *Inactivation of microorganisms and enzymes in pressure-treated raw milk. High pressure food science, bioscience, and chemistry.* The Royal Society of Chemistry; doi:10.1533/9781845698379.3.145

Rowan, N. J. (2019). Pulsed light as an emerging technology to cause disruption for food and adjacent industries – Quo vadis? *Trends in Food Science & Technology, 88*(March), 316–332. doi:10.1016/j.tifs.2019.03.027

Santhirasegaram, V., Razali, Z., & Somasundram, C. (2016). *Safety improvement of fruit juices by novel thermal and nonthermal processing. Food hygiene and toxicology in ready-to-eat foods.* Elsevier Inc.; doi:10.1016/B978-0-12-801916-0.00012-1

Schrader, K., Buchheim, W., & Morr, C. V. (1997). High pressure effects on the colloidal calcium phosphate and the structural integrity of micellar casein in milk. Part 1 phosphate in heated milk systems. *Food / Nahrung, 41*(3), 133–138.

Segat, A., Misra, N. N., Cullen, P. J., & Innocente, N. (2016). Effect of atmospheric pressure cold plasma (ACP) on activity and structure of alkaline phosphatase. *Food and Bioproducts Processing, 98*, 181–188. doi:10.1016/j.fbp.2016.01.010

Şengül, M., Erkaya, T., Başlar, M., & Ertugay, M. F. (2011). Effect of photosonication treatment on inactivation of total and coliform bacteria in milk. *Food Control, 22*(11), 1803–1806. doi:10.1016/j.foodcont.2011.04.015

Shahbaz, H. M., Kim, J. U., Kim, S.-H., & Park, J. (2018). *Advances in nonthermal processing technologies for enhanced microbiological safety and quality of fresh fruit and juice products. food processing for increased quality and consumption.* Elsevier; doi:10.1016/b978-0-12-811447-6.00007-2

Sharma, P., Bremer, P., Oey, I., & Everett, D. W. (2014). Bacterial inactivation in whole milk using pulsed electric field processing. *International Dairy Journal, 35*(1), 49–56. doi:10.1016/j.idairyj.2013.10.005

Styles, M. F., Hoover, D. G., & Farkas, D. F. (1991). Response of Listeria monocytogenes and Vibrio parahaemolyficus to high hydrostatic pressure. *Journal of Food Science, 56*(5), 1404–1407. doi:10.1111/j.1365-2621.1991.tb04784.x

Sui, Q., Roginski, H., Williams, R. P. W., Versteeg, C., & Wan, J. (2011). Effect of pulsed electric field and thermal treatment on the physicochemical and functional properties of whey protein isolate. *International Dairy Journal*, *21*(4), 206–213. doi:10.1016/j.idairyj.2010.11.001

Sun, Y., Chen, J., Zhang, S., Li, H., Lu, J., Liu, L., ... Jiaping, L. (2014). Effect of power ultrasound pretreatment on the physical and functional properties of reconstituted milk protein concentrate. *Journal of Food Engineering*, *124*, 11–18. doi:10.1016/j.jfoodeng.2013.09.013

Trujillo, A. J., Ferragut, B., Juan, B., Roig-Sagués, A. X., & Guamis, B. (2016). Processing of dairy products utilizing high pressure. In V. M. Balasubramaniam, G. V. Barbosa-Cánovas, & H. L. M. Lelieveld (Eds.), *High pressure processing of food* (pp. 553–590). New York: Springer; doi:10.1007/978-1-4939-3234-4_25

Vijayakumar, S., Grewell, D., Annandarajah, C., Benner, L., & Clark, S. (2015). Quality characteristics and plasmin activity of thermosonicated skim milk and cream. *Journal of Dairy Science*, *98*(10), 6678–6691. doi:10.3168/jds.2015-9429 PMID:26233461

Wrigley, D. M., & Llorca, N. G. (1992). Decrease of Salmonella typhimurium in skim milk and egg by heat and ultrasonic wave treatment. *Journal of Food Protection*, *55*(9), 678–680. doi:10.4315/0362-028X-55.9.678 PMID:31084132

Yong, H. I., Kim, H. J., Park, S., Kim, K., Choe, W., Yoo, S. J., & Jo, C. (2015). Pathogen inactivation and quality changes in sliced cheddar cheese treated using flexible thin-layer dielectric barrier discharge plasma. *Food Research International*, *69*, 57–63. doi:10.1016/j.foodres.2014.12.008

Yu, L. J., Ngadi, M., & Raghavan, G. S. V. (2009). Effect of temperature and pulsed electric field treatment on rennet coagulation properties of milk. *Journal of Food Engineering*, *95*(1), 115–118. doi:10.1016/j.jfoodeng.2009.04.013

Zhao, L., Zhang, S., Uluko, H., Liu, L., Lu, J., Xue, H., ... Lv, J. (2014). Effect of ultrasound pretreatment on rennet-induced coagulation properties of goat's milk. *Food Chemistry*, *165*, 167–174. doi:10.1016/j.foodchem.2014.05.081 PMID:25038663

Zhao, W., Yang, R., Shen, X., Zhang, S., & Chen, X. (2013). Lethal and sublethal injury and kinetics of Escherichia coli, Listeria monocytogenes and Staphylococcus aureus in milk by pulsed electric fields. *Food Control*, *32*(1), 6–12. doi:10.1016/j.foodcont.2012.11.029

Chapter 9
Novel Packaging Technologies in Dairy Products:
Principles and Recent Advances

Nazli Turkmen
Ankara University, Turkey

Sebnem Ozturkoglu-Budak
Ankara University, Turkey

ABSTRACT

The packaging process is an important step in maintaining the quality characteristics of foods. Packaging foods protects products from external effects and provides product information to consumers. Due to the various changes occurring during the distribution and storage of the products, some significant quality characteristics can be lost. In recent years, novel packaging technologies have been developed to supply long shelf life, safety, and 'fresh-like' characteristics to the products. These novel technologies include nanotechnology, modified atmosphere packaging, active packaging, and intelligent/smart packaging. Since dairy products are generally vulnerable to biological, physical, and chemical changes, they lose their quality characteristics within a short term. Therefore, the use of these novel techniques in dairy products is greatly important. This chapter informs about general principles of the novel packaging techniques and their current applications in dairy technology.

INTRODUCTION

Containers or cases made of special materials such as metal, glass, and plastic which protect the products against external factors and facilitate the marketing and consumption of foods are called food packaging. To ensure the food safety, the stages of packaging, transportation, and storage until the product reaches consumers are as important as the production of foods (Çelik & Tümer, 2016). The main purpose of food packaging is to ensure food safety by preserving the overall quality throughout the time interval of production and consumption (Cutter, 2006).

DOI: 10.4018/978-1-7998-5354-1.ch009

The UK Packaging Institute defines packaging in three different ways (Gawith & Robertson, 2000):

1. Preparation of products for transportation, distribution, storage, retailing, and final use in a coordinated manner.
2. Safe and cost-efficient delivery way of products to the final consumers.
3. Technological and economic function of the goal of minimizing delivery costs while maximizing sales and profits.

Food packaging is being developed day by day upon the demands of the consumers and the novel trends applied in food industry. There are four important functions to be considered when developing a food package: storage, protection, convenience, and communication. In other words, package should be able to protect the product against external factors such as water, gas, odor, microorganisms, dust, and pressure. In addition, food packages need to contain information about the product and should be constantly improved to adapt to varying living conditions (Gawith & Robertson, 2000). Particularly in milk and dairy products which are prone to physical, chemical, and biological changes in a short time, the packaging technologies have been constantly developed io extend the shelf life of products.

The novel methods used in packaging technology can be listed as follows (Patel, Prajapati, & Balakrishnan, 2015):

1. Nanotechnology
2. Modified Atmosphere Packaging
3. Active Packaging
4. Intelligent/Smart Packaging

NANOTECHNOLOGY

Nanotechnology is an applied science that controls occurrences at atomic or molecular level below 100 nm (Anonymous, 2019). Nanotechnology is implemented in many food fields such as increasing food safety, reducing agricultural inputs, and preventing the nutritional factors (Schnettler et al., 2013). In food science, food packaging is known as the most common field where nanotechnology is applied (Sürengil & Kılınç, 2011).

Nanotechnology can be used in food packaging in three ways (Duncan, 2011):

1. To produce synthetic polymer and biopolymer-based packaging materials for the purpose of developing packages with better barrier and mechanical properties.
2. To develop active packaging materials by using nanoparticles having antimicrobial properties or oxygen absorption such as Ag, ZnO, and TiO_2.
3. To detect the storage conditions in which food products are exposed by use of different nanoparticles such as Fe_2O_3 and TiO_2 in intelligent packaging technology and to produce markers that inform the manufacturer, seller, and consumer.

Nanotechnological applications, which are used in many fields in food technology, have advantages and disadvantages.

The disadvantages and the concerns arising from the lack of scientific data on the subject are mostly related to nanotechnological applications in food products. Therefore, nanotechnological applications in food packaging are considered to be more reliable than the applications in food products.

In a survey that examined the consumers' view about nanotechnological applications in the food industry, panelists stated they would prefer to buy neither nanotechnological foods nor the products packaged with nanotechnological treatments (Siegrist, Cousin, Kastenholz, & Wiek, 2007). However, consumers also believe that the usage of nanotechnology in food packaging is more beneficial than the usage in foods. Siegrist, Stampfli, Kastenholz, & Keller (2008) also investigated the preference of 337 consumers in 19 nanotechnology products. Results showed that nanotechnological packaging materials were determined to be more reliable by consumers than the foods produced by nanotechnological approaches (Siegrist et al., 2008).

Modified Atmosphere Packaging

In the 1930s, the great losses caused by the rapid deterioration of the products in the transportation, especially of fruits and vegetables, led to new searches to increase the shelf life of food products. When CO_2 was supplied to the stores where food products are stored, it was seen that the products could remain stable for a longer period and this has been the starting point for the development of Modified Atmosphere Packaging (MAP) technology (Demir, 1999).

MAP is based on the principle of replacing the air in the food package with a mixture of different gas or gases. This change can be implemented in two ways: active MAP and passive MAP technology. In the Active MAP technology, the air in the package is directly replaced with the desired gas or gases. However, passive MAP technology is based on the occurrence of naturally desired composition in the atmosphere of package over time, depending on the respiration of the food and the permeability of the special packaging material used (Lee, Arul, Lencki, & Castaigne, 1996).

Oxygen (O_2), nitrogen (N_2) and carbon dioxide (CO_2) gases are the main gases used in MAP technology. In addition to these gases, carbon monoxide, ozone, ethylene oxide, nitrous oxide, sulfur dioxide, helium, neon, argon, propylene oxide, ethanol, hydrogen, and chlorine are the gases that can be used in MAP technology. However, they are not preferred because they are costly and impair the sensory properties of the products (Farber, 1991; Sivertsvik et al., 2002).

During the storage of the product, O_2 is consumed and CO_2 is produced by food respiration. N_2 is an inert gas used to prevent shrinkage of packages due to CO_2 absorption (Sandhya, 2010). N_2 is a tasteless and a low solubility gas that is also insoluble in water and oil, which causes it not to be absorbed by foods. Although this gas alone does not have any antimicrobial effect, it indirectly inhibits the development of aerobic microorganisms when used instead of O_2 to delay the oxidative rancidity in oxygen sensitive products (Farber, 1991; Sivertsvik et al., 2002).

It is stated that the development of aerobic bacteria will be supported by using high amounts of O_2 in MAP technology. On the contrary, the reactions of enzymatic discoloration and anaerobic fermentation can be prevented (Van der Steen, Jacxsens, Devlieghere, & Debevere, 2002). In MAP technology, O_2 is mainly used for packaging fresh red meat products so they maintain their bright red color (Farber, 1991).

CO_2, one of the main gases used in MAP technology, is the only gas with a significant direct antimicrobial effect. Easy solubility of CO_2 in water and oil causes the inhibition of microbial growth and also affects the lag phase, maximum growth rate, and maximum population density of microorganisms (Devlieghere & Debevere, 2000). Although the mechanism of action of CO_2 application is not known exactly, this gas penetrates into microbial cell and decreases the pH of microorganisms which inhibits the growth of microorganisms. Using CO_2 also prevents the bad odor that may occur during storage and transportation of the product (Mullan, 2002). CO_2 is also known to have a prevention effect on food respiration (Farber, 1991).

The degree of main gases effect used in MAP technology varies depending on the type of microorganism, temperature, water activity, and characteristics of product (Oliveira et al., 2015). Therefore, combinations and usage rates of double or triple gas mixtures used in packaging change according to the characteristics of the food product (such as pH, water activity, type, and amount of fat) to be maintained during storage. In this way, the product is effectively protected against microbiological, chemical, and enzymatic changes (Devlieghere, Gil, & Debevere, 2002). As a result, the shelf life of a food product packaged by using MAP technology depends on the type and initial quality of the product, storage temperature, gas mixture used inside the package, gas / product volume ratio and the preservation properties of the packaging materials (Sivertsvik et al., 2002; Sivertsvik, Rosnes, & Jeksrud, 2004).

As mentioned above, within the scope of MAP technology, different concentrations of gas mixtures are used during the packaging of different types of foods. If the deterioration is mostly due to microbial spoilage, such as in milk and dairy products, the most important deterioration parameter is generally regarded as high water activity. In this case, the CO_2 value of the gas mixture used in MAP application is recommended to be high. In foods where oxidative rancidity is observed, such as milk and dairy products, all atmosphere in the package must be replaced with nitrogen gas or CO_2/N_2 mixture, and O_2 should not be used in the packaging. In addition to the gas mixture applied in MAP technology, the packaging material also has a crucial effect on the shelf life of foods. Packaging materials such as polyester, polyethylene, nylon, polyvinyldichloride and polypropylene are frequently used in atmosphere modified packaging (Sivertsvik et al., 2002; Kılınç & Çaklı, 2004). When low permeability packaging material is used, the gas remains in the package for a longer period of time and if the permeability of the package increases, this gas escapes and loses its protective effectiveness (Batu, 1994).

Spoilage in milk and dairy products varies according to product properties. For example, it is usual to observe mould in products with low water activity such as hard cheeses. However, mainly yeast, bacterial spoilage, oxidative rancidity, and physical separation are observed in products with higher water activity such as soft type cheeses and cream. It is possible to extend shelf life of products by applying the MAP technology on milk and dairy products (Sivertsvik et al., 2002; Velu et al., 2013). It is stated that the shelf life of cheeses which usually can remain undeteriorated in refrigerator conditions for three weeks, can be extended as far as eight weeks (Anonymous 1998: Batu et al., 2008). Since some types of moulds can grow despite vacuum packaging, application of MAP technology is more effective on milk and dairy products in which mould development is observed. Similarly, the existence of gases used in MAP technology is effective in terms of preservation of integrity of products such as sliced cheese (Taniwaki, Hocking, Pitt, & Fleet, 2001). It is suggested to use the 30/70 proportion of CO_2/N_2 for the sliced cheeses (Farber, 1991). CO_2/N_2 composition is effective on the prevention of mould development, and it is usually used in packaging of hard cheeses. CO_2 proportion used in this stage is desired to be at least 30%, while this proportion can increase as far as 70%. On the other hand, N_2 proportion is suggested to be in the range of 30-100% (Farber, 1991; Fierheller, 1991). Since this gas composition is effective on the prevention of bacterial deterioration and oxidative rancidity, it is similarly used in soft cheeses. MAP technology can also be applied easily on crumbly cheeses which can be deformed when vacuum packaging is applied. It is inconvenient to apply MAP technology on mould-ripened cheeses since the gas composition prevents the mold growth which is desired to occur in the product (Fierheller, 1991). This packaging method is also used on headspace of fresh milk products such as pasteurized milk, yoghurt, ice cream, cream, and sour cream by way of CO_2 application in different amounts for each product type (Hotchkiss & Chen, 1996; Batu et al., 2008).

Active Packaging

Active packaging is accepted as an alternative method to chemical preservatives and MAP technology, which are used for extending the shelf life of foods. With this method, it is made possible to protect the product characteristics and to extend the shelf life of product by specific substances added into headspace, inner side between the different layers or surface of packaging material (Labuza & Breene, 1989; Dobrucka & Cierpiszewski, 2014). Active packaging is a packaging type which has an extra function providing a protective barrier for foods against external factors according to European Union Guidance to the Commission Regulation (EUGCR). The package used in this type of packaging absorbs the unwanted components from food and headspace surrounding the food or on the contrary it enables the release of components, preservatives, and antioxidants which are intended to be supplied to food or the air surrounding the food (Anonymous, 2009). Developed packaging machinery and packaging material of high barrier characteristics are the important advantages of this method over MAP technology (Gutiérrez et al., 2011).

Different systems are used in active packaging technology depending on the product to be protected. These systems can be evaluated under two main headings: 1. Active absorber-scavenger systems, 2. Active release-emitter systems (Üçüncü, 2011). The most commonly used active absorber-scavenger systems are oxygen, carbon dioxide, ethylene, moisture scavenger systems, and the most commonly used active release-emitter systems are carbon dioxide, ethanol, antioxidant, and antimicrobial emitter systems (Hurme, Sipilainen-Malm, & R. Ahvenainen, 2002). More than 15 active packaging products have been used commercially, especially in Japan, Australia, and the United States, with the majority of oxygen scavengers. Among these products, oxygen scavengers are followed by ethylene scavengers, antimicrobial emitters, and moisture scavengers (Biji, Ravishankar, Mohan, & Gopal, 2015).

Oxygen Scavengers

O_2 present in the packages of foods such as dairy products cannot be completely removed even with vacuum packaging and MAP technology, thus it causes an increase in microbial load, aroma losses, unwanted odor, color changes, and nutrition losses in time. The amount of O_2 in the package can be reduced to 0.01% in active packaging systems which O_2 scavengers are used. For this purpose, O_2 scavengers such as iron powder, ascorbic acid, enzymes, and photosensitive dyes are used to absorb O_2 in the pack after packaging (Hurme et al., 2002; Göncü & Özkal, 2017). Another method used in this system is to absorb O_2 in the package by the use of sachets and pads placed inside the packaging material (Huff, 2008). It is possible to prevent rancidity, discoloration and especially mould growth in cheese during storage of milk and dairy products (Kartal, 2010).

Among the O_2-scavenging components, iron-based ones are the most commonly used ones (Vermeiren et al., 1999). In these systems, the iron-based component used during packaging reacts using the O_2 contained in the packaging and is oxidized to the iron oxide after packaging. Iron-based O_2 scavengers are effective in many food products with low, medium, and high moisture content (Özdemir & Floros, 2004). In a study performed by Gomes et al. (2009) active packaging was made for cheese-spread samples using iron-based oxygen scavengers and it was observed that rancidity of samples reduces and all the product properties were preserved for a longer time period.

In addition to iron-based components, some enzymes such as glucose oxidase are also used as active O_2 scavengers during active packaging (Vermeiren et al., 1999). In enzymatic O_2 capture systems, the enzymes react with the O_2 capture substrate present in the package, thereby reducing the amount of O_2 in the package. However, due to the enzymes used, these systems are more expensive than iron-based O_2 scavenging systems. In addition to being costly, these systems are highly sensitive to factors such as temperature, pH, water activity, and solvent/substrate balance in the package, and the use of enzyme-based O_2 scavenging systems is very limited (Özdemir & Floros, 2004).

Carbon Dioxide Scavengers and Emitters

The amount of CO_2 required in the packaging material varies entirely depending on the type of product in the package. In some products, the amount of CO_2 in the package is desired to decrease and in some others it is desired to increase. Therefore, in the active packaging technology, it is possible to use CO_2 scavenger or CO_2 emitting components depending on the purpose.

CO_2 occurs as a result of spoilage and respiration in some foods, and may result in reduced shelf life of the product, deformation of the package, or even explosion (Vermeiren et al., 1999). The use of CO_2 scavengers such as silica gel, calcium hydroxide, sodium hydroxide, potassium hydroxide, and calcium oxide is effective in such products (Fang, Zhao, Warner, & Johnson, 2017).

In some cases, it is aimed to increase the amount of CO_2 in the package because CO_2 has a direct inhibitory effect on many aerobic bacteria and fungi. The rate of this effect varies according to the type of microorganism. For example, while it is possible to inhibit *Pseudomonas* spp. in the presence of about 20% CO_2, only a small proportion of pathogens such as *Clostridium perfringens*, *C. botulinum*, and *Listeria monocytogenes* are inhibited with the presence of less than 50% CO_2 (Fang et al., 2017). It is possible to adjust the amount of CO_2 in the package to desired ratio, according to the type of microorganism which has a risk of occurrence in the product, by using various components in the packages. In such cases, it is aimed to spontaneously consume the O_2 in the package and to produce CO_2, after packaging. Iron carbonate and ascorbic acid/sodium bicarbonate mixtures are generally used for this purpose. In addition to the above-mentioned effects on microorganisms, O_2 scavengers or CO_2 emitters are also used in active packaging technology to increase volume in food packages and to preserve the appearance of bulk packages (Vermeiren et al., 1999).

Ethylene Scavengers

Ethylene has similar effects on fruits and vegetables as a plant hormone, and accelerates respiration and provides ripening. Furthermore, it causes softening in some fruit varieties and leads to yellowing of green vegetables. Therefore, the removal of ethylene from the package atmosphere is very important for fruits and vegetables, and for this purpose various ethylene scavengers are used in the active packaging technology. The most commonly used one is potassium permanganate and the minerals such as zeolite, silica gel, and activated carbon are also used either alone or in combination to remove ethylene in the package (Vermeiren et al., 1999; Dainelli et al., 2008; Pereira de Abreu, Cruz, & Paseiro Losada, 2012; Ergun, 2016). However, the use of ethylene scavengers in milk and dairy products where active packaging technology is applied is not very common.

Moisture Absorbers

As in many foods, high humidity is one of the most important causes of microbial spoilage in milk and dairy products. Since water activity is high in the presence of moisture, microbial growth accelerates in such environments. To increase the shelf life of the product by keeping the moisture content of the packages under control, various moisture scavengers are used in the active packaging technology. Moisture absorbing pads and sheets are generally used in the active packaging of the products in which moisture content is desired to be kept under control. Moreover, active clay, silica gel, and calcium oxide substances are commonly used components due to their moisture-absorbing properties (Brody, Strupinsky, & Kline, 2001; Dobrucka, 2013; Biji et al., 2015).

Antimicrobial Emitters

Antimicrobial active packaging is a very important packaging method in the packaging of foods such as milk and dairy products containing many nutrients which are necessary for the development of microorganisms. The antimicrobial components used in this technique have an inhibitory effect on microorganisms by extending the lag phase and decreasing the expansion section of the microorganisms (Patel et al., 2015). The antimicrobial components are added to the packaging material or the product coating, and the mechanism of action of these components can occur in two ways. These components can migrate through food migration or prevent microbial growth that can be seen on the surface of the food without migration (Irkin & Esmer, 2015; Ergun, 2016). Examples of antimicrobial agents used in antimicrobial active packaging include alcohol, bacteriocin, nisin, natamycin, and various metals such as silver and copper (Nicholson, 1998; Suppakul, Miltz, Sonneveld, & Bigger, 2003). In a study using antimicrobial active packaging in butter, it was determined that the product showed longer resistance to fungi and yeasts (Moraes et al., 2007).

Antioxidant Emitters

Lipid oxidation is one of the most important factors which shortens the shelf life of products such as milk and dairy products. The odor, aroma, and color of the products change and also the nutritional value of food is lost with oxidation, due to the formation of toxic aldehydes and degradation of polyunsaturated fatty acids (PUFA) (Gomez-Estaca et al., 2014). To prevent the changes in the product occurred by oxidation and to prolong the shelf life of the foods, the antioxidants are usually incorporated into the packaging materials and these antioxidants pass into the food or air space around the food during storage. Waxed papers, butylated hydroxy toluene impregnated packaging materials and tocopherols, essential fatty acids, and plant extracts obtained from plants such as rosemary, oregano, and tea have been used in antioxidant spreading systems. Vitamins E and C may be used in these systems in recent years due to their antioxidative effects (Wessling, Nielsen, Leufvén, & Jägerstad, 1998; Tian, Decker, & Goddard, 2012; Yang, Lee, Won, & Song, 2016; Fang et al., 2017). In a study by Granda-Restrepo et al. (2009), it was determined that lipid oxidation decreased in whole-fat milk powder that was active-packaged by using α-tocopherol.

Ethanol Emitters

Ethanol emitters are especially used for active packaging of products with moderate moisture content against microbial spoilage and are particularly effective against mould growth. These components are also stated to be effective against yeasts and reduce staling and oxidative changes when used in high concentrations (Hurme et al., 2002; Suppakul et al., 2003; Dainelli et al., 2008). Ethanol emitters are reported to be particularly effective on bakery products (Dainelli et al., 2008).

The use of ethanol in active packaging technology can be applied in two ways: 1. Direct injection of ethanol into the package, 2. Use of packages with encapsulated ethanol that can release ethanol vapor (Hempel, O'Sullivan, Papkovsky, & Kerry, 2013).

Intelligent/Smart Packaging

Intelligent food packaging is defined as materials that can monitor the conditions of food and the surrounding environment. This technology, also known as smart labels, provides information to the producer, seller, and consumer about changes in food during transport and storage of the product (de Kruijf et al., 2002; Majid, Nayik, Dar, & Nanda, 2018). For this purpose, various sensors and indicators are used by being integrated into the package or directly adhered to the package and they provide information about the product characteristics such as freshness, shelf life and usage conditions. The working principle of these sensors and indicators is generally based on temperature-time measurements and the measurement of changes in chemical and microbiological properties (Yam, Takhistov, & Miltz, 2006; Dobrucka, 2013). Intelligent packaging technology provides information on the product in a short time, thus providing an alternative to time-consuming and costly analysis.

Sensors

Sensors are units that generally detect changes in the atmosphere within the product or packaging itself and transfer it to the manufacturer, seller, and consumer. The sensors consist essentially of a receptor and a transducer. It is possible to examine the sensors used in smart packaging under different headings as biosensors, gas sensors, chemical sensors, and pathogen sensors (Biji et al., 2015).

Biosensors

Devices that detect, record, and transmit the biological reactions occurring in food packages are called biosensors. Biosensors, like other sensors, consist of a bioreceptor and energy-converting devices (transducers). Bioreceptors are responsible for detecting the target parameter, usually organic materials such as various enzymes, antigens, hormones, and nucleic acids. Transducers consist of electrochemical, optical, or calorimetric systems and convert biological signals into measurable electrical messages (Smolander, 2003; Yam et al., 2006; Otles & Yalcin, 2008).

Gas sensors

It is important that the gas mixture in the package does not change until it reaches the consumer, particularly in products packaged using modified atmosphere packaging systems, to maintain the quality of the product. Gas sensors are systems that detect and transmit the presence or absence of gases used in modified atmosphere packaging, packaging integrity, and leaks (Otles & Yalcin, 2008; Robertson, 2012; Heising, Dekker, Bartels, & Van Boekel, 2014). O_2 and CO_2 sensors are the most commonly used gas sensors (Ergun, 2016).

Chemical sensors

Chemical sensors detect the presence of a specific chemical or gas in the packaged product or in the headspace of the package. The substance detected by chemical sensors is converted into signals by transducers and enables the consumer to perceive the presence of the substance (Vanderroost, Ragaert, Devlieghere, & Meulenaer, 2014).

Pathogen sensors

They are used for the detection of pathogenic microorganisms that infect the packaged products after production. Antibodies are generally used for this purpose and visual warning appears in the package as result of the reaction of these antibodies with the pathogens present in the product (Smolander, 2003).

Indicators

Indicators used in intelligent packaging technology indicate the presence, concentration, or deficiency of a particular substance, particularly by color changes. They are generally classified as freshness indicators, time-temperature indicators (TTI), integrity indicators, and Radio frequency information device (RFID) (Hogan & Kerry, 2008).

Freshness indicators

The freshness indicators are generally used in products packaged with modified atmosphere packaging technology, which informs the consumer of the change in gas composition in the package through the label printed on the package. If the necessary conditions are not met during the transportation and storage of foods, some microbiological spoilage may occur in the product and as a result of this deterioration, metabolites such as CO_2, SO_2, NH_3 and ethanol are formed. Freshness indicators identify these metabolites and change the color of the label on the packaging, thus providing information about the quality of food (Smolander, 2003; Smolander, 2008). When classified according to working principles, it is possible to list the most frequently used freshness indicators as indicators; sensitive to pH change, volatile compounds, hydrogen sulfide (H_2S), and various microbial metabolites (Smolander, 2003; Gök, 2007).

Time-Temperature indicators (TTI)

Time-temperature indicators (TTI) detect physical, chemical, enzymatic, and microbial deteriorations in the product due to the exposure of the products to temperatures that they should not be exposed to during transport and storage. They are particularly effective in controlling temperature changes in refrigerated or frozen foods such as milk and dairy products. In case of temperature change, the barcode on the packaging turns into a dark color, thus it prevents the data transfer when the barcode is scanned and prevents the sale of the product. It is possible to classify the most commonly used time-temperature indicators as polymer, diffusion, and enzymatic-based ones (Riva, Piergiovanni, & Schiraldi, 2001; Taoukis & Labuza, 2003; Gök, 2007; Lee & Rahman, 2014; Taoukis & Tsironi, 2016). Time-temperature indicators can be used for all types of food products, including milk and dairy products (Ergun, 2016).

Integrity indicators

The package may be punctured or torn particularly during transport of the products. Such situations can be detected and transferred to the seller and the consumer through integrity indicators. Among the integrity indicators, the most widely used ones are based on O_2. Integrity indicators detect O_2 entering the package when the package is punctured or torn and stain the active substance with redox effect (Mattila-Sandholm, Ahvenainen, Hurme, & Jarvi-Kaariainen, 1995; Davies & Gardner, 1996). Therefore, it can be determined that the integrity of the packaging material is impaired by color change.

Radio frequency information device (RFID)

Radio frequency information device (RFID) is a technology that makes it possible to read labels using radio waves without human intervention. In this system, as in the other methods described above, various changes in food are not detected by physical interaction, but by radio waves, through the microchips inserted into the product (Tajima, 2007; Lee & Rahman, 2014). RFID tags carry the information of all the changes in the food as from the packaging of the product and also allow remote monitoring of this information via radio waves (Karagöz & Demirdöven, 2017). RFID indicators which can be found in many different forms such as disk, glass, capsule, and label can also be combined with other indicators and can be used for all foods including milk and dairy products (Yuksel & Zaim, 2009; Ruiz-Garcia & Lunadei, 2011).

REFERENCES

Anonymous. (2009). *EU Guidance to the commission regulation (EC) No 450/2009 of 29 May 2009 on active and intelligent materials and articles intended to come into contact with food. Version 1.0. European Commission Health and Consumers Directorate-General Directorate E-Safety of the Food chain. E6- Innovation and sustainability.* Retrieved from https://ec.europa.eu/food/sites/food/files/safety/docs/cs_fcm_legis_active-intelligent_guidance.pdf

Anonymous. (2019). *Nanotechnology.* European Food Safety Authority. Retrieved from https://www.efsa.europa.eu/en/topics/topic/nanotechnology

Batu, A. (1994). Properties of modified atmosphere packaging films and application of fruits vegetables. *Gida*, *19*(6), 397–403.

Batu, A., Caglar, A., & Kara, H. H., (2008). Afyon kaymagının raf ömrünün uzatılmasında modifiye atmosferde paketleme önerisi. *Gıda Teknolojileri Elektronik Dergisi, 2008*(2), 43-46.

Biji, K. B., Ravishankar, C. N., Mohan, C. O., & Gopal, T. S. (2015). Smart packaging systems for food applications: A review. *Journal of Food Science and Technology, 52*(10), 6125–6135. doi:10.100713197-015-1766-7 PMID:26396360

Brody, A. L., Strupinsky, E. R., & Kline, L. R. (2001). *Active packaging for food applications.* Boca Raton, FL: CRC Press. doi:10.1201/9781420031812

Buzby, J. C. (2010). Nanotechnology for food applications. More questions than answers. *The Journal of Consumer Affairs, 44*(3), 528–545. doi:10.1111/j.1745-6606.2010.01182.x

Çelik, İ., & Tümer, G. (2016). Gıda ambalajlamada son gelişmeler. *Akademik Gıda, 14*(2), 180–188.

Chau, C. F., Wu, S. H., & Yen, G. C. (2007). The development of regulations for food nanotechnology. *Trends in Food Science & Technology, 18*(5), 169–280. doi:10.1016/j.tifs.2007.01.007

Cutter, C. N. (2006). Opportunities for bio-based packaging technologies to improve the quality and safety of fresh and further processed muscle foods. *Meat Science, 74*(1), 131–142. doi:10.1016/j.meatsci.2006.04.023 PMID:22062722

Dainelli, D., Gontard, N., Spyropoulos, D., Zondervan-van den Beuken, E., & Tobback, P. (2008). Active and intelligent food packaging: Legal aspects and safety concerns. *Trends in Food Science & Technology, 19*, 103–112. doi:10.1016/j.tifs.2008.09.011

Davies, E. S., & Gardner, C. D. (1996). *UK Patent No. GB-2298273.* Oxygen indicating composition, The Victoria University of Manchester.

de Kruijf, N. N., van Beest, M., Rijk, R., Sipilainen-Malm, T., Paseiro, L. P., & De Meulenaer, B. (2002). Active and intelligent packaging: Applications and regulatory aspects. *Food Additives and Contaminants, 19* Suppl, 144-162.

Demir, M. (1999). *Modified atmosphere packaging.* Retrieved from http://www.apack.com.tr/images/userfiles/146705440090949918.pdf

Devlieghere, F., & Debevere, J. (2000). Influence of dissolved carbon dioxide on the growth of spoilage bacteria. *Lebensmittel-Wissenschaft + Technologie, 33*(8), 531–537. doi:10.1006/fstl.2000.0705

Devlieghere, F., Gil, M. I., & Debevere, J. (2002). Modified atmosphere packaging (MAP). In C. J. K. Henry, & C. Chapman (Eds.), *The nutrition handbook for food processors* (pp. 342–370). England: Woodhead Publishing. doi:10.1533/9781855736658.2.342

Dobrucka, R. (2013). The future of active and intelligent packaging industry. *LogForum, 9*(2), 103–110.

Dobrucka, R., & Cierpiszewski, R. (2014). Active and intelligent packaging food - Research and development - A review. *Polish Journal of Food and Nutrition Sciences, 64*(1), 7–15. doi:10.2478/v10222-012-0091-3

Duncan, T. V. (2011). Applications of nanotechnology in food packaging and food safety: Barriermaterials, antimicrobials and sensors. *Journal of Colloid and Interface Science, 363*(1), 1–24. doi:10.1016/j.jcis.2011.07.017 PMID:21824625

Ergun, M. (2016). Taze meyve ve sebzeler için aktif, zeki veya akıllı paketleme teknolojileri. *Alatarım*, *15*(2), 51–60.

Fang, Z., Zhao, Y., Warner, R. D., & Johnson, S. K. (2017). Active and intelligent packaging in meat industry. *Trends in Food Science & Technology*, *61*, 60–71. doi:10.1016/j.tifs.2017.01.002

Farber, J. M. (1991). Microbiological aspects of modified-atmosphere packaging technology - A review. *Journal of Food Protection*, *54*(1), 58–70. doi:10.4315/0362-028X-54.1.58 PMID:31051584

Fierheller, M. G. (1991). Modified atmosphere packaging of miscellaneous products. In B. Ooraikul, & M. E. Stiles (Eds.), *Modified atmosphere packaging of food* (pp. 246–260). Boston, MA: Springer. doi:10.1007/978-1-4615-2117-4_8

Gawith, J. A., & Robertson, T. R. (2000). Wrapping up packaging technology. *Journal of the Home Economics Institute of Australia*, *7*(2), 6–14.

Gök, V. (2007). Gıda paketleme sanayinde akıllı paketleme teknolojisi. *Gıda Teknolojileri Elektronik Dergisi, 2007*(1), 45-58.

Gomes, C., Elena Castell-Perez, M., Chimbombi, E., Barros, F., Sun, S., Liu, J. D., ... Wright, A. O. (2009). Effect of oxygen-absorbing packaging on the shelf life of a liquid-based component of military operational rations. *Journal of Food Science*, *74*(4), 167–176. doi:10.1111/j.1750-3841.2009.01120.x PMID:19490321

Gomez-Estaca, J., Lopez-de-Dicastillo, C., Hernandez-Munoz, P., Catala, R., & Gavara, R. (2014). Advances in antioxidant active food packaging. *Trends in Food Science & Technology*, *35*(1), 42–51. doi:10.1016/j.tifs.2013.10.008

Göncü, A., & Özkal, S. G. (2017). Ekmeklerde aktif paketleme uygulamaları. *Türk Tarım - Gıda Bilim ve Teknoloji Dergisi, 5*(11), 1264-1273.

Granda-Restrepo, D. M., Soto-Valdez, H., Peralta, E., Troncoso-Rojas, R., Vallejo-Córdoba, B., Gámez-Meza, N., & Graciano-Verdugo, A. Z. (2009). Migration of α-tocopherol from an active multilayer film into whole milk powder. *Food Research International*, *42*(10), 1396–1402. doi:10.1016/j.foodres.2009.07.007

Gruere, G. P., Narrod, C. A., & Abbott, L. (2011). Agriculture, food, and water nanotechnologies for the poor: Opportunities and constraints, Policy briefs 19, International Food Policy Research Institute (IFPRI). Retrieved from http://cdm15738.contentdm.oclc.org/utils/getfile/collection/p15738coll2/id/124891/filename/124892.pdf

Gutiérrez, L., Batlle, R., Andújar, S., Sánchez, C., & Nerín, C. (2011). Evaluation of antimicrobial active packaging to increase shelf life of gluten-free sliced bread. *Packaging Technology & Science*, *24*(8), 485–494. doi:10.1002/pts.956

Heising, J. K., Dekker, M., Bartels, P. V., & Van Boekel, M. A. J. S. (2014). Monitoring the quality of perishable foods: Opportunities for intelligent packaging. *Critical Reviews in Food Science and Nutrition*, *54*(5), 645–654. doi:10.1080/10408398.2011.600477 PMID:24261537

Hempel, A. W., O'Sullivan, M. G., Papkovsky, D. B., & Kerry, J. P. (2013). Use of smart packaging technologies for monitoring and extending the shelf-life quality of modified atmosphere packaged (MAP) bread: Application of intelligent oxygen sensors and active ethanol emitters. *European Food Research and Technology, 237*(2), 117–124. doi:10.100700217-013-1968-z

Hogan, S. A., & Kerry, J. P. (2008). Smart packaging of meat and poultry products. In J. Kerry, & P. Butler (Eds.), *Smart packaging technologies for fast moving consumer goods* (pp. 33–59). West Sussex: John Wiley & Sons. doi:10.1002/9780470753699.ch3

Hotchkiss, J. H., & Chen, J. H. (1996). Microbiological effects of the direct addition of CO_2 to pasteurized milk. *Journal of Dairy Science, 79*(Supplement 1), 87. PMID:8675787

Huff, K. (2008). *Active and intelligent packaging: Innovations for the future.* Retrieved from http://www.iopp.org/files/public/VirginiaTechKarleighHuff.pdf

Hurme, E., Sipilainen-Malm, T., & Ahvenainen, R. V. T. T. (2002). Active and intelligent packaging. In T. Ohlsson, & N. Bengtsson (Eds.), Minimal processing technologies in the food industry (pp. 87-123). Cambridge: CRC Press.

Irkin, R., & Esmer, O. K. (2015). Novel food packaging systems with natural antimicrobial agents. *Journal of Food Science and Technology, 52*(10), 6095–6111. doi:10.100713197-015-1780-9 PMID:26396358

Karagöz, Ş., & Demirdöven, A. (2017). Gıda ambalajlamada güncel uygulamalar: Modifiye atmosfer, aktif, akıllı ve nanoteknolojik ambalajlama uygulamaları. *Gaziosmanpaşa Bilimsel Araştırma Dergisi, 6*(1), 9–21.

Kartal, S. (2010). *Çileğin raf ömrünün mikroperfore filmler ve oksijen tutucular kullanılarak denge modifiye atmosfer ile arttırılması.* (Unpublished master's thesis). Çanakkale Onsekiz Mart University, Çanakkale, Turkey.

Kılınç, B., & Çaklı, Ş. (2004). Su ürünlerinin modifiye atmosferde paketlenmesi. *E.U. Su Ürünleri Dergisi, 21*(3-4), 349–353.

Labuza, T. P., & Breene, W. M. (1989). Applications of "active packaging" for improvement of shelf-life and nutritional quality of fresh and extended shelf-life foods. *Journal of Food Processing and Preservation, 13*(1), 1–69. doi:10.1111/j.1745-4549.1989.tb00090.x

Lee, L., Arul, J., Lencki, R., & Castaigne, F. (1996). A review on modified atmosphere packaging and preservation of fresh fruits and vegetables: Physiological basis and practical aspects-Part II. *Packaging Technology & Science, 9*(1), 1–17. doi:10.1002/(SICI)1099-1522(199601)9:1<1::AID-PTS349>3.0.CO;2-W

Lee, S. J., & Rahman, A. T. M. M. (2014). Intelligent packaging for food products. In J. H. Han (Ed.), *Innovations in food packaging* (pp. 171–209). Academic Press. doi:10.1016/B978-0-12-394601-0.00008-4

Majid, I., Nayik, G. A., Dar, S. M., & Nanda, V. (2018). Novel food packaging technologies: Innovations and future prospective. *Journal of the Saudi Society of Agricultural Sciences, 17*(4), 454–462. doi:10.1016/j.jssas.2016.11.003

Mattila-Sandholm, T., Ahvenainen, R., Hurme, E., & Jarvi-Kaariainen, T. (1995). *Finnish Patent No. FI-94802.* Leakage Indicator, VTT Biotechnology, and Food Research.

Momin, J. K., Jayakumar, C., & Prajapati, J. B. (2013). Potential of nanotechnology in functional foods. *Emirates Journal of Food and Agriculture, 25*(1), 10–19. doi:10.9755/ejfa.v25i1.9368

Moraes, A. R. F., Gouveia, L. E. R., Soares, N. F. F., Santos, M. M. S., & Gonçalves, M. P. J. C. (2007). Development and evaluation of antimicrobial film on butter conservation. *Food Science and Technology (Campinas), 27*, 33–36. doi:10.1590/S0101-20612007000500006

Mullan, W. M. A. (2002). *Science and technology of modified atmosphere packaging.* Retrieved from https://www.dairyscience.info/index.php/packaging/117-modified-atmosphere-packaging.html

Nicholson, M. D. (1998). The role of natural antimicrobials in food/packaging biopreservation. *Journal of Plastic Film & Sheeting, 14*(3), 234–241. doi:10.1177/875608799801400306

Oliveira, M., Abadias, M., Usall, J., Torres, R., Teixido, N., & Vinas, I. (2015). Application of modified atmosphere packaging as a safety approach to fresh-cut fruits and vegetables - A review. *Trends in Food Science & Technology, 46*(1), 13–26. doi:10.1016/j.tifs.2015.07.017

Otles, S., & Yalcin, B. (2008). Intelligent food packaging. *LogForum, 4*(3), 1–9.

Özdemir, M., & Floros, J. D. (2004). Active food packaging technologies. *Critical Reviews in Food Science and Nutrition, 44*(3), 185–193. doi:10.1080/10408690490441578 PMID:15239372

Patel, R., Prajapati, J. P., & Balakrishnan, S. (2015). *Recent trends in packaging of dairy and food products.* Paper presented at the meeting National seminar on Indian Dairy Industry - Opportunities and Challenges. Gujarat, India.

Pereira de Abreu, D. A., Cruz, J. M., & Paseiro Losada, P. (2012). Active and intelligent packaging for the food industry. *Food Reviews International, 28*(2), 146–187. doi:10.1080/87559129.2011.595022

Riva, M., Piergiovanni, L., & Schiraldi, A. (2001). Performances of time–temperature indicators in the study of temperature exposure of packaged fresh food. *Packaging Technology & Science, 14*(1), 1–9. doi:10.1002/pts.521

Robertson, G. L. (2012). *Food packaging, principles and practice.* London, UK: CRC Press.

Ruiz-Garcia, L., & Lunadai, L. (2011). The role of RFID in agriculture: applications, limitations, and challenges. *Computers and Electronics in Agriculture, 79*(1), 42–50. doi:10.1016/j.compag.2011.08.010

Sandhya. (2010). Modified atmosphere packaging of fresh produce: Current status and future needs. *Food Science and Technology, 43*, 381-392.

Schnettler, B., Crisostomo, G., Mora, M., Lobos, G., Miranda, H., & Grunert, K. G. (2013). Acceptance of nanotechnology applications and satisfaction with food-related life in southern Chile. *Food Science and Technology (Campinas), 34*(1), 157–163. doi:10.1590/S0101-20612014005000001

Siegrist, M., Cousin, M. E., Kastenholz, H., & Wiek, A. (2007). Public acceptance of nanotechnology foods and food packaging: The influence of affect and trust. *Appetite, 49*(2), 459–466. doi:10.1016/j.appet.2007.03.002 PMID:17442455

Siegrist, M., Stampfli, N., Kastenholz, H., & Keller, C. (2008). Perceived risks and perceived benefits of different nanotechnology foods and nanotechnology food packaging. *Appetite*, *51*(2), 283–290. doi:10.1016/j.appet.2008.02.020 PMID:18406006

Sivertsvik, M., Rosnes, J. T., & Bergslien, H. (2002). Modified atmosphere packaging. In T. Ohlsson & N. Bengtsson (Eds.), *Minimal processing technologies in the food industry* (pp. 61–86). Cambridge: CRC Press. doi:10.1533/9781855736795.61

Sivertsvik, M., Rosnes, J. T., & Jeksrud, W. K. (2004). Solubility and absorption rate of carbon dioxide into non-respiring foods. Part 2: Raw fish fillets. *Journal of Food Engineering*, *63*(4), 451–458. doi:10.1016/j.jfoodeng.2003.09.004

Smolander, M. (2003). The use of freshness indicators in packaging. In R. Ahvenainen (Ed.), *Novel food packaging techniques* (pp. 127–143). Cambridge: Woodhead Publishing. doi:10.1533/9781855737020.1.127

Smolander, M. (2008). Freshness indicators and food packaging. In J. Kerry, & P. Butler (Eds.), *Smart packaging technologies for fast moving consumer goods* (pp. 111–127). West Sussex: John Wiley & Sons. doi:10.1002/9780470753699.ch7

Suppakul, P., Miltz, J., Sonneveld, K., & Bigger, S. W. (2003). Active packaging technologies with an emphasis on antimicrobial packaging and its applications. *Journal of Food Science*, *68*(2), 408–420. doi:10.1111/j.1365-2621.2003.tb05687.x

Sürengil, G., & Kılınç, B. (2011). Gıda - Ambalaj sektöründe nanoteknolojik uygulamalar ve su ürünleri açısından önemi. *Journal of Fisheries Sciences Com*, *5*(4), 317–325.

Tajima, M. (2007). Strategic value of RFID in supply chain management. *Journal of Purchasing and Supply Management*, *13*(4), 261–273. doi:10.1016/j.pursup.2007.11.001

Taniwaki, M. H., Hocking, A. D., Pitt, J. I., & Fleet, G. H. (2001). Growth of fungi and mycotoksin production on cheese under modified atmospheres. *International Journal of Food Microbiology*, *68*(1-2), 125–133. doi:10.1016/S0168-1605(01)00487-1 PMID:11545212

Taoukis, P., & Tsironi, T. (2016). Smart packaging for monitoring and managing food and beverage shelf life. In P. Subramaniam, & P. Wareing (Eds.), *The stability and shelf life of food* (pp. 141–168). Woodhead Publishing. doi:10.1016/B978-0-08-100435-7.00005-8

Taoukis, P. S., & Labuza, T. P. (2003). Time-temperature indicators. In R. Ahvenainen (Ed.), *Novel food packaging techniques* (pp. 103–126). Cambridge: Woodhead Publishing. doi:10.1533/9781855737020.1.103

Tian, F., Decker, E. A., & Goddard, J. M. (2012). Development of an iron chelating polyethylene film for active packaging applications. *Journal of Agricultural and Food Chemistry*, *60*(8), 2046–2052. doi:10.1021/jf204585f PMID:22288894

Üçüncü, M. (2011). *Gıda ambalajlanma teknolojisi*. İstanbul, Turkey: Ambalaj Sanayiciler Derneği.

Van der Steen, C., Jacxsens, L., Devlieghere, F., & Debevere, J. (2002). Combining high oxygen atmospheres with low oxygen modified atmosphere packaging to improve the keeping quality of strawberries and raspberries. *Postharvest Biology and Technology*, *26*(1), 49–58. doi:10.1016/S0925-5214(02)00005-4

Vanderroost, M., Ragaert, P., Devlieghere, F., & Meulenaer, B. D. (2014). Intelligent food packaging: The next generation. *Trends in Food Science & Technology*, *39*(1), 47–62. doi:10.1016/j.tifs.2014.06.009

Velu, S., Abu Bakar, F., Mahyudin, N. A., Saari, N., & Zaman, M. Z. (2013). Effect of modified atmosphere packaging on microbial flora changes in fishery products. *International Food Research Journal*, *20*(1), 17–26.

Vermeiren, L., Devlieghere, F., Van Beest, M., De Kruijf, N., & Debevere, J. (1999). Developments in the active packaging of foods. *Trends in Food Science & Technology*, *10*(3), 77–86. doi:10.1016/S0924-2244(99)00032-1

Wessling, C., Nielsen, T., Leufvén, A., & Jägerstad, M. (1998). Mobility of α-tocopherol and BHT in LDPE in contact with fatty food simulants. *Food Additives and Contaminants*, *15*(6), 709–715. doi:10.1080/02652039809374701 PMID:10209582

Yam, K. L., Takhistov, P. T., & Miltz, J. (2006). Intelligent packaging: Concepts and applications. *Journal of Food Science*, *70*(1), 1–10. doi:10.1111/j.1365-2621.2005.tb09052.x

Yang, H. J., Lee, J. H., Won, M., & Song, K. B. (2016). Antioxidant activities of distiller dried grains with solubles as protein films containing tea extracts and their application in the packaging of pork meat. *Food Chemistry*, *196*, 174–179. doi:10.1016/j.foodchem.2015.09.020 PMID:26593480

Yüksel, M. E., & Zaim, A. H. (2009). *Yeni nesil teknoloji olarak RFID, RFID sistem yapıları ve bir RFID sistem tasarımı yaklaşımı.* Paper presented at the meeting 5th International Advanced Technologies Symposium. Karabük, Turkey.

Chapter 10
Biopreservatives for Improved Shelf–Life and Safety of Dairy Products:
Biopreservatives for Dairy Products

Tejinder Pal Singh
College of Dairy Science and Food Technology, India

Sarang Dilip Pophaly
College of Dairy Science and Food Technology, India

Ruby Siwach
College of Dairy Science and Food Technology, India

ABSTRACT

Globally, there is an increasing demand for minimally processed, easily prepared, and ready-to-eat fresh food, globalization of food trade, and distribution from centralized processing which pose major challenges for food safety and quality because perishable food may get contaminated with undesirable microorganisms. Food spoilage adversely affects the economy and also erodes the consumer's confidence. On other hand, food-borne illness leads to loss of earnings and productivity, unemployment and litigation, and weakens trade and tourism. Another challenge for the food producers is to produce less stable foods by processes that confer less harm to the detrimental microflora. A challenge for food producers is to develop products with a sufficiently longer shelf-life and at a competitive price. This brings them to the most promising approach to this end, the so-called biopreservation. This chapter provides a scientific background, functionality, as well as food applications and further commercial aspects of biopreservatives derived from microbial sources.

DOI: 10.4018/978-1-7998-5354-1.ch010

INTRODUCTION

The concept of biopreservation is not new to us, as we humans have continuously been using this biotechnological approach for preserving food, for many years, without even knowing the underlying mechanisms. In present world, the changing food trends, lifestyle and increasing consumer's awareness has brought up the challenge to food producers to meet totally contradictory trends and demands (Table 1).

Table 1. Highlighting consumer's preferences, changing food trends and demands, and problems associated with them

Preferences	Trends and Demands	Problems Associated
Health trends	Consumers concern for health has raised the demand for food products with reduced levels of salt, sugar and fat.	This also confers an increase in water activity, which provides a much suitable environment for microorganisms.
Taste preferences	In many products, trends are towards a milder (i.e. less acidic) taste.	This results in a higher pH that again is less adverse for microorganisms.
Perception of "natural"	Demand for milder or minimally processed foods (More natural/fresh food). Demand for "preservative-free" products.	Less inactivation of unwanted microorganisms.
Convenience trends ("practically homemade")		Two main risks associated with this trend—namely, more extensive processing, which results in more steps in which contamination with detrimental microorganisms can occur, and the need for proper handling by the consumer (e.g. sufficient heating), which may be neglected.
Durability and open shelf-life	Market access and economically viable logistics require a long shelf-life.	Furthermore, a sufficient open shelf-life is required to ensure customer loyalty.
Ethical issues		Concerns such as corporate social responsibility, carbon dioxide (CO_2) footprint, and fair-trade and organic products put restrictions on which solutions a food producer can employ.

Overall, it has been seen that these trends and demands lead to food formulations that provide conditions much more favourable for microbial growth; milder processing results in minimal reduction, more processing steps increase the risk of contamination, more difficult to maintain longer shelf-life, and pressure to minimize the waste. Moreover, the trendsetters and consumers are not in favour to use conventional preservatives. But the fact is that we cannot meet the demands of growing population and maintain present society living standards, and certainly cannot reduce the global food waste problems, with food that is not preserved.

Normally, many consumers associate the term 'Preservatives' with harmful, modern chemicals in foodstuffs. But, as a brief look back into the past will show that there are possibilities to preserve the food by more natural means (such as, fermentation). Despite a number of misgivings, preservatives have nowadays become an indispensable part of the food we eat; due to increasing demand from consumers for greater choice, ease and convenience of foods, and high food safety standards. Thus, there is a strong market need for natural food preservation methods that can ensure both food safety (i.e. reduce the number and/or outgrowth of pathogenic microorganisms) and longer shelf-life (i.e. delayed development of the

Figure 1. Main categories of biopreservatives that can be produced by using lactic acid bacteria and other suitable microorganisms as "cell factories"

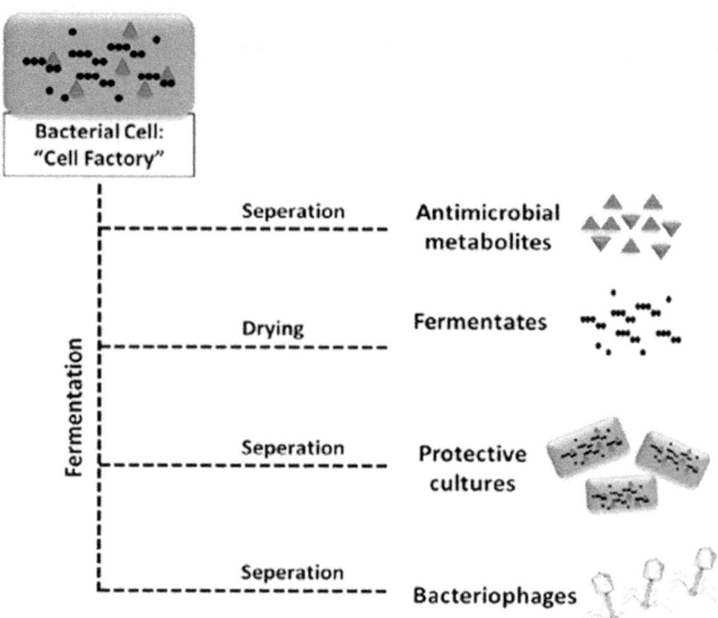

spoilage microflora). One of the few possible solutions is biopreservation based on the concept of using food-grade microorganisms (mainly, Lactic acid bacteria; LAB) as so-called cell factories (Figure 1).

Generally Regarded As Safe (GRAS)/Food-grade microorganisms can be exploited to a great extent for restricting microbial growth as promising means to preserve food. These mechanisms naturally exist to balance the complex microbial ecosystems. Thereby, the naturally occurring fittest microorganisms can be exploited to design preservation methodologies that ensure food safety and shelf life while keeping up the desired quality of the food product.

The biopreservation principles from food-grade microorganisms can be categorized according to the antimicrobial compound (e.g. bacteriocin, other metabolites, bacteriophages, enzymes) as well as product format (purified antimicrobial, fermentate, protective culture), as outlined in Figure 1 (Elsser-Gravesen & Elsser-Gravesen, 2014). Knowing the fact that not all antimicrobial metabolites from food-grade microorganisms have yet been discovered, and even the underlying mechanisms of several well-known antimicrobials are not well understood. Therefore, clear understanding and discoveries of new antimicrobial metabolites will further expand the options for natural food biopreservation systems. Roller (2003) suggested that one should not search for "the silver bullet" for biopreservation systems, as antimicrobial compounds in nature rarely function in isolation. Hence, targeted intelligent strategies based on multifactorial systems are the most likely to succeed for protecting food against detrimental microorganisms.

This chapter aims to provide a scientific background, current knowledge on biopreservatives, functionality, as well as covering solutions that are actually being used industrially today, and points out perceivable directions for future solution development.

BACTERIOCINS

The empirical utilization of microorganisms as well as their metabolites for food security and protection has been a typical practice ever (Rose et al., 2003). Among the wide range of antibacterial metabolites produced by microorganisms, the bacteriocins, particularly those synthesized by lactic acid bacteria (LAB), have pulled in the best consideration as promising means for food safety & biopreservation. Several studies have exclusively been done focusing the pivotal roles that this group of bacteria plays in food and health, structure, biosynthesis, genetics, and food application of LAB bacteriocins (Deegan et al. 2006; Franz et al. 2007; G´alvez et al. 2007).

Ribosomally synthesized antimicrobial peptides or proteins, called Bacteriocins, are nontoxic to eukaryotic cells and thereby, are generally recognized as safe (GRAS) substances. The antimicrobial activity of bacteriocins against pathogenic and saprophytic bacteria has raised significant interest for their application as food preservative. Use of bacteriocins may help decrease the utilization of synthetic additives as well as the intensity of heat and other physical treatments, satisfying customers demand for fresh tasting, ready to eat, and lightly preserved foods. Lately, impressive efforts have been made for applications of different bacteriocins and bacteriocinogenic strains. Depending on the raw materials, processing conditions, distribution, and consumption, the different types of foods offer a great variety of scenarios where food poisoning, pathogenic or spoilage bacteria may proliferate. Therefore, the bacteriocins efficacy needs to be carefully tested in the food systems for which they are intended to be applied against the selected target bacteria (Kaur et al., 2014).

With changing trend, there is also a growing interest in traditional foods and in the adaptation of local production processes to an industrial scale without substantial loss of the original value. Several developing countries have already succeeded but in many others, there is a need to meet the nutritional requirements of the population and to provide a minimal framework of food safety. The need to avoid economic losses due to microbial spoilage of raw materials and food products, to ameliorate the incidence of food borne illnesses, and to meet the food requirements of the growing world population strengthen the relevance of preservation methods in the food industry. In this context, the preservation of foods by natural, biological methods may be a satisfactory approach to solve many of the current food-related issues.

Biopreservation employing bacteriocins is a novel approach aims to eliminate or control pathogens in food while the emergence of resistant variants of the organism remains the major concern and limits their application. Several systematic studies investigating bacteriocin resistance in bacterial pathogens concluded that improved control of the target microorganisms and inhibition of bacteriocin-resistant strains and species can be achieved by using a hurdle concept. Hurdle technology refers to the manipulation of multiple factors (intrinsic and extrinsic) intended to prevent microbial entry, survival and growth in food stuff. In this approach, multiple factors/preservation methods coordinate to provide greater protection than a single method alone, hence the food produced will be more safe and secure. While in some foods intrinsic properties, for example, high salt may provide adequate protection, the conscious addition of an extra hurdle(s) can ensure safety to a greater extent (Leistner, 2000).

Classification and Biosynthesis of Bacteriocins of LAB

There is a wide range of bacteriocins produced by different LAB (Table 2) which can be classified based on their primary structures, molecular weights, post-translational modifications and genetic characteristics (Klaenhammer et al, 1993; Güllüce et al, 2013). However, there is no universally accepted classification

Table 2. Few examples of bacteriocins produced by lactic acid bacteria (LAB)

Type	Characteristic	Example
Class I **(Lantibiotics)**	• Ribosomally synthesized peptides that undergo posttranslational modifications. • Molecular weight 2–5 kDa. • Contain lanthionine and-methyl lanthionine.	• Nisin A from *Lc. lactis* ssp. lactis ATCC114 • Nisin Z from *Lc. lactis* ssp. lactis NIZ022186 • Enterocin A & Enterocin B from *Ent. faecium* T136
Class II	• Heat stable peptides formed exclusively by unmodified amino acids. • Ribosomally synthesized as inactive pre peptides to get activated by posttranslational cleavage of the N-terminal leader peptide. • Molecular weight < 10 kDa.	• Lactococcin A from *Lc. lactis* ssp. lactis LMG2130 • Lactococcin B from *Lc. lactis* ssp. cremoris 9B4 • Lactococcin M from *Lc. lactis* ssp lactis • Pediocin PA-1 from *Ped. acidilactici* PAC1.0
ClassIII	• Nonlantibiotics—Large, Heat-labile Bacteriocins. • Molecular weight >30 kDa.	• Helveticin J from *Lb. helveticus* 481 • Lacticin A from *Lb. delbrukii* JCM1106 • Lacticin B from *Lb. delbrukii* JCM 1248
Class IV	Complex bacteriocins carrying lipid or carbohydrate moieties.	Sublancin from *Bacillus subtilis* 168
Class V	Circular bacteriocins.	• Enterocin RM6 from *Enterococcus faecalis* • Gassericin from *Lactobacillus gasseri* LA39 • Reutericin A from *Lactobacillus reuteri*

scheme for bacteriocins. Most LAB bacteriocins are small (3-6 kDa), cationic, heat-stable, amphiphilic, and membrane-permeabilizing peptides.

Bacteriocinogenic strains of LAB produces bacteriocins throughout the growth phase and production ceases at the end or sometimes before the end of the exponential phase (Parente et al., 1997; Lejeune et al., 1998). Initially, bacteriocins are produced/synthesized as pre-propeptide which are processed/modified before their efflux by dedicated transport machinery (Nes et al., 1996). Bacteriocin production is highly affected by factors like type and level of the carbon, nitrogen and phosphate sources, cations surfactants and inhibitors. For example, nisin can be produced by *Lactococcus lactis* IO-1 from media containing different carbohydrate sources (glucose, sucrose and xylose) but better yield was obtained with glucose compared to xylose (Matsuaki et al., 1996; Chinachoti et al., 1997a,b). Similarly, for production of Pediocin AcH, glucose followed by sucrose, xylose and galactose were the best carbon sources in an unbuffered medium (Biswas et al., 1991).

All bacteriocins are synthesized with an N terminal leader sequence whose function seems to prevent the bacteriocin from being biologically active while still inside the producer and provide the recognition signal for the transporter system (Holo et al., 1991; Muriana and Klaenhammer, 1991; Klaenhammer, 1993; Havarstein et al., 1994). Lantibiotics are well studied upto genetic level and number of genes found in genome includes: (a) *Lan A*, the structural gene, (b) *Lan I* (and in some cases *Lan E, Lan F* and *Lan G*), immunity genes, encodes for proteins that protect the producer from the produced lantibiotic, (c) Lan T gene encodes a membrane associated ABC transporter that transfers the lantibiotic across the membrane, (d) *lan P* gene encodes a serine proteinase which removes the leader sequence of the lantibiotic prepeptide, (e) two genes, *lan B* and *Lan C* (or in some cases only one gene, *Lan M*) encode enzymes involved in the formation of lanthionine and methyl lanthionine, and (f) lan k and lan R genes encodes for two component regulatory proteins that transmit an extracellular signal and thereby induce lantibiotic production.

Bacteriocins: Mode of Action

Bacteriocins recognizes and bind to the specific receptors located on the target microbial cell surface. Once they bind to the cell surface, they alter the functioning of the cytoplasmic membrane (affecting energy synthesis and permeability). The initial electrostatic attraction between the target cell membrane and the bacteriocin peptide is thought to be the driving force for subsequent events whether the case is of broad spectrum bacteriocin or a narrow spectrum bacteriocin. While many bacteriocins, including well studied nisin, have been shown to induce pore formation in sensitive microorganisms. Nisin forms pores that disrupt the proton motive force and the pH equilibrium causing leakage of ions and hydrolysis of ATP resulting in cell death (Figure 2). Lacticin 3147, Pep5, subtilin and epidermin are examples of other lantibiotics that also kill the target cell by pore formation (Schuller et al. 1989; Brotz et al. 1998). Later, it has been recognised that nisin also interferes with cell wall biosynthesis (Reisinger et al. 1980). This was claimed that the nisin has an ability to bind lipid II, a peptidoglycan precursor, thus inhibit cell wall biosynthesis. Such binding is also intrinsic to the ability of nisin to form pores. The possession of dual mechanisms of action renders nisin active at nM concentrations (Breukink et al. 1999). Some other bacteriocins can inhibit nucleic acid synthesis, interference with the protein synthesis and change cell translator mechanism.

Figure 2. Proposed model of cell killing by pore-forming bacteriocins (Jack et al. 1995; Garneau et al. 2002)

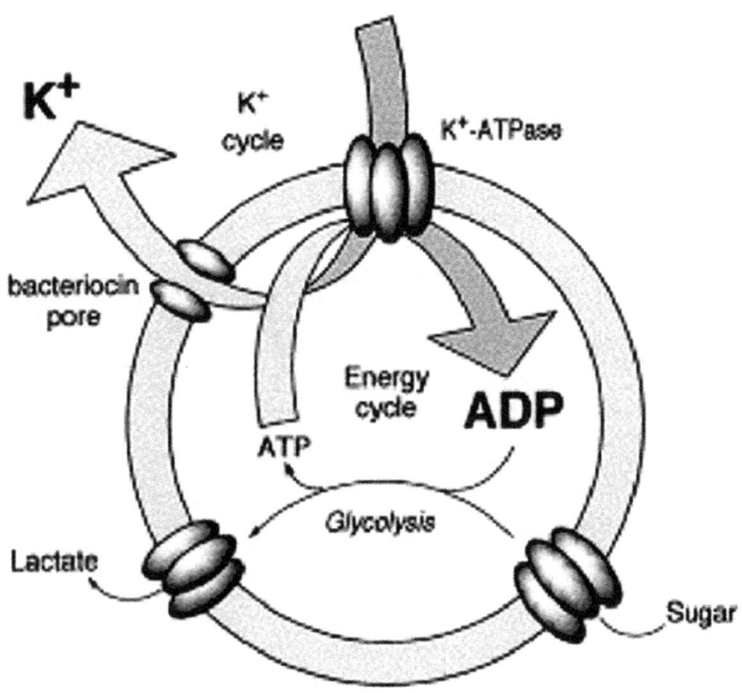

Bacteriocins Applications in Food Safety

In recent years, several studies have indicated that application of bacteriocins in food can offer following benefits: (i) longer shelf-life of foods, (ii) ensure extra protection during temperature abuse conditions, (iii) lower pathogen transmission risk through the food chain, (iv) alleviate economic losses due to food spoilage, (v) less use of chemical preservatives, (vi) permit the application of less severe heat treatments without compromising food safety: better preservation of food nutrients and vitamins, as well as organoleptic properties of foods, (vii) permit the marketing of "novel" foods (less acidic, with a lower salt content, and with a higher water content), and (viii) serve to satisfy industrial and consumers demands from safety and natural aspects (Thomas et al. 2000). The applications of bacteriocins studied in dairy sector/dairy foods are given in Table 3.

Table 3. Applications of bacteriocins studied in dairy sector/dairy foods

Bacteriocin	Producer Strain	Application	Reference
Nisin	*Lactococcus lactis*	prevent gas blowing in cheese caused by *C. tyrobutyricum*	De Vuyst and Vandamme 1994
Nisin	*Lactococcus lactis*	prevent proliferation of surviving endospore formers, mainly the gas-producing clostridia and *Clostridium botulinum*, as well as other post-process contaminating bacteria such as *L. monocytogenes* in processed cheeses and cheese products (e.g., block cheese, soft white cheeses, slices, spreads, sauces, dips)	Thomas and Delves-Broughton 2001
Enterocin AS-48	*Enterococcus faecalis*	added to a rice-based infant formula dissolved in whole milk completely inactivated *B. cereus* and prevented its growth for at least 15 days at 37°C	Grande et al. 2006
Pediocin 5	*P. acidilactici* UL5	Reported to have bactericidal effects against *L. monocytogenes* in milk	Huang et al. 1994
Partially purified Carnocin CP5	*C. piscicola* CP5	Reduced viable counts of *L. monocytogenes* in skim milk	Mathieu et al. 1994
Propionicin PLG-1	*Propionibacterium thoenii* P127	Kill or inhibit several psychrotrophic spoilage or pathogenic bacteria (*L. monocytogenes, P. fluorescens, Vibrio parahaemolyticus, Yersinia enterocolitica, and Corynebacterium sp.*)	Lyon et al. 1993
Jenseniin G	*Propionibacterium jensenii (thoenii)* P126	Control over acidification of yogurt and other fermented products because of its inhibitory activity to *Lactobacillus delbrueckii* ssp. bulgaricus	Weinbrenner et al. 1997
Variacin	*Kocuria varians*	Inhibited the proliferation of B. cereus in chilled dairy products, vanilla, and chocolate desserts in a concentration-dependent way	O'Mahony et al. 2001
Pediocin 34	*Pediococcus pentosaceus* 34	Enhanced the shelf-life of Paneer to about 75 days	Malik et al. 2005

Factors Influencing Bacteriocins Activity in Food System

Food may be commercially sterile, raw or fermented, being nutritionally rich may act as suitable matrix to harbour and support growth of wide variety of microorganisms. Even if commercially sterile foods get post-process contamination, the microorganisms may easily proliferate because of the lack of competitors. Under such conditions, the bacteriocins activity will greatly depend on a number of food-related factors (Table 4) which involve interaction with food components, precipitation, inactivation, or uneven distribution of bacteriocin molecules in the food matrix.

Table 4. Factors affecting bacteriocin efficacy in foods

Food-Related Factors	Food Microbiota	Target Bacteria
Food processing conditions	Microbial load	Microbial load
Food storage temperature, Food pH, and bacteriocin unstability to pH changes	Microbial diversity	
Inactivation by food enzymes	Bacteriocin sensitivity	Bacteriocin sensitivity (Gram-type, genus, species, strains)
Interaction with food additives/ingredients	Microbial interactions in the food system	Physiological stage (growing, resting, starving orviable but non-culturable cells, stressed or sub lethally injured cells, endospores)
Low solubility and uneven distribution in the food matrix and Limited stability of bacteriocin during food shelf life		Protection by physico-che mical barriers (microcolonies, biofilms, slime)
Bacteriocin adsorption to food components		Development of resistance /adaptation

Bacteriocins and Hurdle Technology

The concept of hurdle technology began to apply in the food industry in a rational way after the observation that survival of microorganisms greatly decreased when they were confronted with multiple antimicrobial factors (Leistner 1978; Leistner and Gorris 1995; Leistner 2000). Over 60 potential hurdles have been described to improve food stability and/or quality (Leistner 2000). The application of bacteriocins as part of hurdle technology has received great attention in recent years (Chen and Hoover 2003; Rose et al. 2003; Deegan et al. 2006), since bacteriocins can be used purposely in combination with selected hurdles in order to increase microbial inactivation. Improved control of the target microorganisms and inhibition of bacteriocin-resistant strains and species can be obtained by using a hurdle concept.

FERMENTATES: THE FOOD INGREDIENTS

Fermentates refers to ingredients produced by the fermentation of a variety of raw materials (typically milk, sugar, or plant derived materials such as corn or wheat starch) by food grade microorganisms, typically lactic acid bacteria or propionic acid bacteria (Elsser-Gravesen and Elsser-Gravesen, 2014). Such fermentation gives complex products that inherently do not have a well-defined composition but comprises of high proportion of antimicrobial metabolites, which may include organic acids (lactic, acetic or propionic acid), diacetyl, bacteriocins, and other secondary metabolites, depending on strain(s) used for the fermentation. Fermentates are marketed as a dry, cell-free powder which has very wide applications and thereby, their demand is increasing in food sector but has limited scientific background (Elsser-Gravesen and Elsser-Gravesen, 2014). Therefore, fermentates must be evaluated for their sensory suitability, safety and applicability by *in situ* testing (Crowley et al., 2013).

Currently, MicroGARD range (DuPont) and the DuraFresh range (Kerry) are commercially available fermentates for dairy applications. This also includes the former Alta and Perlac products from Quest, and many other products (namely spray-dried vinegar or fermented wheat flour products) that are claimed to be shelf-life enhancers. Besides wide applications of fermentates very limited scientific reports are available on their functionality in dairy foods. The MicroGARD products (produced by fermenting skimmed milk or dextrose with *Propionibacterium shermanii* or specific lactococci) and Alta (whey-based products prepared by *P. acidilactici*) were demonstrated to inhibit the psychotropic spoilage flora and thereby enhance the shelf-life of cottage cheese (al-Zoreky et al., 1991). Also, these products showed inhibition of *Pseudomonas*, *Salmonella*, *Yersinia*, and certain fungi. In contrast, no such significant effect of the MicroGARD and Alta products was seen against aerobic mesophilic counts, *Escherichia coli* or *Brochothrix thermosphacta* when tested in an acidified chicken meat model stored at 22°C (Lemay et al., 2002). Enhanced anti-listerial effect was reported in liquid cheese whey when nisin was used in combination with MicroGARD fermentate (von Staszewski and Jagus, 2008).

As already stated, there is limited scientific documentation for the fermentates in comparison to bacteriocins. Their wide industrial applications have raised the demands and United States leads the markets for fermentates. Such products are commercially available as ''cultured milk'' or ''cultured sugar'', based on the substrate used for producing the fermentate. A cultured dextrose version of MicroGARD has been evaluated for toxicity and no detrimental effects were observed (Buard et al., 2003). The MicroGARD products are used for a wide range of applications in dairy items including cottage cheese, yogurt, sour cream, dairy desserts. It has been estimated that approximately 30% of the US cheese production is made with MicroGARD (Sani et al., 2005). In 2011, FDA approved Durafresh (labeled as ''cultured grade A skim milk and skim milk powder'') use in cottage cheese to control *Listeria*.

Labelling is a major issue in the European Union (EU), as it would be required to label all active components in the fermentate. This presents two main concerns (i) not all active components are known, and (ii) most of the known ones have E-numbers. Therefore, the use of fermentates as natural preservatives is so far quite limited in the EU.

BIOPROTECTIVE CULTURES

Food preservation can be accomplished either by supplementing the food product with *ex-situ* produced bacteriocins (purified or partially purified), or by using fermentates as food ingredient (raw concentrate). The addition of partially purified or purified bacteriocin concentrates obtained by fermentation at industrial scale; require specific approval as preservatives from the legislative point of view. Till date, nisin is the only bacteriocin licensed as a food preservative. Legally, the raw concentrates/fermentates may also be regarded as food additives or ingredients, since their addition may affect the physico-chemical properties of the food (thickening, protein content etc). Also, the cell-derived antimicrobial metabolites (such as lactic acid, bacteriocins, reuterin etc.) present in these fermentates perform an additional bioprotectant function.

Considering both the processing cost as well as the legal issues related to addition of purified bacteriocins and/or fermentates, the use of bioprotective starter or adjunct cultures in fermented dairy foods is one promising solution. The fermentation of perishable food to enhance their shelf life is one of the oldest known uses of biotechnology. The value addition properties of the fermentation processes includes: (a) enhanced durability through production of antimicrobial metabolites (e.g. organic acids, bacteriocins, ethanol), often in conjunction with decreased water activity (drying and/or salting); (b) enhanced safety by reducing the level of either pathogenic microorganisms or their toxins; (c) enhanced nutritional value; and (d) enhanced organoleptic quality (Bourdichon et al., 2012). Also, there are some unwanted and unacceptable detrimental properties associated with food cultures that include virulence, toxicity, and antibiotic resistance. In the US, acceptable food microorganisms are granted the GRAS status, and in EU they are included in the Qualified Presumption of Safety list. An inventory list of currently used microbial food cultures, comprising 195 bacterial species and 69 fungal species, has recently been compiled (Bourdichon et al., 2012).

Microbial cultures used for fermentation can either be starter cultures (providing nutritional and organoleptic characteristics) or bioprotective cultures (providing durability and safety). All these properties are inherently linked for e.g. Formation of organic acids enhances durability and also contributes to the characteristic taste and texture of fermented product. All starter cultures are per se also protective cultures, but not all protective cultures are also starter cultures. Therefore, it is neither possible nor meaningful to differentiate between starter cultures and bioprotective cultures.

Research activities performed in past decades have aimed to develop cultures that can (i) enhance food safety either by direct killing or inhibiting the growth of pathogens or by suppressing toxin production or (ii) enhance shelf-life by controlling growth of spoilage microorganisms. Comprehensive reviews summarizing research findings including solutions for dairy products are available (Beshkova and Frengova, 2012; Grattepanche et al., 2008). Overall, most of the reports can be allocated to one of the following main categories:

1. **Use of Bacteriocinogenic LAB Cultures:** Mode of action relies on production of bacteriocins. In dairy industries, nisin-producing *L. lactis* strains have been reported to inhibit *L. monocytogenes* in several varities of cheeses, such as cottage cheese (Benkerroum and Sandine 1988) or Camembert (Maisnier- Patin et al. 1992). Also, enterocin producing *Enterococcus faecium* strains in smear of soft cheese controlled outgrowth of *L. monocytogenes* (Izquierdo et al., 2009).
2. **Use of Antifungal LAB and/or PAB to Delay Spoilage of Various Types of Food:** Mode of action relies on production of several antifungal metabolites. For e.g. *Lactobacillus rhamnosus* and *Propionibacterium freudenreichii* ssp. shermanii were used for inhibiting yeast in yogurt (Liptakova et al., 2006). *Lactobacillus harbinensis* was used as an antifungal culture in yogurt (Delavenne et al., 2013).
3. **Use of Non-Bacteriocinogenic LAB With Other Competitive Properties:** Mode of action relies on antimicrobial metabolites other then bateriocins. For e.g. commercial culture had a protective effect by depletion of oxygen, production of organic acids etc (Seibert, 2010).

Protective cultures are produced and marketed in the same way as starter cultures. The protective strains are produced in batch fermenters, subsequently concentrated by centrifugation, and finally formulated either as frozen pellets or freeze-dried powders. Protective cultures are now well established and recognized as an efficient tool to ensure the food safety and security. Few examples of the commercially available protective cultures for dairy products are given in Table 5.

Table 5. Examples of commercially available protective cultures

Protective Function	Microorganisms	Producer
Growth inhibition of *Listeria monocytogenes*	Lactic acid bacteria (e.g. *Lb. sakei, Lb. curvatus, Lb. plantarum*)	Chr. Hansen (Denmark) DuPont (USA)
Inhibition of mold and yeasts	*Lactobacillus* sp. *Lb. rhamnosus, Lb. paracasei, Propionobacterium* sps.	Chr. Hansen (Denmark) DuPont (USA)
Inhibition of *Clostridia tyrobutyricum*; prevention of late blowing	*Lactococcus lactis*	CSK (Netherlands)

BACTERIOPHAGES

Continuously increasing food-borne diseases caused by pathogens, such as *Salmonella, Campylobacter, Escherichia coli, Listeria* and others, shows that the current technologies employed to inactivate bacterial pathogens are not infallible (DuPont 2007). Contaminating bacteria can get access to food during milking, fermentation, processing, storage or packaging. In past decades, several strategies have been tried to minimize the microbial load of raw products, such as the use of antibiotics and physical treatments like steam, dry heat and UV light. But their applications are restricted due to the negative impact of antibiotics on human antimicrobial therapies, development of antibiotic resistant strains and physical treatments deteriorate the organoleptic properties. Also, some approaches used in the dairy industry to reduce contamination cannot be directly applied to dairy products.

Bacteriophages (Greek, meaning ''bacteria-eater'') are viruses that invade bacterial cells (host) and, in the case of lytic phages, disrupt bacterial metabolism and cause the host to lyse. Bacteriophages are host-specific that means the phage recognizes its specific host and can only propagate on a certain bacterial species. Their long history of safe use, relatively easy handling and highly specific antimicrobial activity make them suitable biocontrol tool to ensure food safety (Table 6).

Table 6. Advantages of using bacteriophages as biocontrol tools in food industry

History of safe use	• Ubiquitous in nature including food ecosystems • Natural commensals of humans and animals • Extensive clinical use in Eastern Europe
Highly active and specific	• No adverse effects on the intestinal microbiota • Innocuous to mammalian cells • Autoreplicative • Can be active against biofilms
Genetically amenable	
Versatile use along the food chain	• Phage therapy • Biosanitation • Biopreservation
Tools for detecting pathogens	
Source of potent antimicrobials	Endolysins and other peptidoglycan hydrolases

In the dairy industry, starter cultures failure due to phage attack is a common problem. In contrast, phages which can attack pathogens can be useful in food processing. So to speak, "the enemy of my enemy is my useful friend". Applications of bacteriophages as natural antimicrobials in food industry to inhibit undesirable bacteria have become widely recognized in past years (Hagens and Loessner 2007; Strauch et al. 2007). They have been proposed as biocontrol tool to ensue food safety (Garcı´a et al., 2008).

Bacteriophages can be used for (i) biotherapy (to prevent or reduce colonization and infection in livestock), (ii) biosanitation and biocontrol (to decontaminate raw products and to disinfect equipment and contact surfaces) and (iii) biopreservation (to extend the shelf life of perishable food products). Bacteriophages should also be considered in hurdle technology in combination with different preservation methods (Leverentz et al. 2003; Martı´nez et al. 2008). Several examples of phage application in dairy industry are outlined below.

- *E. coli* O157:H7 remains a continuous public health threat because its ingestion even in small concentration (10–100 cells) may result in potent toxin exposure. Ruminants being the principal reservoir for this strain can release contaminated milk during milking. Raya et al. (2006) observed a 2-log-unit reduction in intestinal *E. coli* O157:H7 within 2 days after oral administration of phage CEV1 in sheep. However, phage KH1 did not show such effect. Sheng et al. (2006) observed significantly less cell count when a combination of phages KHI and SH1 were administered rectally to cattle and maintained at 10^6 PFU ml^{-1} in the drinking water.
- Modi et al. (2001) tested the activity of the *Salmonella* phage SJ2 in cheddar cheese manufacturing. In the presence of phages (MOI 10^4), *Salmonella* did not survive in the pasteurized cheeses after 89 days, whereas about 50 CFU ml^{-1} were still viable in raw milk cheeses.
- Kim et al. (2007a) addressed the issue of *Enterobacter sakazakii* in reconstituted infant milk formula. The authors observed that newly isolated phage at concentration of 10^9 PFU ml^{-1} was able to effectively suppress growth in prepared infant formula, both at 24 °C and 37°C (Kim et al. 2007b).
- Staphylococcal mastitis caused by *Staphylococcus aureus* is a major concern to the dairy industry and infected udder is the most important source of milk contamination by this pathogen. Staphylococcal food poisoning is due to the absorption of preformed staphylococcal enterotoxins (Le Loir et al. 2003). Gill et al. (2006a) evaluated the ability of the lytic *Staph. aureus* bacteriophage K to eliminate bovine *Staph. aureus* intramammary infection during lactation. The authors reported Phage K inactivation in raw milk, likely due to the adsorption of whey proteins to the cell surface that interfere with phage attachment (O'Flaherty et al. 2005; Gill et al. 2006b). However, Garcı´a et al. (2007) found that a cocktail of two lytic phages of dairy origin inhibited *Staph. aureus* in acid and enzymatic curd manufacturing processes.
- Recently, a commercial product named Listex P100 was approved by the FDA as a food biopreservative and granted as GRAS (Federal Register: August 18, 2006. Volume 71, Number 160, pp. 47729–47732). This product is based on the virulent phage P100 (Carlton et al. 2005) and, depending on dosage and treatment, a complete eradication of *L. monocytogenes* on surface-ripened red-smear soft cheese.

Bacteriophages may act as vectors that can transfer virulent and antibiotic-resistance traits, therefore, have raised safety concerns. Also, phages may not show the antimicrobial activity in food systems as observed in laboratory conditions. Several factors such as reduced diffusion rates that decrease the chance of host-phage collisions, the microbial load which might also act as a mechanical barrier by providing unspecific phage binding sites and other adverse factors such as temperature, pH and inhibitory compounds may limit their performance *in situ*.

CONCLUSION

The use of biopreservatives in the dairy industry can help to achieve the target of providing minimally processed, ready to eat, naturally preserved food. Although most efforts have been devoted to find out and understand different approaches to preserve the food products in more natural way but still many limitation to these approaches need to be overcome. Several researches on isolation and characterization of bacteriocinogenic LAB strains and their bacteriocins, their application in food safety preservation of dairy products have already been done. The careful selection of bacteriocinogenic strain with best performance for variety of food type and choice of bacteriocin treatments (either alone or in combination with other hurdles) may greatly help in development of suitable food safety systems. But the developing bacteriocins resistance among the pathogens is of major concern. Therefore, more study is needed to determine the distribution of bacteriocin-resistance phenomena among spoilage causing and pathogenic microorganisms. Also, knowledge of the characteristics of bacteriocin- resistant variants and the conditions that prevent their emergence will help in determining the optimal conditions for application of bacteriocins in foods and minimize the incidence of resistance. Fermentates have limitations as they can affect the organoleptic and physico-chemical properties of the product. No single bioprotective culture can be used for wide range of products i.e. why different bioprotective culture for different products need to be studied. Also, the maintainence of the bioprotective culture and its activity to meet the industrial demand is a challenge in itself. Bacteriophages can act as vector of undesired traits (virulence and antibiotic resistance genes) therefore, have raised safety concerns. Also, their performance *in situ* may not be as good as in laboratory conditions which may be attributed to several factors related to food matrices. Such limiting factors need to be considered while selecting the bacteriophage for particular food product. Lastly, it can be considered that there is no single magic bullet that can be used to preserve the food. With Hurdle technology or manipulation of several factors in combination with the biopreservatives, the aim of natural preservation can only be accomplished.

REFERENCES

al-Zoreky, N., Ayres, J. W., & Sandine, W. E. (1991). Antimicrobial activity of microgard against food spoilage and pathogenic microorganisms. *Journal of Dairy Science, 74*(3), 758–763. doi:10.3168/jds. S0022-0302(91)78222-2 PMID:1906486

Benkerroum, N., & Sandine, W. E. (1988). Inhibitory action of nisin against *Listeria monocytogenes. Journal of Dairy Science, 71*(12), 3237–3245. doi:10.3168/jds.S0022-0302(88)79929-4 PMID:3148644

Beshkova, D., & Frengova, G. (2012). Bacteriocins from lactic acid bacteria: Microorganisms of potential biotechnological importance for the dairy industry. *Engineering in Life Sciences, 12*(4), 419–432. doi:10.1002/elsc.201100127

Biswas, S. R., Ray, P., Johnson, M. C., & Ray, B. (1991). Influence of growth conditions on the prod of a bacteriocin, pediocin AcH, by *Pediococcus acidilactic* H. *Applied and Environmental Microbiology, 57*, 1265–1267. PMID:16348467

Bourdichon, F., Casaregola, S., Farrokh, C., Frisvad, J. C., Gerds, M. L., Hammes, W. P., ... Hansen, E. B. (2012). Food fermentations: Microorganisms with technological beneficial use. *International Journal of Food Microbiology, 154*(3), 87–97. doi:10.1016/j.ijfoodmicro.2011.12.030 PMID:22257932

Breukink, E., Weidemann, I., van Kraaij, C., Kuipers, O. P., Sahl, H. G., & de Kruijff, B. (1999). Use of cell wall precursor lipid II by a poreforming peptide antibiotic. *Science, 286*(5448), 2361–2364. doi:10.1126cience.286.5448.2361 PMID:10600751

Brotz, H., Bierbaum, G., Leopold, K., Reynolds, P. E., & Sahl, H. G. (1998). The lantibiotic mersaci-din inhibits peptidoglycan synthesis by targeting lipid II. *Antimicrobial Agents and Chemotherapy, 42*, 154–160. PMID:9449277

Buard, A., Carlton, B. D., Floch, F., & Simon, G. S. (2003). Subchronic toxicity, mutagenicity and al-lergenicity studies of a cultured dextrose food product. *Food and Chemical Toxicology, 41*(5), 689–694. doi:10.1016/S0278-6915(03)00006-1 PMID:12659722

Carlton, R. M., Noordman, W. H., Biswas, B., de Meester, E. D., & Loessner, M. J. (2005). Bacteriophage P100 for control of *Listeria monocytogenes* in foods: Genome sequence, bioinformatic analyses, oral toxicity study, and application. *Regulatory Toxicology and Pharmacology, 43*(3), 301–312. doi:10.1016/j.yrtph.2005.08.005 PMID:16188359

Chen, H., & Hoover, D. G. (2003). Bacteriocins and their food applications. *Comprehensive Reviews in Food Science and Food Safety, 2*(3), 82–100. doi:10.1111/j.1541-4337.2003.tb00016.x

Chinachoti, N., Matsuaki, H., Sonomoto, K., & Ishikazi, A. (1997a). Utilization of xylose as an alternative carbon source for nisin Z production by *Lactococcus lactis* IO-1. *Fac Agric. Kyushu Univ, 42*, 171–181.

Chinachoti, N., Zaima, T., Masuaki, H., Sonomoto, K., & Ishikazi, A. (1997b). Relationship between nisin Z fermentaire prod and aeration condition using *Lactococcus lactis* I0-1. *Journal of the Faculty of Agriculture, Kyushu University, 43*, 437–448.

Crowley, S., Mahony, J., Morrissey, J. P., & van Sinderen, D. (2013). Transcriptomic and morphological profiling of *Aspergillus fumigatus* Af293 in response to antifungal activity produced by *Lactobacillus plantarum* 16. *Microbiology, 159*(Pt_10), 2014–2024. doi:10.1099/mic.0.068742-0 PMID:23876797

Deegan, L. H., Cotterm, P. D., Hill, C., & Ross, P. (2006). Bacteriocins: Biological tools for bio-preservation and shelf-life extension. *International Dairy Journal, 16*(9), 1058–1071. doi:10.1016/j.idairyj.2005.10.026

Delavenne, E., Ismail, R., Pawtowski, A., Mounier, J., Barbier, G., & Le Blay, G. (2013). Assessment of lactobacilli strains as yogurt bioprotective cultures. *Food Control, 30*(1), 206–213. doi:10.1016/j.foodcont.2012.06.043

DeVuyst, L., & Vandamme, E. (1994). *Bacteriocins of Lactic acid bacteria: microbiology, genetics and application*. London, UK: Chapman & Hill Ltd. doi:10.1007/978-1-4615-2668-1

DuPont, H. L. (2007). The growing threat of foodborne bacterial enteropathogens of animal origin. *Clinical Infectious Diseases*, *45*(10), 1353–1361. doi:10.1086/522662 PMID:17968835

Elsser-Gravesen, D., & Elsser-Gravesen, A. (2014). Biopreservatives. *Advances in Biochemical Engineering/Biotechnology*, *143*, 29–49. doi:10.1007/10_2013_234 PMID:24185748

Franz, C. M. A. P., van Belkum, M. J., Holzapfel, W. H., Abriouel, H., & G'alvez, A. (2007). Diversity of enterococcal bacteriocins and their grouping into a new classification scheme. *FEMS Microbiology Reviews*, *31*(3), 293–310. doi:10.1111/j.1574-6976.2007.00064.x PMID:17298586

G'alvez, A., Abriouel, H., Lucas L'opez, R., & Ben Omar, N. (2007). Bacteriocin based strategies for food biopreservation. *International Journal of Food Microbiology*, *120*(1-2), 51–70. doi:10.1016/j.ijfoodmicro.2007.06.001 PMID:17614151

Garcı'a, P., Madera, C., Martı'nez, B., & Rodrı'guez, A. (2007). Biocontrol of *Staphylococcus aureus* in curd manufacturing processes using bacteriophages. *International Dairy Journal*, *17*(10), 1232–1239. doi:10.1016/j.idairyj.2007.03.014

Gill, J. J., Pacan, J. C., Carson, M. E., Leslie, K. E., Griffiths, M. W., & Sabour, P. M. (2006a). Efficacy and pharmacokinetics of bacteriophage therapy in treatment of subclinical *Staphylococcus aureus* mastitis in lactating dairy cattle. *Antimicrobial Agents and Chemotherapy*, *50*(9), 2912–2918. doi:10.1128/AAC.01630-05 PMID:16940081

Gill, J. J., Sabour, P. M., Leslie, K. E., & Griffiths, M. W. (2006b). Bovine whey proteins inhibit the interaction of *Staphylococcus aureus* and bacteriophage K. *Journal of Applied Microbiology*, *101*(2), 377–386. doi:10.1111/j.1365-2672.2006.02918.x PMID:16882145

Grande, M. J., Lucas, R., Abriouel, H., Valdivia, E., Ben Omar, N., Maqueda, M., ... G'alvez, A. (2006). Inhibition of toxicogenic *Bacillus cereus* in rice based foods by enterocin AS-48. *International Journal of Food Microbiology*, *106*(2), 185–194. doi:10.1016/j.ijfoodmicro.2005.08.003 PMID:16225949

Grattepanche, F., Miescher-Schwenninger, S., Meile, L., & Lacroix, C. (2008). Recent developments in cheese cultures with protective and probiotic functionalities. *Dairy Science & Technology*, *88*(4-5), 421–444. doi:10.1051/dst:2008013

Güllüce, M., Karaday, M., & Barış, Ö. (2013). Bacteriocins: promising natural antimicrobials. In *Microbial pathogens and strategies for combating them: science, technology and education* (pp. 1016–1027). Badajoz, Spain: FORMATEX.

Hagens, S., & Loessner, M. J. (2007). Application of bacteriophages for detection and control of foodborne pathogens. *Applied Microbiology and Biotechnology*, *76*, 513–519.

Håvarstein, H., Holo, H., & Nes, I. F. (1994). he leader peptide of colicin V shares consensus sequences with leader peptides that are common among peptide bacteriocins produced by gram-positive bacteria. *Microbiology*, *140*(9), 2383–2389. doi:10.1099/13500872-140-9-2383 PMID:7952189

Holo, H., Nilssen, O., & Nes, I. F. (1991). Lactococcin A, a new bacteriocin from *Lactococcus lactis* subsp. *cremoris*: Isolation and characterization of the protein and its gene. *Journal of Bacteriology*, *173*(12), 3879–3887. doi:10.1128/jb.173.12.3879-3887.1991 PMID:1904860

Huang, J., Lacroix, C., Daba, H., & Simard, R. E. (1994). Growth of *Listeria monocytogenes* in milk and its control by pediocin 5 produced by *Pediococcus acidilactici* UL5. *International Dairy Journal*, *4*(5), 429–443. doi:10.1016/0958-6946(94)90057-4

Izquierdo, E., Marchioni, E., Aoude-Werner, D., Hasselmann, C., & Ennahar, S. (2009). Smearing of soft cheese with *Enterococcus faecium* WHE 81, a multi-bacteriocin producer, against *Listeria monocytogenes*. *Food Microbiology*, *26*(1), 16–20. doi:10.1016/j.fm.2008.08.002 PMID:19028299

Kaur, M. R. K., & Singh, T. P. (2014). Bacteriocins and their potential applications. In Microbes in the service of mankind: tiny bugs with huge impact (pp. 309-345). JBC Press.

Kim, K., Jang, S. S., Kim, S. K., Park, J. H., Heu, S., & Ryu, S. (2007a). Prevalence and genetic diversity of *Enterobacter sakazakii* in ingredients of infant foods. *International Journal of Food Microbiology*, *122*(1-2), 196–203. doi:10.1016/j.ijfoodmicro.2007.11.072 PMID:18177966

Kim, K. P., Klumpp, J., & Loessner, M. J. (2007b). *Enterobacter sakazakii* bacteriophages can prevent bacterial growth in reconstituted infant formula. *International Journal of Food Microbiology*, *115*(2), 195–203. doi:10.1016/j.ijfoodmicro.2006.10.029 PMID:17196280

Klaenhammer, T. R. (1993). Genetics of bacteriocins produced by lactic acid bacteria. *FEMS Microbiology Reviews*, *12*(1-3), 39–86. doi:10.1111/j.1574-6976.1993.tb00012.x PMID:8398217

Le Loir, Y., Baron, F., & Gautier, M. (2003). *Staphylococcus aureus* and food poisoning. *Genetics and Molecular Research*, *31*, 63–76. PMID:12917803

Leistner, L. (1978). Hurdle effect and energy saving. In W. K. Downey (Ed.), *Food Quality and Nutrition* (pp. 553–557). London, UK: Applied Science Publishers.

Leistner, L. (2000). Basic aspects of food preservation by hurdle technology. *International Journal of Food Microbiology*, *55*(1-3), 181–186. doi:10.1016/S0168-1605(00)00161-6 PMID:10791741

Leistner, L., & Gorris, L. G. M. (1995). Food preservation by hurdle technology. *Trends in Food Science & Technology*, *6*(2), 41–46. doi:10.1016/S0924-2244(00)88941-4

Lejeune, R., Callewaert, R., Crabbé, & De Vuyst. (1998). Modelling the growth and bacteriocin production by *Lactobacillus amylovorus* DCE 471 in batch cultivation. *Journal of Applied Microbiology*, *84*(2), 159–168. doi:10.1046/j.1365-2672.1998.00266.x

Lemay, M. J., Choquette, J., Delaquis, P. J., Claude, G., Rodrigue, N., & Saucier, L. (2002). Antimicrobial effect of natural preservatives in a cooked and acidified chicken meat model. *International Journal of Food Microbiology*, *78*(3), 217–226. doi:10.1016/S0168-1605(02)00014-4 PMID:12227640

Leverentz, B., Conway, W. S., Camp, M. J., Janisiewicz, W. J., Abuladze, T., Yang, M., ... Sulakvelidze, A. (2003). Biocontrol of *Listeria monocytogenes* on fresh-cut produce by treatment with lytic bacteriophages and a bacteriocin. *Applied and Environmental Microbiology*, *69*(8), 4519–4526. doi:10.1128/AEM.69.8.4519-4526.2003 PMID:12902237

Liptakova, D., Valik, L., & Bajusova, B. (2006). Effect of protective culture on the growth of *Candida maltosa* YP1 in yoghurt. *Journal of Food and Nutrition Research*, *45*, 147–151.

Lyon, W. J., Sethi, J. K., & Glatz, B. A. (1993). Inhibition of psychrotrophic organisms by propionicin PLG-1, a bacteriocin produced by *Propionibacterium thoenii*. *Journal of Dairy Science, 76*(6), 1506–1513. doi:10.3168/jds.S0022-0302(93)77482-2 PMID:8326023

Maisnier-Patin, S., Deschamps, N., Tatini, S. R., & Richard, J. (1992). Inhibition of *Listeria monocytogenes* in Camembert cheese made with a nisin-producing starter. *Le Lait, 72*(3), 249–263. doi:10.1051/lait:1992318

Malik, R. K., Rao, K. N., Bandhopadhyay, P., & Kumar, N. (2005). Bacteriocins: Natural and safe anti microbial peptides for food preservation. *Indian Food Industry, 24*(1), 69–70.

Martı'nez, B., Obeso, J. M., Rodrı'guez, A., & Garcı'a, P. (2008). Nisin-bacteriophage crossresistance in *Staphylococcus aureus*. *International Journal of Food Microbiology, 122*(3), 253–258. doi:10.1016/j.ijfoodmicro.2008.01.011 PMID:18281118

Mathieu, F., Michel, M., Lebrihi, A., & Lefebvre, G. (1994). Effect of the bacteriocin carnocin CP5 and of the producing strain *Carnobacterium piscicola* CP5 on the viability of Listeria monocytogenes ATCC 15313 in salt solution, broth and skimmed milk, at various incubation temperatures. *International Journal of Food Microbiology, 22*(2-3), 155–172. doi:10.1016/0168-1605(94)90139-2 PMID:8074969

Matsuaki, H., Endo, N., Sonomoto, K., & Ishikazi, A. (1996). Lantibiotic nisin Z fermentative production by *Lactococcus lactis* IO-1: Relationship between production of the lantibiotic and lactate and cell growth. *Applied Microbiology and Biotechnology, 45*(1-2), 36–40. doi:10.1007002530050645 PMID:8920177

Modi, R., Hirvi, Y., Hill, A., & Griffiths, M. W. (2001). Effect of phage on survival of *Salmonella enteritidis* during manufacture and storage of Cheddar cheese made from raw and pasteurized milk. *Journal of Food Protection, 64*(7), 927–933. doi:10.4315/0362-028X-64.7.927 PMID:11456198

Muriana, P. M., & Klaenhamer, T. R. (1991). Purification and partial characterization of lactacin F, a bacteriocin produced by *Lactobacillus acidophilus* 11088. *Applied and Environmental Microbiology, 57*, 114–121. PMID:1903624

Nes, I. F., Diep, D. B., Håvarstein, L. S., & Brurberg, M. B. (1996). Biosynthesis of bacteriocins in lactic acid bacteria. *Antonie van Leeuwenhoek, 70*, 113–128. doi:10.1007/BF00395929 PMID:8879403

O'Flaherty, S., Coffey, A., Meaney, W. J., Fitzgerald, G. F., & Ross, R. P. (2005). Inhibition of bacteriophage K proliferation on *Staphylococcus aureus* in raw bovine milk. *Letters in Applied Microbiology, 41*(3), 274–279. doi:10.1111/j.1472-765X.2005.01762.x PMID:16108920

O'Mahony, T., Rekhif, N., Cavadini, C., & Fitzgerald, G. F. (2001). The application of a fermented food ingredient containing 'variacin', a novel antimicrobial produced by *Kocuria varians*, to control the growth of *Bacillus cereus* in chilled dairy products. *Journal of Applied Microbiology, 90*(1), 106–114. doi:10.1046/j.1365-2672.2001.01222.x PMID:11155129

Parente, E., Giglio, M. A., Riccardi, A., & Clementi, F. (1998). The combined effect of nisin, leucocin F10, pH, NaCl and EDTA on the survival of *Listeria monocytogenes* in broth. *International Journal of Food Microbiology, 40*(1-2), 65–75. doi:10.1016/S0168-1605(98)00021-X PMID:9600612

Raya, R. R., Varey, P., Oot, R. A., Dyen, M. R., Callaway, T. R., Edrington, T. S., ... Brabban, A. D. (2006). Isolation and characterization of a new T-even bacteriophage, CEV1, and determination of its potential to reduce *Escherichia coli* O157:H7 levels in sheep. *Applied and Environmental Microbiology*, *72*(9), 6405–6410. doi:10.1128/AEM.03011-05 PMID:16957272

Reisinger, H., Seidel, H., Tschesche, P., & Hammes, W. P. (1980). The effect of nisin on murein synthesis. *Archives of Microbiology*, *127*(3), 187–193. doi:10.1007/BF00427192 PMID:6255884

Roller, S. (2003). Introduction. In S. Roller (Ed.), *Natural antimicrobials for the minimal processing of foods* (pp. 1–10). Cambridge, UK: Woodhead Publishing Ltd.

Rose, R. P., Sporns, P., Dodd, H. M., Gasson, M. J., Mellon, F. A., & McMullen, L. M. (2003). Involvement of dehydroalanine and dehydrobutyrine in the addition of glutathione to nisin. *Journal of Agricultural and Food Chemistry*, *51*(10), 3174–3178. doi:10.1021/jf026022h PMID:12720411

Sani, A. M., Ehsani, M. R., & Asadi, M. M. (2005). Effect of *Propionibacterium shermanii* metabolites on sensory properties and shelf life of UF-Feta cheese. *Nutrition & Food Science*, *35*(2), 88–94. doi:10.1108/00346650510585877

Schuller, F., Benz, R., & Sahl, H. G. (1989). The peptide antibiotic subtilin acts by formation of voltage-dependent multi-state pores in bacterial and artificial membranes. *European Journal of Biochemistry*, *182*(1), 181–186. doi:10.1111/j.1432-1033.1989.tb14815.x PMID:2471644

Seibert, T. M. (2010). Protective culture eliminates residual oxygen. *Die Fleischwirtschaft (Frankfurt)*, *90*, 59–61.

Sheng, H., Knecht, H. J., Kudva, I. T., & Hovde, C. J. (2006). Application of bacteriophages to control intestinal *Escherichia coli* O157:H7 levels in ruminants. *Applied and Environmental Microbiology*, *72*(8), 5359–5366. doi:10.1128/AEM.00099-06 PMID:16885287

Strauch, E., Hammerl, J. A., & Hertwig, S. (2007). Bacteriophages: New tools for safer food? *Journal für Verbraucherschutz und Lebensmittelsicherheit*, *2*(2), 138–143. doi:10.100700003-007-0188-5

Thomas, L. V., Clarkson, M. R., & Delves-Broughton, J. (2000). Nisin. In A. S. Naidu (Ed.), *Natural food antimicrobial systems* (pp. 463–524). Boca-Raton, FL: CRC Press.

Thomas, L. V., & Delves-Broughton, J. (2001). New advances in the application of the food preservative nisin. *Advances in Food Sciences*, *2*, 11–22.

von Staszewski, M., & Jagus, R. J. (2008). Natural antimicrobials: Effect of Microgard (TM) and nisin against *Listeria innocua* in liquid cheese whey. *International Dairy Journal*, *18*(3), 255–259. doi:10.1016/j.idairyj.2007.08.012

Weinbrenner, D. R., Barefoot, S. F., & Grinstead, D. A. (1997). Inhibition of yogurt starter cultures by Jenseniin G, a *Propionibacterium* bacteriocin. *Journal of Dairy Science*, *80*(7), 1246–1253. doi:10.3168/jds.S0022-0302(97)76053-3

This research was previously published in Microbial Cultures and Enzymes in Dairy Technology edited by Şebnem Öztürkoğlu Budak and H. Ceren Akal; pages 69-86, copyright year 2018 by Medical Information Science Reference (an imprint of IGI Global).

Chapter 11

Resource–Saving Technology of Dehydration of Fruit and Vegetable Raw Materials:
Scientific Rationale and Cost Efficiency

Inna Simakova
 https://orcid.org/0000-0003-0998-8396
Saratov State Vavilov Agrarian University, Russia

Victoria Strizhevskaya
Saratov State Vavilov Agrarian University, Russia

Igor Vorotnikov
Saratov State Vavilov Agrarian University, Russia

Fedor Pertsevyi
Sumy National Agrarian University, Ukraine

ABSTRACT

Thousands of tons of fruit and vegetables are lost annually during harvesting, transportation, and storage. Meanwhile, there is a problem of insufficient consumption of fruit and vegetables in the diet of modern people which results in an increase in the occurrence of alimentary-dependent diseases. One of the possible solutions to these two interrelated problems is the development of a technology of processing of substandard raw materials directly at the harvesting site. This study aims at the development of the technology of dehydration of fruit and vegetables applicable in a field. The economic effect of the proposed solution is contingent on the reduction of losses at the stage of cleaning and saving water resources and saving transportation and storage costs.

DOI: 10.4018/978-1-7998-5354-1.ch011

INTRODUCTION

Contemporary globalization processes emerge new challenges to food security. Concentration of people in big cities aggravates food supply problems. Since 1950, the share of urban population in the world has increased from 30% up to 54% and is expected to reach 66% by 2050. Megalopolises with population over ten million people are at particular risk in terms of stable food supply due to the complex logistics, high intensity of economic activity, cascade effects in case of failures in functioning of separate elements of infrastructure, critical dependence on food and agricultural products produced outside urban areas.

There are fears of increased food insecurity in different countries including developed ones. One of the reasons of hunger are losses of food and agricultural raw materials which is a complex problem worldwide. For example, in the EU and Russia, major factors of food losses are losses during cleaning (about 11%), consumption (10%), and processing and packaging (4%). Annual losses of vegetables and melon are about 3.5% of the total output. Particular, in 2017, Russia's domestic production vegetables, cucurbits, fruit, and berries totaled 18.6 million tons. At a stage of cleaning, 559.26 thousand tons were lost, not to mention processing and other stages. Reduction of losses is one of the factors of food security improvement and decrease in adverse environmental effects of agriculture and food processing.

Food and Agriculture Organization of the United Nations (FAO) focuses on the development of policies to reduce food losses and spoilage. The methodology elaborated by the FAO as part of a global initiative to reduce food losses and damage in food preservation is the basis of many reports developed to analyze critical points in food value chains and identify possible solutions and strategies to reduce food loss. Considerable losses of food during storage, transportation, and retail trade have different nature and different reasons in developing and developed countries. In developing world, major losses happen during harvesting, transportation, pre-processing, and storage of agricultural products and raw materials due to underdeveloped technologies, lack of availability of expensive modern equipment, as well as organizational issues. In the developed countries, significant losses (up to 30%) happen in retail trade and at end users. In a number of developed countries, governments respond to food losses problem by the implementation of large-scale program actions.

Another global challenge to food security is the problem of hidden hunger associated with the intensification of technological processes and the saturation of food market with refined food. The issue has been becoming common and increasingly relevant for both poorer and richer states. Hidden hunger causes chronic deficiency of vitamins and minerals in diet. Life in environmentally neglected urban zones requires higher consumption of vitamins. Modern technologies of food production do not promote preservation of the most valuable products. Decrease in volume of consumed food and its partial replacement by industrially developed foodstuff lead to the development of year-round deficiency of minor food components in diet. The effect has been registered in many countries worldwide. It may provoke development of a large number of alimentary and dependent metabolic disorders and diseases. The problem becomes even more adverse in the conditions of frigid climate, poverty, stress, location, and shortage of particular elements in soil and water. Hidden hunger has particular negative effect on pregnant and lactating women and children.

Indirectly, the problem of hidden hunger is influenced by the emergence of agro-holdings which strive to every intensification of agricultural production. This process leads to sharp polarization of rural people in employment opportunities and income level. It provokes structural unemployment in rural areas and deterioration in social status of rural dwellers. Rural unemployment is associated with increasing transaction expenses owing to territorial distribution of population and places of application of work; small amount, fragmentariness, and isolation of local labor markets; lateness in the expansion of consumer innovations in rural areas; and rather poor quality of social infrastructure. It leads to decrease in the level of social stability in rural areas and involves outflow of population to the cities.

Large-scale losses of food at storage, transportation, and retail trade, as well as hidden hunger problem, require the search of essentially new technological solutions of food production and processing to achieve the sustainable development and food security goals. This study aims at the development of resource-saving technology of dehydration of fruit and vegetable raw materials and economically expedient design solutions of processing of sub-standard raw materials in field conditions focused on the reduction of food losses during harvesting and storage.

BACKGROUND

In large urban zones, the issue of stable food supply can be solved by means of the development of infrastructure of agricultural production. In developing countries, such modern technologies as vertical farms and robotic greenhouse complexes are not widespread due to their high cost in the conditions of extensive development of agricultural sector and food processing industry.

Dynamic character of business models and technologies implemented in agricultural production and processing is one of the reasons of such social and economic problems as bankruptcy of agricultural enterprises, unemployment in rural areas, reduction of cropland, and degradation of rural infrastructure. Development strategies of large agricultural corporations often create conditions unfavorable for small farmers. Due to higher flexibility at the expense of application of advanced technologies (agrochemicals of new generation, genetically engineered and modified organisms, robots, among others), faster attraction, and geographical redistribution of capital, large multinational corporations are able to solve environmental, social, regulatory, and other problems in more effective manner. Therefore, in the aspiration to gain new market niches and reduce competitive pressure, they are able to operate without profit in the form of hidden dumping, carrying costs of the large-scale modernization programs for later periods, using low-interest rates, and state support whereas small and medium producers, particularly, individual farms, are forced to curtail activity without maintaining competitive pressure.

Technological gap between large agro holdings and small farms is particularly sharp because of low availability of credits to small agribusiness and high risks of investment. Other reason why smaller farms lose to holdings is a lack of advanced processing technologies. Operation of large agro holdings allow solving the problem of hunger, but not that of hidden hunger. The priority direction of development in processing of food raw materials allowing to solve hidden hunger problem is the development of new types of products. Due to their physical and chemical structure, such products are capable to fill the gap of the substances required for the maintenance of human health.

Bioflavonoids and other minor components of natural food are necessary for the increase in the efficiency of immune system of human body, decrease the impact of harmful effects of toxic components in a daily food allowance. Fruit, vegetables, and berries contain a complex of various biologically active agents, sources of vitamins C, P, and E, some vitamins of group B, V-carotene, a number of minerals, carbohydrates and phytoncides available in fresh only (Bessonov, Knyaginin, & Lipetskaya, 2017). Until recently, it has been believed that processing, including canning, allows preserving food substances. It is known that different ways of influencing a product do not allow achieving equal preservation of biologically valuable substances. For example, conservation of vegetables, fruit, and berries promotes only elimination of seasonality in their consumption and also allows supplying industrial centers and remote areas of the planet, for example, the Arctic.

The search for technological solutions of processing of fruit and vegetables without losing their nutritional value continues. There have been explored various ways of processing, including those by ionizing beams, radiation in inert gases, vacuum, low temperatures, antioxidants, conservation by currents of ultrahigh and microwave oven frequency, radiation by ultraviolet rays, and aseptic conservation. In Russia, the Ministry of Health approves various products processed by ionizing radiation. It is possible to apply ionizing radiation, short period of storage of fruit and vegetables which considerably depend on microorganisms. The extension of storage periods even for several days is important. For example, wild strawberry can be kept during 4-5 days in refrigerator and 10-12 days with the use of additional radiation. It is possible to extend storage period of irradiated sweet cherry and red tomatoes twofold. Essential lack of conservation by ionizing radiation is that during processing a product changes its chemical composition and hydrolysis processes. Enzymes are not inactivated which leads to the deterioration in taste, smell, and consistency. The amount of vitamins in comparison with initial phase decreased.

In recent years, much attention has been paid to the selection of the modes of radiation of foodstuff, not defiant changes of organoleptic properties. The most perspective way is radiation in inert gases, vacuum, at low temperatures, and with use of antioxidants. For the extension of storage period of potatoes and some of the vegetables, the allowed norms of ionizing radiation should not exceed 0.10-0.12, which allows complete suppression of germination in onions, garlic, and potatoes during storage. Such way of conservation, however, still has not been applied widely. Its impact on human health and degree of resistance of microorganisms to ionizing radiation has been studied comprehensively, the changes occurring in irradiated foodstuff has been investigated. In some countries, such processing is recognized as unsafe and its application is forbidden.

Conservation by currents of ultrahigh and ultrahigh (microwave oven) frequency is based on the creation of the movement of charged particles in a product. The temperature increases above 100°C. The product is corked in a tight container, placed in ultrahigh-frequency waves, and heated up to boiling during 30-50 seconds. Unlike thermal sterilization, microwave heating happens at the same time in all points, at one speed, warming up heat conductivity of a product does not influence. Microorganisms disappear much quicker than at thermal sterilization due to the oscillating motions of particles in cells. There happens not only allocation of heat but also polarization which influences vital signs of microorganisms. This method is widely used in fruit and vegetable processing for the sterilization of fruit, berries, and vegetable juices.

Radiation by ultraviolet rays (UVR) is a radiation by invisible part of light beams with the length of the waves of 60-400 nanometers. It affects microflora of food. The most effective action is posed by the beams with the length of the waves of 255-280 nanometers. Nucleonic acids and nucleoproteins in microbial cells adsorb UVR that leads to denaturation changes in these substances. Resistance of microorganisms to UVR varies, specifically, bacteria are more sensitive than mold. UVR is used for sterilization of a surface of meat hulks and sausages as their penetration does not exceed 0.1 mm. UVR can be used for sterilization of refrigerators and warehouses. However, this way of conservation requires implementation of tight security measures as UVR are dangerous to people, they affect eyes and skin.

The above-described ways of processing have not been widely used, therefore, the bulk of vegetables used for the production of tinned products and for the extension of seasonality of their processing are processed during summer and autumn in the form of fresh, dried, frozen, semi-finished products, natural purees and juices based on direct extraction, preserved in aseptic way, and concentrated juice and puree.

In aseptic conservation, short-term (dozens of seconds) sterilization of a product in a thin stream layer at high temperature is carried out in combination with rapid cooling, bottling in sterile conditions into a pre-sterilized container with a hermetic seal in aseptic conditions. It allows obtaining high-quality semi-finished products that practically do not differ in its consumer properties (color, taste, smell, vitamin composition, etc.) from non-sterilized one (Barkhatov, Lisitsky, & Kozachenko, 1993). The main advantage of aseptic conservation is the possibility of packaging in sterile conditions into sterile containers of any capacity and its hermetic sealing in aseptic conditions. It allows storing semi-finished product up to a year at a temperature between 0°C and 25°C without sudden fluctuations in temperature and relative humidity of 75% without loss and continue to use it for various types of canned products until new season (Barkhatov et al., 1993).

The most popular way to preserve fruits, vegetables, and berries is freezing. Today, the market of frozen vegetables and berries is one of the largest and fastest-growing segments of food market. In Russia, the share of this segment in food market is 16-17%, which is rather low compared to many developed countries. For example, in the USA, the share of frozen food market is 71%. In Russia, annual average per capita consumption of frozen vegetables is only one kg, while in the developed countries, this parameter reaches 4-6 kg. Russian market of frozen vegetables and berries has almost tripled during previous four years. In the 2000s, the growth rate of the market was about 15%, while in the past few years it has been ranging from 20-25% to 30-40% (Boltavin, 2006). The forecasts expect the continuation of dynamic growth of this market in the future (Vlahovich, 2008).

Freezing, however, is not the best way to preserve natural structure of food product. It partially breaks the intracellular structure of a product which negatively affects its nutritional value. Since there is a re-distribution of moisture, tissues are injured by ice crystals. When freezing fruit, berries, and vegetables, it is almost impossible to achieve maximum reversibility of the phenomena. As water turns into ice, it leads to the compression of fibers and cells which causes additional water outflow and damages outer layers. Increased volume of central freezing layers leads to increased internal pressure in a product. Dense and inelastic outer ice layer is not able to withstand internal pressure and frozen product breaks. In addition to the loss of nutrients, freezing is an energy-intensive process, as it requires maintenance of low temperature during the entire storage cycle.

One of the most promising ways of preserving food products is dehydration which can dramatically reduce the cost of storage, transport, and losses and ensure long-term preservation of organoleptic characteristics of a product. Mass exchange and thermal processes are often accompanied by oxidation reactions, changes in structural and physical properties, formation of polymorphic forms and crystalline hydrates which leads to a partial or complete loss of nutritional value. One of the reasons is the omission of manufacturers and technologists of one of the most important properties of raw materials – thermolability, that is, the instability of essential substances under temperature changes. This leads to intracellular interactions during dehydration and loss of vitamin C, bioflavonoids, and aromatic substances. Loss of nutritional biological value may continue during storage of dehydrated product.

The study of dehydration process of freshly harvested crops should be based on the development of new ways to improve the efficiency of dehydration process using non-traditional energy sources and new types of heat generators. At any scale of drying technologies development, the implementation of a number of technical and economic parameters, such as minimum possible energy consumption, maximum homogeneity of dehydration, minimum time to reach a given humidity, and some other characteristics of dehydration, is considered fundamental (Table 1, Table 2).

Table 1. Comparative characteristics of various methods of dehydration

Type of dehydration	Principle of heat convection	Parameters of final product	Energy consumption, kW•h/kg
Infrared	Heat convection by IR rays	The product quality is as close as possible to the quality of freeze-drying. Up to 90% of the initial product properties are preserved and microbial contamination is reduced.	0.9 – 1.0
Sublimation	Removal of moisture in two stages: sublimation of ice from frozen product and heat finish drying in vacuum	The shape, color, and organoleptic properties are preserved with minimal losses of bioactive substances, the recoverability is 85-95%.	2.7 – 3.0
SHF	Heat generators are water dipoles contained in raw materials that are placed in a microwave electromagnetic field	Uniform heating, almost independent of thermal conductivity of drying material. The most promising combined drying: convection pre-drying and microwave finish drying. No specific effect of the microwave field on the product was found.	1.6 – 1.8
Convective	Heat transfer to raw material with drying agent (heated air or steam-gas mixture)	Reduced product thermal conductivity at the end of drying significantly lengthens the process, degrading the quality of the finished product. Achievement of stable quality is possible by correct cutting and blanching. Convective method produces 90% of dried products.	1.8 – 3.0

Source: Authors' development

Table 2. Parameters of various methods of dehydration

Parameter	Methods			
	Infrared rays	Convective	Sublimation	Microwave heating
Time of dehydration, hours	4-6	8-10	10-20	up to 4
Specific area occupied by evaporated moisture m²/kg	0.04	0.07	0.26	0.18
Recoverability	85-95%	60-70%	85-95%	85-95%
Residual achieved humidity, %	3-4	8.0	3.5	2.5-4.0
Environmental safety of production	safe	safe	unsafe (freon)	unsafe (SHF)
Ability to store	more than 1 year	0.3 – 0.5 years	more than 1 year	more than 1 year

Source: Authors' development

The most effective and safest method of dehydration is IR exposure since it has an optimal dehydration time, minimum specific area of evaporating moisture, and product recoverability at the level of freeze-drying. In addition, this method is environmentally safe and allows obtaining products with a prolonged shelf life.

Chekrygina, Bukreev, and Eremin (2002) proposed a method for drying and disinfection of fruit and berries. It includes four stages: heating by low-frequency currents up to a temperature of 55-65°C until electrolytic disinfection and further drying with IR and microwave energy with a power flow density of not more than 0.2 W/cm² (stage 2), 0.3 W/cm² (stage 3), and 0.4 W/cm² (stage 4). The disadvantages of this method are long period of drying and multi-stage process.

Ivanov and Sapunov (2003) developed alternative method of drying of fruit and vegetables based on blanching of raw materials produced by microwave radiation with a capacity of 0.5-3.0 W/g and a pressure of 200-400 mm Hg at simultaneous centrifugation at a speed of 250-500 rpm. Drying is carried out by supplying microwave energy with a specific radiation power of 1.0-0.25 W/g at a pressure of 30-100 mm Hg. The disadvantages of this method are the inability to obtain dried berries of a certain shape due to significant compression of raw material during centrifugation. The essence of the method is that raw materials are sorted, washed, cut into pieces, blanched, placed on pallets, and placed in a chamber in which raw materials are heated up to 70°C in vacuum, the value of which is cyclically changed in the range of 0.00-0.04 MPa. The moisture obtained during drying is collected for its subsequent processing. The disadvantages of this method are long drying time and low-quality indicators of the final product.

Ermolaev, Fedorov, Sosnina, and Lifentseva (2015) proposed a method of vacuum drying of fruit and berries on the basis of pressure reduction in the chamber to 10-30 kPa during the first stage of dehydration. This leads to self-freezing of a product and sublimation of the resulting ice. After two hours, the chamber pressure is increased up to 3-5 kPa and infrared heating lamps are turned on maintaining a drying temperature of 70-80°C. This invention shortens vacuum drying process while maintaining high quality of dried product.

Antipov, Zhuravlev, Vinichenko, and Kazartsev (2015) offered a technological line for the production of dried berries and powder from them. Production line contains a consistently arranged truck, dump, scraper conveyor, washing machine, inspection conveyor, dryer, cooling chamber, pneumatic conveyor, cooling bin, sifter, screw conveyor, and filling machine. The line has additional installation: calibration vibrating table after dump, fumigation chamber after washing machine; shredder after dryer which is used as vacuum drying chamber. The authors argue that this invention will improve the quality of dried products, increase the shelf life of the finished product, and reduce their cost.

Analyzing the above methods, it should be noted that:

- Energy consumption of the above methods is quite high, especially when vacuum is used;
- None of the given methods can be offered for small businesses;
- The methods do not allow processing of substandard raw materials which are unstable in transportation.

Despite the variety of patents for dehydration of vegetables, fruit, and berries, most manufacturers use convective or combined heating of the working environment for dehydration. For example, ZHAR-KO SPb company produces drying chambers with convective and infrared heating and blowing. Among the advantages is rapid dehydration process, but it is likely to overheat a product in different layers and other defects.

One of the priorities is establishment and development of small and medium enterprises for production of dried fruit and vegetables. For low-power enterprises, the most promising method is IR dehydrogenation in modes that preserve native component by 80-90%. It allows solving food problems: concentration of minor components per kg of food substance increases, while cellulose, hemicellulose, and protopectin remain in native state thus providing a substrate for microorganisms. From a technical point of view, IR dehydrogenation allow solving the problem of high energy consumption inherent in other dehydration methods. The advantages include a small area occupied by the equipment as the heating elements are located parallel to the product under process.

MAIN FOCUS OF THE CHAPTER

In this study, the analysis of the assortment, functional ingredients, main processing methods, and ways of snacks processing recommended as healthy nutrition, different producers, and using mainly regional raw materials has been carried out (Table 3).

Table 3. Comparison of the assortment, functional ingredients, and major processing methods

Product / group of products	Producer	Functional ingredients	Main processing methods	Processing regime
Oranges	Fruits, Saint Petersburg	Circle-shaped oranges	Traditional hydro mechanized processing (washing, cleaning, cutting), drying	Kind and parameters of drying are not stated
Apples		Circle-shaped apples		
Peas		Pea pieces		
Bananas		Banana in the form of oblong slices		
Chestnut –Cranberry – Pea snack	Brainfood, Moscow	Chestnut in the form of halves, pea in the form of segments, cranberry	Nuts' mechanized processing (cleaning from the nutshell) hydro mechanized processing (washing, cleaning, pea cutting), drying	Sublimation drying / Parameters of drying are not stated
Apple – Banana – Spinach snack		All components (apple – banana – spinach) in the form of homogenized mix / solid foam	Traditional hydro mechanized processing (washing, cleaning, apple cutting, crushing in the mashed mass, formation), drying	
Apple – Strawberry snack		Mix: apple in the form of oblong slices, strawberry	Traditional hydro mechanized processing (washing, cleaning, cutting for apple), drying	
Cherry snack		Cherry cut into circles	Traditional hydro mechanized processing (washing, cleaning, cutting), drying	
Apple chips	Yablokoff, Moscow	Circle-shaped apples and peas	Hydro mechanized processing (removal of a core, cutting into circles), drying	Kind of drying is not known / Drying parameters: temperature (60-80°C), drying time – 2.5-3.5 hours
Pea chips				
Carrot snack	C-Fruit Siberia, Omsk	Carrots in the form of straws	Hydro mechanized processing (washing, cleaning, cutting in the form of straw), drying	Drying under moderate temperature regime (according to producer's data), parameters are not stated
Horseradish snack		Horseradish in the form of straws		
Sugar beet snack		Beet in the form of straws		
Candied fruit "Cherry-taste beet"		Beet in the form of a cube and cherry (small cube)		
Candied cherry		Whole cherry		
Pumpkin snack	Ecofarmer, Krasnodar	Pumpkin in the form of slices	Hydro mechanized processing (washing, cleaning, trimming, extracting seeds out of pumpkin, cutting in slices), drying	Drying at low temperature, parameters are not stated
Tomato snack		Tomato in the form of segments	Hydro mechanized processing (washing, trimming, cutting in the form of segments), drying	

Source: Authors' development

Natural sources of ingredients of monocomponent and multicomponent snacks demonstrating functional properties are vegetable raw materials (fruit, berries, nuts, and vegetables) which have food fibers, oligosaccharides, antioxidants, vitamins, and mineral substances. Vegetable raw materials include spinach, carrots, radish, beet, tomato, and pumpkin. Fruit snacks (chips) include oranges, apples, pears, and bananas. They are ranked as high-quality food products with high dietary and flavor properties and useful components (fructose, glucose, apple acid, cellulose, pectin, and iron). Among monocomponent and multicomponent snacks, it is necessary to mention Brainfood snacks which ingredients are different and made in the form of a mixture. Apple-banana-spinach snack is in the form of solid foam.

Fruit raw materials, vegetables, and berries come fresh and undergo traditional hydro-mechanical processing. Cutting is made in various ways, generally in the form of circles for fruit snacks and medium-size cubes for candied fruits. Berries are mainly dried. Sibirskiye Prostory company produces vegetable snacks in the form of straws. In other cases, vegetable chips are produced in the form of segments or slices. It means that such snacks find their application when cooking the first and second courses, namely, being specialized for junk foods. During mechanical action on raw materials, there is a loss of vitamin value. Therefore, it is necessary to consider that when cutting straws loss of nutrients is much higher. The loss is lower when cutting circles, segments, and drying. Therefore, snack mixture by Brainfood has positive sides as the nutritious quality of such snacks is higher compared to monocomponent snacks. It is up-to-date to produce snacks in the form of a mix as they are less commonly presented in the market.

Generally, various ways of drying, such as sublimation by Brainfoods, are applied to produce snacks. At the same time, drying is followed by the processes of warm transfer and mass transfer. Their intensity and depth have significant effect on chemical composition, structure, and physical and organoleptic properties of a product. Only Yablokoff disclosure all of its data, while other producers do not specify time and temperature of drying. The only information provided is that drying takes place at low temperature, presumably, 49°C. The type of sublimation drying of snack products has been specified by Brainfood. It means that data on production of snacks are not authentic. The existing mode of drying by Yablokoff makes it possible stating that at drying temperature above 77°C, duration of processing is reduced minimum to three hours. Other firms presumably use low temperature (minimum value of temperature of process equal to 49°C). At such temperature, standard value of mass fraction of moisture is reached in 20 hours of processing (Demidov, Voronenko, & Bazhanova, 2015; Doymaz, 2007).

Sublimation drying is a hi-tech process which allows keeping up to 95% of nutrients, vitamins, and microelements in their initial form, as well as preserving natural smell, taste, and color of a product. It is one of the most important advantages of sublimation. The way allows avoiding destruction of the structure of a product and restoring sublimated products as they have porous structure. This fact is remarkable because sublimated products are fully suitable for baby and dietary nutrition. However, energy consumption on the organization of sublimation process in vacuum exceeds the cost of thermal drying by 15-20 times. Besides, vacuum sublimation dryers are characterized by high cost, heavy operating costs, and complexity of service (Heredia, Barrera, & Andrés, 2007; Atanazevich, 2000).

In this study, the authors also conducted the analysis of nutrition value declared by producers. The analysis of data on protein content in snack products of different producers demonstrated that among vegetable snacks, more proteins are contained in tomato chips and horseradish and beet snacks. Among monocomponent, it is necessary to distinguish banana fruits from fruit snacks. Among multicomponent snacks, more proteins are contained in walnut snacks consisting cranberry and pear mixture. At the same time, it is necessary to understand that protein content is insignificant and fluctuates in the range from 1% to 9%. Content of fats in various snacks is unequal. Higher content of fats is registered in Brainfood multicomponent snack because walnut contains saturated and nonsaturated fatty acids – palmitic, linoleic, olein, linolenic (according to the producer) are contained in the mixture in the amount of 17.4%. In multicomponent snack (apple, banana, spinach) and tomato chips, fat content is below 2.4%. Other snacks except banana fruit contain minimum quantity of fat.

Most of the carbohydrates are found in banana fruits, candied beetroot with cherry flavor, and candied cherry. Comparing vegetable and fruit snacks, carbohydrates prevail in fruit snack foods due to the fact that fruit snacks contain predominantly glucose and fructose in contrast to vegetable snacks. Regarding multicomponent snacks, they are inferior to fruity in carbohydrate content since it depends on the characteristics of drying and the content of the component. Candied snacks predominate in carbohydrates due to sugars introduced into technological process during processing (Figure 1).

Figure 1. Carbohydrate content in snacks
Source: Authors' development

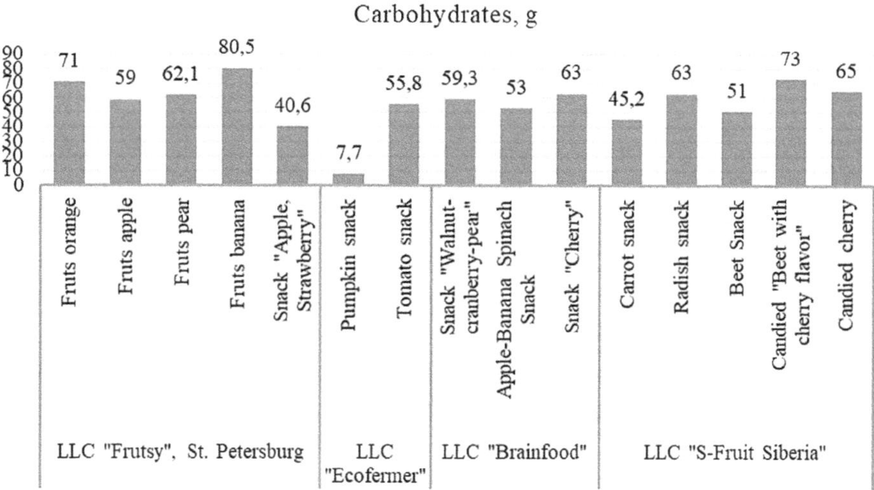

Brainfood multicomponent snacks are those with the highest calorie value as they contain walnuts, cranberries, pears, and bananas. Comparing the calorie value of vegetable snacks, it should be emphasized that candied beet with cherry flavor is higher-calorie product compared to Beet snack. Radish snack is one of the highest in calorie value while pumpkin snack is one of the lowest (Figure 2).

Yablokoff did not provide nutritional value of its snacks, only calorie content, but indicated that the products are obtained by infrared drying at a temperature of 60-80°C during 2.5-3.5 hours.

Protein content in snacks from vegetables and multicomponent snack foods is higher than that in fruit snacks. Multicomponent snacks and tomato chips have high content of fat. Fruit and vegetable snacks have high content of carbohydrates. Analysis of the calorie content demonstrated that multi-component and banana snacks are those with the highest caloric content. Other fruit snacks are low-calorie. At the same time, manufacturers probably do not take into account the digestibility of various carbohydrates. Simple sugars (glucose, fructose, and sucrose) are absorbed in the body, while complex sugars (cellulose and protopectin) are not. Therefore, there is a question if calorie calculation is correct. Some producers indicate the nutrient content values according to which moisture content in a product is 45%. It contradicts the data on dry vegetables and that is why producers misinform consumers about the true nutrient content.

Figure 2. Caloric value of snack foods
Source: Authors' development

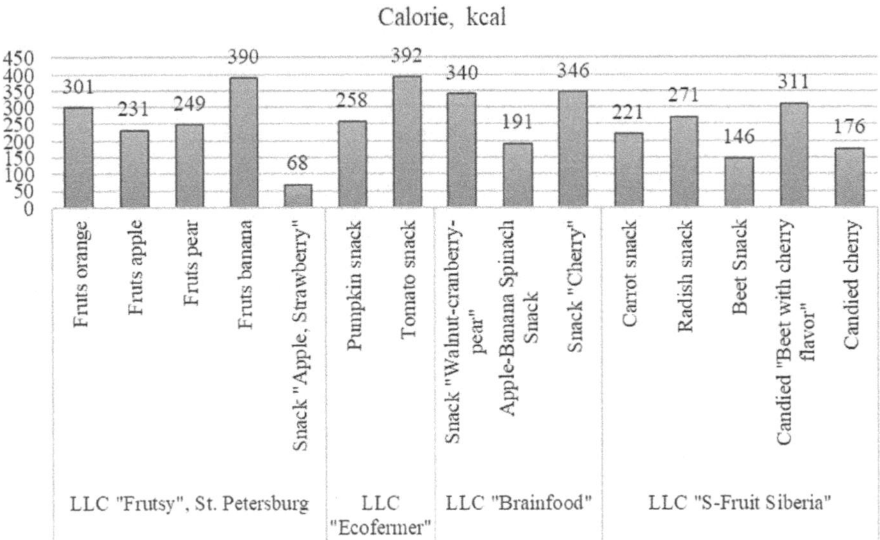

Analysis of labeling data for snack products showed that product information meets the requirements for products intended for the mass segment, but not a functional product and/or a product for a healthy diet. Nutriciological analysis of the preservation of essential and minor components in industrial products offered for a healthy diet is not specified. It is not possible to draw conclusions about the replenishment of the need for necessary substances.

Such conclusions can be made on the basis of the processing modes used. However, the modes of the main process are not fully spelled out, for example, Fruits company has not provided information about drying. Sibirskiye Prostory and Ecofarmer companies also provide incomplete information indicating only that drying is conducted at low temperature. According to this information, it is impossible to understand whether all essential components are really preserved in a product.

Therefore, effective technologies are needed to ensure the safety of minor components in food products (flavonoids and their glycosides, indoles, exogenous peptides, organic acids, and phenolic compounds) with specific biological effects on various functions of individual metabolic systems and the body. One of the potential solutions to this problem is the creation of technologies to preserve natural properties of a product. Focusing on the FAO appeal and the global challenges to food security to reduce food loss and damage, the authors proposed a technological solution that allows processing fruit and vegetable raw materials at harvesting site, including substandard. The focus of the study is increase of the bioavailability of minor components in food by means of gentle processing methods, one of which is IR treatment (dehydrogenation). Not only the preservation of sensory, physical, and chemical properties is achieved but also the ability to increase the availability of substrate for intestinal microorganisms. The work was carried out at Saratov State Agrarian University and the Center for Collective Use (CCU) by scientific equipment in the field of physicochemical biology and nanobiotechnology "Symbiosis" of the Research Institute of Biochemistry and Physiology of Plants and Microorganisms of the Russian Academy of Sciences (IBFRM RAS). Fresh and dehydrated oranges were selected as the objects of the study. Dehydration was carried out by the method of resonant IR-drying at a wavelength of near and middle infrared range of 1.8-3.0 microns. The temperature was lowered from intense (67-75°C) to moderate (32-35°C). In resonant infrared drying, there was used Sator installment equipped with ceramic shell emitters. The study was conducted by comparing the data of the content of bioflavonoids and vitamin C in fresh oranges and dehydrated (immediately after dehydration and during storage for 12 months). The authors also studied a combined snack consisting of chopped tomato, onion, parsley, basil, and coriander, pressed and hydrated.

The analysis was performed by the method of reversed-phase HPLC on a DionexUltimate 3000 chromatograph (ThermoScientific, USA) using a Luna 5u C18 (2) 100A column, 5 μm 4.6 mm × 150 mm (Phenomenex, USA), serial number 125617-12. Components were identified by comparing the retention times of standard flavonoid samples (rutin as a hydrate (≥94%, Sigma-Aldrich, USA), quercetin as a dihydrate (97%, Alfa Aesar, UK), naringin (≥95%, Sigma-Aldrich, USA), apigenin (≥97%, Sigma-Aldrich, USA), and naringenin (≥95%, Sigma-Aldrich, USA).

Analysis of the composition of vitamins was performed by the method of reversed-phase HPLC on a DionexUltimate 3000 chromatograph (ThermoScientific, USA) using a Luna 5u C18 (2) 100A column, 5 μm 4.6 mm × 150 mm (Phenomenex, USA), serial number 125617-12. Analysis time – 15 minutes. The extracts were chromatographed under isocratic elution (Solvent A – methanol, qualification (Ultra) gradient HPLC grade (JTBaker, the Netherlands), solvent B – acetone nitrile qualification HPLC grade (Panreac, Spain), in the ratio 80:20. Speed 1 ml/min flow volume, sample volume 20 μl. Chromatograph control and data analysis was performed by Chromeleon version 7.1.2.1478 (ThermoScientific, Dionex, USA). The detection was performed at the following wavelengths: A, E – 265 nm.

Quantitative calculation of the content of vitamins was performed according to the ratio of the peak areas of the standard and sample.

Analysis of the composition of vitamins was performed by the method of reversed-phase HPLC on a DionexUltimate 3000 chromatograph (ThermoScientific, USA) using a Luna 5u C18 (2) 100A column, 5 μm 4.6 mm × 150 mm (Phenomenex, USA), serial number 125617-12. Analysis time – 25 minutes in a water-acetonitrile gradient.

SOLUTIONS AND RECOMMENDATIONS

A comparative analysis of the content of ascorbic acid (vitamin C) in freshly squeezed orange juice, the residue after extraction and dehydrated orange shows that this method of dehydration allows preserving vitamins (Figure 3). The presence of vitamin C 1.9269 mg per 1 g of dehydrated oranges was registered, which is identical to the content of 10 g of fresh orange. The loss of vitamin C during storage of dehydrated orange for 12 months is 8%.

Analysis of chromatograms of orange juice, chips, and fresh orange residue after separation of juice shows that they all have a similar profile, but differ significantly in the content of certain components. A group of peaks corresponding to polyphenolic compounds, in particular, flavonoids, is observed in the chromatograms of all studied samples. Thus, the most representative flavonoid found in the extracts is pruning which is monoglycoside-naringenin-7-O-glucoside (Figure 4). Retention time (15.00 minutes) and UV-visible spectrum coincide with those of the component obtained as a result of partial acid hydrolysis of naringin sample. The component has an almost identical absorption spectrum with prunin, however, it is characterized by a slightly shorter retention time (14.60 minutes) than the standard naringin sample (14.80 minutes). It suggests that this component is a polymer form of naringin with a low degree of polymerization (dimer, trimer, etc.).

Figure 3. Vitamin C content, mg per g (for juice and residue after pressing mg per 10 g)
Source: Authors' development

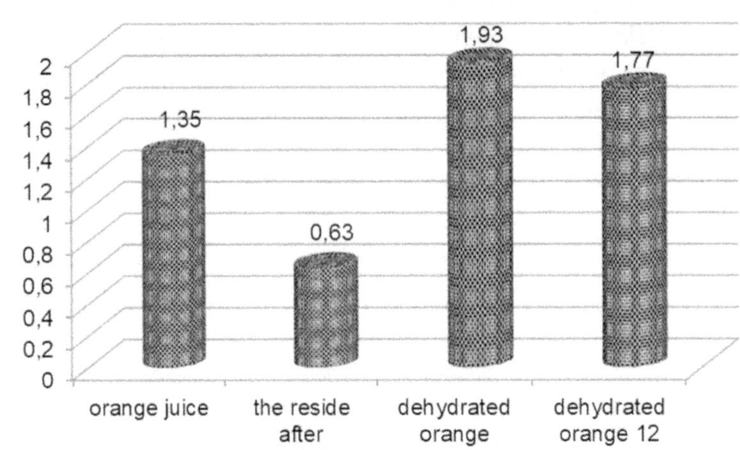

Figure 4. Chromatogram of orange chips extract, integrating at a wavelength of 342 nm
Source: Authors' development

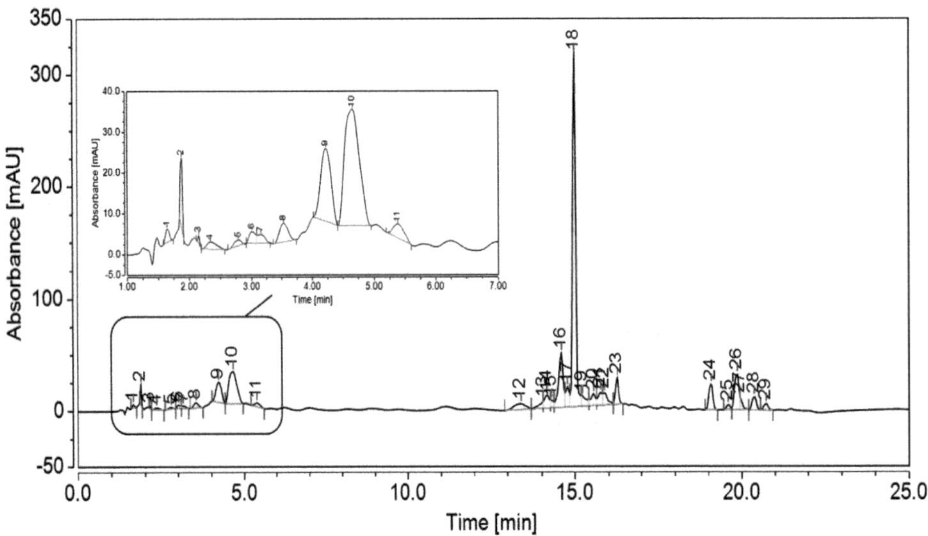

In combined senecah confirmed the safety of chlorophyll (Figure 5). This minor component improves detoxification of the body by quickly removing waste and regulating the level of fluid. In addition, preliminary studies have shown the advantage of chlorophyll in accelerating metabolism which leads to weight loss.

In presented dry and raw (damp) samples, there is found a wide range of phenolic compounds, including flavonol quercetin. However, its content is low compared to other components. The chlorophyll peak is presumably most expressed. In the damp (raw) raw materials, extract concentration of compounds is lower (Table 4).

Figure 5. Chromatogram of chlorophyll peak
Source: Authors' development

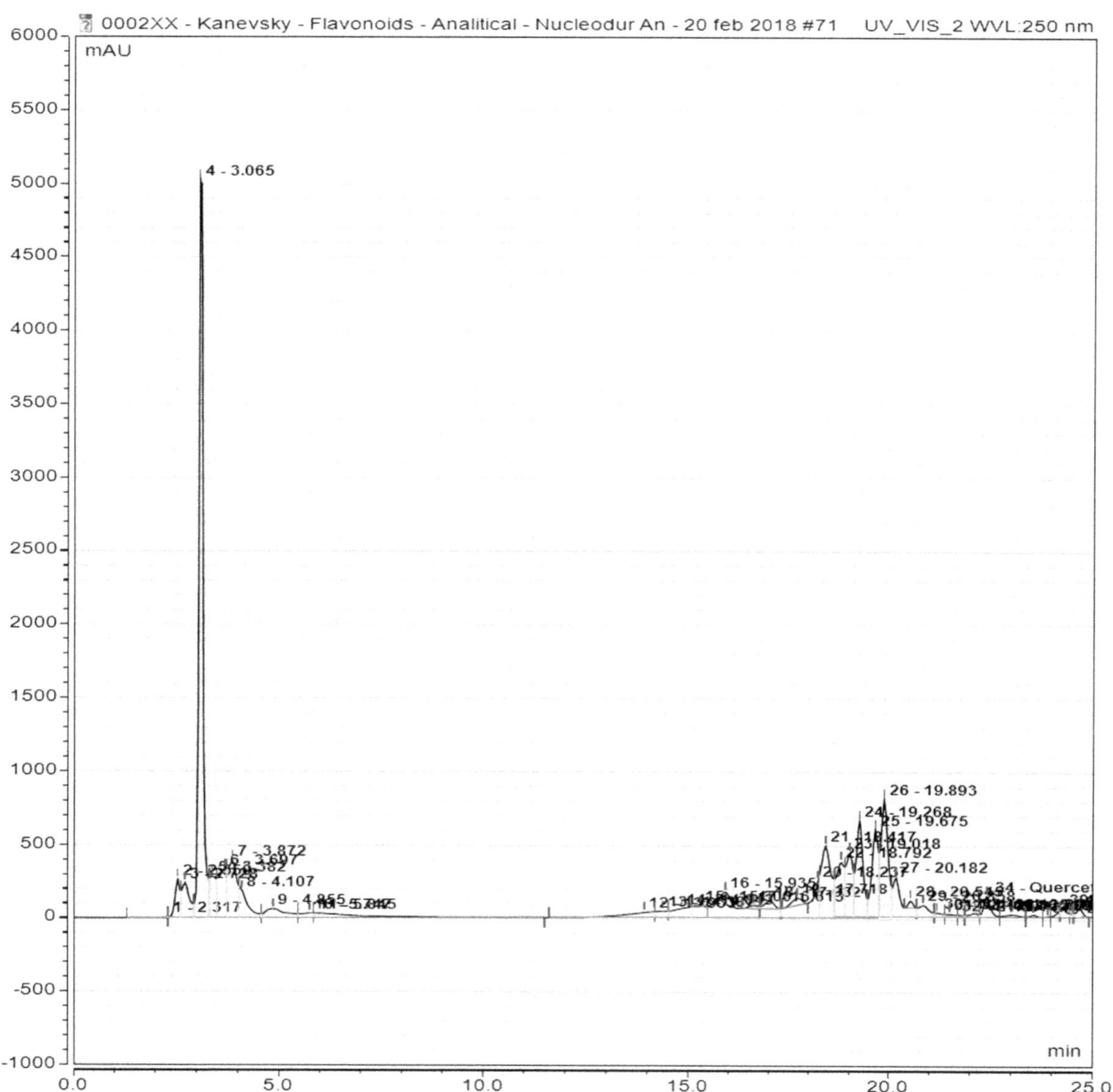

Table 4. Quercetin content in samples

Sample	Peak area, m unit*min	Quercetin content, mkg/g
Damp sample	3.132	6.10
Dry sample	27.619	44.86

Source: Authors' development

Most part of the extract is made by hydrophobic compounds. However, there is a hydrophilic fraction which can be represented by glycosides of flavonoids and free phenolic acids.

The quantitative analysis of content phenolic compounds in a sample (in terms of quercetin) showed the following results (Table 5).

Table 5. Phenolic compounds content in samples

Sample	Total area peaks, m unit. * min	Phenolic connections content, mg/g (in terms of quercetin)
Damp sample	188.10	2.97
Dry sample	1,657.21	26.24

Source: Authors' development

The data on the prescription mixture consisting of tomato, onion, dill, parsley green, basil, and coriander after drying show that vitamin K remains and its content in the dried-up mixture is higher than in damp mixture on 1 g of raw materials. It is proved that the used energy effective and delicate technology of dehydration with the use of long-wave resonant IK-radiation allows keeping the vitamins and other biologically active agents which are contained in a product.

Most small farms and individual farms are not able to organize their own processing facilities. In addition, on-site collection of raw materials is always non-conforming raw materials unsuitable for the long-term storage, losing the quality of fresh raw materials during transportation. It is expensive to keep vegetable and fruit storage facilities while it is convenient to store the packaged dry product in a sealed package and does not require specially prepared premises. The idea is to create a mobile workshop, equipped with resonant IR dryers, collecting evaporated moisture in tanks and used for further washing of raw materials, leaves for the time of collection, thereby minimizing the loss of material and technical resources. A user only needs connect 380 V, water after washing can be used for watering. At the following stage of work, the calculation of the economic efficiency of the mobile workshop for drying of fruits and vegetables was carried out.

The annual output is equal to the product of the designed variable capacity by the number of shifts of the enterprise's work per year.

$$B_{year} = M \cdot * Кст = 120 * 250 = 30,000 \text{ packs} \tag{1}$$

Annual production output will be 30 thousand packs. Annual commodity output is equal to the product of annual output at wholesale prices.

$$TP_{year} = B_{year} \cdot * Ц_{опт} \tag{2}$$

Annual commodity products when connected to a substation:
$$TP_{year} = 30 \cdot * 46.87 = RUB \ 1,406.1 \text{ thousand.}$$
Annual commodity products during the operation of the generator of current on solar oil:
$$TP_{year} = 30 \cdot * 56.78 = RUB \ 1,703.4 \text{ thousand.}$$

Cost of Establishing a Mobile Shop

Capital investments in the creation of production facilities consist of the cost of buildings' construction and equipment cost. The cost of buildings' construction of the main production purpose is calculated by multiplying their areas by the cost of building 1 m^2 of buildings.

Construction $= 18$ m^2 * RUB 25 thousand $=$ RUB 450 thousand.

The cost of equipment specified in the specification is calculated at current wholesale prices for equipment.

Cost of equipment:
Drying chambers – RUB 3-900 thousand.
Vegetable cutting machine – RUB 1-100 thousand.
Other equipment (production table, table with washing tub, sealing machine, rack) – RUB 27 thousand.
Total: RUB 1,027 thousand.
K invest $= 450 + 1,027 =$ RUB 1,477 thousand.

Depreciation (A)

Depreciation rates for equipment – 15%. Depreciation is calculated by producing the cost of equipment by the depreciation rate: $1,027.0 * 0.15 =$ RUB 154.05 thousand. Accrual of depreciation for the annual output: equipment depreciation (dehydrated product) – RUB 154.05 thousand.

Maintenance and Routine Repairs of Equipment (Po)

Deductions for equipment repair accept 20% of its value. The calculation is carried out similarly to the previous section. Deductions for equipment repair: equipment repair (dehydrated product) – RUB 205.4 thousand. The cost prices are calculated in accordance with costing items for the annual production volume.

Raw and Packaging Materials

Since the production of products is carried out from substandard horticultural raw materials, costs are not provided (Table 6).

Table 6. Calculation of the cost of packaging materials

Name	Quantity per shift	Price per unit, RUB	Amount, RUB	Amount per year, RUB thousand
Packaging	120	3	360	90.0

Source: Authors' development

Energy Resource (Ce)

The cost of 1 kW/h of electricity is taken as RUB 9.0 (Table 7, Table 8).

Table 7. Electricity cost for the annual output when connected to the substation

Energy resource	Dehydrated product
Power consumption per shift, kW/h	60.0
Electricity consumption per year, thousand kW/h	15.0
Price 1 kW/h of electricity, RUB	9.0
Electricity cost, RUB thousand	135.0

Source: Authors' development

Table 8. Cost of energy for the annual production with the use of diesel fuel generator

Energy resource	Dehydrated product
Cost of diesel fuel in the shift, RUB	1,171.80
Cost of diesel fuel per year, RUB thousand	292.95

Source: Authors' development

Wage

For the production, one worker per shift is required. Operation mode is single 8-hour shift, 250 shifts are assumed annually. Monthly salary of one employee is RUB 11,280. Annual salary: wages (dehydrated product) – RUB 135.36 thousand. Salary accruals (LF) (30% of salary): dehydrated product – 40.61.

Production Cost

Production cost (SPr) defined as the sum of all previous cost items. Other expenses take 5% of the amount of the previous cost items (Table 9).

Commercial expenses (Ce) take 5% of the product cost. Total cost (Tc) is defined as the sum of production costs and selling expenses.

Product Pricing

The price is determined taking into account the normative profitability of products (40%) and VAT (20%). Dehydrated product when connected to the substation = 27.9 *·1.4 * 1.2 = RUB 46.87. Dehydrated product when operating on the diesel current generator = 33.8 *·1.4 * 1.2 = RUB 56.78.

Table 9. Total annual cost of production

Product	Operation of a substation, RUB thousand	Operation of diesel fuel generator, RUB thousand
Depreciation	154.05	154.05
Deductions for equipment repair	205.40	205.40
Cost of packaging materials	90.00	90.00
The cost of energy	135.00	292.95
Wages	135.36	135.36
Salary accruals	40.61	40.61
Other expenses	38.00	45.90
Production cost	798.40	964.30
Selling expenses	39.90	48.20
Total cost	838.30	1,012.50

Source: Authors' development

Production Efficiency and Sales

The results of the calculations indicate that the effect of the production and sale of annual volume of dehydrated product when the current generator runs on diesel fuel is higher than when connected to the substation and amounted to RUB 690.9 thousand (profit from sales). The construction of a mobile plant for drying fruit and vegetables requires capital investments in the amount of RUB 1,477 thousand. The payback period of capital investments, respectively, with two options of work, is 3.3 years and 2.7 years. The profitability of capital investments is 30.8% and 37.4%, respectively. Efficiency of using fixed assets is higher at the second variant of the mobile production facility of RUB 1.15. This also applies to the indicator of efficiency of labor resources use (labor productivity) – RUB 1,703.4 thousand (Table 10).

At the same time, the parameters of economic efficiency (product profitability and sales profitability) are almost the same for both options of the mobile shop. These figures have a high enough value for the food industry, therefore, production and sales of products are effective from an economic point of view.

FUTURE RESEARCH DIRECTIONS

The proposed technology is simple and allows solving the following tasks on a global scale:

- Obtaining a universal sustainable model for processing of fruit and vegetable raw materials and large-scale reduction of losses at the stages of harvesting and storage.
- Solution to the problems of logistics in promoting the product from producer to consumer, including the storage of raw materials.
- Obtaining products that can be used as an independent product, or as an integral component of food systems.
- Ensuring the safety of the beneficial properties of vegetables and fruit, solving the problem of hidden hunger.

Table 10. Efficiency of production and sales of products at estimated selling prices

Parameters	Operation of a substation	Operation of diesel fuel generator
Selling price of 1 product packaging, RUB	46.87	56.78
Production and sales per year, thousand packs	30.00	30.00
Revenue from sales for the year, RUB thousand	1,406.10	1,703.40
Total cost of 1 product package, RUB	27.90	33.80
Total cost of annual production, RUB thousand	838.30	1,012.50
Profit from sales, RUB thousand	567.80	690.90
Net profit, RUB thousand	454.20	552.70
Product profitability, %	67.70	68.20
Return on sales, %	40.40	40.60
Capital productivity, RUB	0.95	1.15
Capital intensity, RUB	1.05	0.87
Labor productivity, RUB thousand	1,406.10	1,703.40
Return on capital investments, %	30.80	37.40
Payback period of capital investments, years	3.30	2.70

Source: Authors' development

Usage of IR-dehydrogenation allows keeping native components in vegetables and fruit at a level of 80-90% which, in turn, provides concentration of minor components per kg of food substance, allows cellulose, hemicellulose, and protopectin remaining in native state, and thus providing a substrate for microorganisms. Besides, it allows solving complex problems of insufficient consumption of fresh fruit and vegetables and preservation of nutrients during long storage period. Newly developed products are subjected to minimal temperature and time exposure, IR dehydrogenation does not cause a significant effect on the cellular wall of fruits, vegetables, and berries, and thus the technology allows obtaining products of a combined oncology protective and antioxidant action.

Although the production technology with preserved minor components is simple, it requires further studies. It consists of a standard hydro-mechanical treatment of washing, cleaning, and grinding of raw materials. Dehydration is conducted by means of IK resonant drying without compulsory convection. Resonance allows preventing the interaction of molecules of osmotically-bound and physic-mechanically bound moisture prevailing in fruit raw materials with substances in an intact cellular structure.

It is on the basis of these considerations that the most intensive influence of temperature 65-70°C happens in the first hour and allows removing the surface moisture by intensive evaporation. In this case, the main moisture remains in excess. Then the temperature decreases to 45-50°C and most of the moisture removal occurs in this range of 2-3 hours, the last stage of drying occurs at a temperature of 35-38°C, and the remainder of the osmotically retained water is removed. The final moisture of the product is 8-9%. The dehydrated product is cooled in air to 20°C and packed in a sealed package.

The given technologies are applied at different periods of harvesting and a farmer can hand over surplus and non-conforming raw materials for processing or use the opportunity to recycle self-contained for further realization.

CONCLUSION

The authors have proposed a universal technical and economic model of processing of fruit and vegetable raw materials in field conditions. It assumes creating a mobile workshop equipped with resonant IR dryers with devices for collecting evaporated moisture used for washing raw materials. This model is expected to reduce the loss of fruit and vegetables at the stages of harvesting and storage and provide the population with the products with prolonged shelf life and preserved profile of minor components to solve the problem of hidden hunger. The calculation of economic efficiency has shown that there is a potential associated with:

- the possibility of saving water resources, due to the collection of evaporated moisture 96%;
- saving energy consumption (for IR-drying is 3-4 times less energy than for other methods of drying);
- processing of fruit and vegetable raw materials on the spot before receiving the product allowing to get 30% of additional profit.

The production of food products with a prolonged implementation period from substandard and perishable raw materials allows solving the problem of logistics in promoting the product from producer to consumer, including storing raw materials, which also solves the problem of reducing losses and damage to food raw materials, and ensures sustainable development of agricultural production and improvement of food security.

REFERENCES

Antipov, S., Zhuravlev, A., Vinichenko, S., & Kazartsev, D. (2015). *Patent #2548209 "Vacuum Dryer of Continuous Operation with Ultra-High Frequency Power Supply."* Retrieved from https://findpatent. ru/patent/254/2548209.html

Atanazevich, V. (2000). *Drying Food. Reference Manual.* Moscow: DeLi.

Barkhatov, V., Lisitsky, V., & Kozachenko, Z. (1993). Aseptic Preservation of Fruit and Vegetable Puree of Semi-Finished Products from Low-Acid Raw Materials. *News of Institutes of Higher Education. Food Technology, 3-4,* 51–52.

Bessonov, V., Knyaginin, V., & Lipetskaya, M. (Eds.). (2017). *Nutritiology-2040. The Horizons of Science through the Eyes of Scientists.* Saint Petersburg: Center for Strategic Research.

Boltavin, A. (2006). Market for Frozen Convenience Foods from Vegetables. *Ice Cream and Frozen Products, 5,* 16–18.

Chekrygina, I., Bukreev, V., & Eremin, A. (2002). *Patent #2194228 "Method of Drying and Disinfection of Fruits and Berries."* Retrieved from http://www.freepatent.ru/patents/2194228

Demidov, S., Voronenko, B., & Bazhanova, I. (2015). Kinetics of Infrared Drying Shredded Carrots. *Scientific Journal NRU ITMO. Series. Processes and Food Production Equipment, 3,* 158–163.

Doymaz, I. (2007). Air-Drying Characteristics of Tomatoes. *Journal of Food Engineering*, 78(4), 1291–1297. doi:10.1016/j.jfoodeng.2005.12.047

Ermolaev, V., Fedorov, D., Sosnina, O., & Lifentseva, L. (2015). *Patent #2541395 "Method for Vacuum Drying of Fruit and Berries."* Retrieved from http://www.freepatent.ru/patents/2541395

Heredia, A., Barrera, C., & Andrés, A. (2007). Drying of Cherry Tomato by a Combination of Different Dehydration Techniques. Comparison of Kinetics and Other Related Properties. *Journal of Food Engineering*, 80(1), 111–118. doi:10.1016/j.jfoodeng.2006.04.056

Ivanov, V., & Sapunov, G. (2003). *Patent #2195824 "Method of Drying of Fruits and Vegetables."* Retrieved August 11, 2019, from http://allpatents.ru/patent/2195824.html

Vlahovich, S. (2008). Frozen Food Market Today and Forecasts of Its Development for the Future. *Ice-Cream and Frozen Products*, *12*, 28–31.

ADDITIONAL READING

Golovkin, N. (1984). *Refrigeration Food Technology*. Moscow: Consumer Goods and Food Industry.

Kutsakova, V., Rogov, I., Frolov, S., & Filippov, V. (2001). *Examples and Tasks of Food Technology Refrigeration. Part 1: Theoretical Basis of Canning*. Moscow: Kolos.

Makarova, N., & Zyuzina, A. (2011). Investigation of Antioxidant Activity of Juice Production Semis with DPPH Method. *Food Processing: Techniques and Technology*, 22(3), 1–5.

Nariniyants, G., Pacyuk, L., Kostromina, N., Lukashevich, O., & Medvedeva, E. (2005). Technology of Aseptic Canning of Fruit Convenience Foods for Baby Food. *Food Industries*, *3*, 20–21.

Roberfroid, M. B. (1999). Functional Foods and the Intestine: Concepts, Strategies and Examples. In L.A. Hanson & R.H. Yolken (Eds.), Probiotics, Other Nutritional Factors, and Intestinal Microflora (pp. 203-216). Lippincott-Raven, PA: Lippincott-Raven Publishers.

Sacilik, K., Keskin, R., & Elicin, A. K. (2006). Mathematical Modelling of Solar Tunnel Drying of Thin Layer Organic Tomato. *Journal of Food Engineering*, 73(3), 231–238. doi:10.1016/j.jfoodeng.2005.01.025

Zholik, G., & Kozlov, N. (2004). *Technology of Processing of Plant Raw Material: A Tutorial. Gorki*. Belarus State Agricultural Academy.

KEY WORDS AND DEFINITIONS

Bioactive Substances: The chemicals that have high physiological activity at low concentrations in relation to certain groups of living organisms or to certain groups of their cells.

Dehydration of Vegetables or Fruits: Maximum removal of moisture from the product, including osmotic moisture.

Economic Efficiency: A ratio between the obtained results of production – products and services, on the one hand, and the expenditures of labor and means of production, on the other.

Material and Technical Resources: A set of objects of labor (raw materials, materials, fuel, etc.) and tools (machines and equipment), processing objects of labor.

Minor Food Components: Natural food components of an established chemical structure (vitamin-like compounds, some minerals, indole compounds, flavonoids, isoflavones, phytosterols, etc.) present in food in milligrams and micrograms, which play an important and proven role in the adaptation reactions of the body and maintaining health, but not essential nutrients.

Mobile Workshop: A mobile plant processing plant raw materials, including substandard, working independently.

Quercetin: A natural biochemical substance of the flavonoid group, a strong antioxidant.

This research was previously published in the Handbook of Research on Globalized Agricultural Trade and New Challenges for Food Security edited by Vasilii Erokhin and Tianming Gao; pages 296-317, copyright year 2020 by Engineering Science Reference (an imprint of IGI Global).

Section 2
Food Supply Chain Management

Chapter 12
Managing Risk in Global Food Supply Chains:
Improving Food Security and Sustainability

Marco A. Miranda-Ackerman
https://orcid.org/0000-0002-7041-7130
Universidad Autónoma de Baja Callifornia, Mexico

Citlali Colin-Chávez
CONACYT, Centro de Investigación en Alimentación y Desarrollo, Mexico & Centro de Innovación y Desarrollo Agroalimentario de Michoacán, Mexico

Irma Cristina Espitia-Moreno
Universidad Michoacana de San Nicolás de Hidalgo, Mexico

Betzabé Ruiz-Morales
Universidad Michoacana de San Nicolás de Hidalgo, Mexico

Karina Cecilia Arredondo-Soto
https://orcid.org/0000-0002-8929-7319
Universidad Autónoma de Baja Callifornia, Mexico

ABSTRACT

Supply chains have inherent risk given the number of actors that interface. While there are some chains that have low frequencies of unfavorable events, many continuously face uncertainty. Food production has many uncertainties along the global supply chain. The global nature of the large logistical networks increases its complexity. Two main sources of uncertainty arise: External and internal to the SC. External factors mainly come from nature (such as "El Niño" phenomenon) and from human activities (such as food and nutrition policy and standards). Internal factors mainly come from operations such as a cold chain disruption. Thus, one needs to minimize risk and improve resilience in order to achieve food security and sustainability. It is then imperative that risk management practices be integrated into the supply chain design and management process. This chapter presents an overview of the main risks involved in global food supply chains, as well as some techniques for risk management.

DOI: 10.4018/978-1-7998-5354-1.ch012

INTRODUCTION

Supply chains (SC) all have inherent risk given that many actors interface to create the value chain they form a part of. While there are some chains that have low frequencies of unfavorable events, there are many that continuously face uncertainty. The food sector and specially the fresh food segment, have many variables that interact to create many critical uncertainties along the global SC. Many of the food chains are large networks of interacting actors that create a production and logistical network that increases its complexity (see Figure 1). On the upper part of the figure there are two main sources of risk, man-made ones (right side) and those produced by nature (left side). The second layer of flows that stem from the first categorizes each flow into two main groups. For the environmental source, there are risks stemming from biological agents and from geophysical ones. From the human health risks perspective, contamination and handling of food products are paramount risk flows. The environmental risk flows have a stronger effect on the initial stages of the food SC, as is illustrated in the middle section of the figure from top to bottom. This is to say, at the supply side of the chain (e.g. drought and pests). This is not to say that manmade issues don't affect this section, but it is in a progressive scale. On the other end the chain manufacturing and distribution are heavily affected by the potential of contamination (e.g. pathogen contamination at packaging) and mishandling (e.g. disruption in the cold chain). Other external factors that are sources of risk come from the economic and policies that affect the natural and human elements of the food SC (e.g. market volatility and health regulation). Uncertainties arise from the interfaces of these actors. These can be classifies in to two large groups: external and internal to the SC.

External factors are those that come from the environment surrounding the SC system. They can also be grouped in two main categories, those coming from nature and those coming from human activities. The ones from nature range from biotic and abiotic sources in the agro-ecological interaction of a given food producer in its primary form (e.g. eggs, fruits, vegetables, legumes, grains, etc.) with its natural surroundings (Miranda-Ackerman & Colín-Chávez, 2019).

Abiotic aspects range from temperature, sunlight, moisture, precipitation, wind, seasonal changes, earth systems events (e.g. El Niño, La Niña), water flows, geophysical phenomenon (e.g. volcanic events, land erosion, mud slide), etc.

This is not an extensive list, to the contrary, it is just the tip of the iceberg, furthermore each one of these aspect have many elements of risk and uncertainty that interact with the PS (PS) to create vulnerabilities.

Biotic factors, on the other hand, have even higher levels of complexity. Biotic aspects are mainly related to the relationships between the different organisms that interact directly or indirectly with the agrofood PSs in all stages of the SC (Guy, Macdonald, Mackenzie, & Burritt, 2018). In the primary production stage, microorganisms in the soil, air and on plant and animal tissue interact with seeds, roots, plants and fruits, which in turn interact with the food products that are being produced.

In an orchard, chicken farm or greenhouse PS, microbiome of fertilizers, insects, organisms in feed, all interact. Two very important risks related to the biotic aspects of food SCs are the quality and quantity of food to be produced in the primary stages . This has a direct effect on food availability, nutrition, health and other important aspects, one of the most important being food security (Dhankher & Foyer, 2018). On the other hand there is the food safety risks related to the biotic factors. These are mainly related to food contamination with hazardous microorganisms to human and animal health.

Figure 1. Illustration of complexity in food and beverage supply chains

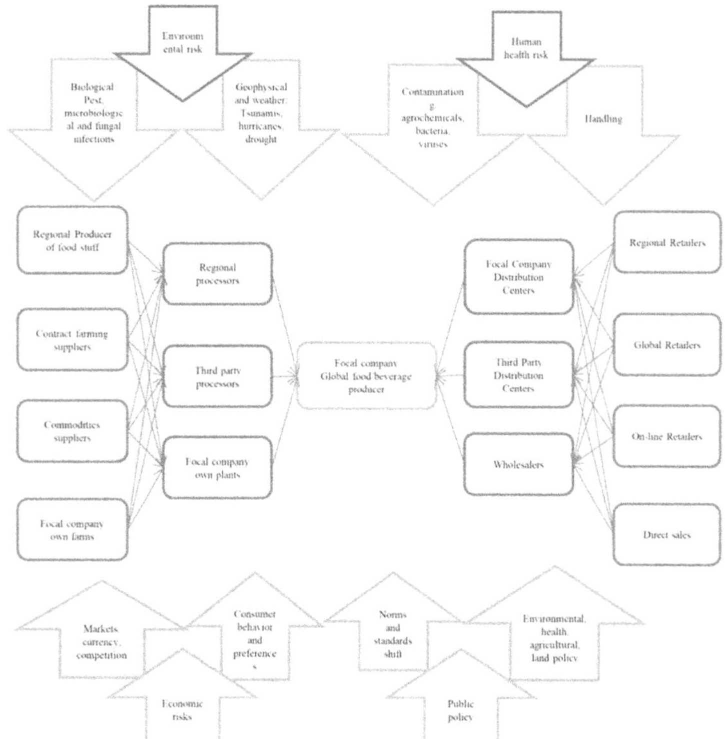

External factors related to the uncertainties caused by human activities, in the global food SC context, are related to commerce and politics (Rahimifard, Stone, & Trollman, 2018). Commercial aspects are mainly related to the forces of the market on supply and demand. These in tern create price variations, which interact with the operational aspects of food SCs, and define the margins to commercially operate and make a profit. Political aspect interacts with the natural and commercial uncertainties. Policies on water use, land use, agrochemical production and use, consumer policies (e.g. nutritional labels), among others, interact with geopolitical uncertainties, such as national production stimulation through subsidies and international import tariffs.

Internal sources of uncertainty in the food SC have to do with the operation. Risk related to supplier disruption, cold chain disruption, logistic disruption, cash flow, information disruption, all form a large chain of operational risk that propagate through the SC. The need for Avoidance and Resilience Strategies have, to both external and internal sources of uncertainty, must be detected, quantifies, planed for and monitored. By doing these activities, one can redesign SCs and their components. Measure risk and quantify in order to face-off losses vs investment in efforts to minimize risk and improve resilience.

Problem Definition

In the case of food SCs the minimization of risk and the improvement of resilience help two important social needs: food security and sustainability. Food security has always been an important issue, yet in recent years, demographic growth and the increase in world wealth has applied new pressures to the existing food SCs. It is estimated that doubling of food production must be achieved (Ray, Mueller, West, & Foley, 2013)in order to feed the population of 9.7 billion by 2050 estimated by(United Nations, Department of Economic and Social Affairs, 2015). While there must be an intensification of food production, another means to increase food availability will be through the minimization of food loss and waste. Food loss and waste are in large part avoidable through operational and logistical improvements (Muriana, 2017; Redlingshöfer, Coudurier, & Georget, 2017). Yet, it is estimated that Mexico, Canada and the USA alone produce close to 170 million tonnes of food waste and loss meant for human consumption, across the food SC each year(CEC, 2017). Food security is one of the SDG, but food SCs also interplay with other SDG such as access to water, working conditions, responsible consumption, human health and nutrition, hunger, etc. It is then important to achieve organizational resilience by improved management practices and innovative redesign along the SC (Zilberman, Lu, & Reardon, 2017).

This book chapter derives from the findings from the Roads to Resilience report (Franken, Goffin, Szwejczewski, & Kutsch, 2014) synthetized in (Hopkin, 2014) the main organizational traits and operational improvements needed to manage risk in the context of food SC. The main ideas that are adapted to food SC organizations are: anticipating unfavorable events, and creating and maintaining warning systems; managing resources to improve flexibility and responsiveness; information sharing, network integrations and relationship development; prevention and planning as a means to reduce vulnerability and increase resilience; and finally, supervision and continues improvement to improve strategic, tactical and operational capabilities in the face of uncertainty.

It is then imperative that risk management practices for diagnosing, monitoring, measuring and planning be integrated into the SC design and management process. These practices is already a key requirement for many national food and health safety government organization, as well as regulatory norm organization that certify and accredit good agricultural and manufacturing practices and food safety of products (e.g. HACCP, Hazard analysis and critical control points). There is a general trend that can be seen in the revision of norms such as ISO 9001 (related to organizational management systems) and ISO 17025 (related to laboratory and metrology organization managed systems) that have updated there model to include Risk Analysis as a key preventive component to how work is done. Yet, other logistic and operational elements in the food SC are not necessarily included in this risk management practices. This book chapter presents an overview of the main risks involved in the agrofood SCs in the context of global food SCs. An overview of techniques to identify, measure, monitor, plan and design based on the risks that may be of interest to a SC practitioner are introduced. And the importance of risk minimizations and resilience development are situated in the context of food security and the sustainable development goals in general.

BACKGROUND

Supply Chain Risk

SCs are systems of systems that interact with unique incentives that coordinate to achieve final customer satisfaction. Because each link in the chain and its interface are systems in themselves complexity irises. In global SCs these links and interfaces can be numerous and heterogeneous. Giving way to risk.

Risk in SC management has evolved. Yet, a well-developed definition based on critical review is provided by (Heckmann, Comes, & Nickel, 2015). Proposing the following definition: "…the potential loss for a SC in terms of its target values of efficiency and effectiveness evoked by uncertain developments of SC characteristics whose changes were caused by the occurrence of triggering-events". This approach to defining and understanding SC risk will be used throughout this chapter. In order to understand the concepts used a description of its components is necessary.

SCs and the organizations that make them up have efficiency and effectiveness targets. Efficiency targets - are based on improvement and the best form of utilizing limited resources. While - effectiveness targets - are focused on accomplishing specific tasks and objectives, fulfilling customer needs. Uncertain events that may have mild or severe consequences may take place. In some cases reducing the ability to maintain efficiency, such as re-routing a delivery trajectory to an alternative route that may take more time or energy. Or, in more severe cases, complete disruptions may occur such that effectivity to delivering customers' demand becomes impossible or unfeasible. Specific issues related to food logistic networks and PSs will be placed in the setting of this definition framework. Indeed these uncertain events are probabilistic in nature. They may or may not occur, or may occur frequently or far apart. SC

In their review (Heckmann et al., 2015) proposes a structure of elements that help understand SC risk. It consists of three components: 1) Risk-affected objective (i.e. Efficiency or effectiveness), 2) Risk exposition (interaction of events, time and SC systems), lastly 3) Risk attitude (i.e. aversion, attraction and neutrality).

Exposure to risk is an interaction of the SCs characteristics, the probability of an undesired event happening and time as a driver of events and actions. SCs may be vulnerable or robust. SC vulnerability is the exposure to risk. One can manage exposure through design and investment. For instance, if a distribution center (DC) is located in a hurricane corridor but is made out of the strongest concrete and metal materials vulnerability to risk is reduced. Alternatively, one can reduce exposure by moving to a different location, and build with cheaper less expensive materials, and obtain similar reduction in vulnerability. In other words, it is a balance between exposure and risk. Exposure to risk likewise relates to the consequences or severity level of the undesired event. Where high frequency of undesired events (e.g. disruptions and disturbances) with very small consequences may be tolerated, might yet be important in terms of operational performances. These are known as High Probability Low Consequence (HPLC) undesired events. While Low Probability High Consequence (LPHC) undesired events invoke the idea of disasters, catastrophes, and crisis. The food SCs operational performance is continuously exposed to risk.

Furthermore, exposure to risk and the level of vulnerability is a result of choice, as illustrated in the DC example previously described. This is especially important in the food SC design and management processes. These are series of choices managers and designers must take. Becoming decision makers that have their own values, objectives, preferences, biases and more importantly attitudes towards risk. Values such as awareness of human and nature wellbeing, religious beliefs, sense of justice are just some that influence the decision-making process. Objectives, too, play a role where long-term economic benefit could be contrasted to short term gains, or even antagonistic objectives paired such as profit versus environmental sustainability. Preferences, biases and attitudes play a similar role. Attitude towards risk is very important in designing and managing SCs for risk. These may be attraction to risk, where the decision maker (be it a group or an individual) ranks threats lower than he does benefits of choosing a risky alternative. While risk averse decision makers, may position the avoidance of undesired events a priority over the possible rewords of risky actions. It is then important that upper, middle and lower management understand and convey the organizational stance in the face of risk.

The vulnerability due to exposure to risk can, as said before, be overcome to a certain measure through design. Design of physical and organizational systems may achieve SC *robustness*. This is to say, "the ability to withstand disruption with an acceptable loss of performance" (Behzadi, O'Sullivan, Olsen, & Zhang, 2018). In many systems this is achieved through redundancy. Take the example of the DC previously discussed, the construction parameters where exaggerated by using concreate and steel to reduce exposure to risk and thereby reducing the DC´s vulnerability to hurricanes. This could have also been solved through numbers redundancy, building two DCs in different sites. Reducing the vulnerability of the DC as a two-unit system to a complete disruption of distribution of goods.

In contrast, *resilience* is the capacity to recover from an undesired event and its effects in a given timeframe. Time is important in risk and recovery given that the extent of loss in efficiency and effectiveness is in most cases a function of time horizons. So, say we build a structurally weaker DC in the hurricane corridor location and suffer extensive roof damage after a hurricane. If we have materials and tools on hand, and a prepared and qualified work force we may be able to recover operations quickly reducing efficiency and effectivity loss. Resilience is then closely linked to planning and access to recovery resources.

Furthermore, the capacity to recover strongly depends on the flexibility of the system. For example, if the DC lost its roof yet we could have access to a nearby facility to serve as a temporary warehouse and an on-hand fleet of moving vehicles, stocks could be moved and loss of efficiency and effectiveness curtailed. Alternatively, if the stock in the DC could not be fully saved, other links in the chain such as the manufacturing echelon could be flexible enough to restock any losses. It is implied in most cases that velocity is playing a role in the response to an undesired event. Rapid response can reduce the effects an unfavorable event has on a system. Velocity of response is subject to the availability of resources, the level of preparedness and the access to information. The later refers to the visibility and understanding of the state of the system. Early warning systems and continues monitoring become an important element of resilience (Wang & Yue, 2017). Along with information flow towards the decision makers, a response has to be coordinated and transmitted to staff, suppliers, customers and support bodies.

The actions to reduce vulnerability to risk can be known as mitigation measures. Mitigation can be categorized in four major strategies: Acceptance, avoidance, limitation (also referred to as mitigation) and transference (Ward & Chapman, 2003). An acceptance strategy consists in deciding to not take mitigating measures, given the cost of action outweighs the relationship between the consequences and the probability of occurrence. Avoidance, on the other hand, opposes this strategy by favoring investing in the reduction of vulnerability and thus mitigating risk. Limitation seeks to limit the exposure and extent of consequence due to vulnerability yet does not curtail it. Lastly, the transference strategy conveys the risk to willing third party bodies such as insurers, business partners, cooperative partners, government agencies, etc. All of these concepts are important to understand in an abstract sense. Yet, food SCs and the organizations that form them need to be understood as a specific set of instances of each concept.

Food Supply Chains

Food SCs come in different forms and sizes. Yet, all types of food SCs have some exposure to risk. Some coming from natural phenomena such as geophysical (e.g. earthquakes, tsunamis and mass movements), meteorological (droughts, floods, storms, wildfires, extreme temperatures) and biological disasters (e.g. epidemics, infestations) (Food and Agriculture Organization of the United Nations, 2018). Risks are also produced from human action such as those branching from economic activity, public policy, consumer/

Figure 2. Food SC classification models

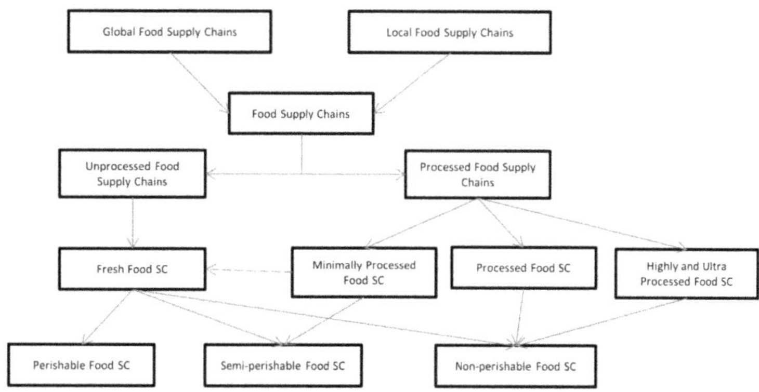

societal behavior to name a few. Depending on the SC type and its unique characteristics its exposure to risk will be different (see Figure 2).

Small business usually construct Local Food SCs that maintain a small network of producers, packers/processors, distributers, retailing outlets and support service providers (e.g. logistic services, materials suppliers, etc.). Due to the integrated nature of Local Food SCs with their natural and human surrounding complexity is reduced. Yet, access to robustness and institutional resilience tools may be limited.

While Global Food SCs are integrated into worldwide logistical networks that are nowadays systems based. Information flows with less personal and community engagements compared to Local Food SCs. Problems that could arise due to this are overcome by information sharing systems. ERP (Enterprise Resource Planning) and CRM (Client Relationship Management) systems helping global food enterprises manage interaction between links.

Different types of product flow in these two types of food SCs. Fresh Food SCs handle perishable and semi-perishable foods. While Processed Food SCs handle both semi-perishable and non-perishable food products (see Table 1).

Table 1. Examples of food by their perishability clarification

Perishable Food	Semi-Perishable Food	Non-Perishable
Meats, poultry and fish	Processed cereals.	Conserved processed foods (cooked, packaged, canned, bottled, salted, dried, pickled)
Eggs and milk	Nuts	Oils and fats.
Some cheeses (fresh and cream)	Some cheeses (semi-cured)	Some cheeses (cured and pasteurized)
Leafy vegetables, some other vegetables.	Some vegetables (e.g. pumpkin, onions, carrots, potatoes, radish, jicama)	Whole cereal, pulses, grains, nuts, oil seeds.
some fruits (tomatoes, strawberries,	Some fruits (e.g. coconuts, apples, oranges, lemons)	Sugar, honey, salt, spices and herbs.

The processing steps that can be applied to food vary widely. The goal of processing is mainly to conserve product in order to maintain or extend its shelf-life, add value through functionality (pre-cooked, microwaveable, single serving, etc.), processing efficiency (e.g. concentration and drying to reduce handling and storage costs) and product diversification and differentiation. The intensity and number of transformation steps change in different degrees the characteristics of food. It is important to state that food in human consumptions have the central role of providing nutrients and energy to the human body while maintaining health and wellbeing. The nutritional characteristics of foods will not be considered in this chapter, yet will be briefly reviewed in the Future Research Direction section.

Sources of Risk in Food Supply Chains

Sources of risk in food SCs. In the beginning of this section the sources of risk where briefly introduced. Yet indeed, it is important to develop these sources in order to better understand their effect on Food SCs. In order to make a connection between the design and managing process needed to construct and maintain a SC many operational and economic objectives are identified. Recently sustainable development goals have started to be incorporated into these design and management process models. By including issues such as environmental impact and social responsibility, through the measurement and inclusion of key performance indicators, the design and management of SCs has started to shift. Yet, has led traction in the paradigm of SC design and management. Many modeling approaches that take uncertainty into account have been widely studied and research continues to develop these ideas (see Figure 3). Nevertheless, the increasing complexity and interrelation of modern SCs demands higher levels of integration of risk in the SC design and management process.

Figure 3. Risk sources classification tree

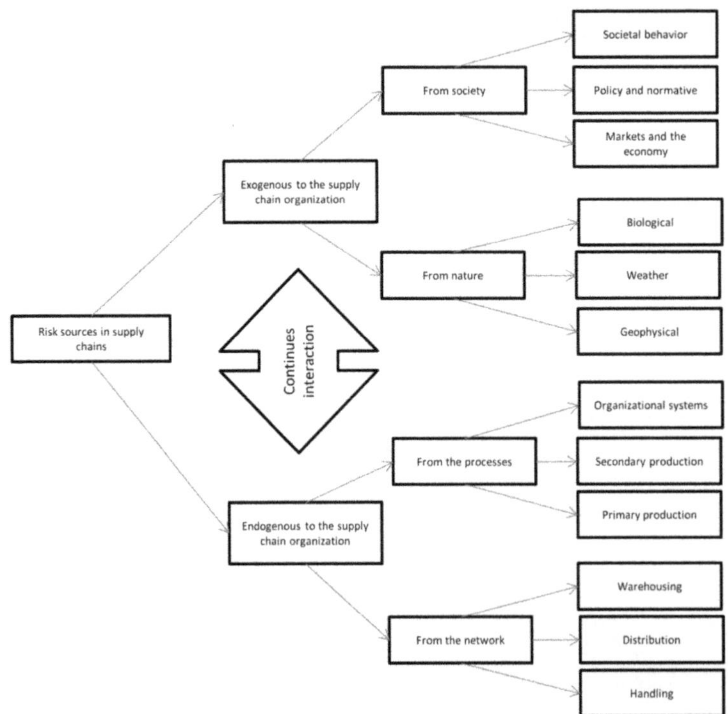

Risk can come from exogenous sources to the SC system. These can be categorized as those due to natural phenomena. Nature is constantly changing, the interaction between abiotic and biotic elements in the system create a series of events that rarely can be foreseen. Nature is one of the most important sources of uncertainty and risk in a SC. Such as in toxic risk, the dose and frequency are key to the severity of the risk or consequence. For instance, salty water or humid weather may not in the short term be a cause for concern, in the case of our concreate and steel DC. But, if protective coating or substitution of material is not performed properly corrosion may yield the DC out of commission or worse cause a health or safety event. This would present itself with due notice, yet workshop blindness could hide chronic issues. While higher dosage yet less frequent events can abruptly appear and cause a crisis. Take for instance a hurricanes or tsunamis. Fisheries and fishing boat fleets may be halted to a stop due to hurricanes and tsunamis.

Indeed, humans are changing nature and have for centuries. The natural landscape has changed dramatically due to humans. Producing interfaces with nature in an agro ecological and urban-ecological sense. Agriculture requires natural resources such as land, water, nutrients, air, energy, all taken from the natural landscape. Transforming the ecological systems that surround them. This many times has created stress in the agro-ecological system. For example, microorganisms encroach and damage agricultural quality and yield. Humans exacerbate these dynamics by the practice of industrial agriculture. Where mono-cultivation and hyper-industrialized PSs (e.g. chicken production) can cause epidemics and outbreak, amplifying health risks. Natural systems maintain a balance where one systems' waste is transformed and used by another in a virtues cycle. Indeed, these equilibrium mechanisms have been produced through millions of years of evolution and systems dynamics. Yet, human development has abruptly (in relative terms changed these systems. It is then understandable to expect uncertainties arise.

Furthermore, human, demographic and economic development worldwide has continuously grown. With positive consequences for many societies, yet at a high cost and heightened risk. Water usage, land change, synthetic intensification of production, among other requirements to satisfy these developmental advancements are expected to cause crisis(Al-Ansari, Korre, Nie, & Shah, 2015). This has already led to protracted crisis, this is to say those "which develop as complex and prolonged emergencies and combine multiple types of conflict with other shocks, such as climate change" (Food and Agriculture Organization of the United Nations, 2018)

The current demographic and economic boom achieved in many regions of the world (e.g. China, India, Mexico and Brazil) has also created new expectations and is expected to demand more food. Furthermore, cultural homogenization and commodities have changed the way consumers behave. Take for example, higher consumption of animal protein. Animal protein require much more resources (energy, water, nutrients, etc.) against other sources of vegetable protein (e.g. pulses) that require much less resources to produce and handle (recall pulses are non-perishable food, while animal flesh requires refrigeration or

another means of conservation) (Miranda-Ackerman & Colín-Chávez, 2019). Moreover, global demand for commodity foods year round have driven a complex network of food providers and PSs. This is important given that many, if not most, agrofood products and food product raw materials, are sensitive to natural environments. Making geographic location of the food SC link a key factor in the ability to continuously supply commodity foods. Taking advantage of phenological cycles and hemispheric seasonal asymmetry to distribute capacity globally.

The dynamic synthesized here produces complexity and interdependency; together with the SC type and its unique characteristics its exposure to risk will be different.

FOOD SUPPLY CHAIN MANAGEMENT AND DESIGN FOR RISK

Designing Food Supply Chain for Risk Management

Supply Chain Network Design in general has the goal of framing organizational and enterprise-wide decisions. Supply Chains are networks of elements that include suppliers, packers, processes/transformation plants/manufacturers, logistical services, warehouses, distributors among other stakeholders. In these networks, materials, information and money exchanges hands in order to provide value to the customer. It is made up of physical infrastructure and material, and intangible systems, organizations and relationships. Physical infrastructure includes trucks, frights, trains, sea vessels, warehouses, extraction facilities, production plants, manufacturing plants, transformation facilities, telecommunications, among others, that are used in coordination to transform, maintain and move products. In the case of Food SCs they include farms, henhouses, refrigerators, extractors, plough machines, silos, greenhouses, dryers, beehives, etc.

It is important to explain that SC Network Design looks at the systems as a whole. Placing especial emphasis on interactions and interphases, and not on a detailed design of the PSs. Looking at general technological decisions that influence strategic outcome. Some examples of the decisions that are framed in a SC Network Design process are:

- PSs strategic design questions:
  - Produce organic, conventional or intensive fruit/vegetables/ livestock?
  - Fresh food presentation, minimally processed, pasteurized?
  - Packaging in plastic film, biofilm, clamshell, micro pore plastic bags?
  - Bottling in glass, aluminum or carton?
  - Bacteriological stabilization through heat treatment, hyperbaric pressure, electric pulse?
- Production capacity:
  - How many head of cattle?
  - What size henhouse?
  - Automated or handpicked egg collection?
  - 100 liter oven? 2 or 3 centrifuges? Copper or stainless steel batch reservoir?
- Location-allocation problem:
  - Productions plant location near raw materials suppliers or near customer? In other word transport raw materials or finished goods?
  - Reconstitution of juice near natural spring or near urban water supply?
- Sourcing decisions:
  - Which suppliers to buy from?
  - How much to buy?
  - Which criteria to use to evaluate supplier performance?
  - What type of contract/arrangement?

SC Network Design involves a decision and model framework that searches "through one or a variety of metrics, for the "best" configuration and operation of all of these (SC network) elements."(Garcia & You, 2015). Given that decision outcome from one part of the SC may influence the outcome of another, it is important that it be simultaneously framed in the same decision structure. Moreover, elements of multiple scales, levels, periods, objectives, attitudes, stakeholders and competitors, creates a higher level of complexity.

The network and design decisions can be modeled through nodes and arcs that connect (see Figure 4). Different routes and configuration can be evaluated by activating arcs and nodes and reviewing the outcome in terms of efficiency and effectiveness to satisfy pre-established objectives.

Figure 4. Network representation of a generic SC model
(Miranda-Ackerman, 2015)

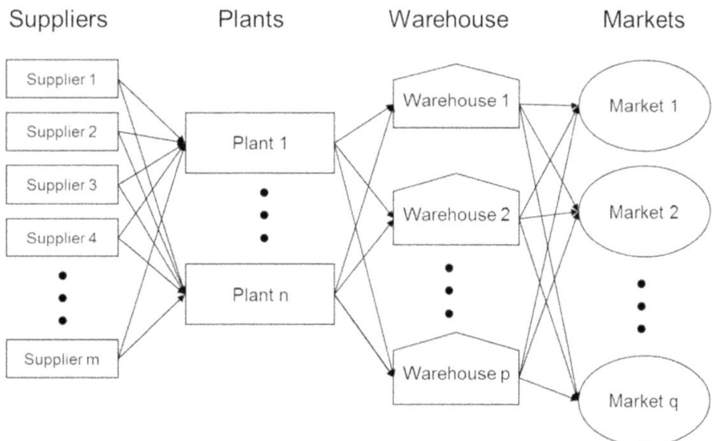

Many layers of arcs and nodes can be placed independently or nested in order to reflect decision interactions. Take for example the nodes and arc modeling of a globally sources and distributed orange juice SC (see Figure 5). In it we see that in level 3 of the SC in the case of process 1 and process 2 technology 1 (out of many) was selected. Yet, other important decisions can be modeled the same way. Type of transport, points of cross-docking, ports of arrival and departure, suppliers, as well as capacity allocation, say for example choosing a silo capacity, equipment capacity, these can all be included in a single model.

Once the initial modeling is done, analytical, heuristic or computational decision making can be performed. Finding the best configuration of the network and its modeled elements to achieve a good or optimal outcome is to optimize the design. Some design optimizations are presented in Design optimization techniques and tools section.

Design Strategies

Nevertheless, this modeling structure rarely included uncertainty. Uncertainty is frequently oversimplified or tried with in an independent set through scenario analysis. Different design strategies have to be places along each other in order to make a "good" decision. One important element to be evaluated is the idea of robustness and resilience.

Figure 5. Network representation of a beverage SC model
(Miranda-Ackerman, 2015)

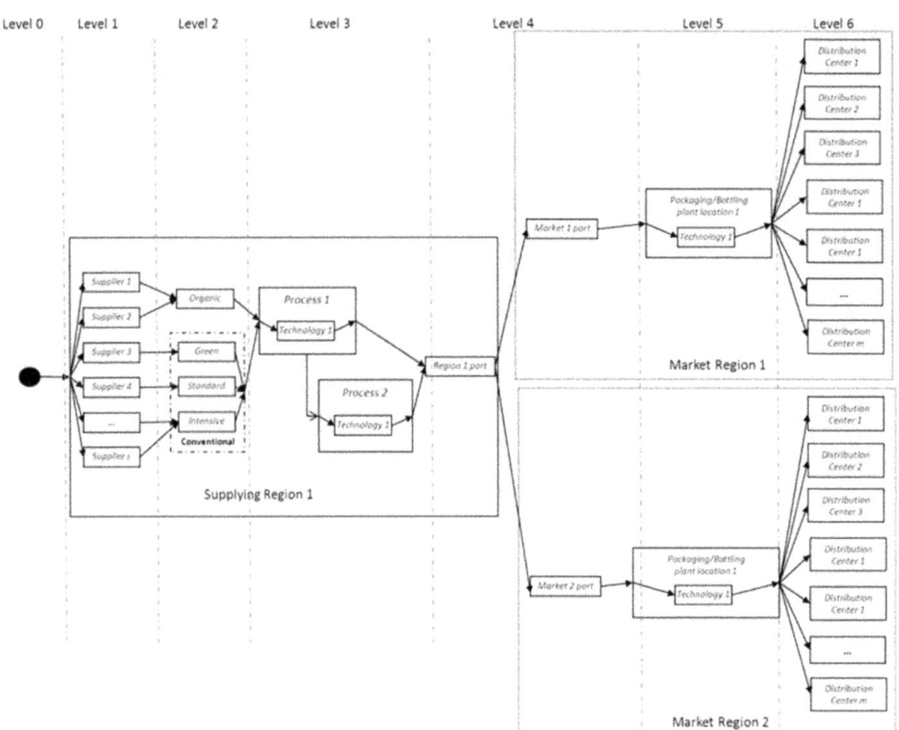

Robustness and Resilience

In recent years LM (LM) principals developed in the automotive and aerospace industries have reached food PSs. One main pillar of LM is the elimination of non-value adding elements of the system and product delivery. This has led to the elimination of redundancies in systems and the reduction of security stocks and extra capacity. Leading to more efficient systems; however at a risk cost. In LM systems visibility of inefficiencies is key. Systems are redesigned to their "Leanest" form where any inconsistency between the elimination of waste with the rhythm of production is observed. This is because they produce intermittent, regularly short disruptions that attracted the attention of engineering and management teams. Yet, the braking down to a "bear bone" system depletes robustness to variability. Let us recall that robustness is the "ability to withstand disruption with an acceptable loss of performance" (Behzadi et al., 2018). Food SCs that adhere to LM principals then have lower levels of robustness. Take for example the principal of Just-In-Time production. It is based on the idea that materials in production process and warehoused either raw materials or finished goods, are waste. They hide inefficiencies and cost to maintain. So, these Food SCs depend on synchronized delivery of raw materials and synchronized shipping of final product, with their cycle time. Suppliers have to follow strict planning and scheduling objectives. In the case of food production raw materials' uncertain nature plays its role. Only in highly protected, controlled and automated systems (e.g. hi-tech greenhouses) it is possible to obtain highly reliable and consistent output. This is because these systems limite environmental uncertainty. Sunlight can be substituted by led lightbulbs, soil by substrate; even microorganisms are used to inoculate roots and seeds for performance. Yet, most agricultural systems, be day livestock or crops, are produces interacting with nature. Thus, uncertainty plays a large role in the quality and yield agricultural systems. To overcome the frailty of LM systems - resilience measures can be used.

Let us recall that resilience is the "potential to recover quickly from disruption" (Behzadi et al., 2018). It is achieved through different approaches. Flexibility for example can be achieved through continues supplier diversification. Focal Companies, this is to say the "owner" or key coordinator of a SC, usually maintains and controls the entry and exit of organizations and stakeholder in a given SC. These include suppliers and customers. By continuously diversifying suppliers and the types of contracting agreements, contingency inclusion in the SC of known yet non-active members can be done. By doing this, capacity that is not part of the system can be tapped with less effort and shorter timeframes. By having a diversified portfolio of suppliers of not only agricultural products, but logistical services, and even clients risk is spread. Risk has an area of exposure, by distributing geographically or organizationally, undesirable events may happen in one area of exposure but not all. This strategy can be costly and difficult to maintain, given that market forces of each player in the SC dynamic has their own objective of reducing risk and being profitable. Yet, it is a feasible and sometimes attractive strategy. Diversification can also increase traceability effort, but the benefits can be great. In the case of food safety issues diversification can help limit the reach of quality or health crises. Contamination of food with human health implications can be limited by geographically or organizationally identifying the source of contaminant. By doing so, the SC as a whole, is not fully disrupted reducing is efficiency. An important downside to this strategy is that relationships between suppliers, focal companies and clients can be strained by doubt.

A different approach to improve resiliency of a SC can also be focusing on the response time. This has two main elements: visibility and preparedness. Visibility consists in continuously assessing known sources of risk and foreseeing future ones. Early warning systems through Statistical Process Control and other time series approaches can help detect when a risky situation occurs. By doing so, the response can be preemptive and curtail any loss of efficiency or effectiveness. For example, say market behavior is pushing food stuff prices up, driving profit margins down in a processed food SC, market awareness and controls can trigger hedging actions through pricing guarantee agreements. While preparedness consists of developing and maintaining procedures and alternatives active. Let us go back to the DC in a hurricane corridor example. If roofing procedures are developed, employees are trained and materials suppliers portfolios are kept, the recovery time after roof failure may be much faster than if unprepared . The simple task of deciding who will coordinate recovery effort in case of an energy prior to it happening may be critical to response time in a crisis situation.

A different tactic is to add robustness to the system. It consists of adding redundant capacity. Continuing with the DC example, having two DCs or having one build from highly resistant materials. This same principle can be applied to many elements of a SC. Take for example having extra equipment, tools or workers ready yet idle. This reduces efficiency as a ratio of capacity used and available capacity. Yet, if uncertain events such as demand spikes, equipment failure, logistical disruptions, redundancy can help reestablish normal operations. It is then, more common to use it as an effectiveness guarantee strategy. This is to say, it is useful to avoid complete or partial disruptions in the flow of goods or information. It relates to availability not only of infrastructure capacity but also on organizational . If client lists and emails are maintained in redundant servers, or food processing is distributed in may plants this may reduce risk. Robustness as a strategy of design can also relate to oversizing alternatives. So, say a warehouse is being built to stock materials that may be stored in ambient temperature, yet Heating, Ventilation, and Air Conditioning (HVAC) systems and wall and sealing insulation may be used. This is a combination of preparedness through redundancy. My choosing this alternative, higher cost may occur in the short term, but this may be outweighed if there is a chance of heatwaves affecting stock. If the food being warehoused is of high value, and the probability of heatwaves or freezing temperatures is at a given level, decisions analysis may yield these as the best choice.

Design Optimization Techniques and Tools

Once the relevant choices in the design process are framed. A solution or choice has to be made. This can be done through different approaches. Some of the most common are: simulation, decisions analysis, optimization and metaheuristics.

Simulation itself has many different paradigm, yet three are common in SC Design: discrete event simulation (series of single path movements and choice nodes), agent based simulation (choice agency is modeled through rules and parameter setting with higher numbers of paths and possibilities) and systems dynamics (focuses on the interrelation of systems components through time at a high level). Simulation uses the principle of simplifying reality through a representation taking key elements of a system and the probabilities that describe behavior. By using this approach different SC Design alternatives can be evaluated without the need of investing in the actual system. By doing so, one can change parameters to find those that have the strongest effect on the outcome. Food SCs can benefit from simulation given that different design and event scenarios can be modeled and understood. The simulation of the effect a smoke plum due to volcanic activity in a logistical route can be simulated to see if the system is robust or resilient enough to withstand the shock. "What if" scenarios can be played out in virtual time in order to find weaknesses and target design effort to overcome them.

Decisions Analysis on the other hand models alternatives of a food SC and the chances a set of events may occur and its effect. These sets are finite and measurements are made through different extraction techniques. Objectives, preferences and attitudes are included in these models in order to capture the organizational or individual decision maker stand in the face of a choice. When using this technique decision threes and influence diagrams can be helpful in understanding and visualizing relationships and possibilities. Decisions Analysis is often used in SC Management and Design given the complexity of choices and their strategic nature. Optimization based on mathematical modeling of Food SCs has become one of the most important strategies for designing SCs under uncertainty (Behzadi et al., 2018). These can be formulated and solved through analytical means such as those the field of Operations Research yields. Or through more computational intensive approaches such as Metahuristic methods. The later is especially important in systems where non-linear behaviors and a high combinatorial nature of the problem require numerical methods to solve efficiently. Furthermore, uncertainty objectives and variables can be integrated as multi-objetive optimization problems that can be solved through different methods (Aqlan & Lam, 2016; Guillén-Gosálbez & Grossmann, 2009).

By using multi-objective optimization, risk, uncertainty and vulnerability can be evaluated and tested. It can be included as part of the objectives, set against the most common objectives of economic and operational performance. Or it can be nested in the model through, for example, time minimization where interruptions and deviations due to uncertain events are reduced or eliminated by evaluating the different alternatives that reduce downtime of a SC link.

Managing Food Supply Chains for Risk

Once a SC in put in place in either case it is or not designed for risk management, it can be managed for risk mitigation. According to findings form an Airmic and Cranfield School of Management study published by (Hopkin, 2014) there is a common pattern found in global reach resilient organizations. These characteristics are useful in Food SCs.

By creating a culture around concepts and practices of risk mitigation, and by creating systems to manage the organizational relationship with uncertainty, risk can be known and controlled, and its harm reduced. The organizational culture has to be developed through many different strategies that will be detailed in the following, yet all strategies have the end goal of allowing and promoting human engagement in the efforts to mitigate risk. While systems are set, to reduce the burden on personal only. By creating systems information flow and organizational robustness can be harnessed as a holistic approach to reducing vulnerabilities that can't be eliminated.

Culture of Risk Reduction

The organization as a whole has to define by action and communication the value it places on risk. Attitudes towards risk have to be communicated as a means to homogenize cultural norms and official policies. By doing so, clarity in the face of doubt can be solved by revisiting communication by management. The organizational culture has to be known by upper management. Where highly innovative food companies, that continuously rollout new products and product lines, have to inspire risk taking as part of a creative and non-punitive culture, while maintaining well established, communicated and understood boundaries. Take for example processed food SCs that aggressively promote newer presentations of processed food, think of yogurt packaging and flavoring. Yogurts continuously change the way packaging is used not only to contain the product but also as a marketing tool. This may seem as relatively innocuous, yet packaging is also a means to preserve the quality and safety attributes as a "for human consumption" product. The loss of packaging or bottling integrate can become a health and quality issue if rolled-out hurriedly. While less innovative, more conservative organizational cultures, which rely on continuity and customer trust have to help workers avoid complacency and reword awareness of the unexpected. Take for example fresh fruit SCs that supply commodity markets.

Culture helps people inside of food companies be empowered and involved beyond normative requirements. Food industry quality and safety requirements worldwide are extensive and ubiquitous. Yet, by definition unfavorable uncertain events are unknown. The culture of risk reduction is especially useful to identify and avoid, when possible, harm from unidentified (a priori) risk events and failure modes.

Leadership has to be the initiator and champion of risk reduction. By setting the example and promoting risk mitigation activities. Risk aversion and attraction is continuously defined. Leadership can promote the use of self-assessment tools in order to understand if the culture of risk is being attained and if the communication is being effective. A review by (De Boeck, Jacxsens, Bollaerts, & Vlerick, 2015) proposes different sets of questioners in order to understand organizational culture in terms of "food safety culture" and "food safety climate".

Leadership must promote collaboration amongst different department and internal SC actors. By maintaining close relationships with customers and suppliers a common understanding of risk attitudes ca be achieved. Furthermore, homogeneity can be improved given that risk can originate at any level of the SC network. A shared set of values and attitudes within the food SCs helps guarantee that there are no "weak links" that place the full SC in danger.

Systems for Risk

Systems can be set and maintained in order to allow for the flow of information. Some of the information systems that can be used are:

- Early warning systems
- Control systems
- Information processing and automated inference systems
- Information routing and distribution systems
- Decision support systems

Other tools to assess systems' risk that are used in food SCs are:

- Failure Mode and Critical Effects Analysis
- Reliability, Availability and Reliability Analysis
- Bow-tie Analysis
- Simulation and Scenario Analysis

Preparedness

In order to guarantee response and recovery times are minimized plans, procedures and organizational structures and hierarchies have to be developed and maintained.

Planning contingency actions and scheduling routine simulations and action plan meetings are important in order to be prepared prior to unexpected events. Response time can greatly be improved by having procedures put in place. And assigning responsibilities among the workers that may be involved in operations at risk. Decision making hierarchies have to be set and communicated through organizational diagrams and action titles. With this simple but important actions recovery after a contingency will be agile and effective.

Review and Improvement

When an undesired event happens, it is important that a Review and Improvement strategy is set in motion after all actions have been done and recovery is set in motion. It is important that proper documentation is registered through forms or information management systems. These registries will allow planners and decision makers to study the actions taken and improve techniques, tools and strategies. Moreover, awareness of future events that are similar to the once that have occur require a well-thought-out knowledge acquisition structure. Historical event must be in the consciousness of workers that join the company and do not yet have tacit knowledge and know-how to be aware of risk.

By documenting the actions executed and the outcomes obtained, the effectiveness of risk analysis tools can greatly be enhanced. In the case of Failure Mode, Effects, and Criticality Analysis (FMECA), a Case-Base reasoning paradigm and technique, actions and outcomes allow to fill-in knowledge gaps by explicitly documenting failure trees and their actual outcomes. Making it easier to find a quick solution to problems that have already occurred and been solved, and by avoiding errors made in the past.

It is especially important to document near miss and incident/accident in reporting systems. As these provide a gauge to visualize tendencies towards actual events. Going back to the DC case study. If each year higher frequency and intensity hurricanes are produced during hurricane season, it may be a trigger to update and simulate action plans, heighten vigilance, acquire resources, among other preventive activities.

DISCUSSION AND RECOMMENDATIONS

Risk Management's Role in Sustainable Food Systems

Sustainable Development Goals have become an important driver and guide towards changes in human activity in a variety of areas and settings. It is an effort to frame general goals and sub-goals that prescribe attention to specific maladies in society and environment. Risk management interacts with many of these goals. In the Appendix a table is provided reviewing some of the most closely related SDG (Sustainable Development Goals) indicators in relation to Food Supply Chain Management and Design for Risk Management. It is important to point out that while (Hopkin, 2014) has provided an outline on risk management in organizations its scope and target is generalized and derived from manufacturing and other sector of industry. While this book chapter has provided parallels that can be applied in the specific context of food SCs illustrated through hypothetical examples and focused discussions related to specific issues in this industry.

Proactive versus Reactive Strategies

It may seem obvious to presume al Food SCs have to take a proactive approach to risk. Yet, proactive strategies have to be accompanied by reactive strategies in order to become adaptive to change and capable of handling adverse events. A company cannot foresee all possible scenarios and outcomes. Thus, it cannot prepare for al contingencies; it must then have a culture that stimulates flexibility and agility during time of crisis.

Robustness versus Resilience

The same case could be made related to de design of a food SC in the face of antagonistic strategies: robustness vs resilience. There cannot be a generalized prescription for the design strategy to be used. Food SCs interact with so many actors and institutional and normative structures that it has to be studies case by case, and link by link. Interfaces between food SC actors must transition and adapt for different nodes in the wide network of connections. Experience helps through tacit knowledge of key managers and decision makers, as well as designers and analyst in order to find the best balance given the available information and attitude towards risk. Furthermore, mathematical modeling and computational methods can help find optimal balance between these two strategies to find the right mix.

FUTURE RESEARCH DIRECTIONS

Nutrition has yet to be incorporated into food SC risk models. As the final function to the customer, nutrition is key to maintaining value in food SCs. Risks related to loss of nutritional value and consumer behavior changes towards what nutrition has to be considered in future research.

CONCLUSION

SCs are systems of systems that interact to achieve final customer satisfaction. Global SCs are complex and have many attributes that contribute to risk and vulnerability. Food SC systems in particular have complexities unique to them given their interactions with nature and given the final use, this is to say human and animal consumption.

Food SCs organizations have efficiency and effectiveness targets that are affected by uncertain events. These may have mild or severe depending on the consequences they have when they occur. Undesired uncertain events are probabilistic in nature. Yet, decisions makers and managers can balance different strategies in order to design and manage a SC.

Furthermore, exposure to risk and the level of vulnerability is a result of choice. These choices have to be made by decision makers that have their own values, objectives, preferences, biases and more importantly attitudes towards risk. It is then important that upper, middle and lower management are able to define the SC's organizational attitude towards risk.

The vulnerability can be overcome through design. Design of physical and organizational systems may achieve SC *robustness* or *resilience* strategies. The former focuses on creating strong and resistant systems, while the later focuses on recovery and is then closely linked to planning. The actions to reduce vulnerability to risk can be known as mitigation measures.

There are many sources of risk in food SCs. Risk can come from exogenous sources to the SC system. Agriculture requires natural resources such as land, water, nutrients, air, energy, all taken from the natural landscape. While human, demographic and economic development worldwide

Moreover, global demand for commodity foods year-round have driven a complex network of food providers and PSs. The dynamic defined here produces complexity and interdependency; together with the SC type and its unique characteristics its exposure to risk will be different.

SC Network Design in general has the goal of framing organizational and enterprise-wide decisions. SC design decisions include suppliers, packers, processes/transformation plants/manufacturers, logistical services, warehouses, distributors among other stakeholders. In these networks' materials, information and money exchanges hands in order to provide value to the customer. We reviewed some of the questions that SC Network Design process related to PSs strategic design, production capacity, location-allocation problem, materials sourcing among many others. In Food SC Design two main strategies can be used: robustness and resilience.

Once a SC designed and deployed organizational actions may help manage risk. One activity is to create a culture of risk reduction and awareness. By doing so, workers and management can create the conditions to be vigilant and prepared, as well as react quickly in the face of an undesired event.

The culture is made through communication and leadership commitment to basic principles and actions as well as a clear understanding of the stance of the organization to risk. Risk averse companies place value on consistency and reliability, while risk attracted ones on reactiveness and agility.

Information systems can be used in order to maintain communications of the state of the food SC, to call to action, coordinate and teach in the aftermath. Preparedness also plays a large role in managing risk. Through plans, procedures and organization, a more resilient and reactive food SC emerges.

Food SCs are unique, each one having a network or interacting actors that need to cooperate in order to handle the uncertainties coming from all types of sources. It is important that Risk Management be integrated into the Food SC Design and Management processes in order to cope with risk. Practitioners and manager will find that by creating a culture of risk management at an enterprise wide scale, overall efficiency and effectiveness to respond to consumers' needs will be achieved successfully.

ACKNOWLEDGMENT

The authors would like to thank the CONACYT Research Network "12.3: To reduce and value food loss and waste: towards sustainable food systems". The book chapter is partially driven by the efforts this research network promotes related to sustainable food systems in Mexico.

REFERENCES

Al-Ansari, T., Korre, A., Nie, Z., & Shah, N. (2015). Development of a life cycle assessment tool for the assessment of food production systems within the energy, water and food nexus. *Sustainable Production and Consumption*, 2, 52–66. doi:10.1016/j.spc.2015.07.005

Albrecht, J. A. (n.d.). Food Storage EC446. Retrieved from http://extensionpublications.unl.edu/assets/pdf/ec446.pdf

Aqlan, F., & Lam, S. S. (2016). Supply chain optimization under risk and uncertainty: A case study for high-end server manufacturing. *Computers & Industrial Engineering*, 93, 78–87. doi:10.1016/j.cie.2015.12.025

Behzadi, G., O'Sullivan, M. J., Olsen, T. L., & Zhang, A. (2018). Agribusiness supply chain risk management: A review of quantitative decision models. *Omega*, 79, 21–42. doi:10.1016/j.omega.2017.07.005

CEC. (2017). *Characterization and Management of Food Loss and Waste in North America*. Retrieved from http://www3.cec.org/islandora/en/item/11772-characterization-and-management-food-loss-and-waste-in-north-america-en.pdf

Christiansen, B. (2001). *Handbook of Research on Global Supply Chain Management*. Retrieved from https://www.igi-global.com/book/handbook-research-global-supply-chain/137126

De Boeck, E., Jacxsens, L., Bollaerts, M., & Vlerick, P. (2015). Food safety climate in food processing organizations: Development and validation of a self-assessment tool. *Trends in Food Science & Technology*, 46(22, Part A), 242–251. doi:10.1016/j.tifs.2015.09.006

Dhankher, O. P., & Foyer, C. H. (2018). Climate resilient crops for improving global food security and safety. *Plant, Cell & Environment*, 41(5), 877–884. doi:10.1111/pce.13207

Food and Agriculture Organization of the United Nations. (2018). *The impact of disasters and crises on agriculture and food security, 2017.*

Franken, A., Goffin, K., Szwejczewski, M., & Kutsch, E. (2014). *Roads to Resilience: Building Dynamic Approaches to Risk.*

Garcia, D. J., & You, F. (2015). Supply chain design and optimization: Challenges and opportunities. *Computers & Chemical Engineering, 81,* 153–170. doi:10.1016/j.compchemeng.2015.03.015

Guillén-Gosálbez, G., & Grossmann, I. E. (2009). Optimal design and planning of sustainable chemical supply chains under uncertainty. *AIChE Journal. American Institute of Chemical Engineers, 55*(1), 99–121. doi:10.1002/aic.11662

Guy, P. L., Macdonald, R., Mackenzie, S., & Burritt, D. J. (2018). Stressed Out: Demonstrating the Effects of Abiotic and Biotic Stress on an Important Food Crop. *The American Biology Teacher, 80*(1), 50–52. doi:10.1525/abt.2018.80.1.50

Heckmann, I., Comes, T., & Nickel, S. (2015). A critical review on supply chain risk – Definition, measure and modeling. *Omega, 52,* 119–132. doi:10.1016/j.omega.2014.10.004

Hopkin, P. (2014). Achieving enhanced organisational resilience by improved management of risk: Summary of research into the principles of resilience and the practices of resilient organisations. *Journal of Business Continuity & Emergency Planning, 8*(3), 252–262.

UNISDR. (2009). UNISDR terminology on disaster risk reduction. Geneva, Switzerland, May.

Miranda-Ackerman, M. A. (2015, Nov. 5). Optimisation multi-objectif pour la gestion et la conception d'une chaine logistique verte: application au cas de la filière agroalimentaire du jus d'orange. Retrieved from http://www.theses.fr/s139158

Miranda-Ackerman, M. A., & Colín-Chávez, C. (2019). Food Supply Chain Demand and Optimization. In P. Ferranti, E. M. Berry, & J. R. Anderson (Eds.), *Encyclopedia of Food Security and Sustainability* (pp. 455–464)., doi:10.1016/B978-0-08-100596-5.22278-6

Muriana, C. (2017). A focus on the state of the art of food waste/losses issue and suggestions for future researches. *Waste Management (New York, N.Y.), 68*(Supplement C), 557–570. doi:10.1016/j.wasman.2017.06.047

Rahimifard, S., Stone, J., & Trollman, H. (2018). Global food security: The engineering challenges. *International Journal of Sustainable Engineering, 11*(2), 77–78. doi:10.1080/19397038.2018.1475091

Ray, D. K., Mueller, N. D., West, P. C., & Foley, J. A. (2013). Yield trends are insufficient to double global crop production by 2050. *PLoS One, 8*(6). doi:10.1371/journal.pone.0066428

Redlingshöfer, B., Coudurier, B., & Georget, M. (2017). Quantifying food loss during primary production and processing in France. *Journal of Cleaner Production, 164*(Supplement C), 703–714. doi:10.1016/j.jclepro.2017.06.173

United Nations. (2016). Report of the Inter-Agency and Expert Group on Sustainable Development Goal Indicators (E/CN.3/2016/2/Rev.1), Annex IV. Retrieved from https://sustainabledevelopment.un.org/content/documents/11803Official-List-of-Proposed-SDG-Indicators.pdf

United Nations, Department of Economic and Social Affairs. (2015). *World Population Prospects: The 2015 Revision, Key Findings and Advance Tables. Working Paper No. ESA/P/WP.241*. Retrieved from https://esa.un.org/unpd/wpp/publications/files/key_findings_wpp_2015.pdf

Wang, J. & Yue, H. (2017). Food safety pre-warning system based on data mining for a sustainable food supply chain. *Food Control, 73*(Part B), 223–229. doi:10.1016/j.foodcont.2016.09.048

Ward, S., & Chapman, C. (2003). Transforming project risk management into project uncertainty management. *International Journal of Project Management, 21*(2), 97–105. doi:10.1016/S0263-7863(01)00080-1

Žiha, K. (2000). Redundancy and robustness of systems of events. *Probabilistic Engineering Mechanics, 15*(4), 347–357. doi:10.1016/S0266-8920(99)00036-3

Zilberman, D., Lu, L., & Reardon, T. (2017). Innovation-induced food supply chain design. *Food Policy*. doi:10.1016/j.foodpol.2017.03.010

ADDITIONAL READING

Accorsi, R., Cholette, S., Manzini, R., Pini, C., & Penazzi, S. (2016). The land-network problem: Ecosystem carbon balance in planning sustainable agro-food supply chains. *Journal of Cleaner Production, 112*(Part 1), 158–171. doi:10.1016/j.jclepro.2015.06.082

Adler, M., & Dumas, B. (1984). Exposure to Currency Risk: Definition and Measurement. *Financial Management, 13*(2), 41–50. doi:10.2307/3665446

Ahumada, O., & Villalobos, J. R. (2009). Application of planning models in the agri-food supply chain: A review. *European Journal of Operational Research, 196*(1), 1–20. doi:10.1016/j.ejor.2008.02.014

Allen, S. J., & Schuster, E. W. (2004). Controlling the Risk for an Agricultural Harvest. *Manufacturing & Service Operations Management: M & SOM, 6*(3), 225–236. doi:10.1287/msom.1040.0035

Aqlan, F., & Mustafa Ali, E. (2014). Integrating lean principles and fuzzy bow-tie analysis for risk assessment in chemical industry. *Journal of Loss Prevention in the Process Industries, 29*, 39–48. doi:10.1016/j.jlp.2014.01.006

Bloemhof, J. M., van der Vorst, J. G. A. J., Bastl, M., & Allaoui, H. (2015). Sustainability assessment of food chain logistics. *International Journal of Logistics Research and Applications, 18*(2), 101–117. doi:10.1080/13675567.2015.1015508

Diabat, A., Govindan, K., & Panicker, V. V. (2012). Supply chain risk management and its mitigation in a food industry. *International Journal of Production Research, 50*(11), 3039–3050. doi:10.1080/00207543.2011.588619

Leat, P., & Revoredo-Giha, C. (2013). Risk and resilience in agri-food supply chains: The case of the ASDA PorkLink supply chain in Scotland. *Supply Chain Management*, *18*(2), 219–231. doi:10.1108/13598541311318845

Validi, S., Bhattacharya, A., & Byrne, P. J. (2014). A case analysis of a sustainable food supply chain distribution system—A multi-objective approach. *International Journal of Production Economics*, *152*, 71–87. doi:10.1016/j.ijpe.2014.02.003

Van der Vorst, J. G., Tromp, S.-O., & van der Zee, D.-J. (2009). Simulation modelling for food supply chain redesign; integrated decision making on product quality, sustainability and logistics. *International Journal of Production Research*, *47*(23), 6611–6631. doi:10.1080/00207540802356747

KEY TERMS AND DEFINITIONS

Focal Company: Companies governing over the supply chains, providing direct contact to end customers, and having bargain power over other actors in the SC (Christiansen, 2001).

Resilience: The ability of a system, community, or society exposed to hazards to resist, absorb, accommodate to and recover from the effects of a hazard in a timely and efficient manner, including through the preservation and restoration of its essential basic structures and functions. (ISDR, 2009).

Robustness: The belief that family is central to wellbeing and that family members and family issues take precedence over other aspects of life (Žiha, 2000).

Risk: The probability of an undesired event happening.

Vulnerability: The conditions determined by physical, social, economic and environmental factors or processes which increase the susceptibility of an individual, a community, assets or systems to the impacts of hazards (ISDR, 2009).

Mitigation: The lessening or minimizing of the adverse impacts of a hazardous event.

Disaster: Serious disruption of the functioning of a community or a society at any scale due to hazardous events interacting with conditions of exposure, vulnerability and capacity, leading to one or more of the following: human, material, economic and environmental losses and impacts.

Early Warning System: An integrated system of hazard monitoring, forecasting and prediction, disaster risk assessment, communication and preparedness activities systems and processes that enables individuals, communities, governments, businesses and others to take timely action to reduce disaster risks in advance of hazardous events (ISDR, 2009).

Exposure: The situation of people, infrastructure, housing, production capacities and other tangible human assets located in hazard-prone areas (ISDR, 2009).

Contingency Planning: A management process that analyses disaster risks and establishes arrangements in advance to enable timely, effective and appropriate responses (ISDR, 2009).

Perishable Food: Includes meat, poultry, fish, milk, eggs and many raw fruits and vegetables. All cooked foods are considered perishable foods. To store these foods for any length of time, perishable foods need to be held at refrigerator or freezer temperatures. If refrigerated, perishable foods should be used within several days (Albrecht, n.d.)

Semi-Perishable Food: If properly stored and handled, may remain unspoiled for six months to about one year. Flour, grain products, dried fruits and dry mixes are considered semi-perishable (Albrecht, n.d.).

Non-Perishable Food: Foods such as sugar, dried beans, spices and canned goods do not spoil unless they are handled carelessly. These foods will lose quality, however, if stored over a long time, even if stored under ideal conditions (Albrecht, n.d.).

This research was previously published in the Handbook of Research on Industrial Applications for Improved Supply Chain Performance edited by Jorge Luis García-Alcaraz, George Leal Jamil, Liliana Avelar-Sosa, and Antonio Juan Briones Peñalver; pages 299-324, copyright year 2020 by Business Science Reference (an imprint of IGI Global).

APPENDIX

Table 2. Contrasting the relationship of risk management in Food SC management with SDGs

SDG Indicators	Risk Management in SCM
Goal 1. End poverty in all its forms everywhere	Risk management in food SCs helps maintain preventive actions in the work place, maintaining food SCs during disasters and other shocks. And help recover from extreme event in order to minimize its impact on human life and well-being.
1.3.1 Proportion of population covered by social protection floors/systems, by sex, distinguishing children, unemployed persons, older persons, persons with disabilities, pregnant women, newborns, work injury victims and the poor and the vulnerable	
1.5 By 2030, build the resilience of the poor and those in vulnerable situations and reduce their exposure and vulnerability to climate-related extreme events and other economic, social and environmental shocks and disasters	
1.5.1 Number of deaths, missing persons and persons affected by disaster per 100,000 peoplea	
1.5.2 Direct disaster economic loss in relation to global gross domestic product (GDP)a	
1.5.3 Number of countries with national and local disaster risk reduction strategiesa	
Goal 2. End hunger, achieve food security and improved nutrition and promote sustainable agriculture	Food SCs play a major role in achieving the end of hunger. By providing reliable food chains access to nutritious and sufficient food sources is maintained. By integrating the straights of the full SC productivity can improve and small farmers can improve quality and yield, key to producing sufficient food. Moreover, information management systems can help secure important information is provided to limit market prices risks.
2.1 By 2030, end hunger and ensure access by all people, in particular the poor and people in vulnerable situations, including infants, to safe, nutritious and sufficient food all year round	
2.3 By 2030, double the agricultural productivity and incomes of small-scale food producers, in particular women, indigenous peoples, family farmers, pastoralists and fishers, including through secure and equal access to land, other productive resources and inputs, knowledge, financial services, markets and opportunities for value addition and non-farm employment	
2.4 By 2030, ensure sustainable food production systems and implement resilient agricultural practices that increase productivity and production, that help maintain ecosystems, that strengthen capacity for adaptation to climate change, extreme weather, drought, flooding and other disasters and that progressively improve land and soil quality	
2.c Adopt measures to ensure the proper functioning of food commodity markets and their derivatives and facilitate timely access to market information, including on food reserves, in order to help limit extreme food price volatility	
2.5.1 Number of plant and animal genetic resources for food and agriculture secured in either medium or long-term conservation facilities	
2.5.2 Proportion of local breeds classified as being at risk, not-at-risk or at unknown level of risk of extinction	
Goal 3. Ensure healthy lives and promote well-being for all at all ages	Risk reduction and preventive actions related to hazardous materials (biological and chemical) that can be emitted to the environment can greatly reduce the number of deaths and illness surrounding food SC actors.
3.9 By 2030, substantially reduce the number of deaths and illnesses from hazardous chemicals and air, water and soil pollution and contamination	
3.9.2 Mortality rate attributed to unsafe water, unsafe sanitation and lack of hygiene (exposure to unsafe Water, Sanitation and Hygiene for All (WASH) services)	
particular developing countries, for early warning, risk reduction and management of national and global health risks	

continues on following page

Table 2. Continued

SDG Indicators	Risk Management in SCM
Goal 6. Ensure availability and sustainable management of water and sanitation for all	By taking into account the limited resources that can be extracted from nature and the surrounding communities, plant locations and resource use efficiencies in the design phase of food SC building can help reduce the effects of water-use competition and other conflicts and harm due to water scarcity.
6.1 By 2030, achieve universal and equitable access to safe and affordable drinking water for all	
6.3 By 2030, improve water quality by reducing pollution, eliminating dumping and minimizing release of hazardous chemicals and materials, halving the proportion of untreated wastewater and substantially increasing recycling and safe reuse globally	
6.4 By 2030, substantially increase water-use efficiency across all sectors and ensure sustainable withdrawals and supply of freshwater to address water scarcity and substantially reduce the number of people suffering from water scarcity	
Goal 8. Promote sustained, inclusive and sustainable economic growth, full and productive employment and decent work for all	Risk mitigation strategies such as diversification and technology and innovation incorporation as means to reduce risk through the food SC also promote sustainable economic growth and wealth to distribute amongst actors in the chains and the communities they serve.
8.2 Achieve higher levels of economic productivity through diversification, technological upgrading and innovation, including through a focus on high-value added and labour-intensive sectors	
8.4 Improve progressively, through 2030, global resource efficiency in consumption and production and endeavor to decouple economic growth from environmental degradation, in accordance with the 10-Year Framework of Programmes on Sustainable Consumption and Production, with developed countries taking the lead	
Goal 9. Build resilient infrastructure, promote inclusive and sustainable industrialization and foster innovation	Building resilient and sustainable industrialization is the foundation of risk management in SCs, and includes food systems. By developing and managing value chains and the markets they serve with risk prevention and resilience perspective improves overall industrialization and SC formation and reliability.
9.1 Develop quality, reliable, sustainable and resilient infrastructure, including regional and trans-border infrastructure, to support economic development and human well-being, with a focus on affordable and equitable access for all	
9.3 Increase the access of small-scale industrial and other enterprises, in particular in developing countries, to financial services, including affordable credit, and their integration into value chains and markets	
9.4 By 2030, upgrade infrastructure and retrofit industries to make them sustainable, with increased resource-use efficiency and greater adoption of clean and environmentally sound technologies and industrial processes, with all countries taking action in accordance with their respective capabilities	
9.a Facilitate sustainable and resilient infrastructure development in developing countries through enhanced financial, technological and technical support to African countries, least developed countries, landlocked developing countries and small island developing States	
9.b Support domestic technology development, research and innovation in developing countries, including by ensuring a conducive policy environment for, inter alia, industrial diversification and value addition to commodities	
Goal 11. Make cities and human settlements inclusive, safe, resilient and sustainable	Resiliency in cities and smaller aggrupation will depend on reliable sources of food. Resilient and efficient food SC systems help cities and town be resilient in terms of access to food and water in disaster situations.
11.b By 2020, substantially increase the number of cities and human settlements adopting and implementing integrated policies and plans towards inclusion, resource efficiency, mitigation and adaptation to climate change, resilience to disasters, and develop and implement, in line with the Sendai Framework for Disaster Risk Reduction 2015-2030, holistic disaster risk management at all levels	

continues on following page

Table 2. Continued

SDG Indicators	Risk Management in SCM
Goal 12. Ensure sustainable consumption and production patterns	Sustainable consumption and production seeks to reduce the materials footprint of food production. In the case of industrial agricultural and processed food, the environmental footprint can be very large. By considering the risk factors through a life cycle approach, waste and loss of food can be minimized. Food SC design can also take into account global companies' willingness to incorporate information that may reduce environmental risks.
12.2.1 Material footprint, material footprint per capita, and material footprint per GDP	
12.3 By 2030, halve per capita global food waste at the retail and consumer levels and reduce food losses along production and SCs, including post-harvest losses	
12.4 By 2020, achieve the environmentally sound management of chemicals and all wastes throughout their life cycle, in accordance with agreed international frameworks, and significantly reduce their release to air, water and soil in order to minimize their adverse impacts on human health and the environment	
12.6 Encourage companies, especially large and transnational companies, to adopt sustainable practices and to integrate sustainability information into their reporting cycle	
Goal 13. Take urgent action to combat climate change and its impacts	Because food SCs depend on animals and plants that are affected by climate, resilience and adaption to hazards due to climate change may be included in risk prevention and resilience strategies during the design and management of food SC systems.
13.1 Strengthen resilience and adaptive capacity to climate-related hazards and natural disasters in all countries	
13.3 Improve education, awareness-raising and human and institutional capacity on climate change mitigation, adaptation, impact reduction and early warning	
Goal 14. Conserve and sustainably use the oceans, seas and marine resources for sustainable development	Fish stocks and sea plants that form a part of the diversity of food products and their respective chains depend on oceans stocks. Foods provided by the sea thus require risk management and recovery strategies to overcome and avoid stock (sourcing) depletion.
14.4 By 2020, effectively regulate harvesting and end overfishing, illegal, unreported and unregulated fishing and destructive fishing practices and implement science-based management plans, in order to restore fish stocks in the shortest time feasible, at least to levels that can produce maximum sustainable yield as determined by their biological characteristics	
Goal 15. Protect, restore and promote sustainable use of terrestrial ecosystems, sustainably manage forests, combat desertification, and halt and reverse land degradation and halt biodiversity loss	Agricultural practices have strained ecosystems due to land use changes. Moreover, industrialization of food PSs has also strained natural resources taken from the earth's landscapes. Creating risk that require design and management strategies to be overcome
15.1 By 2020, ensure the conservation, restoration and sustainable use of terrestrial and inland freshwater ecosystems and their services, in particular forests, wetlands, mountains and drylands, in line with obligations under international agreements	
15.3 By 2030, combat desertification, restore degraded land and soil, including land affected by desertification, drought and floods, and strive to achieve a land degradation-neutral world	

(Data Source:(United Nations, 2016))

Chapter 13
Risks in Sustainable Food Supply Chain Management

Yogesh Kumar Sharma
https://orcid.org/0000-0002-3779-4380
Graphic Era University (Deemed), India

Sachin Kumar Mangla
University of Plymouth, UK

Pravin P. Patil
Graphic Era University (Deemed), India

ABSTRACT

Sustainability is the important factor in the food sector, due to the large demand worldwide. Sustainability in food sector is not accepted globally as per the growing demand of food. Because of business risks, uncertainty, government policy, technology, innovation, etc. So, in this article we will discuss about the risks in adoption of sustainable food supply chain management (SFSCM) and ranking the risks by using Fuzzy Analytic Hierarchy Process (FAHP) technique. We acknowledged various SFSCM related risks and suitable correlation among the identified risks. Ranking the risks by using Fuzzy AHP approach based on their priorities. Nine risks were identified from literature survey and expert's views. Risks like safety, technology, and legal and monetary of food, etc., are barriers in successful adoption of sustainability in the food sector. The risks related some terms which were found according to Indian culture and lifestyle of Indians.

INTRODUCTION

Sustainable manufacturing and distribution are relevant and timely issue in production economics. This is mainly serious for the food industry. In many of the developing or developed countries food is the largest manufacturing sector (Gustavsson, Cederberg, Sonesson, Van Otterdijk, & Meybeck, 2011; Brown, 2012). But still food industries fighting with food wastages, food security and public health. Supply Chain

DOI: 10.4018/978-1-7998-5354-1.ch013

Management (SCM) is a management term in which we manage the whole process from raw material to the final product. SCM has its own limitations so company's moves to sustainable supply chain management (SSCM). Addition of sustainability in the process is the demand of present era. Sustainability is defined as to use the things in a sustainable manner for better future. Sustainability includes three factors like environmental protection, social responsibility and economic practice (Li, Wang, Chan, & Manzini, 2014). SSCM is applied in different industries like food, dairy, medical, automobile and many more.

Sustainable food supply chain management (SFSCM) mainly deals with the forward processes like procurement of materials, manufacturing, packaging and distribution along with reverse processes such as reuse of collected materials, so as to attain the sustainability concept in food supply chain. SFSCM is a powerful tool to reduce the wastages during the whole process and very important for environment protection. But the execution of SFSCM in industry is not so easy because, they are many hurdles in the path. So, the SFSCM is mainly focused on the integration of sustainability concept in food supply chain by removing the risks. Risk is an important factor for the successful adoption of SFSCM. Risks may be of different types in food supply chain, like market risk, operational risk, legal risk, regulatory risk, economic risk and many more. These risks are the hurdles/barriers for the execution of sustainability concept in food supply chain effectively. In addition to this, India is the best example where risks are always at their top in food supply chain. Organization and government are failed to implement sustainability concept in the supply chain successfully. Risk encompasses impacts on company's economic wealth. The probability that an adverse event will occur and the consequences of the adverse event, the combination of these two factors creates risk. The effect of these risks would disturb the sustainability concept in food supply chain (Wang, Chan, Yee, & Diaz-Rainey, 2012). In addition to, it is projected to determine and investigate the risks with an objective to rank them for the successful implementation and understating of SFSCM practices in industry. The first aim of the current study is to determine the risks related to SFSCM adoption. Second, aim of the current study is to analyze the risks and rank them for managing the adoption of SFSCM. But, analyzing of risks is not so easy due to uncertainty in data and decision (Wang, Chan, Yee, & Diaz-Rainey, 2012). To remove the vagueness or uncertainty in the process to analyze the risks, it is planned to use fuzzy theory with (AHP) analytic hierarchy process technique. The AHP technique (Saaty, 1980; Aouam, Lamrani, Aguenaou, & Diabat, 2009) is most common and important to rank the multi criteria decision model but having some limitations regarding the vagueness in the data and judgments. To remove the uncertainty fuzzy set is proposed with AHP to attain the aim of the current research.

The rest of the paper is planned as follows. Literature reviews of SFSCM and their risks; explains about the adopted solution methodology; result and discussion and their managerial implications; explains the conclusions and limitations as well as future scope of the present research.

LITERATURE REVIEW

This section summarizes the literature on sustainable food supply chain management, risks and the use of Fuzzy AHP for the successful adoption of SFSCM.

Sustainable Food Supply Chain Management (SFSCM) Adoption

Increasing demands for food forces the companies to add sustainability in their processes to protect the environment and reduce the wastage of food. SFSCM is a key for food companies to develop climate resilient agricultural sourcing strategies that are free from environmental degradation and negative human impacts. Food companies are already leveraging their influence to help farmers adopt practices that will create healthy soils, conserve water supplies, respect the rights of workers and support biodiversity, as a report by Ceres highlights. Some companies offer technical assistance and incentives while others develop practice and policies to help farmers (Li, Wang, Chan, & Manzini, 2014).

Risks in Adoption of SFSCM

It is difficult to forecast that what will happen in the future, as there is an involvement of risks in all the operations (Gurnani, Mehrotra, & Ray, 2012). For the managerial point of view, risks is a threat in the supply chain that stop and disturb the whole process any time. Failure of machines, failure of government policies, failure of market, failure in packing and failure of logistics are the risks that delay the delivery of products and also affects the economic profit of the organization. So, it is essential to recognize and handle the risks in SFSCM adoption for the preferred aim (Mangla, Madaan, & Chan, 2013). In addition, a number of researchers and scholars have tried to find out the risks and their sources regarding sustainability in food supply chain. Ghadge et al., (2013) provide the potential failure points and overall impact of the risks for the execution of sustainability in food supply chain. They used systems thinking concepts for finding and modeling of risks in supply chain. Gold et al., (2013) applied SSCM to Base of the Pyramid (BoP) projects that can help multinational companies to implement sustainability in food industries. Beske et al. (2014) provided the SSCM practices which allows the organizations to control and manage the supply chain to achieve sustainability in their processes to reduce the risks. Ganguly et al. (2013) used Fuzzy AHP approach for assessing supply risks for product category. The approach is used to establish the supply associated risk and its possible impact on the consumer organization. Kumar and Garg (2017) used Fuzzy AHP approach in automobile industry to rank the indicators to reduce its uncertainty and impreciseness. In the current study, nine risks in the adoption of SFSCM in industries are based on literature and resources. Identified risks were explained in Table 1.

SOLUTION METHODOLOGY

The objective behind the selection of this approach is the identification, assessment and ranking of determined risks to achieve the goal of sustainability adoption in food supply chain. In present work, decision makers include experts from the domain specific and they are highly experienced and qualified and able to take decisions. In addition to 9 risks were identified from the existing literature and expert's opinions (see Table 1). So, we use Fuzzy AHP approach for evaluation of the risks associated with adoption of SFSCM initiatives in food industry. The flow chart of Fuzzy AHP is shown in (Figure 1).

Table 1. Risks in adoption of SFSCM

S. No.	Risks in SFSCM	Description	Authors
1	Regulatory risks (RR)	Regulatory risk is generally the risk in law and regulations which affects an industry or business. These changes can make desirable changes in cost and framework of industry.	Marsden et al., (2014), Montabon et al., (2016) and Scholtenand, (2017).
2	Market risks (MR)	Market risk is also called as "systematic risk" in which investor can meet losses because of factors affecting the performance of the financial markets.	Leat and Revoredo-Giha, (2013), Fayet and Vermeulen, (2014), Kirwan et al., (2017) and Song et al., (2017).
3	Technological Risks (TR)	Technology risk is important for business as it threatens assets and processes. This risk can also affect profitability and company's reputation in the market place.	Freidberg, (2017), Tse and Zhang, (2017) and Zilberman and Reardon, (2017).
4	Legal risks (LR)	Legal risk comprises the risk of reputational or financial resulting from inadequacy of awareness regarding law and regulations.	Gustafson et al., (2016), Berger-Walliser et al., (2016), Carstensen et al., (2016) and Rueda et al., (2017)
5	Economical risks (ER)	Economic risk is the risk in financial condition of the business/ industry. This risk can due to the employee expense, misconduct from the vendor (inflated bills and falsified labor).	Olson et al., (2017) and Kozup, 2017.
6	Logistics and operations risks (LOR)	Logistics and operations risks comprise of damage, delay and piracy and many transportation and logistics companies are lacking in the field.	Accorsi et al., (2017), Mogre et al., (2017) and Qaiser et al., (2017).

Figure 1. Research flowchart

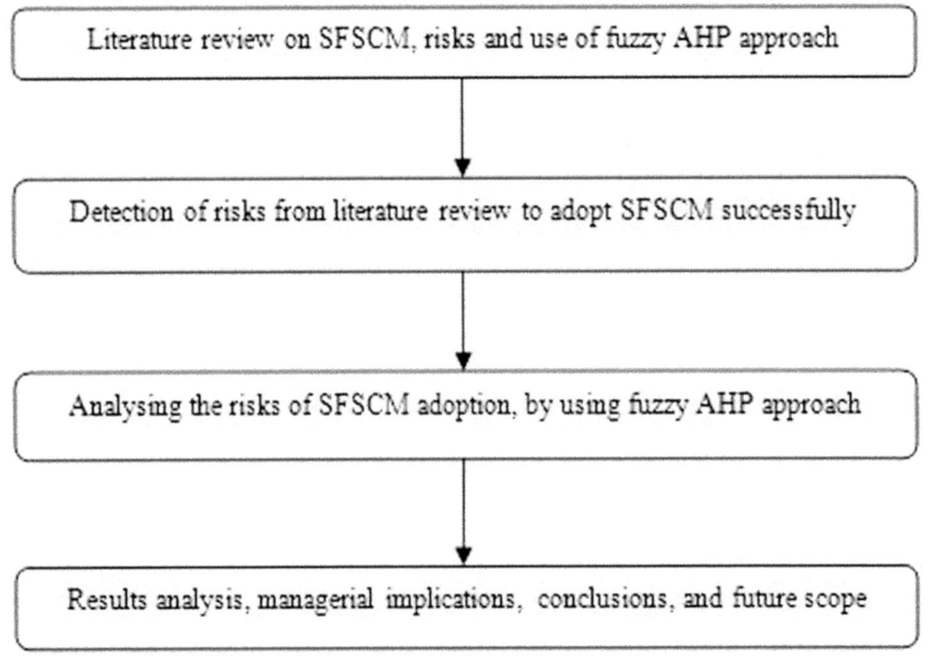

Fuzzy AHP Technique

In the present study AHP approach had been used. AHP is a technique which helps in organizing, decomposing, and analyzing any complex problem. This approach changes the problem into a hierarchical structure (Saaty 1980; Govindan, 2015; Mangla, Madaan, Sarma, & Gupta, 2014). In addition, many other methods like Technique for Order of Preference by Similarity to Ideal Solution (TOPSIS), Decision Making Trial and Evaluation Laboratory Model (DEMATEL), Analytical Network Process (ANP) and ELimination Et Choix Traduisant la REalité (ELimination and Choice Expressing REality (ELECTRE) were used to solve the MCDM problem. The approach is widely accepted by researchers and industrialist because it is ease in use. It is a better tool as compared to other tools presented in the current scenario (Harputlugil, Prins, Tanj Gültekin, & Topçu, 2011). Based on the fineness of (AHP) approach, it is widely used by several practitioners in various sectors like manufacturing, engineering, automobile and education etc. for solving dissimilar MCDM problems (Luthra, Garg, & Haleem, 2013; Govindan, Kaliyan, Kannan, & Haq, 2014; Luthra, Govindan, Kannan, Mangla, & Garg, 2017; Pandey, Garg, & Luthra, 2018). So, judgments for the risks, based on human decisions always full of biasness and vagueness and in this condition, AHP approach is not appropriate. To manage the uncertainty in the decisions, it is planned to use the fuzzy set theory with AHP approach (Chan, Kumar, Tiwari, Lau, & Choy, 2008; Jakhar & Barua, 2013; Mangla, Kumar, & Barua, 2016; Mathivathanan, Kannan, & Haq, 2018). The advantages of fuzzy theory help to use the developed approach Fuzzy (AHP) in the real-world situations for making correct decisions. However, the fuzzy judgments made by experts are converted into the correct numbers with the help of fuzzy numbers. In (Figure 2), (Chan, Kumar, Tiwari, Lau, & Choy, 2008; Baidya, Rahul, Kumar Dey, Ghosh, & Petridis, 2018) the flow chart of Fuzzy AHP based model analysis is explained and describes the various steps in it that are mentioned below.

Figure 2. Flow diagram of Fuzzy AHP analysis

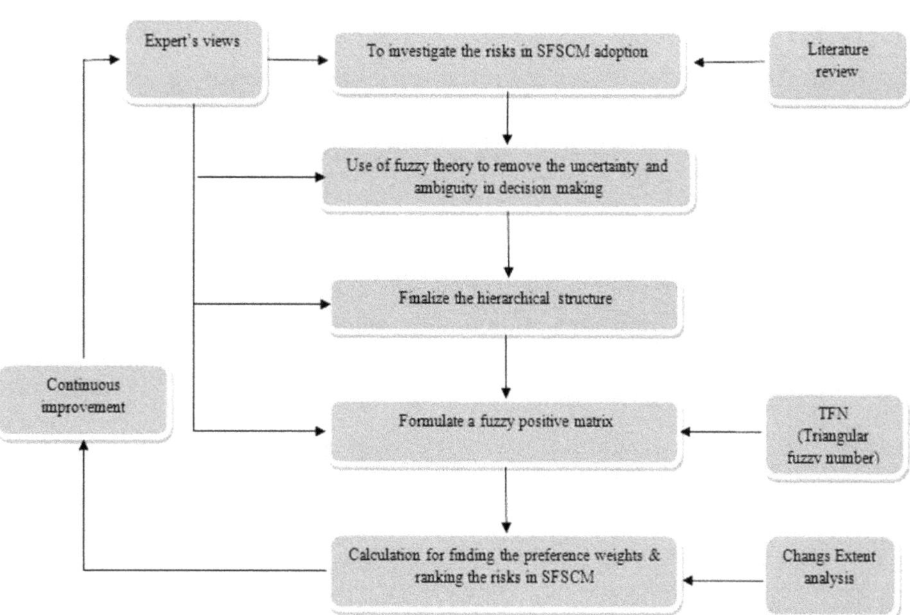

Step One: The objective of the current study is to analyze the risks in adoption of SFSCM, is defined.

Step Two: For analyzing the problem, under the circumstances of uncertainty and biasness in the decision, fuzzy set theory gives the clear and correct information logically (Zadeh, 1965). In fuzzy set theory, if a set of things is mentioned by 'Y', and 'y' having values $\left(y_1, y_2, y_3, y_n\right)$ presents the common element of 'Y', next, the fuzzy set 'N' for this set is denoted by $\{B, \mu_n\left(Y\right)) \mid y \epsilon Y\}$ (Dubois and Prade, 1979). In addition to, N(x) represents its function that operates over a scale of real numbers, mainly between the interval of [0, 1]. Next, a TFN (triangular fuzzy number) is used and is a particular kind of number and frequently used for practical purposes (Zimmerman, 1996). TFN (r, s, t) membership function is mathematically expressed as N(x), given in the Equation (1), where r $\leq$ s $\leq$ t, additionally, (r, s, t) denotes the lower, mean and upper boundary of TFN.

$$\mu_n\left(Y\right) = \begin{cases} 0, & Y \leq r \\ \dfrac{x-r}{s-r}, & Y \in \left[r, s\right] \\ \dfrac{x-t}{s-t}, & Y \in \left[s, t\right] \\ 0, & Y > t \end{cases} \tag{1}$$

Step Three: Obtain the hierarchical arrangement. Consider, the linguistic decision given by experts, the pair wise evaluation matrix is obtained.

Step Four: Formulate the fuzzy positive matrix. To convert the linguistics terms into exact values, the pair-wise evaluation matrix is replaced by equivalent positive TFN, which can be known by, $Y = [C_{ij}]_{nxm}$ next, the fuzzy entities are represents by, $C_{ij} = (r_{ij}, s_{ij}, t_{ij})$ and then positive fuzzy numbers have some properties.

$$r_{ij} = \frac{1}{r_{ji}}, s_{ij} = \frac{1}{s_{ji}}, t_{ij} = \frac{1}{t_{ij}}$$

where, i and j = 1, 2, 3, ..., k

Step Five: Calculations were done for finding the relative weight of the risks. It requires, aggregating the fuzzy numbers into crisp values, which allows the analysts to find out the relative weight of the risks associated to SFSCM implementation. In this study, Chang's extent method is used, and this method is accepted worldwide for finding the aggregate weights for pair wise evaluation matrix.

RESULTS AND DISCUSSION

Data Collection

In the present research, data collection was made i.e., based on literature survey and the expert's opinions. Experts are highly experienced and qualified from the domain specific and they are capable for decision making. In addition to this, nine risks were determined in which six were selected in (Table 1) from literature survey and rest three in (Table 2) from expert opinions. Total nine risks were taken into account to analyze the ranking of the risks for the adoption of SFSCM successfully.

Table 2. Risks added by experts

S. No.	Risks in SFSCM	Description	Authors
7	Governance and cooperation risks (GCR)	Government and cooperation risk is the risk in which government policies are not implemented successfully or they affect the business.	Cagliano et al., (2016), Koopmans et al., (2017) and Zhu et al., (2017).
8	Packaging and contamination risks (PCR)	Packaging and contamination risk is the risk in packaging of food. Packaging of food in vital as it provides protection or resistance, ensuring the freshness and extending the shelf life of food. It should have nutrition facts, manufacturing and expiry date labeled on it.	Verghese et al., (2013), Cruz et al., (2016), Giannakis and Papadopoulos, (2016) and Laszlo and Zhexembayeva, (2017).
9	Quality and safety risks (QSR)	In high risk products like ready to eat food which are manufactured under vulnerable circumstances, there is high risk. As the people are aware about the food safety, efforts are to be made in increasing the food quality.	Bourlakis et al., (2014), Piramuthuand and Zhou, (2016), Lehtinen, (2017) and Starbird and Amanor-Boadu (2017).

Recognition of Common Risks in Adoption of SFSCM

Based on literature survey and experts views, nine risks (RR, MR, TR, LR, ER, LOR, GCR, PCR and QSR) were finalized. These risks were determined for the adoption of SFSCM successfully.

Assessment and Ranking of Determined Risks Using Fuzzy AHP

The risks were ranked according to their weights. In this study we use fuzzy AHP, to remove the biasness in the judgments made by humans. Wang et al., 2007, proposed the pair wise assessment matrix for the risks. A nine point scale is used in the present study to help in the construction of pair wise evaluation matrix.

Construction of Fuzzy Positive Matrix

Fuzzy linguistic scale is given by Wang (Table 3). This scale is used by experts, for the assessment of pair wise matrix for the adoption of SFSCM. Based on the final opinions of experts, a final pair wise evaluation matrix was constructed. However, TFNs were used to transform the pair wise assessment matrix into positive fuzzy number. The formulated fuzzy pair-wise evaluation matrix for risks in SFSCM adoption is given in (Table 4).

Table 3. Fuzzy linguistic scale

Vague Judgment	Fuzzy Score
Approximately equal	1/2,1,2
Approximately a times more important	a − 1, a, a + 1
Approximately a times less important	1/a + 1, 1/a, 1/a − 1
Between b and c times more important	b, (b + c)/2, c
Between b and c times less important	1/c, 2/(b + c), 1/b

Calculation for Relative Weights

Calculation of preference weights was based on the Changs extent analysis method between the risks for the adoption of SFSCM. The preference weights are very useful for the ranking of the risks in the list (Table 5), and these ranks are also useful for the successful adoption of SFSCM.

Priority order of the risks before (RR>MR>LR>TR>ER>LOR>GCR>PCR>QSR) and after (PCR>LOR>GCR>QSR>TR>RR>ER>MR>LR), applying the fuzzy AHP approach. So, the findings of the present work based on their relative weights help the managers to implement the adoption of SFSCM successfully in the organization. The research findings were further discussed with experts in the domain for the successful adoption of SFSCM in food industry to increase their productivity and performance.

Packaging and contamination risk (PCR) attains the highest position in the priority list with value of 1.45. Every time there is a problem of packaging of food products and due to that companies are facing heavy loss (Gaudiano, Manna, Bartolomei, Rodomonte, Bertocchi, Antoniella, & Valvo, 2016). Especially in food industries, packaging and contamination risk which is directly related to human health. So, managers take this risk very seriously.

Logistics and operations risks (LOR) hold the second place in the priority list having value (0.95). Logistics and operations risks (LOR), is also having a good impact on food industries. Piracy, delay and damage are included in this risk (Nakandala, Lau, & Zhao, 2017). Managers should focus on logistic and operational risk for the adoption of SFSCM.

Government and corporation risk comes at the third position in the priority list with value of 0.79. Government and corporation policies (GCR) sometimes became a hurdle in front of companies (Song & Zhuang, 2017). In this risk policies made by governments are not implemented successfully, so the consequences are faced by the organizations and it affects the business as well. Adoption of SFSCM is not easy without fulfilling the requirements of government. So, managers should focus on this as well.

Quality and safety risks (QSR) holds the fourth place in the priority list with value of 0.70. Quality and safety risk (QSR) is always there where the food is ready to eat. Awareness of quality in food among the public is increased now-a-days so they pressurize the companies to make the food of good standards (Cortese, Veiros, Feldman, & Cavalli, 2016). Mangers should consider quality and safety risk very seriously and it is directly related to the packaging risk, for the successful adoption of SFSCM.

Technological risk (TR) attains the fifth place in the priority list with value of 0.50. Technological risk (TR) is always a matter of risk because upgrading of technology directly increases the economic pressure on company. SFSCM requires high technology to manufacture any product sustainably (Fox-Glassman & Weber, 2016). Adoption of SFSCM is a question mark in front of companies because of

Table 4. TFNs based pair-wise evaluation matrix for risks in SFSCM adoption

	RR			MR			TR			LR			ER			LOR			GCR			PCR			QSR		
RR	1.0	1.0	1.0	0.3	0.3	0.5	0.3	0.3	0.5	4.0	5.0	6.0	2.0	3.0	4.0	6.0	7.0	8.0	0.1	0.1	0.2	0.2	0.2	0.3	6.0	7.0	8.0
MR	2.0	3.0	4.0	1.0	1.0	1.0	4.0	5.0	6.0	0.1	0.1	0.2	0.2	0.2	0.3	4.0	5.0	6.0	0.3	0.3	0.5	0.2	0.2	0.3	6.0	7.0	8.0
TR	2.0	3.0	4.0	4.0	5.0	6.0	1.0	1.0	1.0	4.0	5.0	6.0	2.0	3.0	4.0	1.0	2.0	3.0	2.0	3.0	4.0	0.1	0.1	0.2	7.0	8.0	9.0
LR	0.2	0.2	0.3	6.0	7.0	8.0	0.2	0.2	0.3	1.0	1.0	1.0	0.1	0.1	0.2	4.0	5.0	6.0	0.2	0.2	0.3	0.1	0.1	0.1	6.0	7.0	8.0
ER	0.3	0.3	0.5	4.0	5.0	6.0	0.3	0.3	0.5	6.0	7.0	8.0	1.0	1.0	1.0	5.0	6.0	7.0	1.0	2.0	3.0	0.1	0.1	0.2	4.0	5.0	6.0
LOR	0.1	0.1	0.2	0.2	0.2	0.3	0.3	0.5	1.0	0.2	0.2	0.3	0.1	0.2	0.2	1.0	1.0	1.0	0.1	0.1	0.2	0.2	0.2	0.3	2.0	3.0	4.0
GCR	6.0	7.0	8.0	2.0	3.0	4.0	4.0	5.0	6.0	4.0	5.0	6.0	4.0	5.0	6.0	6.0	7.0	8.0	1.0	1.0	1.0	0.2	0.2	0.3	6.0	7.0	8.0
PCR	0.1	0.1	0.2	0.1	0.1	0.2	0.1	0.1	0.1	0.1	0.1	0.2	0.2	0.2	0.3	0.3	0.3	0.5	0.1	0.1	0.2	1.0	1.0	1.0	6.0	7.0	8.0
QSR	0.2	0.2	0.3	0.1	0.1	0.2	0.1	0.1	0.2	0.1	0.1	0.2	0.2	0.2	0.3	1.0	1.0	1.0	0.1	0.1	0.2	0.1	0.1	0.2	1.0	1.0	1.0

Table 5. Ranking of SFs

S. No	Risks in SFSCM	Relative Weights	Ranking
1	RR	0.24	7
2	MR	0.15	8
3	TR	0.50	5
4	LR	0.06	9
5	ER	0.37	6
6	LOR	0.95	2
7	GCR	0.79	3
8	PCR	1.45	1
9	QSR	0.70	4

Source: Fuzzy AHP analysis

high cost of equipment's and there is always a risk of loss. Decision makers should understand the impact of technological risk for the adoption of SFSCM in food industry.

Economic risk (ER) attains the sixth position in the priority list with value of 0.37. Economic risk (ER), directly affects the profits of the company. Proper monitoring and proper uses of statistical tools can help the company to minimize the risk of fraud (Bearth & Siegrist, 2016). Therefore, policy makers should focus their efforts on economic risks for the adoption of SFSCM.

Regulatory risk (RR) comes at seventh the place in the priority list having value of 0.24. Regulatory risk (RR) affects the company's profits. It also affects the business and company structure in many ways (Jain, Ranjan, Dasgupta, & Ramalingam, 2016). So, managers consider this a risk for the successful adoption of SFSCM.

Market risk (MR) comes at the second last in the priority list with value of 0.15. Market is always depending on the investors, if they feel that their investment is not worthy they withdraw their investment (Boyer & Yang, 2017). So, market risk is very important according to the company's point of view. Decision makers should focus on market risk for the successful adoption of SFSCM.

Legal risk (LR) comes at the last with least value of 0.06. Legal risk (LR) is not as much important as other risks. All the risks which were discussed in the section are important for the adoption of SFSCM successfully. Decision makers should focus on these risks for the adoption of SFSCM successfully.

CONCLUSION/ LIMITATIONS

Sustainable food supply chain management (SFSCM) is a tool that helps the food companies to maintain their processes eco-friendly. SFSCM reduces the wastages during the whole processes and helps the companies to achieve their goals. But most of the companies do not agree to adopt SFSCM because of high cost of installation of equipment's, risks like economic, legal, and operational etc. In the present research work, various risks were identified with the help of literature review and expert views. After the discussion with experts, nine risks for the adoption of SFSCM were finalized to reduce the ambiguity in the decisions made by humans regarding risks. The motive of this work is to suggest a structural framework for the evaluation of risks for SFSCM adoption. Fuzzy set theory is used with AHP approach for analyzing these risks. In fuzzy AHP, method the risks were ranked according to their preference weights. Results showing that packaging and contamination risk (PCR) comes at the first place and legal risk (LR) comes at the last place in the priority list of risk. Current research finds that risks have their own impact in SFSCM adoption. Decision makers should focus on the risks according to their rank in the list. The model proposed in this work has some limitations. The identification and evaluation of the risks in SFSCM adoption is not easy. Moreover, some error may occur due to human biasness. In the future we may use some other MCDM tools like decision-making trial and evaluation laboratory (DEMATEL), grey relational analysis (GRA), best worst method (BWM) etc.

ACKNOWLEDGMENT

The authors acknowledge and express the gratitude for the support of the research facilities and funds provided by the Department of Mechanical Engineering, Graphic Era (Deemed to be) University, Dehradun, India.

REFERENCES

Accorsi, R., Manzini, R., & Pini, C. (2017). How Logistics Decisions Affect the Environmental Sustainability of Modern Food Supply Chains: A Case Study from an Italian Large-scale Retailer. *Sustainability Challenges in the Agrofood Sector, 175*.

Aouam, T., Lamrani, H., Aguenaou, S., & Diabat, A. (2009). A benchmark based AHP model for credit evaluation. *International Journal of Applied Decision Sciences, 2*(2), 151–166. doi:10.1504/IJADS.2009.026550

Baidya, R., Dey, P. K., Ghosh, S. K., & Petridis, K. (2018). Strategic maintenance technique selection using combined quality function deployment, the analytic hierarchy process and the benefit of doubt approach. *International Journal of Advanced Manufacturing Technology, 94*(1-4), 31–44. doi:10.100700170-016-9540-1

Bearth, A., & Siegrist, M. (2016). Are risk or benefit perceptions more important for public acceptance of innovative food technologies: A meta-analysis. *Trends in Food Science & Technology, 49*, 14–23. doi:10.1016/j.tifs.2016.01.003

Berger-Walliser, G., Shrivastava, P., & Sulkowski, A. J. (2016). Using Proactive Legal Strategies for Corporate Environmental Sustainability.

Beske, P., Land, A., & Seuring, S. (2014). Sustainable supply chain management practices and dynamic capabilities in the food industry: A critical analysis of the literature. *International Journal of Production Economics, 152*, 131–143. doi:10.1016/j.ijpe.2013.12.026

Bloemhof, J., & van der Vorst, J. G. A. J. (2015). *Sustainable food supply chain networks. Markets, business, and sustainability* (pp. 99–122). The Netherlands: Bentham Books.

Bourlakis, M., Maglaras, G., Gallear, D., & Fotopoulos, C. (2014). Examining sustainability performance in the supply chain: The case of the Greek dairy sector. *Industrial Marketing Management, 43*(1), 56–66. doi:10.1016/j.indmarman.2013.08.002

Boyer, R. R., & Yang, L. L. (2017). Establishing a Food Safe Market: Considerations for Vendors at the Farmers Market. *Food Safety for Farmers Markets: A Guide to Enhancing Safety of Local Foods, 145.*

Brown, R. L. (2012). *Full Planet, Empty Plates: The New Geopolitics of Food Scarcity.* WA, USA: Earth Policy Institute.

Cagliano, R., Worley, C. G., & Caniato, F. F. (2016). The Challenge of Sustainable Innovation in Agri-Food Supply Chains. In *Organizing Supply Chain Processes for Sustainable Innovation in the Agri-Food Industry* (pp. 1–30). Emerald Group Publishing Limited. doi:10.1108/S2045-060520160000005009

Carstensen, P. C., Lianos, I., Lombardi, C., MacDonald, J. M., & Moss, D. L. (2016). Competition law and policy and the food value chain. *Concurrences,* (1), 22-35.

Chan, F. T. S., Kumar, N., Tiwari, M. K., Lau, H. C. W., & Choy, K. L. (2008). Global supplier selection: A fuzzy-AHP approach. *International Journal of Production Research, 46*(14), 3825–3857. doi:10.1080/00207540600787200

Cortese, R. D. M., Veiros, M. B., Feldman, C., & Cavalli, S. B. (2016). Food safety and hygiene practices of vendors during the chain of street food production in Florianopolis, Brazil: A cross-sectional study. *Food Control, 62,* 178–186. doi:10.1016/j.foodcont.2015.10.027

Cruz-Romero, M., & Kerry, J. P. (2016). Packaging systems and materials used for meat products with particular emphasis on the use of oxygen scavenging systems. In *Emerging Technologies in Meat Processing: Production, Processing and Technology* (pp. 231-263).

Dubois, D., & Prade, H. (1979). Fuzzy real algebra: Some results. *Fuzzy Sets and Systems, 2*(4), 327–348. doi:10.1016/0165-0114(79)90005-8

Fayet, L., & Vermeulen, W. J. (2014). Supporting smallholders to access sustainable supply chains: Lessons from the Indian cotton supply chain. *Sustainable Development, 22*(5), 289–310. doi:10.1002d.1540

Fox-Glassman, K. T., & Weber, E. U. (2016). What makes risk acceptable? Revisiting the 1978 psychological dimensions of perceptions of technological risks. *Journal of Mathematical Psychology, 75,* 157–169. doi:10.1016/j.jmp.2016.05.003

Freidberg, S. (2017). Big Food and Little Data: The Slow Harvest of Corporate Food Supply Chain Sustainability Initiatives. *Annals of the Association of American Geographers, 107(6), 1389-1406.*

Ganguly, K. K., & Guin, K. K. (2013). A fuzzy AHP approach for inbound supply risk assessment. *Benchmarking: An International Journal, 20*(1), 129–146. doi:10.1108/14635771311299524

Gaudiano, M. C., Manna, L., Bartolomei, M., Rodomonte, A. L., Bertocchi, P., Antoniella, E., & Valvo, L. (2016). Health risks related to illegal and on-line sale of drugs and food supplements: Results of a survey on marketed products in Italy from 2011 to 2013. *Annali dell'Istituto Superiore di Sanita, 52*(1), 128–132. PMID:27033629

Ghadge, A., Dani, S., Chester, M., & Kalawsky, R. (2013). A systems approach for modelling supply chain risks. *Supply Chain Management, 18*(5), 523–538. doi:10.1108/SCM-11-2012-0366

Giannakis, M., & Papadopoulos, T. (2016). Supply chain sustainability: A risk management approach. *International Journal of Production Economics, 171*, 455–470. doi:10.1016/j.ijpe.2015.06.032

Gold, S., Hahn, R., & Seuring, S. (2013). Sustainable supply chain management in "Base of the Pyramid" food projects—A path to triple bottom line approaches for multinationals? *International Business Review, 22*(5), 784–799. doi:10.1016/j.ibusrev.2012.12.006

Govindan, K. (2015). Embedding sustainability dynamics in supply chain relationship management and governance structures: Introduction, review and opportunities. *Journal of Cleaner Production.* doi:10.1016/j.jclepro.2015.11.036

Govindan, K., Kaliyan, M., Kannan, D., & Haq, A. N. (2014). Barriers analysis for green supply chain management implementation in Indian industries using analytic hierarchy process. *International Journal of Production Economics, 147*, 555–568. doi:10.1016/j.ijpe.2013.08.018

Gurnani, H., Mehrotra, A., & Ray, S. (2012). *Supply chain disruptions: Theory and practice of managing risk.* London: Springer. doi:10.1007/978-0-85729-778-5

Gustafson, D., Gutman, A., Leet, W., Drewnowski, A., Fanzo, J., & Ingram, J. (2016). Seven food system metrics of sustainable nutrition security. *Sustainability, 8*(3), 196. doi:10.3390u8030196

Gustavsson, J., Cederberg, C., Sonesson, U., Van Otterdijk, R., & Meybeck, A. (2011). *Global food losses and food waste* (pp. 1–38). Rome: FAO.

Harputlugil, T., Prins, M., Tanju Gültekin, A., & Ilker Topçu, Y. (2011). Conceptual framework for potential implementations of multi criteria decision making (MCDM) methods for design quality assessment. In *Management and Innovation for a Sustainable Built Environment; CIB International Conference MISBE 2011*, Amsterdam, June 20-23. Delft University of Technology.

Jain, A., Ranjan, S., Dasgupta, N., & Ramalingam, C. (2016). Nanomaterials in food and agriculture: An overview on their safety concerns and regulatory issues. *Critical Reviews in Food Science and Nutrition.*

Jakhar, S. K., & Barua, M. K. (2013). An integrated model of supply chain performance evaluation and decision-making using structural equation modelling and fuzzy AHP. *Production Planning Control: The Management of Operations, 25*(11), 938–957. doi:10.1080/09537287.2013.782616

Kirwan, J., Maye, D., & Brunori, G. (2017). Acknowledging complexity in food supply chains when assessing their performance and sustainability. *Journal of Rural Studies, 52*, 21–32. doi:10.1016/j.jrurstud.2017.03.008

Koopmans, M. E., Rogge, E., Mettepenningen, E., Knickel, K., & Šūmane, S. (2017). The role of multi-actor governance in aligning farm modernization and sustainable rural development. *Journal of Rural Studies.*

Kozup, J. (2017). Risks of Consumer Products. In *Consumer Perception of Product Risks and Benefits* (pp. 23–38). Springer International Publishing. doi:10.1007/978-3-319-50530-5_2

Kumar, D., & Garg, C. P. (2017). Evaluating sustainable supply chain indicators using Fuzzy AHP: Case of Indian automotive industry. *Benchmarking: An International Journal, 24*(6), 1742–1766. doi:10.1108/BIJ-11-2015-0111

Laszlo, C., & Zhexembayeva, N. (2017). *Embedded sustainability: The next big competitive advantage.* Routledge.

Leat, P., & Revoredo-Giha, C. (2013). Risk and resilience in agri-food supply chains: The case of the ASDA PorkLink supply chain in Scotland. *Supply Chain Management, 18*(2), 219–231. doi:10.1108/13598541311318845

Lehtinen, U. (2017). Sustainable Supply Chain Management in Agri-food Chains: A Competitive Factor for Food Exporters. *Sustainability Challenges in the Agrofood Sector, 150.*

Li, D., Wang, X., Chan, H. K., & Manzini, R. (2014). Sustainable food supply chain management. *International Journal of Production Economics, 152,* 1–8. doi:10.1016/j.ijpe.2014.04.003

Luthra, S., Garg, D., & Haleem, A. (2013). Identifying and ranking of strategies to implement green supply chain management in Indian manufacturing industry using Analytical Hierarchy Process. *Journal of Industrial Engineering and Management, 6*(4), 930. doi:10.3926/jiem.693

Luthra, S., Govindan, K., Kannan, D., Mangla, S. K., & Garg, C. P. (2017). An integrated framework for sustainable supplier selection and evaluation in supply chains. *Journal of Cleaner Production, 140,* 1686–1698. doi:10.1016/j.jclepro.2016.09.078

Mangla, S. K., Kumar, P., & Barua, M. K. (2016). An integrated methodology of FTA and fuzzy AHP for risk assessment in green supply chain. *International Journal of Operation Research, 25*(1), 77–99. doi:10.1504/IJOR.2016.073252

Mangla, S., Madaan, J., & Chan, F. T. (2013). Analysis of flexible decision strategies for sustainability-focused green product recovery system. *International Journal of Production Research, 51*(11), 3428–3442. doi:10.1080/00207543.2013.774493

Mangla, S., Madaan, J., Sarma, P. R. S., & Gupta, M. P. (2014). Multi-objective decision modelling using interpretive structural modelling for green supply chains. *International Journal of Logistics Systems and Management, 17*(2), 125–142. doi:10.1504/IJLSM.2014.059113

Marsden, T., & Morley, A. (Eds.). (2014). *Sustainable food systems: building a new paradigm.* Routledge.

Mathivathanan, D., Kannan, D., & Haq, A. N. (2018). Sustainable supply chain management practices in Indian automotive industry: A multi-stakeholder view. *Resources, Conservation and Recycling, 128,* 284–305. doi:10.1016/j.resconrec.2017.01.003

Mogre, R., Mogre, R., Lindgreen, A., Lindgreen, A., Hingley, M., & Hingley, M. (2017). Tracing the evolution of purchasing research: Future trends and directions for purchasing practices. *Journal of Business and Industrial Marketing, 32*(2), 251–257. doi:10.1108/JBIM-01-2016-0004

Montabon, F., Pagell, M., & Wu, Z. (2016). Making sustainability sustainable. *The Journal of Supply Chain Management, 52*(2), 11–27. doi:10.1111/jscm.12103

Nakandala, D., Lau, H., & Zhao, L. (2017). Development of a hybrid fresh food supply chain risk assessment model. *International Journal of Production Research*, *55*(14), 4180–4195. doi:10.1080/0020 7543.2016.1267413

Olson, D. L., & Wu, D. D. (2017). Enterprise Risk Management in Supply Chains. In *Enterprise Risk Management Models* (pp. 1–15). Springer Berlin Heidelberg.

Pandey, H., Garg, D., & Luthra, S. (2018). Identification and ranking of enablers of green lean Six Sigma implementation using AHP. *International Journal of Productivity and Quality Management*, *23*(2), 187–217. doi:10.1504/IJPQM.2018.089156

Piramuthu, S., & Zhou, W. (2016). *RFID and sensor network automation in the food industry: ensuring quality and safety through supply chain visibility*. John Wiley & Sons. doi:10.1002/9781118967423

Qaiser, F. H., Qaiser, F. H., Ahmed, K., Ahmed, K., Sykora, M., Sykora, M., ... Simpson, M. (2017). Decision support systems for sustainable logistics: A review and bibliometric analysis. *Industrial Management & Data Systems*, *117*(7), 1376–1388. doi:10.1108/IMDS-09-2016-0410

Rueda, X., Garrett, R. D., & Lambin, E. F. (2017). Corporate investments in supply chain sustainability: Selecting instruments in the agri-food industry. *Journal of Cleaner Production*, *142*, 2480–2492. doi:10.1016/j.jclepro.2016.11.026

Saaty, T. L. (1980). The analytic hierarchy process: planning. In Priority Setting. Resource Allocation. New York: McGraw-Hill.

Scholten, K., & Fynes, B. (2017). Risk and uncertainty management for sustainable supply chains. In *Sustainable supply chains* (pp. 413–436). Springer International Publishing. doi:10.1007/978-3-319-29791-0_19

Song, C., & Zhuang, J. (2017). Modeling a Government-Manufacturer-Farmer game for food supply chain risk management. *Food Control*, *78*, 443–455. doi:10.1016/j.foodcont.2017.02.047

Song, H., Turson, R., Ganguly, A., & Yu, K. (2017). Evaluating the effects of supply chain quality management on food firms performance: The mediating role of food certification and reputation. *International Journal of Operations & Production Management*, *37*(10), 1541–1562.

Starbird, S. A., & Amanor-Boadu, V. (2017). Managing Food Supply Chains for Safety and Quality. In *Trends in Food Safety and Protection* (pp. 217–250). CRC Press.

Tse, Y. K., & Zhang, M. (2017). Supply chain quality risk. *The Routledge Companion to Accounting and Risk*, 187.

Verghese, K., Lewis, H., Lockrey, S., & Williams, H. (2013). *The role of packaging in minimising food waste in the supply chain of the future*. Melbourne, Australia: RMIT University.

Wang, X., Chan, H. K., Yee, R. W., & Diaz-Rainey, I. (2012). A two-stage fuzzy-AHP model for risk assessment of implementing green initiatives in the fashion supply chain. *International Journal of Production Economics*, *135*(2), 595–606. doi:10.1016/j.ijpe.2011.03.021

Zadeh, L. A. (1965). Information and control. *Fuzzy sets, 8*(3), 338-353.

Zhu, Q., Sarkis, J., & Lai, K. H. (2017). Regulatory policy awareness and environmental supply chain cooperation in China: A regulatory-exchange-theoretic perspective. *IEEE Transactions on Engineering Management*.

Zilberman, D., Lu, L., & Reardon, T. (2017). Innovation-induced food supply chain design. *Food Policy*. doi:10.1016/j.foodpol.2017.03.010

Zimmerman, H. J. (1996). *Fuzzy sets theory and its applications*. Boston: Kluwer Academic Publishers. doi:10.1007/978-94-015-8702-0

This research was previously published in Advanced Fuzzy Logic Approaches in Engineering Science edited by Mangey Ram; pages 117-131, copyright year 2019 by Engineering Science Reference (an imprint of IGI Global).

Chapter 14
Building a Sustainable Food Supply Chain and Managing Food Losses

A D Nuwan Gunarathne
 https://orcid.org/0000-0003-3024-9416
University of Sri Jayewardenepura, Sri Lanka

D. G. Navaratne
University of Sri Jayewardenepura, Sri Lanka

M. L. S. Gunaratne
University of Sri Jayewardenepura, Sri Lanka

Amanda Erasha Pakianathan
University of Sri Jayewardenepura, Sri Lanka

Yasasi Tharindra Perera
University of Sri Jayewardenepura, Sri Lanka

ABSTRACT

With the unprecedented growth in the world's population, the supply of food has already become a major global challenge. The world food crisis highlights a large quantity of food going waste or lost due to many unsustainable practices in the food supply chain. This chapter provides a conceptual model to build a sustainable food supply chain while minimizing the food waste that occurs at different stages. By incorporating stakeholder management and other behavioral aspects while at the same time following a continuous improvement cycle, the model deviates from other techno-oriented or fragmented guidelines available on the subject. For the purpose of better understanding or providing practical applications, real-life case studies are also presented. Hence, the model provides useful guidelines for business organizations and other actors in the food supply chain to incorporate sustainability while minimizing environmental, social, and economic impacts of food losses/waste.

DOI: 10.4018/978-1-7998-5354-1.ch014

INTRODUCTION

As per the United Nations – UN - (2015), the world population will increase by more than one billion people within the next one and half decades to reach 8.5 billion in 2030. This projected population growth, which is concentrated mainly in the developing countries (UN, 2015), raises many challenges for the future of humanity since all the major global problems such as climate change, energy crisis, severe poverty, food scarcity, and economic and political instability relate to population growth in some way (Population Institute, 2017). Uncontrollable population growth has placed millions of people around the world at the risk of hunger leading to a massive and destructive food crisis (Holt-Giménez, 2008; Govindan, 2017). In order to address this global issue, the United Nations Development Program (UNDP) identifies zero hunger as one of its seventeen Sustainable Development Goals (SDGs) to be realized by 2030 (UNDP, 2017).

The world food crisis has many facets and it is pertinent to focus on food supply chain management by emphasizing two extreme consequences: a) food scarcity and b) food waste. According to the Food and Agricultural Organization (FAO) (2011), food waste in rich countries is almost the same as the entire net food production of sub-Saharan Africa. The food crisis in certain parts of Africa is so severe that it can end in famine. Refer Illustration 1 for more details of the food crisis in East Africa. Globally, 28% of the world's agricultural area is used annually to produce food that is lost or wasted. Further, it is estimated that 26% of children in the world are stunted due to malnutrition and two billion people suffer from one or more micronutrient deficiencies. FAO (2011) further states that one third of the edible food produced for human consumption gets lost or wasted along the global food supply chain. The amount of resource inputs to generate this waste and its contribution to greenhouse gas emission intensify the impact of food waste and warns global communities to pay more attention to ensure sustainability of the food supply chains and to minimize food waste by proper management and control. It is evident that the loss of resources in terms of edible food mass, time, energy and cost spent on converting crop into edible food that is being wasted results in direct losses arising from unsustainable food supply chains. Concurrently its environmental impact intensifies the adverse implications of unsustainable food supply chain practices (Nellemann, Macdevetta, Manders, Eickhout, Svihus, Prins, & Kalterrnborn, 2009). Thus, ensuring sustainability throughout the food supply chain has become a major challenge for global communities at present. However, the issue of food waste/loss has not been addressed from a supply chain perspective so far.

Illustration 1: Food Crisis in Africa

In February 2017, a famine was officially declared by the United Nations (UN) in some parts of South Sudan. The present civil war situation, poor economic condition and dry weather are the major contributors of this worst from of food crisis, famine. Due to the war, millions of people are fleeing to the neighbouring countries such as Uganda, abandoning their farms and livestock. In addition to loss of production, this situation also leads to loss of income for millions of families. Poor income coupled with rising cost living is posing a major threat for many families to find food even for survival. In addition, there has not been a rain for years in some parts of the country. As per the UN, not only South Sudan but some other countries in the Africa and Middle East such as Yemen, Somalia and Nigeria are also at risk of famine.

As per the UN sources, in South Sudan alone more than 100,000 people are suffering from starvation while more than a million people are facing an imminent risk starvation. In Yemen the number stands at 18 million people. This situation is similar to which prevailed in Somalia before the famine. The famine in Somalia nearly killed more than 260,000 people between 2010 and 2012. If this situation continues the food crisis in South Sudan will be equal or even worse than the famine in Somalia. In order to help the people in these countries, the UN and other international agencies have sought for help. Despite the significant increase in donor funding, the unprecedented magnitude of the crisis has far overtaken the financial support. Hence the future of millions of people in these countries is very uncertain. (McVeigh & Quinn, 2017; UN, 2017; Plan International, 2017)

Despite the need for sustainable food supply chain management by addressing the issue food waste, support and guidance are lacking for making the food supply chains sustainable. The available guidance is either fragmented (hence, they do not address the issues of the whole food supply chain), or is more techno-oriented (hence, ignores the vital social and behavioural management aspects of the actors in the supply chain) (Govindan, 2017) or non-directional (hence, does not provide direct guidance to instigate management commitment). This paper presents a model for any form of organization for making their food supply chains sustainable.

The rest of the chapter is organized as follows. In the next sections the key concepts and issues are presented. Accordingly, sustainable food supply chain management, food waste and challenges in making the food supply chains sustainable are discussed. In the following section the conceptual model is presented with a description of its elements in detail. In order to explain some aspects of the model, practical case studies are also presented. The last section presents the conclusions.

SUSTAINABLE (FOOD) SUPPLY CHAIN MANAGEMENT

Supply chain management (SCM) has received heightened attention recently (Cooper, Lambert, & Pagh, 1997; Lee & Vachon, 2016; Mentzer, DeWitt, Keebler, Min, Nix, Smith, & Zacharia, 2001). Traditionally a supply chain is defined as "a set of three or more entities (organizations or individuals) directly involved in the upstream and downstream flows of products, services, finances, and/or information from a source to a customer (Mentzer, DeWitt, Keebler, Min, Nix, Smith, & Zacharia, 2001, p.4). SCM aims to deliver superior customer value at least cost by focusing on the upstream and downstream relationships with suppliers and customers (Lee & Vachon, 2016). SCM thus encompasses the planning and management of all activities involved in sourcing, procurement, conversion, and logistics management in coordination and collaboration with channel partners, which may be suppliers, intermediaries, third-party service providers or customers (Council of Supply Chain Management Professionals, CSCMP, 2017). Hence, SCM integrates supply and demand management within and across companies (Grant, Trautrims, & Wong, 2013). In today's global business environment, it is necessary for organizations to work closely with a number of suppliers and customers in a broad system. Lee and Vachon (2016) call this broad network the 'supply network'. Generally, SCM encompasses activities such as sourcing, packaging, handling and transportation, storage and preparation, and consumption (Leon- Bravo, Caniato, Moretto, & Cagliano, 2016). On the other hand, Hines (2004: p76) provides a more customer-focused view of SCM. He suggests that "supply chain strategies require a total systems view of the links in the chain that work together efficiently to create customer satisfaction at the end point of delivery to the consumer". This will result in costs being reduced throughout the chain while mainly focusing on efficiency and value addition. These various definitions and ideas indicate that SCM is a dynamic process spreading across organizational boundaries. Next, the extension of SCM to embrace the principles of sustainable development is discussed.

Guided by the sustainable development definition put forward in the Brundtland Report in 1987[1], Kleindorfer et al. (2005) suggest that sustainable supply chains should focus on triple bottom-line performance including economic, social and environmental performance dimensions, by utilizing and optimizing resources. Seuring and Muller (2008) define sustainable supply chain management as,

the management of material, information and capital flows as well as cooperation among companies along the supply chain while taking goals from all three dimensions of sustainable development, i.e., economic, environmental and social, into account which are derived from customer and stakeholder requirements. (p. 1701)

Extending this definition into sustainable food supply chains, Pothukuchi and Kaufman (1999) suggest that these systems are a collaborative network that integrates several components in order to enhance a community's environmental, economic and social well-being, built on principles that further the ecological, social and economic values of a community and region. In sustainable food supply chains retailers and manufacturers are increasingly expected to take responsibility not only for their own operations and products, but also for everything they buy (Smith, Martino, Cai, Gwary, Janzen, Kumar... Sirotenko, 2007). Aramyan, et al. (2007) highlight three factors that differentiate food supply chains from other types of supply chains. First, is the production being mostly based on biological processes with increasingly complex risks; second is the distinctive product features such as perishability in the supply chain; and third is the growing consumer awareness of the environmental impacts of the production process and the nutritional elements of the products.

The available literature on sustainable food supply chains presents two main approaches to ensure sustainability: a) new product development for sustainability and b) improvement of sustainability in the existing supply chain. The former includes development of healthier products (Hopper, 2007; Maloni & Brown, 2006), design of product for extending the life cycle (Colicchia, Melacini, & Perotti, 2011), investments in research and development and a closer understanding of consumer preferences and expectations for an innovative product. The new product development merits some discussion here. It consists of idea or concept generation and screening, research, development and product testing, and marketing launch activities (Rudder, Ainsworth, & Holgate, 2001). The latter includes the improvements in existing practices related to sourcing, packaging, handling and transportation, storage and preparation, consumption (Leon- Bravo, Caniato, Moretto, & Cagliano, 2016). The next section presents the sources of food waste that occur in the supply chain by disaggregating them into three stages.

SOURCES OF FOOD WASTE

Since food is a biological material, it is subject to degradation within a short period. The longer the food supply chain, the higher the costs and greater the possibilities of food being wasted. The literature provides a range of definitions of food waste which can be used as a basis for describing the impacts and causes of food waste at different stages of the food supply chain. FAO (1981) defines food loss as a change in the availability, wholesomeness or quality of edible material intended for human consumption, arising at any point in the food supply chain (p. 44). More recently, FAO (2011) provided an alternative definition of food waste as the decrease in the edible food mass throughout the human food supply chain. Accordingly, food waste or losses could occur at different stages of the food supply chain.

A thorough understanding of the causes of food waste is vital for developing sustainable food supply chain practices. Disaggregating the food supply chain into distinct stages will help to identify the strategies of, combating food waste (FAO, 2011). Accordingly, the food supply chain is analysed in three stages;

1.   Pre-harvest
2.   Post-harvest
3.   Post-consumption

Pre-harvest food waste arises during the early stage of the food supply chain, predominantly during cultivation and harvesting. During cultivation and husbandry, food loss occurs due to unavoidable factors such as climate changes as well as due to controllable factors such as rodents, parasites, animal damage to crop, poor harvesting techniques, and inappropriate timing of harvests (FAO, 1981; Parfitt, Barthel, & Macnaughton, 2010). The majority of the controllable waste is generated due to underdeveloped agricultural techniques and technologies. In industrialized food supply chains, pre-harvest food waste is minimal compared to developing countries due to technological and infrastructural development along such industrialized food supply chains (FAO, 2011; Papargyropoulou, Lozano, Steinberger, Wright, & Ujang, 2014; Parfitt, Barthel, & Macnaughton, 2010). Hence, action should be taken to overcome the food loss at this stage by the proper integration of suppliers into the food supply chain.

Post-harvest food waste arises from the activities from the point of harvesting until the point the harvest is made available to the customer (FAO, 1981). These activities consist of transportation, packaging, processing, storing and display of food items. Inappropriate handling of food, imbalances in the required temperature, destructive testing, inappropriate packaging, and damage due to poor storing facilities are among factors which give rise to post-harvest food waste (FAO, 2011; Parfitt, Barthel, & Macnaughton, 2010). These losses are caused by improper planning and underdeveloped technologies, which could have been managed with investment in infrastructure development. The developed countries do not contribute much to food waste during the pre-and post-harvest stages of the food supply chain (Papargyropoulou, Lozano, Steinberger, Wright, & Ujang, 2014). FAO (2011) suggests that in developed countries, 40% of the total food waste occur during the consumption stage. On the contrary, Parfitt et al. (2010) suggest that the food supply chains even in developed countries contribute equally to post harvest food waste due to unnecessary quality standards and other controls. This highlights the need for necessary measures to combat food waste in the distribution and storing activities of the supply chain with the coordination of middlemen.

Investment in pre/post-harvest cultivation is also vital for reducing food waste being generated through these channels. These investments are indeed costly. However, through proper integration of the supply chain, it is quite possible to obtain mutual and sustainable benefits for all parties involved with the supply chains. The mini case below provides an example of a successful infrastructure development implemented by PepsiCo in India which had benefitted small scale potato farmers in Bengal while improving quality of the product (refer Illustration 2).

Illustration 2: Environmental and Economic Sustainability Through Improved Cultivation and Post-Harvest Practices

Traditional potato value chain in India is less quality oriented and had zero market premiums for quality. Hence farmers were not motivated to improve quality of their potato produce. However, when Frito-Lay, a product of PepsiCo wanted to buy potatoes from India for the production of potato crisps, they wanted to ensure the potato meets strict quality requirements. To meet Frito-Lay's quality requirements, farmers had to adopt a new potato cultivar ('Atlanta') that is suitable for processing into crisps, adopt new farming practices based on a different and more costly input mix and adopt new post-harvest practices, specifically in terms of handling, grading and sorting, storage and transport.

Clearly, farmers would adopt these upgrading activities only if they resulted in a commercially viable business. A study in West Bengal found that growing potatoes for Frito-Lay resulted in a 20% increase in costs relative to operating in the traditional potato chain, but that this was offset by higher revenues and resulted in gross margins 10–50% higher than those in the traditional chain, depending on yields and market prices. Moreover, the financial incentive was supplemented by capacity-enhancing and risk-reducing elements under a contract growing scheme, a business model that PepsiCo has pioneered in India since 2001. These elements included: free technical extension services; free crop monitoring (i.e. early disease detection); guaranteed markets and prices; on-credit access to quality seed potatoes and other inputs; and weather-based insurance. The model is facilitated by vendors, local people hired by PepsiCo to act as a readily accessible liaison between the farmers and the firm.

This combination of economic incentives drove a rapid growth of the scheme, from 1800 farmers producing 12000 tonnes of potatoes in 2008 to 13000 farmers producing 70000 tonnes of potatoes in 2013. Interestingly, over time the profit motive became less important than the risk-reduction motive. Although the price of 'Atlanta' at times fell to as little as half that of the traditional cultivar, 'Jyoti' (e.g. in 2012), farmers continued to shift to 'Atlanta' because its yields are higher and more stable, and because its prices also more stable, resulting in more-reliable returns. The potatoes that fail to meet PepsiCo's quality standard (commonly 10–20%) can easily be sold by the farmer in the traditional market.

There are clear signals that the traditional potato channel is also modernizing, likely in part as the result of a spill over effect from the development of schemes such as PepsiCo's. This modernization includes the growth of affordable cold-storage technology (linked to extension of the electricity grid), access to price information through cell phones and adoption of improved cultivars. (FAO, 2014)

Post-consumption food waste arises due to consumer activities. Unplanned buying, over cooking or preparation, serving larger quantities, food not being served on time, and food scrap during preparation are a few causes of food waste during the consumption phase. Studies by the Waste and Resources Action Programme (WRAP) (2008) have shown that household food waste in the UK is 8.3 million tons of food with a retail value of GBP 12.2 billion and carbon impact of over 20 million tons of carbon dioxide (Parfitt, Barthel, & Macnaughton, 2010). Hence, consumers should be well educated in making the food supply chains sustainable.

An alternate three-way food waste categorisation associated with household drink and food waste was introduced by WRAP (2008). This categorisation focuses on post-harvest food waste and is based on the controllability of the waste. These categories are avoidable, possibly avoidable and unavoidable. It is interesting to note that 61% of household food waste (post-harvest) could have been avoided and could have been eaten if it had been managed better (WRAP, 2008). Truly unavoidable food waste accounts for only 19% of the post-harvest food waste, which includes vegetable peelings, meat carcasses, tea bags etc. whereas the remaining 20% is categorised as possibly unavoidable, which is wasted due to individual preferences and ways of cooking (WRAP, 2008).

Food waste gives rise to many economic, environmental and social issues. From an economic perspective, the resources consumed to produce the wasted food involve a significant cost. This economic cost is borne by retailers and consumers (Venkat, 2011). Further, the amount of energy expended to produce such wasted food increases the cost of energy. Both such costs together create further economic issues in the form of higher inflation and increased poverty levels. From an environmental perspective, the bulk of food waste is finally disposed of in landfills which results in the emission of greenhouse gases because of natural decomposition. This results in adverse environmental impacts such as increased global warming, climatic changes and depletion of the ozone layer (Papargyropoulou, Lozano, Steinberger, Wright, & Ujang, 2014). The depletion of soil nutrients due to constant agricultural activities, environmental pollution due to fertilizers and damaging the natural habitat exacerbate the adverse environmental impacts of food waste (Papargyropoulou, Lozano, Steinberger, Wright, & Ujang, 2014). From a social perspective food waste implies wasted resources and unnecessary costs. To cover the costs incurred, the remaining output is rated at much higher prices. This will impact the low-income earners as affordability of food can be a problem due to high food costs. Wasted resources due to food losses also threaten the very concept of sustainable development since wasted resources could limit the availability of resources for future generations, causing severe consequences. Thus, it is clear that a strategic systematic approach is required at present to incorporate sustainability aspects within the food supply chain to address these triple bottom line issues.

CHALLENGES/BARRIERS IN MAKING A FOOD SUPPLY CHAIN SUSTAINABLE

The transition to a sustainable food supply chain is a challenging proposition given its numerous barriers/challenges. Such barriers/challenges can be discussed in terms of the three stages of the food supply chain, i.e., pre-harvest, post-harvest and post- consumption.

Changes in climate, scarcity of water and utilization of land are some of the major challenges in the *pre-harvest stage*. Climate change is one of the key barriers faced at the pre-harvest stage of a sustainable supply chain. Garnett (2011) highlights that the food supply chain commencing from agricultural production to food waste, contributes to nearly 15-28% of greenhouse gas emissions. Global warming resulting from such emissions and many other factors has led to serious climate change thereby affecting rain fall patterns and causing extreme weather conditions. These changes pose a great challenge to the agricultural sector in respect of crop yields, food prices and food security. Water scarcity is another grave issue faced at this stage of the food supply chain. The demand for water is increasing with the growth in population, rapid urbanisation and an expanding agricultural sector (UN World Water Assessment Program, (UNWWAP) 2017). OECD (2008) highlights that by 2030, nearly 47% of the global population is expected live in areas where severe water stress will be prevalent. Such situations will undoubtedly threaten the sustainability of the food supply chain. Another barrier faced at this stage is the issue regarding land use. This arises in two ways; soil depletion and demand for land. Smith et al. (2007) specify that agriculture occupies approximately 40 to 50% of the earth's land surface. When the land is continuously used to produce the same food the fertility of the land deteriorates sometimes irreversibly. Forum for The Future (2014) highlights that approximately 60% of the global ecosystem has been degraded so far due to unsustainable land use. Soil depletion results in lower crop yields and reduces the extent of fertile land available and suitable for agriculture. Furthermore, the rising demand for land for both commercial and residential purposes has also created a challenge. As income continually improves and emerging nations develop through rapid urbanisation, the need for commercial and residential space becomes more crucial.

In the *post-harvest stage,* the challenges stem from various sources. As food supply chains become globalised, the complexity and risk of the system increases. Globalised supply chains face the risks created by governments through tariff and non-tariff barriers, natural disasters, economic instability, and rising oil production. These challenges could have negative impacts on farming and transportation of food thereby affecting the long-term sustainability of food supply. Furthermore, post-harvest losses are also driven based on the technological sophistication of the country and the extent to which markets for agricultural produce have developed (Parfitt, Barthel, & Macnaughton, 2010). Barriers such as inadequate storage, infrastructure, and market facilities increase food losses at this stage. FAO (2011) highlights this challenge as one mostly faced more by low income than medium and high-income countries. Parfitt et al., (2010) also supports this claim by clarifying the features of post-harvest infrastructure attributable to each stage of the economic development of a country. Parfitt et al. (2010) further stress that as low-income countries have simple technologies and are more labour-intensive, such countries continue to adopt traditional storage systems and harvesting techniques. Thus, food supply chains are poorly integrated with the local markets and have limited access to international markets, which results in higher food wastage at the post-harvest stage. Rolle (2006) highlights that India reports an estimated post-harvest loss of 40% for fresh fruit and vegetables while loss estimates in Indonesia, Korea, Philippines, Sri Lanka, Thailand, and Vietnam range between 20 to 50%. However, countries such as the USA and UK report 2% and 10% of post-harvest loss for fresh fruit and vegetables respectively (Parfitt, Barthel, & Macnaughton, 2010). Illustration 3 explains the food loss analysis of the rice value chain in Andhra Pradesh, India, an area that contributes significantly to world rice production.

Illustration 3: Food Loss Analysis in the Rice Value Chain in Andhra Pradesh, India

Rice is of national importance in the Indian economy. Andhra Pradesh is the third largest rice producing state in India contributing to 7% of the national rice production and accounting to 1% of the global rice market. A study was conducted to identify main causes of food loss in the rice supply chain in Andhra Pradesh and suggest potential solutions to mitigate these losses. To assess the food losses, field case studies were performed in the selected rice supply chains in east Godavari and Nellore districts as they contribute to approximately 60% of paddy production in the state, and the existence of the entire value chain helps to give a holistic picture.

Paddy supply chain comprises of multiple actors with following actors portraying a major role: Farmers as the producers of paddy, village level aggregators, rice processing industries, warehouse managers, distribution agents and retailers. The key factors affecting the food losses in the rice value chain were categorized at both pre-harvest stage (farmer level) and post-harvest stage (transporter, millers, warehouses and retailing).

The study identified food loss risk factors such as crop varieties, good agricultural practices, rainfall during cultivation and harvest, the timing of harvest and the method of harvesting, at the pre-harvest stage which if managed efficiently could lead to a reduction in losses. The study further revealed that mechanized harvesting and threshing at the pre-harvest stage as one of the critical loss points, where farmers reported a substantial loss of 7-10%.

Similarly, at the post-harvest stage, storage at mills and CWC warehouses were observed as the critical loss points as the qualitative losses for the rice range between 2-4%. The qualitative losses can be further aggravated by the intake of paddy with higher moisture content for mechanical drying and processing, poor storage infrastructure (ventilation and stacking) and in adequate pest control. (Sathguru Management Consultants, 2017)

Challenges in the *post-consumption stage* arise primarily due to changes in consumer demography. Economic growth, urbanization and rising income have led to significant demographic changes. Due to long working hours and a busy lifestyle, a shift in dietary practices is evident as many opt for processed, pre-prepared and fast food (Goyal & Singh, 2007; Habib, Abu, & Zakaria, 2011). This violates the notion of safety and health of a sustainable food supply chain which would ultimately compromise the welfare of the future. Furthermore, the increase in the population growth rate has affected the demand for commodities. This, in turn, has trickled down to higher commodity prices while impacting food security for all people.

The next section of this paper provides the conceptual framework after considering the food waste/losses that occur at different stages of the food supply chain.

CONCEPTUAL MODEL ON SUSTAINABLE FOOD SUPPLY CHAIN MANAGEMENT

There appears to be a lack of proper guidance on sustainable food supply chain management to address the food waste issue and even the little guidance available does not seem to cover a wide enough spectrum as it tends to focus more on the technological and process- related aspects. Hence no attention or only minimum attention has been paid to the stakeholders involved in the supply chain and to the need for continuous improvement. Thus, a proper conceptual model that addresses these aspects is needed.

This conceptual model is primarily based on the stages in the sustainable food supply chain with due consideration for the guiding principles. The proposed model is given below (refer Figure 1).

The elements in the model, i.e., activities and guiding principles are explained next.

Figure 1. Conceptual model on sustainable food supply chain management

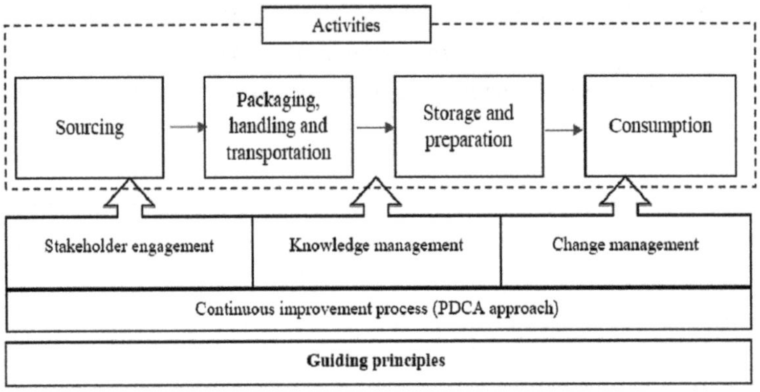

Activities

The model is based on the general sequential stages of a supply chain, i.e., sourcing, packaging, handling and transportation, storage, preparation and consumption. Hence the application/use of this model does not necessitate fundamental changes to the existing supply chains.

Sourcing

There are two sub elements in this initial stage of the sustainable food supply chain: a) sustainable sourcing mechanisms and b) focus areas. There are several sustainable sourcing mechanisms that should be considered in this stage (Leon- Bravo, Caniato, Moretto, & Cagliano, 2016). They are:

Supplier Certifications/Accreditations and Evaluation

One effective sustainable sourcing mechanism is the use of supplier certification/accreditation by a third party to enhance the resource traceability and build trust. These certifications can be in areas such as carbon footprint, water footprint, ecological footprint, and food quality. Supplier evaluation requires consideration of environmental, social, and economic criteria in order to rank the suppliers based on the triple bottom line (Banterle, Cereda, & Fritz, 2013). For example, as shown in Illustration 4, Rainforest Alliance certification ensures that a farm, forest, or tourism enterprise meets standards that address environmental, social, and economic sustainability (Rainforest Alliance, 2016).

Illustration 4: Rainforest Alliance Certification

Rainforest Alliance certification is awarded to organizations that meet the standards of the Sustainable Agriculture Network (SAN). The SAN standard is built on following principles of sustainable farming:

- *Biodiversity conservation*
- *Improved livelihoods and human wellbeing*
- *Natural resource conservation*

- *Effective planning and farm management systems (Rainforest Alliance, 2016)*

Supplier Improvements

Another sustainable sourcing mechanism is supplier improvements. This can be achieved via the enhancement of technical, knowledge and financial assistance of the suppliers, their employees and local communities.

Supplier Collaboration

Supplier collaboration is necessary to build trust, facilitate the knowledge transfer process and further improve the competencies of suppliers in relation to environmental and social welfare.

These mechanisms are not necessarily mutually exclusive and any one of them should focus beyond the traditional *'focus areas'* (such as cost, quality, delivery reliability and technological capability) to incorporate the triple bottom line aspects, i.e., economic, environmental and social (Dickson 1966). The aforesaid mechanisms would ensure natural resource conservation via reduction of food wastage, animal welfare, introduction of sustainable growing and breeding techniques, reduction of water, soil and energy consumption and safeguarding the bio diversity of different geographical locations. As shown in Illustration 5, *Plan A* programme of M&S encompasses supplier improvement, collaboration and many more activities.

Illustration 5: Sustainable Scorecard at M&S

Marks & Spencer (M&S) Plan A is a comprehensive sustainable initiative which encompasses responsible sourcing, waste reduction and community development. Since its launch in 2007, Plan A had shown significant progress with 100 commitments to be achieved in 5 years. Collaborating with suppliers worldwide, M&S seek to set the best quality standards in all products they sell. Accordingly, they have developed their own 'Sustainability Scorecard' to rate existing supplier portfolio.

This scorecard includes categorisation of suppliers into 4 categories depending on their commitment towards sustainability. The categorisation is as follows:

1. *Provisional: suppliers who meet all current minimum requirements for sustainability*
2. *Bronze: suppliers who have the basic systems of governance (policy, measurement and management) in place*
3. *Silver: suppliers who have employed very good governance systems which are consistently applied and trained against. These suppliers apply trials, year-on-year improvements, external collaboration and set-targets.*
4. *Gold: suppliers who lead the industry and demonstrate step change in standards. These suppliers have embedded sustainability throughout the business. (Marks & Spencer, 2015)*

Packaging, Handling, and Transportation

The second stage of SCM involves activities in the delivery process. Packaging, handling and transportation should cover the several aspects discussed below.

In packaging, it is necessary to redesign the primary packaging to reduce food waste while improving food safety throughout the life cycle. This requires the redesign of environmentally friendly packaging while considering the product life cycle, emission of harmful substances and energy utilization (Bevilacqua, Ciarapica, & Giacchetta, 2008). For example, environmentally friendly packaging used by Sainsbury (refer Illustration 6) generates economic benefits while reducing food damage, ensuring food safety and promoting long-term environmental benefits. This will, in turn, contribute to the reduction of food waste during handling and transportation.

Illustration 6: Sainsbury's 2020 Sustainability Plan

Sainsbury 2020 sustainability plan articulates its commitment to sustainability development. Plan 2020 includes 20 different plans covering sustainable sourcing, health and safety, environmental protection and social development to be achieved by 2020. One such plan includes reducing own packaging by 50% compared to 2005. Sainsbury has cut 12 million kilos of packaging material in year 2010/11 through new packaging designs, one bag for life product range, using recycled material for packaging and establishing in-store recycling collection point for customers to discharge separated recyclable waste. The image shows Sainsbury's "eco-friendly" milk bags and jugs that use considerably less amount of plastic than the bottles while saving costs. (Sainsbury, 2015)

Handling food should conform to health and safety standards (HACCP, ISO 22000 etc.) and distributors should be educated in handling food products so as to minimise waste and to ensure the safety of food items.

Sustainable transportation focuses on food safety especially via food safety guidelines. It also focuses on carbon footprint reduction by obtaining food supplies from sources close to the factory while using route optimisation to minimize the number of trips by developing a systematic transportation plan. The dimensions and maximum capacity of the crates, the quantity of crates that can be transported per vehicle, temperature management within vehicles and route optimisation which will reduce time and emissions. In this regard, shipment optimization is another important aspect of rationalizing distribution, coordinating and simplifying logistics processes in the supply chain, and identifying the shortest route for product transportation so as to minimize costs and emissions (Colicchia, Melacini, & Perotti, 2011; Van der Vorst, Tromp, & Zee, 2009).

Storage and Preparation

The next stage involves the "make" of the supply chain process by implementing eco-friendly processes to improve economic and environmental spheres via innovative production and process technologies.

In considering storage, attention should be paid to key optimisation factors such as segregation of food items based on type, perishability of food items, maximum expected period for storage, optimum storage temperatures and guidelines/standards for storage and storage facilities (materials used, ventilation and illumination and energy consumption minimising carbon footprint, etc. (refer Broekmeulen, 1998; Rong, Akkerman, & Grunow, 2010 for more details).

The production process should consider several aspects to adopt eco-friendly processes to optimize water, energy and material consumption, waste management and nutritional quality of the menus prepared. Incorporation of plans such as HACCP to continuously improve the hygiene and quality of food is important (Aruoma, 2006; Sweet, Balakrishnan, Robertson, Stolee, & Karim, 2010). Attention should also be given to the green building aspects in the production plant as it favours green electric power suppliers, cogeneration plants, energy efficiency improvements, and utilization of eco-friendly construction materials. Focus must be extended to the best available techniques for water, energy consumption, waste management and emission control (Catarino et al., 2007). Consideration of health and safety in the workplace should be ensured via providing a favourable working environment, adequate training ensuring gender equality, respecting human rights, and empowering employees to take ownership of sustainability and green initiatives (Maloni & Brown, 2006; Pagell & Wu, 2009).

Sustainable Consumption

This is the stage at which the food prepared is presented to the end-consumer. Traditionally, consumers place a predominant value on attributes such as price, quality and product features. This acts as a constraint in adopting a sustainable supply chain, resulting in increased costs and reduced flexibility in a small, more-sustainable supply base (Smith, 2008). However, there is a growing trend when customers place high value on social and environmental performance in the supply chain with regard to high quality sustainable endorsement (Halweil, 2004).

To promote sustainable food supply chains among consumers, two types of strategies can be adopted: a) regulatory interventions, and b) consumer education. Governments are also involved in this process through various regulatory mechanisms that involve establishing performance standards and mandatory labels to limit damages from products (Organization for Economic Cooperation and Development, OECD, 2008). Labelling is a tool for informing customers especially about their obligation to recycle products and package products for health reasons such as health-declaration requirements for nutritional values of food products, foods with genetically modified content, and organic food.

OECD best practices include education as a most important tool in developing appropriate skills and competencies needed to become sustainable consumers. This was observed by UNESCO designating 2005-2014 as the "Decade of Education for Sustainable Development" (UNESCO, 2005) along with consumer education, communications campaigns are a widely-used strategy by OECD countries to promote sustainable consumption. Some such awareness programmes are Consumption and Environment in Demark, EcoBuyer Campaign in Finland, Green Purchasing Network in Japan, and Consumer Pledge for Sustainable Consumption in Korea (OECD, 2008).

Post-consumption controls should also be in place to ensure that the consumption stage is waste-free or is at a minimum level so that food is not wasted in large quantities to ensure the sustainability of the whole food supply chain. The waste generated within the food supply chain at the consumption stage could be re-used within the supply chain after a little investment to generate energy (bio gas, etc.). This energy can be then used in the sourcing stage as a renewable energy source at the same time enabling curtailment of costs of energy consumption.

As Illustration 7 indicates, Eurest provides a good example of how a restaurant can manage its food waste. There should also be commitment by end-consumers to recycling, reusing or proper disposal of the packaging materials or any food waste.

Illustration 7: Post-Consumption Waste Measurement Programme at Eurest

Taking measures to combat food waste, Eurest, a catering organization, has implemented a waste measurement and awareness campaign in 2010 to showcase the amount of waste generated during the day and publicise the results to guests and employees explaining the impact of food waste and how it can be prevented. These initiatives have engaged customers in the process of reducing food waste which in turn has strengthened the brand image of Eurest in Sweden. Eurest has reached 22,055 guests a month, and within 6 months they have managed to reduce the amount of food waste generated by 23%. (European Commission, 2017)

Guiding Principles

A vital element of the model is its guiding principles. The aims of these guiding principles are primarily two-fold: 1) to address the dynamic nature of sustainable food supply chains by adopting a continuous improvement cycle and; 2) to provide a greater stakeholder-oriented perspective for implementation and continuous sustenance of the model. These principles differentiate the model from other available techno-oriented guidelines. The model incorporates continuous improvement based on the famous "PDCA" cycle while paying attention to stakeholder engagement, knowledge management and change management. These guiding principles are described next.

To ensure successful operationalization and sustenance of a sustainable food supply chain, a sound continuous improvement cycle is required. This assists in continuous evolvement to meet future demands with respect to the sustainability of food supply chains. The suggested approach, PDCA cycle (Plan-Do- Check- Act), is a well-known model of process improvement (Johnson, 2002). There should be continuous planning, implementation, checking and improvement at each stage of the food supply chain. More than being a simple tool, the PDCA cycle/principles emphasizes the embodiment of continuous improvements in the culture of an organization (Sokovic, Pavletic, & Pipan, 2010). Due to the dynamism in the food supply chain it is necessary to continuously improve the standards in the supply chain. The PDCA approach should be adopted in the stages of sourcing, storage and preparation, packaging and transport, consumption in introducing or improving sustainable practises in the business operations.

Each actor, starting from suppliers, producers, intermediaries, consumers, regulators to civil society, plays a significant role in contributing towards sustainability (Beske, Land, & Seuring, 2014; Govindan, 2017). The business community contributes by providing management and technical skills, dissemination and distribution capacity while the public sector offers information, skilled staff, authority to mobilize resources (Tennyson & Wilde, 2000) and the power to create the needed institutional structures. As explained previously, consumers also play a key role in the entire supply chain. Local NGOs offer skills in participatory approaches to change and universities are a source of knowledge, research expertise and local social networks (Smith, 2008).

Another guiding principle for sustainable food supply chains is knowledge management (Beske, 2012; Beske, Land, & Seuring, 2014). Knowledge management ensures that the supply chain partners create internal knowledge, acquire external knowledge, store knowledge as well as update and share knowledge internally and externally (Alavi & Leidner, 2001; Teece 1998). Throughout the supply chain explicit and tacit knowledge should be handled appropriately while achieving single-loop learning and double-loop learning[2] (Rubenstein-Montano, Liebowitz, Buchwalter, McCaw, Newman, Rebeck, & Team, 2001).

Sustainable supply chain management requires management of change throughout the supply chain. It is required to continually renew the direction, structure, and capabilities to serve the ever-changing needs of external and internal customers (Moran & Brightman, 2001). Organizations incorporating a sustainability approach in the existing supply chain and developing innovative sustainable products have to inevitably change prevailing practices. Creation of a shared vision and a common direction whereby sustainability is incorporated into the strategy and vision of the company is fundamental. This is followed by measures to separate from the past where the present level is unfreezed, moving to the new level and refreezing this new level. This model of change recognises the need to discard prevailing sole economic focused structures, processes and culture before successfully adopting new sustainability approaches (Bamford & Forrester, 2003). This will be followed by crafting a sustainability implementation plan for the food supply chain and developing enabling structures. Finally, there is the reinforcement and institutionalizing change which facilitates monitoring and improving strategies in remedying issues arising in the process of changing towards sustainability.

Usefulness of the Model

This model enables individuals, organisations and governments alike to:

- *Identify the elements that exist in a sustainable food supply chain and/ or align existing food supply chains to improve the sustainability by focusing on the food waste/losses*

This model enables an organization to identify the elements that should be incorporated into a sustainable food supply chain to combat food waste. They can assess the gaps in their existing food supply chain and identify the areas which need process improvements. Further, the model presents standard best practices which organisations can directly adopt/merge into their food supply chain or which they can use as guidelines to build their own version of processes that best suit the organisation.

- *Can be used to improve awareness of the supply chain partners on the sustainability of the food supply chain*

In order to ensure the sustainability of food supply chains, support and commitment from all levels of the food supply chain is essential. The model highlights the role and importance of every supply chain partner. If the end-consumers are well educated about the benefits and procedures involved in a sustainable food supply chain, the demand for end-products (food) coming out of a sustainable food supply chain will increase causing the other supply chain partners to strive towards sustainability in their processes. As indicated in Illustration 8, a broad conceptualization of this nature can inform the supply chain partners to get involved in closing the loops of their respective food supply chain through resource recovery and reuse options.

Illustration 8: A Close-Loop Food Sustainable Supply Chain Model in the Meat Industry

A recent study conducted by Sgarbossa & Russo (2017) evaluates how close-loop sustainable food supply chains (CLSFSC) in the the meat industry can be used as a proactive model in achieving triple bottom line benefits. The researchers identify four major areas in meat production. They are; a) farmers/ livestock, b) production c) distribution and d) sales. The study evaluates how the introduction of new loops into CLSFSC that enables to recover resources from the unavoidable waste. The study shows the transformation of waste meat from slaughter into new resources such as electric energy, methane gas or depurated water can be used in minimising the resource consumption, reducing the production of waste, and maximizing the reuse and recycling options. In order to achieve these ends, a major investment has been made to install biogas and cogeneration plants to create new closed loops in the traditional chain by using slaughter wastes as inputs. In this study Sgarbossa and Russo highlight how to activate a circular economy which leads to energy self-efficiency using waste within the sustainable business model. (Sgarbossa & Russo, 2017)

- *Emphasizes the need for change and knowledge management mechanisms in supply chains*

An important aspect of the model is the inclusion of the change and knowledge management concept. When changing to a sustainable food supply chain from an ordinary food supply chain, there will be resistance from almost all stakeholders. The model identifies the importance and provides guidance for organisations willing to incorporate sustainability in their food supply chain. Not only change management, managing knowledge throughout the supply chains by creating, acquiring and preserving new knowledge with regard to sustainability aspects is also essential.

CONCLUSION

The purpose of this paper was to provide a conceptual framework for the organizations involved in the food supply chain to make their supply chains more sustainable by devoting more attention to the food waste that occurs. In developing this model, attention was paid more to combating the food waste/losses that occur at different stages of the supply chain and by different actors. The suggested model is built on activities and guiding principles. The activities follow the sequential steps in the typical supply chain and hence no major deviation from the existing practices is required. At every stage, clear guidelines are provided to build a resilient supply chain. By providing essential guiding principles, the model deviates itself from more techno-oriented guidelines that are currently available. Based on a continuous improvement cycle, the model incorporates stakeholder management, knowledge management and change management in the supply chain in order to bring in the requisite changes or sustain the existing good practices. The paper provide not only guidelines but also practical applications from real life case studies selected from different countries around the globe. This will enable companies to examine these practices further to build a sustainable food supply chain.

REFERENCES

Alavi, M., & Leidner, D. E. (2001). Knowledge Management and Knowledge Management Systems: Conceptual Foundations and Research Issues. *Management Information Systems Quarterly*, *25*(1), 107–136. doi:10.2307/3250961

Aramyan, L., Lansink, A., Vorst, J., & Kooten, O. (2007). Performance measurement in agri-food supply chains: A case study. *Supply Chain Management*, *12*(4), 304–315. doi:10.1108/13598540710759826

Aruoma, O. I. (2006). The impact of food regulation on the food supply chain. *Toxicology*, *221*(1), 119–127. doi:10.1016/j.tox.2005.12.024 PMID:16483706

Bamford, D. R., & Forrester, P. L. (2003). Managing planned and emergent change within an operations management environment. *International Journal of Operations & Production Management*, *23*(5), 546–564. doi:10.1108/01443570310471857

Banterle, A., Cereda, E., & Fritz, M. (2013). Labelling and sustainability in food supply networks: A comparison between the German and Italian markets. *British Food Journal*, *115*(5), 769–783. doi:10.1108/00070701311331544

Beske, P. (2012). Dynamic Capabilities and Sustainable Supply Chain Management. *International Journal of Physical Distribution & Logistics Management*, *42*(4), 372–387. doi:10.1108/09600031211231344

Beske, P., Land, A., & Seuring, S. (2014). Sustainable supply chain management practices and dynamic capabilities in the food industry: A critical analysis of the literature. *International Journal of Production Economics*, *152*, 131–143. doi:10.1016/j.ijpe.2013.12.026

Bevilacqua, M., Ciarapica, F. E., & Giacchetta, G. (2008). Design for environment as a tool for the development of a sustainable supply chain. *International Journal of Sustainable Engineering*, *1*(3), 188–201. doi:10.1080/19397030802506657

Broekmeulen, R. (1998). Operations management of distribution centers for vegetables and fruits. *International Transactions in Operational Research*, *5*(6), 501–508. doi:10.1111/j.1475-3995.1998.tb00132.x

Catarino, J., Mendonc̦, A. E., Picado, A., Anselmo, A., da Costa, J. N., & Partidario, P. (2007). Getting value from wastewater: By-products recovery in a potato chips industry. *Journal of Cleaner Production*, *15*(10), 927–931. doi:10.1016/j.jclepro.2005.12.003

Colicchia, C., Melacini, M., & Perotti, S. (2011). Benchmarking supply chain sustainability: Insights from a field study. *Benchmarking: An International Journal*, *18*(5), 705–732. doi:10.1108/14635771111166839

Cooper, C. M., Lambert, D. M., & Pagh, J. D. (1997). Supply Chain Management: More Than a New Name for Logistics. *International Journal of Logistics Management*, *8*(1), 1–14. doi:10.1108/09574099710805556

Council of Supply Chain Management Professionals (CSCMP). (2017). *CSCMP Supply Chain Management Definitions and Glossary*. Retrieved January, 21, 2017, from https://cscmp.org/imis0/CSCMP/Educate/SCM_Definitions_and_Glossary_of_Terms/CSCMP/Educate/SCM_Definitions_and_Glossary_of_Terms.aspx?hkey=60879588-f65f-4ab5-8c4b-6878815ef921

Dickson, G. W. (1996). An analysis of vendor selection system and decisions. *Journal of Purchasing*, *2*(1), 5–17. doi:10.1111/j.1745-493X.1966.tb00818.x

European Commission. (2017). *Good practices in food waste reduction and prevention*. Retrieved January, 24, 2017, from https://ec.europa.eu/food/safety/food_waste/good_practices/policy_awards_certification_en

Food and Agricultural Organization (FAO). (1981). *Food Loss Prevention in Perishable Crops, Food and Agricultural Service Bulletin, no. 43*. Rome: FAO.

Food and Agricultural Organization (FAO). (2011). *Global food losses and food waste – Extent, causes and prevention*. Rome: FAO.

Food and Agricultural Organization (FAO). (2014). *Developing Sustainable Food Value Chains - Guiding Principles*. Rome: FAO.

Forum for The Future. (2014). *Key challenges for a sustainable food supply*. Forum for The Future. Retrieved January, 18, 2017 from https://www.changemakers.com/sites/default/files/sustainable_food_supply_-_nesta_paper_-_final_version.pdf

Garnett, T. (2011). Where are the best opportunities for reducing greenhouse gas emissions in the food system? *Food Policy*, *36*, 23–32. doi:10.1016/j.foodpol.2010.10.010

Govindan, K. (2017). Sustainable Consumption and Production in the Food Supply Chain: A Conceptual Framework. *International Journal of Production Economics*. doi:10.1016/j.ijpe.2017.03.003

Goyal, A., & Singh, N. P. (2007). Consumer perception about fast food in India: An exploratory study. *British Food Journal*, *109*(2), 182–195. doi:10.1108/00070700710725536

Grant, D.B., Trautrims, A., & Wong. C.Y. (2013). *Sustainable Logistics and Supply Chain Management: Principles and Practices for Sustainable Operations and Management*. New York: Kogan Page.

Habib, F. Q., Abu, D. R., & Zakaria, S. (2011). Consumers' preference and consumption towards fast food: Evidences from Malaysia. *Business & Management Quaterly Review*, *2*(1), 14–27.

Halweil, B. (2004). *Eat here: reclaiming homegrown pleasures in a global supermarket*. New York: WW Norton.

Hines, T. (2004). *Supply Chain Strategies: Customer-driven and customer-focused*. Oxford, UK: Routledge.

Holt-Giménez, E. (2008). *The World Food Crisis: What is Behind it and What We Can Do*. Retrieved February 14, 2017 from http://www.worldhunger.org/world-food-crisis/

Hopper, P. F. (2007). The role of food industry in helping Americans improve the nutritional quality of the diets. *Journal of Food Quality*, *13*(1), 59–67. doi:10.1111/j.1745-4557.1990.tb00006.x

Johnson, C. N. (2002). *The Benefits of PDCA, Quality Progress*. Retrieved February, 12, 2017 from http://asq.org/quality-progress/2002/05/problem-solving/the-benefits-of-pdca.html

Lee, K. H., & Vachon, S. (2016). *Business Value and Sustainability-An Integrated Supply Network Perspective*. London: Palgrave Macmillan.

Leon-Bravo, V., Caniato, F.F.A., Moretto, A., & Cagliano, R. (2016). Innovation for sustainable supply chains for traditional and new products. In Organizing Supply Chain Processes for Sustainable Innovation in the Agri-Food Industry (pp. 31 – 57). Emerald Group Publishing.

Maloni, M. J., & Brown, M. E. (2006). Corporate social responsibility in the supply chain: An application in the food industry. *Journal of Business Ethics*, *68*(1), 35–52. doi:10.100710551-006-9038-0

Manning, L., & Soon, J. M. (2016). Development of sustainability indicator scoring (SIS) for the food supply chain. *British Food Journal*, *118*(9), 2097–2125. doi:10.1108/BFJ-01-2016-0007

Marks and Spencer. (2015). *Sustainability score card.* Retrieved January, 24, 2017 from: http://corporate.marksandspencer.com/plan-a/our-approach/food-and-household/capacity-building-initiatives/sustainability-scorecard

McVeigh, K., & Quinn, B. (2017). Famine looms in four countries as aid system struggles to cope, experts warn. *The Guardian.* Retrieved July, 22, 2017 from https://www.theguardian.com/global-development/2017/feb/12/famine-looms-four-countries-aid-system-struggles-yemen-south-sudan-nigeria-somalia

Mentzer, J. T., DeWitt, W., Keebler, J. S., Min, S., Nix, N. W., Smith, C. D., & Zacharia, Z. G. (2001). Defining Supply Chain Management. *Journal of Business Logistics*, *22*(2), 1–25. doi:10.1002/j.2158-1592.2001.tb00001.x

Moran, J. W., & Brightman, B. K. (2001). Leading organizational change. *Career Development International*, *6*(2), 111–118.

Nellemann, C., Macdevetta, M., Manders, T., Eickhout, B., Svihus, B., Prins, A. G., & Kalterrnborn, B. P. (2009). *The Environmental Food Crises: The Environment's Role in Averting Future Food Crises.* UNEP/GRIP-Arendal, Arendal.

Organization for Economic Cooperation and Development (OECD). (2008). *OECD Environmental Outlook to 2030.* Retrieved from January, 28, 2017 from http://www.oecd.org/env/indicators-modellingoutlooks/oecdenvironmentaloutlookto2030keyresults.htm/

Pagell, M., & Wu, Z. (2009). Building a more complete theory of sustainable supply chain management using case studies of 10 exemplars. *The Journal of Supply Chain Management*, *45*(2), 37–56. doi:10.1111/j.1745-493X.2009.03162.x

Papargyropoulou, E., Lozano, R., Steinberger, J. K., Wright, N., & Ujang, Z. B. (2014). The food waste hierarchy as a framework for the management of food surplus and food waste. *Journal of Cleaner Production*, *76*, 106–115. doi:10.1016/j.jclepro.2014.04.020

Parfitt, J. M., Barthel, M., & Macnaughton, S. (2010). Food waste within food supply chains: Quantification and potential for change to 2050. *Philosophical Transactions of the Royal Society of London. Series B, Biological Sciences*, *365*(1554), 3065–3081. doi:10.1098/rstb.2010.0126 PMID:20713403

Plan International. (2017). *Millions in need as East Africa food crisis worsens.* Retrieved July, 24, 2017 from https://plan-international.org/why-there-food-crisis-east-africa

Population Institute. (2017). *Why Population Matters*. Retrieved January, 22, 2017 from https://www. populationinstitute.org/resources/whypopulationmatters/

Pothukuchi, K., & Kaufman, J. L. (1999). Placing the food system on the urban agenda: The role of municipal institutions in food systems planning. *Agriculture and Human Values*, *16*(4), 213–224. doi:10.1023/A:1007558805953

Rainforest Alliance. (2016). *What Does Rainforest Alliance Certified™ Mean?* Retrieved February 12, 2017 from http://www.rainforest-alliance.org/faqs/what-does-rainforest-alliance-certified-mean

Rong, A., Akkerman, R., & Grunow, M. (2010). An optimization approach for managing fresh food quality throughout the supply chain. *International Journal of Production Economics*, *131*(1), 421–429. doi:10.1016/j.ijpe.2009.11.026

Rubenstein-Montano, B., Liebowitz, J., Buchwalter, J., McCaw, D., Newman, B., Rebeck, K., & Team, T. K. M. M. (2001). A systems thinking framework for knowledge management. *Decision Support Systems*, *31*(1), 5–16. doi:10.1016/S0167-9236(00)00116-0

Rudder, A., Ainsworth, P., & Holgate, D. (2001). New food product development: Strategies for success. *British Food Journal*, *103*(9), 657–671. doi:10.1108/00070700110407012

Sainsbury. (2015). *Sainsbury's 20 by 20 sustainability plan*. Retrieved January, 24, 2017 from https:// www.j-sainsbury.co.uk/media/373272/sainsbury_s_20_by_20_sustainability_plan.pdf

Sathguru Management Consultants. (2017). *Rice value chain- food loss analysis: causes and solutions*. Rome: FAO.

Seuring, S., & Muller, M. (2008). From a literature review to a conceptual framework for sustainable supply chain management. *Journal of Cleaner Production*, *16*(15), 1699–1710. doi:10.1016/j.jclepro.2008.04.020

Sgarbossa, F., & Russo, I. (2017). A proactive model in sustainable food supply chain: Insight from a case study. *International Journal of Production Economics*, *183*, 596–606. doi:10.1016/j.ijpe.2016.07.022

Smith, B. G. (2008). Developing sustainable food supply chains. *Philosophical Transactions of the Royal Society*, *363*(1492), 849–861. doi:10.1098/rstb.2007.2187 PMID:17766237

Smith, P., Martino, D., Cai, Z., Gwary, G., Janzen, H., Kumar, P., ... Sirotenko, O. (2007). *Agriculture*. Cambridge, UK: Cambridge University Press.

Sokovic, M., Pavletic, D., & Pipan, K. K. (2010). Quality Improvement Methodologies – PDCA Cycle, RADAR Matrix, DMAIC and DFSSM. *Journal of Achievements in Materials and Manufacturing Engineering*, *43*(1), 476–483.

Sweet, T., Balakrishnan, J., Robertson, B., Stolee, J., & Karim, S. (2010). Applying quality function deployment in food safety management. *British Food Journal*, *112*(6), 624–639. doi:10.1108/00070701011052718

Teece, D. (1998). Capturing Value from Knowledge Assets: The New Economy, Markets for KnowHow, and Intangible Assets. *California Management Review*, *40*(3), 55–79. doi:10.2307/41165943

Tennyson, R., & Wilde, L. (2000). *The guiding hand: brokering partnerships for sustainable development*. United Nations Staff College and The Prince of Wales Business Leaders Forum.

UNESCO. (2005). *UN Decade of Education for Sustainable Development 2005 – 2014*. UNESCO.

United Nations Development Program (UNDP). (2017). *Sustainable Development Goals*. Retrieved February, 20, 2017 from http://www.undp.org/content/undp/en/home/sustainable-development-goals.html

United Nations (UN). (2015). World Population Prospects - The 2015 Revision. New York: UN.

United Nations (UN). (2017). *Famine declared in region of South Sudan – UN*. Retrieved July, 25, 2017 from http://www.un.org/apps/news/story.asp?NewsID=56205#.WZ_87j4jHDc

United Nations World Water Assessment Programme (UNWWAP). (2017). *The United Nations World Water Development Report 2017-Wastewater: The Untapped Resource*. Paris: UNESCO.

Van der Vorst, J. G., Tromp, S. O., & Zee, D. J. V. D. (2009). Simulation modelling for food supply chain redesign; integrated decision making on product quality, sustainability and logistics. *International Journal of Production Research*, *47*(23), 6611–6631. doi:10.1080/00207540802356747

Venkat, K. (2011). The climate change and economic impacts of food waste in the United States. *International Journal on Food System Dynamics*, *2*(4), 431–446.

Waste and Resources Action Programme. (2008). *The food we waste, Food Waste Report, Banbury*. WRAP.

World Commission on Environment and Development (WCED). (1987). *Our common future*. Oxford, UK: Oxford University Press.

ENDNOTES

[1]   World Commission on Environment and Development (WCED) (1987) in its Brundtland Report defines sustainability as meeting the needs of the present without compromising the ability of future generations to meet their own needs.

[2]   Single-loop learning is that which organizations do for corrective purposes (incremental changes) while double-loop learning is generative; that is, double-loop learning involves learning on a more fundamental level where basic assumptions are changed (Rubenstein-Montano, Liebowitz, Buchwalter, McCaw, Newman, Rebeck, & Team, 2001, p. 10).

This research was previously published in Emerging Applications in Supply Chains for Sustainable Business Development edited by M. Vijaya Kumar, Goran D. Putnik, K. Jayakrishna, V. Madhusudanan Pillai, and Leonilde Varela; pages 261-281, copyright year 2019 by Business Science Reference (an imprint of IGI Global).

Chapter 15

Logistic Strategies to Minimize Losses and Waste in Food Supply Chains

Betzabé Ruiz-Morales
Universidad Michoacana de San Nicolás de Hidalgo, Mexico

Marco A. Miranda-Ackerman
Universidad Autónoma de Baja Callifornia, Mexico

Irma Cristina Espitia-Moreno
Universidad Michoacana de San Nicolás de Hidalgo, Mexico

ABSTRACT

This chapter proposes sustainable supply chains in agrifoods, achieved through logistical strategies to minimize food waste and losses. Proposals will recover organic and inorganic waste and reincorporate it into the supply chain or add it to new chains through new products generated from food waste. A literature review is presented regarding the causes of food losses and waste within the supply chain and the strategic opportunities in the logistical process to reduce such losses. The creation of models that include the three dimensions of sustainability in food logistics is required in order to achieve a reduction in waste and food losses in transport, as well as to minimize costs and environmental impacts. If a correct sustainable logistics is carried out, it would favor the reincorporation of waste into new supply chains.

INTRODUCTION

The relationship between supply chain strategies, food production and the environment derive from their interactions. Climate change, challenges in agriculture need to be addressed, national-level policy drivers and innovation in agricultural processes are required, which are fundamental to fostering sustainable development, an enabling environment for innovation and a sustainable bioeconomy, through the use of clean technologies. (Sarkar, Poon, Lepage, Bilecki and Girard, 2018). Sustainability in agrifood

DOI: 10.4018/978-1-7998-5354-1.ch015

supply chains should be promoted; decisions should be analysed in the competitive environment in which companies operate with regard to the location of their raw material production centres, materials, technologies available to their suppliers, leverage over upstream suppliers and end markets. (Rueda, Garrett, and Lambin, 2016).

Technological changes in the agrifood industry have influenced economic and social development. These changes have also led to new environmental problems, such as those related to the large-scale use and disposal of auxiliary materials. The application of industrial ecology analyzes the potential development of approaches based on a representative context. Efficient solutions can be implemented through material substitution, repair, recycling and exploitation of collaborative strategies between the agro-food and industrial sectors (Simboli, Taddeo, & Morgante, 2015).

The green issue does not figure in the sales and profit objectives of some companies, because they do not have defined strategies for market changes regarding ecology and sustainability, the establishment of a strategic planning model that contemplates objectives and strategies on the environment, is for companies to adopt sustainable proposals and ensure their permanence in the market (Ávila, 2014). The ecological and social circumstances in which food is produced and offered, how the practices of a sustainable supply chain that allow the company to dominate maintain control over its supply chain and achieve a competitive advantage in the implementation of dynamic capabilities (Beske, Land, & Seuring, 2013).

In the case of agrifoods, the application of agroecological principles is sought, that is, the generation of food through environmentally friendly practices, to ensure the sustainability of products. In this commercial sector, producers want to integrate ecological processes and biological controls into the production, as well as make use of available resources at low cost and with less environmental degradation (Dafermos & Vivero, 2015). Towards sustainable agriculture, in Argentina the farmers of this community were able to increase their profits throughout their production chain and in profits, while restoring the ecological balance in their fields, to incursion into ecological practices. Producers can achieve these benefits through the implementation of sustainable strategies, sustainable marketing and the consumer's perception of being socially responsible producers with the environment (Gutiérrez & Suarez, 2014).

Sustainability in agro-industrial supply chains is an issue of great interest to various public and private sectors, due to the progressive deterioration of the environment, one of the great challenges is the design of the supply chain, due to the complexity it represents, many academics choose to take the study of one or parts of the supply chain (Allaoui, Choudhary, & Blormhof, 2016). The first step towards a more sustainable solution to the food waste problem is to adopt sustainable production (Papargyropoulou, Lozano, Steinberger, Wright, Ujang, 2014).

The agrifood supply chain, unlike other chains, implies indicators of food quality, safety, seasonality and a very limited useful life of the products (Alvarenga, Mourinha, Farto, Santos, Palma, Sengo, … Cunha-Queda, 2015). Currently the agricultural sector is under double pressure, first to be sustainable, i.e. to be able to satisfy the needs of the present without compromising the supply capacity of future generations and secondly to provide food, energy and industrial resources to satisfy the needs of the international community. The agricultural market is volatile and extremely sensitive to economic fluctuations (Borodin, Bourtembourg, Hnaien, & Labadie, 2016). Consumers increasingly demand organic and sustainable food, due to this trend the agri-food supply chain considers not only the cultivation of food, but also its distribution from the field to the customer's table, processing, packaging, storage, handling of by-products and waste (Gutierrez & Suarez, 2014).

It is necessary to extend the concept of supply chain management, especially in the food industry, this extension contains the management and recovery of waste, including it as a new loop within the configuration of the sustainable supply chain. A sustainable supply chain is responsible for processing raw materials into final products, managing end-of-life product recovery systems that incorporate useful and less environmentally damaging treatment (Sgarbossa & Russo, 2016). Supply chain management emerges as an area of great importance for the agrifood sector, because the actors involved in the design and execution of the supply chain must systematize the decision-making processes to optimize their waste. The study of supply chains in the agrifood sector has been accepted by the research community, however, systemic approaches are required to support the correct design and planning of the supply chain (Tsolakis, Keramydas, Toka, Aidonis, & Iakovou, 2013).

Environmental concerns and resource scarcity drive decision-making in the sustainable supply chain where alternatives involving the production of waste streams are considered, while simultaneously reusing and recycling waste materials. Closed loops in the supply chain consider improving the economic and environmental performance of waste through two options, the first is to replace it with raw materials and produce less waste, and the second is to reduce the total transport distance (Banasik, Kanellopoulos, Claassen, Bloemhof-Ruwaard, & Van der Vost, 2016). To produce less food waste and replace it as raw material for other products in agriculture, it is necessary to improve and expand infrastructure, technological solutions in harvesting, storage, transport and distribution, to ensure the success of reducing food waste. (Papargyropoulou et al., 2014).

Food waste production covers the entire life cycle, from agriculture to processing industry, retail and domestic consumption. In developed countries 42% of food waste is produced by domestic consumption, 39% in agriculture and food manufacturing, 14% in the restaurant industry and the remaining 5% comes from distribution (Mirabella, Castellani, & Sala., 2013). Harvesting, food preservation, pesticide use and crop protection result in the production of large amounts of waste in agriculture. Waste materials are not only food waste, they can also be auxiliary such as sheets, films, packaging, boxes, damaged pallets, scrap metal, steel and other packaging materials (Simboli et al., 2015). Integrated supply chain waste management in agro-industry is relatively new in the agricultural and food sector, with agricultural waste emerging as a source of pollution (Tsolakis et al., 2013).

Material reuse, recycling and waste have become important aspects of agricultural sustainability (Simboli et al., 2015). Agricultural waste management is based on the organized use of production, for the creation of by-products with sustainable methods to preserve the quality of air, water and soil. The agricultural waste management system covers six phases: production, collection, storage, treatment, distribution and consumption. Agricultural waste can be managed by disposal (incineration and composting) or by added value (for feed, fertiliser or energy). Waste reduction provides environmental benefits and utilities (Tsolakis et al., 2013). If the correct management and implementation of decisions is applied, economic increases of 11% and an environmental improvement of 28% can be presented (Banasik et al., 2016).

More and more citizens, scientists and companies are realizing that the current food system is unsustainable, so changes are required for the world to be able to support the population; reducing and reusing food waste will become an increasingly important strategy, especially for animal livelihoods (Thyberg & Tonjes, 2016). The trend towards sustainable agriculture and the strengthening of the agrifood system represents an opportunity to strengthen and diversify the sector by transforming agriculture into its stages of production and waste, to transform them into high-value bioproducts, through the generation of biofuels derived from non-edible vegetable components (Sarkar et al., 2018).

Food waste management can also be favorably harnessed through bioconversion of ethanol, biodiesel, hydrogen and methane to energy. Although transport to collect and dispose of waste has a high cost, it is estimated that the low or nil cost of food waste, added to the environmental benefits, balances the high costs of investment in biorefineries and the logistics employed (Uckun, Trzcinski, Jern, & Liu, 2014). Another way to take advantage of food wastes derived from fruit and vegetable agriculture in biorefineries is to take advantage of the nutritional properties of antioxidants, fiber, phenols, polyphenols and carotenoids for potential applications in cosmetic and pharmaceutical products (Mirabella et al., 2013).

A global target is that by 2030 global per capita food residues in trade and consumption should be halved, food losses along production and distribution chains, including post-harvest and transportation losses, should be reduced (Govindan, 2018).

BACKGROUND

The marketing and logistics of organizations within their strategies, need to focus on ethics and transparency to best serve consumers who stand out for their ecological awareness and prefer to consume responsibly. There are market segments with consumers who agree to pay a higher price for services and products that prove to be ecological (Ibarra, Casas, Olivia, & Barrasca, 2015). In the long term, companies that do not adopt sustainable business models will be sanctioned by consumers, this needs guidance on processes at the operational level that work with new technologies to consciously use and improve the efficiency of the use of natural resources in the development of sustainable products (Bur, 2013).

The needs of consumers are constantly changing, it is necessary to be clear that now there is the green consumer, who demands ecological, organic and high-quality products because there is a notorious concern for the environment. It was determined that recycling is a highly profitable business and that properly managed and with a well-structured green marketing plan sustainable development is achieved (Andrade, 2017). It shows a need for green marketing in response to a change in consumer behavior, where it seeks to be more environmentally friendly. Companies are concentrating on green packaging rather than green products if they apply green marketing to their entire supply chain, reducing waste and saving money. It has been shown that consumers are willing to pay more money to buy green products (Cherian & Jacob, 2012).

Sustainability in agro-industrial supply chains is an issue of great interest to various public and private sectors, due to the progressive deterioration of the environment, one of the great challenges is the design of the supply chain, due to the complexity it represents, many academics choose to take the study of one or parts of the supply chain (Allaoui, Guo, Choudhary, & Blormhof, 2016). Another proposed solution for non-food waste is the use of substitute materials such as biopolymers, repair of agricultural materials and equipment, to extend their life cycle, and use of waste to create closed loops within the company; development of a recycling platform between companies in the same industry (Simboli et al., 2015). In closed loops it is possible to have a direct connection with suppliers, customers or within the same organization, for the incorporation of waste in the supply chain. There is a growing awareness in society that food waste involves the loss of natural resources, and such losses should be avoided (Sgarbossa & Russo, 2016).

In classic cases of closed loops in the supply chain, products or materials after use are returned by the company or the customer, and are subsequently reused, dismantled and repaired, remanufactured or recycled, for agricultural products, most components cannot be reused or recycled, whereas production inputs that are related to agri-food products can provide a potential to close a nutrient cycle (Banasik et al., 2016). In Italy, biogas and cogeneration plants have been built to create new closed loops in the traditional supply chain, where agricultural waste can be used for energy self-sufficiency and independence (Sgarbossa & Russo, 2016).

Agro-food supply chains extend from producers to consumers, traditionally in the agro-food industry supply chains involve three main stages, 1. Suppliers of materials, 2. In addition to the application of closed loops to take advantage of waste, there is a tendency to reduce these percentages through industrial ecology and the circular economy, in which the main purpose is the use of waste for the production of new products. Another way of reducing waste and recovering it within the supply chain is by applying reverse logistics, returning the products to the supply chain, the valuable parts can be reused and the waste can be recycled or disposed of appropriately (Govindan, 2018). In addition to being a loss of value, the large amount of waste produced poses economic and environmental management problems (Mirabella et al., 2013).

Food production requires large amounts of energy and other resources, which generate an environmental impact and put at risk water, soil and air; agriculture contributes to pollution and eutrophication of water, due to the filtration of nutrients and fertilizers, in addition this activity consumes large amounts of this resource, machinery and transport in agriculture, generate greenhouse gases; the effects on the soil are erosion, nutrient depletion, pollution inside and outside the fields of cultivation, deforestation and loss of biodiversity (Thyberg & Tonjes, 2016). The benefits will depend on the amount of nutrients obtained from the waste, and it is also a sustainable alternative instead of dumping agricultural waste. (Alvarenga et al., 2015).

The generation of food waste is inevitable, especially during the pre-consumption phase, it has been shown that waste is a renewable resource for chemicals with high industrial importance because they can be used as raw material for the production of biofuels and enzymes, used for their use, technologies that allow the production of raw materials and have less impact on the environment, such as intelligent waste separation techniques, biochemical process strategies (fermentation), and biologically active molecule extraction processes for the use of feed and animal feed, which increase producers' interest in their economic benefits. (Ravindran & Jaiswal, 2016).

Agricultural producers are interested in eliminating residues in a more responsible way, with regulatory management in the planning, recycling and monitoring of soil and water to control the emissions that are thrown into these resources, as well as the use of fertilizers and control of ecologically friendly pests with the environment, vegetable producers have greater facilities to measure soil moisture and crop cover, while fruit producers can measure with greater precision the efficiency of water use. (Thorlakson, Hainmueller, & Lambin, 2018). They are also willing to carry out industrial symbiosis, through the collaboration of several companies located in the same community or industry, to share the management of material and energy flows, create solutions for the use of waste from their production processes and obtain by-products that can be included in other processes in order to improve profits (Simboli et al., 2015).

In France and the United States, since 2011 more than 30 companies and non-profit organizations have been created with the mission of fighting against food waste. In France, the leadership of these organizations is on the part of the Ministry of Agriculture, where it seeks to reduce food waste by 50% by 2025, by raising awareness of the formation of associations and regulations that support the proper management of agricultural waste. More and more companies are investing in infrastructure and technology for waste-to-energy conversion processes, however, concern about food waste has not fully entered the realm of agriculture and industrial policies. (Mourad, 2016).

An increasing number of consumers are becoming green consumers, seeking to purchase products that have green certifications and are grown under sustainable practices. A global target is that by 2030 global per capita food residues in trade and consumption should be halved, food losses along production in supply chains, including post-harvest losses, should be reduced (Govindan, 2018). Due to the high degree of homogeneity of agricultural processes and the waste generated, it is feasible to conduct research on waste management and use by researchers (Simboli et al., 2015).

LOGISTIC STRATEGIES TO MINIMIZE LOSSES AND WASTE IN FOOD SUPPLY CHAINS

According to Thyberg and Tonjes (2016), the logistical strategies to be followed to reduce food losses, firstly to invest in logistics equipment and make improvements, to reduce damage to food, secondly, to improve the packaging of food with more resistant products. Similarly, care should be taken to manage stocks in the warehouse for the transfer of goods to retailers. Another way to reduce food losses is the implementation of recovery policies, which encourage the redistribution of food for human consumption, these policies may include fiscal incentives for donors and programs to facilitate and expedite direct contact between donors and people in need of food or to facilitate the logistics of collection and transportation. Another policy is to bring wasted food that is not for human consumption to animal feed. Investment can also be made in improving packaging to prolong the shelf life of food, improving and maintaining warehouses, and properly monitoring stock management.

A large part of food losses are caused by poor logistics processes, especially cold chain management. It is important to use technologies that allow to monitor the useful life of the product, and when this quality falls below the level of acceptance, to develop a plan of the processes of the supply chain to avoid the total loss of food once it expired. Intelligent food logistics is proposed, by improving the quality of food, its containers and packaging, such as gas sensors that can detect ethylene as an index of excess maturation and mold infections, should also monitor chains that include cold chambers for optimal performance. The inconsistency in the quality of fresh products can be explained by the variations in temperature that are found during transportation, to stop these variations requires the measurement of temperatures through a monitoring system in the container and continuous monitoring of fluctuations (Jedermann, Nicometo, Uysal, & Lang, 2014).

Food waste and losses are produced at all stages of the supply chain, the causes are diverse for each stage of the chain. One of the main causes of the loss of food are the policies and quality standards at the international level of food and not for reasons of nutritional value, so that many foods could be used for animal use or composting, maintaining communication between all actors involved in the supply chain, to plan a new appreciation of food and be able to use them, for the long term to achieve a more sustainable food system (Göbel, Langen, Blumentha, Teitscheid, & Ritter, 2015).

Verghese, Lewis, Lockrey, & Williams (2015), in their research identified opportunities to leverage and reduce food waste through logistics:

1. Better protection and shelf life for fresh food with appropriate packaging for retail distribution.
2. Recovering surplus products and distributing them to food rescue supply chains.
3. New packaging with life extension materials and technology, with controlled atmosphere and oxygen absorption.

4. Timely communication between producers, retailers and consumers about the expiry date to ensure that they are distributed properly and avoid waste when it is still edible.
5. Location of food waste hoarding industries for collaboration between producers, transporters, retailers and customers.
6. Optimal packaging for retail, to reduce double handling and damage from stock turnover.

Packaging improvements and technical innovations represent important opportunities to reduce food waste in the supply chain. Although some waste is unavoidable, much of it is due to inefficiencies in the supply chain that damage food through poor handling. In order to reduce such food waste, more awareness-raising and education activities are needed among all stakeholders in the food supply chain.

The levels of residues are mainly due to the natural characteristics of fresh food, such as its useful life, the growing demand for fresh products, the seasonality and variability of demand, most foods with a useful life less than or equal to two weeks have much waste, so it is important that all actors in the supply chain pay special attention to these products and improving the conditions of handling and careful movement, can minimize waste. Opportunities to reduce waste include: sharing shelf-life and food handling information across all actors in the supply chain, measuring performance, forecasting and ordering cold chain management, jointly developing optimal waste management and proper packaging (Menaa, Adenso-Diazb, & Yurt, 2011).

A little studied way to minimize food losses is the just in time delivery adding environmental sustainability, the speed of delivery improves carbon efficiency and extends the useful life of the food, it is important to make structural decisions about the means of logistics, including means of transport, packaging and packaging used, if you invest to implement improvements in these aspects, you can increase product quality and reduce losses. Optimising the amount of waste in each part of the supply chain provides an opportunity to improve the sustainable performance of the supply chain. The faster the deliveries, the more days there are to use the products, and the greater the likelihood of selling the product. The use and development of packaging materials is a way to improve sustainability when packaging sizes are customized enough for different customer needs. Product packaging not only provides information, but also protects food from spoilage (Ala-Harja & Petri, 2014).

Zero Waste is a holistic approach to tackling waste problems in the 21st century. There is a strategy to reduce waste is to prevent their arrival at landfills, through cultural transformation from producers to final consumers, it is proposed that there are government policies that encourage the reduction of food waste (Zaman, 2015). More intense communication between the efforts of governments and charities is probably all that is needed to further reduce food waste and provide the poor with food, with the help of transporters to facilitate the movement of waste that can still be consumed by people, a network of collaboration and information is needed with business associations, businesses, sector policy makers and intermediaries such as food banks to reduce waste (Garrone, Melacini, & Perego, 2014).

Supply network design models and methods have been the subject of several recent literature review studies, but none of them include sustainable development as a major feature of the supply chain design problem. The limited scope of environmental and social measures in current models should go beyond limited greenhouse gas indicators and encompass broader life-cycle approaches that include new parameters with the social indicator. There is also a need for more effective inclusion of uncertainty and risk in models with improved multi-objective approaches (Eskandarpour, Dejax, Miemczyk, & Péton, 2015).

Reverse logistics is a systematic process that manages the flow of products from consumption to the point of manufacture for possible recycling, remanufacturing or disposal. Although the concept of reverse logistics is well known in logistics and supply chain management, the available literature and holistic theory on reverse logistics is scarce. The correct application of reverse logistics requires the planning, design, implementation and control of all activities involved in the logistics process. The strategic decision-making process for reverse logistics starts with the customers and their requirements. Meeting customer requirements for reverse logistics products is a strategic decision and requires an understanding of markets, customers and their potential about a company's strategic values and distinctive competence. Focusing on other strategic factors will do no good if customer needs cannot be met or if customer needs are not compatible with a company's core values. If long-term customer requirements cannot be met or if appropriate changes in business strategy cannot be made to make it compatible with customer requirements, then the reverse logistics process could end at this stage (Dowlatshahi, 2005).

Today, the role of supply chain strategies in the generation of food waste or losses is neglected, because such losses are generally considered an inevitable consequence or the result of accidental events in the logistical process. At present, only operational plans are implemented, the aim of which is to reduce the impact of product losses along the supply chain. This implies that structured analyses and strategic approaches to supply chains are not available for the prevention and minimisation of food waste. The generation of waste and losses depends primarily on supply chain strategies that are often optimized based on market demand. Food waste is an intrinsic feature of the supply chain, which must be linked to market demand and product life, for market conditions such as legal constraints, policy decisions, climatic and microeconomic factors. This should include the study of new demand models dependent on the shelf life of products based on consumer utility, and especially on the redesign of logistics supply chain management models, with specific models for supply chain coordination, planning strategies and pricing models for the prevention and minimization of the foreseeable component of waste (Muriana, 2017).

If the strategic reverse logistics decision-making process advances to the second stage, environmental issues dominate the process. Not only must current regulations and environmental considerations be complied with at this stage, but future trends and possible changes in existing laws and regulations and their impact on reverse logistics operations must also be explored. Reverse logistics is a proactive process that requires scanning the external environment so that the company can respond to external forces in an appropriate and timely manner. This is necessary for the company to practice economic sustainability and operate as a socially responsible company. The final step in the strategic reverse logistics process is to ensure that the quality of the product meets or exceeds the quality of the respective virgin products. Lack of quality and the inability of the product to conform to the design could undermine the entire reverse logistics planning and implementation process. Given customers' typical perception of remanufactured or recycled products, and given the low profit margins these products provide, rigorous compliance with quality standards is mandatory (Dowlatshahi, 2005).

Sustainable supply chain management is a topical issue that continues to grow and evolve. Within supply chains, distribution from producers to customers plays an important role in the environmental performance of production supply chains. With growing consumer awareness in the area of sustainable food supply, food distribution needs to adopt and adapt to improve its environmental performance while remaining economically competitive. A critical component of modern food supply chains is the distribution system, because this is where large amounts of waste can be produced. The sustainable distribution process allows the decision maker in the supply chain to reduce the total carbon emission of the transport involved in the entire distribution process and, at the same time, optimize the total costs, by studying the best types of vehicles are offered taking into account two attributes, CO_2 emissions and costs are the average values of both CO_2 emissions and costs, in the same way the best routes must be traced geographically to obtain the best performance, a distribution of optimal and sustainable products, helping to reduce damage to goods by inefficient logistical design (Validi, Bhattacharya, & Byrne, 2014).

Approximately one third of the edible calories produced for Swiss consumption are lost along the entire food value chain. Reducing food losses is therefore an effective way to increase efficiency and reduce the environmental impact of food consumption. The ecological significance of food losses depends not only on the quantity, but also on the type of food, where it is lost in the food value chain and how it is recycled or disposed of. For example, carrots that remain in fields are ecologically less important than carrots wasted by households after being transported, stored, packaged and processed. Cereals sorted in mills and used for food are less relevant than the same amount of baked bread thrown away in a restaurant. Therefore, food losses should not only be quantified, but also assessed through life cycle assessment. This would allow a more precise quantification of the environmental benefits of reducing food waste and help us define priority areas (Beretta, Stoessel, Baier, & Hellweg, 2012).

The significant causes of food residues in the supply chain according to Raak, Symmank, Zahn, Aschemann-Witzel, and Rohm (2017), are related to logistical handling, product processing and consumption. Potential actions to reduce food waste in the following areas:

1. Product deterioration during transport and storage. Devices such as RFID or GPS technologies, or strategic management processes can help minimize losses along the supply chain through greater control of product shelf life and accelerated product delivery. In this way, excess production could also be reduced because smaller volumes of stock are required to compensate for expired products.
2. Food processing by-products. Parts of the raw materials that are not needed for the product itself still contain functional and/or nutritional compounds. In many cases, the recovery of individual compounds is not cost-effective, so possible applications of the entire by-product should be explored rather than resource-intensive and cost-intensive extraction processes.
3. Consumer perception of quality and safety. Consumers often reject edible foods with changes in visual or sensory quality, or that have passed the expiration date. Intelligent packaging can complement date labels to provide information about edibility.

The causes identified as responsible for food losses and waste can be classified as follows:

a) Losses resulting from treatment operations and quality assurance
b) Products that do not meet the quality requirements of the trade.

Foods that deviate from standards and expectations are often marketed as a second option using alternative trade channels such as specific outlets and special offers. However, it depends on the region and culture to determine what quality requirements are anticipated and how well alternative trade routes are established.

Measures should be taken to prevent food losses at all stages of the food value chain. The implementation of measures requires the participation of all actors, including government. This is particularly true because some food losses do not occur only at the stage at which they occur. Donations alone cannot solve the problem of food losses, mainly due to logistical, political and hygienic constraints. Households are the main source of food losses. Therefore, consumer awareness, good planning and proper food storage are crucial. Since the amounts of food losses depend largely on agricultural infrastructure, food processing technologies, climatic conditions and incomes (Beretta et al., 2012).

SOLUTIONS AND RECOMMENDATIONS

Food waste prevention has not yet become widespread in the United States and abroad. Food waste is widespread around the world and food waste generation is likely to continue to grow if it is not affected by prevention policies. Most of the above authors point out that waste prevention in general has often been ignored in waste management. All authors agree that food waste is a complex issue involving many different actors along the food chain, in order to reduce such food waste, more awareness and education is needed among all stakeholders in the food supply chain. The studies carried out identify that the implementation of improvements in logistics reduce food waste, these improvements can concentrate on the monitoring and optimal operation of cold chambers, on just-in-time delivery, on investment in containers and packaging that allow proper handling of food, on having control over the useful life of products and an efficient network to achieve the transfer of food that is still in good condition to food collection banks, Finally, many authors propose that implementing government policies that encourage and strengthen the return of waste to specific sites for reuse would considerably reduce the amounts of waste and food waste that currently persists.

FUTURE RESEARCH DIRECTIONS

For future lines of research, it is advisable to carry out studies on supply chains for agricultural food, in order to specify the particular problems of the various foods from the field, and provide more exclusive solutions to food losses.

CONCLUSION

Due to the high degree of homogeneity of agricultural processes, their transport and the waste and residues generated, it is important to carry out research on the recovery and use of losses, in order to provide logistical strategies to help achieve the objectives of global food security, according to the contributions of various authors, it is optimal to carry out research on the characteristics of the products and the logistics they carry out. In the same way, it is important to detect the causes of waste and develop a plan of action to reduce or avoid them, by improving packaging, communication and collaboration among all actors in the supply chain in order to take advantage of food waste in compost or cattle feed. It is extremely important to identify strategies that reduce the main causes of losses and provide solutions to identified food loss problems, as food losses affect the amount of food available for consumption, which is reflected in food safety indices.

REFERENCES

Ala-Harja, H., & Helo, P. (2014). Green supply chain decisions – Case-based performance analysis from the food industry. Jornal Elsevier. *Transportation Research Part E, Logistics and Transportation Review*, *69*, 97–107. doi:10.1016/j.tre.2014.05.015

Allaoui, H., Guo, Y., Choudhary, A., & Blormhof, J. (2016). Sustainable agro-food supply chain design using two-stage hybrid multi-objetive decisión-making approach. *Journal Science Direct. Computers & Operations Research, 89,* 369–384. doi:10.1016/j.cor.2016.10.012

Alvarenga, P., Mourinha, C., Farto, M., Santos, T., Palma, P., Sengo, J., … Cunha-Queda, C. (2015). Sewage sludge, compost and other representative organic wastes as agricultural soil amendments: Benefits versus limiting factors. *Journal Waste Management. Science Direct, 40,* 44-52. doi:10.1016/j.wasman.2015.01.027

Andrade, A. (2017). *Plan de marketing de productos fabricados mediante el reciclaje de residuos de vidrio en el barrio de la Viga, con enfoque de género.* Grado: Doctorado en Administración. Instituto Politécnico Nacional. Retrieved from http://tesis.ipn.mx/bitstream/handle/123456789/23631/MAES2017%20A534a%20Ana%20Luc%C3%ADa%20Andrade%20Cevallos.pdf?sequence=1&isAllowed=y

Ávila, O. (2014). La responsabilidad social de la mercadotecnia sobre el medio ambiente. *Journal Contaduría y Administración UNAM, 23,* 178–199. Retrieved from emprendedores.unam.mx/articulo.php?id_articulo=277

Banasik, A., Kanellopoulos, A., Claassen, G., Bloemhof-Ruwaard, J., & Van der Vost, J. (2016). Closing loops in agricultural supply chains using optimization: A case study of an industrial mushroom supply chain. *Journal Production Economics. Science Direct, 183,* 409–420. doi:10.1016/j.ijpe.2016.08.012

Beretta, C., Stoessel, F., Baier, U., & Hellweg, S. (2012). Quantifying food losses and the potential for reduction in Switzerland. *Journal Elsevier, Waste Management 33,* 3, 764-773. doi:http://doi.org.conricyt.remotexs.co/10.1016/j.wasman.2012.11.007

Beske, P., Land, A., & Seuring, S. (2013). Sustainable supply chain management practices and dynamic capabilities in the food industry: A critical analysis of the literature. *Journal of Productions Economics. Science Direct, 152,* 131–143. doi:10.1016/j.ijpe.2013.12.026

Borodin, V., Bourtembourg, J., Hnaien, F., & Labadie, N. (2016). Handling uncertainty in agricultural supply chain managmente: A state of the art. *Journal of Operational Research. Elsevier, 254*(2), 348–359. doi:10.1016/j.ejor.2016.03.057

Bur, A. (2013). Marketing sustentable. Utilización del marketing sustentable en la industria textil y de la indumentaria. En *Journal Scielo. General 45,* 347-358. Retrieved from http://www.scielo.org.ar/scielo.php?pid=S1853-35232013000300012&script=sci_arttext&tlng=pt

Cherian, J. & Jacob, J. (2012). Green Marketing: A Study of Consumers' Attitude towards En *Journal Asian Social Science. General 71,* 68-84. Retrieved from http://www.ccsenet.org/journal/index.php/ass/article/view/20767/13589

Dafermos, J. & Vivero, L. (2015). Agroalimentación Sistema agroalimentario abierto y sustentable en Ecuador. En *Journal Research Gate. General 2.1,* 46-73. Retrieved from https://www.researchgate.net/publication/280566593

Dowlatshahi, S. (2015). A strategic framework for the design and implementation of remanufacturing operations in reverse logistics. *International Journal of Production Research, 43*(16), 3455–3480. doi:10.1080/00207540500118118

Eskandarpour, M., Dejax, P., Miemczyk, J., & Péton, O. (2015). Sustainable supply chain network design: An optimization-oriented review. *Journal Elsevier. Omega, 54,* 11–32. doi:10.1016/j.omega.2015.01.006

Garrone, P., Melacini, M., & Perego, A. (2014). Opening the black box of food waste reduction. *Journal Elsevier. Food Policy, 46,* 129–139. doi:10.1016/j.foodpol.2014.03.014

Göbel, C., Langen, N., Blumenth, A., Teitscheid, P., & Ritter, G. (2015). Cutting Food Waste through Cooperation along the Food Supply Chain. *Sustainability, 7*(2), 1429–1445. doi:10.3390u7021429

Govindan, K. (2018). Sustainable consumption and production in the food supply chain: A conceptual framework. *Journal Production Economics. Science Direct, 195,* 419–431. doi:10.1016/j.ijpe.2017.03.003

Gutiérrez, J. & Suarez, M. (2014). Agrocombustibles y agroalimentos. Considerando las externalidades de la mayor encrucijada del siglo XXI. En *Journal Agroecología. General 4,* 123-134. Retrieved from http://revistas.um.es/agroecologia/article/view/117211/110861

Ibarra, L., Casas, E., Olivas, E., & Barraza, K. (2015). El marketing sustentable como estrategia de posicionamiento global en las franquicias mexicanas que operan en la ciudad de Hermosillo, Sonora. En *Revista internacional administración y finanzas. 133,* 56-78. Retrieved from http://guzlop-editoras.com/web_des/adm01/marketing/pld1870.pdf

Jedermann, R., Nicometo, M., Uysal, I., & Lang, W. (2014). Reducing food losses by intelligent food logistics. *Journal Royal Society. Philosophical Transactions, 372.* doi:10.1098/rsta.2013.0302

Mena, C., Adenso-Diaz, B., & Yurt, O. (2011). The causes of food waste in the supplier–retailer interface: Evidences from the UK and Spain. *Journal Science Direct. Resources, Conservation and Recycling, 55*(6), 648–658. doi:10.1016/j.resconrec.2010.09.006

Mirabella, N., Castellani, V., & Sala, S. (2013). Current options for the valorization of food manufacturing waste: A review. *Journal Cleaner Production. Elsevier, 65,* 28–41. doi:10.1016/j.jclepro.2013.10.051

Mourad, M. (2016). Recycling, recovering and preventing "food waste": Competing solutions for food systems sustainability in the United States and France. *Journal Cleaner Production. Elsevier, 126,* 461–477. doi:10.1016/j.jclepro.2016.03.084

Muriana, C. (2017). A focus on the state of the art of food waste/losses issue and suggestions for future researches. *Journal, Elsevier. Waste Management (New York, N.Y.), 68,* 557–570. doi:10.1016/j.wasman.2017.06.047 PMID:28688545

Papargyropoulou, E., Lozano, R., Steinberger, J., Wright, N., & Ujang, Z. (2014). The food waste hierarchy as framework for the managment of food surplus and food waste. *Journal Cleaner Production. Elsevier, 76,* 106–115. doi:10.1016/j.jclepro.2014.04.020

Raak, N., Symmank, C., Zahn, S., Aschemann-Witzel, J. Y., & Rohm, H. (2017). Processing- and product-related causes for food waste and implications for the food supply chain.

Ravindran, R. & Jaiswal, A. (2016). Exploitation of food industry waste for high-value products. *Journal Trends in Biotechnology.* Elsevier, 34, 1-13. doi:10.1016/j.tibtech.2015.10.008

Rueda, X., Garrett, J., & Lambin, R. (2016). Corporate investments in supply chain sustainability: Selecting instruments in the agri-food industry. *Journal of Cleaner Production. Science Direct, 142*, 2480–2492. doi:10.1016/j.jclepro.2016.11.026

Sarkar, S., Poon, J., Lepage, E., Bilecki, L., & Girad, B. (2018). Enabling a sustainable and prosperous future through science and innovation in the bioeconomy at Agriculture and Agri-food Canada. *Journal New Biotechnology. Science Direct, 40*, 70–75. doi:10.1016/j.nbt.2017.04.001 PMID:28411151

Sgarbossa, F., & Russo, I. (2016). A proactive model in sustainable food supply chain: Insight from a case study. *Journal Elsevier. Science Direct, 183*, 596–606. doi:10.1016/j.ijpe.2016.07.022

Simboli, A., Taddeo, R., & Morgan, A. (2015). The potential of Industrial Ecology in agri-food clusters: A case study based on valorisation of auxiliary materials. *Ecological Economics, 111*, 65–75. doi:10.1016/j.ecolecon.2015.01.005

Thorlakson, T., Hainmueller, J., & Lambin, E. (2018). Improving environmental practices in agricultural supply chains: The role of Company-led standards. *Journal Global Environmental Change. Science Direct, 48*, 32–42. doi:10.1016/j.gloenvcha.2017.10.006

Thyberg, K., & Tonjes, D. (2016). Drivers of food waste and their implications for sustainable policy development. *Resources, Conservation and Recycling, 106*, 110–123. doi:10.1016/j.resconrec.2015.11.016

Tsolakis, N., Keramydas, C., Toka, A., Aidonis, D., & Iakovou, E. (2013). Agrifood supply chain management: A comprehensive hierarchical decisión-making framework and critical taxonomy. *Journal Science Direct. Byosistems Engineering, 120*, 47–64. doi:10.1016/j.biosystemseng.2013.10.014

Uckun, E., Trzcinski, A., Jern, W., & Liu, Y. (2014). Bioconversion of food waste to energy: A review. *Journal Science Direct. Fuel, 134*, 389–399. doi:10.1016/j.fuel.2014.05.074

Validi, S., Bhattacharya, A., & Byrne, P. (2014). A case analysis of a sustainable food supply chain distribution system—A multi-objective approach. *International Journal of Production Economics, 152*, 71-78. doi:http://doi.org.conricyt.remotexs.com/10.1016/j.ipe.2014.02.003

Verghese, K., Lewis, H., Lockrey, S., & Williams, H. (2015). Packaging's Role in Minimizing Food Loss and Waste Across the Supply Chain. *Journal Packag. Technol. Sci., 28*(7), 603–620. doi:10.1002/pts.2127

Zaman, A. (2015). A comprehensive review of the development of zero waste management: lessons learned and guidelines. *Elsevier Journal of Cleaner Production 91*, 12e25. doi:10.1016/j.jclepro.2014.12.013

This research was previously published in the Handbook of Research on Industrial Applications for Improved Supply Chain Performance edited by Jorge Luis García-Alcaraz, George Leal Jamil, Liliana Avelar-Sosa, and Antonio Juan Briones Peñalver; pages 285-298, copyright year 2020 by Business Science Reference (an imprint of IGI Global).

Chapter 16
From Information Sharing to Information Utilization in Food Supply Chains

Kasper Kiil
Norwegian University of Science and Technology, Trondheim, Norway and Aalborg University, Aalborg, Denmark

Hans-Henrik Hvolby
Aalborg University, Aalborg, Denmark and Norwegian University of Science and Technology, Trondheim, Norway

Jacques Trienekens
Wageningen University, Wageningen, The Netherlands

Behzad Behdani
Wageningen University, Wageningen, The Netherlands

Jan Ola Strandhagen
Norwegian University of Science and Technology, Trondheim, Norway

ABSTRACT

Information sharing has been extensively studied as a key enabler for coordination and integration in supply chains. However, exactly how the shared information is utilized for decision making has only received limited scientific attention in the research literature. The aim of this study is to identify the characteristics of information sharing, and conceptualize how to move from information sharing to information utilization in food supply chains. Using a case study methodology together with a review of the existing literature the authors describe the main facets of shared information - which influence the information utilization in a supply chain - and propose a mapping notation for how these facets can be visualized together with a supply chain operations reference (SCOR) model. Information utilization is especially important because more information sharing does not necessarily result in a better supply chain performance unless the shared information is effectively used in the relevant processes in the chain and well-aligned with the requirements for those processes. The proposed notation provides a systematic structure for mapping the information flows, their specific facets, and helps clarify what information is available and how this information can be utilized in different supply chain processes. Four facets of information sharing are identified and elaborated for food supply chains, together with a mapping tool that emphasizes the information flows and the utilization of information in supply chains.

DOI: 10.4018/978-1-7998-5354-1.ch016

1. INTRODUCTION

Information sharing, i.e. the availability of information from other inter-organizational partners has been of interest for more than half a century (Forrester, 1958; Lee, So, & Tang, 2000; Montoya-Torres & Ortiz-Vargas, 2014). It is considered to be one of the key mechanisms for coordination across organizations and has shown to enable more accurate forecasts, lower inventory levels, and reduction of bullwhip effect (Mason-Jones & Towill, 1997; Trapero, Kourentzes, & Fildes, 2012; Zhao & Xie, 2002). However, to fully reap the potential of the shared information, recent studies in the field of supply chain management suggest not only to make information available, but placing a strong focus on how the shared information is and could be utilized at the receiving company (Baihaqi & Sohal, 2013; Jonsson & Mattsson, 2013; Myrelid, 2015).

It has been acknowledged that the utilization and the value of shared information is context specific (El Kadiri et al., 2016; Shaik & Abdul-Kader, 2013). We have chosen food supply chains as the context for this study for two main reasons. Firstly, the characteristics of food supply chains and the products are known to impose special logistical requirements (limited ability to use of buffer inventories, traceability requirements, etc.) (Fredriksson & Liljestrand, 2015; Trienekens & van Der Vorst, 2006). Secondly, due to detailed and fine meshed traceability requirements, starting from the primary producer to the final store, the supply chain as a whole encompasses a vast amount of information (Folinas & Manikas, 2010; Trienekens & van Der Vorst, 2006). Thus, on one hand, food supply chains call for special logistical activities, and on the other hand, the actors in the chain capture valuable information that may be utilized to a higher extent for those logistical activities.

Utilization of shared information is poorly defined in the existing literature (Jonsson & Myrelid, 2016; Kim & Narasimhan, 2002; Myrelid, 2015). Insights from one of the largest wholesalers and retailer in Norway confirms the necessity and potential benefit of utilize the shared information across the whole supply chain to improve coordination further. On one hand, limited transparency or access to information implies that decisions are taken without considering other actors in the chain. On the other hand, the vast amount of information that is captured due to traceability requirements are mostly used for reporting and safety purpose as other areas of usage has not been systematically identified. These challenges have also been stressed in the literature by (Endsley, 2016, pp. 3-4) stating that: "In the face of this torrent of information, many of us feel less informed than ever before. This is because there is a huge gap between the tons of data being produced and disseminated, and our ability to find the bits that are needed and process them together with the other bits to arrive at the actual needed information. That is, it seems to be even harder to find out what we really want or need to know".

To grasp the complexity of all processes and the available and potentially available information in the supply chain and the linkages between processes and information requires a comprehensive and systematic model. According to (Andersson, Jansson, Sandblad, & Tschirner, 2014) visualizing the problem can increase the understanding of the problem - not by reducing the complexity but by coping and recognizing it in the visualization. In operations and supply chain management field several methodologies and mapping tools have been proposed to ease this issue by providing structure and overview of this complexity (Aguilar-Saven, 2004; Alfnes, Dreyer, & Strandhagen, 2008; Thakur et al., 2011). Current solutions seem to either aim towards depicting facets of shared information (timeliness, content, etc.) (Holweg & Pil, 2008) or showing the linkage between the shared information and the decisions processes (Verdouw, Beulens, Trienekens, & Wolfert, 2010). However, no concept nor overview exists to identify what, when, and whom to share information with and more importantly how to utilize the received information (Jonsson & Mattsson, 2013; Sahin & Robinson, 2002). In this study, we seek to address this gab in literature by unraveling the concept of information utilization. We do this by identifying facets of information sharing and conceptualize how to move from information sharing to information utilization in food supply chains by proposing a notation for information flows and utilization. This notation is afterwards tested in a case study to demonstration its relevance and applicability for practitioners.

The remainder of this paper is organized as follows. Section 2 briefly presents how the research was conducted and the interaction of empirical data and literature. Section 3 reviews the relevant literature on food supply chains, information facets and utilization. Common mapping tools are discussed in section 4, while section 5 propose a notation for how to visualize information utilization. Lastly, section 6 includes a discussion and conclusion.

2. METHODOLOGY

An initial literature search revealed that information utilization has only received limited scientific attention despite its connection and importance for information sharing (Jonsson & Myrelid, 2016; Myrelid, 2015). To examine this gap further we adopted an explorative approach that builds on existing literature and empirical data. We applied a case study approach as it is highly applicable for early investigations where the variables and phenomenon are not fully understood (Voss, Tsikriktsis, & Frohlich, 2002; Yin, 2013).

2.1. Case Selection

A Norwegian food supply chain was selected for this study for three main reasons. First, the food industry is known for recording a high amount of data and for fresh food products, decisions need to be made quickly relying on the information available (Taylor & Fearne, 2006; Trienekens & van Der Vorst, 2006). Second, most of the existing literature on information sharing focuses on dyadic relations (Kembro & Näslund, 2014; Kiil, Dreyer, & Hvolby, 2015), which simplify the problem but important non-supplier-buyer interactions in the supply chain might not be observed (Huang, Lau, & Mak, 2003). Thus, we were motivated to study information flows in a complete supply chain to obtain a holistic understanding. Third, the specific Norwegian food supply chain was selected due to ongoing research protocols, and the existing collaborative mindset between the companies in the supply chain. The wholesaler in this study, owns the warehouses, is closely integrated with the stores and has a long history of common improvement projects with its major suppliers and transport providers. Thus, the traditional barriers of information sharing, connectivity and willingness (Fawcett et al., 2007), were not reflected as an issue for this particular setting. Information quality has also been suggested as a prerequisite for effective results of information sharing (Moberg, Cutler, Gross, & Speh, 2002; Myrelid, 2015). However, all actors agreed that the quality of the information was not the main obstacle as the traceability requirement indirectly ensured high standards for all actors.

2.2. Data Collection

The literature on information sharing was studied and in particular literature which aimed to conceptualize information sharing, establish typologies, or which provided descriptive measures to assess the level of information sharing. Additionally, existing mapping tools were reviewed as these are helpful to establish overview and cope with complexity (Gardner & Cooper, 2003).

Four generic facets of information sharing were identified from the literature (this will be elaborated in Section 3.3). These were used to create a questionnaire about the current information flows and ideas for future information flows for the Norwegian food supply chain. The questionnaire was distributed among 25 respondents across the supply chain (see Table 1), if they were from the same company they were allowed to answer together. For each type of information, the company receives or sends, the questionnaire included questions about frequency, aggregation levels, time horizon, source/receivers, and how far in advance the information was shared. Also, questions about how the actual exchange of information took place and how they used the information were included. Response from all involved companies was received.

Table 1. Respondents of questionnaire and their function

Producers	Wholesaler	Warehouses	Transport	Stores
3 Owners 1 Director of supply chain 1 Functional manager	1 Director of logistics development 1 Head of IT 2 Functional mangers	2 Head of warehouse 6 Functional managers	1 Owner 2 Functional mangers	1 Regional manager 4 Store managers

2.3. Data Analysis and Validation

Based on the answers from the questionnaire a high-level flow chart illustrating the involved companies was drawn for each type of shared information and the associated facets were added. Practically, this was done by making one flow chart including stores, transportation providers, regional warehouse, central warehouse, and suppliers were drawn to illustrate the material flow. Afterwards, one type of shared information (e.g. point-of-sales data) was added to the chart which showed how often each tier received the data, in which format, in what level of aggregation, etc. Then, new charts with a new information types were made one by one. This was presented and adjusted accordingly at a common 2-hour workshop with the respondents. For each information type it was discussed how it was used at the companies. Ideas for new information flows, both from the questionnaire and from the ongoing discussion, was elaborated in the end of workshop among all respondents.

3. FOOD SUPPLY CHAINS AND ITS INFORMATION FLOWS

3.1. Characteristics of Food Supply Chains

Food supply chains may be as simple as a local producer selling its products directly to the final consumers, or global supply chains where products flow from farmers, processors, trading units, wholesaler, distributors, and to stores before they reach the consumers (Entrup, 2006). The upstream part of a complete food supply chains typically follows a convergent structure with a high number of suppliers, suppling a variety of different products to a wholesaler. While the downstream part is divergent with a single or few warehouses suppling a high number of stores of different segments (Van der Vorst, Tromp, & Zee, 2009). The presence of both a convergent and a divergent structure within the same supply chain increases the amount of relationships to coordinate and especially for the wholesaler which is in between. The complexity and associated transparency of the supply chain is to a large extent determined by the amount of relationships and the flow of material and information among these relationships (Trienekens, Wognum, Beulens, & van der Vorst, 2012).

The coordination of flow of goods is further complicated in food supply chains due to existence of both supply and demand uncertainty (Romsdal, 2014; Singh, 2014; Taylor & Fearne, 2009). The production of fruit, vegetables, and meat is subject to long throughput times and the exact day, volume, and quality might only be observable at the very end. Additionally, some products like fruit, vegetables, and dairy is subjected to seasonality, and, the quality or availability of those products are not consistent throughout the year (Romsdal, 2014). Regarding uncertainty in demand, at stores, sales have been reported to fluctuate $\pm$ 11% around the mean while it fluctuates up to 115% at the producer (Taylor & Fearne, 2009). This clearly demonstrates the existence of demand amplification and room for improving the inter-organizational coordination. Balancing supply and demand in food supply chains is indeed also present. The availability of products in stores is estimated to range from 93.8% to 96.8% indicating a deficit of supply (Aastrup & Kotzab, 2009). While estimates of food waste along the supply chain ranges from 25% to 35% indicating a surplus of supply (Kummu et al., 2012; Parfitt, Barthel, & Macnaughton, 2010).

Many food products have a limited shelf life and deteriorate over time due their perishable nature, which places unique requirements on logistics (Fredriksson & Liljestrand, 2015; Van der Vorst, Beulens, & van Beek, 2005). For example, storage and transportation in food supply chains has to be accomplished in different temperature zones to account for both ambient, chilled, and frozen products and retained throughout the supply chain to reduce the risk of products perishes. In addition, to provide a long remaining shelf life for the consumers, the products need to move as quickly as possible from the producer to the consumer with limited use of buffer inventories along the supply chain (Kaipia, Dukovska-Popovska, & Loikkanen, 2013). This calls for a flexible and responsive production facilities and planning capabilities (Van der Vorst et al., 2005). The ad hoc solution for incorrect balance of supply and demand is often for stores to mark down products that are close to their expiration date in order to stimulate demand and avoid food waste (Hübner, Kuhn, & Sternbeck, 2013).

Lastly, for several years, companies operating in food supply chains have been obliged to comply with traceability legislation (Trienekens & van Der Vorst, 2006). Traceability can be understood as "the ability to determine the on-going location of products and to trace products back to their origin and used production method" (Trienekens, van der Vorst, & Verdouw, 2014, p. 499). The main purpose and legal argument for implementing a traceability system is due to public food safety and the ability to take prompt actions if required (Thakur et al., 2011; Trienekens & van Der Vorst, 2006). However, as a side effect, of the fine and detailed data capturing along the supply chain, food supply chains are very rich in data which currently may not be fully exploited (Aiello, Enea, & Muriana, 2015).

3.2. Information Sharing and Information Utilization

Information sharing is defined as the availability of operational, tactical, or strategic insights from inter-organizational partners (see e.g. Cao, Vonderembse, Zhang, & Ragu-Nathan (2010); Kembro & Näslund (2014); Moinzadeh (2002)). In a similar vein is "knowledge sharing" and "knowledge management". However, these tend to be prescriptive in nature, while information sharing is descriptive and is used as a basis for future decisions (Kock, McQueen, & Corner, 1997). Information sharing is often discussed as one of the major means to enhance supply chain performance (Baihaqi & Sohal, 2013). It is also known as a key enabler for coordination and integration in a supply chain (Yu, Yan, & Edwin Cheng, 2001). Of course, increased information sharing does not necessarily result in a better performance unless the shared information is effectively used in the relevant processes and well-aligned with the requirements of those processes (Voigt, 2011). Information sharing can be very challenging in practice. Firstly, sharing information needs a level of trust between members in a supply chain (Ebrahim-Khanjari, Hopp, & Iravani, 2012). There is also the need for trust in the sharing technology itself. Companies are willing to share information in a supply chain when they trust both the information sharing system and its alignment with the other companies in the chain. In addition, information sharing is not cost-free and may require significant investment by involved parties (Lee et al., 2000). Accordingly, it is important to clearly understand which information is needed to share, how it can be shared and how it can be utilized in the design and operation of a supply chain (Kim & Narasimhan, 2002). This can be formalized in the term "information utilization". In spite of its importance, the information utilization is a poorly defined concept in the existing literature (Myrelid, 2015). Jonsson & Myrelid (2016) distinguish between four levels of information utilization as presented in Figure 1. At the first two levels the information is available but not connected to processes in the receiving company. At level three the shared information is used at a process, and at level four the information additionally adds value (Jonsson & Myrelid, 2016).

Figure 1. Four levels of information utilization (Adapted from Jonsson & Myrelid (2016))

4	**Efficient and effective usage**	The information adds value to the processes (e.g. more efficient or more accurate planning)
3	**Actual usage**	The information received is being used in the processes at the receiving company but does not necessarily add additional value.
2	**Intended usage**	The receiver has the intention and ability to use the information
1	**Potential usage**	The received information is perceived as useful, no actual usage required

Inspired by the work of Jonsson & Myrelid (2016) we propose the following definition of information utilization in this paper:

Information utilization refers to the inclusion of received information, from the supply chain or surrounding environment, in the internal or collaborative decision processes.

Based on this definition, information sharing (i.e., the availability of information) is a prerequisite for information utilization. The main purpose of information utilization is improving the decision-making process in a supply chain. For example, with sharing information more timely or accurate decisions can be made in managing the inventory levels in the chain. The received information should contribute to a better decision or improving the processes of one actor or the coordination of processes of multiple actors in the chain. Additionally, to benefit from information sharing, different processes (by different actors) may have different requirements which are further discussed as facets in the following.

3.3. Facets of Information Sharing

In the data-information-knowledge-wisdom (DIKW) hierarchy introduced by Ackoff (1989) it can be noticed that structuring of data is necessary to move up the hierarchy (Rowley, 2007). Information utilization is a similar concept and some structure of the shared information is needed before it can be identified where it could be utilized. To characterize and structure information sharing in a supply chain, several descriptive facets are discussed in the existing literature (Barratt & Oke, 2007; Hung, Ho, Jou, & Tai, 2011; Simatupang & Sridharan, 2005; Uusipaavalniemi & Juga, 2008). These facets are summarized in Figure 2. In principle, these facets define different typologies for information sharing in the chain and should be consistent with the (potential) information utilization.

Figure 2. Facets of information sharing, which affect information utilization

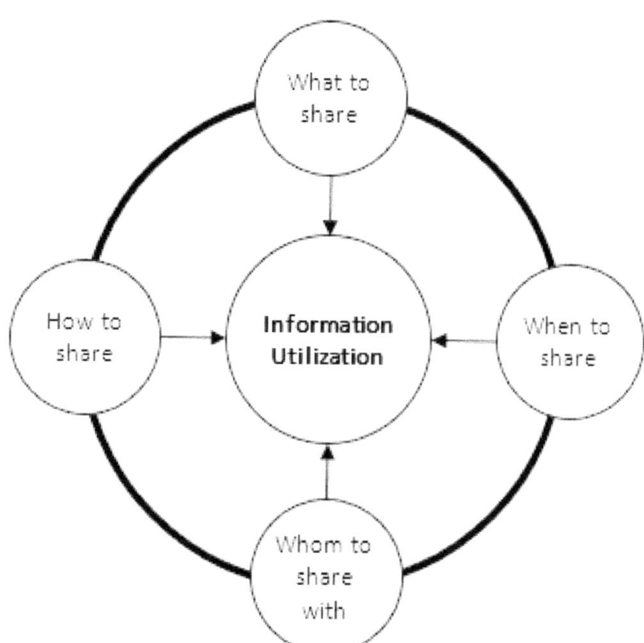

What to share relates to the type and the format in which the information is shared between actors. Common types of shared information include: forecasts, promotions, demand or point-of-sales (POS) data, production schedules, inventory levels, idle capacities, planned orders, and firmed orders (Huang et al., 2003; Jonsson & Mattsson, 2013; Kiil et al., 2015; Montoya-Torres & Ortiz-Vargas, 2014; Sahin & Robinson, 2002). Due to the specific context of food supply chain, additional information types such a temperature logs, remaining shelf life of products, the number of wasted products are also available and can be shared between actors. These context-specific types of information can be used for example in inventory management (Ketzenberg, Bloemhof, & Gaukler, 2015), distribution management (Flamini, Nigro, & Pacciarelli, 2011), and supply chain coordination (Ketzenberg & Ferguson, 2008).

In addition to the type of shared information, the completeness and accuracy of the shared information also influence how the information can be utilized. This is also discussed as information quality in the literature (Gustavsson & Wänström, 2009; Ding, Jie, Parton & Matanda, 2014; Lee, Strong, Kahn, & Wang, 2002). No unambiguous definition or dimensions seem to exist for information quality (Myrelid, 2015). Here, we consider information quality as being "free from deficiencies" (Juran & Godfrey, 2000), which relates to the completeness and accuracy of shared information.

Additionally, it is common in food supply chains to capture information at a very fine level of granularity, but it can be shared in various level of aggregation. The information can be aggregated in different ways, e.g. time, products, and location (Berente, Vandenbosch, & Aubert, 2009; Jin, Williams, Waller, & Hofer, 2015). For instance, the forecasts or POS data can be shared in weekly or monthly "time" format, per stock keeping unit (SKU) or in different product family levels, and additionally by each individual store or a larger regional level. Lastly, some types of shared information may cover a specific time horizon (Barut, Faisst, & Kanet, 2002; Holweg & Pil, 2008). For example, a forecast may cover 12 months of expected sales, or POS data might be shared for the last year.

When to share relates to the timing of exchanging the information between actors. Timeliness consist of two important aspects; firstly, earliness or how far in advance the exchange of information takes place. It is important that the information is delivered in time for the receiving company to react (Gustavsson & Wänström, 2009). The second aspect is the frequency of the exchange of information how frequent the receiving company can expect to get an updated or new set of information (Simchi-Levi & Zhao, 2003). Figure 3 illustrates an example to clarify the relation between earliness, horizon, and frequency.

Figure 3. Relation between earliness, horizon, and frequency

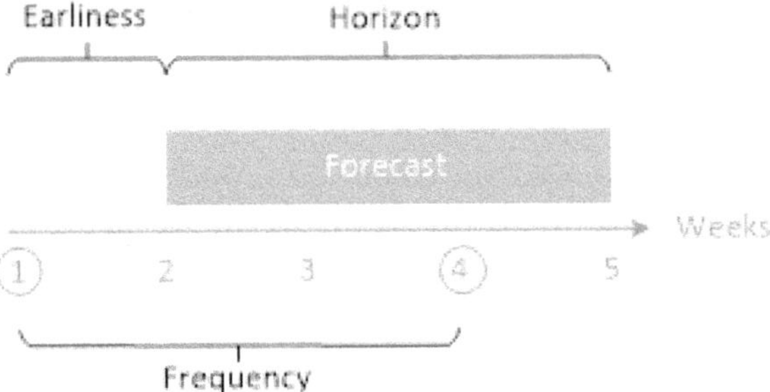

The figure shows a forecast of the expected sales from week 2 to 5 (i.e. end of week 4) which is received in week 1. Thus, the earliness is one week and the horizon covers three weeks. In week 4 a new update of the forecast is expected; thus, the frequency is also three weeks in this case.

The level of aggregation, horizon, and frequency relates to the planning level in food supply chains as illustrated in Figure 4. The figure shows how different facets are related to the hierarchal planning level in the chain. In general, the strategic decisions require information with a longer time horizon and at a higher aggregation level. In this case, the frequency of the information exchange can be yearly or even less frequent. On the other hand, if decisions are on an operational level, the time horizon is shorter, but the level of aggregation is low and the frequency of information exchange increases to continuously

Figure 4. Typical decisions in a food supply chain and its relation to different facets of shared information (Based on Ahumada & Villalobos (2009); Dani (2015); Gu, Goetschalckx, & McGinnis (2007); Hübner et al. (2013); Romsdal (2014); Rouwenhorst et al. (2000); Rushton, Croucher, & Baker (2014); Stadtler et al. (2015); SteadieSeifi et al. (2014))

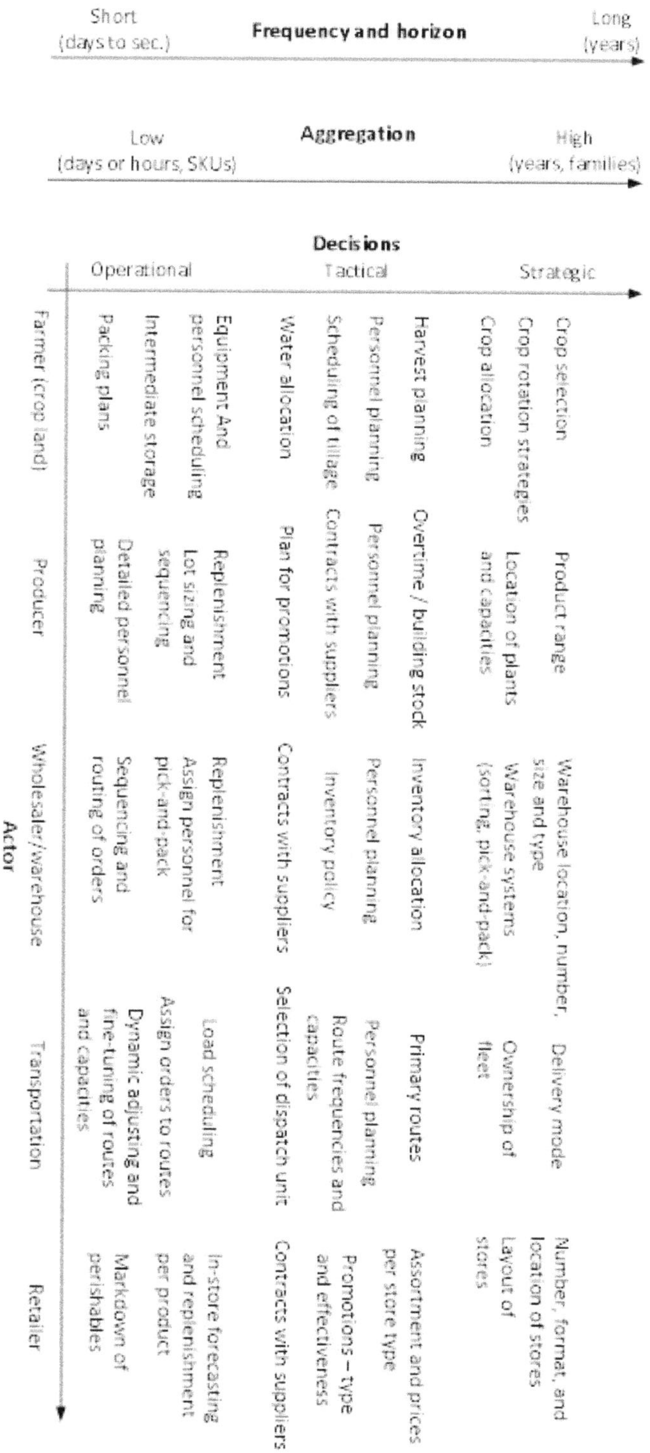

Frequency and horizon: Short (days to sec.) → Long (years)

Aggregation: Low (days or hours, SKUs) → High (years, families)

Decisions

Decisions	Farmer (crop land)	Producer	Wholesaler/warehouse	Transportation	Retailer
Strategic	Crop selection / Crop rotation strategies / Crop allocation	Product range / Location of plants and capacities	Warehouse location, number, size and type / Warehouse systems (sorting, pick-and-pack)	Delivery mode / Ownership of fleet	Number, format, and location of stores / Layout of stores
Tactical	Harvest planning / Personnel planning / Scheduling of tillage / Water allocation	Overtime / building stock / Personnel planning / Contracts with suppliers / Plan for promotions	Inventory allocation / Personnel planning / Inventory policy / Contracts with suppliers	Primary routes / Personnel planning / Route frequencies and capacities / Selection of dispatch unit	Assortment and prices per store type / Promotions – type and effectiveness / Contracts with suppliers
Operational	Equipment And personnel scheduling / Intermediate storage / Packing plans	Replenishment / Lot sizing and sequencing / Detailed personnel planning	Replenishment / Assign personnel for pick-and-pack / Sequencing and routing of orders	Load scheduling / Assign orders to routes / Dynamic adjusting and fine-tuning of routes and capacities	In-store forecasting and replenishment per product / Markdown of perishables

Actor

control the operations (Souza, 2014; Stadtler, Kilger, & Meyr, 2015). It is essential that these facets of the shared information are matched according to the decision level. Too coarse information may not be applicable, and too detailed information might create an overload of information, which brings limited value (El Kadiri et al., 2016; Simchi-Levi & Zhao, 2003). Additionally, increasing the level of detail also increases the cost of data capturing and processing (Aiello et al., 2015).

Whom to share information with specifies how far the information is exchanged in the chain. It is also referred to as "Information Extent" (Barut et al., 2002; Hung et al., 2011) and describes "how far up or down the supply chain a firm exchanges information". Increasing the information extent has been shown to reduce uncertainty in the supply chain (Hung et al., 2011). In a food supply chain, which both holds the convergent and divergent structure, a complete overview of flows between all actors may become substantially complex. From the perspective of the receiving supply chain actor, the important aspect is to understand the 'source', i.e. where the information originates from. In general, the information may originate from other actors in the chain or from the surrounding environment like weather forecasts or similar.

How to share the information relates to the channel in which the information is exchanged. This is also referred to as modality in the literature (Mohr & Sohi, 1995). The modality does not influence the actual content of the information; however, it may influence how it may be utilized (Huang et al., 2003). The likelihood of the receiving actor to utilize the information might be higher if the information is shared directly through their ERP system compared to a case where it is received via telephone. Four general modalities for information sharing include: 1) direct link between databases or EDI, 2) information provided electronically (e.g. email or web portal), 3) information provided physically (fax, mail, or personal handover), and 4) informal meetings and telephone calls (Uusipaavalniemi & Juga, 2008). The choice of sharing method may also indirectly express the formality of the information sharing among actors (Mohr & Sohi, 1995). Figure 1 summaries the four facets and all identified underlying elements of shared information.

4. INFORMATION FLOW AND BUSINESS PROCESS MAPPING

Visualizing, or mapping, information and material flows is known as a key starting point for business process improvements and many mapping tools has been proposed for different purposes (Aguilar-Saven, 2004; Giaglis, 2001). However, there is general tendency to focus on the physical material flow even though it is acknowledged that re-design and process improvement should include the information flow and not only depict the material flow (Berente et al., 2009). As elaborated in Section 3, the facets of the information influence how the information can be utilized in a supply chain. Therefore, we need to visualize the facets of the shared information as well as the current information utilization to support business process improvements. This section assesses the applicability of the most common business process mapping tools and the extensions for visualizing facets of shared information and information utilization (see Table 2).

Several mapping tools, such as flowcharts, role activity diagram, data flow diagram or IDEF maps, support a simple presentation of the type of information flow between supply chain actors. The other facets of shared information are generally neglected in these mapping tools. Furthermore, the utilization is often only considered at a high level, i.e. who the receiver of information is but not the specific processes. The simplicity of these tools might also explain why they are easy to use and effective in

Table 2. Facets of shared information

Facet		Underlying Elements
Content	What to share	Type, aggregation, horizon, quality
Timeliness	When to share	Frequency, earliness
Source	Whom to share with	Supply chain actors, surrounding environment
Modality	How to share	Linked databases or EDI, electronical, physical, and informal

communication (Aguilar-Saven, 2004). Value stream mapping is another common mapping tool, which besides information type and the information source represents the frequency of the information exchange. However, facets such as aggregation, modality, and how information is utilized are not included in a value stream map. The supply chain operations reference (SCOR) model also proposes a methodology to map the processes on three levels of abstraction together with the type of information. As indicated by the name, the SCOR model is a reference model and not an actual mapping tool, but its comprehensiveness continues to receive popularity from practitioners (Huan, Sheoran, & Wang, 2004; Verdouw et al., 2010). However, the focus of SCOR is also mainly on the material flows and the facets of information flows are not usually presented in the standard SCOR model.

Extensions to these tools have also been proposed to include more details or to adapt to specific industries. As an extension of value stream mapping, Alfnes et al. (2008) presents a conceptual model with six complementary views of material flow, processes, information, organizational, layout, and planning and control. The information view clearly specifies the modality, but elements like aggregation, earliness, horizon etc. are not specified. Chibba & Rundquist (2009), Holweg & Pil (2008), and Thakur et al. (2011) present comparable approaches, i.e. to mapping material and information flow consisting of a flowchart and an accompanying table with specifications. The flowchart represents the involved actors, the material flow, and information flow in between them. From the accompanying tables additional elements of each information flow related to frequency and horizon (Holweg & Pil, 2008), aggregation (Thakur et al., 2011), or modality (Chibba & Rundquist, 2009) is presented.

Specifically developed for food supply chains, Olsen & Aschan (2010) present a methodology to map the information flow with respect to traceability. The aggregation of the information is rather important here as the information need to be coupled to a traceable unit (Olsen & Aschan, 2010; Thakur et al., 2011). However, aggregation in respect to location and time is not specified as well as facets related to timeliness or modality. An adaption of value stream mapping for food supply chains is presented by Taylor (2005) where information type, source, and frequency is included, as in the original version. Compared to the other presented mapping tools, Taylor (2005) links some of the shared information to processes, e.g. shared demand and capacity plans are used as an input to the weekly planning. It is, however, not consistent throughout the presentation of the methodology. Lastly, Verdouw et al. (2010) shows how the SCOR model can be used to show the information flows and how to link them to the standard processes from the SCOR model in a fruit supply chain. Nevertheless, not all facets of the shared information is included in the version presented by Verdouw et al. (2010). Table 3 summarizes the enhanced mapping tools presented by various authors elaborated above. The table outlines the degree to which the mapping tools illustrates facets of shared information, information utilization, and its origin.

Table 3. Assessment of enhanced mapping tools

	Content				Timeliness		Source	Modality	Utilization	Origin
	Type	Aggregation	Horizon	Quality	Frequency	Earliness				
Alfnes et al. (2008)	x				x		x	x	R	VSM
Chibba & Rundquist (2009)	x						x	x	R	Flowchart
Holweg & Pil (2008)	x		x	x	x		x		R	Flowchart
Olsen & Aschan (2010)	x	x					x			Flowchart
Taylor (2005)	x				x		x		(x)	VSM
Thakur et al. (2011)	x	x							R	Flowchart
Verdouw et al. (2010)	x						x		x	SCOR

R: Depicts only the receiving company and does not link it directly to a decision-making process. x: supported (x): partly supported

5. VISUALIZING INFORMATION UTILIZATION WITH THE SCOR MODEL

From Table 3 it is clear that various mapping tools have been proposed and each of them is able to present different characteristics of shared information. Only two of the identified mapping tools show the information utilization by fully or partly linking the shared information to decision making or processes (see Taylor (2005) and Verdouw et al. (2010)). Additionally, it appears that all facets of shared information are not included in one single tool. This study proposes a mapping notation which emphasizes all facets and facilitates a shift from information sharing to information utilization.

5.1. Notation for Mapping Information

Similar to the work of Verdouw et al. (2010), we use the SCOR model to map the material and process flow. This is primarily because the SCOR model is acknowledged as one of the most comprehensive frameworks to describe a supply chain and is widely adopted in the industry as a reference model (Huan et al., 2004; Lambert, García-Dastugue, & Croxton, 2005). The SCOR model includes 4 levels with increasing level of details. The first three include standard notation while level 4 is company specific (SCC, 2012). We apply the SCOR model at level 3 for two main reasons. Firstly, when considering a whole supply chain, level 3 provides an appropriate balance between details and complexity (Cheng et al., 2010). Secondly, to communicate across company boundaries, level 3 provides standard processes that all companies are familiar with. If level 4 were applied company specific processes and adaptions will reduce the genericity and the readability across the chain. However, it should be noted that level 3 (and even level 4) describes the processes and not decisions in a supply chain.

To visualize and emphasize information flow with the SCOR model we add an additional layer. Figure 5 depicts the proposed notation for mapping the information flow capturing all four facets from Table 1. For information content the aggregation and horizon (when applicable) is written above the shape, while the type of information is centered in the middle of the shape. The right side shows the timeliness and the left side shows the modality. The form of the shape represents the source (here only showed other inter-organizational supply chain actors).

Figure 5. Proposed notation for mapping information

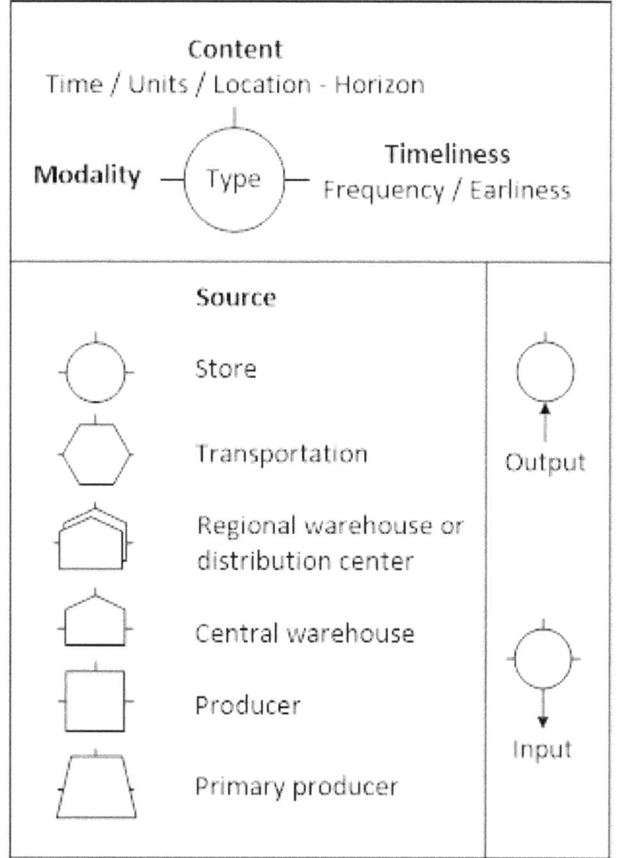

The information is either an "output", meaning that the information is captured somewhere, which is represented by the arrow going towards the shape. Or, the information is an "input" to a process that is represented by the arrow going outwards of the shape. An important distinction between output and input is the modality and timeliness (left and right side of the shape). If the information is depicted as an output, the information is only captured, but not shared with anyone yet. Meaning, the modality and the timeliness cannot be included at that point. Those two facets should only be shown when the information acts as an input.

Figure 6 presents additional notation to highlight differences between the current information utilization (as-is) and a future improved scenario (to-be). If the shape is colored white with a dotted line around it shows that information - which is already captured and maybe used elsewhere - can be further utilized at another process. A black colored shape highlights that some information is captured along the chain, but currently not included in any process. Lastly, a gray colored shape indicates a completely new piece of information, which is not utilized nor captured yet. Thus, the gray shapes should come in pairs – (1) the information needs to be captured (new info. captured) and (2) it should be utilized at a process (new utilization). With the additional notation from Figure 6 traditional as-is and to-be maps can be made and shown at the same time.

Figure 6. Additional notation for highlighting areas of improvement

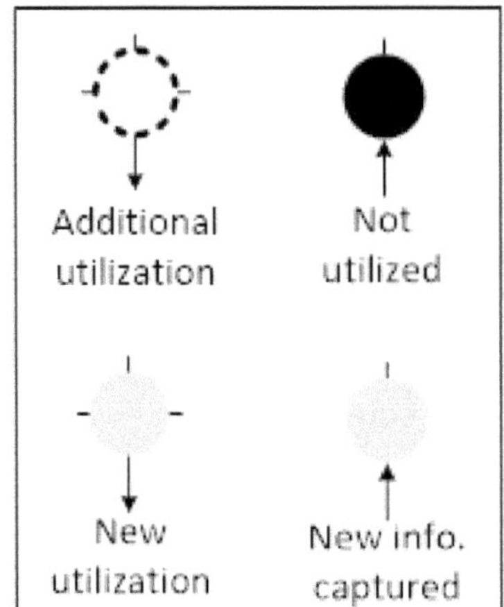

5.2. Combining Information Flows With the SCOR Model

Based on the data from the questionnaire and the workshop, Figure 7 illustrates the Retail Deliver process (SCOR, D4) at the retail store from the Norwegian food supply chain case company. It demonstrates how to combine the proposed notation with the SCOR model. Table 3 includes the abbreviations used in the figure. From left to right it can be observed that to generate the stocking schedule (i.e. the process of scheduling resources to support replenishment) the store receives and uses forecasts for future promotions from the central warehouse. It is received electronically over a portal, the information is shared six weeks in advance and updated every week. The aggregation is weekly (as the promotion is weekly), on a SKU level, and no specific aggregation in location is made. Lastly, the horizon is one week. Besides the promotional forecast, the stores use two other inputs: planned orders and the sales information. First, the planned orders can be viewed electronically in a portal, and is on a daily SKU level for the individual store. The horizon is typically a couple of days or until next delivery. This information is updated daily and orders arriving the following day (1 day early) and forward is possible to see. This information is mainly used to make small adjustments to for the near-future as it only covers the coming days. Second, the sales information is from the store itself, which in this case makes the modality rather informal, but considered every month when the stocking schedule is to be made. The aggregation is daily sales on a SKU level for that particular store. Another example from Figure 7 is the D4.4 process where the shelf is physically replenished. Currently waste is captured on a daily SKU level at each store. But, a potential

Figure 7. Information flow combined with SCOR retail deliver process (D4)

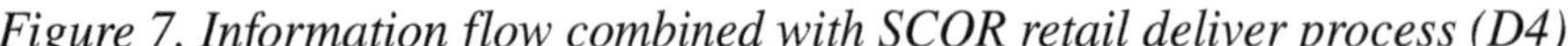

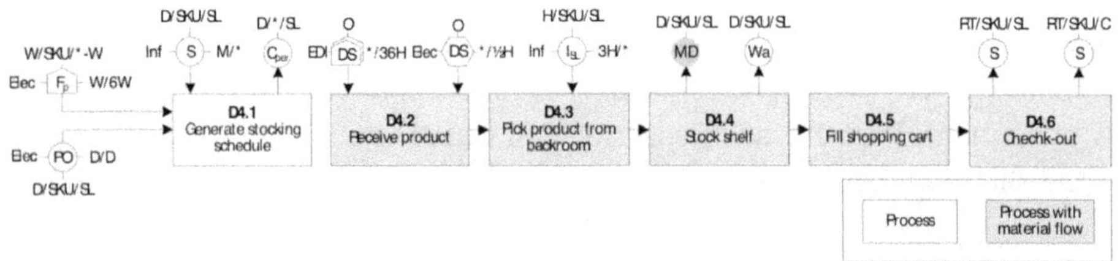

information (as indicated with the gray color of the circle) to capture could be to daily record the SKUs that are markdown because of short shelf life at each store.

By displaying the input and output separately it can be visualized that some information is captured but not yet shared and utilized, or it can be reflected that the information may be shared at a higher level of aggregation that how it was captured. Obviously, a piece of information cannot act as input if it is not captured somewhere, just as the granularity level for the input cannot exceed the granularity level of how it is captured. In Figure 7 (see Table 4) the sales information is captured at D4.6 in real time, but aggregated to daily level before it is used as an input in process D4.1. For the consumers with a loyalty card, the sales information is captured in real time as well and additionally linked to the specific consumer. This is used afterwards at the wholesaler to generate consumer specific promotions.

Table 4. Abbreviations in Figure 7 and Figure 8

Time		Units		Locations		Modality	
RT	Real time	SKU	Stock keeping unit	C	Consumer	Inf	Informal
H	Hourly	B	Batch size (D-pack)			Phy	Physical meeting
D	Daily	O	Order	SLR	Single location Transportation route	Elec	Electronically via SMS, email, portal, etc.
W	Weekly	TG	Temp. group (dry, chilled, frozen)				
M	Monthly					EDI	Linked databases or EDI
Information Type							
C_{per}	Capacity plan, personnel						
C_{tr}	Capacity plan, transportation						
DS	Delivery status (time and quantity)						
FO	Firmed orders						
F	Forecast						
F_p	Forecast, promotion information						
I	Inventory level						
I_{SL}	Inventory level with shelf life						
MD	Markdown						
PO	Planned orders						
PO_p	Planned orders, promotion						
S	Sales						
TL	Temperature log						
Wa	Waste						

Special character: * Not applicable for that given information type

5.3. Interpreting Information Flows in a Food Supply Chain

As the main purpose is to give structure to the information flows in a food supply chain and not just a single entity, Figure 8 illustrates the information and material flow for the regional warehouse, the transport provider, and the store where Figure 7 is the lowest swim lane. The primary producer and the processor is omitted due to space limitations. Figure 8 is also developed based on the data obtained from the questionnaire and the workshop with the Norwegian supply chain. The combination of the SCOR model and the proposed notation provides a structure for the current information utilization at the three actors and highlights areas of improvement simultaneously.

5.3.1. Current Information Flows

All white shapes illustrate the current information flow, all relevant facets of the information, and how the information is utilized for different processes. By focusing on the form of the shapes, information from other supply chain actors can easily be identified. In the lowermost swim lane in Figure 8 the information in circles are from the store itself, and information in other shapes represents information from other actors. For instance, the forecasts from the central warehouse (shaped like a house), the delivery status from the transport provider (hexagon), and delivery status from the regional warehouse (two houses) are clearly emphasized.

The area with gray stripes at the stores indicates a continuous replenishment program (CRP) where the wholesaler receives sales information from the stores to generate a statistical forecast (P4.1). Based on waste information from the stores and previous sales to the stores (P4.2) an estimated inventory balance at the stores are calculated and together with the forecast an order proposal is generated to the stores. The stores review and confirms the order in the end (P4.4). The CRP solution do not handle promotions, thus the planned orders for promotions is made by the stores itself.

5.3.2. Captured But Not Utilized Information

It can be noticed by the black shapes that the temperature log and waste information from the regional warehouse is currently only captured, but not systematically included into any decision-making processes. The temperature registration is due to traceability requirements; however, areas of utilization could be identified for this information.

5.3.3. Additional Utilization of Captured Information

In Figure 8 four areas of further utilization of information - that is already captured - can be identified. If the transport provider could access both primary producers and processors inventory levels through a portal it would enable a better planning of transportation routes. After delivering goods to stores the truck could be scheduled to pick-up goods from producers to increase the utilization of the truck capacity on a round trip. Another type of information is the temperature log from the transportation provider. Currently this is not utilized at any processes, however this type of information can be used to estimate remaining shelf life of perishable products, and act as input for calculating new replenishment quantities (Ketzenberg et al., 2015). Lastly, it became clear that the forecast for the regional warehouse is currently based on previous orders to the stores and not on POS data - even though this data is accessible in the same system. Thus, POS data could be utilized throughout the chain to establish a common forecast and reduce the bullwhip effect (Lee, Padmanabhan, & Whang, 1997).

Figure 8. Information and material flow from regional warehouse to store

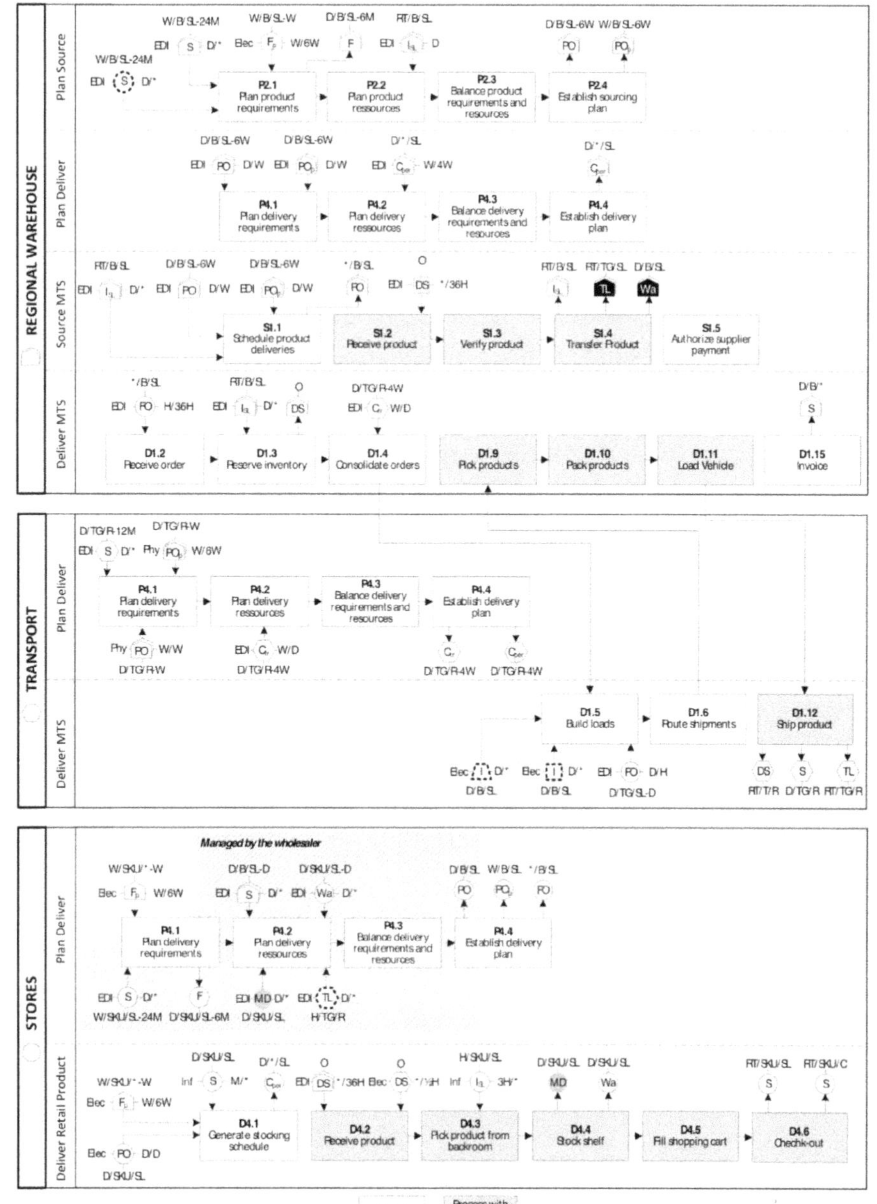

5.3.4. New Information and Utilization

A common practice for perishable products with short remaining shelf life is mark-down of prices in order to stimulate demand and reduce food waste (Hübner et al., 2013; SCC, 2012). However, if this represents a large amount of the products available in the store it needs to be considered for the coming replenishment order. Thus, as illustrated in Figure 8 this number of products, which is mark-downed and soon to expire, should be captured daily and utilized when calculating the next replenishment quantity.

5.3.5. Aligning Information and Processes

With existing knowledge about the individual processes and underlying decisions at each company Figure 8 also provides a structure to align the information and processes, e.g., if a process is executed weekly, but the information is only updated monthly these two can be aligned to have the same frequency. Similar observations can be made for the level of aggregation, if the information should be received some days earlier or if the modality should be changed to facilitate an easier integration and utilization of the information. For example, in Figure 8 it can be observed that the information, which are utilized in P4.1 at the transport provider, comes with different time horizons and frequencies. This could be made more consistent and aligned to fit the process.

6. USAGE AND IMPLICATIONS

From a managerial perspective, the diversity of numerus information flows to and from various actors in the supply chain creates a complex and hazy situation - both of what is needed and what is possible in regard to information utilization in the supply chain (Endsley, 2016). To establish a complete map of information and material flow as in Figure 8 five main steps are proposed in Figure 9. However, a prerequisite before starting with step 1, is to decide how generic or specific the final result should be. I.e. should it reflect the interaction with the main group of suppliers and customers, should it represent all products, or maybe only a specific product family? The SCOR model has specific processes for make-to-stock and make-to-order products, thus making a unique map for each type might be desirable to reduce complexity. Thus, several maps might be necessary if there is a high number of very different supply chains actors and products.

Figure 9. Steps to establish a complete map of information and material flow

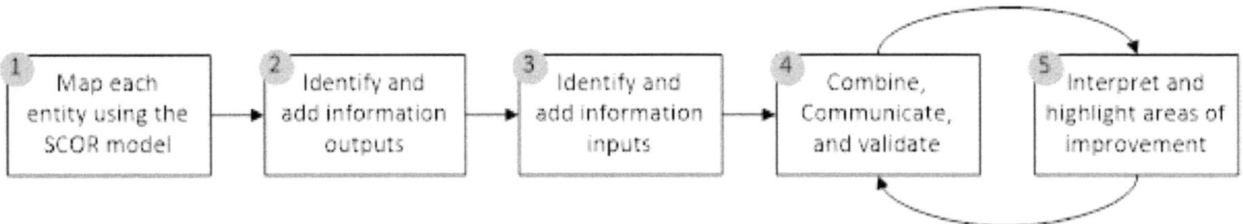

Step 1 - Mapping each supply chain using the SCOR model should be carried out, objectively, by each individual company. Starting with SCOR level 1, progressing down to level 2, and ideally level 4 or at least identify the key decisions made within each level 3 process[1]. Step 2 and 3 – identify the facets of information output and input and add to the SCOR level 3 map. It is beneficial to focus on the output and input separately in the beginning because it makes the mapping process simpler. But, more importantly it will be different personal that should be involved in the two steps, and can provide knowledge about what information that is currently captured in-house (e.g. IT or production department) and how information is utilized (e.g. planning department). *Ideas* for future information flows, i.e. those in

Figure 6, should also be noted at these steps. Step 4 and 5 – establish a common supply chain map with information inputs and outputs based on the individual maps from each company to highlight and discuss areas of improvement. Here, it is essential that each company has its own ideas and reflections on where gabs might exist and how to close these before meeting with representatives from the rest of the supply chain. It is crucial that a valid map of the current situation is established and agreed upon before discussing future scenarios. As indicated in Figure 9 over time, the steps of validating and identifying areas of improvement will be a continuous and iterative process.

The specific context and the facets will provide understandings for how the information can be linked to processes and utilized. However, to ease the identification of this link, between information and processes, it might be useful to group and consider the information types in three generic time periods: past, current, and future as shown in Table 5. Hereafter, at least two approaches to proceed exists.

Table 5. Grouping of information types

Past	**Current**	**Future**
Sales Temperature log Waste	Inventory level Mark-down	Capacity plans Forecasts Planned orders Delivery status Firmed orders

First, depending on the time period each information type can bring different insights. Information in the "past" category is highly applicable to analyze and search for patterns, explanations, and correlations. E.g. identification of seasonal patterns, substitution effect, or promotional effectiveness. Information in the "current" category explains the status as it is now. This is especially true if the information is received in real-time or close to real-time. This does not only include inventory information or products which are marked down, but could also include location information of trucks in a fleet, or current temperature or pressure in a machine. Lastly, information in the "future" category provides insights to what is expected to happen. Clearly, the task with this information is to compare and reconcile with one's own current plans and identify any opportunities or challenges. E.g. is the total volume in the forecast the same or is additional shifts necessary or other actions be initiated? Thus, overall three essential questions relates to each category (1) what happened?, (2) what is happening?, and (3) what is (expected) to happen? By considering the information in this way, i.e. what answers they might bring with them, it might be easier to identify how to utilize it.

The second approach is to use the information in planning processes - which is planning of *future* activities. Thus. information from the "past" and "current" category should be processed or combined to express something about future expected events. Clearly, sales information can be used to generate statistical forecasts. Similar, the temperature log can be used to estimate deterioration rate and together with products that are marked down this can give an estimate of when the products expire and when a new replenishment is required. Another example is to combine the current inventory level with the forecast, which will provide an understanding of if the next replenishment is highly critical or if can be distributed to another actor in case of shortage. Thus, the second approach seeks to process the information to make it express something about future events.

As demonstrated in Figure 8, the proposed mapping tool provides a systematic structure to evaluate the information available and which processes from the SCOR model that is present in the system. Mapping the current information flows will facilitate and secure a common understanding across supply chain actors. This serves as a foundation for enhancing inter-organizational coordination, identify potential valuable pieces of information from other actors, or even from the surrounding environment as well as where to utilize this information.

7. CONCLUSION

The aim of this study was to identify facets of information sharing and conceptualize how to move from information sharing to information utilization in food supply chains. Due to shelf life limitation, perishability of products, seasonality, and wide assortment range, food supply chains have some special logistical requirements. On the other hand, a vast amount of information is regularly collected along the chain – especially due to safety and traceability legislations. The general idea is to use this information - beyond the safety and traceability purposes - for improving the processes along the chain. The information utilization concept strives to emphasize this idea. To facilitate the information utilization, a mapping tool that provide a structure to the vast amount of available information and the linkage to the supply chain processes is proposed in this paper.

7.1. Contribution to Theory

Several studies discuss and quantify the value of sharing information (Baihaqi & Sohal, 2013; Huang et al., 2003; Lee et al., 2000), but how the information is utilized to measure this value has only received very little consideration (Myrelid, 2015). To bring attention to this poorly defined topic Jonsson & Myrelid (2016) propose the very first conceptualization of it. We extend this research by a three-folded contribution.

Firstly, from a scattered amount of literature we synthesized previous identified facets of information sharing (Barratt & Oke, 2007; Hung et al., 2011; Uusipaavalniemi & Juga, 2008) and further elaborated the underlying elements such as aggregation level, horizon, and earliness for food supply chains (Fredriksson & Liljestrand, 2015; Jin et al., 2015). These facets provides structure to move in the DIKW hierarchy (Rowley, 2007). From Figure 4 it is clear that the facets of shared information determine how the information can be utilized for different hierarchical planning decisions. Consequently, it is essential to fully understand these facets of both the current and new potential information flows.

Secondly, we define information utilization to clarify the concept and in order to set the boundaries for further research on the topic itself and against surrounding research topics. Information sharing is the act of making information available to other actors in the supply chain, while information utilization is characterized by inclusion of the shared information into various decision processes. This may appear to conflict with the four phases presented by Jonsson & Myrelid (2016) in Figure 1. They view it as a gradually increase in maturity, where our definition clearly distinguishes between information sharing and information utilization. However, the underlying message is equivalent. It is essential that companies, and supply chains, move from just making information available to include and benefit from the shared information in the planning processes.

Thirdly, to facilitate information utilization we draw on the ideas from various mapping tools and references models. Especially, we build on the ideas by Verdouw et al. (2010) by highlighting information flow together with the SCOR model. Maps are powerful tools because they allow us to see what is too large and too complex to grasp. The proposed mapping tool extend existing mapping tools by (1) showing all facets of the shared information, which is necessary to identify how to utilize the information. (2) Emphasizes the linkage between information and processes. Lastly, (3) it separates information flow to output (capturing) and input (information utilization), which makes it possible to identify available information which may not currently be utilized and the information that is currently being utilized.

7.2. Limitations and Future Research

This study has several limitations and should be used to guide further research. The study has only considered one case; thus, the application of the proposed method has only been tested for this particular case and cannot necessarily be generalized to other cases. However, the SCOR model is rather generic and is developed to fit a variety of settings (SCC, 2012), but it could be investigated if all relevant information types for food supply chains have been identified and considered. Moreover, for the particular food supply chain under investigation information quality was not considered or reported as a challenge. Thus, it was assumed that all information was free of error. It has previously been shown that the quality of shared information affects the performance of food supply chains (Juan Ding et al., 2014), thus it should be studied further and incorporated to a greater extent.

Lastly, we choose to combine the notation for information flows with the SCOR model due to its generic abilities and its adoption in practice. However, for the unfamiliar reader a simple flow chart of the material flow may be easier to interpret than the SCOR model. It could be investigated if the proposed notation combined with other mapping tools, which also depicts the decision processes, would make it even easier visualize the information utilization.

ACKNOWLEDGMENT

The authors gratefully acknowledge the assistance provided by the Norwegian Research Council (NRC) for the financial support of Retail Supply Chain 2020. Also, we thank the participating case companies which together with the NRC enabled this study. Lastly, we thank Peter Falster for his valuable comments and Chris Martin for assistance in editing this paper.

REFERENCES

Aastrup, J., & Kotzab, H. (2009). Analyzing out-of-stock in independent grocery stores: An empirical study. *International Journal of Retail & Distribution Management, 37*(9), 765–789. doi:10.1108/09590550910975817

Ackoff, R. L. (1989). From data to wisdom. *Journal of Applied Systems Analysis, 16*(1), 3–9.

Aguilar-Saven, R. S. (2004). Business process modelling: Review and framework. *International Journal of Production Economics, 90*(2), 129–149. doi:10.1016/S0925-5273(03)00102-6

Ahumada, O., & Villalobos, J. R. (2009). Application of planning models in the agri-food supply chain: A review. *European Journal of Operational Research, 196*(1), 1–20. doi:10.1016/j.ejor.2008.02.014

Aiello, G., Enea, M., & Muriana, C. (2015). The expected value of the traceability information. *European Journal of Operational Research, 244*(1), 176–186. doi:10.1016/j.ejor.2015.01.028

Alfnes, E., Dreyer, H. C., & Strandhagen, J. O. (2008). The operations model: an enterprise mapping framework. In J. S. Arlbjørn, Á. Halldórssen, M. Jahre, & K. Spens (Eds.), *Northern Lights in Logistics and Supply Chain Management* (pp. 201–216). Copenhagen Business School Press.

Andersson, A. W., Jansson, A., Sandblad, B., & Tschirner, S. (2014). *Recognizing complexity: Visualization for skilled professionals in complex work situations. In Building Bridges: HCI, Visualization, and Non-formal Modeling* (pp. 47–66). Springer. doi:10.1007/978-3-642-54894-9_5

Baihaqi, I., & Sohal, A. S. (2013). The impact of information sharing in supply chains on organisational performance: An empirical study. *Production Planning and Control, 24*(8-9), 743–758. doi:10.1080/0 9537287.2012.666865

Barratt, M., & Oke, A. (2007). Antecedents of supply chain visibility in retail supply chains: A resource-based theory perspective. *Journal of Operations Management, 25*(6), 1217–1233. doi:10.1016/j. jom.2007.01.003

Barut, M., Faisst, W., & Kanet, J. J. (2002). Measuring supply chain coupling: An information system perspective. *European Journal of Purchasing & Supply Management, 8*(3), 161–171. doi:10.1016/ S0969-7012(02)00006-0

Berente, N., Vandenbosch, B., & Aubert, B. (2009). Information flows and business process integration. *Business Process Management Journal, 15*(1), 119–141. doi:10.1108/14637150910931505

Cao, M., Vonderembse, M. A., Zhang, Q., & Ragu-Nathan, T. (2010). Supply chain collaboration: Conceptualisation and instrument development. *International Journal of Production Research, 48*(22), 6613–6635. doi:10.1080/00207540903349039

Cheng, J. C., Law, K. H., Bjornsson, H., Jones, A., & Sriram, R. D. (2010). Modeling and monitoring of construction supply chains. *Advanced Engineering Informatics, 24*(4), 435–455. doi:10.1016/j. aei.2010.06.009

Chibba, A., & Rundquist, J. (2009). Effective Information Flow in the Internal Supply Chain: Results from a snowball method to map information flows. *Journal of Information & Knowledge Management, 8*(04), 331–343. doi:10.1142/S0219649209002439

Dani, S. (2015). *Food supply chain management and logistics.* Kogan Page.

Ebrahim-Khanjari, N., Hopp, W., & Iravani, S. M. (2012). Trust and information sharing in supply chains. *Production and Operations Management, 21*(3), 444–464. doi:10.1111/j.1937-5956.2011.01284.x

El Kadiri, S., Grabot, B., Thoben, K.-D., Hribernik, K., Emmanouilidis, C., von Cieminski, G., & Kiritsis, D. (2016). Current trends on ICT technologies for enterprise information systems. *Computers in Industry, 79*, 14–33. doi:10.1016/j.compind.2015.06.008

Endsley, M. R. (2016). *Designing for situation awareness: An approach to user-centered design*. CRC press.

Entrup, M. L. (2006). *Advanced planning in fresh food industries: integrating shelf life into production planning*. Springer Science & Business Media.

Fawcett, S. E., Osterhaus, P., Magnan, G. M., Brau, J. C., & McCarter, M. W. (2007). Information sharing and supply chain performance: The role of connectivity and willingness. *Supply Chain Management, 12*(5), 358–368. doi:10.1108/13598540710776935

Flamini, M., Nigro, M., & Pacciarelli, D. (2011). Assessing the value of information for retail distribution of perishable goods. *European Transport Research Review, 3*(2), 103–112. doi:10.100712544-011-0051-8

Folinas, D., & Manikas, I. (2010). Design and development of an e-Platform for supporting liquid food supply Chain Monitoring and traceability. *International Journal of Information Systems and Supply Chain Management, 3*(3), 29–49. doi:10.4018/jisscm.2010070103

Forrester, J. W. (1958). Industrial dynamics: A major breakthrough for decision makers. *Harvard Business Review, 36*(4), 37–66.

Fredriksson, A., & Liljestrand, K. (2015). Capturing food logistics: A literature review and research agenda. *International Journal of Logistics Research and Applications, 18*(1), 16–34. doi:10.1080/136 75567.2014.944887

Gardner, J. T., & Cooper, M. C. (2003). Strategic supply chain mapping approaches. *Journal of Business Logistics, 24*(2), 37–64. doi:10.1002/j.2158-1592.2003.tb00045.x

Giaglis, G. M. (2001). A taxonomy of business process modeling and information systems modeling techniques. *International Journal of Flexible Manufacturing Systems, 13*(2), 209–228. doi:10.1023/A:1011139719773

Gu, J., Goetschalckx, M., & McGinnis, L. F. (2007). Research on warehouse operation: A comprehensive review. *European Journal of Operational Research, 177*(1), 1–21. doi:10.1016/j.ejor.2006.02.025

Gustavsson, M., & Wänström, C. (2009). Assessing information quality in manufacturing planning and control processes. *International Journal of Quality & Reliability Management, 26*(4), 325–340. doi:10.1108/02656710910950333

Holweg, M., & Pil, F. K. (2008). Theoretical perspectives on the coordination of supply chains. *Journal of Operations Management, 26*(3), 389–406. doi:10.1016/j.jom.2007.08.003

Huan, S. H., Sheoran, S. K., & Wang, G. (2004). A review and analysis of supply chain operations reference (SCOR) model. *Supply Chain Management, 9*(1), 23–29. doi:10.1108/13598540410517557

Huang, G. Q., Lau, J. S., & Mak, K. (2003). The impacts of sharing production information on supply chain dynamics: A review of the literature. *International Journal of Production Research, 41*(7), 1483–1517. doi:10.1080/0020754031000069625

Hübner, A. H., Kuhn, H., & Sternbeck, M. G. (2013). Demand and supply chain planning in grocery retail: An operations planning framework. *International Journal of Retail & Distribution Management, 41*(7), 512–530. doi:10.1108/IJRDM-05-2013-0104

Hung, W. H., Ho, C. F., Jou, J. J., & Tai, Y. M. (2011). Sharing information strategically in a supply chain: Antecedents, content and impact. *International Journal of Logistics Research and Applications, 14*(2), 111–133. doi:10.1080/13675567.2011.572871

Jin, Y. H., Williams, B. D., Waller, M. A., & Hofer, A. R. (2015). Masking the bullwhip effect in retail: The influence of data aggregation. *International Journal of Physical Distribution & Logistics Management, 45*(8), 814–830. doi:10.1108/IJPDLM-11-2014-0264

Jonsson, P., & Mattsson, S.-A. (2013). The value of sharing planning information in supply chains. *International Journal of Physical Distribution & Logistics Management, 43*(4), 282–299. doi:10.1108/IJPDLM-07-2012-0204

Jonsson, P., & Myrelid, P. (2016). Supply chain information utilization–conceptualization and antecedents. *International Journal of Operations & Production Management, 36*(12), 1769–1799. doi:10.1108/IJOPM-11-2014-0554

Juran, J. M., & Godfrey, A. B. (2000). Juran's Quality Handbook (5th ed.). United States of America: McGraw-Hill.

Kaipia, R., Dukovska-Popovska, I., & Loikkanen, L. (2013). Creating sustainable fresh food supply chains through waste reduction. *International Journal of Physical Distribution & Logistics Management, 43*(3), 262–276. doi:10.1108/IJPDLM-11-2011-0200

Kembro, J., & Näslund, D. (2014). Information sharing in supply chains, myth or reality? A critical analysis of empirical literature. *International Journal of Physical Distribution & Logistics Management, 44*(3), 179–200. doi:10.1108/IJPDLM-09-2012-0287

Ketzenberg, M., Bloemhof, J., & Gaukler, G. (2015). Managing Perishables with Time and Temperature History. *Production and Operations Management, 24*(1), 54–70. doi:10.1111/poms.12209

Ketzenberg, M., & Ferguson, M. E. (2008). Managing slow-moving perishables in the grocery industry. *Production and Operations Management, 17*(5), 513–521. doi:10.3401/poms.1080.0052

Kiil, K., Dreyer, H. C., & Hvolby, H.-H. (2015). *Linking Information Exchange to Planning and Control: An Overview. In Advances in Production Management Systems: Innovative Production Management Towards Sustainable Growth* (pp. 391–398). Springer.

Kim, S. W., & Narasimhan, R. (2002). Information system utilization in supply chain integration efforts. *International Journal of Production Research, 40*(18), 4585–4609. doi:10.1080/00207540210000022203

Kock, N. F., McQueen, R. J., & Corner, J. L. (1997). The nature of data, information and knowledge exchanges in business processes: Implications for process improvement and organizational learning. *The Learning Organization, 4*(2), 70–80. doi:10.1108/09696479710160915

Kummu, M., De Moel, H., Porkka, M., Siebert, S., Varis, O., & Ward, P. (2012). Lost food, wasted resources: Global food supply chain losses and their impacts on freshwater, cropland, and fertiliser use. *The Science of the Total Environment*, *438*, 477–489. doi:10.1016/j.scitotenv.2012.08.092 PMID:23032564

Lambert, D. M., García-Dastugue, S. J., & Croxton, K. L. (2005). An evaluation of process-oriented supply chain management frameworks. *Journal of Business Logistics*, *26*(1), 25–51. doi:10.1002/j.2158-1592.2005. tb00193.x

Lee, H. L., Padmanabhan, V., & Whang, S. (1997). The bullwhip effect in supply chains. *Sloan Management Review*, *38*(3), 93–102.

Lee, H. L., So, K. C., & Tang, C. S. (2000). The value of information sharing in a two-level supply chain. *Management Science*, *46*(5), 626–643. doi:10.1287/mnsc.46.5.626.12047

Lee, Y. W., Strong, D. M., Kahn, B. K., & Wang, R. Y. (2002). AIMQ: A methodology for information quality assessment. *Information & Management*, *40*(2), 133–146. doi:10.1016/S0378-7206(02)00043-5

Mason-Jones, R., & Towill, D. R. (1997). Information enrichment: Designing the supply chain for competitive advantage. *Supply Chain Management*, *2*(4), 137–148. doi:10.1108/13598549710191304

Moberg, C. R., Cutler, B. D., Gross, A., & Speh, T. W. (2002). Identifying antecedents of information exchange within supply chains. *International Journal of Physical Distribution & Logistics Management*, *32*(9), 755–770. doi:10.1108/09600030210452431

Mohr, J. J., & Sohi, R. S. (1995). Communication flows in distribution channels: Impact on assessments of communication quality and satisfaction. *Journal of Retailing*, *71*(4), 393–415. doi:10.1016/0022-4359(95)90020-9

Moinzadeh, K. (2002). A multi-echelon inventory system with information exchange. *Management Science*, *48*(3), 414–426. doi:10.1287/mnsc.48.3.414.7730

Montoya-Torres, J. R., & Ortiz-Vargas, D. A. (2014). Collaboration and information sharing in dyadic supply chains: A literature review over the period 2000–2012. *Estudios Gerenciales*, *30*(133), 343–354. doi:10.1016/j.estger.2014.05.006

Myrelid, P. (2015). *Utilisation of shared demand-related information for operations planning and control.* Gothenburg, Sweden: Chalmers University of Technology.

Olsen, P., & Aschan, M. (2010). Reference method for analyzing material flow, information flow and information loss in food supply chains. *Trends in Food Science & Technology*, *21*(6), 313–320. doi:10.1016/j.tifs.2010.03.002

Parfitt, J., Barthel, M., & Macnaughton, S. (2010). Food waste within food supply chains: Quantification and potential for change to 2050. *Philosophical Transactions of the Royal Society of London. Series B, Biological Sciences*, *365*(1554), 3065–3081. doi:10.1098/rstb.2010.0126 PMID:20713403

Juan Ding, M., Jie, F., A. Parton, K., & J. Matanda, M. (2014). Relationships between quality of information sharing and supply chain food quality in the Australian beef processing industry. *International Journal of Logistics Management*, *25*(1), 85–108. doi:10.1108/IJLM-07-2012-0057

Romsdal, A. (2014). *Differentiated production planning and control in food supply chains* [Doctoral Thesis]. Norwegian University of Science and Technology.

Rouwenhorst, B., Reuter, B., Stockrahm, V., Van Houtum, G., Mantel, R., & Zijm, W. (2000). Warehouse design and control: Framework and literature review. *European Journal of Operational Research, 122*(3), 515–533. doi:10.1016/S0377-2217(99)00020-X

Rowley, J. (2007). The wisdom hierarchy: Representations of the DIKW hierarchy. *Journal of Information Science, 33*(2), 163–180. doi:10.1177/0165551506070706

Rushton, A., Croucher, P., & Baker, P. (2014). The Handbook of Logistics and Distribution Management - Understanding the Supply Chain (5th ed.). KoganPage.

Sahin, F., & Robinson, E. P. (2002). Flow coordination and information sharing in supply chains: Review, implications, and directions for future research. *Decision Sciences, 33*(4), 505–536. doi:10.1111/j.1540-5915.2002.tb01654.x

Supply Chain Council (SCC). (2012). *SCOR Supply Chain Operations Reference Model: Revision 11.0.*

Shaik, M. N., & Abdul-Kader, W. (2013). Interorganizational Information Systems Adoption in Supply Chains: A Context Specific Framework. *International Journal of Information Systems and Supply Chain Management, 6*(1), 24–40. doi:10.4018/jisscm.2013010102

Simatupang, T. M., & Sridharan, R. (2005). The collaboration index: A measure for supply chain collaboration. *International Journal of Physical Distribution & Logistics Management, 35*(1), 44–62. doi:10.1108/09600030510577421

Simchi-Levi, D., & Zhao, Y. (2003). The value of information sharing in a two-stage supply chain with production capacity constraints. *Naval Research Logistics, 50*(8), 888–916. doi:10.1002/nav.10094

Singh, R. (2014). Assessing effectiveness of coordination in food supply chain: A framework. *International Journal of Information Systems and Supply Chain Management, 7*(3), 104–177. doi:10.4018/ijisscm.2014070105

Souza, G. C. (2014). Supply chain analytics. *Business Horizons, 57*(5), 595–605. doi:10.1016/j.bushor.2014.06.004

Stadtler, H., Kilger, C., & Meyr, H. (2015). *Supply Chain Management and Advanced Planning - Concepts, Models, Software, and Case Studies* (5th ed.). Springer-Verlag Berlin Heidelberg.

SteadieSeifi, M., Dellaert, N. P., Nuijten, W., Van Woensel, T., & Raoufi, R. (2014). Multimodal freight transportation planning: A literature review. *European Journal of Operational Research, 233*(1), 1–15. doi:10.1016/j.ejor.2013.06.055

Taylor, D. H. (2005). Value chain analysis: An approach to supply chain improvement in agri-food chains. *International Journal of Physical Distribution & Logistics Management, 35*(10), 744–761. doi:10.1108/09600030510634599

Taylor, D. H., & Fearne, A. (2006). Towards a framework for improvement in the management of demand in agri-food supply chains. *Supply Chain Management, 11*(5), 379–384. doi:10.1108/13598540610682381

Taylor, D. H., & Fearne, A. (2009). Demand management in fresh food value chains: A framework for analysis and improvement. *Supply Chain Management, 14*(5), 379–392. doi:10.1108/13598540910980297

Thakur, M., Sørensen, C.-F., Bjørnson, F. O., Forås, E., & Hurburgh, C. R. (2011). Managing food traceability information using EPCIS framework. *Journal of Food Engineering, 103*(4), 417–433. doi:10.1016/j.jfoodeng.2010.11.012

Trapero, J. R., Kourentzes, N., & Fildes, R. (2012). Impact of information exchange on supplier forecasting performance. *Omega, 40*(6), 738–747. doi:10.1016/j.omega.2011.08.009

Trienekens, J., van der Vorst, J., & Verdouw, C. (2014). *Global food supply chains. In Encyclopedia of Agriculture and Food Systems* (2nd ed., pp. 499–517). Academic Press. doi:10.1016/B978-0-444-52512-3.00118-2

Trienekens, J., Wognum, P., Beulens, A. J., & van der Vorst, J. G. (2012). Transparency in complex dynamic food supply chains. *Advanced Engineering Informatics, 26*(1), 55–65. doi:10.1016/j.aei.2011.07.007

Trienekens, J. H., & van Der Vorst, J. G. A. J. (2006). Traceability in food supply chains. In P. A. Luning, F. Devlieghere, & R. Verhé (Eds.), *Safety in argi-food chain*. Wageningen Academic Publishers.

Uusipaavalniemi, S., & Juga, J. (2008). Information integration in maintenance services. *International Journal of Productivity and Performance Management, 58*(1), 92–110. doi:10.1108/17410400910921100

Van der Vorst, J., Beulens, A., & van Beek, P. (2005). *Innovations in logistics and ICT in food supply chain networks. In Innovation in Agri-food Systems: Product Quality and Consumer Acceptance* (pp. 245–292). Wageningen: Wageningen Academic Publishers.

Van der Vorst, J. G., Tromp, S.-O., & Zee, D.-J. (2009). Simulation modelling for food supply chain redesign; integrated decision making on product quality, sustainability and logistics. *International Journal of Production Research, 47*(23), 6611–6631. doi:10.1080/00207540802356747

Verdouw, C., Beulens, A., Trienekens, J., & Wolfert, J. (2010). Process modelling in demand-driven supply chains: A reference model for the fruit industry. *Computers and Electronics in Agriculture, 73*(2), 174–187. doi:10.1016/j.compag.2010.05.005

Voigt, G. (2011). *Supply Chain Coordination in Case of Asymmetric Information*. Springer.

Voss, C., Tsikriktsis, N., & Frohlich, M. (2002). Case research in operations management. *International Journal of Operations & Production Management, 22*(2), 195–219. doi:10.1108/01443570210414329

Yin, R. K. (2013). *Case study research: Design and methods* (5th ed.). Sage publications.

Yu, Z., Yan, H., & Edwin Cheng, T. (2001). Benefits of information sharing with supply chain partnerships. *Industrial Management & Data Systems, 101*(3), 114–121. doi:10.1108/02635570110386625

Zhao, X., & Xie, J. (2002). Forecasting errors and the value of information sharing in a supply chain. *International Journal of Production Research*, *40*(2), 311–335. doi:10.1080/00207540110079121

ENDNOTE

[1] Software like ARIS, Visio, or LucidChart could be potential solutions to draw the actual map.

This research was previously published in the International Journal of Information Systems and Supply Chain Management (IJISSCM), 12(3); edited by John Wang; pages 85-109, copyright year 2019 by IGI Publishing (an imprint of IGI Global).

Chapter 17
IoT–Based Cold Chain Logistics Monitoring

Afreen Mohsin
UTL Technologies, India

Siva S. Yellampalli
UTL Technologies, India

ABSTRACT

This chapter aims to reduce the extent of human presence all along the cold chain by means of a powerful tool in the form of the IoT. It should also be ensured that any details regarding instances of equipment failure leading to product spoilage or an event of a successful delivery must be communicated to the manufacturer's end. It also seeks to fill gaps involving location tracking and environment control by means of a GPS module and an IoT-based sensor platform respectively used here.

INTRODUCTION

A new evolution in technological advancement is happening in the world these days. This increasing evolution permits the world of physical objects close in our surroundings to be connected to the internet. The design of the sensing body within the environment collects the information. Information then collected by sensing body connects itself to the cloud sensing element through a local area network. Later the network hosts information from its surroundings. This whole employment is the ideology behind giving life to IoT.

A cold chain is a temperature-controlled supply chain. It is unbroken and an uninterrupted series of refrigerated production, storage and distribution activities consisting of equipment and logistics, which maintain a desired temperature range. Cold chain logistics needs controlled surrounding environment for sensitive products. These products are suitable to use under the controlled environment. The sole assurance that tells if a certain method has been disbursed with success is the monitoring method. The use of IoT here is to observe cold chain supply leading to higher products handling and management.

DOI: 10.4018/978-1-7998-5354-1.ch017

This book chapter describes a system which consists of a wireless microcontroller-based sensor network and a server which proves to be a perfect system to observe the temperature and humidity of cold chain logistics.

The meeting point between the real and the virtual world through some technologies is referred as "Internet of Things" (IoT). These technologies can be the sensor technology or mobile communication. With the ambition of giving all-pervading computing to automate the tasks or processes and to build a smart world this sort of computing system started a long time ago. The IoT is a trend with powerful technology in shaping the development of the information and communication technology (ICT). Today, the IoT consists of wide variety of items used in our daily lives, including radio frequency identification (RFID) tags, sensors, actuators, and even smart devices like mobile phones. A unique addressing scheme enables these objects to communicate and interact with other items to achieve the respective goals.

The development area like the wireless sensor networks aims at collecting contextual data. Here enhancement is being made in service-oriented architecture (SOA) which is a software approach to expanding web-based services using the capabilities of IoT (Web of Things, WoT) (Shih & Wang, 2016). Further the introduction of sensor technologies can be made doable conjointly together with technologies like artificial intelligence, nanotechnology etc. The sensor technologies create the IoT services as a knowledge domain field. Here most of the human senses are reproduced and replaced within the virtual world.

An electronic identification is given to these objects joining an IoT service. The sensors, for example, are the object/things which are the new electronic devices interacting with the real-world. A lot of chance is given to applications to contribute in building the IoT by combining sensors and mobile communications which seem to be very promising. From privacy, security, scalability and performance points of view these technologies can be improved, though they are already used (Islam, Mukhopadhyay, & Suryadevara, 2017).

The Internet within the IoT may additionally have completely different interpretations on the other hand. The present internet adapted to these new object's connectivity desires is the apparent interpretation which is more direct. With the IP addressing and routing capabilities the current internet is that of connected nodes employing a TCP/IP (internet protocol suite) protocol stack. The likelihood of planning corresponding gateways to specific nodes or networks is designed here in the internet model which runs a TCP/IP stack within the connected device (Islam, Mukhopadhyay, & Suryadevara, 2017). Adapting the TCP/IP stack to the resources of the objects involves the present internet connecting it. Within the long-standing time, the IoT seems among the leading methods to present this goal. IoT challenges the current internet model with new needs of connectivity of objects: like identifying, naming and addressing, measurability, non-uniformity, resource limitation, etc. (TCP Usage Guidance in the Internet of Things, 2018).

Regarding information visibility, IoT is currently running without any concern of autonomous decision-making. To avoid delays between data availability and choices and to alleviate from everyday decision tasks, new technologies and methods have to be compelled so it can be integrated. Autonomous cooperating logistical processes are being researched in logistics. Decentralized and hierarchal designing and management methods are used in the main set up of this idea. The combination of IoT and autonomous control (Autonomous system Internet) is an assortment of IP networks and routers below the control of one entity and additionally the IoT would provide a better level of strength in infrastructure, quantifiability and agility. To achieve subsequent level of user acceptance among the overall public they need to be easy to use and easy to assemble.

With the increasing range of deliveries either smaller or larger is been influenced by e-business in the present economy. IoT can bridge the gap between information technology and objects by the advancement of material handling and monitoring within the past years. Automated monitoring and improved data handling capabilities of the things enable the individual product identification of the product. This makes the monitoring efficient and better, because it was antecedently restricted solely to the kinds of product or a particular identification of batch of products. Massive products recall, which have led to severe monetary and company name mislaying, should be replaced by individual selective product recalls. This improves direct business-to-consumer communication. The IoT persuades to be the lacking connection between logistics and data monitoring. For connecting the things, sensors, actuators, and alternative smart technologies could be foundation for IoT. Hence this enables communication between person-to-object and object-to-object. The current changes in info technology, logistics and electronic (e-)business is aligned with the event of IoT. The IoT in logistics ideas and technologies have been applied to previous issues within the field of logistics. In transport logistics, the autonomous transport of supply objects/things from the sender to the receiver address is considered (Akulwar, 2016).

The IoT goes on the far side communication. The individual object is equipped with intelligence. On the system itself the intelligence can be placed. The product/object is permanently or temporarily linked to the IoT. The proposed system can be used for the transport of fresh fruits like for instance bananas. Traditional Storage of bananas is at 13 degrees Celsius. In Chill mode its 2 degrees Celsius. Whereas at Frozen mode -18 degrees and in deep frozen it's about -29 degrees Celsius. Condition monitoring of this kind are done by the intelligent systems as proposed in the project using ADC values. The small sensors analyze the temperature and humidity data and gather the collected information regarding the fresh products. The monitoring officer will keep a real-time track on the conditions and auto action is taken consequently. Currently, the previously proposed GPS (global positioning systems) consume high energy, they are big and expensive as well does not have the desired accuracy to be maintained (How the Internet of Things Impacts the Logistics Business, 2018).

The location tracker utilized in the proposed system overcomes these difficulties. The modern logistics is growing rapidly with the employment of IoT as the developers are working 24*7 to deal with elementary challenges. The cloud computing on the other hand can access the information using the internet instead of a computer's physical disc drive. Cloud computing and IoT technologies advancement have given vast openings within the logistics industry.

In logistics, the IoT application has for the most part currently taken root. The ability to figure out in times of volatile monetary markets and disruption of supply networks offers supply chain trading a combative advantage over opponents. The data flows in real-time inside the vicinity which is permitted by the cloud. This therefore enhances the economical communication with totally different base stations or trucks having the installed systems. All the operators will exchange data quick, streamlining operations and reducing congestion. The operators may be like fleet managers, drivers, and freight carriers.

Cloud computing can even facilitate with human error recovery. In logistics, cloud computing can even facilitate with disaster recovery as well provides a secure and solid platform to display and store the real-time information. The cloud computing can keep it safe from human error or disasters. The various actions needed to keep up with the optimum monitoring conditions are taken care of. Moreover, technologies having cloud computing even have the capability to reinforce loading and container discharge. The IoT in logistics market worldwide (Ganguli, 2016) throughout the period between 2016-2022 is anticipated to grow at a CAGR of 35.5% to touch an aggregate of $1,050.95 billion by 2022 as shown in Figure 1.

Figure 1. Worldwide IoT in logistics market revenue

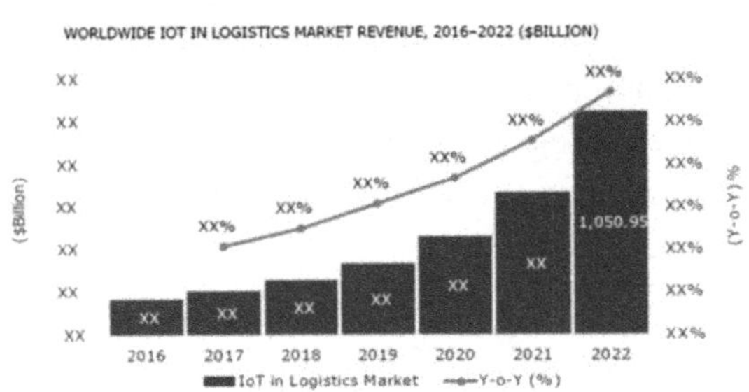

The information exchange with each other over the internet in IoT is a broad framework of inter-connected devices. To come up with a lot of revenue and to open huge opportunities, IoT conjointly helps to scale back prices and employed in places like truck or in tracking the shipment. It is also employed in monitoring parameters in warehouse storage. The sensors are utilized here to monitor and keep track parameters like humidity and temperature. This helps the monitoring officer/driver to provide storage conditions suitable for various containers.

IoT applications usage, like WLAN in several base stations or within the truck ensures transparency in logistics. A safe transit of products from source to their destination is provided by this technology. Using GPS, the monitoring officer are in a position to check the precise location of the container products in the port or throughout transport. The movement of the trucks carrying products inside and outside the vicinity use this IoT based technology to confirm their safe destination. Containers, trucks and ships situated in varied ports with different locations are efficiently handled. Here the IoT interconnects the components situated in different areas. The IoT permits the system to gather and process information for decision-making and performance improvement at a later stage (Verma & Srivastava, 2017).

The thought process of whether the proposed system is an IoT or an WSN can be observed further. Firstly, in IoT routing isn't enforced. The sensors send their information on to the internet. Whereas, WSNs (Wireless sensor networks) nodes route traffic to reach sink node. This sink node is close to the nodes and is often accessed to read the gathered information. In IoT, things are anything ranging from sensors, humans, cameras, PCs and phones. These devices transfer their information to the internet that permits them to use in their applications. Secondly, WSN is an example of ad hoc networks and has its features. However, IoT information is send to the internet in exactly one hop. One hop transmission is against the definition of ad hoc. Thirdly, the sink node in WSN could also be connected to the internet to form IoT. In other words, all of the WSNs is one node in IoT. Hence, WSNs are simply a set of IoT. WSNs solely address the utilization of sensors specifically wirelessly-connected sensors. Major variations between WSN and IoT are shown in the Table 1. Conclusion can be made that the proposed system comes under IoT (Blaisdell, 2018).

The Internet is being exploited to control the virtual world. In IoT, there are direct implications on the physical part of the world. In reference, to being free from public attention, it's necessary for the company's professional/personal information to be treated intrinsically. New legislation is being planned to manage the misuse of personal data by employers. IoT allows additional surveillance potentialities regarding employees and consumers. Laws and regulations are improved and facilitated. However, control mechanisms which are self-regulating are additionally necessary. Power is the foremost vital limitation of the devices connected to the things. Each action taken within which the device used is power driven

Table 1. Major differences between WSN and IoT

Sr.No.	WSN	IoT
1	The foundation of IoT applications are the Wireless Sensor Networks.	The network of physical objects controlled and monitored over internet is IoT.
2	The network of Motes which are formed to observe, study or to monitor the physical parameters in the application desired is WSN.	In IoT application the physical parameters monitoring is done. The desired outcomes are not same but are little different. IoT is a Machine to Machine communication, smartness is brought into daily objects here.
3	For example - In Monitoring Temp-Humidity parameters or checking Soil moisture, motes are deployed in agricultural land. The gathering of data with perfect data analysis produce results about crop yields. This result may be of quality or quantity.	For example - When the device is hooked to the Thermostat, it monitors the surrounding temperature and adjusts it to the most preferred setting for user. It also learns about your habits, and help you build healthy one. All done using data analysis and some quality algorithms.

by batteries like using the wireless trans-receiver for sensing or for running of action devices for the proposed system. All these consume part of the energy. These devices are required to operate for days or months and even years together with an equivalent charge depending upon the battery. The protocols managing the node communication and networking for this reason should be rigorously thought-about. For future work in IoT, clustering would be accustomed to managing the power needed for the devices which represent the objects (Akkerman & Grunow, 2010).

The IoT advantages include new and advanced business opportunities with effectiveness and improved efficiency. In IoT open governance remains a major issue but there are certain levels and problems regarding security, privacy and governance that need to be considered.

Motivation

Getting the proper goods at the correct time and right place at a reduced cost is presently very important within the world market. Visibility is particularly vital in supply chain management of temperature and humidity for transportation and storage. It is of top priority to keep the standard and number of goods in the availability chain at specified levels. In case of transportation of food and medicines, the degrading quality of biodegradable foods and restricted lifespan of medicines contribute considerably to their management complexness. Properly controlled environments are required for biodegradable foods or medicines throughout the production, storage, transportation and sales processes to make sure proper food quality maintenance and cut back on major food losses. This is often referred as "Cold Chain Logistics".

The challenge of keeping perishable foods and pharmaceutical products that have diverse temperature and humidity requirements for storage and distribution environments is being addressed here. A controlled supply chain here senses the humidity and temperature parameter which refers to cold chain. The observation and management are important to maintain an unbroken and sustainable cold chain. To regulate and enhance the standard and safety potency within the cold chain logistics process the issue is taken up by the govt and enterprises and have called it a high priority discussion and crucial topic for analysis. Pharmaceutical merchandise has rigorous temperature and humidity necessities throughout the supply processes whereas in the Food business, the controlled environment varies among variety of food items. Even short amount of exposure like a couple of hours of extreme hot or cold temperatures and high or low humidity will cause a marked decrease in shelf life and loss of harvest. The supply chain is hence very crucial if quality of the merchandise is to be assured. Whereas for the medicine storage, a small variation within the humidity rate within the surroundings might produce bacteria and fungus formation. Real time data need to be communicated between the suppliers and customers to achieve controllability and visibility of each link in a cold chain. Here comes the image of WSNs which is the key element to confirm each and every product throughout its lifecycle visibility. Advanced modeling and analytics identification are the intelligent cold chains. The driver at the wheel and the monitoring staff will be assisted based on necessary safety guidelines. With the advanced choices in the action taken during imbalance of the environmental conditions, the decisions are taken in a sensible and economical way. Therefore, the need to control and monitor the environmental conditions is very crucial. IoT based Cold Chain Monitoring System, seeks to fill gaps involving location tracking and environment control by means of a GPS module and an IOT based sensor platform respectively (Mehta, Sahni, & Khanna, 2018). The sensor data is sent via Wi-Fi transmitter with receiving end involving the driver and the monitoring officer who will receive regular updates on the controlled environment parameters and the location of the transporting vehicle in real-time. The driver and the monitoring officer will have regular updates about the parameters. Automatic swift actions in cases of emergency scenarios are taken. The whole process is explained throughout the course of the book chapter.

Objective of the Product

The goal of this project is to reduce the extent of human presence all along the cold chain by means of a powerful tool in the form of IoT. The proposed idea seeks to fill gaps involving location tracking and environment control by means of a GPS module and an IOT based sensor platform respectively. Swift actions are also taken as per the requirements needed to maintain the exact environmental parameters so that the product/goods are not spoiled under uncontrolled environment conditions. Instead of using an alarm/buzzer to notify the concerned person, taking the precise action upon the condition is proven to be more effective.

Problem Statement

Technology invasion has remained crucial in the modern-day scenario of Logistics due to ever growing global presence and rising capital investments. The modern-day cold logistics companies cannot afford to slack in this ever so competitive market and so ensuring a well-managed and monitored supply chain is crucial throughout. With a rise in the number of immunizations drives and creation of new vaccines, the importance of the logistics behind their transportation cannot be stressed enough. The primary challenges faced are:

1. Increased product sensitivity, quality standards and the volume of goods involved.
2. Ever growing regulations.
3. Infrastructure gaps like location tracking issues and controlled environment monitoring all along the cold chain.

Chapter Outline

This book chapter is structured into 2 sections.
 Section 1 discusses the design specifications for the system.
 Section 2 discusses the IoT Development using Thinkspeak.

SECTION 1

Literature Survey

Over the last few years several techniques and ideas have been implemented for monitoring of cold chain logistics. This chapter provides content and information of previous research papers, which lays the foundation and basis for further work.

IOT is a network framework consisting of various connected real-world objects, which depend on sensors, communication, networking, and information processing technologies. The technology for IOT is RFID. It works by allowing microchips to transfer identifying data to the reader via wireless medium. Using RFID, any person can analyze, trace, and monitor the objects connected with RFID tags. The basic fundamental technology being WSNs, mainly works on intelligent sensors for sensing and monitoring. RFID finds its application in transportation of goods to consumers, production of pharmaceutical goods, retail and applies to traffic, healthcare and industrial monitoring. The advancement in both the technologies accelerate the growth of IoT (Mehta, Sahni, & Khanna, 2018). Cold Chain is the logistics system that provides to the perishable goods from the point of source to the point of consumption through thermal and refrigerated packaging methods and logistical planning to protect the quality and increase the shelf life of these shipments. A Cold Chain is a temperature-controlled supply chain, which involves temperature, and moisture controlled transportation and storage of refrigerated and frozen goods (Chen, Wang, & Jan, 2014).

Temperature is the most often measured parameters because of its critical impact on the quality of food, drugs, volatile chemicals goods transportation and logistics operations. The conventional temperature data loggers are often expensive and have very bulky form. The biggest problem is with their excessive thickness, because in packaging everything thicker than 5 mm is exposed to hazardous situations involving tearing down. High interest has been therefore raised in cost effective, thin and lightweight temperature monitoring smart tags (Pereira, 2018).

Public health care in developing countries are facing poor access to pharmaceutical care and this specific group of population are suffering from "Pharmacy tourism". ePharmacyNet was designed and implemented to meet the challenges caused by the "Pharmacy Tourism". Pharmacies at care units and pharmacies from private health sector are selected to be part of a multidisciplinary remote care system use ePharmacyNet to provide medicine and other pharmaceutical products to remote patients. The question arising here is how to deliver cost effective, secure and safe pharmaceutical products in countries where road-rail networks are in a poor state (Edoh, 2017).

The rise of the IoT paradigm is bringing with it new challenges concerning security and trust. The challenges discussed here are inherent in trust that overcomes for IoT scenarios and have introduced a framework to be used by developers to include trust concerns in IoT systems. The framework proposed here aims to assist developers when adding trust or reputation in IoT systems. Instead of having to implement each trust model from scratch, the framework facilitates the work of the developers by providing them with techniques and guidance for re-using common features of other trust models and following certain steps to carry out the implementation. In developing a framework where different trust management systems for the IoT are present, different aspects of identity management need to be considered. It is particularly crucial to properly define the identity of the 'things'. Their identity could be determined by their context (the set of things that are connected with the user for a specific purpose at a given moment in time) (Fernandez-Gago, Movano, & Lopez, 2017).

The FDA (Food and Drug Administration) and Agriculture Department within the early Nineteen Nineties had started to convey the HACCP rules (Hazard Analysis Critical Control Point) as a scientific stepping stone to safety of food. The pharmaceutical and the food trade industry have adopted identical principle. Both are presently dealing and managing with products which are sensitive to temperature. This system addresses the numerous product safety circumstances coming across. The distribution and handling of the finished product is the foremost necessary concern between them. HACCP has now become an accepted standard and universally recognized for the safety of products. The WHO standards program has adopted HACCP management system. Precautions ought to be taken at each purpose within the cold chain to make sure that the stability of the products are not affected by the any external conditions. A proof of compliance with suggested storage conditions as records of essential temperature and humidity parameters is produced. According to Salin and Nayga (Tennermann, 2012) there are several transnational eating house corporations like Burger King, McDonalds and KFC etc. The technical challenges faced in tight target markets with strict specs and exclusive offer chains are managed in these corporations, whereas the smaller corporations use ample networks to provide foreign frozen potatoes. The added worth within the supply chain and the present net value of the activities will have to be discomposed with the changes in time, temperature and distance within the chain. A thorough investigation performed the perturbation analyses. A steadiness in cold chains is necessary to assure a proper cold chain management. The time delays such as lead times and a few alternative delays will change the behavior of the supply chain.

Cold chain is a process of maintaining medication such as insulin and vaccines with-in counseled temperatures principally between 2°C to 8°C throughout the provision chain. In the pharmaceutical sector, the cold chain is concerned with the transportation, storage, and handling of pharmaceutical merchandise in very safe surrounding environment from the manufacturer end to the user end. Temperatures outside counseled temperature ranges might cut-back efficiency resulting in reduced immunity. Control of storage and transportation temperature is essential in maintaining. At the global perspective, procurement is defined as the procurance of goods, acquisition of services or works from an outdoor external source at the most effective potential price to satisfy the needs of the buyer in terms of the standard of medicines and in serving to shield the patients from sub-standard or ineffective medicines that will result from inadequate management. Lack of awareness by distributors within the management of storage and transportation temperatures will have a serious impact on quality of the goods. A survey by Agyekum (2012), conducted in Ghana, Kenya and Uganda indicates that an average of sixteen percent of the sampled facilities were not compliant to the guidelines laid out by regulatory authorities and fifty percent of these facilities had temperatures 4°c or more outside the recommended temperatures. For example, only four per cent of facilities stored vaccines in cold boxes, while the remainder used refrigerators and storage outside the recommended range. Though significant variation was observed between the countries; twenty six percent, sixteen percent, and eight percent for Ghana, Kenya, and Uganda, respectively there remains significant room to improve cold chain supply in these countries among others in Africa. In a comparison of African countries based on their cold supply chains, it was found that Ghana had developed its supply systems. It is now capable to maintain cold chain for items which are sensitive to temperature than Kenya and Uganda in spite of facing similar challenges (World Health Organization, 2010). The Ghana's regulative authorities were ready to develop validation strategies and guidelines. The aim of providing temperature assurance throughout the produce storage with transportation and delivery of cold chain items within the cold chain is the described cold chain delivery system in Ghana. There are concerned activities that provide cold chain management for foodstuff which source to food security, contract farming, and management of danger, resource and development, on-the-spot trials, coaching and education and project management (Stilmant, 2013). The various management resources were mentioned here which are utmost important while maintaining a good logistics system.

The cold chain management suggests that the combined management of food safety and transportation (Cold chain management). The individuals first judge the full cold chain then organize its transportation. The sourcing ought to be checked to confirm the food security so to contract the farming to debate the detail of contract (Food and Drug Administration, 2018). The danger involved in management is a concern just like the safety and quality of food and whether the source could also be contamination and correctly packed and handled.

Technology invasion has remained crucial in the modern-day scenario of Logistics due to ever growing global presence and rising capital investments. The modern-day cold logistics companies cannot afford to slack in this ever so competitive market and so ensuring a well-managed and monitored supply chain is crucial throughout. With a rise in the number of immunizations drives and creation of new vaccines, the importance of the logistics behind their transportation cannot be stressed enough (Domingo, 2012). The materialistic world objects are bonded with IoT with the help of internet which offers the pliability to simply manage and monitor the them. The cultural, business, social, environmental, etc. along with the environment on multiple levels have been approached with a new perception which brings about this body. The WSNs brings into picture the sensing element which is rising in IoT (Atzori, 2005).

The technological advancement of IoT has led to the rise in the quantity of physical objects being linked to the internet. The two primary entities that allow this technology to flourish are the Sensing entity that senses or collects data and the Cloud Service that plays itself as the host to the data collected (Khemapech, 2005). This meant that there was a rise in combination of wireless sensors and cloud computing strategies. IOT Analytics has emerged as a lifeline to the cold chain logistics industry due to the fact that companies have to rely on third parties (third party logistics) to self-report on performance (Hart & Martinez, 2006). Deployment of a wide array of sensors in storage locations, shipping containers and trucks is crucial in order to monitor the temperature and humidity parameters in Real Time and thereby also ensure that quick and efficient action can be taken in cases of emergencies. Thus, the IOT has offered scope to not just monitor the crucial parameters real time but also aid in preventative and remedial actions if needed through quick intimation (Peng, 2009).

A peak into AVR controller implementation, a system is developed to monitor and humidity of cold chain logistic consisting of Arduino WSN system with Xively sensor cloud service provider (Avitesh, 2017) is discussed briefly. Arduino libraries and hardware designs for connecting to the internet were integrated here. The sensor cloud service provider used here is a paid service provider whose services can be easily availed on yearly payment basis. Email service alert is also mentioned. But this system does not deal with the saving of power and faster processing issues coming across while monitoring.

Testing wireless sensing element motes primarily based within the ZigBee protocol throughout a real cargo is mentioned (Luis & Ruiz-Garcia, 2010). Information regarding water loss and condensation on the merchandise throughout shipments is concisely tested here. These motes offer data regarding temperature and humidity in a very closed container. The motes utilize the RF power isn't robust which is enough to travel along the pallets owing to the content having large amount of water of the merchandise transported. There is higher energy consumption by the readying of higher range of motes that use RF power. As well there is no mention of testing in deep trouble long run conditions.

A monitoring system using a with ZigBee WSN and GPS positioning, according to the characteristics of cold chain logistics is discussed (Mei & Wu, 2015). ZigBee has a disadvantage over WiFi. ZigBee is not secure based system. It is prone to attack from unauthorized people. Replacement cost will be high when any problem occurs in ZigBee compliant appliances and the coverage is limited. The disadvantage of this system is it requires very long battery life. An unsecure network is also a drawback.

The importance of temperature monitoring in perishable articles has been discussed (Aung & Chang, 2014). A sample dataset is included of products that have different temperatures ranging from 0 degree Celsius to 21 degrees Celsius. Methods to improve temperature control are presented and investigated to manage the cold storage of multi-temperature commodities. The author here has given light upon the Multi-commodity cold stores and mentioned the rapid growth of food delivery multi-temperature trailers, particularly for freelance grocery stores and fast food. Three methods were proposed which are used as a tool for decision making associated with cold chain logistics of perishable foods. The storage and transport facilities for a temperature-controlled supply chain require transporting a product which is temperature-sensitive from the producer to the end user. However, this provides chain management was found to be quite advanced, coping with food merchandise having completely different temperatures.

A proposed model to make a system, using IoT, which senses the room temperature and sends this data to an online cloud (Thinkspeak) for further analysis in a graphical form using API keys is presented (Mali, & Akshay, 2016). Here only the temperature is measured and tested in a room. This application can be used either for home automation, lab monitoring, etc. Humidity is not monitored and there is no mention of remedies to be taken when there is an uncontrolled environment condition in the room.

Proposed System Level Description

The System Block Diagram of IoT based Cold Chain Logistics Monitoring is as shown in Figure 2.

Figure 2. System Block Diagram

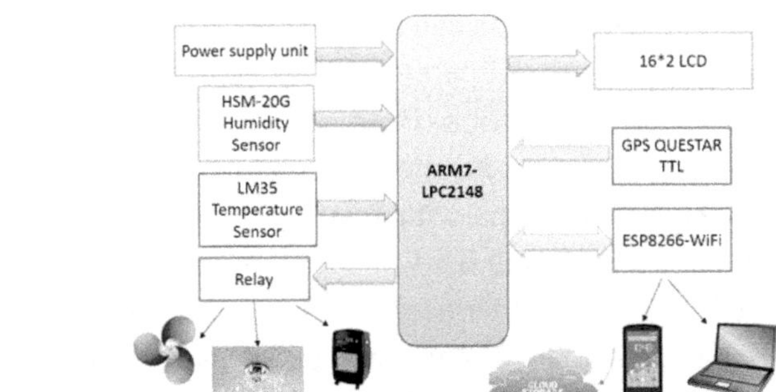

Figure 2 consists of components such as Humidity sensor (HSM-20G), Temperature sensor (LM35) and GPS (QUESTAR TTL) given at the input side of the microcontroller whereas 16*2 LCD and ESP8266 Wi-Fi module is given at the output side. The microcontroller used here is ARM7/TDMI (LPC2148). Relay circuit is connected to the devices depending upon requirement such as fan, sprinkler and heater. A Smartphone/Laptop (with TCP/IP client app) is used for real-time data acquisition.

1. Workflow of the Monitoring System

Every package should have distinctive tag name or number to spot the goods being transported which may be registered with the monitoring staff. Within the truck, the designed system consists of Temperature and Humidity Sensors installed at multiple places. Each system installed is termed as a node. Multiple nodes within the truck yield an additional sturdy observation because it can cater for various Temperature and Humidity points within the section. The monitoring officer at the specified monitoring centres or the driver at the wheel can read the information which can either be a laptop, computer, smartphone or a tablet. The block diagram can be explained in this manner by considering Figure 2, initially sensors in the nodes are going to sense the surrounding temperature and humidity. These sensors then feed the analog value to the ADC which is present in LPC2148 microcontroller. The ADC is approximation type ADC which converts analog value to digital values. The ADC values are set to specific limit depending on the environmental conditions, either displaying High/Low/Normal Temperature and High/Low/Normal Humidity Concentration. The respective action is taken on the sensed values by switching ON the fan for High Temperature or by simply switching ON the sprinkler for Low Humidity by the command given by the microcontroller.

2. IoT Implementation

The nodes embrace a WiFi Module that permits to constantly send Temperature and Humidity values to the monitoring centres or driver at the wheel can read the information which can either be a laptop, computer, smartphone or a tablet in real-time. The information gathered from the nodes at the centre or in the hand-held device(s) is transferred to the sensor cloud alongside with the location obtained from the GPS. The inventory information that is ready are sent to the respective personnel with the assistance of the TCP/IP client app within the Smartphone and using the ESP-link firmware in Laptop. The data input values from the sensor nodes given to the controller is stored as a CSV format in the server. Concurrently, the data is sent from server to client side on thingspeak.com portal using HTTP protocol.

3. Proposed System Safety

ESP-link firmware is employed that connects the micro-controller to the net using an ESP8266 WiFi module. The ESP-link's role is to facilitate communication over wireless local area network. It's doable to visualize the respective real-time data on-line. Humidity and Temperature position of the motion truck is unbroken in track to keep up with the optimum conditions needed. The location information is employed to find and trace the transport facility that calculates the coordinates by GPS. This ensures the protection of the commodities within the truck. Real-time data plotted in the graph can be observed to keep in track of the temperature and humidity with respect to the date and time of the truck.

System Requirements

The aim of this project is to implement an ARM7 based Cold Chain Logistics System using the IoT platform. The system is used to monitor the temperature and humidity through the controller. The GPS location with Real-time data readings is captured in a smartphone/laptop with the help of the WiFi module. The complete overview of our architecture is defined in the diagram shown in Figure 3. In the proposed system 32-bit microcontroller (LPC2148 from NXP) is used.

Figure 3. Architectural Block Diagram

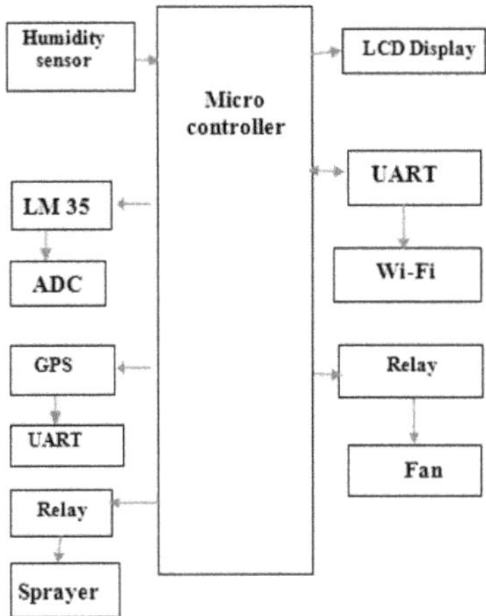

Both the hardware and software specification requirements are very necessary before any development of a system. The following specifications will be explained. Based on this, the respective requirements are needed to design the system.

Table 2. Hardware specification table

Hardware	Specification
ARM7	60 MHz, v=3.3v, max 100mA capacity
RS232 USB to UART	Data rate=115.2 kbps
LM35	-55 to 150 Celsius, 60uA
HSM-20G	20-95% RH, max 2mA
LCD	16 char x 2 lines, max 3mA
GPS QUESTER TTL	3.3v, max 60-40mA
ESP8266-12E	3.6v, 2.4-2.5GHz Frequency Range, 3 power modes
RELAY FOR CONNECTED DEVICES	12v to 240v devices
ADAPTER FOR POWER SUPPLY	12v

1. Hardware Requirements

The availability of the specific part numbers in hardware and Keil IDE µvision4.0 are the ideal requirements needed for the project. Flash Magic tool in software and USB to Serial Converter for dumping
the code in microcontroller is a part of hardware is used.

2. Software Requirements

The project is designed with the software module using Embedded C language and unit integration testing done with independent modules. All the initialization and operation of ADC, UART, LCD, WiFi are
done by using Embedded C. IDE tool used for this software design is Keil IDE µvision4.0.

Table 3. Software requirements table

Software	Requirements
IDE	Keil µvision v4
Flash Magic tool for programming	LPC2000 Flash Magic
TCP/IP client App	From Sollae systems v1.1 for Android
ESP-link firmware	Jeelabs v2.2.3

3. Specification Matching With the Proposed System

As observed the use of specified requirements mentioned in Table 2 must be matched with the proposed
system. The following components are described briefly depending upon their application in the system.

a. Power Supply

The provision of electrical power is through power supply. It is a device that gives electrical energy
to output load(s). This is termed as power supply unit or PSU. A 230V, 50Hz Single phase AC power
supply is given to a transformer to urge 12V supply. By employing a Bridge Rectifier this voltage is
regenerated to DC voltage. The capacitor filters the DC voltage and gives to LM7805 voltage regulator.
This gives the constant 5V supply which further provides it to all parts within the circuit which require
maximum 5V to power up the device. To make sure the power is in ON state an LED is provided for
indication purpose.

Figure 4. Power supply unit

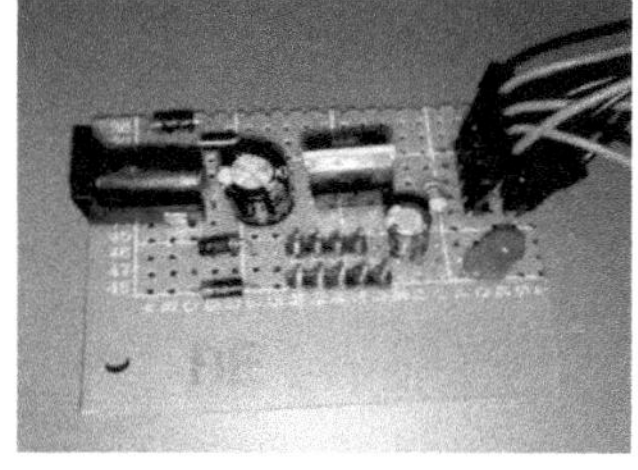

b. LPC 2148

In the proposed system ARM7 TDMI-S CPU based LPC2148 microcontroller board is used. Flash memory ranges from 32 kB to 512 kB (Datasheet of ARM 7[LPC2148]. The crystal oscillator frequency is 12MHz and has 32-bit code execution. It is a "Low Power Low-Cost microcontroller".

Figure 5. LPC 2148 Board

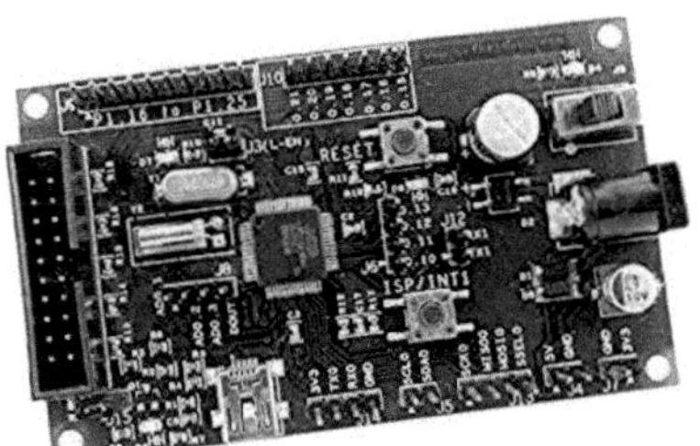

LPC2148 is a 32-bit microcontroller manufactured by Philips semiconductors (NXP). It is very small in size as compared to other ARM controllers. Its power utilization is the lowest among other controllers. Miniaturization is a key requirement nowadays. In this case, LPC2148 based ARM7 Controller is the best fit. By disabling the peripheral functions and by peripheral clock scaling, it is possible to handle power optimization feature in this controller.

Table 4. Differences between different microcontrollers

Features	8051	PIC	AVR	ARM
Bus Width	8-bit	8/16/32-bit	8/32-bit	32/64-bit
Communication Protocols	UART, USART, SPI, I2C	PIC, UART, UASART, LIN, CAN, Ethernet, SPI, I2C	UART, USART, SPI, I2C,	UART, USART, LIN, I2C, SPI, CAN, USB, Ethernet, I2C, DSP, SAI (serial audio interface) IrDA
Speed	12 Clock/Instruction cycle	4 Clock/Instruction cycle	1 Clock/Instruction cycle	1 Clock/Instruction cycle
Memory	ROM, SRAM, FLASH	SRAM, FLASH	Flash, SRAM, EEPROM	Flash, SDRAM, EEPROM
ISA (Instruction Set Architecture)	CLSC	Some feature of RISC	RISC	RISC
Memory Architecture	Von Neumann architecture	Harvard Architecture	Modified	Modified Harvard architecture
Power consumption	Average	Low	Low	Low
Cost (as compared to features provide)	Very Low	Average	Average	Low
Other features	Known for its standard	Cheap	Cheap, effective	High speed operation Vast

All industry level applications use ARM controllers. From the above comparison table, it can be observed that, power consumption is very low in ARM as compared to other controllers. Each pin in LPC2148 consumes only 3.3v and has maximum capacity of 100mA. This is best suitable industrial controller; the required remedial active devices or additional sensors can be used without worrying about huge power consumption as compared to other controllers.

c. ADC Conversion in LPC2148

For the microcontroller to process the signal/voltage and make it human readable, ADC is required which converts the analog signal into its counterpart digital number. The resolution indicates the number of digital values in ADC. A 10-bit ADC is present in LPC2148. The maximum value will be 2 raised to 10 which is equal to 1024. The digital numbers lie between 0-1024. The ADC in this controller is a 10-bit successive approximation ADC. There are two ADCs in LPC2148, namely ADC0 and ADC1 having 6-channels between AD0.1 to AD0.6 and 8-channels between AD1.0 to AD1.7 respectively. The 4.5 MHz is the max operating freq. which divides the conversion time. The ADC related channel pins used in the proposed system is AD0.1 which is the pin P0.28 for LM35 and AD0.2 which is pin P0.29 for HSM-20G; both present in the 6-channel ADC port 0.

d. LCD Module (16*2 Character)

An LCD is an electronic display module. LCDs are better than 7-segment displays which consume huge power. They are economical and easily programmable. Command and Data are the registers present in LCD. There are three control signals namely, register select, read/write, enable and eight address/data pins, command register is an9instruction given to the LCD. A pre-defined task is done by the LCD by the command instruction. Data is stored by the data register which is to be displayed on the LCD. The pins P0.15 to P0.21 from LPC2148 are connected to the pins of LCD module. Figure 6 is the LCD module used in the project.

Figure 6. LCD Module

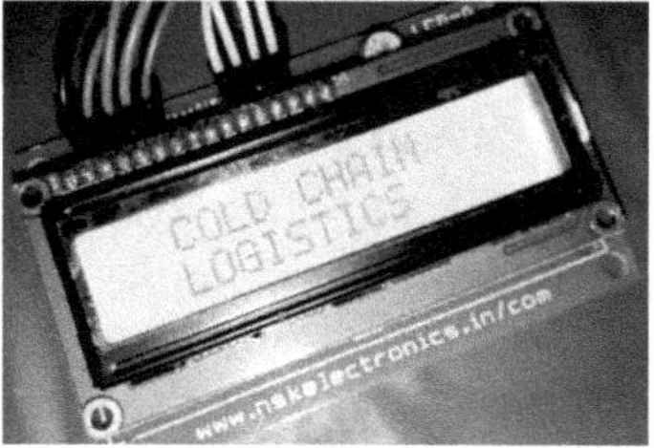

e. LM35: Temperature Sensor

The LM35 is calibrated in Kelvin. This is considered one of the most advantageous over other temperature sensors. There is no requirement of subtraction of a large constant voltage to obtain centigrade scaling. The LM35 provides typical accuracies of one-fourth degree Celsius at room temperature and about three-fourth degree Celsius. The temperature ranges between $-55°C$ to $150°C$ (National Semiconductor, 2000).

Figure 7. LM35

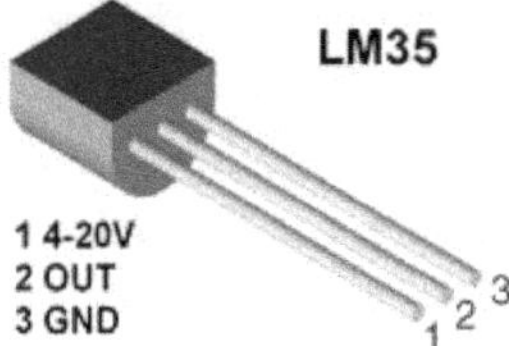

LM35 temperature sensor is used in the proposed system as seen in Figure 8. It has precise inherent calibration, low output impedance and a linear. Readout is very easy in LM35. The device is used with single power supply between 2.7v and 5.5v. Only 60 µA from the supply is drawn because of its self-heating capacity is low in still air.

Figure 8. Temperature sensor

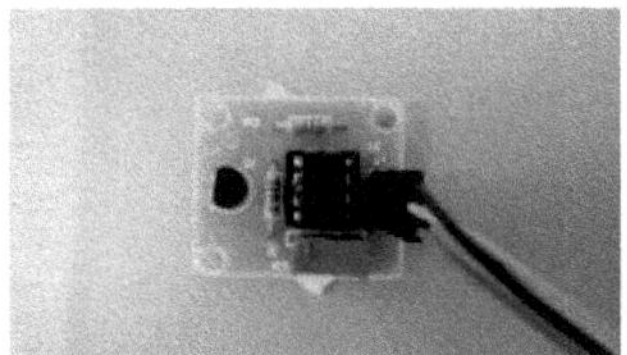

In LM35, the output voltage is 10mV per degree centigrade. LM35 is precise and work under many environmental conditions. This proves it to be consistent between sensors and readings. They are also very inexpensive and quite easy to use. Supply voltage of 3.3v is given from the controller to the sensor and grounded accordingly. The Vout (output pin) of LM35 is connected to ADC pin AD0.1.

- **LM358 – Low Power Dual Amplifier:** It is a low power OPAMP IC which can amplify low level signals to readable high levels. It works on 5V supply and can give a maximum. saturated output of ~4V. It has a very low supply current drain of approximately 500 µA. It is fundamentally independent of supply voltage. Connect Pin8 to 5 V rail and Pin4 to ground rail. Connect 10kOhms variable POT pin to pin 1 and any fixed pin to pin 2 of LM358 op-amp. By setting the position of the variable by turning the pot, the temperature in the truck/room can be sensed accordingly.

Figure 9. LM358 with schematics

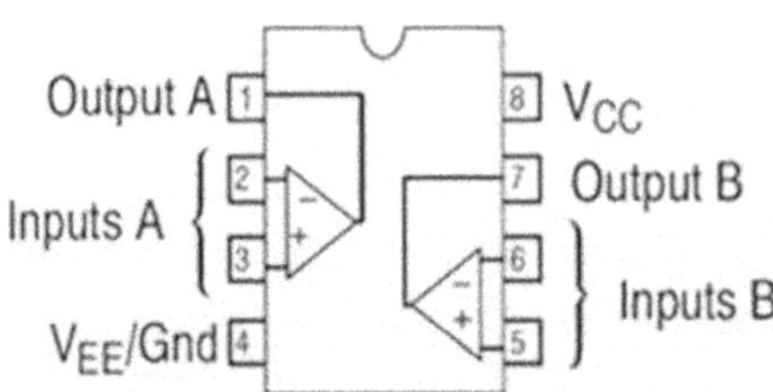

f. HSM-20G: Humidity Sensor

HSM-20G is a humidity sensor which can sense, measure and report the moisture and air temperature jointly. Relative humidity (RH) is the proportion of moisture content in the air to the amount of moisture which is higher in content at a distinct temperature of air. The HSM-20G used in the proposed model is an analog humidity as well as senses temperature which gives voltage which is analog with output with respect to relative humidity and temperature (Department of Atmospheric Sciences, 2010). The Storage range is from -20°C to 70°C and the Operating range is from 0°C to 50°C. As compared to other humidity sensors, HSM-20G is one of the most used operating sensors. This sensor is used for weather forecasting. The Storage RH Range is about 0-99% RH and the Operating RH range is between 20-95% and only about 2mA of operating current, which is the required specification met for the system. The 3 basic kinds of humidity sensors are Resistive, Thermal and Capacitive sensors. A Capacitive humidity sensor is used here. A thin strip of metal oxide (whose electrical capacity changes with atmosphere's RH) is placed to measure the RH between the two electrodes. The H-out of the Humidity sensor is connected to ADC pin AD0.2. Max operating current is 2mA, hence this module consumes less current.

- **LMV324 – Single, Dual, Quad Low-Voltage, Rail-to-Rail Operational Amplifiers:** This is a cost−effective solution for the developed system application. This amplifier uses lower power consumption and saves the package space. This amplifier covers covering different voltage ranges. It includes many combinations of power consumption and gain bandwidth. Industrial temperature Range is from −40°C to +85°C. Operates from 2.7 V to 5.0 V as a Single−Sided Power Supply. Maximum input current is 10mA. Best performance for appropriate accuracy is gained from this amplifier. It requires very low supply voltage range (Texas Instruments, 2014).

Figure 10. Humidity Sensor (Front view)

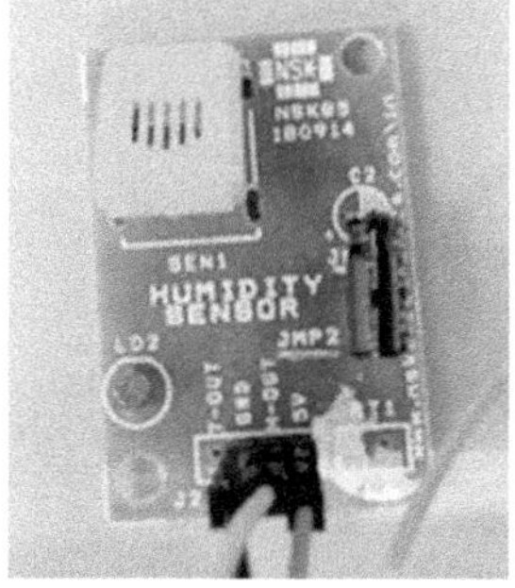

Figure 11. Humidity Sensor (Back view)

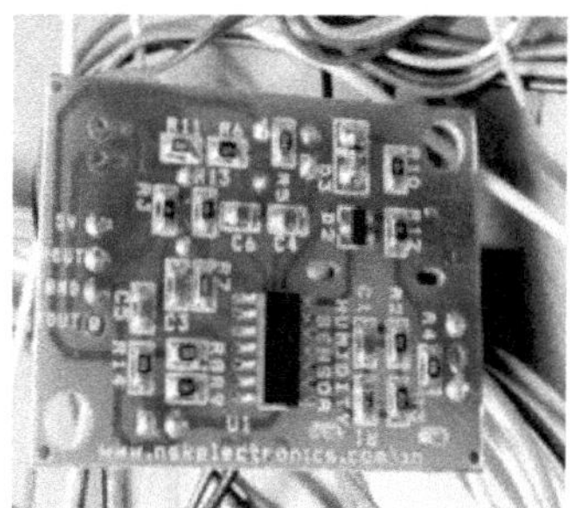

g. GPS QUESTAR TTL

The GPS QUESTAR TTL is a compact all-in-one GPS module solution used to locate the exact location of the object using the help of satellite it uses the 3D parameter i.e. the longitude, latitude, and attitude of the object and hence gives the position of the object. In areas having limited sky this GPS offers good navigation. Maximum. supply of 3.3v to 5.0v is supported which is perfect power saving module for the system. Operating temperature is from -30 °C to 80 °C. Supports lower power consumption of about 55mA at acquisition and 40mA while tracking which makes it an ideal power saving device. It has a built in RTC and EEPROM for accurate timings and storage (Datasheet of GPS QUESTAR TTL]. The UART1 pin RX1 of LPC2148 is connected to UART pin TX pin of the GPS module. Here only transmitting the coordinate values to the controller be read in the LCD. The 5V supply and ground from controller is given to GPS pins respectively.

Figure 12. GPS Module

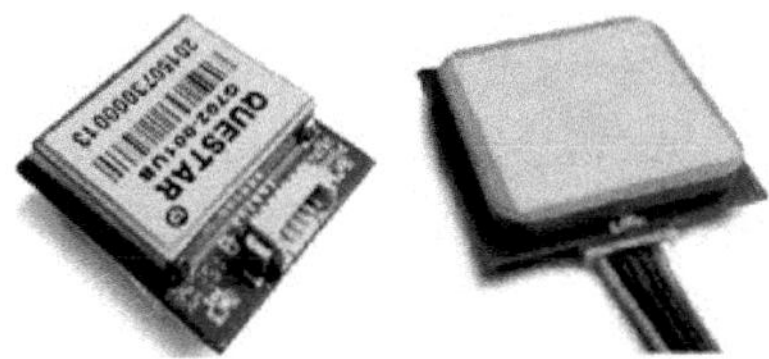

h. USB-UART

USB-UART is a hardware device used for asynchronous serial communication. Serial data is sent from transmitter to receiver. 115200bits per second (bps) is the maximum speed of UART, here in the system baud rate of 9600 bps is used. The signal is transmitted in the form of data packets or chunks and are called as transmission characters. Each data packet consists of start bit, parity, and stop bit. Data packet is transmitted to the output serially bit by bit from Transmit (TX) and Receive (Rx) pin. MAX232 transceiver IC is present on a board where the RS232 serial port is connected to TTL converter module which is a board. Serial communication between both the ports becomes easier by allowing the required electrical signal conversion. Here is used 4 header pins with jumper cables at one end and DB9 connector is soldered at the opposite end. The microcontroller is connected to converter module through jumper cables. The DB9 connects directly to a COM port of the PC. Used to dump the code to the controller from PC/Laptop. Figure 13 shows the usage of USB-UART device in displaying name on 16*2 LCD.

Figure 13. USB-UART module

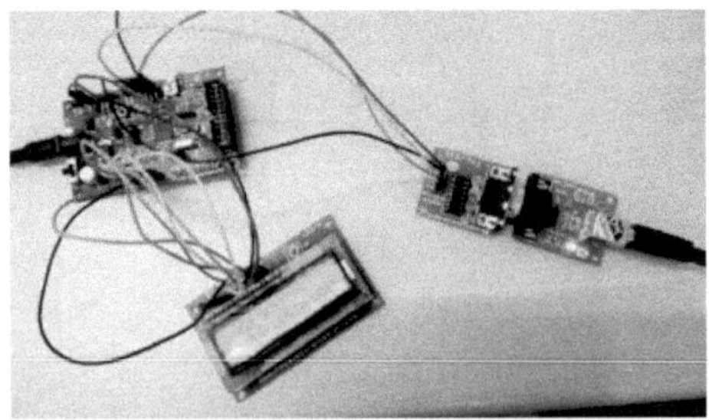

i. WiFi Module - ESP8266

It is a low-cost Wi-Fi chip with a microcontroller unit and an enabled TCP/IP stack. Its range is upto 2.4 GHz. ESP series modules use lower power. It has 11 GPIO pins and a single ADC converter (ADC) present is with a 10-bit resolution. The WiFi Module used in the system for easy access of real time data is shown in Figure 14.

Figure 14. ESP8266 – AI THINKER

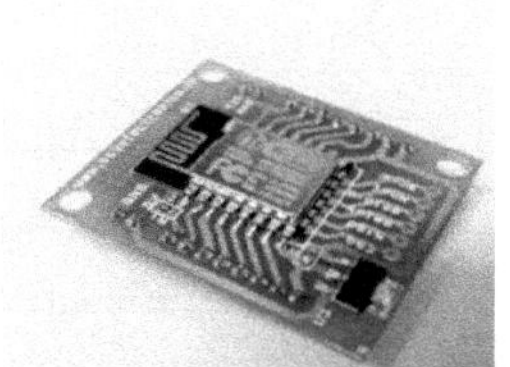

- **Why ESP8266?** The following points specifies the reasons:
  - It has good storage capabilities and processing in the board itself.
  - Permits to be integrated with application specific devices and sensors.
  - The GPIOs present have minimal loading during runtime, development is up-front.
  - Have minimal external circuitry which is designed to occupy minimal PCB area.
  - A larger server, which responded to multiple requests.
  - It offers low-level control and a very large programming memory space.
  - It executes faster and uses less resources.
  - The board is given 5v and the terminals of power connector is given to the regulator to have 3.3v resulting in minimal power requirement.
  - As per the survey and usage, a 2.4 GHz is considered better choice over 5 GHz depending upon its wireless range. 5 GHz range has limited support by devices and is of higher cost.
- What are the issues faced with ESP8266?
  - Challenges faced:
    - Endless reset on power-up
    - Power drain issues
  - Preventive measures taken:
    - Sufficient current was given. The current requirements for other components were also considered aside from the 300mA peak current needs of ESP8266. Normally, a regulated 3.3V source of at least 500ma is essential.
    - Connections were rechecked.
    - Clearing the memory. The code gets stuck somewhere in the loop and hence never returns resulting in a watchdog timer reset. Memory can be cleared by flashing the blank. bin file which comes with the nodemcu flash programmer.
    - The module needs to flash AT command set. It should respond to the "AT" command with "OK". This is the hello world for the device.
    - It can easily configure deep-sleep mode which lets the module run for 3 years on two AA batteries to rectify the power issues. The antenna is a track on the PCB which delivers good results for Wi-Fi sensitivity.

ESP8266 draws almost 1 Amp of power which is very huge, but the transmission capability is from 500 meters to about few miles which is very large horsepower for such low-cost device which is in hundreds. As shown in the table above, a solution for power saving can still be rectified to an extent by using the power modes available in the module. The Wi-Fi Modem circuit shuts down to save power but requires the CPU to work in the Modem-sleep mode power mode. This is implemented with no data transmission

Table 5. Power consumption modes of ESP8266

Parameters	Power Consumption
Modem Sleep	15 mA
Light Sleep	0.9 mA
Deep Sleep	10 mA

with secure Wi-Fi connection. To maintain a 300ms of sleep time, about 15mA is the current rating. For example, in a Wi-Fi switch, the Light-sleep power mode is suspended. Without the data transmission, Wi-Fi modem circuit can be turned off and CPU is suspended to save power. To maintain a sleep of 300ms the current is 0.9mA. For Wi-Fi connection in Deep-Sleep mode is not required to be sustained. As in system developed, the temperature and humidity sensor sense the temperature and humidity at every 100s, then sleep for 300s and wakes up to connect to the Access Portal which takes about 0.3 to 1second. The total average current will come down to less than 1mA. Deep sleep is for long time between data transmission. As for the mobility of operation, with the help of a LiPo connector it can be battery operated from any PC also very useful for IoT devices which can be further enhanced in the system.

- **TCP/IP Client App for Smartphone/Tablet:** The main protocols of the IP (Internet Protocol) suite is the TCP (Transmission Control Protocol. TCP complements the IP. Hence, the TCP/IP refers to the entire suite (Fairhurst, 2003). World Wide Web, remote administration, email, and file transfer depend on TCP which are the major internet applications. By using TCP/IP communication, transmitting and receiving data after accessing specific server is allowed. The App shown in Figure 15 is used in the application.

Figure 15. TCP/IP Client App

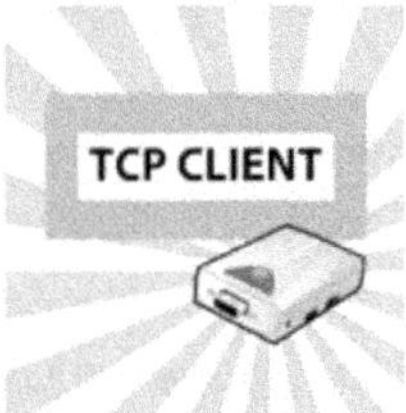

- **What Is ESP-Link?** It is a WiFi Serial Bridge which is transparent. This is useful for inputting or debugging into a microcontroller. Communication over WiFi is done by ESP-link. The ESP-link connects TCP/UDP sockets through to the attached microcontroller. It applies most of the higher-level functionality to offload the attached microcontroller because the latter has much less flash and memory than ESP-link.
- **Role of ESP-Link in Proposed System:** The ESP-link is a platform for independent applications and supports the connected temperature and humidity sensors directly to it. The WiFi is configured for the ESP-link for the network needed. After attaching the microcontroller to ESP8266 module via a serial port the program can be uploaded. All the controller details are fed into as

shown in the Figure 16. The microcontroller can use REST and MQTT which are the forthcoming functionalities requests to services. One of the online free service namely, thingspeak.com which is a sensor cloud uses the sensor values. These values get stored, then the data obtained is plotted in a graph. This can be part of the future work when the functionalities are available in the firmware. RX of ESP8266 is connected to TX of the controller and visa-versa for unit testing.

Figure 16. Configuring for ESP-link

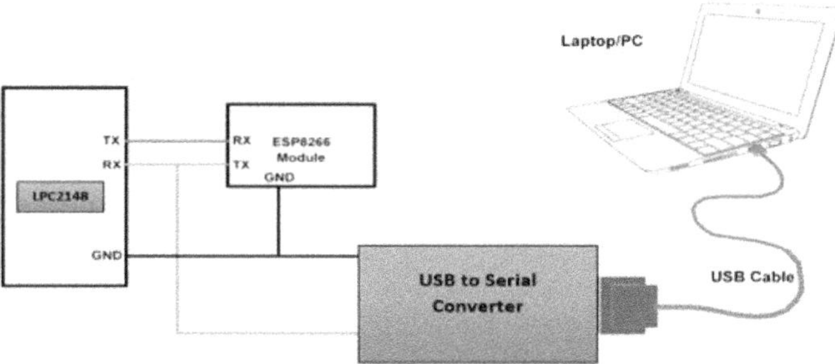

j. Other Requirements to Be Considered

- **System Maintenance and Placement During Transportation:** The proposed active system is used in a dedicated portable container of the vehicle. The nodes with the designed system in the containers are powered by on-board batteries such as the LiPo batteries which can be used to an extend of 10-12 hours per day. An external electrical power source from the vehicle can also be used to run the fans and sprinklers or if required, heaters. The microcontroller controls the activation of the cooling or heating (if required) mechanism and circulating fans and sprinklers at distributed places which help to monitor and conserve the temperature and humidity levels within specified limits around the enclosed environment.

To support the operation of those specialized vehicles, it is essential for the proper infrastructure. To have a compatible electrical connection to power the system specifically at all regular drop-off points is needed, if not using any battery supply. Particularly when the smaller vehicles are used where the system designed unit is power-driven off the vehicle engine generator. In case of battery operated connections, the batteries must be replaced after every 10-12 hours depending upon requirement. During overnight stops, these settings are critically important. In instances wherever the system is power-driven exclusively by the vehicle's engine, the engine should stay running in the slightest degree at times to avoid interruptions in maintaining correct temperature and humidity. Hence, the vehicles are equipped with an integrated continuous temperature and humidity monitoring with real-time data monitoring system. In addition, data is retrievable by logging into any PC/Laptop/Tablet/Smartphone used by the monitoring staff. The proposed system should preferably be packed to the shipped products individually to keep track of the monitoring parameters as well as the GPS location of the product or can be placed inside the truck containing all the similar products.

Flowchart of the Proposed System

Once the specification requirements are met, the system needs to be designed as proposed. The flowchart of the proposed model is as shown in Figures 17-20.

Figure 17. Flowchart of the real-time display part

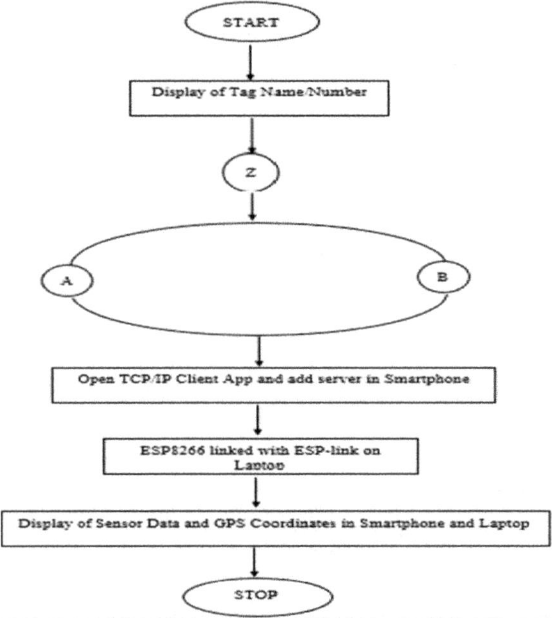

Figure 18. Flowchart of the data storage part

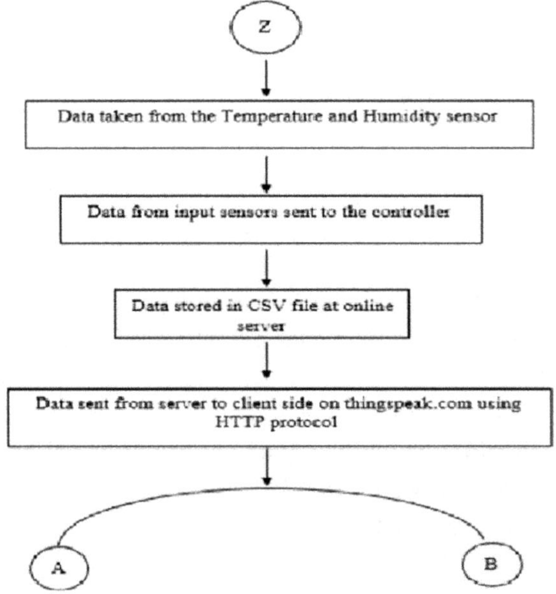

Figure 19. Flowchart of Humidity Sensor *Figure 20. Flowchart of Temperature Sensor*

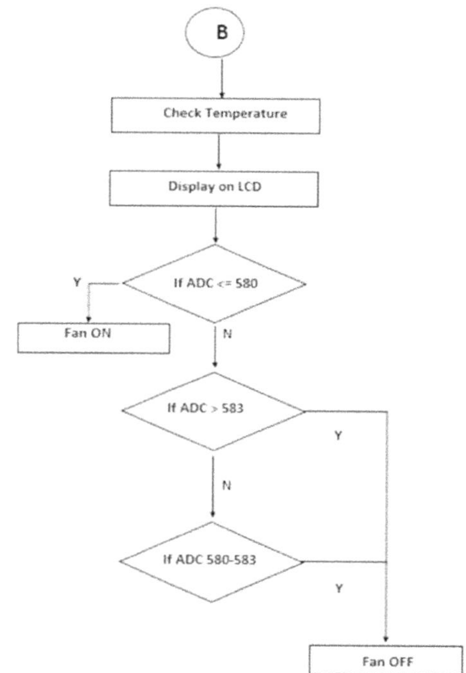

The commodity/products need to be transported are placed in the truck and the system/nodes are physically fixed at areas where the parameters can be recorded whereas the devices such as Fan and Sprinkler are also placed appropriately at necessary places. The system or node when powered by the power supply unit first displays the respective tag name or number provided to it by the manufacturer. Initialization settings are done. Temperature and Humidity sensor begin their operation by converting the ADC values obtained to respective degrees Celsius and relative humidity in percentage by using required calculations. Parallelly, the GPS module and ESP8266 sets up their platform and starts initialization. The threshold ADC values for the sensors are set accordingly beforehand depending upon the type of logistic products being transported. Here a predefined set of values have been taken for demonstration as shown in Table 6.

Table 6. Parameter values set for LM35 and HSM-20G

Parameter	Range	Value	Action Taken
Temperature	High Low Normal	ADC<=580 ADC>583 ADC 580-583	Turn ON Fan Turn OFF Fan Turn OFF Fan
Humidity	High Low Normal	ADC>848 ADC<845 ADC 845-848	Turn OFF Sprinkler Turn ON Sprinkler Turn OFF Sprinkler

According to Table 6, as per the set ADC values when the Temperature sensor (LM35) reads ADC value less than or equal to 580 the fan turns ON to set the environment to required temperature. When the temperature read is either less than 583 or between 580 and 583 the fan turns OFF by the command given by the controller. Simultaneously, when the ADC value read from the Humidity sensor (HSM-20G) is less than 845, this turns ON the Sprinkler which brings the humidity under control. When the relative humidity is either greater than or in between 845 to 848, the Sprinkler turns OFF. The ADC values of both are displayed in the 16x2 LCD. The system is designed to display the ADC values. These values can be adjusted as per the specific requirement. The ADC to degree Celsius values for temperature are done internally in the Embedded C program. Calculation of Relative Humidity (RH) formula is shown in equation (1) as shown,

Humidity (in %) = (ADC value * 100) / 1023 (1)

For example, an ADC value less than 522 (RH 51%) in a humid summer season results in significant reductions in allergen and mite levels for specific medications.

While the sensor operation is going on, the ESP8266 connection is set and GPS coordinates are calculated. The driver in the front wheel can keep track of the monitoring taking place with the help of the LCD display. With the help of the pre-installed app and preferred WiFi ESP_F086C selected in the smartphone/tablet a real-time data of the temperature and humidity values is monitored along with the action taken. The GPS coordinates is calculated, and the position is displayed on the app. Along with this facility the same can be seen on a PC by the monitoring officer, an online firmware called ESP-link which is a stand-alone application that support the connected sensors and GPS, displays the values on its console. By entering the IP address on the http bar of internet explorer/google chrome; by connecting to the ESP_F086C on a new page, the real-time data can be observed easily in the range of within few miles.

Results and Discussion

Results

Stepwise results obtained from the designed project is as follows:

Step 1: Turn on the Cold Chain Logistics System. The tag name is displayed.

Figure 21. Tag name(Title name) displayed on 16x2 LCD

Step 2: Temperature (LM35) and Humidity sensor(HSM-20G) will activate and sense the environmental conditions inside the truck respectively and the data is displayed on LCD.

Figure 22. Temperature range displayed on 16x2 LCD

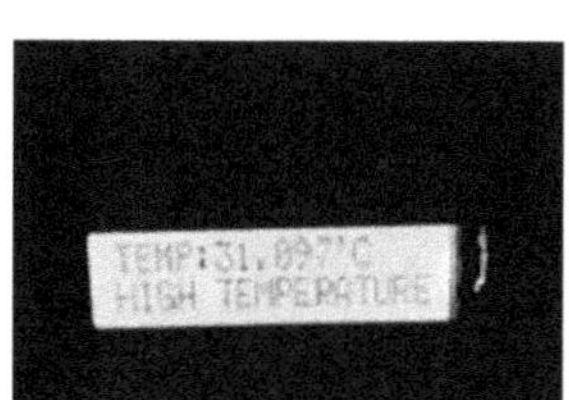

Figure 23. Humidity range displayed on 16x2 LCD

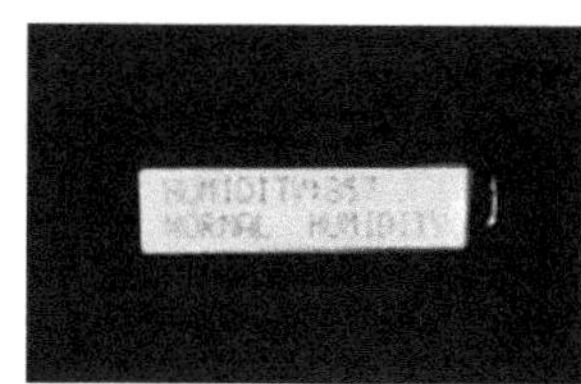

The Figures 22 and 23 show the three ranges namely Normal, High and Low Temperatures and Low, High and Normal Humidity content for the Temperature and Humidity sensors respectively which are set according to decided ADC values. As per the products/commodities placed in the cold chain truck the values can be set.

Step 3: According to the Table 6, the test values set for High Temperature is when ADC is less than or equal to 580 and for Low Humidity is when ADC is less than 845. As per the proposed system, when temperature is high, fan turns on to reduce the heat developed in the atmosphere. When there is low humidity, sprinkler (denoted by a 10mm LED) turns on to bring the condition back to normal humidity. This happens inside the container of the truck either on the move or stationary. In either condition, the changes can occur mostly due to the outside temperature and humidity imbalance. The following figures (Figure 24 and 25) shows the developed set-up.

Figure 24. System set-up with LM35 and HSM-20G

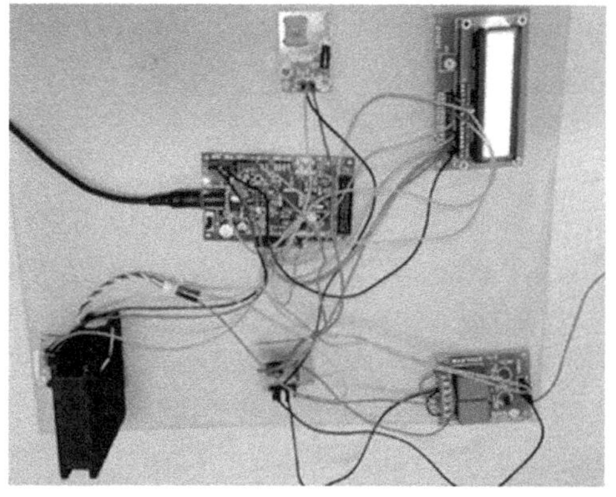

Figure 25. Complete set of proposed system model

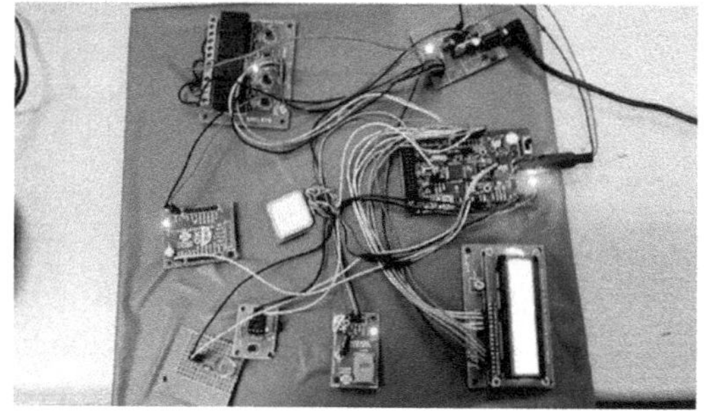

Step 4: The set-up is done, readings are displayed on LCD and respective actions are taken accordingly. While displaying on LCD, real-time data readings are obtained on the smartphone/tablet by setting up the platform as follows. TCP/IP client is downloaded free from playstore for any android smartphone.

Figure 26. TCP/IP Client App adding server and setting connection

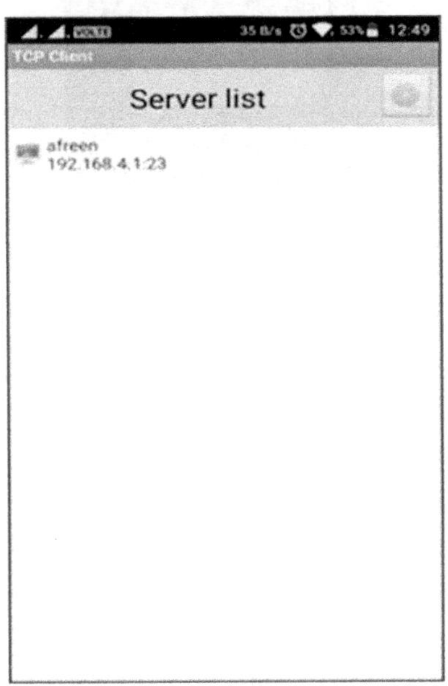

Figure 27. Real-time readings on Smartphone

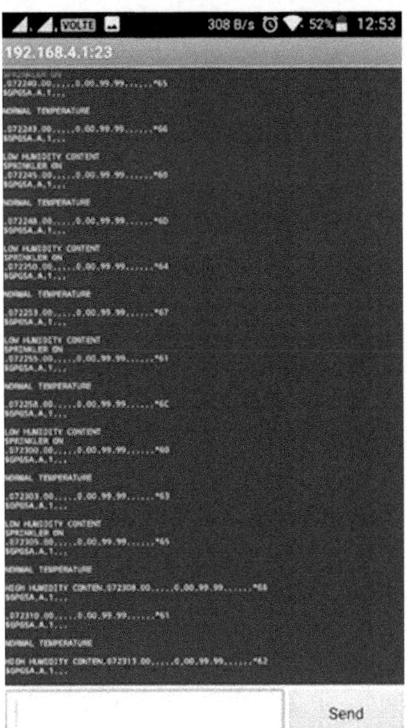

Step 5: In the PC/Laptop add and connect to ESP_F086BC connection available in the network and internet settings. For real-time data readings the IP address on PC/Laptop, the IP address of the Wireless LAN adapter Wi-Fi needs to be entered on the http bar. This will direct to the ESP-link Homepage. Click on the microcontroller console to check the real-time readings obtained. The IP address used in the proposed system is 198.168.4.2.

Figure 28 and 29 shows the home and microcontroller page console respectively in the ESP-link firmware displaying real-time values with GPS location, Sensor data and the respective action taken. This data can be obtained at the base station by the monitoring officer or can be monitored by the truck driver at the wheel.

The cold chain market in India is expected to reach INR 624 billion by the end of 2017 (Penumarthi, 2017). Cold Storage in the Indian Cold Chain Industries are the major revenue contributors. Our country's Cold Chain market is estimated to grow rapidly in the following years to come. For the cold chain infrastructure in the country to grow, private investments and favorable initiatives should be undertaken by the government on the account of rising food transportation demand.

1. **Challenges Faced:** If the solution proposed are not applied effectively this would lead to the reduction in the produce life which may affect the product nutrients to be affected.
    a. Cost involved in maintenance and monitoring. Inadequate knowledge and training of the staff in handling temperature and humidity sensitive products with the system installed is also a concerning factor.

Figure 28. Home page on ESP-link

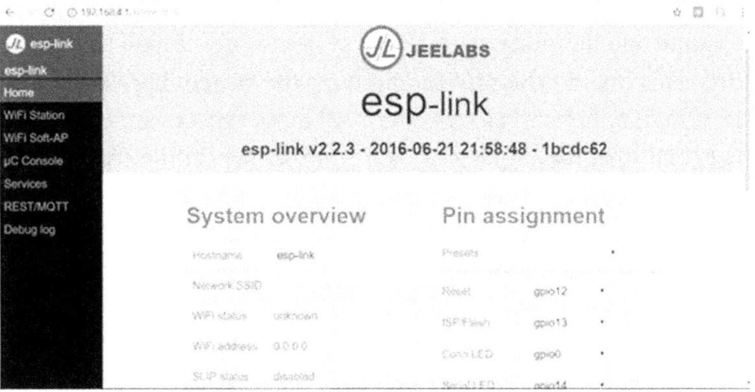

Figure 29. Microcontroller Console page on ESP-link

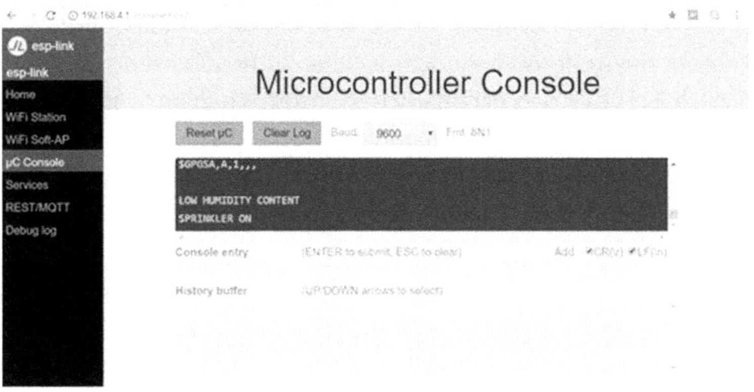

    b.   Issues with power back-ups and steady power supply is a longstanding problem pushes the capital investment requirement. Power issues with ESP8266 may come up during operation. Heating problem may also be faced.

    c.   The devices used here like the fan and sprinklers; continuous running or simultaneous ON/OFF will put a huge load on the system control.

2.   Advantages of proposed system:

    a.   Wireless operated via WIFI and be installed or made detachable system as required and light weight. Battery powered lasting up to 10-12hrs per day depending on conditions. Can be re-used as necessary.

    b.   Temperature accuracy of about one-fourth degree Celsius at room temperature and three-fourth degree Celsius over the temperature ranges between $-55°C$ to $150°C$. The temperature accuracy is from positive to negative values of degree Celsius. Humidity operating RH range is between20-95%.

    c.   Real time reports of location, temperature and humidity with respective action taken notification on display.

    d.   Maximum capacity of 100mA by the controller to run the proposed system.

SECTION 2: IoT DEVELOPMENT

This IoT based temperature and humidity monitoring system is developed using powerful development platform ARM 7 board. This board is helpful to minimize the system hardware. This system uses Temperature (LM-35) and Humidity Sensor (HNM-20G). All these sensors are interfaced with GPIO header of ARM7 board. To get real time monitoring of data from sensors ESP8266 WiFi Module is used.

In literature, there are showcased communication using either ZigBee WSN or and BLE module where both lack security and have less frequency range compared to WiFi. The microcontroller uses the REST and MQTT functionality request for services. REST (Representational State Transfer protocol) is a scalable architecture that allows things to communicate over Hyper Text Transfer Protocol and is easily adaptable for IoT applications to provide a communication from things to a central web server. Here client is a web browser and application running on the computer or system is a server. HTTP (Hyper Text Transfer Protocol) is an application protocol used for data communication for the World Wide Web. It is the protocol which is used to exchange or transfer hypertext. HTTP functions as request-response protocol in the client-server computing model. In this system LPC2148 interfaced with the ESP8266 itself act as a server. HTTP request is sent by the client to the server. Then response message is sent by the server to the client. In the response completion status of request and requested content is sent. In that web technology such as HTTP was originally designed for human to machine communication and now utilized for machine to machine communication.

It is useful to use REST calls to update or retrieve data from a ThingSpeak channel and MQTT to update data to a ThingSpeak channel. TCP/IP client app downloaded from playstore keeps real-time values of sensors posted every 100ms.

REST (Representational State Transfer protocol) is a scalable architecture that allows things to communicate over Hyper Text Transfer Protocol and is easily adaptable for IoT applications to provide a communication from things to a central web server. Interoperability between computer systems on the internet is provided by the web services like REST or RESTful. Web service is a service offered via World Wide Web by an electronic device to another electronic device, communicating with each other.

On the system developed the WiFi module operates as a data acquisition mode and as a web server mode. It collects data from Temperature and Humidity sensor. This data is then sent to the client side using HTTP protocol. On client-side real-time data can be seen from anywhere in the world on thingspeak.com. Internet connection to the board is given by using LAN through ESP8266 module. Results on thingspeak.com are shown in graphical format. On this website one channel is created and all six fields are placed in this channel. Field 1 shows temperature, Field 2 shows humidity, Realtime data of the two fields are shown in the Figures 30 and 31.

FUTURE RESEARCH DIRECTIONS

The system proposed here is Real-Time data communication received on Smartphone and PC. Data is displayed only when the device is running and not when it is switched off. By registering for a paid gateway service, data can be accessed whenever required by the monitoring officer at any part of the world. There are two on-board relays, one for Fan when encountered with high temperatures and other for Sprinklers when there is a condition of low humidity in the container. Similarly, few other sensors and devices can be added which can maintain the optimum conditions required for the commodities/

Figure 30. Real-time Temperature monitoring in graph

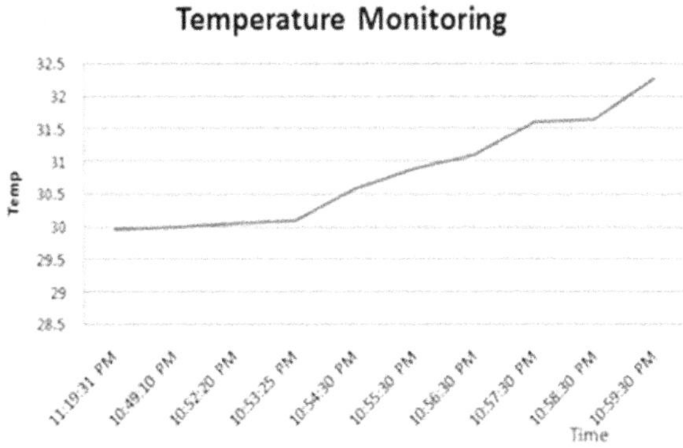

Figure 31. Real-time Humidity monitoring in graph

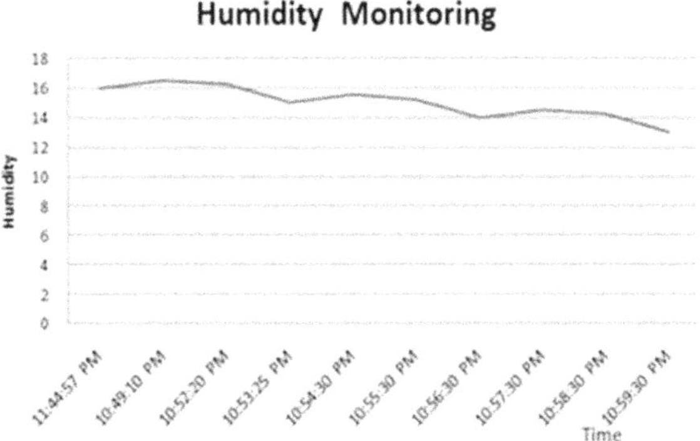

products. LEDs for indication purposes can be added such as Red LED for power on, Blue LED for breach in temperature (Fan turns on), Yellow LED for breach in humidity (Sprinkler turns on), Yellow LED for communications (On-going real-time data transfer). It can be wall mountable or placed as a tag on the commodity box in the truck.

Along with the existing features, vehicle speed/drive/idle time, fuel level efficiency and engine diagnostics can also be introduced for more precise monitoring. Alarms/buzzers can also be added for alerting the driver/officer in charge in-case of breakdown of the devices such as fan and sprinklers to receive faster and efficient service. Storage of the data can be done by external storage devices such as SD cards or EEPROMs to retrieve data log of months or years.

CONCLUSION

An Effective Cold Chain is a complete combination of three main elements which should ensure proper transport, storage and handling of the products/commodities being transported. They are namely, Trained Personal, Transport with Storage Equipment and Efficient management procedures are important to maintain cold chain logistics. The Cold Chain Logistics System within distribution centres generate wireless monitoring solution specifically for end to end cold chain protection. It is a complete cold chain standalone system whose data is monitored at distribution centres and by the driver at the wheel. It is automated temperature and humidity data collection which can run up to 10-12 hrs on battery which are replaceable. This system maintains product quality and company reputation. It reduces wastage. A greater involvement of railways and airports can also strengthen the cold chain infrastructure. There is a large scope of public partnerships in this sector. Some of the industries which use cold chain facilities are Fruits and vegetables, Floriculture, Meat and Fish products, Pharmaceutical products, Diary products, Ice cream sector and confectionaries.

REFERENCES

Akkerman, F., Farahani, P., & Grunow, M. (2010). Quality, safety and sustainability in food distribution: A review of quantitative operations management approaches and challenges. *OR-Spektrum*, *32*(4), 863–904. doi:10.100700291-010-0223-2

Akulwar, K. (2016). *5 ways Internet of Things is helping logistics industry around the globe*. DreamOrbit. Retrieved from: http://dreamorbit.com/5-ways-internet-of-things-is-helping-logistics-industry-around-the-globe/

Atzori, L., Iera, A., & Morabito, G. (2005). The Internet of Things: A survey. *Journal of Computer Networks*, *54*(15), 2787–2805. doi:10.1016/j.comnet.2010.05.010

Aung, M. M., & Chang, Y. S. (2014). Temperature Management for The Quality Assurance of a Perishable Food Supply Chain. *Journal of Food Control*, *40*, 198–207. doi:10.1016/j.foodcont.2013.11.016

Avitesh, A. (2017). A Method of WSN and Sensor Cloud System to Monitor Cold Chain Logistics as Part of The IoT Technology. *International Journal of Multimedia and Ubiquitous Engineering*, *9*(10), 145–152.

Blaisdell, R. (2018). *The risks of IoT. Rick's Cloud*. Retrieved from: https://rickscloud.com/the-risks-of-iot/

Chen, W., Wang, Y.-J., & Jan, J.-K. (2014). A novel deployment of smart cold chain system using 2G-RFID-Sys. *Journal of Food Engineering*, *141*, 113–121. doi:10.1016/j.jfoodeng.2014.05.014

Department of Atmospheric Sciences. (2010). *Relative Humidity*. University of Illinois at Urbana-Champaign. Retrieved from: http://ww2010.atmos.uiuc.edu/%28Gh%29/guides/mtr/cld/dvlp/rh.rxml

Domingo, M. C. (2012). An overview of the Internet of Things for people with disabilities. *Journal of Network and Computer Applications*, *35*(2), 584–596. doi:10.1016/j.jnca.2011.10.015

Edoh, T. (2017). Smart Medicine Transportation and Medication Monitoring System in EPharmacyNet. *2017 International Rural and Elderly Health Informatics Conference (IREHI)*, 1-9.

Fairhurst, G. (2003). *Transmission Control Protocol (TCP)*. Retrieved from: https://erg.abdn.ac.uk/users/gorry/course/inet-pages/tcp.html

Fernandez-Gago, M., Moyano, F., & Lopez, J. (2017). Modelling trust dynamics in the Internet of Things. *Information Sciences*, *396*, 72–82. doi:10.1016/j.ins.2017.02.039

Food and Drug Administration. (2018). *Hazard Analysis Critical Control Point System (HACCP)*. Food and Drug Administration. Retrieved from http://www.who.int/foodsafety/fs_management/haccp/en/

Ganguli, S. (2016). *Worldwide IoT in Logistics Market: Drivers, Opportunities, Trends, and Forecasts*. Infoholic Research LLP. Retrieved from https://www.infoholicresearch.com/worldwide-iot-in-logistics-market-to-grow-at-a-cagr-of-35-5-over-the-period-2016-2022-to-aggregate-1050-95-billion-by-2022/

Hart & Martinez. (2006). Environmental Sensor Networks: A revolution in the earth system science. *Journal of Earth-Science Reviews, 78*(3), 177–191.

How the Internet of Things impacts the logistics business. (2018). Softweb Solutions. Retrieved from: https://www.softwebiot.com/iot-use-cases/how-iot-impacts-transportation-and-logistics-industry/

Instruments, T. (2014). *Single, Dual, and Quad General Purpose, Low-Voltage, Rail-to-Rail Output Operational Amplifiers. Datasheet of LMV321/358/324*. Texas Instruments.

Islam, M., Mukhopadhyay, S. C., & Suryadevara, N. K. (2017). Smart Sensors and Internet of Things: A Postgraduate Paper. *IEEE Sensors Journal, 17*(3), 577–584. doi:10.1109/JSEN.2016.2630124

Khemapech, I. (2005). *A Survey of Wireless Sensor Networks Technology. 6th Annual Postgraduate Symposium on the Convergence of Telecommunications, Networking and Broadcasting*, Liverpool, UK.

Mali, A. R. (2016). A novel approach for temperature sensing and monitoring through wireless sensor using IoT. *Journal of Engineering and Computer Science, 5*(12), 19657–19659.

Mehta, S., Sahni, J., & Khanna, K. (2018). Internet of Things: Vision, Applications and Challenges. *Procedia Computer Science, 132*, 1263–1269. doi:10.1016/j.procs.2018.05.042

National Semiconductor. (2000). *Precision Centigrade Temperature Sensors*. National Semiconductor.

Peng, J. (2009). Comparison of several cloud computing platforms. *Information Science and Engineering (ISISE), 2009 Second International Symposium on*, 23-27. 10.1109/ISISE.2009.94

Penumarthi, H. (2017). *Indian Cold Chain Industry – Challenges and Opportunities*. Food Marketing & Technology. Retrieved from http://fmtmagazine.in/indian-cold-chain-industry-challenges-opportunities/

Pereira, A., Bergeret, E., Benzaim, O., Routin, J., Haon, O., Tournon, L., ... Depres, G. (2018). Near-field communication tag development on a paper substrate—application to cold chain monitoring. *Flexible and Printed Electronics, 3*(1), 014003. doi:10.1088/2058-8585/aaaeca

Ruiz-Garcia, L., Barreiro, P., Robla, J. I., & Lunadei, L. (2010). Testing ZigBee Motes for Monitoring Refrigerated Vegetable Transportation Under Real Conditions. *Journal of Sensors, 10*(5), 4968–4982. doi:10.3390100504968 PMID:22399917

Shih, C.-W., & Wang, C.-H. (2016). Integrating wireless sensor networks with statistical quality control to develop a cold chain system in food industries. *Computer Standards & Interfaces, 45*, 62–78. doi:10.1016/j.csi.2015.12.004

Stilmant. (2013). *Pharmaceutical Cold Chain*. Retrieved from http://www.coldchain.be/guidelines-and-regulations/some-history.html

Tennermann, J. (2012). *Cold Chain for Beginners*. Vaisala. Retrieved from https://www.rdmag.com/article/2012/06/cold-chain-beginners

Tools.ietf.org. (2018). *TCP Usage Guidance in the Internet of Things (IoT)*. Retrieved from: https://tools.ietf.org/id/draft-ietf-lwig-tcp-constrained-node-networks-01.html

Verma, R., & Srivastava, K. (2017). Middleware, Operating System and Wireless Sensor Networks for Internet of Things. *International Journal of Computers and Applications*, *167*(11), 11–17. doi:10.5120/ijca2017914356

World Health Organization. (2010). *WHO guide to good storage practices for pharmaceuticals. WHO Expert Committee on Specific cations for Pharmaceutical Preparations (WHO Technical Report Series, No. 920)*. World Health Organization.

Wu, M. M. (2015). The Design and Implementation of Food Cold Chain Monitoring System Based on ZigBee. *Journal of Applied Mechanics and Materials*, *751*, 281–286. doi:10.4028/www.scientific.net/AMM.751.281

ADDITIONAL READING

Dong, H. (2009). China's agricultural products Cold-chain logistics status, Problems and Solutions. *Journal of Ecological Economy*, *10*, 255–257.

Lei, Y., Cheng, L., Zhang, Z., Guosheng, L., & Jun, L. (2009). livestock product supply chain safety control studies based on RFID traceability system. *Zhongguo Xumu Zazhi*.

Liu, L., & Li, J. (2008). Summary of Development Pattern and Government Behavior of Cold Chain Logistics of Agricultural Products. *Journal of Food Science*, *29*(9), 680–683.

Singh, A., & Singh, G. (2016). Review on Temperature & Humidity Sensing using IoT. *International Journal of Advanced Research in Computer Science and Software Engineering*, *6*(2).

KEY TERMS AND DEFINITIONS

AVR: Is a family of microcontrollers developed by Atmel beginning in 1996.

GPS: The global positioning system enables to locate the latitude and longitude coordinates of the location.

HACCP: Is a management system in which food safety is addressed through the analysis and control of biological, chemical, and physical hazards from raw material production, procurement and handling, to manufacturing, distribution, and consumption of the finished product.

HTTP: The hypertext transfer protocol (HTTP) is an application protocol for distributed, collaborative, and hypermedia information systems. HTTP is the foundation of data communication for the world wide web.

IDE: An integrated development environment is a software application that provides comprehensive facilities to computer programmers for software development.

TCP/IP: The transmission control protocol/internet protocol is a suite of communication protocols used to interconnect network devices on the internet.

ZigBee: Is newly developed technology that works on IEEE standard 802.15.4, which can be used in the wireless sensor network (WSN).

This research was previously published in Predictive Intelligence Using Big Data and the Internet of Things edited by P.K. Gupta, Tuncer Ören, and Mayank Singh; pages 144-179, copyright year 2019 by Engineering Science Reference (an imprint of IGI Global).

Chapter 18

An Exploratory Study on Blockchain Application in a Food Processing Supply Chain to Reduce Waste

Emily Anne Carey
Samsung Electronics, UK

Nachiappan Subramanian
Independent Researcher, UK

ABSTRACT

This chapter aims to explore the feasibility of using blockchain in the beef supply chain to reduce waste. A mono-method, qualitative, inductive, single case study approach was taken on a cross-sectional scale from June 2018 to August 2018, with two individuals interviewed: a beef and a blockchain expert. The case study also involved observations, a field visit, and other secondary source data. Beef is a high demand, valuable food product with a limited shelf life. By using blockchain in conjunction with RFID and sensor technologies, farming and processing stages in the beef supply chain can be streamlined. Firstly, using the technology to monitor the animals on the farm and during transportation can reduce the amount of water and energy wasted. Secondly, blockchain can be used to establish exactly when and where the meat is cut and packaged, improving the accuracy of information between supply chain entities, resulting in improved inventory management, specifically more accurate delivery times and lengthened product shelf lives.

INTRODUCTION

Beef Supply Chain and Waste

The British meat market consists of poultry, beef, pork, lamb and others. Beef is a high value, high demand food product, with global popularity and its supply chain is complex. Cattle are raised on beef

DOI: 10.4018/978-1-7998-5354-1.ch018

farms from 3 months to 30 months dependent on breed and market demand. When they reach the required age, they are sent to the abattoir and processor, where they are butchered, boned, and processed into different beef products, such as mince, steak, burger, joint, stir fry, etc. then the processed products are packaged and labelled (Mishra & Singh, 2016). There is a preferential bias in developed countries like the UK towards the more expensive cuts of beef such as the hindquarters, for example sirloin and rump steaks (Traill, 1997). This carcass imbalance causes an oversupply of the lower-value forequarter cuts, which is a problem for beef processors. This issue is especially prominent because of the foodservice industry, where high-value cuts of meat are a common menu component. Food suppliers tend to over-produce to be able to cope with demand at short-notice, to avoid the possibility of being delisted from large retailers (Parfitt et al., 2010).

WRAP (2007) estimates that each household throws away edible food worth £4.80 to £7.70 each week, which adds up to £15,000 to £24,000 in a lifetime. Whilst the UK Food Standards Agency has published a figure, estimating that food fraud, such as the Salmonella Peanut Butter Outbreak in 2009 and the Horsemeat Scandal of 2013, costs families £1.17 billion a year (National Food Crime Unit, 2017). Moreover, food waste that is sent to landfill that produces methane and carbon dioxide in its decomposition, which contributes to global warming. Also contributing to the negative environmental impact of food waste, are natural resource depletion and embedded carbon from previous life cycles of food before it becomes waste. There is also the ethical note in terms of food waste, which is the lack of balance between food waste and food poverty. The World Health Organisation (WHO) estimates 420,000 people die and a tenth of people fall ill each year after eating contaminated food (National Food Crime Unit, 2017). The two most advantageous options for food waste reductions according to Papargyropoulou et al., (2014) are food surplus prevention and reduction of avoidable food waste, as waste is largely from by-products and unsold prepared food products.

Blockchain Technology

Blockchain is a decentralised, distributed ledger and a single database where every member with access has an identical copy, allowing every database entry to be shared. Continual crosschecking also ensures the integrity of existing entries. One party does not own it and records made in the database are perma-nent and unalterable (Abeyratne & Monfared, 2016).

Blockchain technology is known to improve visibility, productivity and security for businesses. A blockchain ledger acts as a single location where all members of the business supply chain record their actions. It simplifies record keeping, it is updated in real-time and it is readily accessible by all parties with permission. As a distributed ledger, blockchain allows many kinds of business transactions to be decentralised, preventing any one party from exclusively owning all the information within the supply chain. This enables reductions in cost and complexity, facilitates faster transactions and disintermediates the supply chain. Businesses carry legal liability for their services and products and are therefore, with blockchain, more interdependent than ever before (Johnson, 2018).

Blockchain is already popular in financial business, but only since 2016 has blockchain had the abil-ity to work in a supply chain function. The technology is increasing in popularity and IBM currently has 400 companies trailing their blockchain service including Unilever, Nestlé, Tyson Foods and on the largest scale, Walmart (Supply Management, 2017a). However, doubts about the operational feasibility of blockchain have been highlighted in Supply Management (2017b) such as blockchain is decentralised and there is uncertainty about who will pay for it.

Potential to Reduce Supply Chain Waste Using Blockchain Technology

Blockchain can record every interaction a product has from the farm to the shop with cryptography, making the supply chain fully transparent (Creasy, 2017). Faulty products can individually be identified using blockchain and removed from the shelves without the need for large-scale costly recalls (Steiner et al., 2015). In addition, consumers receive transparency and security with the knowledge that they know exactly what they are buying and where it came from, improving customer loyalty. Food safety and food quality consumer information asymmetry has been a problem for years. Traceability can ultimately be cost saving, reduce risk and strengthen liability incentives for food safety (Hobbs, 2003).

Common problems that cause waste in food supply chains include: food fraud, illegal production, foodborne illness and food recalls. Blockchain technology can be used to resolve these problems by providing transparency, efficiency and food safety. Brigid McDermott, the Vice President of blockchain business development at IBM shares how currently, identifying the precise point of contamination that has caused a food scare and it can take weeks without blockchain (Creasy, 2017). Blockchain implementation to a food supply chain digitises tracking and storage of all information at every stage of the supply chain, avoiding food fraud and increasing consumer confidence. Blockchain technology improves how food is tracked, transported and sold, eliminating inaccuracies caused by paper tracking and manual inspections. Retailers can better manage shelf life and distribution processes can be streamlined, improving competition between online retailers like Amazon. Additionally, costs can be cut and food waste and foodborne illness can be reduced if few batches of contaminated food product can be recalled as opposed to recalling the entire supply of food product from every retailer (Koonce, 2017).

Academic Rationale

The food supply chain comprises of countless players that are functionally and geographically diverse, with many of these entities largely unaware of each other. The fragmented structure of current food supply chains inhibits the flow of information up and down the supply chain. These long-standing structural issues in food supply chains pose challenges that lend themselves to blockchain-based supply chain solutions. Despite the obstacles of implementing blockchain, supply chains in the food industry represent one of the most important applications of the technology. Given the potential benefits and promise offered by blockchain-based applications, the question is not whether it will be implemented, but when (Material Handling and Logistics (MHL News), 2017). However, this statement is very presumptuous that blockchain will be successful and widespread. Therefore, it is important that the feasibility of blockchain application is properly assessed.

Creasy (2017), looks at the potential for blockchain in the food industry. As well as preventing food counterfeit and fraud, blockchain can play an important role in quickly addressing food scares and emergency product recalls. It has been found by IBM, that as customers are becoming more digital, they are expecting more information about the origin and journey that their product took to get to the retailer, and blockchain can certify this information. Consumers would be able to receive the entire desired product and supply chain information by scanning an icon (such as a QR code) on the product, enabling packaging space to be freed.

There is a gap in the literature involving the reduction of waste in beef supply chains and also little research about reducing waste using blockchain. The major contributions to the research area that this study will provide, will be a full assessment into the feasibility of using blockchain technology in a beef supply chain and in addition, if blockchain can be used to reduce waste in a beef supply chain.

The primary research question in this study is "can the application of blockchain reduce waste in a beef supply chain" and the following questions will support the investigation, "what kind of waste occurs in a beef supply chain" and "can blockchain technology be applied to beef supply chains". To achieve answers to these questions, the following research objectives are to be investigated; "identify all waste in a beef supply chain" and "identify how blockchain be applied to a beef supply chain".

LITERATURE REVIEW

Beef Supply Chain Waste

A definition found in a review by Parfitt et al., (2010) defines waste in the food supply chain as "wholesome edible material intended for human consumption, arising at any point in the food supply chain that is instead discarded, lost, degraded or consumed by pests". Food loss occurs at the production, post-harvest and processing stages of a food supply chain and refers to the loss of edible food mass throughout the part of the supply chain that leads to edible food, excluding feed and parts of the supply chain not for human consumption. Food waste occurs at the retail and consumption end of the food supply chain and relates to the retailer and customer behaviour (FAO, 2011). For the duration of this study, I will be referring to the food losses and food waste along a food supply chain as the collective term 'food waste'.

Results from interviews conducted by Mena et al., (2011) showed that based on actual waste records, more than 7% of beef products are wasted by consumers. One reason for this relatively high level of waste is due to the short shelf life of the beef products. The tight selling deadline gives beef supply chains little room to manoeuvre, in order to maximise the product use by date for customers. Another cause of consumer waste of beef products is volatile demand related to the weather.

Improving beef product characteristics is important in order to meet consumers' demand for specific attributes, such as fat content, colour, flavour and texture. Different attributes are important to different consumers; colour, leanness, type of cut, price, sell-by-date, country of origin, production methods used (i.e. halal, kosher), and farm of origin (Fearne et al., 2001).

Garrone et al., (2014) reveals that livestock farming involves overproduction at the farming stage as the main source of surplus food waste. However, livestock farming has a low degree of recoverability regarding surplus product, as the products are unable to be consumed immediately. In addition to high management intensity, as products are perishable and require refrigeration during storage and transportation.

FAO (2011) identifies five system boundaries to distinguish different types of food waste for beef, as seen in Table 1.

According to Mishra and Singh (2016) and the maximum amount of waste has shown to be produced at the consumer end of the supply chain. Consumers expect their beef products to be a fresh red colour, of the correct fat content, tender when cooked, not to have a bad smell and not to contain any foreign bodies. Some reasons for the generation of waste include discolouration before expiry date, lack of tenderness, the presence of extra fat and inefficient trimming procedures in the boning hall of the abattoir. Additionally, the oxidation of beef, the presence of foreign bodies in beef product and inefficient cold chain management can generate waste.

Table 1. End-to-end food waste or loss

Type of Food Waste/Loss	Beef Supply Chain Case
Agricultural production	Food losses refer to animal death during breeding
Post-harvest handling and storage	Losses refer to death during transport to slaughter and condemnation at slaughterhouse
Processing	Losses refer to trimming spillage during slaughtering and additional industrial processing
Distribution	Losses and waste in the market system, for example, at wholesalers or supermarkets
Consumption	Losses and waste at the household level

Source: FAO, 2011

According to 'Improving efficiency, generating better returns & tackling environmental impacts in beef supply chains' (2017), if beef carcases are too fat, yields and returns are adversely affected, and it is estimated that beef carcases that are out of the specification range cost British farmers £12.5 million per year. The beef industry is known for its lack of integration, and improvements to quality standards and cost savings could be made by better communications between retailers and producers, as a result of the two supply chain ends working more closely together 'Improving efficiency, generating better returns & tackling environmental impacts in beef supply chains' (2017).

To improve residual material waste, to benefit both the environment and finances, material edible by humans must be maximised and residual materials that are not fit for human consumption must be minimised. The material waste not fit for human consumption is split into two categories; category one, which includes cattle that are dead on arrival to the slaughterhouse, post-mortem failures, and soiled or medicine-contaminated materials. The second category, category one includes high risk waste material, and material unsuitable for human or animal consumption. Methods to reduce residual material waste include providing sufficient bins in the slaughterhouse to enable better segregation of the different categories of material, exploring alternative waste outlets or engaging with producers to reduce avoidable carcase rejections (Improving efficiency, generating better returns & tackling environmental impacts in beef supply chains, 2017).

Blockchain Application

Blockchain gained prominence in 2009, but researchers and practitioners are still at the beginning of trying to fully understand its potential, especially the technical challenges and limitations of the technology (Fridgen et al., 2017). According to DecisionNext (2018), every stage of the value chain in a food supply chain estimates demand. Information distances could be shortened and visibility increased between different stages of the supply chain by applying blockchain. In addition, streamlining supply chains and increasing accurate information sharing can reduce food waste.

According to Authenticate (2018), some challenges associated with the application of blockchain to a food supply chain include sourcing data, data duplication, reasonable transparency and the implications of the majority of food being disassembled rather than assembled. In regards to data sourcing, additional data capture is viewed as a burden by most food producers, as they see no immediate benefit. Existing ERP systems may not support blockchain entries and making separate entries can cause additional costs as well as receiving little support. Commercially, extra transparency may not be desirable and the right balance must be created between traceability and transparency and protecting individual businesses.

Furthermore, the common disassembly of food products means that it becomes harder to trace a product after it has been processed. Therefore, in the meantime, single animal commodities are likely to be the products taken on by blockchain strategies first (Authenticate, 2018).

Blockchain provides an enormous task for management, as tools must be developed to manage the vast quantity of devices and extra data that this technology brings (Haddud et al., 2017). Tian (2016), looks at how blockchain can be combined with RFID and used in a traceability system in an agri-food supply chain. There are benefits of this in tracking and traceability management, enhancing the credibility of food safety information and fighting against food fraud. Some disadvantages mentioned in this study include the high cost of RFID and the current immaturity of blockchain. In addition, a study by Saberi et al., (2018) listed four potential barriers for block chain implementation and they are intra and inter organisational, technical and external barriers.

Moreover, research shows that in order for blockchain to be implemented effectively across the supply chain, IT infrastructures must be in place from end-to-end. Digital profiles must be updated at every stage of the supply chain using technology such as RFID. Blockchain-run 'smart contracts' should also be integrated into the system to improve the security of transactions and give the ability to monitor the progress of a business process (Abeyratne & Monfared, 2016).

Pilot Trials

The food industry is one of the next big targets for blockchain technology. With multiple pilot tests happening in big retailers, and food contamination and fraud outbreaks in the news, it is a good time for blockchain technology to make an impact in the food industry (Food Logistics, 2017).

Last year Walmart, IBM and Tsinghua University piloted blockchain technology in tracing a pork supply chain in China and mango sourcing in the US. The pilot investigated whether blockchain could be a viable alternative to paper tracking and manual inspections. Data such as farm details, batch numbers, factory data, processing data, shipping data and expiry dates were added to the blockchain supply chain data collection and matched to each product. Certificates and testing and auditing documentation were also added to the blockchain. The results from the pilot tests were positive, with a mango being traced within two seconds, compared to the multiple days it would have taken with the previous method. Walmart said using blockchain in this way could improve supply chain efficiency, promote sustainability and reduce food waste. There were some concerns during the pilot about information sharing but the trail ultimately led to the formation of the Blockchain Food Safety Alliance, comprising of IBM, JD.com, Walmart and Tsinghua University. The alliance has a goal to improve food tracking, traceability and safety in China. In addition, the alliance has created a standards-based method of collecting data about food safety, origin and authenticity, using blockchain technology (Supply Management, 2018).

In a pilot trial, JD.com rolled out a blockchain platform for Chinese customers to track their beef orders from overseas (specifically Australia). The customers were able to see where their beef product has been, how it was transported and how the cow was raised. China currently has 292.5 billion active users of blockchain, and the Chinese middle class place an importance of knowing where their beef has come from (Medium, 2018). The high levels of transparency in this beef supply chain and success from the project will surely encourage others in the Chinese market and even around the world to follow suit. The Chinese beef market is especially important to the UK because China has lifted the ban on exports of British beef, with estimates of £250 million to be made from the market in the next five years (GOV. UK, 2018).

To demonstrate the importance of food waste reduction in the UK, in July 2018 the FSA (Food Standards Agency) trialled the first use of blockchain as a regulatory tool to ensure compliance in the food industry. Blockchain technology was used in a cattle slaughterhouse during the pilot, due to the amount of inspections and collation of results that take place in a slaughterhouse. Further blockchain pilots have been planned with cattle and subject to the pilot successes and industry backing, blockchain technology will become a permanent fixture in the food industry (Food Standards Agency, 2018).

Ripe.io is a leading start-up that uses blockchain technology and the Internet of Things to enable data transparency from farm to fork, focussing on agriculture (Ripe.io, 2018). A podcast interview with Raja Ramachandran, the CEO of Ripe.io, revealed that one of the reasons for starting the company was finding out that food spoilage is a \$250 billion problem globally and 25% of our water goes to spoiled food. As well as finding out that the top 50 food suppliers make up less than 20% of all sales. Ripe.io want to enable consumers and businesses to improve upon this \$4 trillion industry (Wolf, 2017).

In another interview, Raja Ramachandran gives his perspective on blockchain as a method to reduce waste in a food supply chain. He said food waste from the USA is mainly from consumer waste, at the farm level and a little bit from transportation. Contributing factors to the waste include temperature control, bacteria formation, and produce that is discoloured or misshapen. He does not believe that blockchain will be able to solve the problem of food waste and says consumer waste will be the hardest to reduce. Blockchain gives analytics and the ability to identify how to improve systems in order to reduce waste. Therefore, the first solution to waste reduction could be to use blockchain analytics to investigate problems such as temperature mismanagement, or to monitor water usage. Secondly, market spaces should be created to specifically sell 'non-perfect' food products that are still safe and edible. Thirdly, involving scientific invasive technologies in the blockchain can reduce the bacteria formation problem. Finally, improving the time taken to trace the food products will also allow for better detection of food waste problems. However, if these identified problems are isolated, there will only be a partial solution, the problems must be solved altogether. A system of records shared by the industry will be required, and this is where blockchain can provide the level of visibility required and a full longitudinal look at the supply chain (Hammerich, 2018). In addition, blockchain's development is constant and does not fit into a single artefact and specifically further researchers need to investigate the type of blockchain fit for particular food supply chain (Treiblmaier, 2018).

From this literature review it can be seen that there are few studies about waste reduction in the supply chain and specifically in a beef supply chain. There are also few studies that relate blockchain technology to reduction of waste in food supply chains and no studies relating reduction of waste to blockchain technology in a beef supply chain. Therefore, this study paper will attempt to assess the feasibility of waste reduction in a beef supply chain as a result of the application of blockchain. This will be done by explaining what waste is found in a beef supply chain, how blockchain technology can be applied, and then a link between blockchain application and waste reduction in a beef supply chain will be explored.

METHODOLOGY

Philosophy and Approach

This research will be carried out using a qualitative design. The research philosophy associated with a qualitative research design is interpretivism, using a subjective ontological approach. The interpretivist approach is taken so that the researcher can investigate the subjective and socially constructed meanings around the research area (Saunders, Lewis, & Thornhill, 2012). The approach to conducting this research project will be induction; looking at numerous specific events leading to general conclusions or relationships. This approach is best used for the exploratory nature of the research questions as the research topic is immature, and also to produce a richer theoretical perspective in the literature (Saunders, Lewis, & Thornhill, 2012).

Methodological Choice, Strategy and Time Period

This research will be carried out as a mono-method qualitative investigation. The mono-method methodological choice uses a single data collection technique and a qualitative research design (Saunders, Lewis, & Thornhill, 2012). The mono-method approach was chosen due to the nascent nature of the research topic and the lack of current research on the topic. Focussing on a mono-method will easily allow for conclusions to be drawn in a clear and concise manner, on a topic that can sometimes be perceived as complex. Multiple-methods are not required for this particular investigation and along with mixed-methods, would be difficult to adopt given the time and resource constraints.

In the literature, a case study approach was implemented for a study about blockchain integration in the supply chain (Korpela et al., 2017). Case studies can provide multiple perspectives of a situation in a specific context (Järvensivu & Törnroos, 2010) and in this case, different perspectives on the ability of blockchain to reduce waste in beef supply chains. A case study approach is often adopted in exploratory research therefore the research strategy for this study will be based on the use of a singular case study.

The unit of analysis for the case studies will be a supply chain professional from the beef supply chain for a firm-level perspective, and also a professional with expertise in blockchain in food supply chains. Interviewing a beef industry professional will provide evidence to address the research objective to identify all waste in a beef supply chain. Whereas interviewing a blockchain expert will address the research objective about identifying how blockchain can be applied to a beef supply chain, from a supply chain and technology perspective. Yin (2013) emphasize the importance of case study context with the distinctiveness between the context and the phenomenon. A single case study design can be justified due to the nascent technology and new phenomenon of the research topic.

In terms of a time horizon, investigations into the research questions and primary data collection was conducted on a cross-sectional scale, between June 2018 and August 2018. This timescale is more suited to the research question than a longitudinal study, due to the fast-pace of technological development and business implementation processes (Saunders, Lewis, & Thornhill, 2012).

Data Sample

In order to fully understand beef supply chain waste and also properly assess the feasibility of blockchain application, it was necessary to interview more than one partner from different areas of a beef supply chain. A butcher was approached as this individual produced, processed and sold the beef themselves, so could give a deep insight into the beef supply chain on a local level. An employee from blockchain technological company was approached as this individual could give a high level insight into the beef supply chain from a business and large-scale perspective, as well as insight into blockchain application.

Qualitative Procedure

Within an exploratory, qualitative single case study research design, interviews will be the primary mode of data collection. Non-standardised, in-depth individual unstructured interviews will take place, either in person, or on the phone with an inductive approach. The interviews for a qualitative study must be flexible, the questions must be open and an interview guide should not be too structured (Bryman & Bell, 2011).

The informant interviews will be audio-recorded where permission is given, and then transcribed. NVIVO software will not be used in this study as only two interviews will be conducted and the creation of codes and themes will not be necessary for the ability to analyse the data thoroughly. NVIVO data analysis can also fragment and decontextualize the data, therefore it is of the judgement of the researcher to instead transcribe and analyse data directly from the interviews (Bryman & Bell, 2011).

Several measures must be overcome to prevent researcher and interviewee bias in the in-depth interviews. For example, careful consideration of initial question and approach to questioning, appropriateness of time, place and appearance at the interview, the impact of researcher's general behaviour in the interview and ability of researcher to accurately record data (Saunders, Lewis, & Thornhill, 2012).

The individual interviews will be taken from two candidates, firstly, a supply chain professional from the beginning of the beef supply chain, who is a farmer and butcher. The second interview will be conducted with the president and founder of technological company that provides blockchain solutions to food supply chains. It is important to select candidates for interviews from each of the food and technology sectors in order to determine what wastes are found in the beef supply chain, and also if blockchain technology has the potential to be applied to a beef supply chain.

The delphi technique was implemented in some of the literature. This group communication method was used to allow groups of individuals to tackle the complex problem of blockchain integration in supply chain (Korpela et al., 2017). Triangulation was also used in various studies to increase validity and reliability. However, this study investigates using a mono-method technique. Perhaps if interview data is requiring further validation, triangulation using multiple sources of evidence could then be used as a follow-up post-interview.

Data Quality Checks

Interviewing a supply chain professional from the beef supply chain and also interviewing a blockchain professional with an expertise in food supply chains will benefit the study by providing a more balanced argument, with the benefits, negatives and details of potential blockchain solutions and beef supply chain waste. Inevitably, there may be limitations around the level of detail that interviewees are able to or want to share, in regards to their company's supply chain strategies. Due to the popular nature of blockchain research at the current time, many potential interviewees were unable to provide the time for even a short interview. Therefore, in the given timeframe, it was not possible to interview any further professionals from different areas of the beef supply chain.

Constraints experienced during the study may be around company accessibility - there may be no response to the request for an interview. A minor constraint in data acquisition would be if permission were not to be given to audio-record the interviews. This would impact the validity of responses, as physical note taking would have to occur instead. Therefore, to prevent the data becoming inaccurate and to ensure reliability in the data, interview transcripts will be sent back to the interviewees, to check the accuracy of their responses.

To further increase reliability of the data, variables in the interview guides will be clearly laid out to prevent researcher or participant bias. Also, the researcher will try to be objective during the interview, which will increase the reliability of the data. In addition, ethical approval was granted before approaching the individuals for an interview. A consent form was created, and a sample information sheet and interview guide were also sent off and granted approval by the Business School.

FINDINGS

Beef Supply Chain Perspective

The first interview involved interviewing the CEO of Butcher and Grazier in the UK. The firm owns their own farm, where they rear the cattle (and other animals) and then they process and sell the meat. They supply meat at the butcher shop and also to select retailers and restaurants across the county.

Regarding issues around carcass yields or excess fat, CEO does not buy cattle that are too fat and there are strict specifications to which he abides by. Residual material use is low and this is their biggest source of waste. Waste due to appearance standards is only an occasional problem and animal loss on the farm happens only rarely. Other issues regarding the meat quality was a subject that was brushed over, as case farm, processes and sells the meat directly, so the person is in control and sure of the meat quality. There's also low mileage and a fast processing speed as the person's farm is local, therefore waste during transportation is not a significant problem.

Residual material refers to the bones and trimmings amongst other bits, which are discarded when the meat is processed and turned into the final product. These discarded materials are thrown out constantly in the business but are rendered down. Residual material cannot be helped though, so perhaps an alternative disposal method is required, but EU law is selective about the disposal methods used for raw meat. Appearance standards refer to discolouration in this case. Often when the meat does not turn out the way it should, such as discolouration or bruising, it is due to circumstances that are not observed, such as knocks to the cattle or carcasses. However, these are few and far between.

CEO supplies to select retailers and local restaurants as well as selling in his own butcher shop. The products to the retailers are sold in packaging with dates and the meat he sells in his butcher shop aren't packaged or dated in this way. However, CEO says that the packaging and labelling is the only difference between the meat he sells and the meat he supplies retailers and that the meat is cut the exact same way. He says that customers from his butcher shop either buy meat to eat on the same day or else they buy in bulk and freeze it, and he verbally advises his customers over the use by date.

Regarding traceability, each cattle carries an ear tag and is also assigned a 'passport', in which the numbers in these are used to identify the animal and relate to its ancestral history. Asked if he thinks the current systems are good enough for traceability, CEO replies rather defensively that he does not see why there would be a problem with the current system and that there is not a problem on his behalf.

The butcher was reluctant to be interviewed for very long. He was reluctant and dismissal at the idea of change, not seeing any problem with the current systems and processes. He was unsure and slightly defensive when it came to asking about waste. He did not seem to know much or was not willing to share information about the different technology currently used or for potential use, nor have any figures to hand.

Table 2. Firm level issues

Waste Type	Causes
Residual materials at the processing stage	The bones and trimmings amongst other bits, which are discarded when the meat is processed and turned into the final product. These discarded materials are thrown out constantly, but this cannot be helped.
Beef products below appearance standards	Discolouration can be caused by knocks to the animals or carcasses. Often the cause of the discolouration is unknown.
Animal loss before slaughter	Not specified.
Damage to beef products during transportation	Poor temperature control during transportation, meat can travel long distances along the supply chain.

Technology Perspective

The second interview was with the president and founder of an emerging technological company, a company specialising in blockchain for food supply chains. The interview began with the founder saying that meat supply chains, including beef, are highly inefficient. He said that the beef supply chain could be improved at the beginning, middle and end of the supply chain, and proceeded to explain his thoughts.

Waste at the end of the supply chain is simply about the ability of consumer facing entities to better manage their inventories. The link between the producer, distributor and consumer facing entity is that they all have their data in silos. There is not a lot of information that comes from the slaughterhouse, into the processor, all the way through. Shelf life and sell by dates are "a load of rubbish", they do not really mean anything. If the retailers have more insight into the timestamps of the processing in the slaughterhouses, then they have more data that can time the delivery, in terms of inventory to the grocery store or other consumer facing entity. For example, more data can enable more accurate deliveries, which can prevent late food deliveries due to a poorly connected supply chain. It is about having more data available, which then gives an easier decision as to when the shelf life runs out. These statements are contrary to Beef supply chain (Interview One), who was adamant that there was no waste in the process. However, founder of technological company was speaking on a higher macro level than CEO of beef supply chain and founder of technological company has experience of a lot of different beef supply chains, rather than CEO, who only has experience of his own small-scale beef supply chain.

Data in terms of ownership of the consumer-facing brand, like supermarkets, is shared on a really sensitive basis. Data from the distributor, the farm, and the slaughterhouse does not always get into the hands of the supermarkets or grocery store in time, it might be two or three days late. By collapsing the data, as it is available in relatively real time, the supply chain should see improved inventory management and a better sense of shelf life and waste at the end point.

At the beginning of the supply chain, waste can be measured in terms of how water is used, how energy is used, how feed is used, and how the animals are kept healthy. When we look at waste, it is not just a piece of meat that comes from a cow; it is also all of the periphery things around the creation of that piece of meat that can also be reduced. So, by tagging individual cows, which can be done through RFID tags or other technology, we are now able to make sure that the animals can stay healthy, because there is a better way to make sure that they are kept well and healthy. Making sure that they are up to date with all of their vaccinations, the medical records are kept up to date and they are receiving the correct quantity of feed does this. Hence, a lot of those processes can be streamlined to reduce the amount of water consumption that is also going in. Waste is not just about food that is thrown away from the supermarket shelf, we define waste also basically around sustainability. All of those dimensions that go into raising and growing an animal can be improved and waste can be reduced in the cattle.

In the middle of the supply chain, at the processor and slaughterhouse, there is a void of data. This information is very relevant to understand the real shelf life of a piece of meat. The inventory does not work as it should for an animal that is slaughtered on a Tuesday and shipped out on a Thursday. There is a lot of waste where bits of meat are being thrown off the shelf because they are past their sell by date, when in fact they technically have two more days of shelf life than what is stated on the label. It is important, in order to reduce this waste, to establish exactly when the meat gets cut and packaged, to enable a more accurate and probably longer shelf life. What blockchain can do is to bring all of these data sets together and share more information along the supply chain, which is very difficult to do in a traditional silo of data.

When asked about how accepting he thinks different members of the supply chain will be, Founder responded that technology companies are working on this problem on a global basis. The company has projects in pork, beef, chicken, dairy, fruits, vegetables, all over the world and in many different categories. The right condition for his company to work is where there is a willing collaboration of supply chain partners to achieve something. The company ask the supply chain partners what it is they want to achieve, whether it is ensuring the quality of the meat, exposing to the consumer that the product is grown sustainably, or is it organic. It is currently very hard to quantify and get evidence for these statements, especially 'local'. The people that the company work with all have a common goal that they want to achieve, either exposing quality, traceability, or authenticity, etc.

Technology company have seen great traction from the innovators, but there is going to be older, more traditional food companies that are going to resist this transformation, as is human nature. However, seeing their market share drop, no more questions will be asked and they will have to make the change. For example, if you look at all of the companies that did not get on the e-commerce bandwagon and continued selling different services with just brick and mortar, brands that have been wiped off the face of the earth. It will be a very similar chain of events, if something is not blockchain certified then people are not going to buy it, so this is a very good comparison to make.

Blockchain certification will be the future of everything you buy, not just food. We are already seeing that first hand in the USA. Based on the two interviews and literature review, we listed the causes and mitigation strategies for waste in the food supply chain in Tables 3 and 4.

Table 3. Supply chain and technology related issues

Waste Type	Causes
Beginning of SC	
Water and energy throughout every step	Lack of monitoring consumption.
Animal loss before slaughter	Poor health.
Middle of SC	
Waste caused by poor inventory Management	Void of data at the processor and slaughterhouse.
End of SC	
Shelf-life waste	Data in silos down the supply chain and lack of data from the slaughterhouse leads to inaccurate shelf life dates.
Waste caused by poor inventory Management	Lag in data retrieval from farm, slaughterhouse and distributor.

Table 4. Mitigation Strategies for end to end supply chain

Waste	Blockchain Mitigation
Beginning of SC	
Water and energy throughout every step	Processes can be streamlined to reduce the amount of water and energy consumption.
Animal loss before slaughter	Ensuring animals stay healthy by tagging individual animals with RFID tags, and through these, keeping vaccinations up to date, medical records up-to-date and consumption of the optimal quantity of feed.
Middle of SC	
Waste caused by poor inventory Management	Establish exactly when the meat gets cut and packaged, to enable a more accurate and probably longer shelf life, by bringing all of these data sets together and sharing more information along the SC.
End of SC	
Shelf-life waste	Processing timestamps in the slaughterhouse will allow for more accurate delivery times to retailers and hence better product shelf life.
Waste caused by poor inventory Management	Collapsing the data as it is available in relatively real-time should improve inventory management and give a better sense of shelf life and waste at the end of the SC.

DISCUSSION

Interview one with CEO of beef supply chain identified several causes of waste, although the identified types of waste were said to be minimal or rare, these are highlighted in Table 5.

Table 5. Mitigation strategies (interview one)

Waste	Blockchain Mitigation
Residual materials at the processing stage	N/A
Beef products below appearance standards	An end-to-end blockchain system would provide customers with a detailed view of the product's timeline in an easy to access format, which customers would trust and realise that the product is of equal quality to the others. In addition, detailed data, for example concerning temperature control could indicate why product is discoloured.
Animal loss before slaughter	When the farmer is not sure what caused the loss, blockchain data logs would be able to prove the history and assist with route causing the problem, i.e. potential hereditary diseases or weaknesses to certain infections.
Damage to beef products during transportation	Quickly identify where the meat quality of a particular product might have been tarnished.

The different types of beef waste identified by FAO (2011) were confirmed in the findings in Interview One and Two. However, beef waste due to below-standards appearance was not mentioned in FAO (2016) but was highlighted by CEO of beef supply chain in Interview One. Furthermore, loss and waste in the market system was mentioned in FAO (2016), but poor inventory management and shelf life waste were not specifically identified as root causes of waste. Therefore, this study further advances empirical base in the literature about beef supply chain waste identification.

Founder of technology company in Interview Two confirmed that blockchain can be used to reduce waste in beef supply chains in his explanation of how each waste can be mitigated or significantly reduced using blockchain technology. Echoing Raja Ramachandran in an interview by Hammerich (2018), the Food Standards Agency (2018) and Brigid Mcdermott from IBM (Creasy, 2017).

Tian (2016) looked at how blockchain and RFID could be used in combination in an agri-food supply chain. This study, which focuses on the beef supply chain, supports research by Tian in statements about the combination of blockchain and RFID bringing tracking and traceability management benefits to food supply chains. Furthermore, research by Abeyratne and Monfared (2016) shows IT infrastructure must be in place from end to end in the supply chain for blockchain to be implemented effectively, which supports blockchain mitigation strategies proposed in this study. Mitigation strategies supported by Abeyratne and Monfared include having an end-to-end blockchain infrastructure and streamlining all processes throughout the supply chain using blockchain. These mitigation strategies would help reduce waste from beef below appearance standards, in addition to reducing water and energy waste, amongst other wastes.

Referring to Interview Two, in which Founder talks about acceptance of the application of blockchain to the beef supply chain, there are links to the literature under lean supply chain concepts that can support his statements. Vitasek, et al., (2005), said that cultural change is the biggest recurring obstacle to successfully applying lean supply chain concepts. Cultural change in this instance is referring to resistance from people who will be asked to embrace and implement the change to learn new lean supply chain concepts.

In addition, to tie in to when Founder was speaking about how there must be more data sharing up and down the supply chain to streamline processes, Taylor (2006) supports this point. Taylor (2006) says that the full cooperation of all value chain partners is required for a really efficient value chain. In addition, cooperation can contribute to a stable, dedicated and competitive supply chain, by improving on quality, cost and delivery year on year. Additionally, DecisionNext (2018) supported this point, believing that streamlining supply chains and increasing accurate information sharing can reduce food waste.

However, as demonstrated in Interview One by the reluctance of CEO of Beef supply chain to accept the possibility and need for change from current processes, Taylor (2006) also backs up this behaviour. Taylor (2006) says that such improvements to the red meat sector will require a significant change in attitude for every member of the value chain, to overcome some of the lack of trust and hostility between value chain members. In addition, improvements will require the desertion of many long held business norms, which could be a cause of reluctance to improvement.

Differences between firm level views and supply chain views can be explained through Ignorance Theory. Firm level views can be seen as ignorant, arising from the absence of knowledge; this can be explained when a firm refrains from acquiring knowledge when the cost of education exceeds the potential benefit of what the knowledge would acquire (Roberts, 2012). For example, CEO of beef supply chain could be reluctant to learn about blockchain any further because he does not know enough about it to see its potential and only views the technology as an added cost. Whereas Founder of technology company, has a supply chain perspective and is knowledgeable about the technology, therefore, his views are not tainted by ignorance.

Furthermore, Founder of technology company ends the interview with the statement about blockchain certification being essential for every purchase in the future. This cements his and his company's belief in the blockchain technology and in its successful application in food and beef supply chains.

Weaknesses and Limitations

One weakness of the research is the lack of exploration into other processes and technologies that are currently used in beef supply chains and their ability to reduce waste. We believe, with further research, the extra information could balance our argument and lead to a more rounded conclusion. In addition, if more professionals from different parts of the beef supply chain were interviewed, further detail and insight could have been provided on beef supply chain waste, increasing the validity of the study.

Contribution to Knowledge

The findings in this study provide a good insight into the feasibility of blockchain application to a beef supply chain and the consequential waste reduction. Wastes in the beef supply chain were identified and general knowledge was increased compared to the current literature. An additional contribution to supply chain literature is that blockchain has been shown to have the potential to reduce different waste in a beef supply chain. Now that the feasibility of blockchain application to a beef supply chain has been acknowledged, this study could be used as a platform for further research into waste reduction in the beef supply chain. Eventually all food supply chains will utilise blockchain technology in various forms and to various extents, and food waste will be reduced on a global scale, as a result.

CONCLUSION AND RECOMMENDATIONS

The key takeaway of the chapter is to confirm the feasibility of blockchain technology application in beef supply chain. The affirmation that waste can be reduced in a beef supply chain by the application of blockchain technology. All areas of the beef supply chain can be streamlined by increasing data sharing between the different entities and adopting various blockchain enabled processes. Finally, even though the global direction of food supply chains is to become leaner, more cost effective and more visible and traceable, there is resistance especially from the farming area of the beef supply chain for any change in regards to technology and improving current practices.

Beef supply chain waste was identified, including residual materials at the processing stage, animal loss before slaughter, use of water and energy throughout the supply chain, damage to beef products during transportation, beef products below appearance standards, and waste caused by poor inventory management. Targeted blockchain mitigation strategies were then proposed. Using blockchain and other technologies combined in the farm, transportation and slaughterhouse supply chain stages, animal loss, damaged meat products and water and energy use can be reduced. Exactly where and when the meat is cut and packaged can be determined and communicated between supply chain entities more accurately with the support of blockchain. This will improve inventory management, improve the accuracy of delivery times and lengthen product shelf lives for the benefit of consumers and retailers alike.

Problems faced in this study included difficulty in collecting substantial data through interviews from relevant individuals. It was difficult to secure interviews that would provide the necessary data due to the nascent research topic and few companies that could provide relevant data. In order to overcome this difficulty, further research was required to identify companies that linked to the research topic. It was also necessary to think carefully about access available to other parts of the beef supply chain, and this was where the butcher was identified and brought into the study. In order the extract the necessary data from the interviewees, questions had to be posed concisely and often with further explanation. This was difficult as the individuals interviewed had very different levels of knowledge on the topic already, but analysis after the interviews and linking to the literature ensured that enough conclusions could be made to support the study.

The research question, to understand the feasibility of blockchain application in relation to beef supply chain waste reduction was answered by the combination of interviews and current literature review. Types of waste in a beef supply chain were identified and the cause of each type of waste was identified. For each type of waste, the extent to which blockchain could mitigate the waste was discussed, and that answered the question about whether blockchain could be applied to a beef supply chain and also if blockchain could be used to reduce waste in a beef supply chain. Furthermore, acceptance of blockchain technology in a beef supply chain was touched upon, as well as current processes and the future of blockchain application. Therefore, the gap in the literature around waste reduction in a beef supply chain and also waste reduction by using blockchain technology, has been narrowed.

The link between blockchain and the reduction of waste in a beef supply chain was researched in this study, as this research had not been carried out previously. Further studies should include more research on the acceptance of blockchain technology on a widespread level for beef supply chains, as this arose as an important point in this study. Further studies should also include the feasibility of blockchain to reduce waste in other meat and food substance supply chains, as blockchain is a technology that is only increasing in popularity and the benefits it brings are only increasing in importance. Finally, research must be done on how to increase the awareness, education and adoption of streamlining technology amongst the various stakeholders in the supply chains.

Stakeholders in beef supply chains must be aware of the importance of including blockchain technologies in future strategies and they must also be aware that waste reduction is a topic that is increasing in importance as supply chains look to become more sustainable as well as more cost-effective.

REFERENCES

Abeyratne, S., & Monfared, R. (2016). Blockchain Ready Manufacturing Supply Chain Using Distributed Ledger. *International Journal of Research in Engineering and Technology*, *05*(09), 1–10. doi:10.15623/ijret.2016.0509001

Arc-net. (2018). *Arc-net and PwC join forces to use blockchain in combating food fraud*. Available at: https://arc-net.io/blog/arc-net-pwc-blockchain-food-fraud/

Authenticate. (2018). *Blockchain Technology for the Global Food Supply Network: Transformation or Hype?* Whitepaper.

Bryman, A., & Bell, E. (2011). *Business Research Methods*. New York: Oxford University Press.

Creasey, S. (2017). *The potential for blockchain in the food industry - just-food global news*. Aroq Limited.

Davies, G. (1992). The two ways in which retailers can be brands. *International Journal of Retail & Distribution Management*, *20*(2). doi:10.1108/09590559210009312

DecisionNext. (2018). *The Missing Link in the Food Chain: Blockchain*. Whitepaper.

FAO. (2011). Global food losses and food waste – Extent, causes and prevention. Rome: FAO.

Fearne, A., Hornibrook, S., & Dedman, S. (2001). The management of perceived risk in the food supply chain: A comparative study of retailer-led beef quality assurance schemes in Germany and Italy. *The International Food and Agribusiness Management Review, 4*(1), 19–36. doi:10.1016/S1096-7508(01)00068-4

Food Standards Agency. (2018). *FSA trials first use of blockchain*. Available at: https://www.food.gov.uk/news-alerts/news/fsa-trials-first-use-of-blockchain

Fridgen, G., Radszuwill, S., Urbach, N., & Utz, L. (2017). Cross-Organizational Workflow Management Using Blockchain Technology – Towards Applicability, Auditability, and Automation. *51st Annual Hawaii International Conference on System Sciences.*

Garrone, P., Melacini, M., & Perego, A. (2014). Opening the black box of food waste reduction. *Food Policy, 46*, 129–139. doi:10.1016/j.foodpol.2014.03.014

Good Logistics. (2017). *Blockchain Next on Food Supply Chain Menu*. Available at: https://www.food-logistics.com/technology/article/12382466/blockchain-next-on-food-supply-chain-menu

gov.uk. (2018). *China lifts ban on exports of British beef*. Available at: https://www.gov.uk/government/news/china-lifts-ban-on-exports-of-british-beef

Haddud, A., DeSouza, A., Khare, A., & Lee, H. (2017). Examining potential benefits and challenges associated with the Internet of Things integration in supply chains. *Journal of Manufacturing Technology Management, 28*(8), 1055–1085. doi:10.1108/JMTM-05-2017-0094

Hammerich, T. (2018). *Blockchain and the Internet of Food*. Future of Agriculture.

Hobbs, J.E. (2003). *Consumer demand for traceability*. Academic Press.

Improving efficiency, generating better returns & tackling environmental impacts in beef supply chains. (2017). WRAP. Available at: http://www.wrap.org.uk/sites/files/wrap/Tackling%20hotspots%20in%20the%20beef%20value%20chain_Published%20March%202017%20(2).pdf

Järvensivu, T., & Törnroos, J. (2010). Case study research with moderate constructionism: Conceptualization and practical illustration. *Industrial Marketing Management, 39*(1), 100–108. doi:10.1016/j.indmarman.2008.05.005

Johnson, E. (2018). *Blockchain: shaking up logistics*. Epicor.

Koonce, L. (2017). *Blockchains & Food Security in the Supply Chain*. Academic Press.

Korpela, K., Hallikas, J., & Dahlberg, T. (2017, January). Digital Supply Chain Transformation toward Blockchain Integration. *Proceedings of the 50th Hawaii International Conference on System Sciences.* 10.24251/HICSS.2017.506

Management, S. (2017a). *Case study: Walmart*. Available at: https://www.cips.org/en/supply-management/analysis/2017/june/case-study-walmart/

Management, S. (2017b). *Six things wrong with blockchain*. Available at: https://www.cips.org/en/supply-management/analysis/2017/december/six-things-wrong-with-blockchain-/

Management, S. (2018). *Blockchain for supply chains: From hype to reality*. Available at: https://www.cips.org/supply-management/analysis/2018/june-/blockchain-hype-reality/

Management, S. (2018). *Unilever and Sainsbury's testing blockchain for supply chain data*. Available at: https://www.cips.org/supply-management/news/2017/december/unilever-and-sainsburys-testing-blockchain-for-small-farmers/

Material Handling and Logistics (MHL News). (2017). *Blockchain Can Improve Visibility in Food Supply Chain*. Available at: http://www.mhlnews.com/technology-automation/blockchain-can-improve-visibility-food-supply-chain

Medium. (2018). *The Amazon of China has Adopted Blockchain to Track high-end Beef Imports*. Available at: https://medium.com/@Michael_Spencer/the-amazon-of-china-has-adopted-blockchain-to-track-high-end-beef-imports-bf927671191a

Mena, C., Adenso-Diaz, B., & Yurt, O. (2011). The causes of food waste in the supplier–retailer interface: Evidences from the UK and Spain. *Resources, Conservation and Recycling, 55*(6), 648–658. doi:10.1016/j.resconrec.2010.09.006

Mishra, N., & Singh, A. (2016). Use of twitter data for waste minimisation in beef supply chain. *Annals of Operations Research*, 1–23.

National Food Crime Unit. (2017). *Food Crime Annual Strategic Assessment - A 2016 Baseline*. Food Standards Agency and Food Standards Scotland.

Papargyropoulou, E., Lozano, R., Steinberger, J.K., & Wright, N., & bin Ujang, Z. (2014). The food waste hierarchy as a framework for the management of food surplus and food waste. *Journal of Cleaner Production, 76*, 106–115. doi:10.1016/j.jclepro.2014.04.020

Parfitt, J., Barthel, M., & Macnaughton, S. (2010). Food waste within food supply chains: Quantification and potential for change to 2050. *Philosophical Transactions of the Royal Society of London. Series B, Biological Sciences, 365*(1554), 3065–3081. doi:10.1098/rstb.2010.0126 PMID:20713403

Ripe.io. (2018). *Ripe – Let's Talk About the Quality of our Food*. Available at: http://www.ripe.io

Roberts, J. (2012). Organizational ignorance: Towards a managerial perspective on the unknown. *Management Learning, 44*(3), 215–236. doi:10.1177/1350507612443208

Saberi, S., Kouhizadeh, M., Sarkis, J., & Shen, L. (2018). Blockchain technology and its relationships to sustainable supply chain management. *International Journal of Production Research*, 1–19.

Saunders, M., Lewis, P., & Thornhill, A. (2012). *Research methods for business students* (6th ed.). Harlow, UK: Pearson.

Steiner, J., Baker, J., Wood, G., & Meiklejohn, S. (2015). *Blockchain: the solution for transparency in product supply chains*. Project Provenance Ltd.

Taylor, D. H. (2006). Strategic considerations in the development of lean agri-food supply chains: A case study of the UK pork sector. *Supply Chain Management, 11*(3), 271–280. doi:10.1108/13598540610662185

Tian, F. (2016, June). An agri-food supply chain traceability system for China based on RFID & blockchain technology. In *Service Systems and Service Management (ICSSSM), 2016 13th International Conference on* (pp. 1-6). IEEE.

Traill, B. (1997). Structural changes in the European food industry: Consequences for innovation. In *Products and Process Innovation in the Food Industry* (pp. 38–60). Boston, MA: Springer. doi:10.1007/978-1-4613-1133-1_2

Treiblmaier, H. (2018). The impact of the blockchain on the supply chain: A theory-based research framework and a call for action. *Supply Chain Management, 23*(6), 545–559. doi:10.1108/SCM-01-2018-0029

Vitasek, K. L., Manrodt, K. B., & Abbott, J. (2005). What makes a lean supply chain? *Supply Chain Management Review, 9*(7), 39–45.

Wolf, M. (2017). *How Could Blockchain Be Used With Food*. Smart Kitchen Show.

World Health Organization. (2017). *WHO's first ever global estimates of foodborne diseases find children under 5 account for almost one third of deaths*. Available at: http://www.who.int/mediacentre/news/releases/2015/foodborne-disease-estimates/en/

WRAP. (2007). *Understanding the Food Waste*. Research Summary.

Yin, R. K. (2013). *Case study research: Design and methods*. Sage publications.

This research was previously published in Industry 4.0 and Hyper-Customized Smart Manufacturing Supply Chains edited by S.G. Ponnambalam, Nachiappan Subramanian, Manoj Kumar Tiwari, and Wan Azhar Wan Yusoff; pages 61-85, copyright year 2019 by Business Science Reference (an imprint of IGI Global).

Chapter 19
Performance Evaluation of Food Cold Chain Logistics Enterprise Based on the AHP and Entropy

Yazhou Xiong

Research Centre of Mining and Metallurgy Culture & Socio-economic Development in the Middle Reaches of the Yangtze River, Hubei Polytechnic University, Huangshi, China

Jie Zhao

School of Economics and Management, Hubei Polytechnic University, Huangshi, China

Jie Lan

School of Economics and Management, Hubei Polytechnic University, Huangshi, China

ABSTRACT

This article evaluates the performance of food cold chain logistics enterprises based on the analytic hierarchy process (AHP) and entropy method. Based on the analysis of the present situation, an evaluation system of food cold chain logistics enterprises is established from four aspects, including the financial management, cold chain logistics process, development ability and customer service. The AHP method is used to determine subjective weights, and entropy method is used to get experts' own weights. Finally, a comprehensive index fusion weight is conducted. In addition, the result of an empirical analysis proved to be valid.

INTRODUCTION

With the development of economy and the improvement of living standards in China, social demand for low-temperature frozen food products is increasing, and people's demand for low-temperature frozen food products is higher and higher. Therefore, what measures should be taken to ensure the safety, rest assured, nutrition of frozen food by the government and related employees, which has become the primary problem of cold chain food logistics (Zhang, 2004; Xiao & Zhang, 2008). At present, most of

DOI: 10.4018/978-1-7998-5354-1.ch019

low-temperature frozen food products belong to the agricultural and sideline products, and they have a characteristic of strict seasonal and freshness, which lead to a demand of timeliness, constant temperature and diversity for logistics. A complete cold chain logistics system usually includes raw materials procurement, frozen food processing, frozen food storage, frozen food transportation, frozen food distribution and frozen food sales (Deng, 2007).

In the study of existing literature, there are a lot of evaluation methods for the performance of the enterprise, such as fuzzy comprehensive evaluation method, the BP neural network algorithm and the analytic hierarchy process (AHP) and so on (Ren & Wang, 2006; Xu et al., 2005; Shang & Ning, 2005; Xiong, 2015; Kengpol & Tuominen, 2006). All these evaluation methods have certain applicability, but they still have some limitations. Some methods are too simple, and too much information is missing, so the evaluation results are unconvincing; some methods are too complex and there are too qualitative evaluation indexes, which lead to weak operability and the lack of practical value.

At present, there exist many methods to determine weight (Diego et al., 2012; Biju et al., 2017; Xiu & Chen, 2011; Guo & Wang, 2015; Huo & Wei, 2008); Chen et al., 2014; Wang et al., 2012; Bazulin, 2010; Hertog et al., 2007). The current methods mostly only consider one side of the subjective evaluation, such as analytic hierarchy process (AHP); or they only consider one side of the objective evaluation, such as the entropy value method and the variation coefficient method, etc. Due to one-sided character of the subjective and objective method, they may cause some influence on decision-making results. In order to eliminate or avoid these influences, this study combines the analytic hierarchy process (AHP) with entropy value method to make an evaluation of food cold chain logistics enterprise. In this paper, the analytic hierarchy process is used to determine subjective weights, and entropy value method is used to get experts' own weight, which are given information quality by the all the evaluation experts, finally comprehensive index fusion weights are conducted.

MEANING AND COMPOSITION OF FOOD COLD CHAIN LOGISTICS

Food cold chain refers to a special supply chain system, in which perishable food which is processed, stored, transported, distributed, retailed, until transferred to the final consumer from the place of origin after being purchased or fished. In order to ensure food quality and safety, reduce wastage, and prevent pollution, its various links are always at the required low temperature of the product.

In China's logistics industry standards, these cold chain foods always consist of the following three categories: First, primary agricultural products, mainly poultry, eggs, milk, meat, aquatic products, fruits and vegetables. Second, processing agricultural and sideline food, mainly egg processing, slaughtering and meat processing, aquatic products processing and fruits and vegetables processing and so on. Third, manufacturing food, mainly dairy products, frozen food, canned food and edible ice, quick-frozen food, soft beverages.

Food cold chain logistics refers to a logistics system, in which the fresh or perishable food always is kept in the specified low temperature environment in the production, storage, transportation, sales to the final consumer hands of each link, the best logistics means to ensure food for reducing food loss and product quality.

Food cold chain includes frozen processing, frozen storage, refrigerated transportation and distribution, refrigerated sales and cold chain reverse.

Food cold chain is composed of five aspects, which including all aspects from food collected in the production area through pre-cold-processing storage packaging to the sales terminal for sale to the end consumer, and finally to the whole process of waste recycling.

Five specific aspects of food cold chain are as follows:

- **Frozen processing:** It mainly includes pre-cooling, cooling and freezing of frozen food, as well as processing operations and so on in low temperature environment. As the first link of food cold chain logistics, the quality of precooling and cooling has an important influence for the whole to the quality of the cold chain. After obtaining the raw materials, timely and rapid cooling and freshness preservation are of great importance to ensure the original quality of food;
- **Refrigerated storage:** It includes cold storage and frozen storage of food, as well as air-conditioned storage of fruits and vegetables. At present, there are mainly four refrigeration storage technologies, including Modified Atmosphere Packaging (MAP) storage technology, decompression storage technology, ice-temperature storage technology, and gas conditioning storage technology in China;
- **Refrigerate transportation and distribution:** It mainly includes medium and long-distance transportation and regional distribution of frozen food. During refrigerated transportation, the degree of temperature fluctuation is one of the main causes of the decline of food quality. Therefore, the means of transport must be good performance, not only maintain the specified low temperature, but also avoid large temperature fluctuations, especially for long-distance transportation;
- **Frozen sales:** The manufacturers, distributors and retailers mainly accomplish the frozen sales together. With the rapid development of all kinds of self-selected supermarkets, they gradually become the main sales channel of cold chain food. In the construction process of food cold chain logistics, we should take into account various issues concerning production, sales, logistics, economy and technology in a comprehensive manner and address each other's concerns, effective coordination to ensure high quality consumption of perishable fresh food;
- **Cold chain reverse logistics:** It mainly consists of recycling logistics and waste logistics. Recycling logistics mainly refers to the physical flow of goods, the return of food and the packaging container used in the turnover shall return from the demander to form by the supplier. Waste recycling refers to the resulting physical flow of goods; in the process of cold chain logistics, the corrosion of food or other goods have lost economic value, according to actual collection, classification, processing, packaging, handling, storage, and distribution to a special processing site.

CONSTRUCTION OF EVALUATION INDEX SYSTEM

Index system refers to a series of interrelated indicators composed of the whole. Every evaluation indicator can comprehensively reflect various aspects of objects from the characteristics of objects with different profiles. The performance evaluation of food cold chain logistics enterprises must construct several specific indicators for enterprises, these indices are the basis and standard of evaluation. Whether the index system constructed is comprehensive, the choice is scientific and reasonable, the index value, the accuracy of the measurement affects the evaluation results of food cold chain logistics performance.

Evaluation method refers to the specific means of performance evaluation of food logistics enterprises. Performance appraisal means passing a certain amount, the mathematical model combines several evaluation indexes into a comprehensive evaluation value. If the evaluation method is not enough scientific and rational, the evaluation index system and evaluation criteria will become an isolated evaluation element, and they will lose the meaning of itself.

Performance evaluation criteria depend on the evaluation purpose of the enterprise. Because of the different scope, target and starting point of enterprise evaluation, we need to have corresponding appraisal standard to adapt to it. The evaluation criterion is the benchmark to evaluate the performance of the evaluation object.

Overall evaluation index system of food cold chain logistics includes cold chain value indicators and customer value indicators (Luo et al., 2008). Due to the particularity of food, the requirements of cold chain logistics are extremely high in the collection transmission of information, mastery of time and temperature control. On the basis of it, this paper combining them with the characteristics of cold chain logistics to design 16 key indicators to build the overall performance evaluation index system of food cold chain logistics enterprise, which contains 4 first-level indicators and 17 second-level indicators shown on the Table 1 (Xue, 2010).

Table 1. Performance evaluation index system of food cold chain logistics enterprise

First-Level Indicators	No.	Weight(w_j)	Second-Level Indicators	No.
Financial management	U_1	w_1	Rate of return on total assets	u_{11}
			Increase rate of business revenue	u_{12}
			Current ratio	u_{13}
Cold chain logistics process	U_2	w_2	Unit transportation cost of cold chain	u_{21}
			Utilization rate of refrigerator car	u_{22}
			Cargo damage rate of refrigerated transport	u_{23}
			Utilization rate of cold storage	u_{24}
			Inventory carry rate	u_{25}
			Food defect rate	u_{26}
Customer service	U_3	w_3	Delivery rate on time	u_{31}
			Accuracy of delivery	u_{32}
			Customer satisfaction	u_{33}
			Quality and safety of food	u_{34}
Development ability	U_4	w_4	Ability to develop new customers	u_{41}
			The new service income rate	u_{42}
			Quality of employees	u_{43}
			Employee training rate	u_{44}

COMPREHENSIVE EVALUATION MODEL

This paper presents a comprehensive weighting method; its basic principle of the method is as follows: firstly, we use AHP to determine the subjective weight, and then establish the judgment matrix via the pair wise comparison according to various experts' opinion. In addition, entropy method is applied to get experts' own weight, which are given information quality by the all the evaluation experts, finally two methods are combined to draw the index fusion weight (Huang & Xie, 2009).

Calculation of Index Subjective Weights via Based on AHP Method

The main steps are as follows:

- To construct the hierarchical structure model via literature review;
- To establish all judgment matrices of every level via the pair wise comparison;
- To conduct the sorting and consistency test of each single hierarchical;
- To perform sorting and consistency test of total hierarchy;
- If necessary, the judgment matrix and hierarchical ranking model may be corrected and readjusted (Jiang et al., 2009).

Calculation of Experts' Own Weight via Transfer Entropy

In the course of information theory, entropy is used to measure the uncertainty, the greater the amount of information, the less the uncertainty is, and the smaller the entropy, the smaller the amount of information, the greater the uncertainty is, the greater the entropy is. According to the characteristics of entropy, randomness and disorder of an event can be judged by calculating the entropy value, and discrete degree of the index can be judged by entropy values. The greater the discrete degree of the index, the greater the index has the influence on the comprehensive evaluation.

In the process of constructing the judgment matrix, there are many experts who construct the judgment matrix simultaneously. Now it is assumed that there exists an ideal optimal expert, whose judgment matrix is the fairest and most accurate in all judgment matrixes. In the actual calculation and determination, this study can choose the expert that has the highest consistency of the knowledge to the evaluation object and the expert group, that is to say, the optimal expert has the smallest overall difference between the experts. Moreover, the entropy can be used to measure the difference, which can be indicated as the following model (Ren and Wang, 2011).

Supposing the symbols Z_1, Z_2, ..., Z_m represent m experts, they constitute the evaluation group G. In addition, the symbols T_1, T_2, ..., T_n represent the targets to be evaluated. The symbol $x_{ij}(i=1,2,...,m, j=1,2,...,n)$ represents the evaluation value of the ith expert to the jth target. The vector $x_i = (x_{i1}, x_{i2}, L, x_{in})^T \in E_n$ and matrix $X = (x_{ij})_{m \times n}$ is the conclusion of the experts group in an assessment. Let Z_* represent the optimal expert, and his evaluation score vector is $x_* = (x_{*1}, x_{*2}, L, x_{*n})^T \in E_n$. The difference value between the evaluation score of each expert and Z_* is used to measure the pros and cons of the selected experts.

So the horizontal vector of experts is shown on the Equation (1):

$$E_i = (e_{i1}, e_{i2}, L\ , e_{in})$$

(1)

where, $e_{ij} = 1 - |x_{ij} - \overline{x_{ij}}|/\max x_{ij}$, $(i = 1,2,L\ ,m;\ j = 1,2,L\ ,n)$, which reflects the level of the evaluation conclusion of the expert Z_i to the target $T_1, T_2, \ldots, T_n$, $\overline{x_{ij}} = \sum_{i=1}^{m} x_{ij}/m$, $\max x_{ij} = \max\{x_{ij}\}$, $(i=1,2,\ldots,m)$. and the transfer entropy can be indicated as the following Equation (2) (Qiu, 2002):

$$h_{ij} = \begin{cases} -e_{ij}\ln e_{ij} & \left(1/e \le e_{ij} \le 1\right) \\ 2/e - e_{ij}\left|\ln e_{ij}\right| & \left(-1/e - 1 \le e_{ij} \le 1/e\right) \end{cases}$$

(2)

Therefore, the evaluation model of the expert results can be established via the entropy as following Equation (3):

$$H_i = \sum_{j=1}^{n} h_{ij}$$

(3)

In this model, the evaluation ability of the experts to the given problem is measured by the uncertainty of the given problem, and the size of entropy value H_i represents the degree of uncertainty. The smaller the entropy value, the higher the decision-making level of experts is, and the more scientific the ratings given by experts is; on the other hand, the bigger the entropy value is, the lower credibility of the experts to give the evaluation conclusion is.

Therefore, the following Equation (4) can be used to express the weight of the experts in each target, in other words, the weight of the ith expert is:

$$q_i = \frac{1/H_i}{\sum_{i=1}^{m} 1/H_i}$$

(4)

where, the greater the value q_i, the greater the proportion of experts' opinion should be accounted for in the evaluation.

Calculation of Weighted Fusion Weight of Evaluation Index

Supposing n is the number of the indicators, m is the number of the experts. $W_j' = \left[w_{j1}', w_{j2}', L\ , w_{jn}'\right]^T$ is subjective weight given by the jth expert, $E = [E_1, E_2, \ldots, E_m]^T$ is expert weight vector, $W = [w_1, w_2, \ldots, w_n]^T$ is weighted fusion weight, and $0 < w_i < 1$, $\sum_{i=1}^{n} w_i < 1$, $i=1,2,\ldots,n$.

In addition, weighted fusion weight of evaluation index can be calculation via the following Equation (5):

$$W = \sum_{j=1}^{m} w_j' \times E_j, \, j=1,2,\ldots,m \tag{5}$$

CASE STUDY

According to the above described and analysis, some surveys of a food cold chain logistics enterprise are made and six experts are asked about the performance evaluation about the enterprise. Then judgment matrix of the first-level indicators is obtained, the index fusion weights are calculated as follows.

Establishing the Judgment Matrix A_i (i = 1, 2, …, 6) From the Six Experts

$$A_1 = \begin{pmatrix} 1.0000 & 7.0000 & 5.0000 & 3.0000 \\ 0.1429 & 1.0000 & 0.3333 & 0.2000 \\ 0.2000 & 3.0000 & 1.0000 & 0.5000 \\ 0.3333 & 5.0000 & 2.0000 & 1.0000 \end{pmatrix}$$

$$A_2 = \begin{pmatrix} 1.0000 & 5.0000 & 4.0000 & 3.0000 \\ 0.2000 & 1.0000 & 0.5000 & 0.3333 \\ 0.2500 & 2.0000 & 1.0000 & 0.5000 \\ 0.3333 & 3.0000 & 2.0000 & 1.0000 \end{pmatrix}$$

$$A_3 = \begin{pmatrix} 1.0000 & 4.0000 & 3.0000 & 2.0000 \\ 0.2500 & 1.0000 & 0.3333 & 0.2000 \\ 0.3333 & 3.0000 & 1.0000 & 0.5000 \\ 0.5000 & 5.0000 & 2.0000 & 1.0000 \end{pmatrix}$$

$$A_4 = \begin{pmatrix} 1.0000 & 3.0000 & 3.0000 & 1.0000 \\ 0.3333 & 1.0000 & 2.0000 & 0.2000 \\ 0.3333 & 0.5000 & 1.0000 & 0.5000 \\ 1.0000 & 5.0000 & 2.0000 & 1.0000 \end{pmatrix}$$

$$A_5 = \begin{pmatrix} 1.0000 & 3.0000 & 2.0000 & 1.0000 \\ 0.3333 & 1.0000 & 0.5000 & 0.3333 \\ 0.5000 & 2.0000 & 1.0000 & 2.0000 \\ 1.0000 & 3.0000 & 0.5000 & 1.0000 \end{pmatrix}$$

$$A_6 = \begin{pmatrix} 1.0000 & 2.0000 & 3.0000 & 4.0000 \\ 0.5000 & 1.0000 & 3.0000 & 5.0000 \\ 0.3333 & 0.3333 & 1.0000 & 2.0000 \\ 0.2500 & 0.2000 & 0.5000 & 1.0000 \end{pmatrix}$$

Calculation Process of Subjective Weight via AHP Method

Based on the judgment matrices from the six experts, feature vector method is used to calculate the maximum feature root λ_{max} and feature vector of the judgment matrix $A_i(i=1,2,\ldots,6)$, all consistency checking results (CR) are smaller than 0.1, which are in line with the requirements of consistency checking. All the subjective weight calculation and consistency check outcomes are shown on the Table 2.

Table 2. Calculating results of the subjective weight via AHP method

Experts No.	U_1	U_2	U_3	U_4	λm_{ax}	CR
Z_1	0.5738	0.0563	0.1310	0.2388	4.0776	0.0288
Z_2	0.5462	0.0838	0.1377	0.2323	4.0511	0.0189
Z_3	0.4543	0.0743	0.1693	0.3021	4.1023	0.0379
Z_4	0.3560	0.1343	0.1182	0.3915	4.2277	0.0843
Z_5	0.3557	0.1074	0.2816	0.2553	4.2072	0.0767
Z_6	0.4505	0.3336	0.1360	0.0799	4.0961	0.0356

Calculation Process of the Experts' Own Weight via Entropy Method

Based on the above theory and analyses, calculation process of experts' own weight via entropy method is as following Table (3). On the Table 3, the first column is experts' number, including six experts; the second column is the horizontal vector of experts. According to Equation (2) and (3), the third column is the sum of transfer entropy. Based on Equation (4), expert weight values are shown on the fourth column; finally, the weights are sorted from large to small, and outcomes are seen on the last column on the Table 3.

Table 3. Calculating results of experts' own weight via entropy method

Experts No.	$E=(e_1, e_2,\ldots, e_n)$	H_i	q_i	Rank
Z_1	(0.7948, 0.7742, 0.8888, 0.9714)	0.5135	0.1570	③
Z_2	(0.8429, 0.8567, 0.9126, 0.9548)	0.4041	0.1995	②
Z_3	(0.9969, 0.8282, 0.9751, 0.8669)	0.3076	0.2620	①
Z_4	(0.8256, 0.9920, 0.8434, 0.6385)	0.5963	0.1352	⑤
Z_5	(0.8251, 0.9274, 0.5763, 0.9864)	0.5596	0.1440	④
Z_6	(0.9903, 0.3945, 0.9066, 0.5656)	0.7878	0.1023	⑥

As can be shown on the Table 3, the entropy of expert Z_6 is the maximum, so his accuracy of the opinion is the worst; and the entropy of expert Z_3 is the minimum, so his accuracy of the opinion is the highest. At the same time, expert Z_3 is the closest to the group expert opinions, so expert Z_3 has the maximum weight. On the contrary, the opinion of expert Z_6 is the most deviation from the group expert opinions, so the weight of expert Z_6 is the smallest, which also illustrates the rationality of using the entropy method for solving the weights of experts.

Calculation Process of Weighted Fusion Weight of Evaluation Index

Based on Equation (5), the subjective weight of expert evaluation index is conducted to get weighted sum with the experts' own weight, and the final weight of the index is shown on the following Equation (6):

$$w = \begin{pmatrix} w_1 \\ w_2 \\ w_3 \\ w_4 \end{pmatrix} = \begin{pmatrix} 0.5738 & 0.5462 & 0.4543 & 0.3560 & 0.3557 & 0.4505 \\ 0.0563 & 0.0838 & 0.0743 & 0.1343 & 0.1074 & 0.3336 \\ 0.1310 & 0.1377 & 0.1693 & 0.1182 & 0.2816 & 0.1360 \\ 0.2388 & 0.2323 & 0.3021 & 0.3915 & 0.2553 & 0.0799 \end{pmatrix} \times \begin{pmatrix} 0.1570 \\ 0.19995 \\ 0.2620 \\ 0.1352 \\ 0.1440 \\ 0.1023 \end{pmatrix} = \begin{pmatrix} 0.4635 \\ 0.1128 \\ 0.1628 \\ 0.2609 \end{pmatrix} \qquad (6)$$

As can be seen from the above analysis, the final index fusion weights are a combination of both the all experts' opinions and main opinions of the authority experts in the final result, so the final index weight of the results is closer to reality.

In the same way, the internal evaluation weights of second-level indicators in the evaluation system can be calculated.

There are several results summarized from data of the case analyses. First, besides the four factors (financial management, cold chain logistics process, customer service and development ability) that are commonly regarded as critical success factors in the performance evaluation index system of food chain logistics enterprise, financial management are rated as one of the highest factors. It is obvious that the development ability is also important for its big subjective weight. Second, every expert has different scoring preferences, which can be corrected by the entropy method. However, according to our case study, customer service only rated security in the fourth importance group, which is not fit for some firms. Third, most of the big companies prefer adopting financial management while some small logistics companies prefer improving the customer service.

CONCLUSION

For the performance evaluation of food cold chain logistics enterprises, this paper proposes a comprehensive evaluation model combining entropy weighting and analytic hierarchy analysis from four aspects. The analytic hierarchy process is used to subjectively evaluate the evaluation indicators. At the same time, the entropy weight method is applied to the expert's evaluation. The uncertainty of subjective determination of weights in multi-index evaluation is overcome, and the index system for performance evaluation of chain logistics enterprises is established from four aspects. In addition, this study takes the

quantitatively process and compare evaluation indicators and comprehensive ranking of performance evaluation of cold chain logistics enterprises. Finally, the case proves that the model reduces the influence of subjective factors and improves the objectivity and accuracy of the evaluation conclusions, And the result of an empirical analysis proved to be valid. For food cold chain logistics corporate performance evaluation, this paper provides a new approach.

ACKNOWLEDGMENT

The study is partially supported by the open fund project of Research Centre of Mining and Metallurgy Culture & Socio-economic Development in the Middle Reaches of the Yangtze River Grant No. 2014kyz01, the scientific research project of the Hubei Polytechnic University Grant No.15xjr03A, National college students' innovation and entrepreneurship training projects Grant No. 201710920009 & No. 201810920011.

REFERENCES

Bazulin, E. G. (2010). Application of the maximum entropy method in ultrasound nondestructive testing for scatterer imaging with allowance for multiple scattering. *Acoustical Physics*, *56*(1), 96–104. doi:10.1134/S1063771010010148

Biju, P. L., Shalij, P. R., & Prabhushankar, G. V. (2017). An evaluation tool for sustainable new product development using analytic hierarchy process approach. *International Journal of Innovation and Sustainable Development*, *11*(4), 393. doi:10.1504/IJISD.2017.086874

Chen, T., Jin, Y., Qiu, X., & Chen, X. (2014). A hybrid fuzzy evaluation method for safety assessment of food-waste feed based on entropy and the analytic hierarchy process methods. *Expert Systems with Applications: An International Journal*, *41*(16), 7328–7337. doi:10.1016/j.eswa.2014.06.006

Deng, R. C. (2007). *Operation practice of cold chain logistics*. Beijing: China Logistics Publishing House.

Falsini, D., Fondi, F., & Schiraldi, M. M. (2012). A logistics provider evaluation and selection methodology based on AHP, DEA and linear programming integration. *International Journal of Production Research*, *50*(17), 4822–4829. doi:10.1080/00207543.2012.657969

Guo, Z., & Wang, X. (2015). Selection and evaluation of e-commerce enterprises logistics operation models based on F-AHP method. In *International Conference on Mechatronics, Robotics and Automation*. 10.2991/icmra-15.2015.3

Hertog, M. L. A. T. M., Lammertyn, J., Ketelaere, B. D., Scheerlinck, N., & Nicolaï, B. M. (2007). Managing quality variance in the postharvest food chain. *Trends in Food Science & Technology*, *18*(6), 320–332. doi:10.1016/j.tifs.2007.02.007

Huang, X. R., & Xie, R. H. (2009). Performance evaluation of food cold chain logistics enterprise based on entropy and gray relevant. [Natural Science Edition]. *Journal of Guangzhou University*, *8*(4), 87–90.

Huo, H., & Wei, Z. (2008). Grey Multi-Hierarchical Evaluation of Third Party Logistics Providers in the Environment of Supply Chain. In *International Conference on Wireless Communications, NETWORK-ING and Mobile Computing* (pp. 1-4). IEEE.

Jiang, C. B., Wang, H., & Chen, L. (2009). Evaluation research of automobile logistics informationization based on AHP. *Journal of WUT, 31*(5), 792–795.

Kengpol, A., & Tuominen, M. (2006). A framework for group decision support systems: An application in the evaluation of information technology for logistics firms. *International Journal of Production Economics, 101*(1), 159–171. doi:10.1016/j.ijpe.2005.05.013

Luo, Y. L., Li, J. H., & Bai, L. (2008). Study on integrated performance evaluation index system of food cold chain. *Market Modernization, 17*(2), 156–157.

Qiu, W. H. (2002). *Management decision making and entropy application.* Beijing: Machinery Industry Press.

Ren, C. Y., & Wang, X. B. (2006). Study on the third party logistics performance evaluation system based on FCE. *Logistics Science Technology, 29*(6), 40–42.

Ren, Y.H., & Wang, N. (2011). Study on the evaluation system of brand competition ability of food enterprise based on Fuzzy AHP-Entropy. *Journal of Dezhou University, 27*(5), 30-34, 39.

Shang, H. Y., & Ning, X. X. (2005). The performance evaluation of 3PL enterprises based on the AHP model of multiplicative synthesis. *Science & Technology Progress and Policy, 22*(11), 94–96.

Wang, K., Zhu, Y., & Zhang, X. (2012). Index System of Construction Safety Evaluation Based on Analytic Hierarchy Process. In *The Twelfth COTA International Conference of Transportation Professionals* (pp.2469-2473). 10.1061/9780784412442.251

Xiao, J., Zhang, D. J., Liu, Z. Y., & Ma, Z. S. (2008). Research on construction of food cold chain logistics management system of our country. *Journal of Agriculture Mechanics Research, 7*(2), 13–17.

Xiong, Y. Z. (2015). A comprehensive quality evaluation on the College Students via DEA. *Journal of Interdisciplinary Mathematics, 18*(5), 639–648. doi:10.1080/09720502.2015.1047595

Xiu, G., & Chen, X. (2011). Research on the third party logistics supplier selection evaluation based on AHP and entropy. In *International Conference on Mechatronic Science, Electric Engineering and Computer* (pp.788-792). IEEE.

Xu, X. Q., Chen, J. M., & Yang, B. L. (2005). Study of choosing third party logistics serves based on BP neural network. *East China Economic Management, 19*(9), 85–88.

Xue, H. (2010). *Research on Performance Measurement of Food Cold Chain Logistics Enterprise on Green Supply Chain* [M.S. Thesis]. Chongqing University.

Zhang, Q. (2004). Status quo of farm produces logistics in the foreign countries. *World Agriculture, 47*(11), 11–13.

This research was previously published in the International Journal of Information Systems and Supply Chain Management (IJISSCM), 12(2); edited by John Wang; pages 57-67, copyright year 2019 by IGI Publishing (an imprint of IGI Global).

Chapter 20
A Circular Economy Perspective for Dairy Supply Chains

Christina Paraskevopoulou
https://orcid.org/0000-0001-6141-7721
Aristotle University of Thessaloniki, Greece

Dimitrios Vlachos
Aristotle University of Thessaloniki, Greece

ABSTRACT

The environmental issues and the projected world population increase have brought into light many different terms and concepts. For over 20 years, sustainability attracts the main focus of most researchers; however, recently the concept of circular economy (CE) is considered to be its successor. CE is based on a closed loop supply chain, where waste is minimized and reintroduced into the supply chain, thus requiring a systemic change. In the agri-food sector, the CE principles have many possible applications. This chapter provides a CE perspective for the dairy supply chain by identifying and analyzing the associated technologies and strategies through a literature review taxonomy based on the related stage of the supply chain.

INTRODUCTION

Over the past few years, the emerging environmental issues have been in the center of attention of people, cities, countries and organisms all around the world. In 1992, when the United Nations Framework convention on Climate Change was adopted, the problems of climate change came to light, leading to the Kyoto Protocol in 1997 and the Paris Agreement in 2015 (United Nations, 2017a). Thus, the idea of sustainability was born. It is based on three pillars: the environmental, the social and the economical. In order to be sustainable, a product, company or country needs to balance these three aspects.

At the same time, Circular Economy (CE) has recently gained in importance, with the academic world, policymakers and companies realizing its worth (Geissdoerfer, Savaget, Bocken, & Hultink, 2017) and the EU promoting it (Korhonen, Honkasalo, & Seppälä, 2018). This concept gives life back

DOI: 10.4018/978-1-7998-5354-1.ch020

to the product after its use, aiming to reduce, reuse, recycle and recover materials, as the 4R Framework suggests (Kirchherr, Reike, & Hekkert, 2017). It is an alternative model to the traditional Linear Economy following the 'take-make-dispose' pattern resulting to environmental and economic impacts (Ellen MacArthur Foundation, 2012).

CE is considered to be a means to achieve sustainability (Ellen MacArthur Foundation & McKinsey Center for Business and Environment, 2015), but there are major differences as well, e.g. their purpose, priorities and beneficiaries (Geissdoerfer et al., 2017). Their main connection is their way of thinking; CE combines sustainability and closed-loop supply chains into the business model of the industry (Preston, 2012), with sustainable development being its main goal (Kirchherr et al., 2017). Thus, while the two have common ground, CE focuses more on the environmental and economic aspects.

Along with the environmental issues, by 2050 the World's population will have reached 9.5 billion people according to UN's projections of 2017 (United Nations, 2017b). This will result in an increase of agricultural production, which is affected by the existing climate change but can also have a negative impact on the environment. The sector is developing globally, with 28.06% production growth in 2016 compared to the 2004-2006 period (FAO, 2018), while it employs 30.7% of the total workforce (World Bank, 2019). Agri-food supply chains, technological solutions for energy production and waste management are only some of the main challenges today. As a result, the term Circular Agriculture, i.e. Circular Economy in Agriculture, has been introduced.

One of the basic types of agriculture is livestock farming. Animal products, by-products and co-products are important for human nutrition and the economy, with the annual consumption achieving an annual growth of 1.2, 0.4 and 1.5% for meat, milk and eggs respectively (FAO, 2013). Dairy products in particular have a critical role, as they are important for human nutrition and development throughout life and represent around 14% of total calorie consumption (FAO, 2013). However, they have an undeniable impact to the environment. According to FAO, more than 10% of Dairy products are lost or wasted in Europe, a lower percentage than most regions but significant nonetheless (FAO, 2011). Most of that percentage is during the consumption period (40-60% of the total), however the percentage during agriculture is also high. Other than waste, there are other important issues; the animals themselves and their feed, the production and distribution of products, but most importantly what happens with leftover products and wastewaters. Considering the above-mentioned population increase, all these challenges present an opportunity for the development of CE.

However, despite the importance of the dairy industry and the considerable amounts of produced waste, there is a lack in the research literature of a holistic framework that analyses the CE perspective of the dairy supply chain, while identifying state-of-the-art technologies that can contribute to this objective. This has been the key motivation for this chapter. To that end, in this chapter, the circular dairy processing system is presented as well as its additional components with respect to the conventional system. Different technologies and solutions are analyzed and discussed along with the resulting classification of relevant literature. This allows for the identification of existing gaps, overlaps and future research areas of CE in dairy supply chain.

The objectives of this chapter are to determine:

- Which are the state-of-the-art technologies aligning with the CE principles?
- How can CE be applied in Dairy Supply Chains?
- What is the future of the CE in Dairy Supply Chains?

BACKGROUND

As mentioned in the Introduction, CE has been gaining ground the past few years as a concept that can reshape the Economy and the environment. The term has been analyzed in multiple occasions, with more than 114 definitions by 2017 (Kirchherr et al., 2017), while the European Union promotes it on its "Roadmap to a Resource Efficient Europe" in order to achieve resource efficiency (Commission Staff, 2014). The material flows are the main concern CE policies address. In the case of biological nutrients, after they are discarded they can be reintroduced into the natural cycle, while the rest are designed to be circulated by being reused and recycled (Haas, Krausmann, Wiedenhofer, & Heinz, 2015).

Through this process, there is value creation in the material's supply chain. There are four principles that govern this value creation (Ellen MacArthur Foundation, 2013):

- Inner circles: when the material is circled in tighter circles, less resources are being used for its repurposing.
- Longevity of the circle: a product with a longer life, either in the same or in different product circles, keeps creating value for as long as it is being repurposed.
- Product remarketing: the material can be repurposed as a part of a completely different product.
- Better Inputs: cleaner, purer and higher quality materials, chosen in the concept of CE, result in products that can be recycle and reprocessed.

Winans, Kendall, & Deng (2016) categorized the bibliography of the current applications of the CE concept into three categories:

1. **Policies:** The authors review the applications of CE according to the definition and components of policy as defined by Jiao & Boons (2014, 2017). This category includes eco-industrial parks and networks industrial symbiosis networks in Denmark, Sweden, the Netherlands, Italy, United Kingdom, United States of America, China, Thailand and South Africa, most of them promoted by government laws and initiatives. Ghisellini, Cialani, & Ulgiati (2016), however, further taxonomize the bibliography in accordance to the level where the policies are implemented:
   a. **Micro Level:** The smaller companies or the consumer constitute this category, where "Green Consumption", recycling and "Cleaner Production" are the main players.
   b. **Meso Level:** Hubs, parks, clusters and districts with an ecological with ecological consciousness.
   c. **Macro Level:** Wider regions e.g. cities, provinces, networks, countries, or waste management systems and programs.
2. **Value Chains, Material Flows and Product Applications:** In this category, the systems are reviewed according to the product's resource i.e. wood products and by-products, plastics, metals chemicals, agricultural products and waste, water and land.
3. **Innovations in Technological, Organizational and Social Context:** This category includes all the current trends and new technologies that are in harmony with the CE principles.

Consequently, the CE concept can be adopted by businesses, systems or regions of different sizes and of a multitude of products and value chains. The optimal technologies and organizational models that are applicable on each case differ. In 2014, Naustdalslid stated that the decoupling of resources, i.e. energy and materials, and the environment, was an idealistic strategy to implement CE in China, whereas "relative decoupling", which is a less aggressive and slower solution. In 2015 Wijkman & Skånberg further studied the delinking by simulating decoupled systems in order to determine the effects of reducing energy use, of increasing the use of Renewable Energy Sources (RES) and of the more efficient use of materials separately. In a system as such, the economic progress does alter the use of resources but optimizes their use and therefore does not affect the ecosystem. After simulations on the effects of CE in Finland, France, the Netherlands, Spain and Sweden, the authors concluded that the countries could reduce their carbon emissions, while achieving improvements in trade and employment (Wijkman & Skånberg, 2015a, 2015b).

This chapter focuses on smaller scale businesses of micro or meso level as they were defined above, producing agricultural goods and in particular dairy products, by-products and co-products. To this end, there have been several studies focusing on evaluating the economic feasibility of producing bioenergy from different agricultural products and manure using Anaerobic Digestors (AD) (Blades et al., 2017; Vega-Quezada, Blanco, & Romero, 2017) or wastewaters (Ferreira et al., 2018). In 2014, Ghisellini et al. compared an Italian and a Polish Dairy Farming Systems. The Italian farm had installed Solar Photovoltaic (PV) and a manure AD to produce energy, while the Polish used manure as a fertilizer. The transition to an energetically self-sufficient system was, according to the authors, efficient, however energy is not the only concern and a balance needs to be sustained for optimal results.

In terms of the design of dairy supply chains in line with the CE concept, Stanchev, Vasilaki, & Katsou (2017) demonstrated a dairy processing farm in the South-West of United Kingdom that produces 42 million liters of milk and 80,000 m³ of wastewater per year. The linear economy system consists of the Farm stage (1), where the livestock grazes freely or from produced crops (1a), is milked (1b) and then the raw product is sent to the processing industry (1c), and the Manufacturing stage (2), where the product is being processed (2a), packaged (2b) and then distributed (2c) in order to reach the consumer. The systems inputs are materials (ex. packaging), fuels, electricity, chemicals and water, while the outputs are emissions to air, soil and water, and the resulting dairy product, co-product and by-product.

In case of the equivalent circular system, Stanchev et al. (2017) added two more stages aiming to minimize the system inputs and emissions and maximize its production; the Wastewater Treatment stage (3), during which the wastewater is repurposed for production of energy, water and nutrient recycling through Anaerobic Digestion, and Recycling (4).

However, there are many different technologies that can make use of bio-waste in order to produce energy, fertilizers or other products, in order to close the loops and create a supply chain based on the CE principles.

THE CIRCULAR ECONOMY CONCEPT IN THE DAIRY SUPPLY CHAIN

In order to categorize the technologies and strategies associated with CE, the dairy supply chain shall be thoroughly investigated. According to Lowe & Gereffi (2009), the dairy value chain can be separated into four main stages, as shown in Figure 1:

- **Inputs**: According to the authors, this stage consists of forage and animal feed, veterinary services and genetics (breeds). However, the supply chain has even more inputs, the main ones being: (a) materials e.g. packaging, (b) energy e.g. fossil fuels for transportation or electricity for the factory,

(c) water for the livestock, crops and factory and (d) chemicals e.g. fertilizers. These resources cost money and impose an environmental burden by polluting and reducing natural resources.

- **Production**: This stage consists of the production of milk as a raw material and takes place in the farm. Through water and food consumption, in the stables and with veterinary support, the animals reproduce and produce milk and meat. Lowe & Gereffi (2009) mention there are alternative types of producing systems such as Dairy Cooperatives. These are especially important for smaller scale farms, where the construction of dairy factories is expensive and cannot be carried out by a single farmer and where the competitiveness creates the need and the opportunity for teamwork from smaller farmers. In this stage, animal manure and agricultural residues can be gathered from the farm to be processed as biomass or to produce fertilizers, saving resources and money and protecting the aquifer from chemical contamination.

- **Processing/ Manufacturing Stage**: This is the main field of application of the CE concept. During the Dairy Processing, which includes all the chemical and industrial processes, the dairy products, co-products and by-products are produced with the use of the previous stage's raw material resulting in waste, i.e. wastewaters and unusable whey. This waste however can be used for electricity, heat, transportation fuel, and fertilizers production with the use of the appropriate technologies. The products are later on packaged in order to be transported to the next stage.

- **Distribution & Marketing**: This is the most important stage of all in the value chain in general, as the product is being sold to the consumer through Supermarkets, Foodservice Suppliers and Restaurants, or even directly through vending machines. From the above and according to Lowe & Gereffi (2009), supermarket is the most important middleman accounting for almost half of the total sales. On this stage, waste is created both by the consumer, who throws away the packaging or does not use all the product, but also the intermediaries who throw away a lot of the packaging and also have unsold product that can be reused and recycled in accordance to the CE principles.

Figure 1. The dairy supply chain adapted from Lowe & Gereffi (2009)

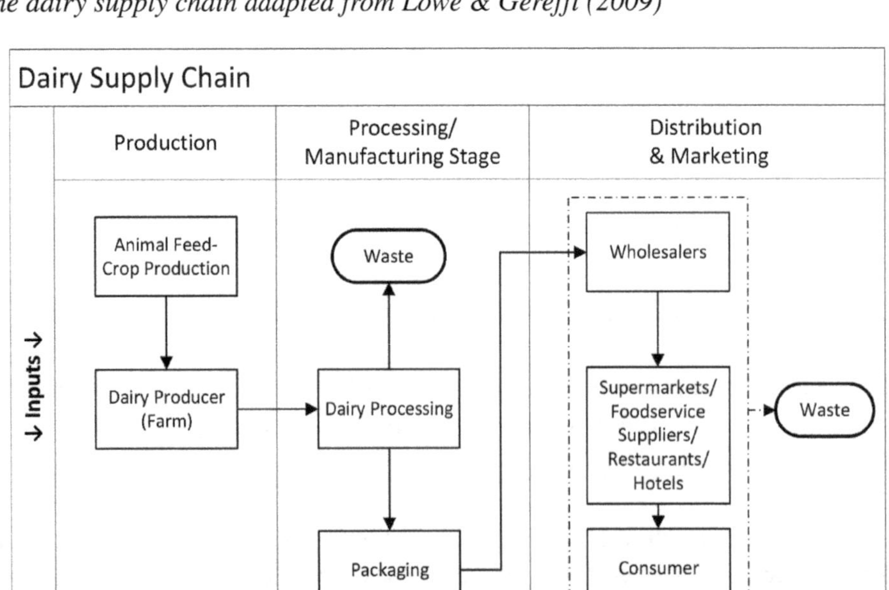

The main outputs of the dairy supply chain are (a) waste and (b) emissions to air, soil and water mainly during the dairy processing. There are two types of waste: one is the organic waste i.e. milk residues, dairy products that go to waste, damaged goods, out-of-date products and wastewaters and the inorganic waste which is the packaging. In order to better understand the first, the dairy production process is presented in Figure 2 based on the relevant bibliography (Durham & Hourigan, 2007; Fenyvessy, Csanádi, & Eszes, 2007; Peacock, 1996). There are three main production phases:

Phase One: The raw milk, after being transported from the farm, is received and stored in the facility.
Phase Two: The milk is separated and standardized producing yogurt, butter, milk powder and certain types of cheese.
Phase Three: Pasteurization occurs, producing cheese and milk products.

Depending on the type of raw milk (it can be from cattle, sheep, goat or even other mammals), there are deferent types of products produce, thus the above phases match accordingly. For example, in the case of cattle milk, whole and skimmed milk products, cheese, milk powder, butter, yogurt, ice-cream, yoghurt desserts are derived.

All these products lead to two types of residues: wastewater and whey. Wastewater, depending on its consistency, is treated in several ways that will be analyzed in the "Wastewater Treatments" subsection of this section. Whey however, can be evaporated, electrodialyzed or ultrafiltrated and produce by-products that can be used back in the processing facilities to produce other dairy products, can be used as a product on its own, sold as a supplement or can even be used for other, non-dairy products (Durham & Hourigan, 2007; Fenyvessy, Csanádi, & Eszes, 2007).

Figure 2. The dairy processing

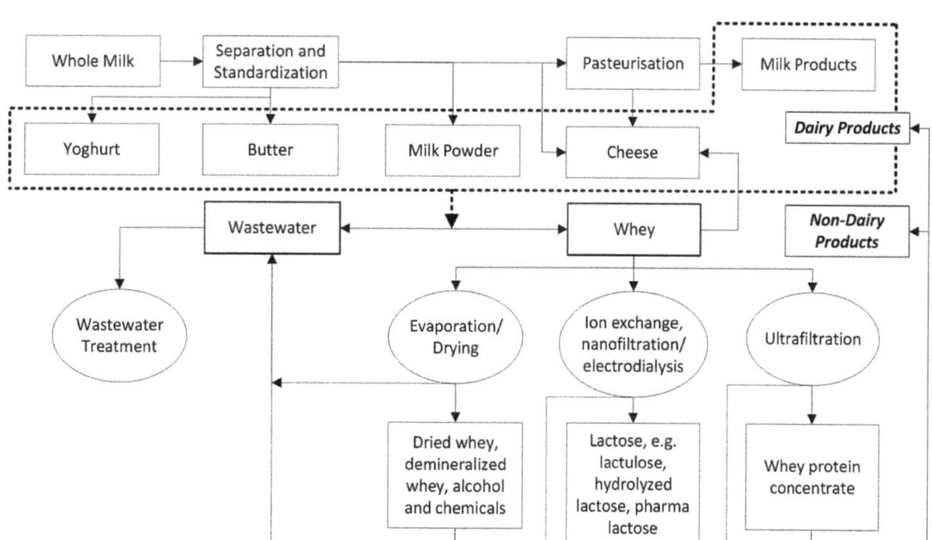

In the concept of CE, the open ends are transformed into closed-loops through technologies and recycle of materials (Murray, Skene, & Haynes, 2017; Urbinati, Chiaroni, & Chiesa, 2017; Winans et al., 2017). This system uses and restores waste in order to produce:

- materials e.g. using whey as an ingredient to produce cheese
- energy via the transformation of biomass into biofuel, electricity or heat
- water through wastewater management and
- feed for the livestock either directly (with the use of unneeded products and whey), or indirectly (by using it as a fertilizer)

In the case of the use of waste indirectly for the livestock nourishment, the chemicals needed as fertilizer or soil-amendment are reduced, possibly decreasing the business' expenses, while protecting the aquifer and reducing the waste produced from the packaging of such chemical substances.

As a result, the system's inputs and outputs are minimized, creating a more productive, sustainable and self-sufficient system where the produced waste is reduced or/and transformed into other products, by-products and co-products. In the following sections and subsections, a classification of relevant literature on technologies that can be implemented in the realms of the CE concept - according to the stage of the dairy supply chain as shown in Figure 1 - will be presented and analyzed.

Milk Production and Processing of Dairy Products

Anaerobic Digestion

Anaerobic digestion(AD) is the key element in a developing Circular Economy (European Biomass Association (EBA), 2015). First the manure, slurry or wastewater is being collected and placed pasteurized in a pre-storage tank in order to be used by the anaerobic digester, where in absence of oxygen and with the aid of its bacteria, the organic matter is broken down. This process results in two products: the biogas and the digestate (Mason & Burns, 2017).

Biogas can be used to produce electricity and/or heat or as a transport fuel. One of the most common uses is combined heat and power generation (CHP), resulting in electric power and hot water (Kılkış & Kılkış, 2017), which can be used by the farm's and the plant's facilities. There is also a possibility for the biogas to be fed into the natural gas system of the area after meeting certain standards (Kaltschmitt, Thrän, & Smith, 2003), while part of the heat can be reused from the anaerobic digestor, the stables and the factory. Biogas can also be used as a transport fuel and when enriched with CH4 it is a renewable biofuel with a competitive edge (Murphy & Power, 2006).

In the case of animal manure, for the production of energy, AD is preferable due to their high moisture (Gomez, Zubizarreta, Rodrigues, Dopazo, & Fueyo, 2010). For wastewaters from cheese processing, many researchers consider AD as the only method that is sustainable, while some suggest the use of another anaerobic treatment: the Upflow Anaerobic Sludge Blanket (UASB) reactors that can be applied to cheese whey wastewater whether it is diluted or not (Carvalho, Prazeres, & Rivas, 2013). This type of wastewater has a difficult composition due to the whey and cannot be easily processed.

Direct Combustion

Direct Combustion is the process of burning biomass without prior treatment, producing gases in high temperatures (Mckendry, 2002a). Although different types of biomass can be burned, a moisture content of less than 50% is essential, although biomass can be pre-dried (Iakovou, Karagiannidis, Vlachos, Toka, & Malamakis, 2010). The released heat has a number of applications; it can be used on the spot or be transported to another place of consumption as heat or be converted with a combined heat and power process (CHP) (Kaltschmitt et al., 2003).

Gasification

During gasification, biomass is converted to a gaseous fuel called synthesis gas (better known as syngas) by thermal decomposition in a limited oxygen environment (Kaltschmitt et al., 2003; Prapaspongsa, Poulsen, Hansen, & Christensen, 2010; Wu, 2013). It can produce two types of gas, Low Energy Gas and Medium Energy Gas which can result into different products, e.g. heat, steam, electricity, fuel gases, used for Internal Combustion Engines (Mckendry, 2002a) .

There are two basic types of gasifiers; the fixed bed and fluidized bed. The fixed bed method relies upon gravity for the feed of biomass, which slowly moves downward surpassing the mentioned above stages (Kaltschmitt et al., 2003). The biomass is (a) dried to remove moisture, (b) devolatilized (pyrolysis) resulting in tar gases, (c) combusted at around 1000 °C depending on the type of the gasifier producing carbon dioxide and heat, and while the hot gases pass upwards they are (d) reduced and hot gas leaves the system (Mckendry, 2002b). The issues with this gasifier are the bad temperature distribution, the time it needs to process and the high costs (Warnecke, 2000).

In the case of fluidized bed gasifiers, the temperature rise increases the produced gas and energy in general. The reactor is open ended and as the name suggests, the bed consists of a fluid material, such as sand or soil (Wu, 2013).

Pyrolysis

Pyrolysis is the process of decomposing biomass and breaking down the matter into smaller molecules in total absence or in a limited supply of air, producing gases, bio-char and bio-oil that can be used as a biofuel (Basu, 2018). Pyrolysis is also a part of other processes e.g. gasification (Mckendry, 2002b). There are also different types of pyrolysis' reactors, the most important being according to Nachenius, Ronsse, Venderbosch, & Prins (2013):

- **Fast pyrolysis Reactors:** in this case, the heating rates are high, the vapor residence time is low and the temperature is around 500 °C, producing bio-oil (Bridgwater, 1999; Sharma, Pareek, & Zhang, 2015).
- **Slow pyrolysis Reactors:** as the name suggests, this technology has significantly lower rates compared to fast pyrolysis, while it takes place at similar temperatures and produces mainly char and tar (Fahmy, Fahmy, Mobarak, El-Sakhawy, & Abou-Zeid, 2018)
- **Torrefaction Reactors:** these reactors convert the biomass at a much lower temperature ranging between 200-300 °C and can produce a high quality biofuel (van der Stelt, Gerhauser, Kiel, & Ptasinski, 2011).

Pyrolysis Coupled With AD

During the AD, a lot of the heat converted which is produced by the CHP system along with electricity is being lost due to the location of the farms, as they are usually isolated (Monlau, Sambusiti, Antoniou, Barakat, & Zabaniotou, 2015), thus it not as easily transportable near residential areas. At the same time, solid digestate from the anaerobic process is mostly used as a fertilizer (El-Mashad & Zhang, 2010; Tambone et al., 2010) or biofertilizer (Nizami et al., 2017; Stiles et al., 2018) with applications on-site (Ghisellini et al., 2014).

However, in order to intensify energy recovery from biomass and manure, Monlau et al. (2015) decided to use the produced digestate as a fuel for pyrolysis. The system is designed to take advantage of the produced heat from the CHP system that was untapped in order to dry out the digestate form AD, resulting in a solid digestate that can be used in Pyrolysis. With this method, syngas, bio-oil and bio-char were produced. The first two can be used for electrical production and the latter as a soil amendment.

The results were an increase of 42% in the produced kWh from the coupling of AD and Pyrolysis compared to stand-alone AD. Another benefit is that the bio-char can be used in the soil, which due to its composition of highly stable carbon (Hübner & Mumme, 2015; Monlau et al., 2016) which is a means of natural storage, thus further helping the environment by protecting it from the atmospheric Carbon Dioxide. Bio-char can also be used as a bio-absorbent, i.e. as a detoxifier of lignocellulosic hydrolysate, mainly from furans, in order for them to be used as biofuels (Monlau, Sambusiti, Antoniou, Zabaniotou, et al., 2015).

Wastewater Treatments

Wastewater is one of the most important wastes produced during dairy processing. Wastewater treatments can result not clean water that can be used again in the industry or the farm. Slavov (2017), outlines three types of wastewater:

- **Processing Wastewater:** This category mainly includes the wastewater produced from the cooling and drying procedures of dairy products.
- **Cleaning Wastewater:** As the name suggests, this wastewater is usually the water used to clean equipment that was in contact with the milk or other dairy products.
- **Sanitary Wastewater:** This is like the municipal wastewater and can be treated as such.

Depending on the type of wastewater and its consistency, different treatments are advised. Examples of such treatments are presented in the following subsections.

Discharge to the Municipal Sewage Treatment

Municipal Sewage Treatment facilities are the ones treating wastewater from municipal waste but can treat certain amount of organic substances (Britz, van Schalkwyk, & Hung, 2006). However, although sanitary wastewater is similar to municipal wastewater and is often directly connected to the same sewage treatment plant (Kolev Slavov, 2017), for cleaning and processing dairy wastewater that is not always the case, thus pre-treatment is often advised.

Reverse Osmosis

Reverse Osmosis (RO) for water treatment is a process where a membrane collects and rejects particulates dissolved in the water which is pressured through said membrane (Malaeb & Ayoub, 2011) RO treatment of the dairy wastewaters can produce water that can be used by the processing facilities as well as a milk-based by-product that can be used for dairy products e.g. dulce de leche (Brião, Vieira Salla, Miorando, Hemkemeier, & Cadore Favaretto, 2019). Vourch, Balannec, Chaufer, & Dorange (2008) consider that an extra stage of RO could be added to achieve drinking water requirements to the 11 French dairy plants they investigated. Thus, depending on the method of RO, the facility can retrieve water of satisfactory quality for the processing facilities or consumption and components for dairy products.

Aerobic Processes

Aerobic processes, unlike the anaerobic, take place in the presence of oxygen. In this case there are aerobic micro-organisms that break down organic matter such as manure, wastewaters and other types of biomass. Different types of aerobic processes exist and are applicable in the case of the production of dairy products.

Aerobic Composting

The aerobic composting process starts by piling the organic matter, whose temperature increases as micro-organisms are metabolizing the matter, and is followed by a "curing stage", where temperature decreases. In the end, the material becomes darker and more soil-like (Misra, Roy, & Hiraoka, 2003). Passive composting is also a very common practice, where the organic waste is simply left to compost over a long period of time with slow aeration rate.

In the case of dairy farms, this technology can be utilized mainly for the animal manure. It is important to state here that passive composting has been a common practice for many years as in farms manure is being directly used as a fertilizer.

Activated Sludge Process (ASP)

This method is applicable to both industrial and domestic wastewaters, is space-saving and results in a satisfactory quality outflow (von Sperling, 2007). The inflow originates from the primary treatment, where the wastewater enters and the first sludge is removed (Ahansazan, Afrashteh, Ahansazan, & Ahansazan, 2014). According to van Sperling (2007), in the aeration tank the biochemical reaction takes place in the presence of oxygen and with the growth of organisms such as bacteria, fungi and protozoa (Bhargava, 2016). Afterwards, the secondary sedimentation tank is where the solid biomass settles, and the remaining wastewater is the clarified effluent. The biomass is recirculated where feasible, acting as a new influent to the system, while the unusable sludge will be treated in the sludge treatment stage.

This process is important for the treatment of wastewater from the factory is of dairy products, the farm or a slaughterhouse. The result is reusable water, which can be repurposed in the farm or factory operations, while the reuse of the secondary sludge in the aeration is in accordance to the principles of CE. Further looking into the treatment or use of the excess sludge is necessary in order to make it more sustainable.

Dairy Wastewater Treatment Using Water Treatment Sludge as Coagulant

In a study using synthetic dairy wastewater, Suman, Tarique, & Kafeel (2018) attempt to utilize waste and residue for water treatment plants in order to process wastewaters from dairy. This resulted in significant removal of pollutants and turbidity, proving that at the same time dairy wastewater can be treated and sludge from the water treatment plants can be disposed.

Marketing/Consuming

At the last stage of the dairy supply chain, the product has been transported to the wholesalers who then sell the dairy goods to supermarkets, foodservice suppliers, restaurants and hotels in order for them to be bought and/or consumed by the final customer. During this process, both organic and inorganic waste is generated and should be treated. Thus, although in the supply chain of dairy products the main products are all the dairy products, by-products and co-products, there is also the packaging, which in many cases is excessive and usually plastic. In the concept of CE both types of waste should be treated.

Dealing With the Organic Waste

In the case of the wholesalers and the retailers, the expired or spoiled products are the main source of waste (Nizami et al., 2017). A possibility is the return of said products to the dairy processing facility in order to be treated like the onsite remaining products, i.e. as organic waste, or to produce other dairy products. However, this solution is not viable in the case of bigger supply chains, as transportation uses resources and pollutes the environment. In those cases, marketing strategies may be adopted e.g. lowering the prices of products that are close to be out-of-date in order to avoid having to throw away these products.

The consumer may have a similar waste profile; however alternative measures are advised. The usual routes to the household organic waste are (a) the sewer, (b) curbside collection of residual waste, (c) food waste collections, (d) home composting and (e) using it as feed for their pets (Parfitt, Barthel, & Macnaughton, 2010). From these methods of discarding waste, food waste collections, home composting and use of it as pet food are sustainable practices and in accordance to the CE principles since they restore natural resources, thus preserving and enhancing the natural capital (Ellen MacArthur Foundation & McKinsey Center for Business and Environment, 2015).

Packaging

As with most products, packaging is a part of the dairy supply chain, whether it is bought in bulk, e.g. cheese from a cheese shop, or pre-packaged e.g. from the fridges at the supermarket. Over the past few years, the reduction, the weight, the recyclability and the renewability of packaging has gathered interest (Vasilaki, Katsou, Ponsá, & Colón, 2016). The amount of packaging of products is proportionate to the dairy product's environmental impact (Finnegan, Goggins, & Zhan, 2018), thus the packaging plays an important role to the sustainability and the environmental profile of the product. At the same time, the quality and type of packaging affects the food security and shelf life of the product which should not be compromised (Conte, Cappelletti, Nicoletti, Russo, & Nobile, 2015), as it affects the human health and can produce waste i.e. the product will be thrown away and be wasted if due to the incorrect packaging it gets spoiled.

To that end, a strategic design of the supply chain in terms of packaging is necessary for dairy products. In the literature review, there are two categories of packaging that are in harmony with the CE principles:

- **Recyclable Packaging**: In this category different types of packaging are suggested depending on the product: glass bottles (which are 100% and indefinitely recyclable), aluminum caps, polyethylene labels, polystyrene caps, cartons (Vasilaki et al., 2016), complete propylene, tin or carton and polyethylene (Conte et al., 2015) are only some of the types of packaging found in the bibliography. It is also important to point out that, when sold to the wholesalers, the shops and eating establishments, they are usually in cardboard boxes and/or plastic protective films to be easily transported. Plastics, cardboard and glass can be recycled (Vasilaki et al., 2016), while thinner products are more sustainable (Conte et al., 2015), thus during package design they both recyclability and thickness of the material should be taken into account.
- **Biobased Packaging**: During the past few years, bio based materials for limited shelf-life products have been introduced and research, product development and investments on biopolymers have made (Jacobsen, Holm, & Mortensen, 2008). Biobased packaging is renewable and sometimes compostable and can be a solution on waste management issues from disposable packaging and can represent a CE system on its own (Casarejos, Bastos, Rufin, & Frota, 2018).

SOLUTIONS AND RECOMMENDATIONS

In the previous section, the technological and strategical solutions that can help design a dairy supply chain from a CE perspective by closing the open ends and creating a closed loop system were analyzed based on the stage they can be applied at. In Figure 3, the desired system is presented.

As shown in Figure 3, the dairy supply chain from a CE perspective, based on Figure 1 and maintaining the same four categories has new product and material flows. The waste created during the Processing/Manufacturing stage, often combined with the dairy waste created during the consumption period, can be used to produce energy, water and fertilizer using the technologies of the previous section of this chapter. This results in less inputs for the system during the production stage, both for animal feed production and the farm, thus creating a more sustainable and self-sufficient supply system.

During the Distribution and Marketing period, waste can be divided to dairy waste and packaging waste. Dairy waste can be processed along with the waste created during the previous stage, as mentioned above. Packaging can recycled or be biodegradable when possible in order to reduce pollution.

During the Processing/Manufacturing stage, Dairy Processing produces waste which can be divided into four categories in order of preference in a CE Framework:

1. Reusable: this category includes all the products, co-products and by-products that can be reintroduced as materials in order to produce products.
2. Suitable for energy or water production: biomass and wastewaters can be treated through a vast number of technologies to produce energy e.g. through A.D. or provide usable water. This energy and water can be used by the facilities or the farm.

3.   Treatable: the materials and wastewaters that cannot be treated for energy should be processed in order to be environmentally safe e.g. with wastewater management.
4.   Untreatable: in the end, there are materials that cannot be otherwise treated and have to be discarded.

During the Distribution and Marketing Stage, the waste is produced from Packaging and from Products that are out of date or thrown away:

1.   Packaging: the dairy products are packaged both to be bought from the consumer as well as to be transported to be sold in bulk. During the product design, the company should aim to the minimization, recyclability and renewability/biodegradability/compostability of packaging when possible. Informing the shoppers on how to properly recycle or bring the packaging back to the sellers for reimbursement in the case of returnable packaging, e.g. glass milk bottles, is also necessary to ensure optimal results.
2.   Wasted Dairy Products: The dairy waste produced from the sellers (whether they are wholesalers, retailers or eating establishments) should be minimized. Two possible strategies are:
     a.   Selling the products close to the expiration date at a lower cost to attract more customers.
     b.   Giving the products close to the expiration date to organizations thus demonstrating social responsibility.

If none of the above choices are eligible, the remaining products can be sent back to the processing facilities to produce other products or be treated along with the facility's waste.

Figure 3. A CE perspective of the dairy supply chain

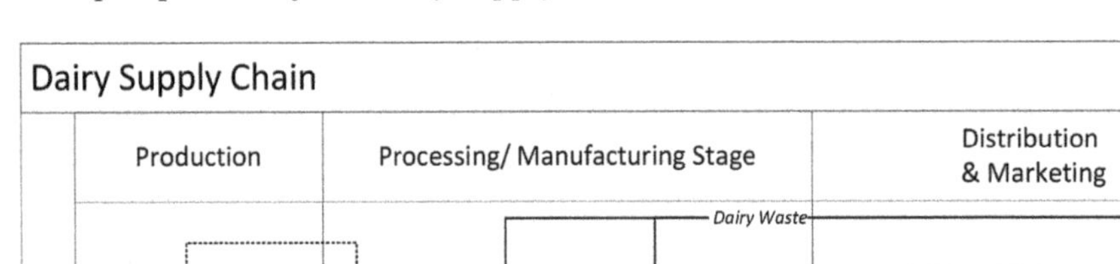

FUTURE RESEARCH DIRECTIONS

The CE concept is an emerging topic over the past few years due to the irrational use of Earth's natural capital causing resource depletion, especially after World War II. In combination with the projections of International Organisms that show a sharp increase of the world population by the year 2050, which will lead to the need of more land, food and water, the CE concept is for many the sustainable solution to a possible socio-economic crisis on the rise, thus recently it has been thoroughly studied by many researchers, companies and countries.

At this point, sustainability, waste management, closed-loop models and practices have been more thoroughly investigated and applied in businesses. At the same time, applications of CE in supply chains are minimal, due to the fact that the term is relatively new. In the case of agro-food supply chains and especially dairy supply chains, there are only a few recorded cases. In the future, such models should be designed, simulated and applied in order to optimize the performance and circularity of supply chains. With the progress of technology, more solutions can be developed in order to provide greener, more efficient and lower cost CE solutions.

CONCLUSION

The pressing need to resolve the emerging environmental issues has led researchers, businesses, organizations and countries to search for solutions that can balance the protection of the environment and the satisfaction of people's wants and needs. This has created the sustainability concept, which has been in the center of attention for over 20 years. There are many papers theoretical frameworks as well as implementation examples of sustainable supply chains, sustainable design and development and sustainable business practices; the research however is far from over.

More recently, CE has emerged as sustainability's successor and has received a lot of attention, especially in the European Union and China. Many researchers see similarities between the two concepts since they are both aiming to the protect the environment. However, in bibliography CE is applied specifically by closing the loops of the overall supply chain of a product and applying the 4R framework i.e. "reducing, reusing, recycling and recovering" the waste in the supply chain.

At the same time, world population is continuously rising and thus issues with food and water security arise. In order to cover the increased needs is a sustainable way, CE principles can be applied on agri-food supply chains. This chapter focuses on a category of products of wide consumption; the dairy products. This particular supply chain consists of a variety of products, with different consistencies, shelf lives and temperatures of storage, that are produced from various types and sizes of businesses. In order to close the loops, there are several different technologies and available strategies.

During the production stage, where the raw material i.e. milk is produced, and the processing/manufacturing stage, there are alternative ways to treat biomass in order to produce energy, fertilizer, with AD getting most commonly mentioned, and materials that can make other products, by-products and co-products. Wastewater treatment is also an important procedure which can provide the supply chain with water and extra biomass. During the marketing and consuming stage, the main source of waste is packaging, which in a CE should be recycled; thus, when designing such a supply chain the amount of packaging as well as it recyclability, reusability or biodegradability should be taken into consideration during the product's design and the consumer should be informed on how to appropriately dispose of it. However, during this stage there is leftover product that either expires or gets spoiled. To avoid this, close-to-expire products should be sold at a lower price or made available to humanitarian organizations, while the rest should be treated as biomass.

In conclusion, although in theory there are many technological and strategical solutions applicable from a CE perspective on the dairy supply chain, in practice there are not many examples of such applications which constitutes a real challenge. In the future, the design, simulation and implementation of such practices is necessary as different combinations of technologies could bring different results, while the technological evolution could bring new solutions. At the same time, further research on waste management and in particular biomass management and packaging materials is necessary. Following these recommendations could further improve and optimize CE and the dairy supply chain.

REFERENCES

Ahansazan, B., Afrashteh, H., Ahansazan, N., & Ahansazan, Z. (2014). Activated Sludge Process Overview. *International Journal of Environmental Sciences and Development*, *5*(1), 81–85. doi:10.7763/IJESD.2014.V5.455

Basu, P. (2018). *Biomass gasification, pyrolysis and torrefaction : practical design and theory* (3rd ed.). Academic Press.

Bhargava, A. (2016). Activated Sludge Treatment Process - Concept and System Design. *International Journal of Engineering Development and Research*, *4*(2), 890–896. Retrieved from www.ijedr.org

Blades, L., Morgan, K., Douglas, R., Glover, S., De Rosa, M., Cromie, T., & Smyth, B. (2017). Circular Biogas-Based Economy in a Rural Agricultural Setting. *Energy Procedia*, *123*, 89–96. doi:10.1016/j.egypro.2017.07.255

Brião, V. B., Vieira Salla, A. C., Miorando, T., Hemkemeier, M., & Cadore Favaretto, D. P. (2019). Water recovery from dairy rinse water by reverse osmosis: Giving value to water and milk solids. *Resources, Conservation and Recycling*, *140*, 313–323. doi:10.1016/j.resconrec.2018.10.007

Bridgwater, A. V. (1999). Principles and practice of biomass fast pyrolysis processes for liquids. *Journal of Analytical and Applied Pyrolysis*, *51*(1-2), 3–22. doi:10.1016/S0165-2370(99)00005-4

Britz, T. J., van Schalkwyk, C., & Hung, Y.-T. (2006). Treatment of Dairy Processing Wastewaters. In L. K. Wang, Y.-T. Hung, H. H. Lo, & C. Yapijakis (Eds.), *Waste Treatment in the Food Processing Industry* (pp. 1–28). CRC Press. doi:10.1201/9781420037128.ch1

Carvalho, F., Prazeres, A. R., & Rivas, J. (2013). Cheese whey wastewater: Characterization and treatment. *The Science of the Total Environment*, *445-446*, 385–396. doi:10.1016/j.scitotenv.2012.12.038 PMID:23376111

Casarejos, F., Bastos, C. R., Rufin, C., & Frota, M. N. (2018). Rethinking packaging production and consumption vis-à-vis circular economy: A case study of compostable cassava starch-based material. *Journal of Cleaner Production*, *201*, 1019–1028. doi:10.1016/j.jclepro.2018.08.114

Commission Staff. (2014). *Towards a circular economy: a zero waste programme for Europe*. Retrieved from http://ec.europa.eu/transparency/regexpert/

Conte, A., Cappelletti, G. M., Nicoletti, G. M., Russo, C., & Del Nobile, M. A. (2015). Environmental implications of food loss probability in packaging design. *Food Research International*, *78*, 11–17. doi:10.1016/j.foodres.2015.11.015 PMID:28433271

Durham, R. J., & Hourigan, J. A. (2007). Waste management and co-product recovery in dairy processing. In K. Waldron (Ed.), *Handbook of waste managment and co-product recovery in food processing* (pp. 332–387). Cambridge, UK: Woodhead Publishing Limited and CRC Press LLC. doi:10.1533/9781845692520.4.332

El-Mashad, H. M., & Zhang, R. (2010). Biogas production from co-digestion of dairy manure and food waste. *Bioresource Technology*, *101*(11), 4021–4028. doi:10.1016/j.biortech.2010.01.027 PMID:20137909

Ellen MacArthur Foundation. (2012). *Towards the Circular Economy: Economic and business rationale for an accelerated transition*. Retrieved from http://circularfoundation.org/sites/default/files/tce_report1_2012.pdf

Ellen MacArthur Foundation. (2013). *Towards the Circular Economy Economic and business rationale for an accelerated transition* (Vol. 1). Author. doi:10.1162/108819806775545321

Ellen MacArthur Foundation, & McKinsey Center for Business and Environment. (2015). *Growth Within: a Circular Economy Vision for a Competitive Europe*. Author. Retrieved from https://www.ellenmacarthurfoundation.org/assets/downloads/publications/EllenMacArthurFoundation_Growth-Within_July15.pdf

European Biomass Association (EBA). (2015). *Contribution of anaerobic digestion to the European Circular Economy*. Brussels. Retrieved from www.european-biogas.eu

Fahmy, T. Y. A., Fahmy, Y., Mobarak, F., El-Sakhawy, M., & Abou-Zeid, R. E. (2018). Biomass pyrolysis: Past, present, and future. *Environment, Development and Sustainability*. doi:10.100710668-018-0200-5

FAO. (2011). Extent of food losses and waste. In *Global food losses and food waste – Extent, causes and prevention* (pp. 4–9). Rome: Food and Agriculture Organization of the United Nations. Retrieved from http://www.fao.org/docrep/014/mb060e/mb060e02.pdf

FAO. (2013). *MILK and dairy products in human nutrition*. Rome. Retrieved from www.fao.org/

FAO. (2018). *FAOSTAT- Production Indices*. Retrieved January 12, 2019, from http://www.fao.org/faostat/en/#data/QI

Fenyvessy, J., Csanádi, J., & Eszes, F. (2007). Product Development Utilising Sheep Milk Whey. *Review of Faculty of Engineering: Analecta Technica Szegedinensia*, 37–41. Retrieved from http://acta.bibl.u-szeged.hu/11758/1/engineering_2007_037-041.pdf

Ferreira, A., Marques, P., Ribeiro, B., Assemany, P., de Mendonça, H. V., Barata, A., ... Gouveia, L. (2018). Combining biotechnology with circular bioeconomy: From poultry, swine, cattle, brewery, dairy and urban wastewaters to biohydrogen. *Environmental Research*, *164*, 32–38. doi:10.1016/j.envres.2018.02.007 PMID:29475106

Finnegan, W., Goggins, J., & Zhan, X. (2018). Assessing the environmental impact of the dairy processing industry in the Republic of Ireland. *The Journal of Dairy Research*, *85*(3), 396–399. doi:10.1017/S0022029918000559 PMID:30088466

Geissdoerfer, M., Savaget, P., Bocken, N. M. P., & Hultink, E. J. (2017). The Circular Economy – A new sustainability paradigm? *Journal of Cleaner Production*, *143*, 757–768. doi:10.1016/j.jclepro.2016.12.048

Ghisellini, P., Cialani, C., & Ulgiati, S. (2016). A review on circular economy: The expected transition to a balanced interplay of environmental and economic systems. *Journal of Cleaner Production*, *114*, 11–32. doi:10.1016/j.jclepro.2015.09.007

Ghisellini, P., Protano, G., Viglia, S., Gaworski, M., Setti, M., & Ulgiati, S. (2014). Integrated Agricultural and Dairy Production within a Circular Economy Framework. A Comparison of Italian and Polish Farming Systems. *Journal of Environmental Accounting and Management*, *2*(4), 372–391. doi:10.5890/JEAM.2014.12.007

Gomez, A., Zubizarreta, J., Rodrigues, M., Dopazo, C., & Fueyo, N. (2010). Potential and cost of electricity generation from human and animal waste in Spain. *Renewable Energy*, *35*(2), 498–505. doi:10.1016/j.renene.2009.07.027

Haas, W., Krausmann, F., Wiedenhofer, D., & Heinz, M. (2015). How Circular is the Global Economy?: An Assessment of Material Flows, Waste Production, and Recycling in the European Union and the World in 2005. *Journal of Industrial Ecology*, *19*(5), 765–777. doi:10.1111/jiec.12244

Hübner, T., & Mumme, J. (2015). Integration of pyrolysis and anaerobic digestion – Use of aqueous liquor from digestate pyrolysis for biogas production. *Bioresource Technology*, *183*, 86–92. doi:10.1016/j.biortech.2015.02.037 PMID:25725406

Iakovou, E., Karagiannidis, A., Vlachos, D., Toka, A., & Malamakis, A. (2010). Waste biomass-to-energy supply chain management: A critical synthesis. *Waste Management (New York, N.Y.)*, *30*(10), 1860–1870. doi:10.1016/j.wasman.2010.02.030 PMID:20231084

Jacobsen, M., Holm, V., & Mortensen, G. (2008). Biobased Packaging of Dairy Products. In E. Chiellini (Ed.), *Environmentally Compatible Food Packaging* (pp. 478–495). Cambridge, UK: Woodhead Publishing Limited and CRC Press LLC. doi:10.1533/9781845694784.3.478

Jiao, W., & Boons, F. (2014). Toward a research agenda for policy intervention and facilitation to enhance industrial symbiosis based on a comprehensive literature review. *Journal of Cleaner Production*, *67*, 14–25. doi:10.1016/j.jclepro.2013.12.050

Jiao, W., & Boons, F. (2017). Policy durability of Circular Economy in China: A process analysis of policy translation. *Resources, Conservation and Recycling*, *117*, 12–24. doi:10.1016/j.resconrec.2015.10.010

Kaltschmitt, M., Thrän, D., & Smith, K. R. (2003). Renewable Energy from Biomass. In *Encyclopedia of Physical Science and Technology* (pp. 203–228). Academic Press. doi:10.1016/B0-12-227410-5/00059-4

Kılkış, Ş., & Kılkış, B. (2017). Integrated circular economy and education model to address aspects of an energy-water-food nexus in a dairy facility and local contexts. *Journal of Cleaner Production*, *167*, 1084–1098. doi:10.1016/j.jclepro.2017.03.178

Kirchherr, J., Reike, D., & Hekkert, M. (2017). Conceptualizing the circular economy: An analysis of 114 definitions. *Resources, Conservation and Recycling, 127*(September), 221–232. doi:10.1016/j.resconrec.2017.09.005

Kolev Slavov, A. (2017). Dairy Wastewaters – General Characteristics and Treatment Possibilities – A Review. *Food Technology and Biotechnology, 55*(1), 14–28. doi:10.17113/ftb.55.01.17.4520 PMID:28559730

Korhonen, J., Honkasalo, A., & Seppälä, J. (2018). Circular Economy: The Concept and its Limitations. *Ecological Economics, 143*, 37–46. doi:10.1016/j.ecolecon.2017.06.041

Lowe, M., & Gereffi, G. (2009). *A Value Chain Analysis of the U.S. Beef and Dairy Industries.* doi:10.13140/RG.2.1.1502.9523

Malaeb, L., & Ayoub, G. M. (2011). Reverse osmosis technology for water treatment: State of the art review. *Desalination, 267*(1), 1–8. doi:10.1016/j.desal.2010.09.001

Mason, S., & Burns, C. (2017). *Biomass Supply Chain Evaluation.* Retrieved from: http://multisite.iris.cat/agrocycle/files/2017/11/D6.2-Biomass-Supply-Chains.V3.compressed.pdf

Mckendry, P. (2002a). Energy production from biomass (part 2): Conversion technologies. *Bioresource Technology, 83*(1), 47–54. doi:10.1016/S0960-8524(01)00119-5 PMID:12058830

Mckendry, P. (2002b). Energy production from biomass (part 3): Gasification technologies. *Bioresource Technology, 83*(1), 55–63. doi:10.1016/S0960-8524(01)00120-1 PMID:12058831

Misra, R. V., Roy, R. N., & Hiraoka, H. (2003). *On-farm composting methods.* Retrieved from http://www.fao.org/3/a-y5104e.pdf

Monlau, F., Francavilla, M., Sambusiti, C., Antoniou, N., Solhy, A., Libutti, A., ... Monteleone, M. (2016). Toward a functional integration of anaerobic digestion and pyrolysis for a sustainable resource management. Comparison between solid-digestate and its derived pyrochar as soil amendment. *Applied Energy, 169*, 652–662. doi:10.1016/j.apenergy.2016.02.084

Monlau, F., Sambusiti, C., Antoniou, N., Barakat, A., & Zabaniotou, A. (2015). A new concept for enhancing energy recovery from agricultural residues by coupling anaerobic digestion and pyrolysis process. *Applied Energy, 148*, 32–38. doi:10.1016/j.apenergy.2015.03.024

Monlau, F., Sambusiti, C., Antoniou, N., Zabaniotou, A., Solhy, A., & Barakat, A. (2015). Pyrochars from bioenergy residue as novel bio-adsorbents for lignocellulosic hydrolysate detoxification. *Bioresource Technology, 187*, 379–386. doi:10.1016/j.biortech.2015.03.137 PMID:25863902

Murphy, J. D., & Power, N. M. (2006). A Technical, Economic and Environmental Comparison of Composting and Anaerobic Digestion of Biodegradable Municipal Waste. *Journal of Environmental Science and Health. Part A, 41*(5), 865–879. doi:10.1080/10934520600614488 PMID:16702064

Murray, A., Skene, K., & Haynes, K. (2017). The Circular Economy: An Interdisciplinary Exploration of the Concept and Application in a Global Context. *Journal of Business Ethics, 140*(3), 369–380. doi:10.100710551-015-2693-2

Nachenius, R. W., Ronsse, F., Venderbosch, R. H., & Prins, W. (2013). Biomass Pyrolysis. In G. B. Marin, D. H. West, J. Li, & S. Narasimhan (Eds.), *Advances in Chemical Engineering* (Vol. 42, pp. 75–139). Academic Press. doi:10.1016/B978-0-12-386505-2.00002-X

Naustdalslid, J. (2014). Circular economy in China – the environmental dimension of the harmonious society. *International Journal of Sustainable Development and World Ecology*, *21*(4), 303–313. doi:10.1080/13504509.2014.914599

Nizami, A. S., Rehan, M., Waqas, M., Naqvi, M., Ouda, O. K., Shahzad, K., ... Pant, D. (2017). Waste biorefineries: Enabling circular economies in developing countries. *Bioresource Technology*, *241*, 1101–1117. doi:10.1016/j.biortech.2017.05.097 PMID:28579178

Parfitt, J., Barthel, M., & Macnaughton, S. (2010). Food waste within food supply chains: Quantification and potential for change to 2050. *Philosophical Transactions of the Royal Society of London. Series B, Biological Sciences*, *365*(1554), 3065–3081. doi:10.1098/rstb.2010.0126 PMID:20713403

Peacock, C. (1996). Processing and marketing goat products. In *Improving Goat Production in the Tropics: A manual for development workers* (pp. 307–363). Oxfam and FARM-Africa. doi:10.3362/9780855987732.007

Prapaspongsa, T., Poulsen, T. G., Hansen, J. A., & Christensen, P. (2010). Energy production, nutrient recovery and greenhouse gas emission potentials from integrated pig manure management systems. *Waste Management & Research*, *28*(5), 411–422. doi:10.1177/0734242X09338728 PMID:19723830

Preston, F. (2012). *A Global Redesign? Shaping the Circular Economy*. Retrieved from www.mckinseyquarterly.com/The_second_economy_2853

Sharma, A., Pareek, V., & Zhang, D. (2015). Biomass pyrolysis—A review of modelling, process parameters and catalytic studies. *Renewable & Sustainable Energy Reviews*, *50*, 1081–1096. doi:10.1016/j.rser.2015.04.193

Stanchev, P., Vasilaki, V., & Katsou, E. (2017). Multilevel Environmental Assessment of Dairy Processing Industry in the Context Of Circular Economy. *5th International Conference on Sustainable Waste Management*. Retrieved from https://pdfs.semanticscholar.org/66a1/8671926cf493cc8f1d2a3d92e2082c6e818f.pdf?_ga=2.145837748.1221711423.1542979831-205321401.1542979831

Stiles, W. A. V., Styles, D., Chapman, S. P., Esteves, S., Bywater, A., Melville, L., ... Llewellyn, C. A. (2018). Using microalgae in the circular economy to valorise anaerobic digestate: Challenges and opportunities. *Bioresource Technology*, *267*, 732–742. doi:10.1016/j.biortech.2018.07.100 PMID:30076074

Suman, A., Ahmad, T., & Ahmad, K. (2018). Dairy wastewater treatment using water treatment sludge as coagulant: A novel treatment approach. *Environment, Development and Sustainability*, *20*(4), 1615–1625. doi:10.100710668-017-9956-2

Tambone, F., Scaglia, B., Schievano, A., Orzi, V., Salati, S., & Adani, F. (2010). Assessing amendment and fertilizing properties of digestates from anaerobic digestion through a comparative study with digested sludge and compost. *Chemosphere*, *81*(5), 577–583. doi:10.1016/j.chemosphere.2010.08.034 PMID:20825964

United Nations. (2017a). *UN Climate change - Annual Report 2017*. Retrieved from http://unfccc.int/resource/annualreport/media/UN-Climate-AR17.pdf

United Nations. (2017b). *World Population 2017. United Nations. Department of Economic and Social Affairs*. Population Division. doi:10.1093/nar/gkl248

Urbinati, A., Chiaroni, D., & Chiesa, V. (2017). Towards a new taxonomy of circular economy business models. *Journal of Cleaner Production*, *168*, 487–498. doi:10.1016/j.jclepro.2017.09.047

van der Stelt, M. J. C., Gerhauser, H., Kiel, J. H. A., & Ptasinski, K. J. (2011). Biomass upgrading by torrefaction for the production of biofuels: A review. *Biomass and Bioenergy*, *35*, 3748–3762. doi:10.1016/j.biombioe.2011.06.023

Vasilaki, V., Katsou, E., Ponsá, S., & Colón, J. (2016). Water and carbon footprint of selected dairy products: A case study in Catalonia. *Journal of Cleaner Production*, *139*, 504–516. doi:10.1016/j.jclepro.2016.08.032

Vega-Quezada, C., Blanco, M., & Romero, H. (2017). Synergies between agriculture and bioenergy in Latin American countries: A circular economy strategy for bioenergy production in Ecuador. *New Biotechnology*, *39*, 81–89. doi:10.1016/j.nbt.2016.06.730 PMID:27287049

von Sperling, M. (2007). *Activated Sludge and Aerobic Biofilm Reactors*. London: IWA Publishing. Retrieved from https://www.iwapublishing.com/sites/default/files/ebooks/9781780402123.pdf

Vourch, M., Balannec, B., Chaufer, B., & Dorange, G. (2008). Treatment of dairy industry wastewater by reverse osmosis for water reuse. *Desalination*, *219*(1-3), 190–202. doi:10.1016/j.desal.2007.05.013

Warnecke, R. (2000). Gasification of biomass: Comparison of fixed bed and fluidized bed gasifier. *Biomass and Bioenergy*, *18*(6), 489–497. doi:10.1016/S0961-9534(00)00009-X

Wijkman, A., & Skånberg, K. (2015a). *The Circular Economy and Benefits for Society, Jobs and Climate Clear Winners in an Economy Based on Renewable Energy and Resource Efficiency*. Retrieved from https://www.clubofrome.org/wp-content/uploads/2016/03/The-Circular-Economy-and-Benefits-for-Society.pdf

Wijkman, A., & Skånberg, K. (2015b). *The Circular Economy and Benefits for Society, Swedish Case Study Shows Jobs and Climate as Clear Winners*. Retrieved from http://wijkman.se/wp-content/uploads/2015/05/The-Circular-Economy-and-Benefits-for-Society.pdf

Winans, K., Kendall, A., & Deng, H. (2017). The history and current applications of the circular economy concept. *Renewable & Sustainable Energy Reviews*, *68*, 825–833. doi:10.1016/j.rser.2016.09.123

World Bank. (2019). *Employment in agriculture (% of total employment) (modeled ILO estimate) | Data*. Retrieved January 12, 2019, from https://data.worldbank.org/indicator/SL.AGR.EMPL.ZS?end=2017&start=1991&view=chart

Wu, H. (2013). *Biomass Gasification: An Alternative Solution to Animal Waste Management*. University of Nebraska-Lincoln. Retrieved from http://digitalcommons.unl.edu/biosysengdiss/34

ADDITIONAL READING

Bark, R., Achimescu, A., Neumann, C., & van Wijk, D. (2017). Supporting the circular economy transition: The role of the financial sector in the netherlands. Retrieved from https://www.oliverwyman.com/content/dam/oliver-wyman/v2/publications/2017/sep/CircularEconomy_print.pdf

Kiørboe, N., Sramkova, H., & Krarup, M. (2015). *Moving Towards a circular economy-successful Nordic business models. Nordic co-operation* (Vol. 771). Nordic Council of Ministers; doi:10.6027/ANP2015-771

Way, T. K., Ong, M., Kai, J., Ho, S., & Kan, M. (2016). Is your Waste a Waste? Rethinking the linear economy. Industry Watch, 3(2), 62–69. Retrieved from https://www.ellenmacarthurfoundation.org

KEY TERMS AND DEFINITIONS

Anaerobic Digestion: A process where in absence of oxygen and with the aid of its bacteria, the organic matter is broken down, resulting in biogas and digestate.

Bioenergy: The energy produces by processing the biomass.

Biomass: Organic matter that is usually used for energy production.

Circular Agriculture: The circular economy concept applied in agriculture.

Manure Management: The collection, storage, and processing of manure in order to provide mainly energy and fertilizer.

Wastewater Management: The processing of wastewater in order to be suitable to be discharged back to the environment or reused.

Whey: The effluent at the end of milk production which can be used as a product or be used for the production of other dairy products.

Whey Management: The storage and treatment of whey in order to provide new products or be processed as biomass.

This research was previously published in the Handbook of Research on Interdisciplinary Approaches to Decision Making for Sustainable Supply Chains edited by Anjali Awasthi and Katarzyna Grzybowska; pages 73-93, copyright year 2020 by Business Science Reference (an imprint of IGI Global).

Chapter 21
Consumer Purchase Preference for the Perception of Quality of Perishable Products in a Smart City

Iván Alonso Rebollar-Xochicale
Universidad Autónoma de Querétaro, Mexico

Fernando Maldonado-Azpeitia
Universidad Autónoma de Querétaro, Mexico

ABSTRACT

Freshness, flavor, presentation, and nutritional value of fruits and vegetables deteriorate as time passes. That is why the correct implementation of supply chains is a subject of great interest for companies dedicated to the rotation of food marketing. Consumers play a particularly important role: the interaction between the retailer and the consumer determines the waste of food along the supply chain. The consumer's choice behavior and the perception of what is acceptable (or not) affect the management of the offer in the different points of sale dedicated to this line of business, as well as the aesthetic standards to be applied when distributing the products. This chapter explores consumer purchase preference for the perception of perishable products in a smart city.

INTRODUCTION

Natural and desirable properties of fruits and vegetables are at their best just after harvesting; in the same way, it can be said that prepared foods have the same aspects mentioned just after finishing their preparation. These values decrease as time goes until that food products lose them entirely. It can be said that the quality is 100% when the load can be sold without losses at the current market price (Osvald and Stirn, 2007). The difficulty in preserving the nutritional characteristics of fresh foods during transportation presents a direct problem for distributors and food traders where the perishability of the

DOI: 10.4018/978-1-7998-5354-1.ch021

product requires that it be handled in ways not necessarily conducive to the traditional view of profitable distribution activities. Highly perishable products play an essential role in the process of operational distribution, particularly in the planning task of supply chains. Supply chains are a topic of great interest for companies dedicated to the marketing of food, where an effort is required in the coordination of the actors, activities, and resources to meet the requirements of customers. Food Supply Chains (FSC), are integrated by networks of organizations that work together in different processes and activities to deliver products or services to the market and meet the demands of customers (Christopher, 2011), always caring the quality. The main problems encountered in the operation of the FSC are: 1) demand forecasting, 2) production planning, 3) inventory management and 4) transportation. Several factors affect the management of FSC, such as the management of information, the territory, the forms of organization and the types of the configuration according to how the demand is met.

The waste of food has been identified as a problem with different facets and levels in the food sector (AschemannWitzel, Hooge, Amani, Bech-Larsen, and Oostindjer, 2015) with an impact on aspects such as environmental, social and economic (Alexander, Brown, Arneth, Finnigan, Moran, Rounsevell, 2017). Especially in the economic sphere, in our country, micro and small businesses (MiPYMES) represent a significant source of employment and economic development for many Mexicans, according to official data provided by INEGI, there are 4.2 million commercial units in our country. Of all these companies, 99.8% are considered Micro, Small and Medium Enterprises (SMEs), they contribute 42% of the Gross Domestic Product (GDP) and currently generate 78% of employment in the country, according to information analyzed in the National Survey on Productivity and Competitiveness of Micro, Small and Medium Enterprises, (ENAPROCE) (ENAPROCE, 2015). The highest amount in the segment of microenterprises was registered in groceries and retail foods with 44.9% participation in economic units, occupying a critical place in the economy of the country since they present the characteristic of generating a lot of employment.

On the other hand, consumers play a particularly important role in the cause of food waste in industrialized countries, since around 40% of food waste is related to consumer households (FAO, 2013). Also, consumer behavior affects food wasted in homes (Stuart, 2009); and the interaction between the retailer and the consumer determines the waste of food along the supply chain (AschemannWitzel, Jensen, Jensen, and Kulikovskaja, 2017). An ordinary panorama in our country: stores offer a diversity of products and, in doing so, they influence how consumers are accustomed to seeing certain foods and picturing that the products are in "optimal" conditions to be consumed. There is also the possibility that changes in the FSC can also change the perception of the consumer. The consumer's choice behavior and the understanding of what is acceptable —or not— affect the management of the offer in different points of sale or business dedicated to this line, as well as the aesthetic standards to be applied when distributing the products, either by wholesale orders or home services. This is a reason to

1. Investigate the perception of the consumer regarding the quality of the food and what aspects are decisive at the time of purchase; and
2. Design strategies for MiPYME to standardize their FSC to maintain high standards of quality and aesthetics towards the consumer.

The present research focuses on obtaining and studying data to know the importance for consumers of the quality of the food products they consume, their confidence level of purchase in the different points of sale and what aspects they consider essential at the moment of shopping.

METHODOLOGY

The research consists in carrying out an analysis of consumers' perception of the population of the municipality of San Juan del Río, in the state of Querétaro, with the objective to obtain data that will allow us to know how important freshness is for consumers. Good presentation is the first perception of the quality of food products; but, which other factors are considered for the decision of purchase? For the determination of the sample, INEGI data were taken, which indicate that the number of inhabitants for 2015 of people between 18 and 60 years old is 268,408 people that we can consider as the total number of potential consumers in our population. The calculation was made with a confidence level of 90% and a margin of error of 10%, the sample size is at least 68 to obtain significant conclusions.

As a measuring instrument, a questionnaire was designed with the purpose of assessing whether the quality, freshness, and presentation of the food are relevant to the people when purchasing raw and prepared foods. In the same way, we seek to know how much consumers trust in the different types of businesses of market food: raw foods which we call "basic basket" in the questionnaire and prepared foods. This questionnaire was applied online via the "google surveys" platform for consumers in the state of Querétaro at random.

The first part of the questionnaire consists of four questions to know the demographic data of the participants which help us categorize them according to:

1. Age range
2. Gender
3. The maximum degree of studies
4. Current occupation

The second part of the questionnaire is focused on obtaining data that will provide us with an overview and better understand the following:

5. How concerned are you with the quality of the prepared or raw foods you eat?
6. How much confidence do you have in market-food businesses in terms of managing the FSC?
7. How do you perceive market-food businesses in terms of the information they have about their food management?
8. What aspects are more relevant to consumers and affect the decision to purchase food?
9. What is the preference level of the sales channels for raw foods?
10. What is the preference level of the sales channels for prepared foods?

From the questions described above, responses were established with Likert scales, depending on the subject they were evaluated according to the following parameters.

For question number five the parameters are:

1. Nothing worried
2. Something worried
3. Worried
4. Very worried
5. Pretty worried

For question number six the parameters are:

1. Very distrustful
2. Something distrustful
3. I am indistinct
4. Something trusting
5. Very confident

For question number seven the parameters are:

1. Not informed
2. Little informed
3. Informed
4. Somewhat informed
5. Very informed

For question number eight the parameters are:

1. Irrelevant
2. Little irrelevant
3. Relevant
4. Very relevant
5. Fairly relevant

For question number nine and ten, the parameters are:

1. No preference
2. Low preference
3. Preference
4. Total preference.

RESULTS AND DISCUSSION

According to the results obtained (shown in Table 1), it was found that, of the 68 participants in the survey, 69.1% are women and of which the vast majority (with 63.2%) is in an age range between 29 and 38 years old.

Table 2 shows that 63.2% of the participants have university studies and 47.1% work for companies that are owned by private investors. With this information, it can be established that the profile of the consumers with the highest interest in quality and presentation of food is professional women between 29 and 38 years'old who are employed in the private sector.

Table 1. Age range / gender

			Gender Type		Total
			Female	Male	
Age range in years	18 - 28	Count	11	3	14
		% within Age range in years	78.6%	21.4%	100.0%
		% within Gender type	23.4%	14.3%	20.6%
		% of the total	16.2%	4.4%	20.6%
	29 - 38	Count	30	13	43
		% within Age range in years	69.8%	30.2%	100.0%
		% within Gender type	63.8%	61.9%	63.2%
		% of the total	44.1%	19.1%	63.2%
	39 - 48	Count	5	1	6
		% within Age range in years	83.3%	16.7%	100.0%
		% within Gender type	10.6%	4.8%	8.8%
		% of the total	7.4%	1.5%	8.8%
	49 - 60	Count	1	2	3
		% within Age range in years	33.3%	66.7%	100.0%
		% within Gender type	2.1%	9.5%	4.4%
		% of the total	1.5%	2.9%	4.4%
	60 o más	Count	0	2	2
		% within Age range in years	0.0%	100.0%	100.0%
		% within Gender type	0.0%	9.5%	2.9%
		% of the total	0.0%	2.9%	2.9%
Total		Count	47	21	68
		% within Age range in years	69.1%	30.9%	100.0%
		% within Gender type	100.0%	100.0%	100.0%
		% of the total	69.1%	30.9%	100.0%

After knowing the profile of the respondents, an interesting fact (see Figure 1) describes that the vast majority, 39.7%, is "somewhat concerned" about the quality of food they consume. However, 29.4% are "very worried" and 23.5% are only "worried. According to the data, it can be concluded that the level of concern is high. So, if they are concerned about aspects such as nutritional value, freshness, and taste, such features are not crucial for consumption.

Another interesting fact reflected in Figure 2 is that for 36.7% of the participants the level of confidence in the food businesses is "indistinct" (only 32.3% are "somewhat distrustful"). For consumers, the confidence level of purchase in these businesses is relatively low, even more so if we consider that none of the respondents indicated that they felt "very confident" in buying their food at different points of sale.

Regarding the aspects that consumers consider relevant as a purchase decision, we can see the data described in Table 3. It was found that among consumers with a high level of concern, 65% considered that the quality can be perceived visually. In other words, that they can make judgments about the texture, color and presentation of the products to be consumed.

Table 2. Occupation / maximum degree of studies

			Maximum Grade of Studies			Total
			High School Degree	College Degree	Master's Degree	
Occupation of respondents	Public sector employee	Count	1	9	6	16
		% within Occupation of respondents	6.3%	56.3%	37.5%	100.0%
		% within Maximum grade of studies	25.0%	20.9%	28.6%	23.5%
		% of the total	1.5%	13.2%	8.8%	23.5%
	Private sector employee	Count	1	24	7	32
		% within Occupation of respondents	3.1%	75.0%	21.9%	100.0%
		% within Maximum grade of studies	25.0%	55.8%	33.3%	47.1%
		% of the total	1.5%	35.3%	10.3%	47.1%
	Freelance	Count	0	2	2	4
		% within Occupation of respondents	0.0%	50.0%	50.0%	100.0%
		% within Maximum grade of studies	0.0%	4.7%	9.5%	5.9%
		% of the total	0.0%	2.9%	2.9%	5.9%
	Entrepreneur / Independent	Count	2	8	6	16
		% within Occupation of respondents	12.5%	50.0%	37.5%	100.0%
		% within Maximum grade of studies	50.0%	18.6%	28.6%	23.5%
		% of the total	2.9%	11.8%	8.8%	23.5%
Total		Count	4	43	21	68
		% within Occupation of respondents	5.9%	63.2%	30.9%	100.0%
		% within Maximum grade of studies	100.0%	100.0%	100.0%	100.0%
		% of the total	5.9%	63.2%	30.9%	100.0%

Another critical aspect for the purchase decision is that the aesthetics or integrity of the packaging is in excellent condition since for 48.1% of the respondents this aspect was "quite relevant" (see Table 4).

Table 5 and 6 describe as consumers have little confidence in different points of sale. The "preference" to buy raw foods or basic food in small businesses is 59.1% (and 27.3% for "Little preference"). As for prepared foods, "the preference" for small businesses is 40.9%.

In the first instance, the level of confidence does not affect too much the purchase preference for small food businesses, but we do compare (see Figures 3 and 4) the purchase preference for the basic basket between small businesses and supermarkets, the latter are slightly preferred.

Figure 1. Level of concern

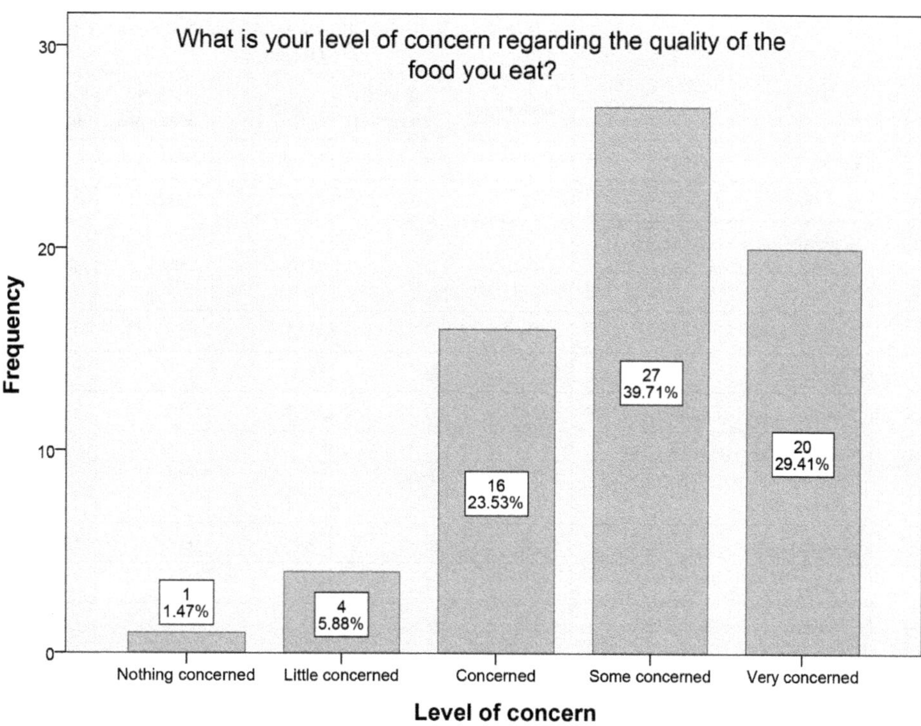

Figure 2. Confidence level

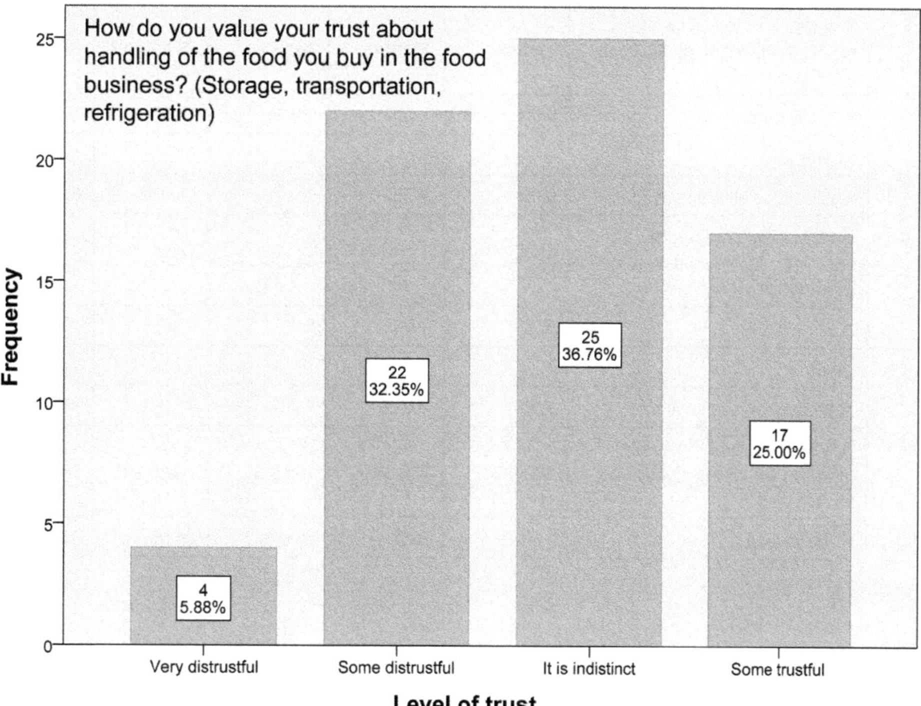

Table 3. Level of concern / Purchase relevance – Visual check

			Purchase Relevance Based on Which the Product Can Be Observed					Total
			Irrelevant	Little Relevant	Relevant	Very Relevant	Quite Relevant	
Level of concern	Nothing concerned	Count	0	0	0	1	0	1
		% within Level of concern	0.0%	0.0%	0.0%	100.0%	0.0%	100.0%
		% within Purchase relevance based on which the product can be observed	0.0%	0.0%	0.0%	5.9%	0.0%	1.5%
		% of the total	0.0%	0.0%	0.0%	1.5%	0.0%	1.5%
	Little concerned	Count	0	0	3	0	1	4
		% within Level of concern	0.0%	0.0%	75.0%	0.0%	25.0%	100.0%
		% within Purchase relevance based on which the product can be observed	0.0%	0.0%	17.6%	0.0%	3.8%	5.9%
		% of the total	0.0%	0.0%	4.4%	0.0%	1.5%	5.9%
	Concerned	Count	1	4	6	3	2	16
		% within Level of concern	6.3%	25.0%	37.5%	18.8%	12.5%	100.0%
		% within Purchase relevance based on which the product can be observed	100.0%	57.1%	35.3%	17.6%	7.7%	23.5%
		% of the total	1.5%	5.9%	8.8%	4.4%	2.9%	23.5%
	Some concerned	Count	0	3	4	10	10	27
		% within Level of concern	0.0%	11.1%	14.8%	37.0%	37.0%	100.0%
		% within Purchase relevance based on which the product can be observed	0.0%	42.9%	23.5%	58.8%	38.5%	39.7%
		% of the total	0.0%	4.4%	5.9%	14.7%	14.7%	39.7%
	Very concerned	Count	0	0	4	3	13	20
		% within Level of concern	0.0%	0.0%	20.0%	15.0%	65.0%	100.0%
		% within Purchase relevance based on which the product can be observed	0.0%	0.0%	23.5%	17.6%	50.0%	29.4%
		% of the total	0.0%	0.0%	5.9%	4.4%	19.1%	29.4%
Total		Count	1	7	17	17	26	68
		% within Level of concern	1.5%	10.3%	25.0%	25.0%	38.2%	100.0%
		% within Purchase relevance based on which the product can be observed	100.0%	100.0%	100.0%	100.0%	100.0%	100.0%
		% of the total	1.5%	10.3%	25.0%	25.0%	38.2%	100.0%

Table 4. Level of concern / Purchase relevance - Quality packaging

			Purchase Relevance Based on the Quality of the Packing				Total
			Little Relevant	Relevant	Very Relevant	Quite Relevant	
Level of concern	Nothing concerned	Count	0	0	1	0	1
		% within Level of concern	0.0%	0.0%	100.0%	0.0%	100.0%
		% within Purchase relevance based on the quality of the packing	0.0%	0.0%	5.3%	0.0%	1.5%
		% of the total	0.0%	0.0%	1.5%	0.0%	1.5%
	Little concerned	Count	1	2	0	1	4
		% within Level of concern	25.0%	50.0%	0.0%	25.0%	100.0%
		% within Purchase relevance based on the quality of the packing	33.3%	10.5%	0.0%	3.7%	5.9%
		% of the total	1.5%	2.9%	0.0%	1.5%	5.9%
	Concerned	Count	1	9	3	3	16
		% within Level of concern	6.3%	56.3%	18.8%	18.8%	100.0%
		% within Purchase relevance based on the quality of the packing	33.3%	47.4%	15.8%	11.1%	23.5%
		% of the total	1.5%	13.2%	4.4%	4.4%	23.5%
	Some concerned	Count	1	4	9	13	27
		% within Level of concern	3.7%	14.8%	33.3%	48.1%	100.0%
		% within Purchase relevance based on the quality of the packing	33.3%	21.1%	47.4%	48.1%	39.7%
		% of the total	1.5%	5.9%	13.2%	19.1%	39.7%
	Very concerned	Count	0	4	6	10	20
		% within Level of concern	0.0%	20.0%	30.0%	50.0%	100.0%
		% within Purchase relevance based on the quality of the packing	0.0%	21.1%	31.6%	37.0%	29.4%
		% of the total	0.0%	5.9%	8.8%	14.7%	29.4%
Total		Count	3	19	19	27	68
		% within Level of concern	4.4%	27.9%	27.9%	39.7%	100.0%
		% within Purchase relevance based on the quality of the packing	100.0%	100.0%	100.0%	100.0%	100.0%
		% of the total	4.4%	27.9%	27.9%	39.7%	100.0%

CONCLUSION

The data obtained with this research indicates that there is a high level of concern about the quality of the food consumed and therefore the level of confidence in the handling of these products by suppliers or marketers is low. Likewise, there are indications that the purchase decision is based mainly on what the product pretends to be makes the most significant plus value (judgments about appearance are more decisive than actual freshness and nutritional properties). In line with this idea, the integrity and aesthetics are essential too. On the other hand, we find that the purchase preference in small businesses is lesser than that of the supermarket chains, which have better tools and resources to ensure food handling during the supply chain. As a consequence, the design of a strategy that guides how to guarantee consumer preference standards in terms of storage, distribution and presentation of products to small businesses will improve their levels of purchase preference.

Table 5. Level of confidence / Preference of purchase basic basket - small businesses

			Purchase Cannel Preference for the Basic Basket of Foodstuffs in Small Food Businesses				Total
			Nothing of Preference	Low Preference	Preference	Total Preference	
Level of trust	Very distrustful	Count	0	1	1	2	4
		% within Level of trust	0.0%	25.0%	25.0%	50.0%	100.0%
		% within Purchase cannel preference for the basic basket of foodstuffs in small food businesses	0.0%	5.6%	2.6%	18.2%	5.9%
		% of the total	0.0%	1.5%	1.5%	2.9%	5.9%
	Some distrustful	Count	0	6	13	3	22
		% within Level of trust	0.0%	27.3%	59.1%	13.6%	100.0%
		% within Purchase cannel preference for the basic basket of foodstuffs in small food businesses	0.0%	33.3%	34.2%	27.3%	32.4%
		% of the total	0.0%	8.8%	19.1%	4.4%	32.4%
	It is indistinct	Count	0	7	15	3	25
		% within Level of trust	0.0%	28.0%	60.0%	12.0%	100.0%
		% within Purchase cannel preference for the basic basket of foodstuffs in small food businesses	0.0%	38.9%	39.5%	27.3%	36.8%
		% of the total	0.0%	10.3%	22.1%	4.4%	36.8%
	Some trustful	Count	1	4	9	3	17
		% within Level of trust	5.9%	23.5%	52.9%	17.6%	100.0%
		% within Purchase cannel preference for the basic basket of foodstuffs in small food businesses	100.0%	22.2%	23.7%	27.3%	25.0%
		% of the total	1.5%	5.9%	13.2%	4.4%	25.0%
Total		Count	1	18	38	11	68
		% within Level of trust	1.5%	26.5%	55.9%	16.2%	100.0%
		% within Purchase cannel preference for the basic basket of foodstuffs in small food businesses	100.0%	100.0%	100.0%	100.0%	100.0%
		% of the total	1.5%	26.5%	55.9%	16.2%	100.0%

Table 6. Confidence level / Preference for buying prepared foods - small businesses

			Purchase Cannel Preference for Prepared Foods in Small Food Businesses				Total
			Nothing of Preference	Low Preference	Preference	Total Preference	
Level of trust	Very distrustful	Count	1	0	2	1	4
		% within Level of trust	25.0%	0.0%	50.0%	25.0%	100.0%
		% within Purchase cannel preference for prepared foods in small food businesses	50.0%	0.0%	5.1%	7.1%	5.9%
		% of the total	1.5%	0.0%	2.9%	1.5%	5.9%
	Some distrustful	Count	1	6	9	6	22
		% within Level of trust	4.5%	27.3%	40.9%	27.3%	100.0%
		% within Purchase cannel preference for prepared foods in small food businesses	50.0%	46.2%	23.1%	42.9%	32.4%
		% of the total	1.5%	8.8%	13.2%	8.8%	32.4%
	It is indistinct	Count	0	6	14	5	25
		% within Level of trust	0.0%	24.0%	56.0%	20.0%	100.0%
		% within Purchase cannel preference for prepared foods in small food businesses	0.0%	46.2%	35.9%	35.7%	36.8%
		% of the total	0.0%	8.8%	20.6%	7.4%	36.8%
	Some trustful	Count	0	1	14	2	17
		% within Level of trust	0.0%	5.9%	82.4%	11.8%	100.0%
		% within Purchase cannel preference for prepared foods in small food businesses	0.0%	7.7%	35.9%	14.3%	25.0%
		% of the total	0.0%	1.5%	20.6%	2.9%	25.0%
Total		Count	2	13	39	14	68
		% within Level of trust	2.9%	19.1%	57.4%	20.6%	100.0%
		% within Purchase cannel preference for prepared foods in small food businesses	100.0%	100.0%	100.0%	100.0%	100.0%
		% of the total	2.9%	19.1%	57.4%	20.6%	100.0%

Figure 3. Preference to buy basic basket small businesses

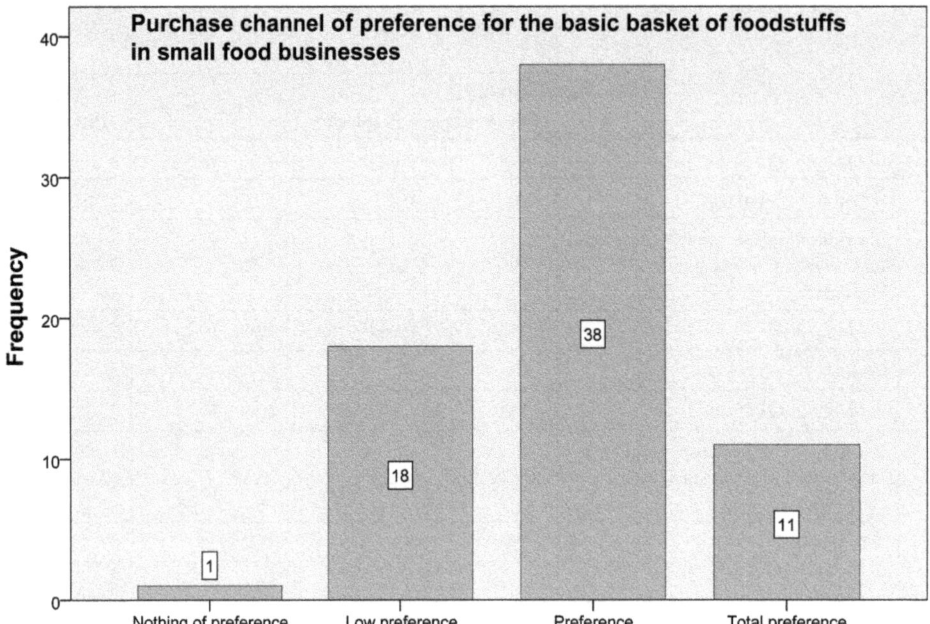

Figure 4. Shopping preference supermarket basket

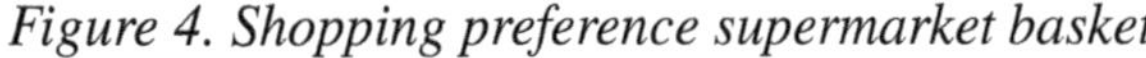

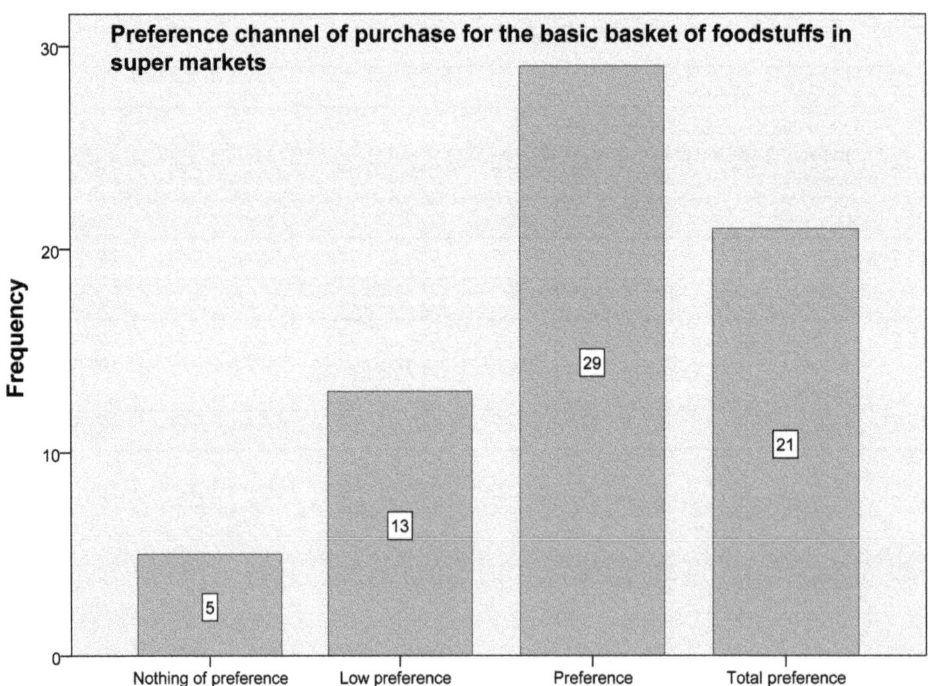

ACKNOWLEDGMENT

The authors would like to acknowledge Alberto Ochoa Ortiz-Zezzatti for his assistance with this chapter.

REFERENCES

Alexander, P., Brown, C., Arneth, A., Finnigan, J., Moran, D., & Rounsevell, M. D. A. (2017, February). Losses, inefficiencies and waste in the global food system. *Agricultural Systems, 153*, 190–200. doi:10.1016/j.agsy.2017.01.014 PMID:28579671

Aschemann-Witzel, de Hooge, Amani, Bech-Larsen, & Oostindjer. (2015). Consumer-Related Food Waste: Causes and Potential for Action. *Sustainability, 7*, 6457-6477.

Aschemann-Witzel, J., Jensen, J. H., Jensen, M. H., & Kulikovskaja, V. (2017). Consumer behaviour towards price-reduced suboptimal foods in the supermarket and the relation to food waste in households. *Appetite, 116*, 246–258. doi:10.1016/j.appet.2017.05.013 PMID:28487247

FAO. (2013). *Food wastage footprint: Impacts on natural resources - Summary report*. Retrieved from http://www.fao.org/docrep/018/i3347e/i3347e.pdf

INEGI. (2016). Encuesta Nacional sobre Productividad y Competitividad de las Micro, Pequeñas y Medianas Empresas ENAPROCE (2015). *Censo Económicos 2014, 1*, 1-221.

Matin, C. (2011). *Logistics & supply chain managment*. Reino Unido: Pretince Hall.

Osvald & Stirn. (2007). A vehicle routing algorithm for the distribution of fresh vegetables and similar perishable food. *Journal of Food Engineering, 85*, 285-295.

Stuart, T. (2009). *Waste: Uncovering the Global Food Scandal. Inglaterra*. Penguin.

Chapter 22
Methodology for the Design of Traceability System in Food Assistance Supply Chains:
Case Bienestarina, Colombia

Feizar Javier Rueda-Velasco
https://orcid.org/0000-0002-0109-9204
Universidad Distrital "Francisco José de Caldas", Colombia

Angie Monsalve-Salamanca
Universidad Nacional de Colombia, Colombia

Wilson Adarme-Jaimes
Universidad Nacional de Colombia, Colombia

ABSTRACT

The food assistance programmes (FAP) has the mission to guarantee minimum nutrition requirements in a vulnerable population. Nevertheless, the small deliveries for a spread population, the social conditions, and the limited technological infrastructure could make it difficult to adequately aid supply. To solve these limitations, this chapter proposes a methodology for the design of traceability systems in FAP which allows increasing supply chain visibility, coordination between deliveries and social conditions, and therefore, possible impacts on public policy implications. A qualitative and quantitative comparison of the conventional frameworks is carried out and contrast with the needs of the programmes studied. Also, new criteria are also added to adapt the design to the technological infrastructure and the socio-demographic conditions of the territory. The methodological proposal is applied to the Bienestarina nutritional programme in Colombia, where the technologies and tools to subsequently design the traceability system are proposed.

DOI: 10.4018/978-1-7998-5354-1.ch022

INTRODUCTION

The Food Assistance Programmes (FAP) aims to reduce social inequities, address the specific needs of vulnerable populations and improve their living conditions. For example, a set of these programmes seeks to improve food security through direct transfers of products (Tiwari et al., 2016).

Some examples of direct transfer programmes can be found in Argentina such as the Remediar programme that supplies medicines to the needy population (Argentina, 2015), in Mexico where dairy products are supplied (Liconsa, 2015) and in the United States through The Emergency Food Assistance Programme (TEFAP) which provides food to the vulnerable population. Those programmes set up supply chains that link the supply, production, storage and transport of aid with final beneficiaries.

Remediar programme distributed 76.082 first-aid kits and 16.721.152 treatments in the first semester of 2018, reducing four times the retail price (Ministerio de la Salud Presidencia de la Nación, 2018). The government investment overcome 34 million to supply the demand, covered 70% of the population (Secretaria de promoción y programas sanitarios, 2013). The Liconsa programme coverage is similar, in 2017 the government invested 2.845 million pesos to server more than 6.370 million of beneficiaries, among them: children between 0 and 12 years, teenagers between 13 and 15 years, nursing mothers, elderly and disabled people (Secretaria de Desarrollo Social - SEDESOL, 2018). These numbers represent the huge impact generated by SAP in society.

Within the supply chain management, traceability systems focus on managing the flow of information throughout the chain, thus preventing potential loss to the product (Aung & Chang, 2014; Opara, 2002; Wilson & Clarke, 1998), measuring the environmental impacts (Wilson & Clarke, 1998) and guaranteeing the delivery to the final customer. Systems and procedures are used to access information in real time and measure the performance of the system (Comunidades Europeas, 2002).

The traceability systems design requires technical and social factors. Nevertheless, social factors are not explicit in literature. For instance, Ringsberg(2014) and Mattevi & Jones (2016) considered factors as information management, production, quality and logistics as critical elements. Bosona & Gebresenbet (2013) refer to more specific guidelines such as regulation, quality and safety, technology, efficiency, competitive advantage, corporate image, product characteristics and internationalization. Note, the authors did not include social factors.

In the other hand, within scientific literature there are numerous attempts to quantify the effects of implementing traceability systems as can be seen in the works of (Alfaro & Rábade, 2009; Dabbene, Gay, & Tortia, 2014; Mithas, Krishnan, & Fornell, 2016; Opara, 2002). However, those papers focus on the impacts of an already implemented or ready-to-use traceability system, and not on the conditions and design elements to take into account in the system development. Those facts occur because the traceability systems are mainly related to manufactured goods which distribution chains, parcel and pallet transport and inventory management.

The implementation of a traceability system involves all decisional system levels (see Figure 1). In the strategy level must evaluate the supply chain structure, including not only their taxonomy, operational means and modes available, also idiosyncratic features or common customs that can be changed in one geographical area than another. In the same way, tactical and operational levels are implicated in the traceability context, being the principal input to redefine the inventory policy, freight consolidation, stakeholder coordination, evaluate coverage, establish indicators, so on (Balcázar-Camacho, D. A et al., 2016; Castrellón-Torres, J. P. et al., 2015).

Figure 1. Traceability in the planning levels

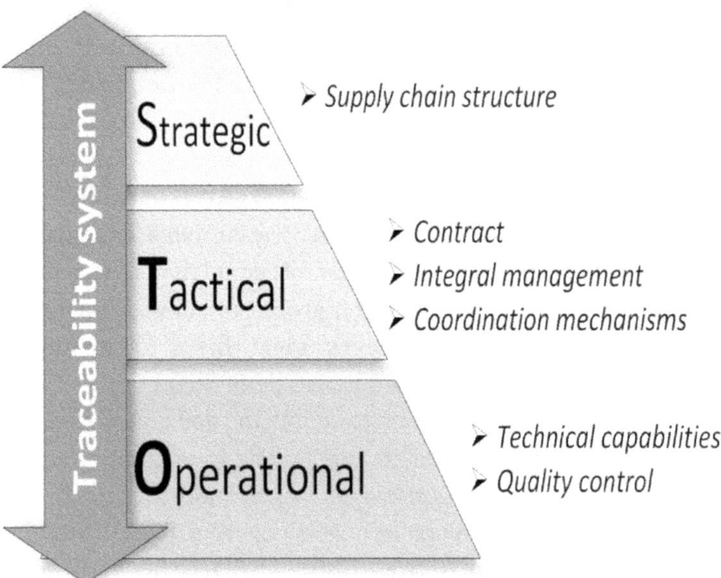

In food distribution, and mainly in local food production and distribution in developing countries like Colombia, with specific geographic, climate and demographic conditions, it seems relevant to deploy specific traceability systems that consider those conditions. Especially, in these systems where people without technical skills, majority volunteers, interact with the distribution and delivery process.

Countries like Colombia has many problems related to social conditions and by then, limited access to information technologies. For instance, just 48% of the population can manage a computer with Internet (Departamento Administrativo Nacional de Estadísticas - DANE, 2017b). Also, 41% of children under five years look after in community homes, child development center or public school, 62% of the rural zones have not water access (Departamento Administrativo Nacional de Estadísticas - DANE, 2017a), and 34.7% of the people consider that their incomes are not enough to cover the minimum expenses. These aspects affect the performance of the traceability systems when some of these people could execute the distribution process.

This paper will present a methodology for the traceability systems design, supporting in the Quick Scan methodology (Naim, M. M. et al., 2002), which includes social factors and allows the involvement of the distribution system and the population benefiting from the programme. First, an analysis of tracking and tracing technologies and their articulation in traceability systems is presented. Subsequently, the criteria to be considered for the design of a traceability system in social programmes are outlined and in the following section, the limitations for implementation are described. Finally, the methodology was validated in the nutritional assistance programme in Colombia called Bienestarina.

BACKGROUND

The concept of traceability was defined as "The ability to trace the history, application or location of an entity using recorded identifications" (International Organization for Standardization, 1994), quoted by European Commission (2002); Moe (1998); Wilson & Clarke (1998). This notion arises from the need to create a collaborative work environment between suppliers, producers and customers throughout the logistics system. Previously, most operations depended on the manual information flow at each stage, which generated a lack of shared information (Renfroe, Mcdonald, & Bradshaw, 1988).

Table 1. Information system and technologies in supply chain management

Information System	Technology and Tools
Document exchange systems	Fax, electronic data exchange tools (web-based or Internet-based), Internet, Smartphone applications, could computing.
Communications systems	Onboard radio, onboard/portable terminals, fixed-line phone, mobile phone, a multifunction portable terminal, Wi-Fi, GSM.
Tracking systems	Identification/codification, electronic lecture, barcodes, RFID, sensors, waymarks, recorders, memory system, IoT.

(Feng Tian, 2016; Gnimpieba, Nait-Sidi-Moh, Durand, & Fortin, 2015; Zhang et al., 2015)

The development of traceability systems is intrinsically related to the use of Information and Communication Technologies (ICT), using technologies and tools as shown in Table 1. Through making the complete information about a product available at any time, ICT allows the optimization of production and distribution costs leading to increase in market competitiveness and achieve supply chain efficiencies and the integration of the members of the chain (Loebbecke & Powell, 1998).

Some of the parameters to be considered for the traceability design are: product data, calibration (standards for evaluating product quality), IT and physical integrity. Those allow ensuring the accuracy of the traceability (Jansen-Vullers, van Dorp, & Beulens, 2003; Moe, 1998).

The frameworks for the design of traceability systems proposed by Aung & Chang (2014); Bosona & Gebresenbet (2013); Kumar, Heustis, & Graham (2015); Regattieri, Gamberi, & Manzini (2007) consider factors such as: product identification, data tracking, product tracking and selection of measurement devices. These frameworks are generic, i.e. they do not make explicit recommendations for each supply chain. Likewise, the European Union (Comunidades Europeas, 2002) designs its standard which proposes guidelines for food supply chains, but only at the conceptual level.

In contrast, other authors propose more complex and specific traceability systems for certain products, for example Bosona & Gebresenbet (2013); Thakur & Hurburgh (2009) design traceability systems that in addition to product tracking between different echelons of the chain, establish specific requirements for the control of internal management and conservation conditions.

Models focused on the strict control of food quality and security (Dai, Ge, & Zhou, 2015; Mattevi & Jones, 2016), use a combination of statistical and technological tools to find a design that fits the needs of the system.

Based on the above it can be noted that it is necessary to design systems adapted to the specific requirements of each supply chain. Specifically, in the case of social assistance, success means that more aid is given thanks to the control and follow-up that takes place in the delivery of the products to the end user. One example is the Remediar programme in Argentina where a multiphase traceability scheme with real-time control was implemented (Fernandez et al., 2012).

Programmes like one implemented in Argentina have been proposed in countries such as Brazil, Colombia, the Philippines, India and the United States. These have been promoted through public policy emphasizing the importance of traceability systems to control adulteration, improve inventory control and dispatch times and ensure that the patient receives the appropriate medication (Argentina, 2015).

There are other programmes focused on counteracting malnutrition such as Liconsa and Diconsa in Mexico, whose objective is to guarantee the right to food for optimal physical and cognitive development of beneficiaries that are below the established indexes (Gonzalez-Feliu, Osorio-Ramirez, Palacios-Arguello, & Talamantes, 2018; Liconsa, 2015). For this program, a need to implement georeferencing tools has been identified in order to guarantee the effective delivery of the product and allow the evaluation of the socio-demographic conditions of the population (Talamantes, 2016).

Other particularities of the supply chains for social assistance, a traceability system was designed that includes technological aspects, based on the geographical location conditions, education level and the penetration level of the service provided to the target population.

METHODOLOGICAL FRAMEWORK

Some essential elements for the design of traceability systems are related to the integration level, the technological devices, actors involved, the sector complexity, size of the company and specificity of the system.

The integration level refers to the connection between the traceability scheme and the chain processes. Zhang et al. (2015) explain the importance of the interoperability between the tracking system and manufacturing information schemes. The integration requires the link between sensors and physical devices, manufacturing data processing and application services.

Thus, technological devices can be located within a process, which is called internal traceability or can be located between the links in the chain, which is considered as external traceability (Aung & Chang, 2014; Ringsberg, 2014). In terms of the complexity of the sector and the size of the company (Aung & Chang, 2014; Scholten, Verdouw, Beulens, & van der Vorst, 2016), social problems are related to the coverage of the system, which is reflected in the number of beneficiaries, the geographic scope, the availability of communications infrastructure and the final devices that are used to interact with the system.

Other actors add factors related to the management of the supply chain. For example: efficient distribution and storage processes; inventory policies; the complexity of the traceability type; unique identification of the product, where the traceability parameters are specified; the information management relying on technological tools; transparency that involves the visibility of information along the chain; interoperability to ensure the operation of traceability system regardless of the heterogamous technologies (Feng Tian, 2016); production management and quality and safety requirements (Ringsberg, 2014).

According to Regattieri et al. (2007), the most important technical parameters for the design of traceability systems are: product identification, physical characteristics (volume, weight, dimensions and packaging); data tracking, level of detail of information, storage needs, reliability and availability; product tracking; technological tools (RFID, TAGs, GPS) (Costa et al., 2013; Feng Tian, 2016); identification of all the ingredients and the all products (where the products are and what its status is) and data linkage system (Aung & Chang, 2014; Ringsberg, 2014).

Table 2. Traceability system methodologies

Methodology Approach	Authors
Information system	Aung & Chang (2014); Renfroe et al. (1988); Ringsberg (2014)
Technology	Feng Tian (2016a); Gnimpieba et al. (2015); Jansen-Vullers et al. (2003); Regattieri et al. (2007); Wilson & Clarke (1998); Zhang et al. (2015)
Logistics management	Bosona & Gebresenbet (2013); Scholten et al. (2016)

Based on the parameters proposed by these authors, the main guidelines in the traceability system have a technical nature as shown in Table 2, spite of the fact that these methodologies are not enough to design a system focused on programmes with social impact. To define the technological tools required, it is not enough to study the technological development of the country, it is necessary to regard socio-demographic, geographic and educational level characteristics; to determine the possible penetration level that the system would have in the target population.

The proposed framework for designing traceability systems of programmes with a social focus begins with the evaluation of the characteristics of the context. The complete methodology with its stages is presented in Figure 2. It is possible to identify the factors that affect the system, based on this characterization. Once the evaluation is done, the scope of the scheme should be delimited, defining the type of desired traceability, the stakeholders involved and the parameters of product identification by their physical characteristics.

The methodology proposed in this article is composed of four stages, which are executed sequentially as follows:

Stage 1: System Assessment

In this phase the evaluation of the geographical, demographic, social and technological development conditions, is carried out; in order to identify the initial conditions before the development of the design. According to evaluate whole aspects is required a supply chain diagnostic, including supply chain structure, planning and control mechanisms and company material flows (Naim, M. M et al., 2002).

As a result, the traceability design needs to determine the actual stage of the communication architecture, penetration of Internet service, use of terminals and mobile devices. This data will be used to select the best technological solution.

Figure 2. Framework traceability system

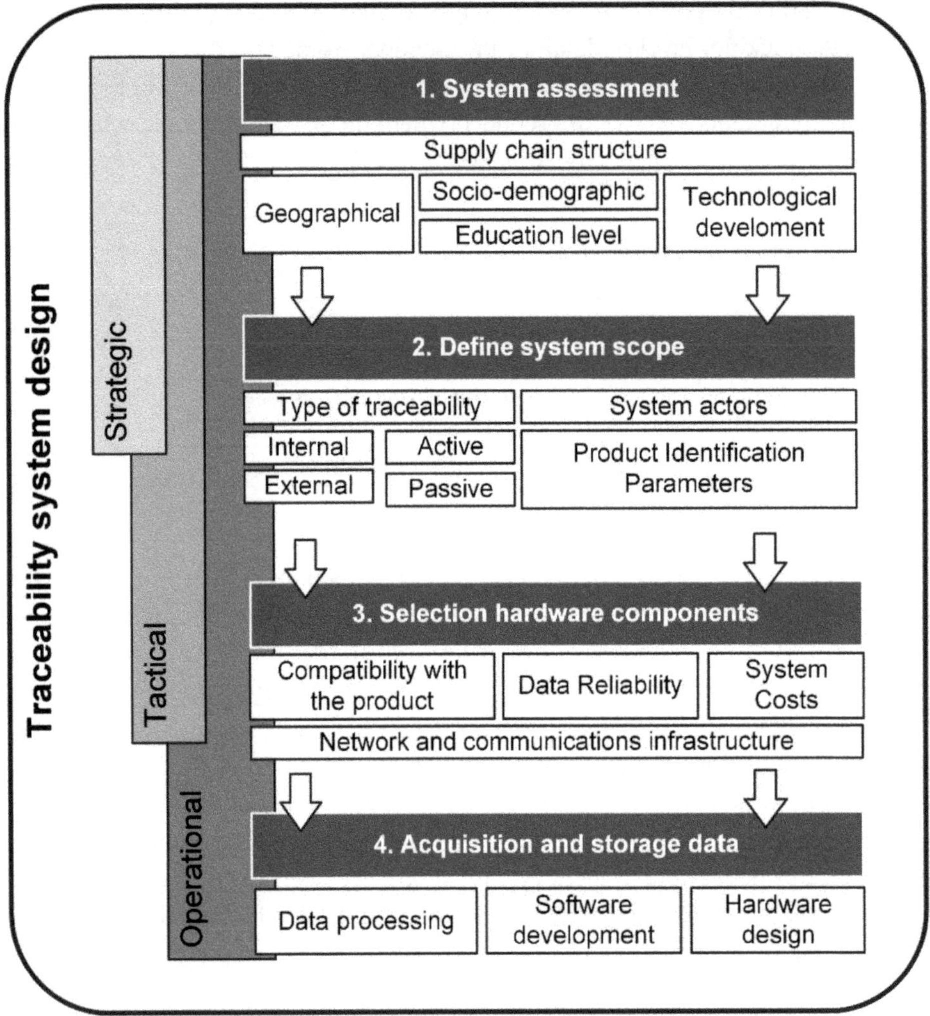

Stage 2: Define System Scope

In this phase, the requirements of the design are defined. Some of these requests are the traceability type (Aung & Chang, 2014), the actors involved, the product parameters and the identification parameters (Regattieri et al., 2007).

As mentioned earlier, the type of traceability depends on system coverage. If just need to track the good in a specific echelon, require internal traceability. In contrast, if the requirement is covered more than one echelon of the supply chain, talking external traceability (Aung & Chang, 2014; Ringsberg, 2014). The active and passive traceability rely on the dynamic that interacts the sensors and technological devices, sending and requesting data.

The identification and interaction between actors, determine the dimensions of the storage and process equipment. The amount of data to flow in the system, the format and weight of the transported data, are relevant parameters to calculate the capacity.

When all parameters are defining, the following step is the selection of the sensors and physical devices.

Stage 3: Selection of Technology Tools

In this phase, the technological devices are selected to perform traceability based on product specifications and the compatibility with the selected tool (Costa et al., 2013; Feng Tian, 2016). The reliability of data depends on the degree of accuracy of the measurement devices and the environment where it will be implemented (Abad et al., 2009) This stage includes the costs of implementing the proposed system and the description of the current infrastructure related to networks and communications.

Within the selection of the sensors and physical devices, the conditions of the environment where the system will be installed should be noted, as well as the technical specifications of each device (communication protocol, power consumption, scope, type of data collected) (Hashem Eiza, Ni, & Shi, 2016; JiaJu Wu, Gang Liu, Peng Liu, & ChuanYu Xi, 2005; Shi, Ding, Zuo, & Zillante, 2016; Wang & Xiao, 2010; Yuvaraj & Sangeetha, 2016). The necessary infrastructure to support the selected technological tool will depend on the factors mentioned.

Stage 4: Acquisition and Storage Data

Once the technical specification is done, the next step is to select the method to process and store the data according to the amount of data, the information availability, frequency that the devices and actors interact with the system. Techniques like business analytics, big data, could computing, and blockchain (Feng Tian, 2016).

In the final step is required to design the devices with sensors and electronic components for the data acquisition (G.-Escribano, Garcia, Wissendheit, Loffler, & Pastor, 2010). Also, develop all software components, databases, interfaces, data processing, interoperable with the hardware design (G.-Escribano et al., 2010).

IMPLEMENTATION CONSTRAINTS

Some factors that obstruct the implementation of a traceability system are: lack of regulation, management between suppliers, lack of interoperability of systems between supplier and customer (Kumar et al., 2015), lack of standards, high costs of financing, lack of accessibility, lack of reliable technological devices, lack of final customer information and ethical and privacy issues (Mattevi & Jones, 2016).

Other significant drawbacks that can occur in the implementation of traceability schemes are the lack of guidelines to determine what data should be captured within the system, which makes it difficult to define the parameters of the product (Ramesh & Jarke, 2001). This flaw generates a more significant impact in systems where it is intended to track a product or a service related to a social programme, due to the data from the beneficiaries in most of these systems are segmented because of the restrictions of the handling of personal information (Canavari, Centonze, Hingley, & Spadoni, 2010).

One of the main challenges is the availability of supporting technological infrastructure. This infrastructure may restrict the implementation of real-time traceability systems and thus decision-making (Aung & Chang, 2014).

In the Colombian context, the implementation of a traceability system involves more challenges than technological infrastructure. The huge differences between the qualification levels, means availability, accessibility, communication, coverage, some aspects like cultural and ancestral according to the region; make the difference and represent the barries for the system implementation and development.

Based on the methodology proposed in this article for the design of traceability systems in Social Assistance Programmes and considering the limitations may be present in the stage of the implementation, this methodology is applied in the case of the Bienestarina nutritional program. Bienestarina is a strategy managed by the Colombian Institute of Family Welfare (ICBF), whose shortcomings have been identified in terms of the administrative procedures for delivering the product and in the current technological infrastructure which prevent the recognition of the beneficiary and the authorized Delivery Points (DPs).

CURRENT SCHEME OF THE BIENESTARINA PROGRAMME

Colombian Institute of Family Welfare (ICBF) manages direct transfers of food to the vulnerable population through the program called Bienestarina. The programme encompasses the production and distribution of a cereal mix food supplement entirely financed by the Colombian Government (Instituto Colombiano de Bienestar Familiar, 2014). As well, the programme is a strategy to attack the problems of malnutrition, especially in the cases of children and young people living in poverty (Departamento Nacional de Planeación; Departamento para la Prosperidad Social; Instituto Colombiano de Bienestar Familiar; Ministerio de Hacienda & Crédito Público, 2015).

Also, the program is closely related to strengthening the fundamental right to food security and is aligned with the ICBF policy of children and family protection (Departamento Nacional de Planeación - DNP, 2006). The annual budget allocation of around 40 US million has been set aside to cover a programmed quota of six million users annually until 2019 (Departamento Nacional de Planeación; Departamento para la Prosperidad Social; Instituto Colombiano de Bienestar Familiar; Ministerio de Hacienda y Crédito Público, 2015).

The structure of the Bienestarina Más® distribution system includes public and private actors. Among these actors are: the Colombian Institute of Family Welfare (ICBF), as the public entity in charge of leading the program, and about 15 private companies working as suppliers of goods.

Bienestarina Más® is a nutritional supplement of high nutritional value, composed of: flour, cereal starch, soy flour, whole milk powder, vitamins and minerals, whose expiration date is 6 months; this is produced by the ICBF to combat the malnutrition problem in the Colombian population (Instituto Colombiano de Bienestar Familiar, 2017). The distribution process starts at the factories and ends at the Service Units (SUs) that can be located: in associations, community mothers, homes of children or Child Development Centers (CDI); there, the aid is delivered to the vulnerable population that is enrolled in any of the programmes provided by the ICBF.

The distribution structure is composed of two manufacturing plants located in Sabanagrande (Atlántico) and Cartago (Valle del Cauca) as shown in Figure 3, once the production stage has culminated, the freight is distributed to 21 warehouses depending on the estimated demand in each region of the country. In 2017, the program delivered nearly 18 thousand tons produced in two factories, distributed through 21 warehoused and nearly 4.200 delivery points to about 2.5 million beneficiaries (Instituto Colombiano de Bienestar Familiar, 2018a). In the distribution process the Stock Keeping Unit (SKU)

Figure 3. Scheme Bienestarina supply chain

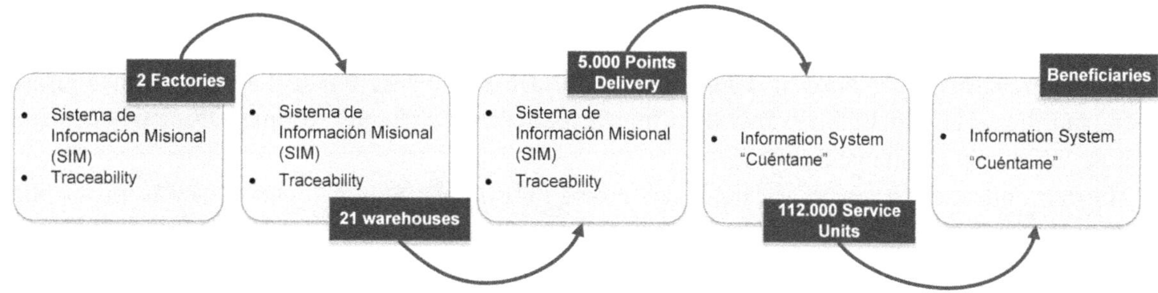

used through the supply chain until the Delivery Points is sacks, in the last mile change the SKU to bags that contain 900 grams of Bienetarina.

The production and distribution processes use a technological tool called Missionary Information System (SIM). With this tool, traceability takes place from the reception of the raw materials to the programming of shipments to DPs. This information system is supported by a network and communications infrastructure (Instituto Colombiano de Bienestar Familiar, 2016). In the next two echelons in the chain, there is an information system called Cuéntame which allows to record information about the beneficiaries and the SUs representatives, as shown in Figure 3.

CURRENT TECHNOLOGICAL INFRASTRUCTURE

At the technological level, the ICBF has several technological tools that support some processes related to the production and distribution of Bienestarina. For data management, there are two Information Systems mentioned previously. The SIM guarantees the effective delivery of the product to the DP, through the programming of orders. For this programming it is necessary to register the data of the freight receptors and their coverage, in order to calculate the rations dispatched and compare them with the Social and Financial Goals (SFG) proposed by the Nutrition Management (Instituto Colombiano de Bienestar Familiar, 2016).

This system allows controlling the inventories, estimating the delivery times and monitor the freight until the arrival to each DP, guaranteeing the traceability of the product until this echelon of the chain.

However, the process does not end in the DP because this echelon also sends products to beneficiaries or the SUs. Since the information flow can take these two possible ways, the product tracking to the final consumer is not easy. Furthermore, considering that the programme has nationwide coverage, it becomes necessary to subcontract logistics operators, to reach all destinations, which brings a coordination problem between multiple actors.

As an ICBF plan to counteract these shortcomings, the Institution is implementing the information system Cuéntame, which aims to record information concerning the programmes of the different modalities of the Early Childhood Division, in the two last echelons of the chain. This system collects and digitizes the information related to: data of the administrative entity of the service and its legal representative; contracts with each of these entities; human talent team involved in each SU, beneficiary data, the SU data and nutritional status of beneficiaries enrolled in the programmes provided by ICBF (Dirección de Primera Infancia - ICBF, 2017). However, even with the implementation of this new system, there are still gaps in terms of traceability, as there is no constant updating of information, likely resulting in the use of incomplete information in the medium and long term.

Additionally, in this system, the amounts of Bienestarina delivered to the beneficiaries are not recorded. Without this information, it is impossible to validate the impact of nutrition programmes despite having nutritional control for everyone. Also, this factor makes it difficult to estimate the actual demand, limiting the supply chain management.

The data collection that is being carried out in both Information Systems is necessary as an essential requirement for the recognition of the population. However, this is only the beginning of a unified system. Although these information systems cover all the supply chain as shown in Figure 4, the integration is required to enable interoperability between them.

Figure 4. Bienestarina supply chain information systems

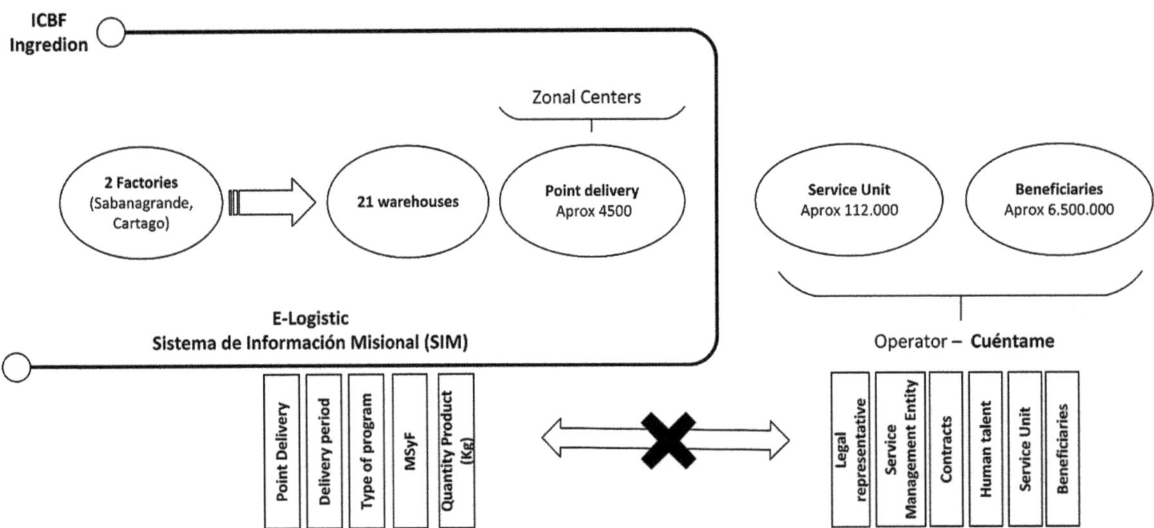

Information systems are supported by the infrastructure of communications and network, which allows the connectivity between the interfaces with the devices where the information is managed (servers). To achieve this interconnection, the ICBF has an infrastructure with coverage from the general direction to the Zonal Centers. Zonal Centers can also act as a DP. At the general level, there are computer centers, physical and virtualized servers, storage equipment and databases. In terms of the communications infrastructure, there are fixed-line and mobile Internet service and local wired and wireless networks, which connect the main headquarters with the sub-directorates (Dirección Informacion y Tecnologia - ICBF, 2015).

Accordingly that, although there is infrastructure that supports information systems in the first echelons of the chain (until DP), there is no full coverage of the actors involved, nor tracking to the final consumer. In other words, the Bienestarina programme still has only partial traceability.

APPLICATION OF THE PROPOSED METHODOLOGY TO THE BIENESTARINA CASE

In order to apply the proposed methodology to generate a traceability scheme in the Bienestarina programme, the evaluation of the current system and the definition of its scope (stages 1 and 2 Figure 2) is carried out in order to select the appropriate technological tools that allow the unification of existing information systems. The application of stages 1 and 2 of the proposed methodology is mandatory, because these are differentiating stages of the analysis of social assistance supply chains. The remaining stages will be described in future publications and correspond to the application of the frameworks exposed in Aung & Chang (2014); Regattieri et al. (2007); Scholten et al. (2016) once social needs have been revealed.

System Assessment (Stage 1)

Given the Colombian geographical and socio-demographic diversity, it is necessary to carry out an evaluation considering rural and urban environments, since the parameters to be taken into account for the design of the traceability system vary considerably between them (see Table 3). For instance, in the socio-demographic area, there are differences in the degree of vulnerability in dispersed regions where there is a lack of entities who promote and control solutions to the population's social problems. In turn, there are differences in access to public services, especially in rural regions where only 60% of the population has access to the aqueduct service (Departamento Administrativo Nacional de Estadistica, 2017).

Table 3. Scenario assessment

Scope	Parameter	Urban	Rural
Sociodemographic	Demographic concentration	High	Low
	Geographical dispersion	Low	High
	Education Level	High	Medium/Low
	Access to public services	High	Low
	Degree of vulnerability	Low	High
	Malnutrition level	Medium	High
Technological development	Technological appropriation	Medium	Low
	Internet Penetration (Mobile/Fixed-line)	Medium	Low
	Access to terminals	High	Low
Communications infrastructure	Internet Coverage (Mobile/Fixed-line)	High	Medium
	Diversity mobile operators	High	Medium
	Diversity transmission means	High	Low

In terms of technological development, there is still a lack of access to end-user devices in rural areas, especially in the Pacific, Caribbean and San Andrés regions, where only 14.7% of the population in rural areas have a desktop, laptop and/or tablet computer (Departamento Administrativo Nacional de Estadistica, 2017). The penetration of Internet service in general is low, for example, in Bogota it is scarcely 21.7%, and in regions such as Guainía, Vaupés and Amazonas, the percentage of use of the service is less than 1% (Ministerio de las Tecnologías de la Información y Comunicaciones, 2016).

Regards to communications infrastructure, there is evidence of coverage by mobile operators in most of the national territory. In contrast, according to the survey presented by the (Departamento Administrativo Nacional de Estadistica, 2017), only 45.8% of households have access to the fixed-line Internet. Hence, in some dispersed regions is not possible to access to various transmission media, such as: cable, XDSL, optical fiber, satellite, WiMax, microwave, among others; significantly restricting access to the Internet (Ministerio de las Tecnologías de la Información y Comunicaciones, 2016).

In order to attend the different social and technical country conditions, the traceability system design is divided in twofold: one oriented to the dispersed regions, considered as non-interconnected zones, and the other one focused on concentrated regions, which have a higher degree of use of technological tools and therefore knowledge about their usage.

For technological development analysis, technological characteristics associated with the two proposed scenarios were identified as shown in Figure 5. In dispersed regions it is important to consider the lack of permanent Internet connection due to the limitations of wire connections. In contrast, in concentrated regions such as urban areas, consideration should be given to whether fixed-line and mobile Internet access guarantee an available and reliable connection.

Figure 5. Technological features according to the region

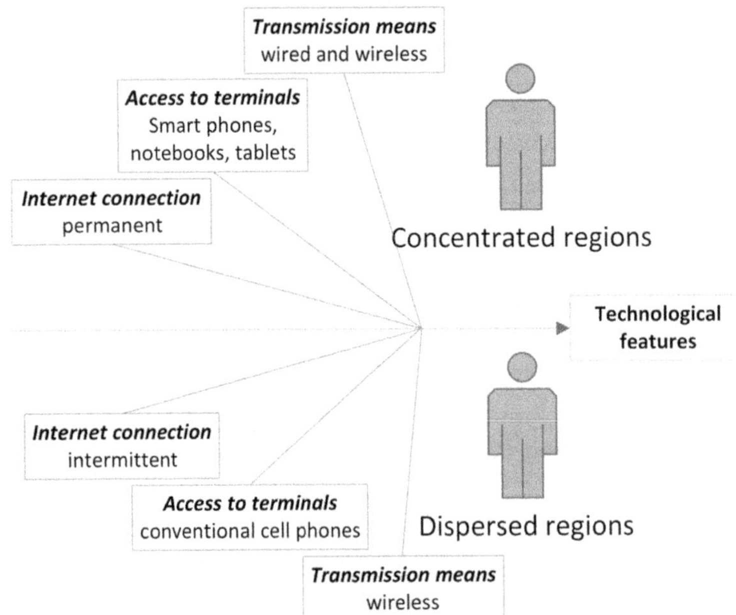

To evaluate the current conditions of fixed-line Internet access in the DP, it begins with the identification of municipalities in Colombia that do not have Internet access through conventional technologies (Cable, XDSL). In these municipalities, access is only available through satellites or microwave links, which are expensive and difficult to access, generating a subscriber number of less than 50 per municipality (Ministerio de las Tecnologías de la Información y Comunicaciones, 2016). This data was extracted in the statistics made by the Ministry of Information Technologies and Communications.

Once the municipalities with limited alternatives to access the fixed-line Internet are identified, the contrast is made regarding the location of the DPs. The analysis obtained that around 35.08% of DPs cannot access to a fixed-line internet. Thus, in departments such as Guainía and Vichada located in dispersed regions, there is no fixed Internet access, as shown in Figure 6. On the other hand, in regions with greater urban concentration such as Bogotá, Antioquia, Tolima and Caldas; the fixed-line Internet coverage reaches approximately 95% of the DPs.

Based on the technical evaluation, the reach of the existing infrastructure in terms of connecting dispersed populations is analyzed, as shown in the matrix of Figure 7. In dispersed regions, the implementation of a traceability system design needs to consider the lack of infrastructure for fixed-line Internet connection, as well as the connection to a mobile internet as an alternative for the system update in cases of intermittent connectivity.

Figure 6. Delivery point without access to a fixed-line Internet

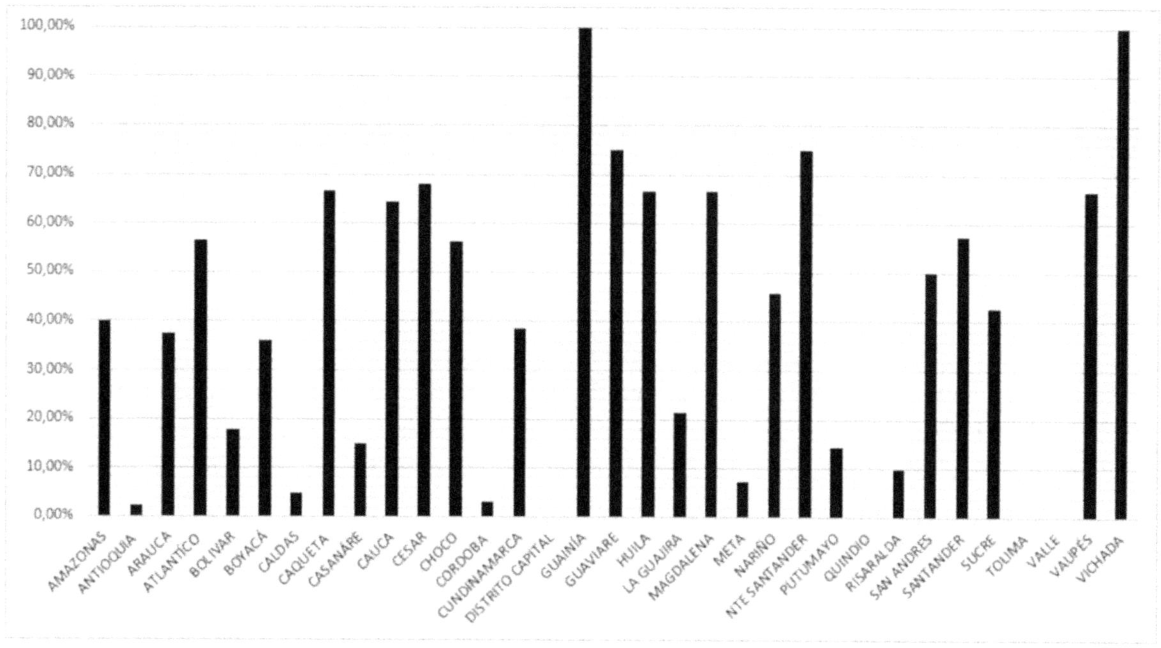

The twofold design has different implications for a system such as the one analyzed, because it requires having at least two designs of technological architecture, one for dispersed or non-connected areas and another for interconnected zones. While this distinction may seem obvious, in practice one-off traceability systems are usually designed, omitting the conditions of availability and fixed-line Internet access.

Figure 7. Type of scenarios

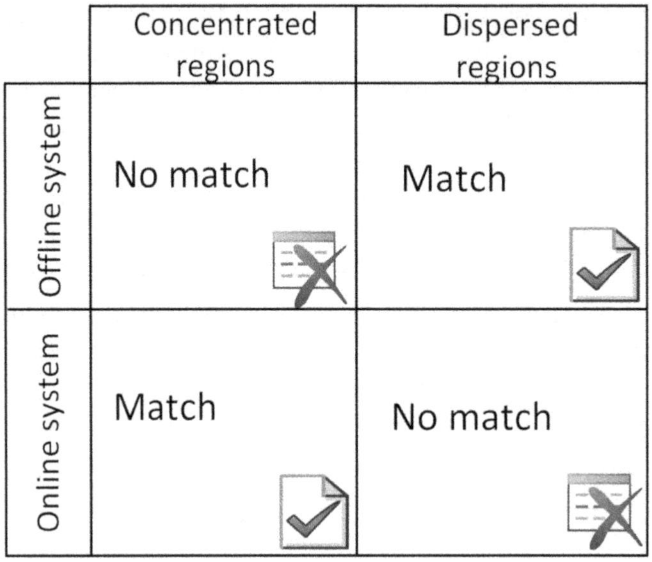

	Concentrated regions	Dispersed regions
Offline system	No match	Match
Online system	Match	No match

Define the System Scope (Stage 2)

The social assistance programmes can compromise its effectivity if the access level of the freight and technology for traceability are not coherent. This situation is evident in the system distribution of Bienestarina, where traceability of the freight covers the supply chain until the DP, omitting the connection between DPs and rough 4.5 billion of beneficiaries. In order to guarantee the coherence between the scope of freight and the beneficiaries who received the product the Bienestarina distribution process in the last mile was evaluated and the involved actors were identified.

System Process and Stakeholders

Based on the system characterization in the previous stages, there is a feasible solution to implement the traceability system in the last mile. The distribution process starts with the registration of the inventory that arrives at the PD, through the barcode printed on the Bienestarina sacks. Each sack contained 25 bags of Bienesatrina with 900 grams per bag (Departamento Nacional de Planeación- DNP, Departamento para la Prosperidad Social, Instituto Colombiano de Bienestar Familiar, & Ministerio de Hacienda y Crédito Público, 2015). This condition inhibits the possibility of carrying out adequate control of the product, thus tracking each product is difficult. Therefore, SKU should be modified from sacks to bags in this echelon of the chain.

Once the delivery request is received, either by SU or beneficiary, the user authentication is performed, so that the person responsible for delivery can validate the registration of beneficiary in the databases and the amount of product to deliver. In this point of the process has two alternatives, one is directly transferred to the beneficiary, the other is to deliver to the SU and they transfer the product from there to the beneficiary, as shown as in Figure 8.

Figure 8. Bienestarina last mile distribution process

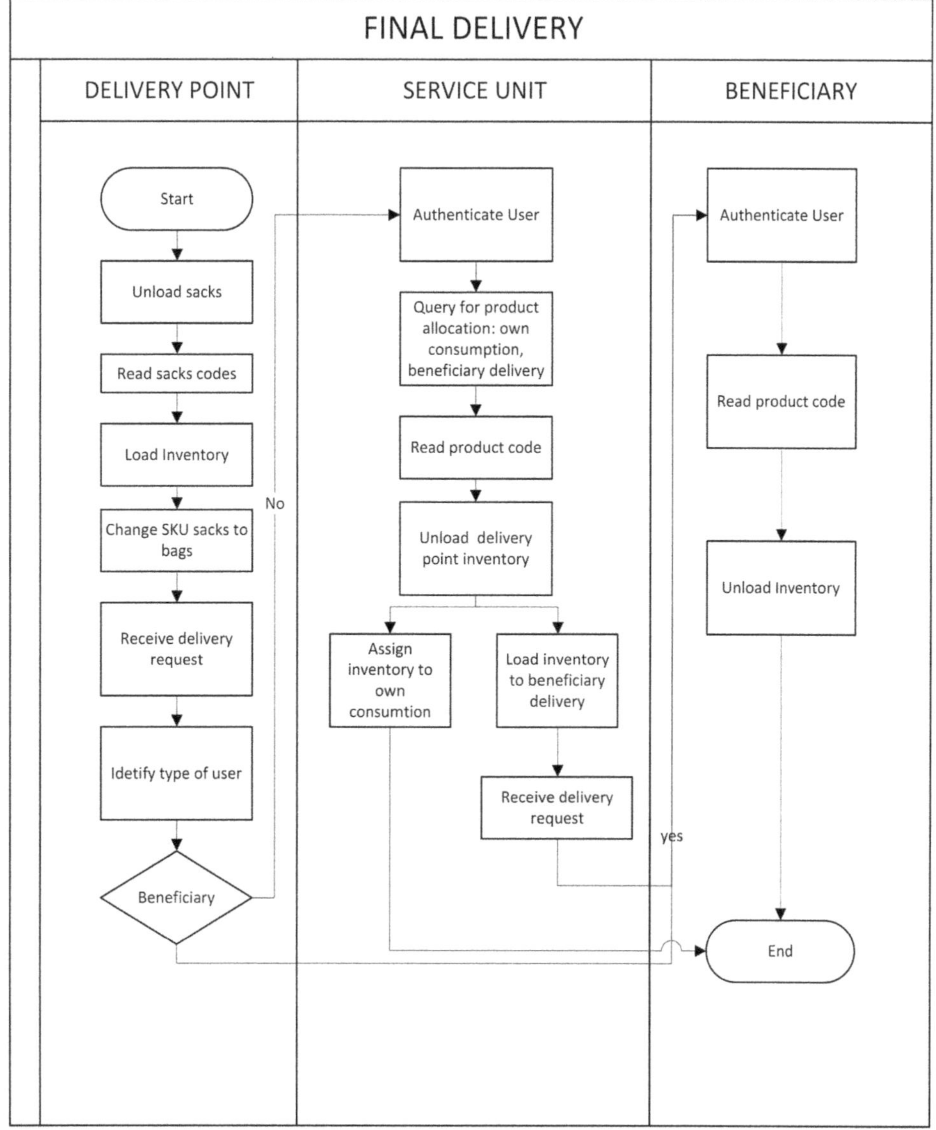

Given the importance to performing traceability in the last mile, it is necessary to consider DP, SU and beneficiaries as actors in the system, especially in the last segment in the supply chain as shown as in Figure 8. Some actors like a DPs and SUs can register beneficiaries, schedule Bienestarina deliveries, make inventory control and update information of the anthropometric profile of beneficiaries. Some anthropometries parameters are: weight, height, age, gender and so on.

The DP and SU actors should have a profile that can access the databases with records of the product's delivery and the users, to consult data before to be registered in order to avoid duplicate entries. In contrast, the beneficiary should be able to display its nutritional evolution and registered delivery. For this reason, is necessary to create three types of profile with role permissions with the follow features: the SU can register the beneficiaries, change the status of the beneficiaries, deliver product and inven-

Figure 9. System actors, traceability in the last mile

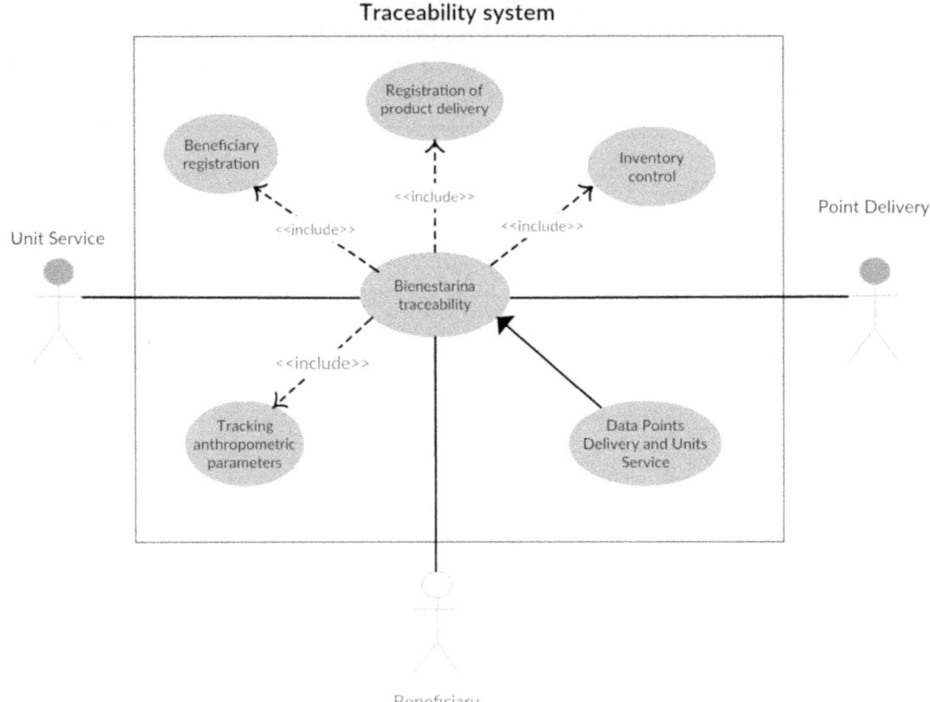

tory control; the DP have to transfer the inventory and deliver the product of beneficiary and beneficiary profile as described in Figure 9.

Once the process and actors identification were done (Figure 8 and 9), will propose a possible technological solution. To identify each actor that interact with the system, is necessary the use of ID card or biometric devices, so validate their authenticity. Other device requirements are the barcode lector to load or unload the product, depending on the process. Other elements that have to define are: the communication system, storage equipment and data processing method.

CONCLUSION

Through the methodology proposed in this paper shown particular aspects required in the complex systems. Each stage includes relevant factors that impact the strategic, tactical and operational levels in the organization. In the literature review researches like Jansen-Vullers et al. (2003); Regattieri et al. (2007) and Wilson & Clarke (1998) proposed methodologies to implement traceability systems that including technological features, being this important but not the only element to determine the implementation feasibility.

The guidelines of the traceability system design mainly based on the technical requirements, depending on where the process will be implemented (characteristics of the product, environmental conditions and stakeholders). Before selecting technology, it is relevant to assess the system, especially when the traceability involves Social Assistance Programmes.

The identification of the geographical dispersion of beneficiaries, heterogeneous conditions of communication networks and different educational level of the population, represent the complexity of the system. For that, emerge the importance to perform the system assessment along the supply chain structure, including all organization planning level, being these impacted with the traceability system.

In the evaluation of the case of Bienestarina above, the first stage included the current diagnosis of the context. With this analysis it was possible to identify technical requirements needed in the implementation phase. It was found that Internet access and technological appropriation are considered relevant factors. Also, if there is no previous assessment, it is difficult to have a homogeneous system that adjusts to all requirements.

The fixed-line Internet connection in the Delivery Point is 65% due to it is necessary to complement the technological infrastructure with alternative solutions such as a mobile Internet connection in order to guarantee the coverage of the system. Within the traceability system design it is crucial to consider two connection status for the storage of the database, online and offline. This way, it can be used the local storage in the final devices where there is no Internet connection. In terms of technology, it is necessary to incorporate tools such as: bar-codes and digital fingerprint scanners, smartphones or computers; in order to be sure that the actors have access to the system.

The implementation of traceability technologies in social assistance programmes as here presented is the first step to integrating information technologies around the user approach. In countries as Colombia is usual to have independent programmes around different necessities of vulnerable populations, as many views of the same subject.

Fully integrated information, data analytics, freight traceability around the same subject could improve the basic necessities fulfillment for instance in education, health, security, and food assistance. Hence the user approach in social assistance programmes requires further research and further technologies development, especially in collaborative aspect.

ACKNOWLEDGMENT

We would like to thank Dr. Jesus Gonzalez-Feliu for their assistance in the creation of this chapter. Also, we would like to acknowledge to COLCIENCIAS-Colombia for finance the project which results are here presented.

REFERENCES

Abad, E., Palacio, F., Nuin, M., Zárate, A. G., Juarros, A., Gómez, J. M., & Marco, S. (2009). RFID smart tag for traceability and cold chain monitoring of foods: Demonstration in an intercontinental fresh fish logistic chain. *Journal of Food Engineering*, *93*(4), 394–399. doi:10.1016/j.jfoodeng.2009.02.004

Alfaro, J. A., & Rábade, L. A. (2009). Traceability as a strategic tool to improve inventory management: A case study in the food industry. *International Journal of Production Economics*, *118*(1), 104–110. doi:10.1016/j.ijpe.2008.08.030

Argentina, G. (2015). *Tecnologías y modelos de «seguimiento y localización» existentes y que los estados miembros vayan a desarrollar*. Academic Press.

Aung, M. M., & Chang, Y. S. (2014). Traceability in a food supply chain: Safety and quality perspectives. *Food Control, 39*, 172–184. doi:10.1016/j.foodcont.2013.11.007

Balcázar-Camacho, D. A., López-Bello, C. A., & Adarme-Jaimes, W. (2016). Strategic guidelines for supply chain coordination in healthcare and a mathematical model as a proposed mechanism for the measurement of coordination. *Dyna (Bilbao), 83*(197), 203–211. doi:10.15446/dyna.v83n197.55596

Bosona, T., & Gebresenbet, G. (2013). Food traceability as an integral part of logistics management in food and agricultural supply chain. *Food Control, 33*(1), 32–48. doi:10.1016/j.foodcont.2013.02.004

Canavari, M., Centonze, R., Hingley, M., & Spadoni, R. (2010). Traceability as part of competitive strategy in the fruit supply chain. *British Food Journal, 112*(2), 171–186. doi:10.1108/00070701011018851

Castrellón-Torres, J. P., García-Alcaraz, J. L., & Adarme-Jaimes, W. (2015). Freight consolidation as a coordination mechanism in perishable supply chains: A simulation study. *Dyna (Bilbao), 82*(189), 233–242. doi:10.15446/dyna.v82n189.48551

Costa, C., Antonucci, F., Pallottino, F., Aguzzi, J., Sarriá, D., & Menesatti, P. (2013). *A Review on Agrifood Supply Chain Traceability by Means of RFID Technology.* Academic Press. doi:10.100711947-012-0958-7

Dabbene, F., Gay, P., & Tortia, C. (2014). Traceability issues in food supply chain management: A review. *Biosystems Engineering, 120*, 65–80. doi:10.1016/j.biosystemseng.2013.09.006

Dai, H., Ge, L., & Zhou, W. (2015). A design method for supply chain traceability systems with aligned interests. *International Journal of Production Economics, 170*, 14–24. doi:10.1016/j.ijpe.2015.08.010

Departamento Administrativo Nacional de Estadisticas. (2017). *Encuesta nacional de calidad de vida - ECV 2016.* Retrieved from https://www.dane.gov.co/files/investigaciones/condiciones_vida/calidad_vida/Boletin_Tecnico_ECV_2016.pdf

Departamento Administrativo Nacional de Estadísticas - DANE. (2017a). *Encuesta Nacional de Calidad de Vida (ECV) 2017.* Author.

Departamento Administrativo Nacional de Estadísticas - DANE. (2017b). *Indicadores básicos de tenencia y uso de Tecnologías de la Información y Comunicación en hogares y personas de 5 y más años de edad.* Author.

Departamento Nacional de Planeación, Departamento para la Prosperidad Social, Instituto Colombiano de Bienestar Familiar, & Ministerio de Hacienda y Crédito Público. (2015). *CONPES 3843 Importancia estratégica de los alimentos de alto valor nutricional que serán entregados por el ICBF en las vigencias 2016-2019.* Authors.

Departamento Nacional de Planeación - DNP. (2006). Conpes 3443 Contratación del operador para la producción y distribución del componente nutricional (Bienestarina) en el Instituto Colombiano de Bienestar Familiar - ICBF. Author.

Departamento Nacional de Planeación- DNP, Departamento para la Prosperidad Social, Instituto Colombiano de Bienestar Familiar, & Ministerio de Hacienda y Crédito Público. (2015). *Importancia estratégica de los alimentos de alto valor nutricional que seran entregados por el ICBF en las vigencias 2016-2019 CONPES 3842.* Authors.

Dirección de Primera Infancia - ICBF. (2017). *Sistema de Información Cuéntame - Primera Infancia ICBF V2.* Author.

Dirección Informacion y Tecnologia - ICBF. (2015). *Ficha de condiciones técnicas especiales para la prestación del servicio y/o entrega del bien.* FCT.

Escribano, J., Garcia, A., Wissendheit, U., Loffler, A., & Pastor, J. M. (2010). Analysis of the applicability of RFID & wireless sensors to manufacturing and distribution lines trough a testing multi-platform. In *2010 IEEE International Conference on Industrial Technology* (pp. 1379–1385). IEEE. 10.1109/ICIT.2010.5472510

European Commission. Regulation (EC) No 178/2002 of the European Parliament and of the Council of 28 January 2002 laying down the general principles and requirements of food law, establishing the European Food Safety Authority and laying down procedures in matters of food saf, 31 Official Journal of the European Communities 1–24 (2002). European Commission Brussels, Belgium.

Comunidades Europeas. (2002). *Reglamento (CE) no 178/2002 del Parlamento Europeo y del Consejo del 28 de enero de 2002.* Author.

Fernandez, C., Manzur, J. L., Diosque, M. A., Ventura, G., Monsalvo, M., La cava, G., & Grinblat, E. (2012). *Remediar + Red 10 años comprometidos con la salud pública.* Academic Press.

Gnimpieba, Z. D. R., Nait-Sidi-Moh, A., Durand, D., & Fortin, J. (2015). Using Internet of Things Technologies for a Collaborative Supply Chain: Application to Tracking of Pallets and Containers. *Procedia Computer Science*, *56*, 550–557. doi:10.1016/j.procs.2015.07.251

Gonzalez-Feliu, J., Osorio-Ramirez, C., Palacios-Arguello, L., & Talamantes, C. A. (2018). Local Production-Based Dietary Supplement Distribution in Emerging Countries: Bienestarina Distribution in Colombia. In Establishing Food Security and Alternatives to International Trade in Emerging Economies (pp. 297–315). IGI Global.

Hashem Eiza, M., Ni, Q., & Shi, Q. (2016). Secure and Privacy-Aware Cloud-Assisted Video Reporting Service in 5G-Enabled Vehicular Networks. *IEEE Transactions on Vehicular Technology*, *65*(10), 7868–7881. doi:10.1109/TVT.2016.2541862

Instituto Colombiano de Bienestar Familiar. (2014). *Distribución, cuidado y uso de un alimento de alto valor nutricional. Bienestarina precocida.* Author.

Instituto Colombiano de Bienestar Familiar. (2018a). *Informe de Gestión 2017.* Retrieved from https://www.icbf.gov.co/sites/default/files/informe_de_gestion_2017_-_30_de_enero_de_2018_1.pdf

Instituto Colombiano de Bienestar Familiar. (2018b). *Instituto Colombiano de Bienestar Familiar Cecilia De la Fuente de Lleras.* Retrieved from http://www.icbf.gov.co/portal/page/portal/PortalICBF/EiInstituto

International Organization for Standardization. (1994). *ISO 8402: 1994: Quality Management and Quality Assurance-Vocabulary*. International Organization for Standardization.

Intituto Colombiano de Bienestar Familiar. (2016). *Macroproceso Gestión para la Nutrición - Manual SIM V2*. Author.

Jansen-Vullers, M., van Dorp, C., & Beulens, A. J. (2003). Managing traceability information in manufacture. *International Journal of Information Management*, *23*(5), 395–413. doi:10.1016/S0268-4012(03)00066-5

Kumar, S., Heustis, D., & Graham, J. M. (2015). *The future of traceability within the U.S. food industry supply chain: A business case*. Academic Press. doi:10.1108/IJPPM-03-2014-0046

Liconsa, S. A. D. C. . (2015). *Programa Institucional 2016*. Academic Press.

Loebbecke, C., & Powell, P. (1998). Competitive advantage from IT in logistics: The integrated transport tracking system. *International Journal of Information Management*, *18*(1), 17–27. doi:10.1016/S0268-4012(97)00037-6

Mattevi, M., & Jones, J. A. (2016). Traceability in the food supply chain: Awareness and attitudes of UK small and medium-sized enterprises. *Food Control*, *64*, 120–127. doi:10.1016/j.foodcont.2015.12.014

Ministerio de la Salud Presidencia de la Nación. (2018). *Trasferencia monetarias por medicamentos*. Retrieved from http://186.33.221.24/medicamentos/index.php?option=com_content&view=article&id=1092&catid=79&Itemid=206

Ministerio de las Tecnologías de la Información y Comunicaciones. (2016). *Ministerio TIC - Estadísticas Sectoriales*. Author.

Mithas, S., Krishnan, M. S., & Fornell, C. (2016). Information Technology, Customer Satisfaction, and Profit: Theory and Evidence. *Information Systems Research*, *27*(1), 166–181. doi:10.1287/isre.2015.0609

Moe, T. (1998). Perspectives on traceability in food manufacture. *Trends in Food Science & Technology*, *9*(5), 211–214. doi:10.1016/S0924-2244(98)00037-5

Naim, M. M., Childerhouse, P., Disney, S. M., & Towill, D. R. (2002). A supply chain diagnostic methodology: Determining the vector of change. *Computers & Industrial Engineering*, *43*(1–2), 135–157. doi:10.1016/S0360-8352(02)00072-4

Opara, L. U. (2002). Traceability in agriculture and food supply chain: A review of basic concepts, technological implications, and future prospects. *Journal of Food Agriculture and Environment*, *1*(1), 101–106.

Ramesh, B., & Jarke, M. (2001). Toward reference models for requirements traceability. *IEEE Transactions on Software Engineering*, *27*(1), 58–93. doi:10.1109/32.895989

Regattieri, A., Gamberi, M., & Manzini, R. (2007). Traceability of food products: General framework and experimental evidence. *Journal of Food Engineering*, *81*(2), 347–356. doi:10.1016/j.jfoodeng.2006.10.032

Renfroe, M., Mcdonald, E., & Bradshaw, K. (1988). Integrated tracking of components by engineering and logistics utilizing logistics asset tracking system. *2nd Space Logistics Symposium*. 10.2514/6.1988-4729

Ringsberg, H. (2014). *Perspectives on food traceability: A systematic literature review*. Academic Press. doi:10.1108/SCM-01-2014-0026

Scholten, H., Verdouw, C. N., Beulens, A., & van der Vorst, J. G. A. J. (2016). *Defining and Analyzing Traceability Systems in Food Supply Chains*. Elsevier Inc. doi:10.1016/B978-0-08-100310-7.00002-8

Secretaria de Desarrollo Social - SEDESOL. (2018). *Programa institucional 2018*. Author.

Secretaria de promoción y programas sanitarios. (2013). *Impacto Redistributivo del programa Remediar en el gasto de medicamentos*. Author.

Shi, Q., Ding, X., Zuo, J., & Zillante, G. (2016). Mobile Internet based construction supply chain management: A critical review. *Automation in Construction*, *72*, 143–154. doi:10.1016/j.autcon.2016.08.020

Talamantes, C. (2016). *Análisis de los procesos de acopio, producción y distribución de leche Liconsa en México*. Chihuahua, Mexico: Ciudad Juárez.

Thakur, M., & Hurburgh, C. R. (2009). Framework for implementing traceability system in the bulk grain supply chain. *Journal of Food Engineering*, *95*(4), 617–626. doi:10.1016/j.jfoodeng.2009.06.028

Tian, F. (2016). An agri-food supply chain traceability system for China based on RFID & blockchain technology. In *2016 13th International Conference on Service Systems and Service Management (ICSSSM)* (pp. 1–6). IEEE. 10.1109/ICSSSM.2016.7538424

Tiwari, S., Daidone, S., Ruvalcaba, M. A., Prifti, E., Handa, S., Davis, B., ... Seidenfeld, D. (2016). Impact of cash transfer programs on food security and nutrition in sub-Saharan Africa: A cross-country analysis. *Global Food Security*, *11*, 72–83. doi:10.1016/j.gfs.2016.07.009

Wang, Z., & Xiao, L. (2010). Modern logistics monitoring platform based on the internet of things. In *2010 International Conference on Intelligent Computation Technology and Automation, ICICTA 2010* (Vol. 2, pp. 726–731). IEEE. 10.1109/ICICTA.2010.650

Wilson, T. P., & Clarke, W. R. (1998). Food safety and traceability in the agricultural supply chain: Using the Internet to deliver traceability. *Supply Chain Management*, *3*(3), 127–133. doi:10.1108/13598549810230831

Wu, J. J., Liu, G., Liu, P., & Xi, C. Y. (2005). The study on attemperment arithmetic based on neural network of logistics distribution tracking and attemperment system used GSM cellular phone (July 2005). In *2005 IEEE International Conference on Granular Computing* (p. 284–287). IEEE. 10.1109/GRC.2005.1547286

Yuvaraj, S., & Sangeetha, M. (2016). Smart supply chain management using internet of things(IoT) and low power wireless communication systems. *2016 International Conference on Wireless Communications, Signal Processing and Networking (WiSPNET)*, 555–558. 10.1109/WiSPNET.2016.7566196

Zhang, Y., Zhang, G., Wang, J., Sun, S., Si, S., & Yang, T. (2015). Real-time information capturing and integration framework of the internet of manufacturing things. *International Journal of Computer Integrated Manufacturing*, *28*(8), 811–822. doi:10.1080/0951192X.2014.900874

Chapter 23
Analyzing Sustainable Food Supply Chain Management Challenges in India

Yogesh Kumar Sharma
Graphic Era University, India

Sachin Kumar Mangla
Graphic Era University, India

Pravin P. Patil
Graphic Era University, India

Surbhi Uniyal
Graphic Era University, India

ABSTRACT

The demand of food is increasing day by day, innovative agricultural practices and sustainable food supply chain management (SFSCM) has gained an emergent importance. Food industries across the globe mainly focus on the manufacturing of their own products to achieve sustainability. The importance of sustainable food supply chain management is to overcome the wastage in food manufacturing industries. In the present research, we identified eleven challenges in the SFSCM on the basis of literature review and expert opinion. The approach is an integration of fuzzy with DEMATEL which can be used for dividing the challenges into cause and effect group. Fuzzy DEMATEL method has continuously been used for the analysis of challenges and is the novel approach for decision making. Thus, this method can be implemented in many fields including automobiles, food industries, retail market etc. From the fuzzy DEMATEL results, it can be confirmed that the Safety and Security is one of the most influencing challenge and has the strongest association with other challenges.

DOI: 10.4018/978-1-7998-5354-1.ch023

INTRODUCTION

Since from the past decades, there is a development of green and sustainable supply chain management methods for reducing the environmental concerns and issues. Also the food production and consumption processes have been changed to overcome some of the major problems of the environment (Genovese and Acquaye, 2017). According to the report of India brand equity foundation (IBEF), 2017, the world food trade is rising day-by-day with the increase in the establishment of new food industries. The Indian food industries have evolved as a high income and growth area because of its enormous potential for value addition, especially in food processing industries. The current value of food industries is US\$ 39.71 billion and it will be increase at a Compounded Annual Growth Rate (CAGR) of 11% to US\$ 65.4 billion by 2018. The Government of India has constantly making efforts for the development of food processing industries which will account for approximately 32% of the country's total food market. The Ministry of Food Processing Industries (MOFPI) has already taken and is still taking many initiatives to increase investments in this business. Many proposals had been approved for foreign collaborations, joint ventures and export oriented units and in industrial licenses. Indian food processing industry is one of the largest industries accounting for 32% of the country's total food market and it secures fifth rank among other industries. The food industry accounts for around 14% of GDP (Gross Domestic Product), 13% of exports and 6% of total industrial investment. In context with organic food market, India is projected to increase its production by three times in next 3-4 years. The current value of Indian gourmet food market is US\$ 1.3 billion which is continuously growing at a CAGR (Compound Annual Growth Rate) of 20%. Idea of fuzzy approach was used by (Bellman and Zadeh, 1970) in decision making theory. Fuzzy set theory is very useful for removing the uncertainty in the supply chain (Lee et at., 2004). According to the literature or researchers point of view it is clearly mentioned that fuzzy set theory is capable of managing the supply chain inventory (Petrovic et al., 1998, 2001). In the current problem Fuzzy DE-MATEL is used to remove the biasness in the human judgments. Fuzzy approach is used for the better implementation of SFSCM in Indian food industry. To manage the increased demand of food throughout the world, SFSCM is very important. Supply Chain Management (SCM) is an upcoming and wide area and has been considered by scientists, researchers and academicians in the last years. One prominent research field is sustainability in SCM, namely Sustainable Supply Chain Management (SSCM). Both research and practical implementation have been growing steadily in the last decade in this specific area (Ahi and Searcy, 2013, 2014). The role of the food industry (retailers, manufacturers and food service) in helping consumers eat healthily and sustainably has been receiving considerable attention in recent years. Consumer perceptions thus show an increasing concern about food safety and about properties of the food they buy and eat. As the country experiences more pressure from globalization, the food industry sector is also subjected to the increased competition in the domestic market. The processors have to meet those challenges by responding very fast to avoid delays which can take them out of the business. If we combine both supply chain management and sustainability together one more interesting filed emerges i.e., sustainable food supply chain management (SFSCM), which is applied in recent years as a reaction to stakeholder pressures (Gold and Hahn, 2013). The consumers are very cautious about the food they eat and this is the duty of producers, retailers and manufacturers to provide them healthy and sustainable food. Also the consumers are well educated and they know what to eat and what not to, thus the food industry has to fulfill the consumer's demands in less time due to increase in globalization. For the analysis of SFSCM based challenges in Indian food industry, we used Fuzzy DEMATEL approach.

The paper is planned as follows: investigated the literature review related to SFSCM; solution methodology apply to solve the present problem in the paper; data collection for Fuzzy DEMATEL; results and discussion of identified challenges in SFSCM implementation; explained the conclusions, limitations and future opportunities of the present research in the food industry sector.

LITERATURE REVIEW

The literature review mainly focuses on SFSCM and analysis of challenges in the Indian food industry.

SFSCM

SFSCM means all the processes in the food industries such as production, procurement of materials and distribution, and also their inverse processes for collecting, returning of unused products to avoid wastage and a *socioeconomically* and *ecologically* sustainable recovery (Bloemhof, 2017). SSCM not only includes information about the food products, their management and capital flows but also maintains the cooperation between different companies. SSCM also results in taking goals of three dimensions of sustainable development viz; social, economic and environmental (Seuring and Mueller, 2008). In the modern food industry, processes have become developed, characterized by mass production. In addition, production, financing, and marketing have become globally incorporated to form global food supply chains (Manning et al., 2006; Trienekens et al., 2012). SSCM is an increasingly main topic in sustainability and (SCM), as companies respond to internal and external pressures from stakeholders, policymakers, and consumers, and from governments, and profit and non-profit organizations dedicated to ecological, public, and commercial responsibility (Ageron et al., 2012; Seuring and Müller, 2008). Managing food supply chains is a well-known problem due to the scale of this industry, the quantity of global food waste, and the relationship between food waste and global malnutrition (Parfitt et al., 2010). In the past years there were many food scandals and incidents which make consumers more attentive towards food products thus food products should be more sustainable to retain and regain consumer's trust. Consumer wants all the knowledge about the food products right from its origin to its delivery which includes safety and expiry date of the product. Sustainability is a broad area which comprises of social issues, environmental issues and expected returns. By this work we aim to discover the status of information technology which supports sustainability in the food supply chains and communication between stakeholders (Wognum et al., 2011).

Challenges in SFSCM

For the successful implementation of SFSCM in Indian food industries we identified eleven challenges based on experts opinion and literature review.

Table 1. Identified challenges to implement SFSCM in Indian food industry

S.No.	Challenges	Description	References
1	Food safety and security (CH1)	In the food production, food safety is an important issue and needs to be considered by stakeholders. From a safety point of view, food chains have numerous vulnerabilities.	(Beulens, 2005, Whipple, 2009 and Bloemhof, 2017)
2	Food quality (CH2)	Food quality means physical properties of food until the food is finally reached to the consumer. It not only includes microbial aspects but also flavors or texture.	(Grunert, 2005, Akkerman et al., 2010, Beta et al., 2017)
3	Transparency (CH3)	Transparency means that all the stakeholders have to share all the information regarding the product without delay and alteration.	(Hofstede, 2004, Trienekens, 2012 and Soysal, 2012)
4	Food wastage (CH4)	Food wastage is the major concern for our country now-a-days and is becoming a cause of global food security. This issue needs to be solved for protecting India's economy.	(Liu et al., 2013 Papargyropoulou et al., 2014, Girotto et.al., 2015)
5	Regulations and standards (CH5)	There should be strict rules and regulations for both food producers and stakeholders. Standards mean well-known norms or necessities for a product like material and packaging specifications. Standards should be maintained by industry associations, regulatory agencies and public organizations.	(Marucheck et al., 2011, Havinga and Verbruggen, 2017)
6	Traceability (CH6)	Keeping consumer's protection in view traceability is an essential and potential factor. Consumers can trace the food products and eliminate non-consumable food products thus can prevent from food safety issues.	(Badia et al., 2015, Souquet et al., 2017, Thomas et. al., 2017)
7	Transportation (CH7)	The food products should be transported well so that it reaches to consumers with all the nutritional qualities. The specific food should be transported in specific conditions to increase their shell life.	(Gustavsson et al., 2011, Egilmez and Park, 2014, Boukherroub et.al., 2017)
8	Supplier selection (CH8)	The relationship between buyer and supplier should be close enough so that buyer gets guaranteed by the food quality. Also supplier should not be fraud in any ways including financial matter and other issues regarding food.	(Liao and Rittscher, 2007, Van Weele and Van Tubergen, 2017)
9	Benchmarking (CH9)	The organizational products, services and processes should be evaluated in relation to its best practice and this is called benchmarking. Benchmarking is often used as a significant tool for the improvement of performance of an organization, competitive advantage and quality management.	(Yakovleva et.al., 2012, Swinburn et.al., 2013, 2015)
10	Information Technologies (CH10)	Efficiency, safety, globalization, refrigerants and efficiency are the most important constrains in the food delivery system. In recent years the market is based on information technology.	(Zailani et al., 2010, and Attaran, 2012)
11	Product life cycle management (CH11)	The management of the products lifecycle is crucial step for manufacturing any food and it is difficult to predict the lifecycle of the product. This includes the time from manufacturing to the final disposal. The data regarding products design, support and ultimate disposal of manufactured goods is hard to manage and it is important for improving safety and security of food product.	(Marucheck and Greis, 2011 and Stark 2015)

SOLUTION METHODOLOGY

Fuzzy Set Theory

Fuzzy set theory is mainly used where there is an inaccuracy in the information or knowledge present in the nature. According to Zadeh (1965), a fuzzy set theory was proposed in the decision making process where the information is insufficient in context with the problem (Bellman and Zadeh, 1970, Zimmermann, 2011). Fuzzy set theory evaluates the method for linguistic and vague terminology by capturing human injustice (Kumar et al., 2013). There are various examples in real world where decisions of decision makers are full of incorrectness and biasness. Linguistics variables are suitably expressed by fuzzy numbers and the fuzzy numbers like trapezoidal and triangular are suitable and commonly used as fuzzy numbers (Mangla et al., 2015).

Fuzzy Set

A fuzzy set is denoted as:

$$\tilde{E} = \left\{ x, \mu_E(X) \right\}, \qquad x \in X \tag{1}$$

where $\mu_E(x)$: $X \rightarrow [0,1]$ is the membership function of $\tilde{E}$ and $\mu_E(x) = 0$ then (x) does not belong to the fuzzy set $\tilde{A}$. $\mu_E(x) = 1$ then (x) completely belongs to the fuzzy set $\tilde{E}$.

Though, unlike the classical set theory, if $\mu(x)$ has a value between 0 and 1 then x partially belongs to the fuzzy set $\tilde{E}$. That is, the pertinence of x is true with the degree of membership given by $\mu_E(x)$.

Fuzzy Numbers

A fuzzy number is a fuzzy set in which the membership function satisfies the conditions of normality

$$\sup \tilde{E}(X)_{x \in X=1} \tag{2}$$

and of convexity $C_1 C_2 C_j C_m$

$$\tilde{D} = \begin{matrix} E_1 \\ E_2 \\ E_3 \end{matrix} \begin{matrix} \tilde{X}_{11} & \tilde{X}_{12} & \tilde{X}_{13} & \tilde{X}_{14} \\ \vdots & \vdots & \vdots & \vdots \\ \tilde{X}_{n1} & \tilde{X}_{n2} & \tilde{X}_{nj} & \tilde{X}_{nm} \end{matrix} \tag{3}$$

For all x_1, $x_1 \in X$ and all $\lambda \in [0,1]$. The triangular fuzzy number is usually used in decision making because to its instinctive membership function,

$$\widetilde{W} = \left[\widetilde{W_1} + \widetilde{W_2} + \widetilde{W_3} + \widetilde{W_4} \right], \text{given by,}$$

For practical applications a unique type of fuzzy number i.e., triangular fuzzy number (TFN) is generally chosen [Dubois and Prade, 1979]. In any (TFN) (p, q, r) its function is given by mathematically equation $\mu E_t x)$ as given in Eq. (4), where $p \leq q \leq r$. Also, (p, q, r,) represents the lower, mean and upper boundary of the TFN:

Mathematical Operations with Fuzzy Numbers

Given any real number K and two fuzzy triangular number $\tilde{E} = \left(p_1, q_1, r_1 \right)$ and $\tilde{F} = \left(p_2, q_2, r_2 \right)$, the main mathematical operations are given as follows: [Pedrycz and Gomide, 2007].

1. Addition of 2 TFNs

$$\tilde{E}(+)\tilde{F} = \left(p_1 + p_2, q_1 + q_2, r_1 + r_2 \right) \quad p_1 \geq 0, p_2 \geq 0 \tag{5}$$

2. Subtraction of 2 TFNs

$$\tilde{E}(-)\tilde{F} = \left(p_1 - p_2, q_1 - q_2, r_1 - r_2 \right) \quad p_1 \geq 0, p_2 \geq 0 \tag{6}$$

3. Multiplication of 2 TFNs

$$\tilde{E}(*)\tilde{F} = \left(p_1 * p_2, q_1 * q_2, r_1 * r_2 \right) \quad p_1 \geq 0, p_2 \geq 0 \tag{7}$$

4. Division of 2 TFNs

$$\tilde{E}(\div)\tilde{F} = \left(p_1 \div p_2, q_1 \div q_2, r_1 \div r_2 \right) \quad p_1 \geq 0, p_2 \geq 0 \tag{8}$$

5. Inverse of a TFN

$$\widetilde{E^{-1}} = \left(\frac{1}{r_1}, \frac{1}{q_1}, \frac{1}{p_1} \right) \geq 0 \tag{9}$$

6. Multiplication of a TFN by a constant

$$k * \tilde{A} = \left(k * p_1, k * q_1, k * r_1 \right) \tag{10}$$

7. Division of a TFN by a constant

$$\frac{\tilde{E}}{k} = \left(\frac{p_1}{k}, \frac{q_1}{k}, \frac{r_1}{k} \right) \tag{11}$$

Figure 1. Research flow chart

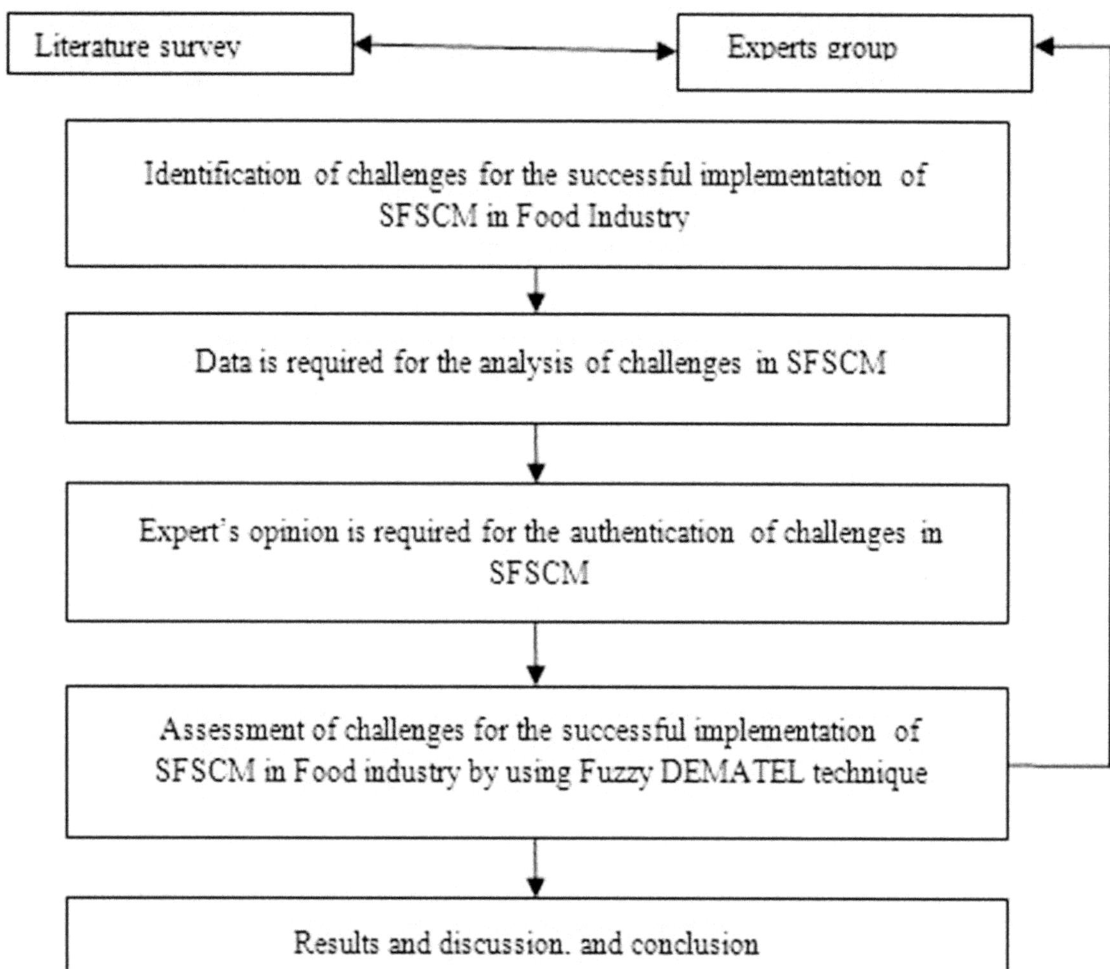

Fuzzy DEMATEL

The Geneva Research Centre of the Battelle Memorial Institute who use DEMATEL method for the first time to solve MCDM problem (Gabus, and Fontela, 1972). DEMATEL approach is mainly used to detect the interrelationship among the factors and it is capable to solve complex problems (Tsai and Chou, 2009, Xia et al., 2015, Govindan et al., 2014, Jia et al., 2015). It is not able to handle the human bias and ambiguity in the data (Patil and Kant, 2013, Hsu et al., 2013). Fuzzy DEMATEL is a powerful tool to handle such situations. Presently many researchers and professionals used DEMATEL to find out the solutions of complex problems successfully (Wu WW, 2011, Mangla et al., 2015). Fuzzy DEMATEL is used in the present work to analyze the identified challenges in the implementation of SFSCM in Indian food industry; in this approach we combine fuzzy logic theory and the benefits of DEMATEL. Fuzzy DEMATEL is very useful to find out the causal relations among the challenges and also helps the managers to construct policies for the successful implementation of SFSCM in food industries. In the given literature DEMATEL has been proved as a powerful tool to solve the complex MCDM problems.

In many cases it is very difficult to decide the human decisions and its preferences into crisp values due to the fuzziness. For the present problem we applied fuzzy theory to the DEMATEL in order to measure the qualitative decisions on the interrelationships among challenges. Steps and equations used in Fuzzy DEMATEL are listed below ((Govindan et. al., 2013, 2015, Mangla et al., 2014 and Hernandez et al., 2014). Defining aim and assessment of factors: To collect the data and to attain the purpose of the problem, literature assessment and experts opinion is required. Possible associated factors that are important for the application of SFSCM are listed as assessment factors.

Step One: To define an experts opinion and evaluation criteria.

In the present step group of experts was created to give experts opinion on associated issues. The important challenges of SFSCM implementation in food sector were determined from literature and were finalized as the evaluation criteria.

Step Two: Formulate fuzzy direct evaluation matrix (F)

Once the assessment criteria are established, pair wise comparison is performed. For the comparison between challenges we need to design a five point linguistic scale in Table 2 which will helps the experts to identify the interrelation. For evaluating and transforming the linguistic information obtained from expert's judgments, the positive triangular fuzzy number (TFN) is used (see Table 2).

The TFN is denoted by quadruplet i.e., (pij, qij, rij), where p $\leq$ q $\leq$ r. Suppose $x^{k}_{ij=p^{k}_{ij}, q^{k}_{ij}, r^{k}_{ij}}$ where $1\leq$ k $\leq$ K, is the fuzzy evaluation that the kth expert gives about the degree to which i has an impact on factor j.

Table 2. Linguistic scale (Mangla et al., 2015)

Linguistic Values (TFN)	Linguistic Terms
No effect	(0,0,0.25)
Very low effect	(0,0.25,0.5)
Low effect	(0.25,0.5,0.75)
High effect	(0.5,0.75,1.0)
Very high effect	(0.75,1.0,1.0)

Step Three: To construct fuzzy initial direct relation matrix

Defuzzification is compulsory for the conversion of fuzzy numbers into crisp number. We can easily defuzzify the fuzzy evaluation matrix with the help of bisection area method. Equation 12 helps in the formation of fuzzy initial relation matrix (F). For fuzzy average matrix (A) we calculate the average of k fuzzy initial relation matrix (F) of n x n experts vies, where k is the number of experts.

Step Four: To attain the normalized initial direct relation matrix (D)

$$S = \min \left| \frac{1}{\max \sum_{j=1}^{n}\{m_{ij}\}}, \frac{1}{\max \sum_{i=1}^{n}\{m_{ij}\}} \right| \tag{12}$$

$$D = M \times S \tag{13}$$

Step Five: To obtain the total relation matrix

$$T = D(I - D)^{-1} \tag{14}$$

where, T= total relation matrix; I= Identity matrix

$$T = [t_{ij}] \, nxn$$

Step Six: To find the total of rows (R) and the total of columns (C)

$$R = \sum_{j=1}^{n} t_{ij} \Big|_{nx1} \tag{15}$$

$$C = \sum_{j=1}^{n} t_{ij} \Big|_{1xn} \tag{16}$$

Step Seven: To sketch a cause and effect graph with the help of *(r+c, r-c)* values.

If the value of *(r-c)* is positive, that challenge come in to the cause group, and if the value of *(r-c)* is negative that challenge come under effect group. A flowchart is given in the Figure 2. In which all steps are explained in Fuzzy DEMATEL approach.

Data Collection

In the current work, the data is collected in 3 steps:

1. Detection of significant challenges for the execution of SFSCM in Indian food industry.
2. Giving ranks to the challenges according to the calculated values and also numbering them accordingly.
3. All the challenges were divided into cause and effect group according to their value of *(r+c* and *r-c)*.

Eleven challenges (CH1, CH2, CH3, CH4, CH5, CH6, CH7, CH8, CH9, CH10, and CH11) were identified on the basis of literature survey and experts opinion in the beginning of the data collection. Experts from industries, academician in the particular field give their opinion for the identification of challenges. Among all, nine challenges were identified by literature survey and two from expert's opinion which were explained in Table 1.

Figure 2. Fuzzy DEMATEL flowchart for the successfully implementation of SFSCM in Indian food industry

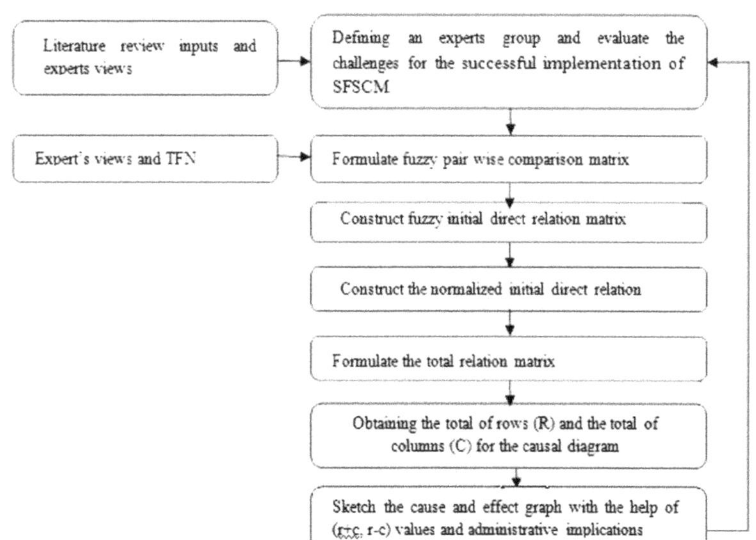

RESULTS AND DISCUSSIONS

Step One: A group of experts (two senior members, one from the food industry and one from the academician) has created the aim of this present research, to find out the key challenges in the implementation of SFSCM in Indian food industries. Selected members were very much capable in their respective areas and good in decision making. Expert's selection was made on the basis of their knowledge and expertise in their particular area. Eleven challenges were identified from the given literature for the successful implementation of SFSCM in Indian food industry and validated by expert's views.

Step Two: Pair wise evaluation was made by experts between the key challenges for the implementation of SFSCM in Indian food industries using the linguistic scale given in the Table 2.

Table 3. Fuzzy direct evaluation matrix (F)

CH	CH1			CH2			CH3			CH4			CH5			CH6			CH7			CH8			CH9			Ch10			Ch11		
CH1	0.0	0.0	0.3	0.0	0.3	0.5	0.0	0.3	0.5	0.5	0.8	1.0	0.8	1.0	1.0	0.8	1.0	1.0	0.5	0.8	1.0	0.3	0.5	0.8	0.0	0.3	0.5	0.3	0.5	0.8	0.8	1.0	1.0
CH2	0.8	1.0	1.0	0.0	0.0	0.3	0.3	0.5	0.8	0.8	1.0	1.0	0.3	0.5	0.8	0.0	0.3	0.5	0.5	0.8	1.0	0.5	0.8	1.0	0.0	0.3	0.5	0.5	0.8	1.0	0.0	0.3	0.5
CH3	0.8	1.0	1.0	0.5	0.8	1.0	0.0	0.0	0.3	0.5	0.8	1.0	0.3	0.5	0.8	0.5	0.8	1.0	0.0	0.3	0.5	0.5	0.8	1.0	0.3	0.5	0.8	0.0	0.3	0.5	0.0	0.3	0.5
CH4	0.5	0.8	1.0	0.8	1.0	1.0	0.8	1.0	1.0	0.0	0.0	0.3	0.5	0.8	1.0	0.5	0.8	1.0	0.0	0.3	0.5	0.8	1.0	1.0	0.8	1.0	1.0	0.5	0.8	1.0	0.5	0.8	1.0
CH5	0.3	0.5	0.8	0.0	0.3	0.5	0.5	0.8	1.0	0.3	0.5	0.8	0.0	0.0	0.3	0.8	1.0	1.0	0.5	0.8	1.0	0.5	0.8	1.0	0.8	1.0	1.0	0.8	1.0	1.0	0.0	0.3	0.5
CH6	0.8	1.0	1.0	0.5	0.8	1.0	0.3	0.5	0.8	0.5	0.8	1.0	0.5	0.8	1.0	0.0	0.0	0.3	0.8	1.0	1.0	0.5	0.8	1.0	0.3	0.5	0.8	0.8	1.0	1.0	0.5	0.8	1.0
CH7	0.5	0.8	1.0	0.8	1.0	1.0	0.0	0.3	0.5	0.3	0.5	0.8	0.5	0.8	1.0	0.8	1.0	1.0	0.0	0.0	0.3	0.8	1.0	1.0	0.8	1.0	1.0	0.3	0.5	0.8	0.8	1.0	1.0
CH8	0.8	1.0	1.0	0.3	0.5	0.8	0.3	0.5	0.8	0.0	0.3	0.5	0.5	0.8	1.0	0.0	0.3	0.5	0.3	0.8	1.0	0.0	0.0	0.3	0.5	0.8	1.0	0.5	0.8	1.0	0.5	0.8	1.0
CH9	0.8	1.0	1.0	0.5	0.8	1.0	0.5	0.8	1.0	0.8	1.0	1.0	0.3	0.5	0.8	0.5	0.8	1.0	0.3	0.5	0.8	0.5	0.8	1.0	0.0	0.0	0.3	0.5	0.8	1.0	0.3	0.5	0.8
CH10	0.8	1.0	1.0	0.8	1.0	1.0	0.3	0.5	0.8	0.8	1.0	1.0	0.3	0.5	0.5	0.0	0.3	0.5	0.3	0.5	0.8	0.0	0.3	0.5	0.0	0.3	0.8	0.0	0.0	0.3	0.8	1.0	1.0
CH11	0.8	1.0	1.0	0.8	1.0	1.0	0.3	0.5	0.8	0.8	1.0	1.0	0.0	0.3	0.5	0.0	0.3	0.5	0.3	0.5	0.8	0.3	0.5	0.8	0.5	0.8	1.0	0.3	0.5	0.8	0.0	0.0	0.3

Step Three: To formulate the initial direct matrix, defuzzification process is used in which fuzzy number is converted into crisp number. Table 4 explained the initial direct relation matrix of key challenges for the implementation of SFSCM in Indian food industries.

Table 4. Fuzzy initial direct relation matrix

Challenges	CH1	CH2	CH3	CH4	CH5	CH6	CH7	CH8	CH9	CH10	CH11
CH1	0.04	0.25	0.3	0.8	1.0	1.0	0.8	0.5	0.3	0.5	1.0
CH2	1.0	0.0	0.5	1.0	0.5	0.3	0.8	0.8	0.3	0.8	0.3
CH3	1.0	0.8	0.0	0.8	0.5	0.8	0.3	0.8	0.5	0.3	0.3
CH4	0.8	1.0	1.0	0.0	0.8	0.8	0.3	1.0	1.0	0.8	0.8
CH5	0.5	0.3	0.8	0.5	0.0	1.0	0.8	0.8	1.0	1.0	0.3
CH6	1.0	0.8	0.5	0.8	0.8	0.0	1.0	0.8	0.5	1.0	0.8
CH7	0.8	1.0	0.3	0.5	0.8	1.0	0.0	1.0	1.0	0.5	1.0
CH8	1.0	0.5	0.5	0.3	0.8	0.3	0.7	0.0	0.8	0.8	0.8
CH9	1.0	0.8	0.8	1.0	0.5	0.8	0.5	0.8	0.0	0.8	0.5
Ch10	1.0	1.0	0.5	1.0	0.5	0.3	0.5	0.3	0.3	0.0	1.0
Ch11	1.0	1.0	0.5	1.0	0.3	0.3	0.5	0.5	0.8	0.5	0.0

Step Four: Explains about the fuzzy normalized initial direct relation matrix of identified important challenges for the implementation of SFSCM in Indian food industries which is illustrated in Table 5.

Table 5. Normalized initial direct relation matrix (D)

Challenges	CH1	CH2	CH3	CH4	CH5	CH6	CH7	CH8	CH9	CH10	CH11
CH1	0.005	0.029	0.029	0.086	0.109	0.110	0.086	0.057	0.029	0.057	0.110
CH2	0.109	0.005	0.057	0.109	0.057	0.029	0.086	0.086	0.029	0.086	0.029
CH3	0.109	0.086	0.005	0.086	0.057	0.086	0.029	0.086	0.057	0.029	0.029
CH4	0.086	0.109	0.109	0.005	0.086	0.086	0.029	0.109	0.109	0.086	0.086
CH5	0.057	0.029	0.086	0.057	0.005	0.109	0.086	0.086	0.109	0.109	0.029
CH6	0.109	0.086	0.057	0.086	0.086	0.005	0.109	0.086	0.057	0.109	0.086
CH7	0.086	0.109	0.029	0.057	0.086	0.109	0.005	0.109	0.109	0.057	0.109
CH8	0.109	0.057	0.057	0.029	0.086	0.029	0.081	0.005	0.086	0.086	0.086
CH9	0.109	0.086	0.086	0.109	0.057	0.086	0.057	0.086	0.005	0.086	0.057
CH10	0.109	0.109	0.057	0.109	0.052	0.029	0.057	0.029	0.033	0.005	0.109
CH11	0.110	0.110	0.057	0.110	0.029	0.029	0.057	0.057	0.086	0.057	0.005

Step Five: Provides the total direct relation matrix of identified important challenges for the implementation of SFSCM in Indian food industries was obtained by equation 5 which is shown in Table 6.

Table 6. Total relation matrix

Challenges	CH1	CH2	CH3	CH4	CH5	CH6	CH7	CH8	CH9	CH10	CH11
CH1	0.328	0.183	0.328	0.238	0.207	0.181	0.328	0.207	0.328	0.203	0.256
CH2	0.236	0.196	0.206	0.300	0.216	0.185	0.244	0.270	0.198	0.263	0.188
CH3	0.211	0.262	0.152	0.273	0.211	0.230	0.191	0.264	0.216	0.209	0.178
CH4	0.200	0.349	0.300	0.268	0.286	0.328	0.244	0.346	0.317	0.319	0.281
CH5	0.200	0.250	0.253	0.283	0.189	0.281	0.269	0.295	0.293	0.311	0.212
CH6	0.211	0.326	0.247	0.336	0.284	0.203	0.313	0.321	0.270	0.335	0.283
CH7	0.230	0.344	0.222	0.311	0.283	0.297	0.219	0.341	0.315	0.292	0.213
CH8	0.230	0.251	0.209	0.238	0.243	0.190	0.247	0.198	0.253	0.268	0.241
CH9	0.210	0.311	0.263	0.343	0.248	0.266	0.253	0.307	0.205	0.301	0.243
CH10	0.218	0.298	0.209	0.309	0.211	0.186	0.221	0.222	0.204	0.190	0.259
CH11	0.213	0.301	0.212	0.312	0.194	0.189	0.224	0.251	0.252	0.244	0.166

Step Six: Total of rows (r) and total of columns (c) of the challenges for the implementation of SFSCM in Indian food industries was obtained by equation 15 and 16.

Step Seven: The value of *(r+c)* and *(r-c)* of the important challenges for the implementation of SFSCM in Indian food industries is explained in the Table 7.

Table 7. Assessment of cause and effect challenges

Challenges	Sum= ri	Sum= cj	r+c	Rank	r-c	Cause/effect
CH1	2.787	2.487	5.27	1	**0.30**	Cause
CH2	2.503	3.071	2.50	10	**-0.57**	Effect
CH3	2.398	2.601	2.40	11	**-0.21**	Effect
CH4	3.238	3.212	3.24	2	**0.03**	Cause
CH5	2.836	2.571	2.84	6	**0.27**	Cause
CH6	3.128	2.536	3.13	3	**0.59**	Cause
CH7	3.067	2.754	3.07	4	**0.31**	Cause
CH8	2.565	3.023	2.57	7	**-0.46**	Effect
CH9	2.950	2.849	2.95	5	**0.10**	Cause
CH10	2.528	2.936	2.53	9	**-0.4**	Effect
CH11	2.559	2.521	2.56	8	**0.04**	Cause

The weight of eleven challenges in the perspective of SFSCM implementation in Indian food industry through the sum of *(r+c)* is given as CH1-CH4-CH6-CH7-CH9-CH5-CH8-CH11-CH10-CH2-CH3 given shown in the Table 7. (CH1) food safety and security, (CH4) food wastage, (CH5) regulations and standards, (CH6) traceability, (CH7) transportation, (CH9) benchmarking, (CH11) product life cycle management were grouped into cause group and (CH2) food quality, (CH3) transparency, (CH8) supplier selection, (CH10) information technology were grouped into effect group by using *(r-c)* values.

Cause Group Challenges

Challenges that come under cause group are having more importance and they are crucial so that focus should be made on them. In the cause group (CH6) traceability has higher (r-c) value (0.59), which directly affects the other challenges in the whole process. But the value of *(r+c)* of (CH6) is 3.13 which is very low as compared to other challenges. It is clearly seen from the picture that traceability affects the other challenges in the list but they receive very less influence in the return. Similarly other challenges in the cause group are ranked according to the *(r-c)* values affect the other challenges but not getting more influence in the return.

Effect Group Challenges

Effect group challenges gets easily influenced by the other challenges in the list, these challenges are not having that much of impact on other challenges but still they contribute significantly. In the effect group (CH2) food having the least *(r-c)* value of -0.57, which confirms that this challenge attain the maximum impact. (CH2) is a very important challenge in the food industry in terms of sustainability establishment, (CH2) directly affect the cause group. The other challenges in the effect group are sequentially arranged according to their priority. (CH8) transparency with *(r-c)* value of -0.46, (CH10) information technology with *(r-c)* value of -0.40 and transparency (CH3) with (r-c) value of -0.21. If industries and government give more emphasis on cause group challenges it automatically affect the effect group challenges.

CONCLUSION

In the present work, challenges were discussed for the successful implementation of SFSCM in Indian food industries. In SFSCM we combined three pillars of sustainability i.e. social, economic and environment. For achieving sustainability in the food sector it is mandatory for all the companies to consider environmental factors, and also ensures that the product which they are making does not have any harmful effect on the environment. The companies are considering the whole product life cycle for the measurement of environment impact of the particular product. Also in future the production of the food depends on the consumers demand or priorities. There is a lot of pressure on food manufacturing companies by consumers, governments, retailers and suppliers for the development of sustainable products. Although the insufficient amount of natural resources, companies should consider the sustainability for making the product environmentally safe. The environmental safe products can be made by change in labeling, packaging types, size, weight and making initiatives to increase recycling and reuse. Indian food industry is still having many challenges in respect of sustainable implementation such as food safety and security, food wastage, food quality, information technology and regulations and standards etc. Researchers and

Figure 3. Cause and effect diagram of challenges for the implementation of SFSCM in Indian food industry

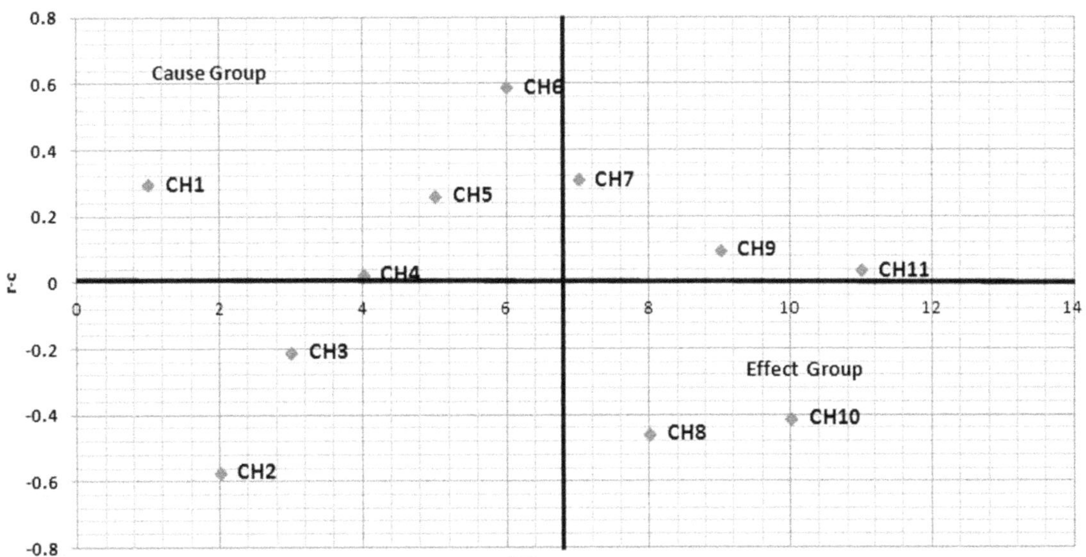

academicians are still working to handle the major problem of food globally. Selected challenges in the current research work mainly focused to achieve sustainability in the food supply chain. It was suggested that SFSCM is an emerging tool for the sustainable, durable and healthy food supply for all. This works mainly focused on the challenges in Indian food industries for the implementation of SFSCM. In this research an effort has been made to put practical use of SFSCM in Indian food industries by identifying the challenges. Here, it can be suggested that Fuzzy DEMATEL, a decision model can be used to clarify the relationship among the challenges as well as causal interactions related to the implementation of SFSCM in Indian food industries. Fuzzy set theory is used for the human biasness or judgment and DEMATEL is used for the interrelation between challenges. Based on the proposed model Fuzzy DEMATEL we analyzed eleven challenges for the implementation of SFSCM in Indian food industry. Challenges namely (CH1) food safety and security, (CH4) food wastage, (CH5) regulations and standards, (CH6) traceability, (CH7) transportation, (CH9) benchmarking, (CH11) product life cycle management are grouped into cause group and more attention is required by the higher management for better results. The remaining challenges are (CH2) food quality, (CH3) transparency, (CH8) supplier selection, (CH10) information technology and they come under effect group, if these challenges are improved it can automatically increase the success rate of SFSCM in Indian food industry.

LIMITATIONS AND FUTURE SCOPE

Present work has its own limitations as well. The eleven challenges were identified which were related to SFSCM implementation in Indian food industry. The other challenges were not identified. On the basis of present work challenges were identified as a future perspective. All identified challenges are made a pair wise comparison by Fuzzy DEAMATEL and experts views. Fuzzy DEMATEL is modified according to the situations in many foreign countries. For the future aspects these eleven challenges were also analyzed by Fuzzy analytic hierarchy process (AHP), analytical network process (ANP) approach to solve multi criteria decision making (MCDM) problem. Total interpretive structural modeling (TISM) is also used for the challenges for successful decision making in Indian food industry.

ACKNOWLEDGMENT

The authors acknowledge and express the gratitude for the support of the research facilities and funds provided by the Department of Mechanical and Automobile Engineering, Graphic Era University, Dehradun, India.

REFERENCES

Ageron, B., Gunasekaran, A., & Spalanzani, A. (2012). Sustainable supply management: An empirical study. *International Journal of Production Economics*, *140*(1), 168–182. doi:10.1016/j.ijpe.2011.04.007

Ahi, P., & Searcy, C. (2013). A comparative literature analysis of definitions for green and sustainable supply chain management. *Journal of Cleaner Production*, *52*, 329–341. doi:10.1016/j.jclepro.2013.02.018

Ahi, P., & Searcy, C. (2014). A stochastic approach for sustainability analysis under the green economics paradigm. *Stochastic Environmental Research and Risk Assessment*, *28*(7), 1743–1753. doi:10.100700477-013-0836-5

Akkerman, R., Farahani, P., & Grunow, M. (2010). Quality, safety and sustainability in food distribution: A review of quantitative operations management approaches and challenges. *Spectrum (Lexington, Ky.)*, *32*(4), 863–904.

Attaran, M. (2012). Critical success factors and challenges of implementing RFID in supply chain management. *Journal of Supply Chain and Operations Management*, *10*(1), 144–167.

Badia-Melis, R., Mishra, P., & Ruiz-García, L. (2015). Food traceability: New trends and recent advances. A review. *Food Control*, *57*, 393–401. doi:10.1016/j.foodcont.2015.05.005

Bellman, R. E., & Zadeh, L. A. (1970). Decision-making in a fuzzy environment. *Management Science*, *17*(4), B-141–B-164. doi:10.1287/mnsc.17.4.B141

Beta, T., Nam, S., Dexter, J. E., & Sapirstein, H. D. (2017). Phenolic content and antioxidant activity of pearled wheat and roller-milled fractions. *LWT-Food Science and Technology*, *78*, 151–159.

Beulens, A. J., Broens, D. F., Folstar, P., & Hofstede, G. J. (2005). Food safety and transparency in food chains and networks Relationships and challenges. *Food Control*, *16*(6), 481–486. doi:10.1016/j.foodcont.2003.10.010

Bloemhof, J. M., & Soysal, M. (2017). Sustainable food supply chain design. In *Sustainable Supply Chains* (pp. 395–412). Springer International Publishing. doi:10.1007/978-3-319-29791-0_18

Boukherroub, T., Bouchery, Y., Corbett, C. J., Fransoo, J. C., & Tan, T. (2017). Carbon footprinting in supply chains. In *Sustainable Supply Chains* (pp. 43–64). Springer International Publishing. doi:10.1007/978-3-319-29791-0_3

Dubois, D., & Prade, H. (1979). Fuzzy real algebra: Some results. *Fuzzy Sets and Systems*, *2*(4), 327–348. doi:10.1016/0165-0114(79)90005-8

Egilmez, G., & Park, Y. S. (2014). Transportation related carbon, energy and water footprint analysis of US manufacturing: An eco-efficiency assessment. *Transportation Research Part D, Transport and Environment*, *32*, 143–159. doi:10.1016/j.trd.2014.07.001

Gabus, A., & Fontela, E. (1972). *World problems, an invitation to further thought within the framework of DEMATEL*. Geneva, Switzerland: Battelle Geneva Research Center.

Genovese, A., Acquaye, A. A., Figueroa, A., & Koh, S. L. (2017). Sustainable supply chain management and the transition towards a circular economy: Evidence and some applications. *Omega*, *66*, 344–357. doi:10.1016/j.omega.2015.05.015

Girotto, F., Alibardi, L., & Cossu, R. (2015). Food waste generation and industrial uses: A review. *Waste Management (New York, N.Y.)*, *45*, 32–41. doi:10.1016/j.wasman.2015.06.008 PMID:26130171

Gold, S., Hahn, R., & Seuring, S. (2013). Sustainable supply chain management in Base of the Pyramid food projects—A path to triple bottom line approaches for multinationals? *International Business Review*, *22*(5), 784–799. doi:10.1016/j.ibusrev.2012.12.006

Govindan, K., Kannan, D., & Shankar, K. M. (2014). Evaluating the drivers of corporate social responsibility in the mining industry with multi-criteria approach: A multi-stakeholder perspective. *Journal of Cleaner Production*, *84*, 214–232. doi:10.1016/j.jclepro.2013.12.065

Govindan, K., Kannan, D., & Shankar, M. (2015). Evaluation of green manufacturing practices using a hybrid MCDM model combining DANP with PROMETHEE. *International Journal of Production Research*, *53*(21), 6344–6371. doi:10.1080/00207543.2014.898865

Govindan, K., Khodaverdi, R., & Jafarian, A. (2013). A fuzzy multi criteria approach for measuring sustainability performance of a supplier based on triple bottom line approach. *Journal of Cleaner Production*, *47*, 345–354. doi:10.1016/j.jclepro.2012.04.014

Grunert, K. G. (2005). Food quality and safety: Consumer perception and demand. *European Review of Agriculture Economics*, *32*(3), 369–391. doi:10.1093/eurrag/jbi011

Gustavsson, J., Cederberg, C., Sonesson, U., Van Otterdijk, R., & Meybeck, A. (2011). Global food losses and food waste. *Food and Agriculture Organization of the United Nations, Rom.*

Havinga, T., & Verbruggen, P. (2017). Understanding complex governance relationships in food safety regulation: The RIT model as a theoretical lens. *The Annals of the American Academy of Political and Social Science*, *670*(1), 58–77. doi:10.1177/0002716216688872

Hernandez, R. R., Easter, S. B., Murphy-Mariscal, M. L., Maestre, F. T., Tavassoli, M., Allen, E. B., ... Allen, M. F. (2014). Environmental impacts of utility-scale solar energy. *Renewable & Sustainable Energy Reviews*, *29*, 766–779. doi:10.1016/j.rser.2013.08.041

Hofstede, G. J., Spaans, L., Schepers, H., Trienekens, J. H., & Beulens, A. J. M. (2004). *Hide or confide: the dilemma of transparency*. Academic Press.

Hsu, C. W., Kuo, T. C., Chen, S. H., & Hu, A. H. (2013). Using DEMATEL to develop a carbon management model of supplier selection in green supply chain management. *Journal of Cleaner Production, 56*, 164–172. doi:10.1016/j.jclepro.2011.09.012

Jia, P., Govindan, K., & Kannan, D. (2015). Identification and evaluation of influential criteria for the selection of an environmental shipping carrier using DEMATEL: A case from India. *International Journal of Shipping and Transport Logistics, 7*(6), 719–741. doi:10.1504/IJSTL.2015.072684

Kumar, S., Singh, B., Qadri, M. A., Kumar, Y. S., & Haleem, A. (2013). A framework for comparative evaluation of lean performance of firms using fuzzy TOPSIS. *International Journal of Productivity and Quality Management, 11*(4), 371–392. doi:10.1504/IJPQM.2013.054267

Lee, H. L., Padmanabhan, V., & Whang, S. (2004). Information distortion in a supply chain: the bullwhip effect. *Management Science, 50*(12), 1875-1886.

Liao, Z., & Rittscher, J. (2007). A multi-objective supplier selection model under stochastic demand conditions. *International Journal of Production Economics, 105*(1), 150–159. doi:10.1016/j.ijpe.2006.03.001

Liu, G., Liu, X., & Cheng, S. (2013). Food security: Curb Chinas rising food wastage. *Nature, 498*(7453), 170–170. doi:10.1038/498170c PMID:23765482

Mangla, S., Kumar, P., & Barua, M. K. (2014). An evaluation of attribute for improving the green supply chain performance via DEMATEL method. *International Journal of Mechanical Engineering & Robotics Research, 1*(1), 30–35.

Mangla, S. K., Kumar, P., & Barua, M. K. (2015). Flexible decision modeling for evaluating the risks in green supply chain using fuzzy AHP and IRP methodologies. *Global Journal of Flexible Systems Management, 16*(1), 19–35. doi:10.100740171-014-0081-x

Mangla, S. K., Kumar, P., & Barua, M. K. (2015). Prioritizing the responses to manage risks in green supply chain: An Indian plastic manufacturer perspective. *Sustainable Production and Consumption, 1*, 67–86. doi:10.1016/j.spc.2015.05.002

Manning, L., Baines, R. N., & Chadd, S. A. (2006). Quality assurance models in the food supply chain. *British Food Journal, 108*(2), 91–104. doi:10.1108/00070700610644915

Marucheck, A., Greis, N., Mena, C., & Cai, L. (2011). Product safety and security in the global supply chain: Issues, challenges and research opportunities. *Journal of Operations Management, 29*(7), 707–720. doi:10.1016/j.jom.2011.06.007

Papargyropoulou, E., Lozano, R., Steinberger, J. K., & Wright, N., & bin Ujang, Z. (. (2014). The food waste hierarchy as a framework for the management of food surplus and food waste. *Journal of Cleaner Production, 76*, 106–115. doi:10.1016/j.jclepro.2014.04.020

Parfitt, J., Barthel, M., & Macnaughton, S. (2010). Food waste within food supply chains: Quantification and potential for change to 2050. *Philosophical Transactions of the Royal Society of London. Series B, Biological Sciences, 365*(1554), 3065–3081. doi:10.1098/rstb.2010.0126 PMID:20713403

Patil, S. K., & Kant, R. (2014). A hybrid approach based on fuzzy DEMATEL and FMCDM to predict success of knowledge management adoption in supply chain. *Applied Soft Computing*, *18*, 126–135. doi:10.1016/j.asoc.2014.01.027

Pedrycz, W., & Gomide, F. (2007). *Fuzzy systems engineering: toward human-centric computing*. John Wiley & Sons. doi:10.1002/9780470168967

Petrovic, D. (2001). Simulation of supply chain behaviour and performance in an uncertain environment. *International Journal of Production Economics*, *71*(1), 429–438. doi:10.1016/S0925-5273(00)00140-7

Petrovic, D., Roy, R., & Petrovic, R. (1998). Modelling and simulation of a supply chain in an uncertain environment. *European Journal of Operational Research*, *109*(2), 299–309. doi:10.1016/S0377-2217(98)00058-7

Seuring, S., & Müller, M. (2008). From a literature review to a conceptual framework for sustainable supply chain management. *Journal of Cleaner Production*, *16*(15), 1699–1710. doi:10.1016/j.jclepro.2008.04.020

Souquet, J., Liu, H., Liu, J., Fan, X., Liddell, J., Levison, P., ... Thomas, O. R. T. (n.d.). Tracking the movement of individual adsorbent particles in expanded beds. In *Book of Abstracts* (p. 76). Academic Press.

Soysal, M., Bloemhof, J., & van der Vorst, J. G. (2012). A Review of Quantitative Models for Sustainable Food Logistics Management: Challenges and Issues. *Proceedings in Food System Dynamics*, 448-462.

Stark, J. (2015). Product lifecycle management. In *Product Lifecycle Management* (pp. 1–29). Springer International Publishing. doi:10.1007/978-3-319-17440-2_1

Swinburn, B., Kraak, V., Rutter, H., Vandevijvere, S., Lobstein, T., Sacks, G., ... Magnusson, R. (2015). Strengthening of accountability systems to create healthy food environments and reduce global obesity. *Lancet*, *385*(9986), 2534–2545. doi:10.1016/S0140-6736(14)61747-5 PMID:25703108

Swinburn, B., Vandevijvere, S., Kraak, V., Sacks, G., Snowdon, W., Hawkes, C., ... & L'abbé, M. (2013). Monitoring and benchmarking government policies and actions to improve the healthiness of food environments: a proposed Government Healthy Food Environment Policy Index. *Obesity Reviews*, *14*(S1), 24-37.

Thomas, A. M., White, G. R., Plant, E., & Zhou, P. (2017). Challenges and practices in Halal meat preparation: A case study investigation of a UK slaughterhouse. *Total Quality Management & Business Excellence*, *28*(1-2), 12–31. doi:10.1080/14783363.2015.1044892

Trienekens, J. H., Wognum, P. M., Beulens, A. J., & van der Vorst, J. G. (2012). Transparency in complex dynamic food supply chains. *Advanced Engineering Informatics*, *26*(1), 55–65. doi:10.1016/j.aei.2011.07.007

Tsai, W. H., & Chou, W. C. (2009). Selecting management systems for sustainable development in SMEs: A novel hybrid model based on DEMATEL, ANP, and ZOGP. *Expert Systems with Applications*, *36*(2), 1444–1458. doi:10.1016/j.eswa.2007.11.058

van Weele, A., & van Tubergen, K. (2017). Responsible purchasing: moving from compliance to value creation in supplier relationships. In *Sustainable Supply Chains* (pp. 257–278). Springer International Publishing. doi:10.1007/978-3-319-29791-0_11

Whipple, J. M., Voss, M. D., & Closs, D. J. (2009). Supply chain security practices in the food industry: Do firms operating globally and domestically differ? *International Journal of Physical Distribution & Logistics Management, 39*(7), 574–594. doi:10.1108/09600030910996260

Wognum, P. N., Bremmers, H., Trienekens, J. H., van der Vorst, J. G., & Bloemhof, J. M. (2011). Systems for sustainability and transparency of food supply chains–Current status and challenges. *Advanced Engineering Informatics, 25*(1), 65–76. doi:10.1016/j.aei.2010.06.001

Wu, W. W. (2012). Segmenting critical factors for successful knowledge management implementation using the fuzzy DEMATEL method. *Applied Soft Computing, 12*(1), 527–535. doi:10.1016/j.asoc.2011.08.008

Wu, W. W., Lan, L. W., & Lee, Y. T. (2011). Exploring decisive factors affecting an organizations SaaS adoption: A case study. *International Journal of Information Management, 31*(6), 556–563. doi:10.1016/j.ijinfomgt.2011.02.007

Xia, X., Govindan, K., & Zhu, Q. (2015). Analyzing internal barriers for automotive parts remanufacturers in China using grey-DEMATEL approach. *Journal of Cleaner Production, 87*, 811–825. doi:10.1016/j.jclepro.2014.09.044

Yakovleva, N., Sarkis, J., & Sloan, T. (2012). Sustainable benchmarking of supply chains: The case of the food industry. *International Journal of Production Research, 50*(5), 1297–1317. doi:10.1080/0020 7543.2011.571926

Zadeh, L. A. (1965). Fuzzy sets. *Information and Control, 8*(3), 338–353. doi:10.1016/S0019-9958(65)90241-X

Zailani, S., Arrifin, Z., Abd Wahid, N., Othman, R., & Fernando, Y. (2010). Halal traceability and halal tracking systems in strengthening halal food supply chain for food industry in Malaysia (a review). *Journal of Food Technology, 8*(3), 74–81. doi:10.3923/jftech.2010.74.81

Chapter 24
Wastage and Cold Chain Infrastructure Relationship in Indian Food Supply Chain:
A Study From Farm to Retail

Saurav Negi
https://orcid.org/0000-0002-5553-0098
University of Petroleum and Energy Studies, India

Neeraj Anand
https://orcid.org/0000-0002-2243-434X
University of Petroleum and Energy Studies, India

ABSTRACT

India, the world's second-largest producer and one of the centers of origin of Fruits and Vegetables is also one of the biggest food wasters in the world. The challenge of feeding India's billion plus people is not really about agriculture and food production but getting the quality food to the concerned people in a right time. The biggest contributors to this waste are lack of temperature controlled transport and inadequate quality of cold storage facilities for both Farmers and Food sellers i.e. retailers. What India lacks, and needs, is a well-developed, world-class cold chain infrastructure. Without it, India's problems are vast and likely to grow. In this chapter, the authors tries to outlines the extent of Fruits and Vegetables waste in India (at various stages from farm to retail) and its ramifications on food production and safety. Authors also highlighted the challenges faced by cold chain sector in India and a roadmap for improvements. As Indian economy is based on agriculture, development of Cold Chain infrastructure from farm to retail points will play a crucial role.

DOI: 10.4018/978-1-7998-5354-1.ch024

INTRODUCTION

Fruit and Vegetables is a very growing sector and constitute of around 90% of horticultural produce in India. Production of horticultural crops in India has increased as compared to the situation a couple of decades ago. Several factors like globalization, Increasing urbanization, Nuclear families, working women, disposable income, changing lifestyles, and rise of organized retails are gearing up the Indian fruits and vegetables supply chains for a better future. Supply chain plays a very vital role in this sector. This area becomes even more important because of perishability and very short shelf life. Supply Chain Management not only helps to cut costs, but also adds to maintain and improve the quality of produce delivered, which are perishable in nature.

India the second-largest producer of Fruits and Vegetables is also one of the biggest food wasters in the world-wasting INR 2 Lakh crore per annum worth of Fruits and Vegetables every year (ASSO-CHAM, 2013).

The challenge of feeding India's billion plus people is not really about agriculture production but getting the proper food to the individuals. The biggest contributors to waste are the lack of cold chain facilities, required infrastructure and temperature controlled transportation system which is hindering the overall growth of this sector and making the supply chain inefficient.

What India lacks, and needs, is a well-established cold chain facilities and infrastructure. Without it, India's problems are vast and likely to grow. The most prone food category to a lack of cold chain infrastructure is Fruits and Vegetables where annual wastage is estimated to be around 35-40% of the total production. Various studies on Fruits and Vegetables supply chain found Poor Cold chain system as a major problem in the Supply chain of F&V which are resulting in various inefficiencies and leads to losses sand wastage across the chain.

From various studies on post-harvest losses in India, it is evident that the amount of food wasted in a year in India is equivalent to annual food consumption in some countries like UK (Rathore, Sharma, & Saxena, 2010) and the total production of the Great Britain (Khan, 2005). Controlling the level of waste is beyond the capabilities and scope of individual farmers. The problem is widespread and proper controlled temperature to maintain and sustain the quality to increase the shelf life of the produce and makes them easily available to the customer in a quality manner is a major concern. The weak and ill equipped cold chain infrastructure (Rathore, Sharma, & Saxena, 2010), improper marketing systems and facilities (Gauraha & Thakur, 2008; Singh, Kushwaha, & Verma, 2008) of the country has become the major impediments in the growth of the sector.

This chapter outlines the extent of Fruits and Vegetables waste in India and highlights where wastage occurs across the supply chain stages starting from farm to retail and its ramifications on food production and safety. The present study undertakes a thorough review of basic and contemporary literature available to explain the present status of post-harvest losses and cold chain infrastructure. It focuses on Fruits and Vegetables since India wastes more of this item than any other food product. In this chapter authors also highlighted the challenges faced by the cold chain sector in India and a roadmap for improvements, including greater use of proven technologies.

BACKGROUND

This section discusses the current Scenerio of Fruits and Vegetables production in India and its world-wide status. It has been seen that India is among the world's largest food producer and serving the food consumer all across the globe.

Cold chain system has gained an importance to the growth of international trade in perishable food items and to the global availability of food supplies. Each year, billions of tons of fresh food items with millions of dollars' worth are lost due to poor cold chain system in developing market (International Trade Administration, 2013). As per the list of World Economic Forum, food crises is the fourth top global risks of highest concern for the next 10 years (World Economic Forum, 2016). Globally, billions of dollars are spent on improving agricultural processes to create higher food produces, but the fact is that nearly half of all food produce never reaches to the consumer's plate (World Economic Forum, 2013).

Global losses in the food sector total more than $750 billion annually (FAO, 2013). These losses are majorly the outcome of lack of proper facilities, inadequate food safety handling procedures and lack of training for those human resources working in the cold chain sector.

The Current State of Fruits and Vegetables Production and Wastage in India

During 2014, India's contribution in the world production of F&V was 13.6% and 14% respectively (NHB, 2014). India is the second largest food producer in the world, after China and one of the centers of origin of F&V with the total production of 91.44 million metric tonnes of Fruits and 166.60 million metric tonnes of vegetables till the year end 2016 (NHB, 2016). The production of F&V in India has been shown in Figure 1 from the year 1991-2016 which has increased from 28.63 million metric tonnes to 91.44 million metric tonnes in fruits and 58.53 million metric tonnes to 166.60 million metric tonnes in vegetables from the year 1991-2016.

Figure 1. Fruits and Vegetables production in India
Source: Indian Horticulture Database, NHB, 2016

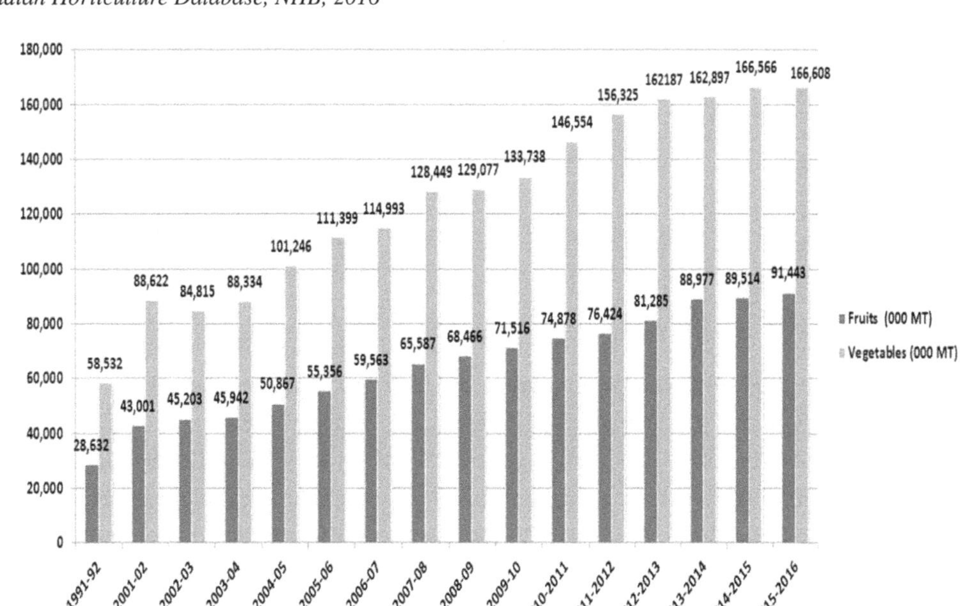

Despite high production and an existing distribution network, India finds it difficult to feed its own people. The main reason for that is high amount of food wastage due to ill-equipped and weak cold chain infrastructure of the country. Because of lack of cold chain infrastructure, poor post harvesting technology, inadequate storage and transportation & lack of food processing industry, about 20 -30 percent of all foods produced in India (Rs. 500 b) gets wasted annually (Mishra & Anjani, 2010; Viswanadham, 2007; Jain, 2007).

There are many studies pertaining to quality and quantity losses during and post-harvest (Negi and Anand, 2016a; Turan, 2008; Murthy, Gajanana, Sudha and Dakshinamoorthy 2009; Troger, 2007; Ozcan, 2007; Karabulut et al., 2005; Kumar et al., 2004; Lawande, 2004; Reddy, 2004; Singh, Banerjee, Singh, Pandey, Sudhakar, & Rai, 2004; Tatlidil, Kiral, Gunes, Demir, Erdemir, and Fidan 2003; Klein and Lurie, 1991; Ozcan and Baklaya, 1995; Ozcan, Balkaya and Ceyhan (1997; Dokuzoguz, 1997; Gunduz, 1997; Kaynas, Celikel, Türkes and Surmeli 1988). It has been reported that a huge amount of fresh produce is wasted in various operational stages of the F&V Supply Chain (Murthy, Gajanana, Sudha and Dakshinamoorthy 2009). According to the calculation of (ASSOCHAM, 2013) India, the producers have to forgo every year Rs. 2.13 lakh crore due to losses in the supply chain of fruits and vegetables.

The Fruits and Vegetables loss among major producing states in India has been shown in Table 1.

Table 1. Fruits and vegetables losses among the major producing state

State	Total Loss (Rs. Crore)
Maharashtra	10100
Andhra Pradesh	5633
Tamil Nadu	8170
Gujarat	11398
Karnataka	7415
Uttar Pradesh	10312
Bihar	10744
Madhya Pradesh	5332
West Bengal	13657
All India	**212552**

Source: ASSOCHAM India

According to CIPHET, Ludhiana, the post-harvest losses of major agricultural produces at national level was of the order of Rs 44,143 crore per annum at 2009 wholesale prices and most of the wastage is happening in fruits and vegetables of about 5.8-18% worth value of Rs 7,437 crore in fruits and Rs 5,872 crore in vegetables (GOI, 2012) due to the lack of cold chain facilities and infrastructure. Poor cold chain infrastructure not only affects the quality of fresh produce but also affects the prices due to the non-availability of products and lack of supply due to losses and wastage.

Negi & Anand (2014) discusses that supply chain of Fruits and Vegetables in India is highly inefficient which is leading to huge losses and wastages and less income to the stakeholders in return. Apart from the loss of revenue to the farmers, it leads to increased additional costs in the supply chain which ultimately enforces the final consumers to pay high charges from his pocket.

COLD CHAIN: PRESENT STATUS

A cold chain protects a wide variety of food produce to get deteriorate in the whole supply chain by providing temperature controlled facility. It is a logistic system that provides a series of controlled temperature storage and transport conditions from the point of origin to the point of consumption, i.e. from farm to fork. It saves fresh produce from degradation, humidity, improper expose to temperature and keeps them frozen, fresh and chilled (Saurav and Potti 2016; Bishara, 2006). Fresh foods, like vegetables, fruits, dairy, confectionary items, meat and poultry requires continuous and uninterrupted temperature controlled atmosphere known as cold chain due to their perishable nature. By controlling proper temperature throughout the chain can improve the shelf life of the products for days, weeks and even for months (for some products) and minimize the chances of losses. The basic concept of cold chain is depicted in Figure 2.

Figure 2. A cold chain
Source: Sapra, and Joshi (2011)

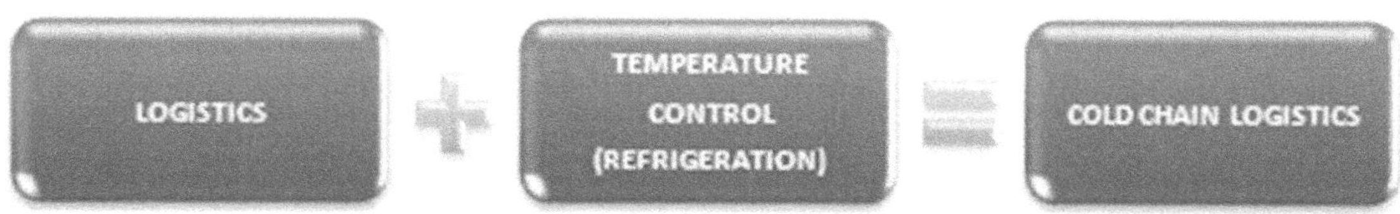

The basic difference between the supply chain of non-perishable items and the temperature controlled supply chain i.e. cold chain is the possibility of degradation in quality and value of the product, which start from the farms to the customer (Joshi et al., 2009). The basic difference between supply chain of non-perishables and cold chain is shown in the Table 2.

Table 2. Difference between supply chain of non-perishables and cold chain

Supply Chain of Non Perishable	Cold Chain.
Includes temperature-insensitive products like nuts, bolts, m/s and equipments.	Includes temperature-sensitive items like plant and animal-based product
Produce information regarding transaction (order, shipment, payment) and location (warehouse, traffic, inventory)	Cold chain includes "condition" and "time" along with transaction and location.
Can bear being stuck in traffic jam.	Require keeping the refrigeration system in a running state, which devours more cost.
Less transportation cost as ordinary trucks, vehicles are used.	Refrigerated vehicles are mandatory for transportation.
Different products can be loaded based on the space available	Different temperature is required for different products, e.g. milk is to be kept at 48C to 108C, whereas ice-cream requires- 18 degree Celsius.
No degradation in value while in transport.	Continuous degradation in value right from the producer till final consumption.
Stops as the product reaches customer.	Includes customer practices related to temperature sensitivity.

Source: Rohit Joshi, Devinder Kumar Banwet, Ravi Shankar, (2009)

The cold chain starts at farm level and covers up to the consumer level in a temperature controlled practices and behavior. Cold chain infrastructure generally consists of grading, sorting, packing, storage, processing and transportation facilities. A typical cold chain infrastructure is shown in Figure 3.

Figure 3. The Cold supply chain infrastructure
Source: Sapra & Joshi (2011)

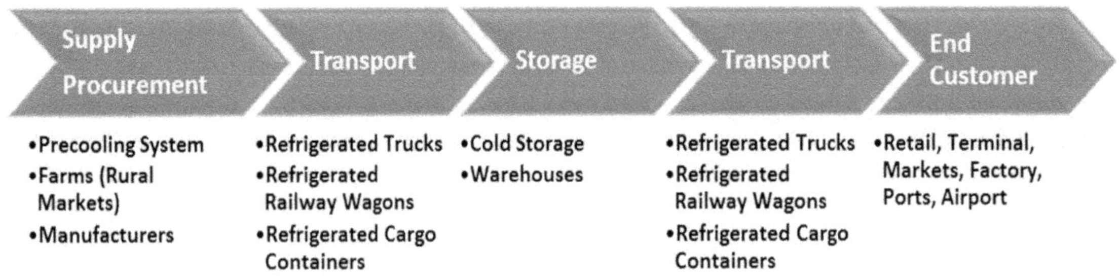

It contains Precooling system at farms to keep the produce fresh and refrigrated vehicles and containers for the effective and efficient movement of Fruits and Vegetables from the point of origin, i.e Farm to the point of consumption, i.e Fork. It also requires cold storage facilities to store the fresh produce in a temeprature controlled warehouse to maintain the quality of Fruits and Vegetables so they couldnot get deteriorated. The cold supply chain pertaining to Fruits and Vegetables is complex as compared to other supply chain due to the perishable nature of the produce, high fluctuations in demand and prices, increasing consumer concerns for food safety & quality (Vorst & Beulens, 2002), and the most important is its dependence on climate conditions (Salin, 1998).

Stakeholders in Cold Chain

Some of the Stakeholders like User Industries, Authorities and Associations, Cold chain Infrastructure sector and Intermediaries using cold chain in India are as follows:

User Industries

- *Fruit and Vegetable Businesses*
- *Food Processing Businesses*
- *Horticulture*
- *Livestock Producers*
- *Seafood Companies*
- *Pharmaceutical Companies*
- *Hotels and Restaurants*
- *Large Format Retailers and Wholesalers*
- *Small Retailers*
- *Laboratories/Healthcare Centers*
- *Medical Equipment Manufacturers*
- *Oil Refineries and Chemical Industries*

- *CRO's (Contract Research Organisations)*

Authorities and Associations

- *Government Agencies (Planning commission, customs, etc.)*
- *DCGI (Drugs Controller General of India)*
- *CDSCO (Central Drug Standard Control Organization)*
- *IARW (International Association of Refrigerated Warehouses)*
- *Global Cold Chain Alliances*
- *Academic and Research Institutions*
- *Growers Association of Fruits and Vegetables*

Infrastructure

- *Warehouse/Cold Storage Owners*
- *Refrigeration and Cold Chain Equipment*
- *Technology suppliers*
- *Refrigeration Solution Providers*
- *Specialized Equipment Providers*
- *ICD's (Inland Containers Depots)*
- *Sea / Air Ports*
- *Transport Vehicles*
- *Security*

Intermediaries

- *Logistics Service Provider*
- *Cold Logistics Players (Shipping Lines, Transporters, Container Companies) Warehousing Agents*
- *Supply Chain Solution Providers*
- *Packaging Service Providers*
- *Banks and Financial Institution*
- *Consultants From the Relevant Spheres Who Are Interested in Knowledge Building.*

Others

- *Power/Electricity*
- *Shelf Life*
- *Temperature*
- *Humidity*
- *Distance*
- *Seasonal Changes*
- *Roads Connectivity*

CHALLENGES

The trend for fresh fruits and vegetables is gaining acceptance in India and is growing at a steady rate. This increasing trend has raised various issues associated with quality, safety and availability of these fresh produce. To make the fresh produce available and achieve the quality and safety it requires proper cold chain management. The Cold chain industry in India is estimated to be presently worth over Rs.13, 000 crores (US$2.6 Billion) per annum (Narula, 2011) with various opportunities in the F&V segment in terms of trade and value addition. Despite the huge opportunities, the cold chain industry is at a nascent stage with various challenges discussed below.

India stores only two percent of its horticulture products in temperature-controlled conditions, while China stores 15 percent and Europe and North America stores 85 percent of their products in such conditions. Adequate cold storage facilities are available for just about 10 percent of India's horticulture production. Of the total annual production, 30-40 percent is wasted before consumption. During the peak production period, the gap between the demand and supply of cold storage capacity is approx. 25 million tonnes (ONICRA, 2012). Although cold storage capacity of over 30 million tonnes has been created in the country, the concept of cold-chain is still in its infancy in India. Considering the fact that India is producing about 240 million tonnes of Fruits and Vegetables every year, the development of cold-chain networks assumes high priority. Owing to the tremendous pressure on improving supply chain and reducing losses during produce handling and movement, the need for creation of a cold chain network is crucial for perishable food commodities. The cold chain sector involved in the business of Fruits and Vegetables have wide opportunities as India is the largest and second largest producer of many F&V such as Mango, Guava, Banana, Papaya, Okra, Potato, Onion, Tomato, Cabbage etc. in world production (NHB, 2016).

Regionally, the existing cold storage capacity is concentrated in terms of both number and capacity in the northern region. Uttar Pradesh and West Bengal contain over 65 percent of the cold storage units in the country and the rest are spread across India. The Region wise Number and Capacity of Cold Storages in India has been shown in Table 3.

Table 3. Region wise number and capacity of cold storages in India (2011)

	Central	East/North East	North	South	West	All India
Number	430 (7.0%)	975 (15.8%)	2895 (47.0%)	866 (14.1%)	990 (16.1%)	6156 (100%)
Capacity (Million MT)	1.71 (6.0%)	7.82 (27.3%)	14.95 (52.1%)	1.95 (6.8%)	2.25 (7.9%)	28.68 (100%)

Source: ONICRA (2012)

The existing cold storage facilities are available only in the wholesale market or nearer to that market. The local market or regional market does not have the cold storage facility where the major fresh produce is sold by the farmer. Cold storage in India has been largely adopted for long-term storage of potatoes, onions and high value crops like apples, grapes and flowers. 75 percent of the cold storage capacity is used to store potatoes, while only 23 percent fall in the multi-product category (ONICRA, 2012).

The major challenges which are found from the various literatures in the cold supply chain are Lack of cold storage and warehousing facilities (Veena *et al.*, 2011; Bhardwaj & Palaparthy, 2008; Dharni

& Sharma, 2008), Inadequate capacities to serve the needs (Narula, 2011), Inadequate usage/improper management of cold storage (Bhardwaj & Palaparthy, 2008); Halder & Pati, 2011), Irregular supply of power or shortage of power to run cold chain (Kapoor, 2009; Shukla D., 2010), Poor post-harvest cold chain technology (Kapoor, 2009), lack of temperature controlled vehicle for the movement of goods (Negi & Anand, 2015a) and non-availability of cold chain infrastructure in traditional retail supply chain of F&V (Negi and Anand 2016b).

Maheshwar & Chanakwa (2006) also highlighted various gaps in cold chain such as poor infrastructure, unavailability of cold storage in close proximity to farms, insufficient cold storage capacity, poor transportation infrastructure etc. Because of these bottlenecks in cold supply chain this sector is suffering from maximum inefficiency and decreases the returns of F&V which affect the income of the farmers and their livelihood. It plays a very vital role and is the backbone for the supply chain of F&V industry but due to the bottlenecks it becomes a very weak link and one of the main reasons for Supply chain losses in food. Negi & Anand (2015b) in his study on cold chain also highlighted that the cold chain infrastructure from farm to retail stage in India has emerged as one of the weakest link in the supply chain of fruits and vegetables sector resulting to losses.

Around 95% of the cold storages are in private hands and because of high charges, an average Indian farmer is not able to avail the facilities of cold storage (Dharni & Sharma, 2008). There is a lack of ownership within the chain and all the players are concerned with their own revenue maximization with limited attention towards the overall profit of the chain. This lack of a holistic view of a supply chain is leading to the post-harvest waste (Shukla & Jharkharia, 2013).

The magnitude of losses is also depends on the infrastructure such as road connectivity and network (Kader & Rolle, 2004). In India most of the northern and eastern region is covered with hilly terrain areas and are the major sources of Fruits and Vegetables but losses and wastage is also one of the major problems of fresh supply chain in hilly areas (Negi and Anand 2015c). The road connectivity for cold chain and network infrastructure in such areas are very poor which takes a long time to take the fresh fruits and vegetables product to the market and deteriorate the quality and condition of the produce which results in wastage. Modi *et al.* (2009) highlighted that the villages, farms and the markets in the Uttarakhand state (Hilly region) are not well connected as well as there are lack of cold chain facilities and the farmers had to somehow bring their harvests to the nearby road for transportation, which increased the wastage of their produce. On its way to market, a lack of proper cold chain facilities results in greater wastage of the fresh produce. Prompt measures are required by the government and other stakeholders in India to improve the state of cold chains and to reduce the huge losses of fruits and vegetables and large amount of money. A lot is yet to happen in the industry with respect to development of technology, Government plans, and strategy before it can transform the lives of farmers and the growth of Indian economy.

According to ASSOCHAM (2013) in his study "Opportunities in Cold Chain: Emerging Trends and Market Challenges-2013", during the period of 2009-2017, the cold chain industry in India is expected to grow at a CAGR of around 25.8 per cent to reach INR 64 billion. The National Horticulture Board (NHB) recommends that investments worth INR 550.74 billion in new cold storage capacity are needed by 2015–16 to keep up with the increasing production of fruits and vegetables.

If the projected growth in Fruits and Vegetables production becomes a reality and cold chain industry investments are not made, the current food waste scenario will only become worse. Despite initiatives by the Government of India and investments by private players to develop efficient cold chain infrastructure, the cold storage industry continues to face a lot of challenges. Further enhancement in the cold storage capacity for Fruits and Vegetable would be very beneficial to both the farmer and the consumer as it minimizes wastages and provides fresher and off-seasonal food items to the consumers.

NEED GAPS

- Lack of backward and forward linkages to supplement cold chain (High VDC- Variable Distribution Cost).
- Needs to study the potential risks and the return on investment (RoI) with reference to Cold Chain Infrastructure like Coolers, warehouses, refrigerated trucks, carriers, shopping malls and others.
- High cost of power: Agricultural sector is offered subsidized power tariffs by the Government of India; Cold chain industry is instead subjected to industrial power tariffs.
- Lack of knowhow and trained manpower.
- 104 million metric tons Perishable produce is transported between cities each year. Only 4 million metric tons moves via reefer mode.
- Lack of Optimization Practice/Technique in reefer transport
- Lack of two-way cargo movement/ back haulage.
- Poor timely deliveries and inefficient utilization of fleets.
- Reefer location tracking challenges (Technology effectiveness and low penetration)
- Third-party logistics:
  - Manual- handling reduces the product quality and life.
  - Lack of 3 Party solution providers for small players. Geographical and service range expanding on project basis from big players. Logistics providers with air conditioned trucks, automatic handling equipment and trained manpower will provide end-to-end support.
  - Lack of end-to-end solutions. One can also adapt state-of-the-art techniques such as cross docking that will reduce the transit times and inventory.
- **FP Industry:** The Central government allows 100% FDI in this sector to promote food processing and increase the shelf life of the product.
- Discontinuous Energy Supply for hours (Backup power is very expensive)
- Education and awareness. Low acceptance due to high costs.

Further the identified challenges in cold chain infrastructure pertaining to Fruits and Vegetables supply chain in India may be graphically represented as shown in Figure 4.

ROADMAP FOR IMPROVEMENTS

India can take further its economic growth by embarking upon strategies and measures to improve its cold chain infrastructural facilities which will reduce the losses and wastage in food and also helps to develop the Indian economy. Prevalent and yielding practices from the developed countries may be adopted and replicated for the betterment of this sector. On the basis of studies, the following measures are suggested to enhance the agribusiness of Fruits and Vegetables sector, curb huge amount of losses and wastage and improve the livelihood of farmers, rural areas and Indian economy as a whole.

Figure 4. Challenges in cold chain in India
Source: Negi and Anand (2015), Cold Chain in India

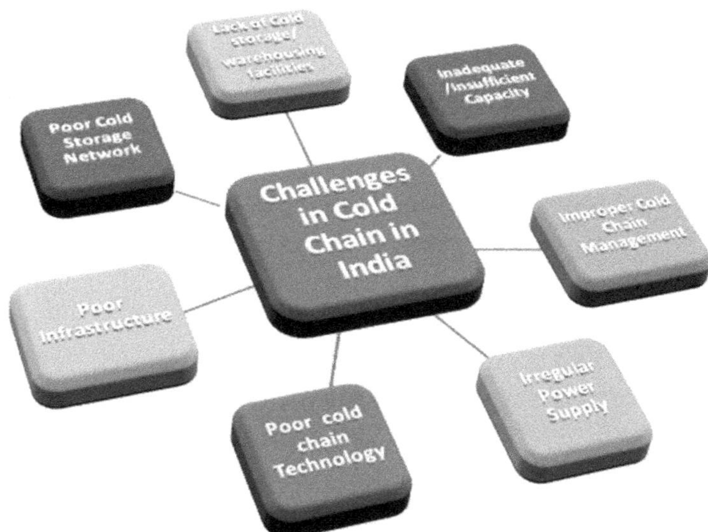

What we require is an integrated cold chain infrastructure covering major production areas, processing units and distribution centers which will call for the following:

- Strong fleet of refrigerated transport vehicles to connect the farm level storage facilities, the processing units and the various distribution centers.
- At retail outlets, display cabinets for marketing of frozen food products are to be provided.
- Need to augment cold storage facilities and container handling facilities at major ports as also an air cargo complex for targeting the global market.
- Infrastructure should be improved in terms of connectivity to farms, grading and packaging facilities etc.
- Cold chain facilities can be developed at the central areas of major Fruits and Vegetables production belt by Government, NGOs or any private firm.
- The adoption of various proven technology solutions can help bring down operating costs and improve quality of Fruits and Vegetables by increasing the shelf life.
- Multipurpose cold storage facilities can be designed to store a range of commodities such as fruit, vegetables, dry fruits, spices, pulses and milk throughout the year. These facilities may have separate chambers that operate at various temperatures and are simultaneously maintained. This makes them more cost and space efficient and delivers higher profitability. This method helps to increase shelf life while ensuring the quality and freshness of the produce.
- Concerned government ministries and authorities like Ministry of Food Processing, National Horticulture Board and NCCD should encourage entrepreneurship in agribusiness by providing subsidies, grants, and assisting (providing technical support) in setting up of cold chain infrastructure/facilities and processing units.
- Strong fleet of refrigerated transport vehicles to connect the farm level storage facilities, the processing units and the various distribution centers.

- Losses due to poor storage and transportation can be minimized by use of Refrigerated Containers which can be used to supplement the existing conventional cold storages.
- Developing efficient and effective cold chain infrastructure has to be the concerted effort of the entire stakeholder present in the supply chain of Fruits and Vegetables sector. There has to be structural changes at different levels of the supply chain-Farmers, Local Intermediaries, Wholesale, Retailers and Consumers. The government, private, public-private partnership, cooperative societies, technology providers, educational institutions dealing in agricultural studies and NGOs can play a very important role in improving the cold chain situations.

TOP PLAYERS IN INDIA

Some of the Top players in India pertaining to cold chain are discussed in this section. Same are as follows:

Snowman Frozen Foods

- A joint venture between Gateway Distiparks, Mitsubishi Corp & Nichirei Logistics Group. Nichirei of Japan is the fourth largest in this business in the world.
- Income $10.2 million in 2010.

Fresh and Healthy Enterprises

- A subsidiary of the state-owned Container Corporation of India (CONCOR), which deals in transporting containers via rail.
- India's largest CA store with capacity of 12,000 MT at Rai in Sonepat, Haryana.

Coldstar Logistics

- Incubated by Tuscan Ventures, a $ 50 million venture capital fund in 2010.
- 3 existing and 9 WIP warehouses across India.

RK Foodland

- A 35 year old 3pl company with pan-India presence.
- Clients include Domino's, Abbott, GSK, and Cadbury.

GATI RedSun

- A leading cold chain company for perishable goods and frozen items.
- The Hyderabad-based Gati recently bought a majority stake in the company. Gati plans to scale up operations in cold chain logistics.

Adani Agrifresh

- A logistics venture formed by the Gujarat-based $ 6 Billion Adani Group.
- Has invested $ 40 Million in setting up 3 CA stores in HP.
- Promotes FARMPIK Brand in North India.

IMPLICATION AND DIRECTION FOR FUTURE RESEARCH

The study has highlighted the cold chain infrastructure and its relationship with losses and wastages of F&Vs. In this chapter, major factors pertaining to cold chain infrastructures are also determined which are leading to losses and wastage in the F&V supply chain. The measures that have been adopted in various cases to minimize the losses and wastage are also discussed. The study will be helpful to the various stakeholders involved in the supply chain of F&V like Farmers, Retailers, Transporters, Local traders, Commission Agents, Cold storage providers etc. to identify and map the factors leading to losses and wastage due to the lack of cold chain infrastructure, and to also adopt appropriate suggested measures to offset the risk of losses and wastage. Prompt measures are required by the Government, related authorities and regulatory bodies in India to improve the situation of cold chain and to mark down the existing losses.

This study will be helpful for the researcher to further empirically test and validate the challenges pertaining to cold chain infrastructure in various regions of the country. A similar research can be carried out with the help of identified challenges with reference to other industries which are associated with cold chain. Researches can also be carried out to overcome the issues pertaining to Cold chain infrastructure like "Return on Investment (ROI) models for establishing a cold chain infrastructure". It can be carried out separately for hilly as well as plain areas.

CONCLUSION

The Fruits and Vegetables sector is seen as an emerging and fast growing business sector in India. With the present food wastage, food shortage, food security and safety are issues taking on growing prominence in India. Considering the current levels of Fruits and Vegetables wasted, cold chain facilities will play an important role in feeding the country populations.

The study and research conducted on the supply chain of F&V in India suggest that there is a dearth of cold chain infrastructure and it becomes a weak link in the supply chain of fruits and vegetables. Cold chain which is known as a backbone for the F&V supply chain is suffering from various bottlenecks which results in the losses of huge quantity and money. These losses and efficiency can be improved by providing proper cold chain facilities such as cold storage, processing facilities, and refrigerated transportation system to the farmers in the local or regional markets and by attracting large number of private Agri business players to set up infrastructural facilities. To develop a world-class cold chain infrastructure, the government and industry bodies need to join hands to adopt better and more efficient technologies to prolong the shelf life of food products and to bring commensurate economic returns to the farmers. This will not only ensure year-round availability of perishable food products and reasonable prices to the consumers but also equitable distribution to other parts of the country.

REFERENCES

ASSOCHAM. (2013a). *Horticulture Sector in India- State level experience*. New Delhi: The Associated Chambes of Commerce and Industry of India.

ASSOCHAM. (2013b). *Opportunities in Cold Chain: Emerging Trends and Market Challenges-2013*. New Delhi: ASSOCHAM Publication.

Bhardwaj, S., & Palaparthy, I. (2008). Factors Influencing Indian Supply Chains of of Fruits and Vegetables: A Literature Review. *The Icfai University Journal of Supply Chain Management, V*(3), 59–68.

Bishara, R. H. (2006). *Cold chain management – an essential component of the global pharmaceutical supply chain*. Retrieved from American Pharmaceutical Review: www.americanpharmaceuticalreview. com/life_science/Bishara_APR.pdf

Dharni, K., & Sharma, S. (2008). Food Processing in India: Opportunities and Constraints. *The Icfai University Journal of Agricultural Economics, V*(3), 30–38.

Dokuzoguz, M. (1997). *Developments on Storage of Horticultural Products in Turkey*. First Symposium of Storage and Marketing in Horticultural Products, Yalova, Turkey. (in Turkish)

Gauraha, A., & Thakur, B. (2008). Comparative economic analysis of post-harvest losses in vegetables and foodgrains crops in Chhattisgarh. *Indian Journal of Agricultural Economics, 63*(3), 376.

GOI. (2012). *Annual Report- Ministry of Food Processing Industries*. New Delhi: Government of India.

Gunduz, M. (1997). Market Structure, Storage, Marketing Systems and Foreign Trade Relations in Horticulture Products. *First Symposium of Storage and Marketing in Horticultural Products*, 9-14. (in Turkish)

Halder, P., & Pati, S. (2011). A Need For Paradigm Shift to Improve Supply Chain Management of Fruits & Vegetables in India. *Asian Journal of Agriculture and Rural Development, 1*(1), 1–20.

Jain, N. (2007). *International Conference on Agribusiness and Food Industry in Developing Countries: Opportunities and Challenges*. Retrieved February 19, 2013, from IIM Lucknow: http://www.iiml.ac.in/events/Program.html

Kader, A., & Rolle, R. (2004). *In the role of post harvest management in assuring the quality and safety of horticultural produce*. Rome: FAO Food and Agricultural Organizations of the United Nations.

Kapoor, P. (2009, July 28). *Doctoc-International Summit on Food Processing and Agribusiness*. Retrieved January 22, 2014, from Docstoc.com: http://www.docstoc.com/docs/127265667/ENTREPRENEURIAL-OPPORTUNITIES-IN-THE-AGRI-BUSINESS

Karabulut, O. A., Kuruoglu, G., Ilhan, K., & Arslan, U. (2005). Using of Heat Treatments against Post-harvest Diseases, J. Ondokuz Mayıs Univ. [in Turkish]. *Facul. Agric., 20*(1), 94–101.

Kaynas, K., Celikel, F. G., Türkes, N., & Surmeli, N. (1988). *Studies on Maturity Physiology of Storage Facilities and of Some Tomato Varieties Grown in Yalova and Iznik Regions. In Vegetable Breeding in Open Research Project Report* (pp. 415–423). Ataturk Horticulture Research Institute. (in Turkish)

Khan, A. (2005, September 5). *The domestic food market: is India ready for food processing?* Retrieved January 26, 2014, from India Development Foundation: http://www.idfresearch.org/pdf/dommarket.pdf

Klein, J. D., & Lurie, S. (1991). Postharvest Heat Treatment and Fruit Quality. *Postharvest News Inf.*, *2*, 15–19.

Kumar, S., Pal, S., & Joshi, P. K. (2004). Vegetable Sector in India: An Overview. Impact of Vegetable Research in India, National Centre for Agricultural Economics and Policy Research, ICAR.

Lawande, K. E. (2004). Status of Onion and Garlic Research in India. Impact of Vegetable Research in India, National Centre for Agricultural Economics and Policy Research, ICAR.

Maheshwar, C., & Chanakwa, T. S. (2006). Postharvest losses due to gaps in cold chain in India-A solution. *ISHS Acta Horticulturae 712: IV International Conference on Managing Quality in Chains - The Integrated View on Fruits and Vegetables Quality.* Retrieved January 26, 2014, from Acta Horticulturae: http://www.actahort.org/books/712/712_100.htm

Mishra, P. K., & Anjani, S. (2010). *Supply Chain Management of Agricultural Commodities through Electronic Spot Exchanges.* Retrieved from http://ssrn.com/abstract=1728686

Modi, P., Mishra, D., Gulati, H., & Murugesan, K. (2009). Uttarakhand state cooperative federation: Can it help the horticulture farmers? *Vision—The Journal of Business Perspective, 13*(2), 53-61.

Murthy, D. S., Gajanana, T. M., Sudha, M., & Dakshinamoorthy, V. (2009). Marketing and Post harvest losses in fruits: Its implications on Availability and economy. *Indian Journal of Agricultural Economics, 64*(2), 259–275.

Narula, S. A. (2011). Reinventing cold chain industry in India: Need of the hour: Interview with Mr Sanjay Aggarwal. *Journal of Agribusiness in Developing and Emerging Economies, 1*(2), jadee.2011.52401baa.001. doi:10.1108/jadee.2011.52401baa.001

Negi, S., & Anand, N. (2016a). Factors Leading to Losses and Wastage in the Supply Chain of Fruits and Vegetables Sector in India. *Energy Infrastructure and Transportation Challenges and Way Forward-Conference Proceedings, International Conference on Management of Infrastructure* (pp. I 89 - I 105). Dehradun.

Negi, S., & Anand, N. (2016b). An Overview of Fruits and Vegetable's Retail Supply Chain Models in India. In N. Kamath, & S. Saurav (Eds.), Handbook of research on strategic supply chain management in the retail industry (pp. 170-187). Hershey, PA: Business Science Reference, IGI Global.

Negi, S., & Anand, N. (2015a). Issues and challenges in the supply chain of fruits & vegetables sector in India: A Review. *International Journal of Managing Value and Supply Chains, 6*(2), 47–62. doi:10.5121/ijmvsc.2015.6205

Negi, S., & Anand, N. (2015b). Cold Chain: A Weak Link in the Fruits and Vegetables Supply Chain in India. *The IUP Journal of Supply Chain Management*, 48-62.

Negi, S., & Anand, N. (2015c). Supply Chain of Fruits & Vegetables' Agribusiness in Uttarakhand (India): Major Issues and Challenges. *Journal of Supply Chain Management Systems, 4*(1 & 2), 43–57.

Negi, S., & Anand, N. (2014, December). Supply Chain Efficiency: An Insight from Fruits and Vegetables Sector in India. *Journal of Operations and Supply Chain Management, 7*(2), 154–167. doi:10.12660/joscmv7n2p154-167

NHB. (2014). *Horticulture Statistics at a glance.* Retrieved February 21, 2017, from National Horticulture Board: http://nhb.gov.in/PDFViwer.aspx?enc=3ZOO8K5CzcdC/Yq6HcdIxC0U1kZZenFuNVXacDLxz28=

NHB. (2016). *3rd Advance Estimate of Area and Production of Horticulture Crops (2015-2016).* Retrieved March 21, 2017, from National Horticulture Board: http://nhb.gov.in/PDFViwer.aspx?enc=3ZOO8K5CzcdC/Yq6HcdIxC0U1kZZenFuNVXacDLxz28=

ONICRA. (2012). *Indian Cold Chain Industry.* Retrieved January 25, 2015, from ONICRA: http://www.onicra.com/images/pdf/publications/coldchainindustryreportjune2014.pdf

Ozcan, M. (2007). *Affects on Quality and Durability of Harvest and Post-Harvest Practices in Horticultural Products.* Retrieved September 18, 2013, from http://www.carsambaziraatodasi.com/ab1_1.asp

Ozcan, M., & Balkaya, A. (1995). Causes of Harvest and Post-Harvest Losses on Fruits and Vegetables Product Grown in Amasya Province. *J. Ondokuz Mayıs Univ.* [in Turkish]. *Facul Agric., 10*(1), 51–61.

Ozcan, M., Balkaya, A., & Ceyhan, V. (1997). Analysis of Vegetable Marketing Activities in the Black Sea region. *First Symposium of Storage and Marketing in Horticultural Products,* 229-234s. (in Turkish)

Rathore, J., Sharma, A., & Saxena, K. (2010). Cold Chain Infrastructure for Frozen Food:A Weak Link in Indian Retail Sector. *The IUP Journal of Supply Chain Management, 7*(1-2), 90–103.

Reddy, P. P. (2004). Vegetable Research in India-An IIHR Perspective. Impact of Vegetable Research in India, National Centre for Agricultural Economics and Policy Research, ICAR.

Salin, V., & Nayga, R. M. Jr. (2003). A cold chain network for food exports to developing countries. *International Journal of Physical Distribution & Logistics Management, 33*(10), 918–933. doi:10.1108/09600030310508717

Sapra, R., & Joshi, S. (2011, Nov-Dec). *Cold Chain Logistics Sector Analysis Nov-Dec.* Retrieved February 4, 2014, from Business Design: http://www.businessdesign.co.in/webfiles/Project/312313092332Cold%20Chain%20Logistics_Jan.2011.pdf

Saurav, S., & Potti, R. (2016). Cold Chain Logistics in India: A Study. In A. Dwivedi (Ed.), Innovative Solutions for Implementing Global Supply Chains in Emerging Markets (pp. 159-172). IGI Global. doi:10.4018/978-1-4666-9795-9.ch011

Shukla, D. (2010). *UNCTAD.* Retrieved January 22, 2014, from http://unctad.org/sections/wcmu/docs/ettcp05_en.pdf

Shukla, M., & Jharkharia, S. (2013). Agri-fresh produce supply chain management: A state-of-the-artliterature review. *International Journal of Operations & Production Management, 33*(2), 114–158. doi:10.1108/01443571311295608

Singh, B., Banerjee, M. K., Singh, K. P., Pandey, P. K., Sudhakar, P., & Rai, M. (2004). *AICRP on Vegetables in India: Evolution andAchievements Impact of Vegetable Research in India.* New Delhi: National Centre for Agricultural Economics and Policy Research,ICAR.

Singh, R., Kushwaha, R., & Verma, S. K. (2008). An economic appraisal of post-harvest losses in vegetable in Uttar Pradesh. *Indian Journal of Agricultural Economics, 63*(3), 378.

Tatlidil, F., Kiral, T., Gunes, A., Demir, K., Erdemir, G., & Fidan, H. (2003). *Economic Analysis of Crop losses during Pre-Harvest and Harvest Periods in Tomato Production in the Ayaşand Nallıhan Districts of Ankara Province.* Academic Press.

Troger, K., Hensel, O., & Burkert, A. (2007). Conservation of Onion and Tomato in Niger - Assessment of Post-Harvest Losses and Drying Methods. In *Conference on International Agricultural Research for Development.* University of Kassel-Witzenhausen and University of Gottingen.

Turan. (2008). *Post-harvest Practices on Fruits.* Author.

Veena, Babu, K. N., & Venkatesha, H. R. (2011). Supply Chain: A Differentiator in Marketing Fresh Produce. *The IUP Journal of Supply Chain Management, 8*(1), 23-36.

Viswanadham, N. (2007). *Can India be the food basket for the world?* Working Paper series, IBS, Hyderabad. Retrieved from http://www.cccindia.co/corecentre/Database/Docs/DocFiles/Can_India_be.pdf

Vorst, J. V., & Beulens, A. (2002). Identifying sources of uncertainty to generate supply chain redesign strategies. *International Journal of Physical Distribution & Logistics Management, 32*(6), 409–430. doi:10.1108/09600030210437951

World Economic Forum. (2016). *The Global Risks 2016* (11th ed.). Geneva: World Economic Forum.

World Economic Forum. (2013). *Outlook on the Logistics and Supply Chain Industry 2013.* Geneva: World Economic Forum.

ADDITIONAL READING

Aneesh, M., & Arnav, S. (2011). Cold chain: Finally warming up to India. *Infrastructure Today*, 22-25.

Blanco, A. M., Masini, G., Petracci, N., & Bandoni, J. A. (2005). Operations management of a packaging plant in the fruit industry. *Journal of Food Engineering, 70*(3), 299–307. doi:10.1016/j.jfoodeng.2004.05.075

Bogataj, M., Bogataj, L., & Vodopivec, R. (2005). Stability of perishable goods in cold logistic chains. *International Journal of Production Economics, 93/94*, 345–356. doi:10.1016/j.ijpe.2004.06.032

Bourlakis, C., & Bourlakis, M. (2005). Information technology safeguards, logistics asset specificity and fourth-party logistics network creation in the food retail chain. *Journal of Business and Industrial Marketing, 20*(2), 88–98. doi:10.1108/08858620510583687

Bourlakis, M. A., & Weightman, P. W. (Eds.). (2008). *Food supply chain management.* John Wiley & Sons.

Derens, E., Palagos, B., & Guilpart, J. (2006). The cold chain of chilled products under supervision in France. In *13th World Congress of Food Science & Technology 2006* (pp. 823-823). 10.1051/IU-FoST:20060823

Donk, D. P. V., Akkerman, R., & Vaart, T. V. (2008). Opportunities and realities of supply chain integration: The case of food manufacturers. *British Food Journal, 110*(2), 218–235. doi:10.1108/00070700810849925

Donselaar, K., Woensel, T., Broekmeulen, R., & Fransoo, J. (2006). Inventory control of perishables in supermarkets. *International Journal of Production Economics, 104*(2), 462–472. doi:10.1016/j.ijpe.2004.10.019

Emond, J. P. (2008). The cold chain. *RFID-Technology and applications*, 144-156.

Fearne, A., & Hughes, D. (2000). Success factors in the fresh produce supply chain: Insights from the UK. *British Food Journal, 102*(10), 760–772.

Fearne, A., Barrow, S., & Schulenberg, D. (2006). Implanting the benefits of buyer-supplier collaboration in the soft fruit sector. *Supply Chain Management: An International Journal, 11*(1), 3–5. doi:10.1108/13598540610642402

Fernie, J., & Sparks, L. (2014). *Logistics and retail management: emerging issues and new challenges in the retail supply chain*. Kogan Page Publishers.

Goldman, A., Ramaswami, S., & Krider, R. E. (2002). Barriers to the advancement of modern food retail formats: Theory and measurement. *Journal of Retailing, 78*(4), 281–295. doi:10.1016/S0022-4359(02)00098-2

Hahn, K. H., Hwant, H., & Shinn, S. W. (2004). A returns policy for distribution channel coordination of perishable items. *European Journal of Operational Research, 152*(3), 770–780. doi:10.1016/S0377-2217(02)00753-1

Heap, R. D. (2006). Cold chain performance issues now and in the future. *Bulletin of the IIR, 4*.

Hingley, M. K. (2005). Power imbalanced relationships: Cases from UK fresh food supply. *International Journal of Retail & Distribution Management, 33*(8), 551–569. doi:10.1108/09590550510608368

International Trade Administration. (2016). Retrieved March 30, 2017, from 2016 Top Markets Report Cold Chain: http://trade.gov/topmarkets/pdf/Cold_Chain_Executive_Summary.pdf

Jedermann, R., Ruiz-Garcia, L., & Lang, W. (2009). Spatial temperature profiling by semi-passive RFID loggers for perishable food transportation. *Computers and Electronics in Agriculture, 65*(2), 145–154. doi:10.1016/j.compag.2008.08.006

Joshi, R., Banwet, D. K., & Shankar, R. (2009). Indian cold chain: Modeling the inhibitors. *British Food Journal, 111*(11), 1260–1283. doi:10.1108/00070700911001077

Kuo, J. C., & Chen, M. C. (2010). Developing an advanced multi-temperature joint distribution system for the food cold chain. *Food Control, 21*(4), 559–566. doi:10.1016/j.foodcont.2009.08.007

Kittipanya-ngam, P., Shi, Y., & Gregory, M. J. (2011). Exploring geographical dispersion in Thailand-based food supply chain (FSC). *Benchmarking: An International Journal, 18*(6), 802–833. doi:10.1108/14635771111180716

Likar, K., & Jevšnik, M. (2006). Cold chain maintaining in food trade. *Food Control, 17*(2), 108–113. doi:10.1016/j.foodcont.2004.09.009

Mahajan, R., Garg, S., & Sharma, P. B. (2016). Food Cold Chain Management: An Indian Perspective. In A. Dwivedi, Innovative Solutions for Implementing Global Supply Chains in Emerging Markets (pp. 187-202). IGI Global.

Mahajan, R., Garg, S., & Sharma, P. B. (2011). Indian frozen peas market: A case study on FPIL. *International Journal of Globalisation and Small Business, 4*(2), 154–169. doi:10.1504/IJGSB.2011.042250

Marsden, T., Banks, J., & Bristow, G. (2000). Food supply chain approaches: Exploring their role in rural development. *Sociologia Ruralis, 40*(4), 424–438. doi:10.1111/1467-9523.00158

Mingfei, L., & Ting, Y. (2011, July). The cold chain logistics performance evaluation on sideline products based on data envelopment analysis. In *Product Innovation Management (ICPIM), 2011 6th International Conference on* (pp. 371-374). IEEE. 10.1109/ICPIM.2011.5983679

Ovca, A., & Jevšnik, M. (2009). Maintaining a cold chain from purchase to the home and at home: Consumer opinions. *Food Control, 20*(2), 167–172. doi:10.1016/j.foodcont.2008.03.010

Punt, H., & Huysamer, M. (2005). Supply chain technology and assessment—temperature variances in a 12 m integral reefer container carrying plums under a dual temperature shipping regime. *Acta Horticulturae, 687*(687), 289–296. doi:10.17660/ActaHortic.2005.687.35

Ren, Y., Hu, Q., & Huang, X. (2011, August). Researching on benefit assignment of logistics system in cold chain for food. In *Emergency Management and Management Sciences (ICEMMS), 2011 2nd IEEE International Conference on* (pp. 513-515). IEEE.

Ruiz García, L., & Lunadei, L. (2010). *Monitoring cold chain logistics by means of RFID.* In-Tech. doi:10.5772/8006

Viator, C. L., Fang, W. Y., Hadley, J. L., Aiew, W., Salin, V., & Nayga, R. (2001), *Infrastructure Needs Assessment for Distribution of Frozen Processed Potato Products in Southeast Asian Countries,* Final report on Cooperative Agreement No. 5599-109, prepared for US Department of Agriculture, Foreign Agriculture Service, available at: http://agecon.tamu.edu/faculty/salin/research/aptapg.html

Xiaohong, X. U., Lan, H., & Wang, R. (2010, January). Identification of critical control points of the food cold chain logistic process. In *Logistics Systems and Intelligent Management, 2010 International Conference on* (Vol. 1, pp. 164-168). IEEE. 10.1109/ICLSIM.2010.5461444

KEY TERMS AND DEFINITIONS

Cold Chain: A cold chain is a temperature-controlled supply chain. An unbroken cold chain is an uninterrupted series of storage and distribution activities which maintain a given temperature range. It is used to help extend and ensure the shelf life of products such as fresh agricultural produce, seafood, frozen food.

Cold Storage: It refers to a form of refrigerated storage.

Food Loss and Wastage: Food loss and food waste refer to the decrease of food in subsequent stages of the food supply chain intended for human consumption.

Horticulture: Horticulture is the branch of agriculture that deals with the art, science, technology, and business of growing plants. It includes the cultivation of medicinal plants, fruits, vegetables, nuts, seeds, herbs, sprouts, mushrooms, algae, flowers, seaweeds and non-food crops such as grass and ornamental trees and plants.

Infrastructure: The basic physical and organizational structures and facilities (e.g. buildings, roads, and power supplies) needed for the operation of a society or enterprise.

Local Intermediaries: Firm or person (such as a broker or consultant) who acts as a mediator on a link between parties to a business deal, investment decision, negotiation, etc.

Metric Ton (MT): Equal to 1000 kilogram. Also called tonne.

NGO: A non-governmental organization (NGO) is a not-for-profit organization that is independent from states and international governmental organizations.

Post-Harvest: In agriculture, postharvest handling is the stage of crop production immediately following harvest, including cooling, cleaning, sorting and packing.

Reefer Trucks: A refrigerator truck is a van or truck designed to carry perishable freight at specific temperatures. Like refrigerator cars, refrigerated trucks differ from simple insulated and ventilated vans (commonly used for transporting fruit), neither of which are fitted with cooling apparatus. It can be ice-cooled, equipped with any one of a variety of mechanical refrigeration systems powered by small displacement diesel engines, or utilize carbon dioxide (either as dry ice or in liquid form) as a cooling agent.

Refrigerated Container: A refrigerated container or reefer is an intermodal container (shipping container) used in intermodal freight transport that is refrigerated for the transportation of temperature sensitive cargo.

Shelf Life: The length of time a product may be stored without becoming unsuitable for use or consumption.

Supply Chain: The sequence of processes involved in the production and distribution of a commodity from the point of origin to the point of consumption.

This research was previously published in Supply Chain Management Strategies and Risk Assessment in Retail Environments edited by Akhilesh Kumar and Swapnil Saurav; pages 247-266, copyright year 2018 by Business Science Reference (an imprint of IGI Global).

Chapter 25
Perishable Goods Supply Cold Chain Management in India

Anju Bharti
Maharaja Agrasen Institute of Management Studies, India

Arun Mittal
Birla Institute of Technology, India

ABSTRACT

India has seen a phenomenal growth and occupies the top three positions in production from last decades in production of horticulture produce, dairy and meat products over the last decade. But at present, India's share in global farm trade is still very small even with such large production volumes. This is mainly caused due to lack of cold chain infrastructure which includes both storage and transportation facilities. The cold chain industry in India is still at a nascent stage and despite large production of perishables, the cold chain potential still remain untapped due to high share of single commodity cold storage, high initial investment (for refrigerator units and land), lack of enabling infrastructure like power & roads, lack of awareness for handling perishable produce and lapse of service either by the storage provider or the transporter leading to poor quality produce. Cold chain systems are crucial to the growth of global trade in perishable products and to the worldwide availability of food and health supplies.

INTRODUCTION

India has seen a phenomenal growth and occupies the top three positions in production from last decades in production of horticulture produce, dairy and meat products over the last decade. But at present, India's share in global farm trade is still very small even with such large production volumes. India is also one of the world's largest consumers of food. According to Top Markets Report, 2015, on Cold Chain by International Trade Administration, it is the third largest producer of agriculture. India is one of the largest producers of milk in the world with the largest livestock population. India is the second largest producer of fruits and vegetables in the world with production of 81.3 million MT and 162.2 million MT respectively but its share in global export of fruits and vegetables is around 1.4% only. Approximately,

DOI: 10.4018/978-1-7998-5354-1.ch025

18% of fruits and vegetables get wasted in the country. This is mainly caused due to lack of cold chain infrastructure which includes both storage and transportation facilities.

Food processing methods refers to value addition to agricultural or horticultural produce. The food processing sector is composed of two segments:

1. Primary food processing sector (62% in value, packaged fruits and vegetables, milk, etc.) and
2. Value added food processing sector (38% in value, processed fruits and vegetables, juices, jam & jelly etc.).

Specifically in India, around 40% of produce gets wasted due to inadequate cold chain infrastructure, and one third of losses incur during storage and transit as it has less than half the capacity to meet its current cold chain needs(www.coolingindia.in, 2016).

Now, the Indian agriculture sector is on the threshold of a major shift from traditional farming to horticulture, meat and poultry and dairy products, all of which fall under perishables. As the consumption habit is changing drastically, the demand for fresh and processed fruits and vegetables is also increasing with urban population. It is expected that Indian cold chain industry will attract more overseas partners to learn more about the market to position themselves to take full advantage of emerging opportunities. Cold chains are primarily for fruits and vegetables, meat and marine products, dairy products, ice creams and confectionery, which are perishable. The markets for cold chain have been sub-divided into a number of sectors. These are, for example, agriculture, horticulture, fisheries aquaculture, dairy, processed food for ready-to-eat together with the packaging companies, retailers, wholesalers, etc.

There is an arising increase in demand, diversification and value addition which are the dominating factor in the Indian agriculture today. The emergence of an organised retail food sector coupled with changes in FDI laws has created fresh opportunities in domestic perishables and food industry which includes the cold chain sector. The Indian government needs to focus more on food preservation so the cold storage sector may undergo a major breakthrough. The government is giving full support and has introduced various incentives and policy changes in order to eliminate production wastage and decide on fair price for harvest, increase PPP and improve the country's rural infrastructure. It is expected that Indian cool chain industry will attract more overseas partners to learn more about the market to position them to take full advantage of emerging opportunities (www.itln.in, 2014).

The success totally relies upon effective management of the 'cold chain', a term used to describe the series of interdependent operations in the production, distribution, storage and retailing of chilled and frozen foods. Control of the cold chain is vital to preserve the safety and quality of refrigerated foods and comply with legislative directives and industry 'codes of practice' (EU Commission).

REQUIREMENTS OF COLD CHAIN

Cold chain for perishable foods is becoming increasingly important. As, a study done by the United Nations Environment Program conveyed that over half of the food produced globally is lost, wasted or discarded as a result of inefficiency in the human-managed food chain. Now a day, proper temperature monitoring and management throughout the cold chain is no longer a luxury but have become a necessity. Even relatively a small variation in temperature can significantly impact the shelf life of fresh produce and its value. The cold chain requires the monitoring of temperature monitoring throughout the cold chain providing the ability to act on changes in temperature in real-time. It enables documented delivery quality which in turn provides increased customer satisfaction.

It has become a responsibility of manufacturer to maintain the quality of goods and to ensure their preservation by maintaining the correct temperature inside the vehicles so as to follow the cold chain system and its guidelines. It is, therefore, essential to track goods accurately in real time to monitor the temperature at all times.

The world has seen the impact of poor food preservation and global food supply which is undoubtedly far greater than the observed food losses alone. It is noteworthy that the loss of hundreds of millions of tonnes of foodstuffs exerts an additional effect on global warming due to wasting of the scarce or non-renewable resources required to produce and transport them. The costs of the cold chain, both economic and environmental, can often be more than offset by the economic and environmental benefits due to reduced post-harvest losses.

Table 1 shows the range of temperature of the food product storage:

Table 1. Predicted loss of fresh food storage in developing countries

Food Product Storage	At Optimum Cold Temperature	Optimum Temperature + 10° C	Optimum Temperature +20°C	Optimum Temperature + 30°C
Fresh Fish	10 days at 0° C	4-5 days at10°C	1-2 days at 20°C	A few hours at 30° C
Milk	2 Weeks at0°C	7 days at 10°C	2-3 days at 20°C	A few hours at 30° C
Fresh Green Vegetables	1Month at 0°C	2 weeks at 10°C	1 week at 20°C	Less than 2 days at 30° C
Potatoes	5-10 months at 4-12° C	Less than 2 months at 22°C	Less than 1 month at 32° C	Less than 2 weeks at 42° C
Mangoes	2-3 weeks at 13° C	1 week at 23°C	4 days at 33° C	2 days at 43° C
Apples	3-6 months a - 1°C	2 months at 10°c	1 month at 20°C	A few weeks at 30° C

Adapted from Kitinoja (2013)

The sector of cold storage is undergoing a massive transformation, with the government focusing on food preservation. A lot of stress is being laid on energy efficiency as the cold stores are energy intensive. With the advent of newer materials / equipments, every part of a cold chain rendering itself for improvement. As a result, all of them are witnessing changes like the type of construction, insulation, refrigeration equipment, and other type of controls.

Table 2. Temperature requirement of selected fresh food

Fresh Food	Temperature Requirement (°C)
Fresh fish (in ice), crustaceans and shellfish (excluding live ones)	+2
Meat and cooked meats pre-packaged for consumer use	+3
Cooked meats other than those which have been salted, smoked, dried or sterilized	+6
Butter and edible fats, including cream to be used for butter making	−14
Deep frozen foods	−18
Fishery products	−18

Source: Alexandria Engineering Journal, Volume 55, Issue 2, June 2016, Pages 1359–1365

Cold chain systems are very important to the growth of global trade in perishable products providing worldwide availability of food and health supplies. Each year, billions of tons of fresh food products and millions of dollars' worth are lost due to poor cold chain systems in developing markets. The World Economic Forum lists food crisis as fourth on its top global risks of highest concern for the next 10 years. Though globally, billions of dollars are spent on improving agricultural processes to create higher food yields. But the fact is that nearly half of all food never gets consumed by the consumer and this fact was totally getting ignored.

By controlling parameters of temperature, humidity and atmospheric composition, along with utilizing proper handling procedures, cold chain service providers can increase the product life of fresh foods for days, weeks or even months. The cold chain management system allows fresh products to hold their value longer while increasing their transportability and provide better opportunities expanding horizon of market reach.

LITERATURE REVIEW

All food company and supermarket is committing itself to provide better products. To provide good quality fresh food products, the logistics part has to be considered (Hsiao et al., 2008).The quality and safety of the fresh foods is largely influenced by the logistics (Smith, 2006). However, the researches and studies on fresh food logistics are few (Liu et al., 1999).Many perspectives can be adapted to discuss the fresh food logistics, however, the literature study indicates that analyzing the problem via the perspective of cost and effectiveness is main (Liu et al., 1999, Joshi et al., 2009; Boronico et al., 1995; Manning et al., 2006; Beardsell et al., 1999; Kelepouris et al., 2007; Henderson, 1994; Manikas et al., 2009; Manning et al., 2006).

The cost of the fresh food logistics is viewed as one of the key elements (Kelepouris et al., 2007; Henderson, 1994; Fearne et al., 1999). Hsiao et al. (2008) claim that the fresh food logistics cost is decided based on several factors, e.g. transportation, warehousing, value-added activities, and inventory management. But they also view the asset specificity, core closeness, and supply chain complexity is the determinant issues (Hsiao et al., 2008).

Logistics effectiveness is very important in maintaining cold chain. Manikas et al. (2009) point out in their survey that the bottleneck of the fresh food logistics in England is the unimproved efficiency, which results in low utilization of the facilities and space. Logistics effectiveness not only influences the quality of the fresh food, but also determines the safety of fresh food, especially in the process of primary production (Manning et al., 2006).

According to the definition proposed by Smith (2006), perishable products are: live plants, fresh or chilled vegetables, fresh mushrooms, fresh fruits, fresh cut flowers, and concentrated citrus juice. Marsden et al (1998) consider the definition of fresh food includes a wide range-- the products that need to be kept in a refrigerator can be called fresh or perishable food, such as fruits, vegetables, meats, and fish. The fresh food in this paper refers to the perishable food that should be stored in fridge, including dairy products, meats, fish, vegetables, and concentrated citrus juice. In addition, fresh food, fresh products, perishable food, and perishable products refer to the same thing in this paper.

According to Smith (2006), fresh products require much more in the logistics conditions. Many details should be considered in the fresh foods logistics procedure, such as the air quality, the temperature, the humidity, the room pressure, and even the lighting level. For example, lighting directly affects the quality of the fresh products, while the bacterial growth will be out of control without appropriate temperature and humidity.

Manikas et al (2009) discussed that automatic machines are invented to improve the efficiency of the fresh foods logistics as the general efficiency is not high. Since, the products types of the fresh foods are various and hard to be controlled by machines, so a large part of the logistics process, especially the picking process, is handled manually.

As there is no specific guideline for the foods storage so the standards in different countries can vary, though the storage environment is very important for maintaining the quality of fresh food (Smith, 2006). Manikas et al. (2009) believe that it is quite demanding to reach the storage requirements of the agricultural perishable foods, because the requirements for the storage of those products are rare and so its facilities. Most of the regional distribution centers or supermarkets still lack those facilities. But merely purchasing the facilities is not enough for satisfactory food logistics. Smith (2006) states that in order to keep the environment suitable for fresh food storage, the facilities that are used in fresh food logistics should be easy to clean or it will cost a lot to remove the bacteria and dust.

Hsiao (2008) explains that logistics outsourcing is a good choice for many supermarkets or food companies which are involved in the fresh food business. It means the fresh food logistics can be handled by an external logistics company or shipper. Hsiao et al. (2008) also argue that the decision making process for conducting outsourcing logistics is very important. Items like asset specificity, uncertainties measurement, core closeness, supply chain complexity, and logistics strategies are suggested to be evaluated in the decision making process.

Liu et al. (1999) pointed out that their survey report that the relationship between a third party logistics or outsourcing logistics company and the fresh food company should be defined clearly. But they also believed that companies should not rely too much on one or more distributors.

Rathore et al (2010) compared that the amount of food wasted in India is equivalent to annual food consumption in UK. The study done by ASSOCHAM (2013), claimed that India producers are losing Rs. 2.13 lakh crore due to supply chain loss in of fruits and vegetables.

Viswanadham (2007) mentioned that waste of food is due to lack of adequate infrastructure of processing, cold storage and transportation in India. It has resulted in loss of fresh vegetables ranged from 20 to 50% (Verma and Singh, 2004).

As reported by Capellán-Pérez (2014), there is a need of continuous power supply for overall maintenance of cold chain. Cold storage are purposely for preserving the quality of raw food. In developing countries, there is enormous shortfall in power generation and also lack of technical know-how to explore environmental friendly energy, fossil fuel is highly explored as alternative means of energy. This convectional fuel source has been widely reported as global emission of carbon dioxide which is a major contributor to global warming. Full-size table.

PROBLEMS AND VULNERABILITIES

There are various challenges faced by manufacturers and distributors of frozen products that how they will be able to maintain the cold chain of refrigerated zones within distribution centers and equipments like refrigerated docks and multi-temperature trailers.

The frozen food product's safety is a priority for every reputable distributor as it's often taken for granted by customers. Maintaining the cold chain from farm to fork is challenging. All these food products must be loaded correctly to prevent cross-contamination with raw product and damage by heavier items at the bottom of a stack. And, they must be stored at the correct temperatures (frozen, refrigerated or dry) in the truck to maintain quality and safety. During the harsh summer season, the 'reefers' (truck refrigeration units) have to work extra-hard to maintain temperature so that perishable products could retain its chillness throughout the multi-stop delivery process. Although, food distribution companies must adhere to government rules and regulations calling for greater food protection scrutiny.

In India, the production volumes of most of the fruits and vegetables are uneven. The fruits and vegetables need cold storages during the peak months of the years. However, there is a lack of cold storages. The report from Emerson food wastage and cold storage cites studies that have pegged the value of fruits, vegetables and grains wastage in India at INR 440 billion annually. From which the fruits and vegetables account for the largest portion of that wastage. The wastage is valued at INR 133 billion which is eighteen per cent of India's fruit and vegetable production go waste annually, according to data from the Central Institute of Post-Harvest Engineering and Technology (CIPHET).

The recent data published by the Ministry of Food Processing Industries is estimated at Rs 92,651 crore for loss of perishables due the wastage of agricultural produce at the national level (Naqvi Ghufran,2016). India's major agricultural goods is almost three times as high as the new budget for the agriculture sector. Though, there were food shortage issues and the constant rising food inflation, there was heavy harvest and post-harvest loss of perishables, which shown 44% increase from Rs 24,909 crore in 2015-16 to Rs 35,984 crore in 2016-17.

Table 3. Central Institute of Post-Harvest Engineering and Technology (CIPHET),Ludhiana,2016

Commodity/Crop	Losses During Transportation(%)	Losses During Farm Operations(Including Transportation loss(%)	Losses During Storage (%)	Overall Total Loss(%)	Monetary Value of Loss(in Rs. Crores)
Milk	0.02	0.71	0.21	0.92	4409
Meat	0.00	1.99	0.72	2.71	1235
Marine Fish	0.91	9.61	0.91	10.52	4315
Inland Fish	0.17	4.18	1.05	5.23	3766
Egg	0.36	4.88	2.31	7.19	1320
Poultry Meat	0.66	2.76	4.00	6.74	3942
Cereals				4.65-5.99	20698
Pulses				6.36-8.41	3877
Oilseeds				3.08-9.96	8278
Fruits &Veg				4.58-15.88	40811

Further, effective cold chains and cold stores need latest technology and the major problem here is the cost of that technology. Similarly some of the fruits and vegetables are expected to be cheaper (oranges, papaya, tomatoes, onion, potato) in price as compare to the others (apples, plums, litchi, peas etc.). The cold storage cost (carrying cost) sometimes is too high that it is not commercially feasible for farmers or middlemen supply them through an effective cold chain. It results in perishablility of the goods and finally in the hike of their price in the consumer market.

COLD CHAIN MANAGEMENT SYSTEM

Following are different ways of managing cold chain system (Aung MM et al, 2012):

- Quality Management System
- Risk Assessment Process
- Temperature Monitoring System
- Handling frozen food products

Although, cold chain is composed of various stages though it can also be seen as a single entity since a breakdown in temperature control in any of the stage can impact the final quality of the product. In a cold chain, the shelf life, quality, and safety of perishable food throughout the supply chain is greatly impacted by environmental factors especially temperature (Aung MM et al, 2012).

For storage and distribution of perishable food, the proper temperature condition is needed as they are time and temperature sensitive in nature and are of higher value and more vulnerable to temperature disturbances. Cold chains are very common in the food as well as in pharmaceutical industries and also some chemical shipments. It is required in order to retain high quality and good nutritional value. So, to maintain the quality, there should be increasing concerns for supply chain through quality control and monitoring of goods during the cold chain. In this sector, there is a presence of commercial systems which can monitor containers, refrigerated chambers and trucks, but they typically measure only a single or very limited number of points as they do not give complete information about the cargo. The quality can degrade depending on time and environmental conditions, it is beneficial to know and act appropriate planning when the quality and safety problems arise. As soon as the current quality status is known, the shelf life and price is adjusted dynamically and decision support to management and competitive advantages could be achieved. The fresh food highly demands proper temperature control in the whole logistics process. Therefore, to control food safety efficiently in the cold chain process, and to improve the quality monitoring and management system of cold chain logistics process, become concerns of government and enterprises.

Due to the development of telecommunication, information technology and information system, there is the rise of wireless sensing technologies which is being used in cold supply chain. Such technology like Radio Frequency Identification (RFID) and wireless sensors provides a feasible way to enhance the safety and quality of food cold chain. Integrating RFID systems with condition-monitoring systems will enhance existing track and trace applications, not only the location and movement history, but also the condition of perishable products.

Management of Cold Chain

Cold chain management refers to maintaining the proper temperature of the products through all the handoffs in the cold chain until it reaches the ultimate consumer (Aung MM et al, 2012). The aim of cold chain management is to preserve quality of perishables and deliver them to market in safe and good condition.

Quality and Safety of Frozen Foods

The process of frozen food involves reducing food temperatures to below ambient temperatures, but above −1°C. Reducing the food temperatures results in retarding many of the microbial, physical, chemical and biochemical reactions associated with food spoilage and deterioration. This is found to be effective short-term preservation of food materials. The growth of microorganism occurs slowly at chilled temperatures (generally between 0°C and +5°C) and food spoilage and deterioration reactions are inhibited to such an extent that food safety and quality is preserved for extended periods (EU commission).

Frozen foods are perishable and they deteriorate progressively throughout their life. The growth and activity of microorganisms, which may be present in the food ingredients or may be introduced when the food is handled or processed, may cause deterioration. Safe and high quality chilled foods require minimal contamination during manufacture (including cross-contamination), rapid chilling and low temperatures during storage, handling, distribution, retail display and consumer storage.

Freezing preserves the storage life of foods by making them more inert and slowing down the detrimental reactions that promote food spoilage and limit quality shelf life (EU Commision). There are major attractions with the freshness, quality, safety and convenience of frozen foods. In frozen food industry, there is an increased sophistication which has led to many breakthroughs in frozen food technology, but diligent controls are needed at all times. This technology ensures microbiological safety, extended quality shelf life, temperature control, and the retention of nutrients.

Quality and Safety Food and Agriculture Organisation (FAO) stated that managing food safety and quality is also the responsibility of governments, industry and the consumers (FAO, 2003). Quality defined by ISO is 'the totality of features and characteristics of a product that bear on its ability to satisfy stated or implied need' (Reeuwijk LP, 1998). Also, quality can be defined as 'conformance to requirement', 'fitness for use' or, more appropriately for foodstuffs, 'fitness for consumption'. Thus, quality can be described as the requirements necessary to satisfy the needs and expectations of the consumer (Ho SKM, 1994) (Peri C, 2006).

However, food quality is very general, implying many expectations which can be different from consumer to consumer. Quality includes attributes that influence a product's value to the consumer. The class of quality attributes is following:

Table 4. Classes of food quality attributes (scholar.waset.org, 2012)

External	Internal	Hidden
Appearance (Sight)	Odour	Wholesomeness
Feel (touch)	Taste	Nutritive Value of Product
Defects	Textures	Safety

Sensors can either be simply associated directly with the items or produce of interest or attached to a Returnable Transport Item (RTI) that is being used to transport the goods (Bowman et al, 2009). There is a problem to know the quality of the product inside containers or refrigerated rooms in cold chain without visual inspection. Therefore, quality evaluation can be considered based on the environmental factors which have direct impact on the quality of the products during their storage and distribution. The role of wireless sensors plays a very important role in this kind of sensory evaluation.

TEMPERATURE MONITORING

Temperature monitoring is very important component of cold supply chain. Throughout the food supply chain, many kinds of products have to be handled under controlled environmental quantities, such as temperature, humidity, vibrations and light exposure. The temperature is one of the major concerns among all these parameters due to its huge variety of effects. As the rise in temperature in frozen food may lead to microbial growth which will deteriorate the quality and may increase the risk of food poisoning(Carullo et al,2008). Therefore, perishable food products must be continuously monitored for safety and quality concerns throughout the whole supply chain to avoid the breakdown in temperature control which will impact on the final quality of the product (SARDI, 2006).

The International Institute of Refrigeration (IIR) indicated that about 300 million tonnes of produce were wasted annually through deficient refrigeration worldwide (Flores and Gormley, 2000).Therefore, the key to managing the cold chain is to monitor and maintain the product temperature in each stage of the supply chain. Temperature control in cold chain preserves both sensory and nutritional qualities. Most of the mechanisms of quality loss are determined by storage temperature and are accelerated with time spent above the recommended value. They are also promoted by temperature fluctuations (George M, 2000).

RISK ASSESSMENT PROCESS

In cold supply chain logistics, various risks are involved regarding the maintenance of quality of food. There are a number of common elements that will exist in logistics routes like

1. The type of cartons/packaging being used.
2. The type of routes to be used like by road, sea or the air as it does has an impact on products in cold van.
3. The way the products are being handled(i.e hand-offs and human elements)
4. The location and the time of year in the world where the products are going to be shipped
5. The size and the quantity of products to be shipped
6. The type of tools applied for monitoring the shipment like USB, RFID etc.
7. The procedures for storing and collection of data applied for the products to be shipped.

Risk Assessment

The risk must be identified from the past experience which mostly occurs during transportation, product handling etc. We must focus on the potential risk generating events which are commonly encountered in this sector (Peter D. Norton, 2013):

1. The point where we have human intervention in handling products
2. The point where we have product handoff point
3. When high value products are being sent on a high route
4. Transfer of products from one country to another
5. Storing the outsourced data
6. To check the carton packet before receiving at the end point.

Risk Mitigation

Various strategies must be included (Peter D. Norton, 2013):

1. We must review the supply chain to assess the scope of risk that may exist
2. Impact of assessment of the risks which can be evolved
3. Documenting the strategies to be implemented
4. Defining risk mitigation strategies

Risk management tools support enterprises to plan, implement and optimise the cold chain. Risk management ensures the integrity of the cold chain.

Food enterprises have to translate food safety requirements of new government regulations, recommendations, guidelines, customer (retailer) requirements as well as requirements of audit standards etc. into enterprise-internal specific product and process criteria.

Risk Management Methods

Strategies must be developed to avoid failures like the deterioration in the quality of perishables in any steps of cold supply chain (Schmitz Thomas, 2006). Like,

1. For maintenance of quality of perishables, temperature controlled vans should be used.
2. To correctly assess the quality of perishables through strong monitoring and to minimize the losses.
3. There should be use of approved carriers only to maintain the standard
4. Packaging must be according to the need for protecting the products
5. Placements of monitoring devices inside the shipping boxes to avoid business risk

A comprehensive risk assessment of the transportation logistics process must be continued to identify and implement adequate solutions and improvements to assure a successful shipment of the perishables satisfying consumer needs.

HANDLING FROZEN FOOD PRODUCTS

The rapid growth of sales reflects consumer satisfaction in the high quality of products, its availability throughout the year, and general convenience in product use. It is actually the preferences and appreciation by the consumer that the product values and that's why frozen foods are sold and new products are being introduced for enhancing sales.

Proper care is to be taken to maintain the quality of frozen foods which depends fundamentally on the quality of raw materials used and product manufacture. It can be at risk if failed to maintain product temperature at a suitable low level in any part of the cold chain, including storage, transport, distribution, and display in retail stores, or by faulty inventory control at all levels that would allow product to be retained for unduly long periods in the cold chain. It must be handled with utmost care to avoid operational failures which may lead to customer dissatisfaction and harm to the entire industry, not only those who may be at fault (www.cold.org.gr,2008). As the freezing process does not actually kill harmful bacteria and other organisms that were present in the food before freezing but, while frozen, bacteria populations do not continue to grow, although they will resume doing so once your food is thawed (www. foodsafety.com.au,2012).

STORAGE PERIOD

As various types of frozen foods have different stabilities in frozen storage so they develop abnormal flavors and decolorize accordingly. It has also been noticed that different lots of the same type of frozen food may have different stabilities, depending on many factors including the quality of raw material and product ingredients, processing, and packaging materials. According to the need storage life can be extended significantly as storage temperatures become colder.

TIME AND TEMPERATURE TOLERANCE (TTT)

The quality of the frozen food depends upon the integrated effects of time and temperature that affect their color, flavor and texture. The degree to which individual products tolerate the time & temperature effects is called the Time-Temperature Tolerance (TTT). Regulations or company quality-assurance standards must specify and control both the time and temperature factors to guarantee product quality.

There is an utmost importance of maintaining the frozen food quality in all segments of the frozen food industry to prevent conditions as it could lead to product deterioration in any part of the cold chain and would cause consumer dissatisfaction.

HANDLING

There can be a serious contributing factor to quality loss in frozen foods if exposed to elevated temperatures. Though, very short periods of exposure may not be serious, unless often repeated, but prolonged exposure may cause severe damage. However, for some particularly sensitive products, even a short exposure to temperatures warmer than 10-15 °F will result in marked loss in quality which will only become apparent after further storage. In cold supply chain, temperature fluctuations should be avoided because they will cause migration of moisture from the product or within the package causing formation of ice crystals and partial dehydration of the product. In general, the product temperature is more important than the air temperature. A change in air temperature for a short period may not affect the product temperature significantly (www.cold.org.gr, 2008).

There are parameters to maintain the temperature within the van while in transit. The Refrigeration equipment used in transportation of frozen foods has been designed in such a way so that it removes heat that may leak into the load compartment of the container. It should be noted that the refrigeration capacity does not provide for removal of much heat from the load. Therefore, if products are loaded with the temperature warmer than 0 °F (-18 °C), there is little or no opportunity for the product temperature to be reduced to the desired level during transit.

OPPORTUNITY

The cold chain management for perishables is envisaging a rapid growth in Indian market. The entry of the New Economic Policy of 1991 have ushered a huge prospect in the Indian market. Liberalization policy has transformed the protected economy into one of a land of opportunities for investors. According to the WTO commitments, globalization intends to integrate the Indian economy with the world economy (Bose SK and Chatterjee J, 2008).

The cold chain is required not only for the raw material but also for the frozen and ready to eat food. Avoiding spoilage and wastage of perishable products can certainly enhance the economy in direct or indirect ways. The market possesses enormous opportunities for the cold chain sector due to massive demand from consumer as their food eating habits are changing. The time has come for bridging gaps in appropriate infrastructure development, adoption of energy efficient technologies, moving from mass storage to direct access storage and use of latest equipments for the cold chain management. The cold supply chain can provide opportunity to various service providers, infrastructure designers, refrigerated vehicle manufacturers, alternate energy experts, shipping and international trade companies, temperature controlling equipment providers etc. (www.asiacoldchainshow.com, 2015).

CONCLUSION

The cold chain industry in India is still at a nascent stage and despite large production of perishables, the cold chain potential still remain untapped due to high share of single commodity cold storage, high initial investment (for refrigerator units and land), lack of enabling infrastructure like power & roads, lack of awareness for handling perishable produce and lapse of service either by the storage provider or the transporter leading to poor quality produce. However, increasing urbanization and growth of organized retail, food servicing and food processing sector are boosting the growth of cold chain industry in India. The trend is shifting towards establishing multipurpose cold storages and providing end to end services to control parameters throughout the value chain.

REFERENCES

Adekomaya, O., Jamiru, T., Sadiku, R., & Huan, Z. (2016, June). Sustaining the shelf life of fresh food in cold chain – A burden on the environment. *Alexandria Engineering Journal*, *55*(2), 1359–1365. doi:10.1016/j.aej.2016.03.024

Aung, M. (2012). Quality Monitoring and Dynamic Pricing in Cold Chain Management. *Mechatronic and Manufacturing Engineering*, *6*(2).

Bishara, R. H. (2006). Cold chain management – an essential component of the global pharmaceutical supply chain. *American Pharmaceutical Review*. Available at: www.americanpharmaceuticalreview.com/life_science/Bishara_APR.pdf

Bose, S.K., & Joydeep, C. (2008). *Challenges faced by the Indian tinplate packaging industry: An analysis*. Retrieved from file:///C:/Users/Anju%20Bharti/Desktop/paper%20for%20IGI/5_Bose_Chatterjee.pdf

Bowman, Ng, Harrison, López, & Illic. (2009). *Sensor based condition monitoring*. Building Radio Frequency Identification for the Global Environment (Bridge) Euro RFID Project.

Capellán-Pérez, M., Mediavilla, M., de Castro, C., Carpintero, Ó., & Miguel, L. J. (2014). Fossil fuel depletion and socio-economic scenarios: An integrated approach. *Energy*, *77*, 641–666. doi:10.1016/j.energy.2014.09.063

Carullo, A., Corbellini, S., Parvis, M. L., & Vallan, A. (2008). A measuring system for the assurance of the cold-chain integrity. *Proceedings of the IEEE International Instrumentation and Measurement Technology Conference*, 1598-1602. 10.1109/IMTC.2008.4547298

Cold Chain sea of opportunities for emerging markets. (2015). Retrieved from http://www.asiacoldchain-show.com/2015/03/13/cold-chain-sea-of-opportunities-for-emerging-markets/

FAO. (2003). *FAO's strategy for a food chain approach to food safety and quality: a framework document for the development of future strategic direction*. Retrieved from http://www.fao.org/DOCREP/MEETING/006/Y8350e.HTM

Flores, S. E., & Tunner, D. (2008, July). RFID technologies for cold chain applications. *International Institute of Refrigeration Bulletin*, 4-9.

George, M., & Gormley, R. (2000). *Managing the cold chain for quality and safety*. Retrieved from http://www.teagasc.ie/ashtown/research/preparedfoods/managing_the_c old_chain.pdf

Ghufran, N. (2016). *Food loss! A Big Challenge for Modi Government, Agro & Food Processing*. Retrieved from http://agronfoodprocessing.com/food-loss-a-big-challenge-for-modi-government/

Ho, S. K. M. (1994). Is the ISO 9000 series for Total Quality Management? *International Journal (Toronto, Ont.)*, *11*(9), 74–89.

Indian Cold Chain – An Emerging Industry. (2016). Retrieved from http://www.coolingindia.in/blog/post/id/13496/indian-cold-chain--an-emerging-industry

ITLN. (2014). *India on fast track to shape perishables logistics trends*. Retrieved from http://www.itln.in/india-on-fast-track-to-shape-perishables-logistics-trends/

Joshi, R., Banwet, D. K., & Shankar, R. (2009). Indian cold chain: Modeling the Inhibitors. *British Food Journal*, *111*(11), 1260–1283. doi:10.1108/00070700911001077

Kelepouris, T., Pramatari, K., & Doukidis, G. (2007). RFID-enabled traceability in the food supply chain. *Industrial Management & Data Systems*, *107*(2), 183–200. doi:10.1108/02635570710723804

Kovacs, G. (2008). Corporate environmental responsibility in the supply chain. *Journal of Cleaner Production*, *16*(15), 1571–1578. doi:10.1016/j.jclepro.2008.04.013

Lisa, K. (2013). *Table 1: Predicted loss of fresh food storage in developing countries – Use of cold chains for reducing food losses in developing countries* (PEF White Paper No. 13-03). The Postharvest Education Foundation (PEF).

Liu, H., & Wang, I.P. (1999). Co-ordination of international channel relationships: four case studies in the food industry in China. *Journal of Business & Industrial Marketing, 14*(2), 130-150.

Manikas, I., & Terry, L. A. (2009). A case study assessment of the operational performance of a multiple fresh produce distribution centre in the UK. *British Food Journal, 111*(5), 421–435. doi:10.1108/00070700910957276

Manning, L., Baines, R. N., & Chadd, S. A. (2006). Quality assurance models in the food supply chain. *British Food Journal, 108*(2), 91–104. doi:10.1108/00070700610644915

Maxwell, D., Sheate, W., & Vorst, R. V. D. (2006). Functional and systems aspects of the sustainable product and service development approach for industry. *Journal of Cleaner Production, 14*(17), 399–416. doi:10.1016/j.jclepro.2006.01.028

Peri, C. (2006). The universe of food quality. *Food Quality and Preference, 17*(1-2), 3–8. doi:10.1016/j.foodqual.2005.03.002

Rathore, J. (2010). Cold chain infrastructure for frozen food- a weak link in Indian retail sector. *The IUP Journal of Supply Chain Management, 7*(1-2), 90-103.

Salin, V., & Nayga, R.M. (2002). A cold chain network for food exports to developing countries. *International Journal of Physical Distribution & Logistics Management, 33*(10), 918-933.

SARDI. (2006). *Maintaining the cold chain: air freight of perishables*. South Australian Research and Development Institute. Retrieved from http://www.australianairfreight.com/vac/pdfs/airfreight_perish.pdf

Smith, D. (2006). Design and management concepts for high care food processing. *British Food Journal, 108*(1), 54–60. doi:10.1108/00070700610637634

Thomas. (2006). *Using risk management tools to manage the integrity of the cold chain*. Cold Chain-Management, 2nd International Workshop, Bonn, Germany. Retrieved from http://ccm.ytally.com/fileadmin/user_upload/downloads/12_SCHMITZ.PDF

Van Reeuwijk, L. P. (n.d.). *Guidelines for quality management in soil and plant laboratories*. Rome Publication #M-90. Retrieved from http://www.fao.org/docrep/w7295e/w7295e00.HTM

Verma, A., & Singh, K. (2004). An economic analysis of post harvest losses in fresh vegetables. *Indian Journal of Agricultural Marketing, 18*(1), 134–139.

Viswanadham, N. (2007). *Can India be food basket for the world?* Working Paper Series, IBS, Hyderabad. Retrieved from http://www.cccindia.co/corecentre/Database/Docs/Docfiles/Can_india_be.pdf

KEY TERMS AND DEFINITIONS

Cold Chain: A cold chain is a temperature-controlled supply chain. An unbroken cold chain is an uninterrupted series of refrigerated production, storage and distribution activities, along with associated equipment and logistics, which maintain a desired low-temperature range.

Cross Contamination: The process by which bacteria or other microorganisms are unintentionally transferred from one substance or object to another, with harmful effect. 'Cross-contamination between raw and cooked food is the cause of most infection'.

Frozen Food: Food preserved by a freezing process and stored in a freezer before cooking. Freezing food preserves it from the time it is prepared to the time it is eaten. Freezing food slows down decomposition by turning residual moisture into ice, inhibiting the growth of most bacterial species.

Non- Renewable Resource: A non renewable resource is a resource of economic value that cannot be readily replaced by natural means on a level equal to its consumption. Most fossil fuels, such as oil, natural gas and coal are considered non renewable resources in that their use is not sustainable because their formation takes billions of years.

Perishables: A perishable is also a type of food with a limited shelf life if it's not refrigerated. Since perishing is dying, anything perishable could die or is likely to die. Perishable foods are those likely to spoil, decay or become unsafe to consume if not kept refrigerated at 40 F° (4.4 °C) or below or frozen at 0 F° (-17.8 °C) or below. Examples of foods that must be kept refrigerated for safety include meat, poultry, fish, dairy products, and all cooked leftovers. Refrigeration slows bacterial growth and freezing stops it. There are two completely different families of bacteria that can be on food: pathogenic bacteria, the kind that cause food borne illness, and spoilage bacteria, the kind of bacteria that cause foods to deteriorate and develop unpleasant odors, tastes, and textures.

RFID: RFID (radio frequency identification) is a technology that incorporates the use of electromagnetic or electrostatic coupling in the radio frequency (RF) portion of the electromagnetic spectrum to uniquely identify an object, animal, or person. RFID is a technology similar in theory to bar codes.

Sensor: A device which detects or measures a physical property and records, indicates, or otherwise responds to it.

This research was previously published in Supply Chain Management Strategies and Risk Assessment in Retail Environments edited by Akhilesh Kumar and Swapnil Saurav; pages 232-246, copyright year 2018 by Business Science Reference (an imprint of IGI Global).

Chapter 26

Factors that impact Quality during the Transportation of Tomatoes:
Evidence from India

Saurav Negi

https://orcid.org/0000-0002-5553-0098

University of Petroleum and Energy Studies, Dehradun, India

Neeraj Anand

University of Petroleum and Energy Studies, Dehradun, India

Shantanu Trivedi

University of Petroleum and Energy Studies, Dehradun, India

ABSTRACT

This paper examines the factors that impact the quality of tomatoes during the transportation through the supply chain. This is motivated by the criticality transportation in north India region. Primary data was collected through a survey using a questionnaire with responses from 140 transporters from the Himachal Pradesh and Uttarakhand states of India. The data were analyzed using factor analysis to identify the factors that are impacting the quality of tomatoes during the transportation stage. Based on the analysis, three factors were identified that impact quality: Operational, Preservation and Infrastructure. The identification of these factors will benefit the stakeholders involved in the process of decision-making, like the state government, food processing units, transporters, and the farmers. This will help us to understand the current status of transportation and related issues and challenges which enable them to make better planning and management to improve efficiency in the transportation stage of the supply chain.

DOI: 10.4018/978-1-7998-5354-1.ch026

1. INTRODUCTION

Transportation is one of the most important elements of supply chain management. It plays a crucial role in moving goods from one place to another and without its presence the supply chain cannot run successfully. It plays a more important role in supply chain of perishable commodities where the goods needs to be reached to its destination a lesser time as compared to other products (i.e., the customers) in a limited period due to high perishability and shorter shelf-life of the products. Supply chains connect each stage of production and distribution starting from the farms to the consumers and helps to move the fresh produce from farm gate to local markets, often called mandis in India, to wholesale markets, then to retailers, and then ultimately to the end-consumers.

Faster transportation with less damage in transit is vital for successful supply chain of perishable products. In India, transportation through roadways is preferred for shipping fresh produce because of the rapid movement of items and advantages of door step services.

The rising significance of vegetables in the Indian economy can be seen in terms of the increasing national demand on description of increase in population and per capita income; their growing export potential; the need for providing employment prospects in the rural area, and vegetables being relatively more remunerative crops. While national and export demand is progressively rising, the distribution and logistics of vegetables face tremendous uncertainties on numerous counts.

Tomatoes are one of the most popular and extensively grown vegetables in the world ranking second in importance to potatoes in many countries. It is the second most extensively grown vegetable crop in India which provides a healthy perspective on the post-harvest encounters facing the Indian agriculture sector. India is second highest producer of tomatoes in the world after China, with the total production of about 19.40 million tons in 2013-14 (NHB, 2015). They are widely grown in the Himalayan region of north India, especially in Himachal Pradesh and Uttarakhand. Like the rest of the nation, the economies of Himachal Pradesh and Uttarakhand are predominantly agrarian. About 80% of the employment is directly or indirectly linked with agriculture and allied activities. Most growers in Himachal Pradesh and Uttarakhand state are of marginal and are small businesses. However, tomato crops have gained importance as they provide sustainable income, nutritional security and for providing employment opportunities to lots of people in these states. Agro-climatic situations in the states provide opportunity for production of off-season vegetables for sustainable income to the farmer.

Tomatoes grown in these areas have its own importance as they are produced in the foothills of Himalayas and are considered as some of the best quality produce having high demand in the plain areas. It is widely used as vegetable, consumed both as raw and cooked form. Tomatoes, being perishable in nature and produced in excess, must be either processed or stored in cold storage for further consumption, which otherwise would lead to glut resulting in wide price fluctuations. Owing to the limited shelf life and high perishability, these items require appropriate transportation and handling system so they can travel from farm to plate in a fresh manner. Transportation also connects the parties responsible for efficient production and supply of fresh items from farmer to final consumers, to consistently meet the need of the customer in terms of required quantity, fresh quality and right price. Over India, tomatoes are widely grown but the supply chain is characterized by inefficiencies which consequently results in poor price realization for the producers of tomato on one hand and high purchase prices to consumers due to improper quality of tomatoes at the final point of sale. In these states, the transportation stage of perishable fruits and vegetables is suffering from maximum inefficiency leading to significant loss and waste.

Tomatoes were selected for this research as they are one of the most perishable fresh produce and there are significant losses of value during transportation (Singh, Kushwaha, & Verma, 2008; Hazarika, 2008; Gajanana, Murthy, Sudha, & Dakshinamoorthy, 2006; Parkan & Dubey, 2009). Hence, the present study has been conducted with the objective of identifying the factors that are impacting the quality of tomato's supply chain majorly focusing on the criticality of transportation.

According to a FCI report, an average of 20-30% of agricultural produce is lost during transportation stage from farm to processors (Bhardwaj & Palaparthy, 2008). These post-harvest wastage leads to loss of revenue to the farmers due to reduction in the final price paid by the consumer. There is low motivation for the growers in perishable food produce as it results in lowering the bargaining control for the growers. On the demand side of the chain, losses in transportation results in lesser availability of the produce and thus higher amounts of the commodity. It also rigorously reduces the quality of the existing produce and the choices available for the final consumers. Increasing issues and amount of losses during the transportation stage has motivated this research to identify the factors impacting quality during the transportation stage of tomato.

The rest of this article is structured as follows. First, a review of relevant literature on transportation of perishable products in developing nations is presented. Second, the research methodology is presented. Third, the results are outlined and discussed. Fourth, a conclusion and opportunities for future research are presented.

2. LITERATURE REVIEW

Agriculture is one of the most significant and thrust sector of Indian economy, the transportation stage in the supply chain of fruits and vegetables, especially in tomatoes. Tomatoes are one of the most perishable commodities in agri-sector and are laden with the major issue of post-harvest losses and wastages due to various factors impacting quality (Verma & Singh, 2004; Singh, Banerjee, Singh et al., 2004; Hazarika C., 2006; Gajanana, Murthy, Sudha & Dakshinamoorthy, 2006; Sharma & Singh, 2011; Parkan & Dubey, 2009). The identification of the factors leading to wastage may pave a path for planning and implementation of effective mitigation strategies. This review focuses on developing nations as they will exhibit characteristics different to those of supply chains in developed nations. Furthermore, research from the developing nations will be most relevant to the setting of this research in rural and hilly regions of India.

Losses and wastage in fresh produce have been highlighted as one of the major causes of the food problem in most developing countries (Ojo, 1991; Babalola, Megbope, & Agbola, 2008). The major concern for fruits and vegetables supply chain management is the post-harvest wastage. A huge amount of fruits and vegetables are lost in various operational phases (Murthy, Gajanana, Sudha, & Dakshinamoorthy, 2009). Negi and Anand (2014) discussed supply chain inefficiency in fresh produce and highlighted inefficiency as the major reasons contributing to huge amount of losses in the supply chain of fruits and vegetables which ultimately results in less income to the stakeholders.

Globally, the average loss of perishable fresh produce over the entire chain from farm to the retail shelf and to the consumers' end is estimated to be around 35% (Parfitt, Barthel, & Macnaughton, 2010); in other terms, one-third of the fresh items produced for human beings is wasted (Gustavsson, Cederberg, Sonesson, & van, 2011). Dagar (2007) found 25-40% of fresh produce amounting US$12 billion (Rs 50,400 crore) deteriorates every year even before it reaches to the end customers, thereby squeezing both sides of the chain, from farm to the customer. The amount of loss after harvesting ranges from

20% to 60% of the total amount of production across the countries (Widodo, Nagasawa, Morizawa, & Ota, 2006). Singh, Sikka, and Singh (2009) found losses during transportation and storage as one of the existing problems in the Indian fresh produce supply chain. Negi and Anand (2015), in their study on cold chains in India, discussed the importance of temperature controlled transportation system in the supply chain of perishables agri-commodities in India.

Rehman, Khan, and Jan (2007) conducted a study of tomato crop in Peshawar valley (Pakistan) to estimate the amount of losses during post-harvest. It was found that 20% of the total production gets wasted during picking of tomatoes, handling, and transportation. Hazarika (2006) estimated and analyzed the losses (post-harvest) of major perishable horticulture products in Assam and maximum post-harvest loss was found 22.62% for tomatoes. Adeoye, Odeleye, Babalola, and Afolayan (2009) conducted an economic loss analysis in tomato supply chains and found a high level of post-harvest damages on tomatoes. Sharma and Singh (2011) studied the nature and amount of losses (post-harvest) in the supply chain of vegetables widely grown in the Kumaon region of Uttarakhand and found maximum post-harvest losses in tomatoes. Negi and Anand (2015) also discussed the issue of transportation in supply chain of perishable agri-commodities in Uttarakhand region and suggested various mitigation strategies.

Bhardwaj and Palaparthy (2008) carried a thorough review of available literature and explain the factors that are influencing fruit and vegetable markets in India and their effects on the various partners involved in the supply chain. As per NCCD (National Centre for Cold Chain Development), India, the excess amount of waste in the fresh produce occurs during its transportation from the farm to wholesale mandis and thereafter. Verma and Singh (2004) assessed the post-harvest losses of vegetables in quantitative terms at transportation, storage and sorting level and found overall losses vary up to 25% in vegetables; viz., tomato, cabbage, cauliflower, and chili. Hazarika (2006) also found post-harvest loss was greater during the storage and transportation of the product. Sharma and Singh (2011) estimated the losses in Uttarakhand state of India with respect to different activities at producer-level (e.g., harvesting, sorting, grading & packaging, handling, transportation, and marketing) and trader-level (e.g., transportation, loading-unloading of loads, sorting and grading, and selling). Maximum post-harvest losses have been found in tomatoes with 23.19% and minimum in radishes with 6.52% at producer; this includes both the wholesale- and retail-level. Gajanana, Murthy, Sudha, and Dakshinamoorthy (2006) undertook a study in the major tomato growing state of Karnataka to assess the post-harvest loss at different level of handling. The total post-harvest loss was observed to be about 19%, consisting of 9.43% at the field-level, 4-5% at market-level, and about 5% at the retail-level.

Transportation related challenges are high in India due to reasons including a lack of integrated transportation mode, lack of temperature controlled vehicle, and high cost of transportation (Negi & Anand, 2015). It has been witnessed that losses in transportation are the major operational causes of losses and wastage in the supply chain of perishable horticultural produce (Murthy, Gajanana, Sudha, & Dakshinamoorthy, 2009; Rehman, Khan, & Jan, 2007), followed by inventory management (Shukla & Jharkharia, 2013). Negi and Anand (2016) also found that transportation was one of the most important factors leading to losses and wastage in the supply chain of perishable food produce. Poor and insufficient transportation amenities contribute more to this problem (Gauraha & Thakur, 2008; Sharma & Singh, 2011; Kader, 2005; and Kader, 1992).

Singh, Kushwaha, and Verma (2008) attempted to assess the extent and magnitude of post-harvest losses in Uttar Pradesh and found transportation and distribution of agricultural commodities as the factors responsible for such losses. They found that the transit loss contributed to around 24% of the total loss. In logistics and transportation of perishable commodities, time is a critical factor as the fresh produce must reach the customer in a timely manner with proper handling. Verma and Singh (2004) found delays in moving the harvested fresh produce to the market as the reason of losses at the farm-level.

In the Indian scenario, there are inherent difficulties associated with gathering and transporting small amounts of fresh produce from the various small farms and this results in high post-harvest losses (Verma & Singh, 2004). Rehman, Khan, and Jan (2007) observed that most farmers picked their crops in the morning, packed them in wooden crates, and used pickup trucks or trucks as a mode of transportation to transport their produce to the outside market. Loss at the market-level is primarily due to the transportation and handling practices followed in marketing channels (Verma & Singh, 2004). Mathi (2007) studied supply chains of perishable fresh produce in Allahabad (Uttar Pradesh, India) and found ordinary transportation, irresponsible driving, and the rough roads are the reasons for post-harvest losses. Some crops required special facilities like controlled temperature transportation and unavailability of such is the reason for the marketing loss (Ozcan, 2007). Negi and Anand (2016) examined the various supply chain models of fruits and vegetables in Indian retail sector wherein they discussed the importance of transportation in retail sector. In India, produce is handled roughly and transported in the open atmosphere in trucks. It takes approximately twenty-four hours, and sometimes even more, to reach the retailer (normally an open-market vendor or a pushcart) after harvesting. Fresh produce is stacked into large cane baskets or on to truck beds without any primary packaging or cushioning, which leaves it exposed to sun in hot temperature and contributes to the rapid deterioration of the fresh produce quality (Jain, 2007). Faulty systems of transport and delayed delivery of fresh produce causes wastage in the retail market (CEAGESP, 2002). At retailer's end, it arrives too late and with a very short remaining shelf life, contributing to the wastage in the perishable food supply chain at the retailer-level (Mena, Adenso-Diaz, & Yurt, 2011), and additionally results to the penalty (Shukla & Jharkharia, 2013). The bulkiness in transportation of fresh produce makes the management and handling a difficult task which leads to losses and wastage of around 35% of the total production amounting to around INR 23,000 (CII, 1997).

It has been seen from the literature review that losses and wastage of fruits and vegetables is a matter of concern for every country. In developing countries, the extent of losses is higher than the developed ones. This paper identifies the factors which are impacting the quality of tomatoes during the transportation activity in the supply chain. The transportation activity is the backbone of supply chain which helps to move the goods from the point of source to the point of consumption. Better transportation therefore plays a very important role in case of perishable's supply chain by delivering the goods to the consumer at a right point of time and in a proper quality.

Based on this literature review, a gap was identified as there was a dearth of literature available on the factors contributing to supply chain inefficiency in terms of quality in the transportation stage of Tomato's supply chain with reference to Himalayan state of Himachal Pradesh and Uttarakhand in India.

This leads to the research question we address: What are the factors contributing to quality losses during the transportation stage of Tomato's supply chain in Himachal Pradesh and Uttarakhand? Answering this question allows us to identify the factors contributing to quality losses during the transportation stage of Tomato's supply chain in Himachal Pradesh and Uttarakhand

3. RESEARCH METHODOLOGY

Secondary literature for this research was collected from various research papers, case studies published in peer-reviewed journals and conference proceedings, presentations and white papers from the industry.

Primary data was collected from Himachal Pradesh and Uttarakhand states where the production of Tomato is higher and one of the important source of income for the farmers of hilly areas. The selected districts for data collection are Solan, Sirmaur, Lakha-Mandal, Purola, Uttarkashi, Chakrata and Nainital. These regions have high potential of tomato production in both the states.

The mode of investigation used for the study was the use of a survey using predominantly close-ended questions; therefore, the quantitative research methodology was used for analysis. A questionnaire was designed on the basis of variables extracted through the literature review. Both descriptive analysis and factor analysis were carried out to analyze the data in detail.

Sampling Frame: Initially, the questionnaire was sent to 8 respondents and experts and based on their inputs, the questionnaire was modified. The questionnaire was handed over primarily in person. The following ten parameters or variables were used after modifications of questionnaire to detect the factors that are impacting the quality of tomato during transportation stage:

1. Fungal infection during transit
2. Jerks in Transit, by which pack structure get loose
3. Overburden and Overloading
4. Hitchhiking pests during transit
5. Packaging boxes of different weight, size, commodity in the same carrier
6. Non-Usage of Temperature-controlled Transportation system
7. Improper stacking during transportation
8. No control on Temperature/ Humidity during transit
9. Compression of produce due to putting weight on the load
10. Poor road conditions

Pilot testing: Based on the final list of the variables, a questionnaire was prepared and pre-tested with 30 respondents to check its reliability.

Administration of the survey: The questionnaire was administered to a total of 140 transporters who are closely involved in the transportation of fruits and vegetables, and specifically tomatoes, from the selected areas of Himachal Pradesh and Uttarakhand during the peak seasons. They were then responsible for delivering the goods to the Asia's largest Fruits and Vegetables Mandi (i.e., Azadpur Mandi at Delhi). Based on initial contacts, the snowball sampling technique was used to identify further respondents. This approach was used as there is no list of transporters that could be used. In total, 190 questionnaires were distributed; 140 valid and complete responses were received, giving a 74% response rate. This was judged to be a sufficient number for analysis, as the general norm to conduct factor analysis is to have five respondents for each variable (Hair, Black, Babin, Anderson & Tatham 2008). Bryant and Yarnold (1995) state that, one sample should be at least five times the number of variables. The subjects-to-variables ratio should be no lower than 5 (Garson, D, 2008; Gorsuch, 1983; MacCallum, Widaman, Zhang & Hong, 1999; Everitt, 1975; Arrindell & van der Ende, 1985, p. 166). It was satisfied in the study.

The operators are both individual owners and registered firms. For example, individual owners that have their own truck that they drive while making deliveries; registered firms may have a manager or owner and multiple truck drivers. However, the owner of any firm or any other person does not necessarily know the operational problem as well as the driver does. The driver who is directly involved in transportation activity can only tell about the problems. Therefore, the drivers were the actual respondents because they are aware of the exact situations and issues which impact the goods during transport.

A five-point Likert-type scale was used to identify the significance of particular variable impacting the quality during transportation, where 1 refers to 'Not Significant', 2 refers to 'Less Significant', 3 refers to 'Neutral', 4 refers to 'Significant' and 5 refers to 'Highly significant'. Factor analysis was carried out using SPSS: Statistical Package for the Social Sciences (version 21) to analyze the data and determine the factors.

4. DATA ANALYSIS AND DISCUSSION

The results and discussions related to the study are presented in the following two sub-sections. The first section includes the summary of the profile of respondents in which descriptive analysis was used. The second section discussed an analysis on the factors impacting the quality of tomatoes in the transportation stage.

4.1. Descriptive Analysis

140 transporters were interviewed. Table 1 shows the age, education and experience profile of the transporters from two selected states. Table 1 illustrates that 53% (more than half) of the transporters were in the age category between 36-50 years. 44% of the transporters were ranging 25-30 years old category, only about 3% of the transporters were ranging the age category of 51 or above. In terms of education, the profile showed that out of 140 transporters, 16 (11%) of the transporters have never been to school, 82 (59%) of the total respondents passed primary education, whereas 34 (24%) of the respondents went to secondary school and only 8 (6%) of them did their education till tertiary level. In terms of experience in transportation sector 6% of the total respondent have 20 years or above experience, 41% of the transporters have 15-20 years of experience, 63% of the respondents have 10-15 years of experience, 38% transporters have 5-10 years of experience and 8% of the transporters have 0-5 years of experience.

4.2. Reliability Analysis

Reliability test needs to be conducted and it is very essential before going for any discussion on factor generated by the factor analysis. In reliability analysis, the Cronbach's alpha is an 'index of reliability' related with the 'variation accounted for' by the true score of the 'underlying construct'. The construct is the hypothetical variable that is being measured (Hatcher, 1994).

From the analysis based on the primary data collection, the internal reliability for all the variables has been tested and the score representing alpha is presented in Table 2. The result of the test shows that the alpha score is more than 0.7. It meets the criterion outlined by Peter (1979) and Churchill and Peter (1984); the criterion is that those reliability levels that are greater than 0.5 are acceptable in social sciences. In this case, the Cronbach alpha is 0.785 which is greater than 0.5. Hence, the data is reliable to proceed with Factor Analysis.

Table 1. Sample distribution of respondents on the basis of age, educational qualifications, and experience in transportation sector

Stage	Respondent	Age	Total	Percentage
	Transporter	20-35	62	44%
		36-50	74	53%
		51-above	4	3%
	Grand Total		**140**	**100%**
	Respondent	**Education**	**Total**	**Percentage**
	Transporter	No Education	16	11%
		Primary	82	59%
		Secondary	34	24%
Transportation/ In Transit Stage		Tertiary education	8	6%
	Grand Total		**140**	**100%**
	Respondent	**Experience**	**Total**	**Percentage**
	Transporter	0-5 Yrs	12	8%
		5-10 Yrs	38	24%
		10-15 Yrs	63	39%
		15-20 Yrs	41	26%
		20< above	6	4%
	Grand Total		**140**	**100%**

Table 2. Reliability statistics

Cronbach's Alpha	Cronbach's Alpha Based on Standardized Items	N of Items
.785	.798	10

4.3. Factor Analysis

Factor analysis was used to examine the interconnection and interrelationship among the explanatory variables and to determine the important factors that are impacting the quality of tomatoes during transportation. Factor analysis refers to a "variety of statistical techniques whose common objective is to represent a set of variables in terms of a smaller number of hypothetical factors". The basic assumption of factor analysis is a linear combination of the factors that are not actually observed.

The factor analysis of the ten variables was conducted using the 'principal component method'.

i.   Criterion for the extraction of number of factors: Eigenvalue of each factor had to be equal or higher than one.
ii. The numbers of extracted factors were then rotated by the varimax method.
iii. Each of ten variables was assigned to the factor which had the highest correlation.

4.4. Measure of Sampling Adequacy

Table 3 explains the Kiaser-Meyer-Olkin (KMO) and Bartlett's test of sphericity test which was carried to check the sampling adequacy. It was initially performed on the data and confirmed the appropriateness of conducting the PCA (Principal Component Analysis) (Tabachnick & Fidell, 2001). The Bartlett's test showed that the correlation matrix was at suitable level to perform the factor analysis. The Kiaser-Meyer-Olkin static value differs between 0 and 1. Small values for the Kiaser-Meyer-Olkin shows that the factor analysis of the variables may not be suitable, since the associations (correlations) between the variables cannot be described by the other variables (Norusis 1993). The values which are higher than 0.6 are considered as satisfactory to carry out factor analysis. The KMO test here in this case is more than 0.6 and reached the value of 0.788, so it is judged to be acceptable. After the confirmation of sampling adequacy, it is clear that the sample is adequate and factor analysis can be carried out as an appropriate analysis.

Table 3. KMO and Bartlett's Test

Kaiser-Meyer-Olkin Measure of Sampling Adequacy.		.788
	Approx. Chi-Square	782.901
Bartlett's Test of Sphericity	df	45
	Sig.	.000

5. RESULTS AND DISCUSSION

Table 4 lists the Eigen value connected with each linear component and the factor before extraction and after rotation. Ten linear components were identified. The Eigen value connected with the factor represents the amount of variance explained by that particular linear component. In this case, SPSS extracts three factors having Eigen value greater than one and mutually they account for 75.16% of the variation across the sample. In isolation, component one or Factor one explained 37.40% of the total variance; Factor two explained 23.08% of the total variance and Factor three explained 14.69% of the total variance.

The subsequent factor loadings are described in Table 5 in which the factor loadings for each variable/reason into each factor have been calculated after rotation through SPSS. The factor analysis discovered three broad issues (factors) which are impacting the quality of tomatoes in the transportation stage of its supply chain. These issues and factors are labelled and inferred below.

Factor 1– Operational Factor: Factor one can be named as 'Operational factors' which impacts the quality of tomatoes as the issues/variables underling in this factor/category are directly related to operational issues. The variables which are underling in this factor/category and explained 37.39% of the variation, are 'Non-Usage of Temperature-controlled Transportation system', 'Jerks in Transit by which pack structure get loose', 'Packaging boxes of different weight, size, commodity in the same carrier', 'Compression of produce due to putting weight on the load', 'Overburden and Overloading' and 'Improper stacking during transportation'. Non-Usage of Temperature-controlled Transportation system ensures the maximum factor loading (0.925) followed by Jerks in Transit by which pack structure get loose (0.838), Packaging boxes of different weight, size, commodity in the same carrier (0.829), Com-

Table 4. Total variance explained

Component	Initial Eigenvalues			Rotation Sums of Squared Loadings		
	Total	% of Variance	Cumulative %	Total	% of Variance	Cumulative %
1	4.185	41.855	41.855	3.739	37.395	37.395
2	2.314	23.137	64.991	2.307	23.075	60.469
3	1.016	10.165	75.156	1.469	14.687	75.156
4	.672	6.720	81.876			
5	.475	4.753	86.629			
6	.411	4.109	90.738			
7	.327	3.269	94.007			
8	.276	2.765	96.772			
9	.178	1.782	98.555			
10	.145	1.445	100.000			

Extraction Method: Principal Component Analysis.

Table 5. Summary-Factor analysis on issues impacting quality of tomatoes in Transportation

Factors	Factor Name	Variable	Factor Loading	Variance (% of explained) eigenvalues
F1	Operational	Non Usage of Temperature controlled Transportation system	.925	37.395
		Jerks in Transit, by which pack structure get loose	.838	
		Packaging boxes of different weight, size, commodity in the same carrier	.829	
		Compression of produce due to putting weight on the load	.741	
		Overburden and Overloading	.676	
		Improper stacking during transportation	.636	
F2	Preservation	Fungal infection during transit	.927	23.075
		No control on Temperature/ Humidity during transit	.880	
		Hitchhiking pests during transit	.779	
F3	Infrastructure	Poor road conditions	.913	14.687

pression of produce due to putting weight on the load (0.741), Overburden and Overloading (0.676) and Improper stacking during transportation (0.636). It appears that most of the issues are arising from operational factors which can be controlled and improvised by providing proper training to the workforce.

Factor 2 – Preservation: Factor two can be named as 'Preservation issues' which are impacting the quality of tomatoes as the issues/variables underling in this factor/category are directly related to preservation and atmospheric controlled issues in transit. The variables which are underling in this factor/category and explained 23.08% of the variation, are 'Fungal infection during transit', 'No control on Temperature/Humidity during transit' and 'Hitchhiking pests during transit'. Fungal infection during transit ensures the maximum factor loading (0.927) in the said factor which is followed by No control on Temperature/ Humidity during transit (0.880) and Hitchhiking pests during transit (0.779). The respondents indicated that due to improper preservation during the transportation, the quality of tomatoes undergoes rapid deterioration. Pest and infections due to poor preservation techniques and no control on temperature were the main reasons impacting the quality.

Factor 3 – Infrastructure: Factor three can be named as 'Infrastructure issue' which is impacting the quality of tomatoes as the issues underlying in this factor/category are directly related to the problems associated with transportation infrastructure. For example, where in the road condition is not good it hampers the delivery of high-quality tomatoes. The variable which is underling in this factor/category and explained 14.69% of the variation is 'Poor road conditions'. A poor road condition is the only one variable lying in this factor with the loadings 0.913. Respondents indicated that poor road conditions in hilly areas is one of the most important issue which impacting the quality of tomatoes during in transit. Due to poor road conditions, it generally takes hours for the goods to reach their destination and mostly these items are transported in open/non-refrigerated trucks, which hamper the transportation atmosphere required for perishable items. Due to poor road conditions, the vehicles take a significant amount of time to reach market and this also contributes to the deterioration of the fresh items.

The identified factors impacting the quality of Tomatoes during the transportation are shown below in Figure 1.

Figure 1. Factors impacting quality of tomatoes during transportation

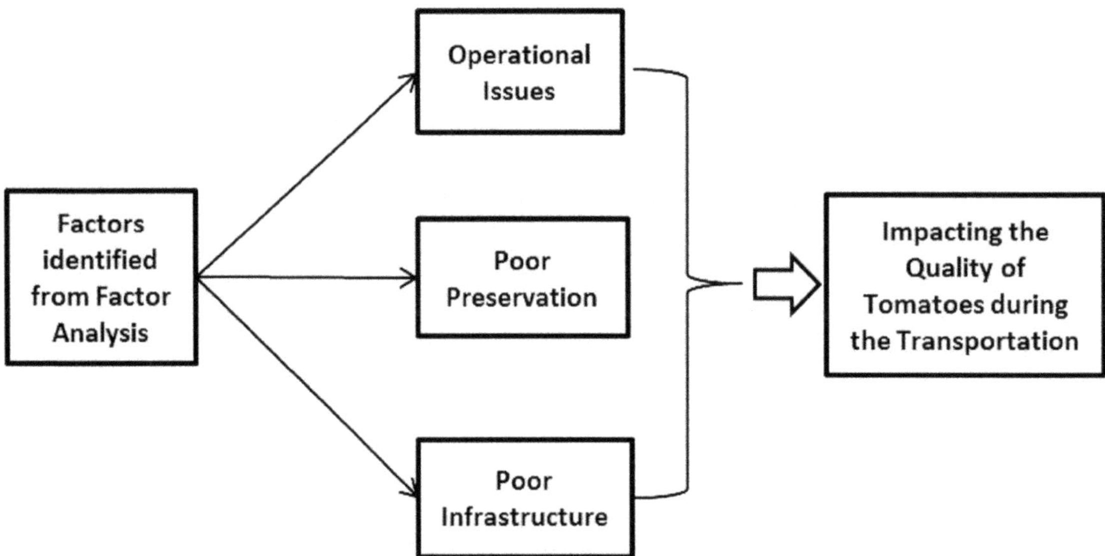

5.1. Managerial Contributions

The necessities for atmosphere during transportation of fresh produce are proper control of temperature and humidity and suitable ventilation. In addition, the fresh produce should be immobilized by proper packaging and stacking, to avoid unnecessary movement or trembling. These situations during transportation may cause severe bruising or other types of mechanical damage.

Temperature controlled/refrigerated containers and trailers should be used for long distance shipping. Shipping by refrigerated trucks is not only convenient, but also effective in stabilizing the quality of produce. However, both the initial investment and the operating costs are very high. Another best option in this case is insulated or properly ventilated trailer trucks.

Pre-cooled items can be transported through well-insulated non-refrigerated trucks for up to several hours without any substantial increase in product temperature. For short-distance shipping, only insulated trucks can be used rather than refrigerated trucks to save significant cost without any sacrifice of quality. If the product is not pre-cooled or the shipping distance is long, a ventilated truck is a better alternate than an insulated truck. The use of only ventilation does not usually provide a constant cool temperature, but it may help to eradicate excessive field heat and respiration heat, and thus avoid damage due to high temperatures.

Implementation of better-quality transportation methods, which strengthens the need for dedicated transportation vehicles like reefer trucks to transport perishable commodities, needs to be emphasized for perishable food produce like tomatoes and other crops. The use of this type of transportation will add value in the quality of fresh produce, enhance the shelf life, and will also results in reducing the transit losses.

The Government of Himachal Pradesh and Government of Uttarakhand can provide refrigerated transportation van service to the farmers of state in low price, so they can avail the services and use temperature controlled transportation system.

Loading and unloading are very important steps in the logistical handling of fruits and vegetables but are often neglected. The individual handling of packaged produce in India leads to mishandling and to high post-harvest losses. With the introduction of CFB boxes, serious consideration should be given to the introduction of palletization and mechanical loading and unloading of produce particularly with the use of fork-lift trucks. Loading and unloading practices need to be addressed to take greater care while handling the perishable items. The goods should be stacked properly so during transit it does not damage the other items which are placed in other crates. A continuous and time-to-time training and development program on skill development and capacity development needs to be organized to overcome the operational issues driven by staff actions.

The packing during transit should not allow pests to access the produce as this may damage the quality of an entire load. The crates should be properly tied and stacked so pests and another unwanted nuisances cannot entered the vehicle.

The identified factors must be addressed properly by the stakeholders so the chances of losses can be reduced and fulfill the requirements of the customer by providing quality food item. As transportation is one of the most important activities in the supply chain and acts as a bridge between the demand and fulfillment of supply, this activity must be properly planned and executed as per the nature of product, required lead time, distance to be covered so the goods can be transported in a properly manner without impacting the quality of fresh items.

6. CONCLUSION

In this study, important factors contributing to supply chain inefficiency in terms of quality during the transportation stage are identified which are ultimately leading to losses and wastage in the fresh food supply chain. The most important factor that contributes more towards the reduction in quality during transportation is 'Operational factors' followed by poor preservation techniques, and then poor Infrastructure. The evidence showed that most of the issues are related to operations and one of the most important reason impacting the quality is non-usage of temperature controlled transportation system followed by jerks in transit; non-uniformity of packaging boxes; compression; overburden; overloading and improper stacking. The poor road condition which is a critical element of road infrastructure is also one of the key impediments in the supply chain of fresh produce. It has been evident that non-usage of temperature controlled transportation system, poor transportation infrastructure, lack of operational efficiency and carelessness by the human resource involved in the processes are the main reasons impacting quality during the transportation of tomatoes which is resulting into huge amount of losses and wastage to farmers and state government.

This research is important as the identification of these factors will benefit the stakeholders involved in the process of decision making like Government of Himachal Pradesh and Government of Uttarakhand, Department of food processing industries, Policy makers, transportation and logistics companies, private agri-business companies and ultimately the farmers in planning and executing their operations accordingly. This will help to understand the current status of transportation and related challenges which enables them to make better planning and management to improve efficiency in the transportation stage of Tomato's supply chain.

This research will also pave a path for the state government to make their policies to improve the infrastructural facilities in a way that they can address the situation of significant losses and wastage due to the improper transportation of fresh produce. It will also help to identify the operational measures required to perform the duties by the human resource while transporting and performing the activity of loading and unloading of perishable goods at various stages of the supply chain.

The present paper has some limitations. It is limited to only one item (i.e., tomatoes) with reference to the Himalayan states in India and the identified factors may vary from the transportation of other food items depending upon its perishability, handling, and types of vehicle. The result may also vary depending upon the geography and region.

Therefore, there are several opportunities for future research. Factors identified through the study may further be used and tested on the supply chain of other perishable food items such as mangoes, apples, litchi, onions, and potatoes. Similar studies can also be carried out in other major agricultural producing states in India like Andhra Pradesh, UP, and Bihar. A detailed study can be carried out to find out the solutions to improve the logistics situation of perishable items in India. Also, identification of the impact level of the variables through regression model can be a very interesting area of study.

REFERENCES

Adeoye, I., Odeleye, O., Babalola, S., & Afolayan, S. (2009). Economic analysis of tomato losses in Ibadan Metropolis, Oyo State, Nigeria. *African Journal of Basic & Applied Sciences, 1*(5-6), 87–92.

Arrindell, W. A., & van der Ende, J. (1985). An empirical test of the utility of the observations-to-variables ratio in factor and components analysis. *Applied Psychological Measurement, 9*(2), 165–178. doi:10.1177/014662168500900205

Babalola, D., Megbope, T. A., & Agbola, O. P. (2008). Post-harvest losses in pineapple production: A case study Of Ado-Odo Otta Local Government Area Of Ogun State. *Bowen Journal of Agriculture*, *5*(1 & 2), 55–62.

Bhardwaj, S., & Palaparthy, I. (2008). Factors Influencing Indian Supply Chains of Fruits and Vegetables: A Literature Review. *The Icfai University Journal of Supply Chain Management*, *5*(3), 59–68.

Bryant, F. B., & Yarnold, P. R. (1995). Principal components analysis and exploratory and confirmatory factor analysis. In L. G. Grimm & R. R. Yarnold (Eds.), *Reading and understanding multivariale statistics* (pp. 99–136). Washington, DC: American Psychological Association.

CEAGESP. (2002). *Diganao ao desperdicio. Disponivelem.* Retrieved July 28, 2013, from http://www.ceagesp.com.br

Churchill, G., & Peter, P. J. (1984). Research design effects on the reliability of rating scales: A meta-analysis. *JMR, Journal of Marketing Research*, *21*(4), 360–375. doi:10.2307/3151463

CII. (1997). *The Fruit and Vegetable Opportunity:Food and Agriculture Integrated Development (FAID) Action Report.* Mckinsey Report.

Dagar, S. S. (2007, May 20). Agriculture's Second Wind. *Business Today*.

Everitt, S. (1975). Multivariate analysis: The need for data, and other problems. *British Journal of Psychiatry*, *126*, 2S7-240.

Gajanana, T. M., Murthy, D. S., & Sudha, M., & Dakshinamoorthy. (2006). Marketing and estimation of post-harvest losses of tomato crop in Karnataka. *Indian Journal of Agricultural Marketing*, *20*(1), 1–7.

Garson, D. G. (2008). Factor Analysis: Statnotes. Retrieved March 22, 2008, from http://www2.chass.ncsu.edu/garson/pa765/factor.htm

Gauraha, A., & Thakur, B. (2008). Comparative economic analysis of post-harvest losses in vegetables and foodgrains crops in Chhattisgarh. *Indian Journal of Agricultural Economics*, *63*(3), 376.

Gorsuch, R. L. (1983). *Factor analysis* (2nd ed.). Hillsdale, NJ: Erlbaum.

Gustavsson, J., Cederberg, C., Sonesson, U., & van, R. O. (2011). *Global food losses and food waste.* Rome: Food and Agriculture Organisation of the United Nations, (FAO).

Hair, J. F., Black, W. C., Babin, B. J., Anderson, R. E., & Ronald, T. L. (2008). Multivariate Data Analysis (6ed.). New Delhi: Pearson Education.

Hatcher, L. (1994). A Step-by-Step Approach to Using the SAS[R] System for Factor Analysis and Structural Equation Modeling. Cary: SAS Institute.

Hazarika, C. (2006). Post-harvest loss and food security — A study on fruits and vegetables in Assam. *Indian Journal of Agricultural Economics*, *61*(3), 418–419.

Hazarika, C. (2008). Extent of post-harvest losses of ginger in Assam – A micro level analysis. *Indian Journal of Agricultural Economics*, *63*(3), 370–371.

Jain, N. (2007). *International Conference on Agribusiness and Food Industry in Developing Countries: Opportunities and Challenges.* Retrieved February 19, 2013, from IIM Lucknow: http://www.iiml.ac.in/events/Program.html

Kader, A. (2005). Increasing food availability by reducing postharvest losses of fresh produce. *Proceedings of the International Post-harvest Symposium*, International Society for Horticultural Science. Italy: Verona. 10.17660/ActaHortic.2005.682.296

Kader, A. A. (Ed.). 1992. Postharvest Technology of Horticultural Crops (2nd ed.). Oakland, California: University of California.

MacCallum, R. C., Widaman, K. F., Zhang, S., & Hong, S. (1999). Sample size in factor analysis. *Psychological Methods*, *4*(1), 84–99. doi:10.1037/1082-989X.4.1.84

Mathi, K. M. (2007). A Study on the Supply Chain Management of Guava in Allahabad District of Uttar Pradesh. *Proceedings of the International Conference on Agribusiness and Food Industry in Developing Countries: Opportunities and Challenges.* Retrieved February 19, 2013, from http://www.iiml.ac.in/events/Program.html

Mena, C., Adenso-Diaz, B., & Yurt, O. (2011). The causes of food waste in the supplier-retailer interface: Evidences from the UK and Spain. *Resources, Conservation and Recycling*, *55*(6), 648–658. doi:10.1016/j.resconrec.2010.09.006

Murthy, D. S., Gajanana, T., Sudha, M., & Dakshinamoorthy, V. (2007). marketing losses and their impact on marketing margins: A case study of Banana in Karnataka. *Agricultural Economics Research Review*, *20*, 47–60.

Murthy, D. S., Gajanana, T. M., Sudha, M., & Dakshinamoorthy, V. (2009). Marketing and post harvest losses in fruits: Its implications on Availability and economy. *Indian. Journal of Agricultural Economics*, *64*(2), 259–275.

Negi, S., & Anand, N. (2014, December). Supply chain efficiency: An insight from fruits and vegetables sector in India. *Journal of Operations and Supply Chain Management*, *7*(2), 154–167. doi:10.12660/joscmv7n2p154-167

Negi, S., & Anand, N. (2015). Cold Chain: A Weak Link in the Fruits and Vegetables Supply Chain in India. *The IUP Journal of Supply Chain Management*, *12*(1), 48-62.

Negi, S., & Anand, N. (2015). Issues and challenges in the supply chain of fruits & vegetables sector in India: A review. *International Journal of Managing Value and Supply Chains*, *6*(2), 47–62. doi:10.5121/ijmvsc.2015.6205

Negi, S., & Anand, N. (2015). Supply chain of fruits & vegetables' agribusiness in Uttarakhand (India): Major issues and challenges. *Journal of Supply Chain Management Systems*, *4*(1 & 2), 43–57.

Negi, S., & Anand, N. (2016). Factors leading to losses and wastage in the supply chain of fruits and vegetables sector in India. In T. Dhingra (Ed.), *Energy Infrastructure and Transportation Challenges and Way Forward-Conference Proceedings International Conference on Management of Infrastructure* (pp. I 89-I 105). Dehradun: UPES.

Negi, S., & Anand, S. (2016). An overview of fruits and vegetables' retail supply chain models in India. In N. Kamath & S. Saurav (Eds.), *Handbook of Research on Strategic Supply Chain Management in the Retail Industry* (pp. 170–187). United States of America: Business Science Reference (an imprint of IGI Global). doi:10.4018/978-1-4666-9894-9.ch010

National Horticulture Board (NHB). (2015). *Area and Production Statistics.* Retrieved July 21, 2016 from http://nhb.gov.in/area%20_production.html

Norusis, M. J. (1993). *SPSS for Windows Advanced Statistics, Release 6.0.* Chicago: SPSS Inc.

Ojo, M. O. (1991). Food policy and economic development in Nigeria for Central Bank of Nigeria. Page Publishers Services Limited.

Ozcan, M. (2007). *Affects on Quality and Durability of Harvest and Post-Harvest Practices in Horticultural Products.* Retrieved September 18, 2013, from http://www.carsambaziraatodasi.com/ab1_1.asp, Parfitt, J., Barthel, M., & Macnaughton, S. (2010). Food waste within food supply chains: Quantification and potential for change to 2050. *Philosophical Transactions of the Royal Society B-Biological Sciences, 365*(1554), 3065-3081.

Parkan, C., & Dubey, R. (2009). Recent developments in the practice of supply chain management and logistics in India. *Portuguese journal of management studies, 14*(1), 71–87.

Peter, J. (1979). Reliability: A review of psychometric basics and recent marketing practices. *JMR, Journal of Marketing Research, 16*(1), 6–17. doi:10.2307/3150868

ur Rehman, M., Khan, N., & Jan, I. (2007). Post harvest losses in tomato crop (A case of Peshawar Valley). *Sarhad Journal of Agriculture.*

Sharma, G., & Singh, S. (2011). Economic analysis of post-harvest losses in marketing of vegetables in Uttarakhand. *Agricultural Economics Research Review, 24*, 309–315.

Shukla, M., & Jharkharia, S. (2013). Agri-fresh produce supply chain management: A state-of-the-art literature review. *International Journal of Operations & Production Management, 33*(2), 114–158. doi:10.1108/01443571311295608

Singh, B., Banerjee, M. K., Singh, K. P., Pandey, P. K., Sudhakar, P., & Rai, M. (2004). *AICRP on Vegetables in India: Evolution andAchievements Impact of Vegetable Research in India.* New Delhi: National Centre for Agr"cultural Economics and Pol"cy Research,ICAR.

Singh, R., Kushwaha, R., & Verma, S. K. (2008). An economic appraisal of post-harvest losses in vegetable in Uttar Pradesh. *Indian Journal of Agricultural Economics, 63*(3), 378.

Singh, S. P., Sikka, B. K., & Singh, A. (2009). Supply chain management and Indian fresh produce supply chain: Opportunities and challenges. *Proceedings of the International Food & Agribusiness Management Association 19th Annual World Symposium.*

Tabachnick, B. G., & Fidell, L. S. (2001). *Using Multivariate Statistics* (4th ed.). Boston: Allyn and Bacon.

Tatlidil, F., Kiral, T., Gunes, A., Demir, K., Erdemir, G., Fidan, H., ... (2003). Economic Analysis of Crop losses during Pre-Harvest and Harvest Periods in Tomato Production in the Aya∫and Nall″han Districts of Ankara Province. Ankara.

Verma, A., & Singh, K. (2004). An economic analysis of Post harvest losses in Fresh Vegetables. *Indian Journal of Agricultural Marketing, 18*(1), 134–139.

Widodo, K. H., Nagasawa, H., Morizawa, K., & Ota, M. (2006). A periodical flowering-harvesting model for delivering agricultural fresh products. *European Journal of Operational Research, 170*(1), 24–43. doi:10.1016/j.ejor.2004.05.024

This research was previously published in the International Journal of Applied Logistics (IJAL), 7(1); edited by Lincoln C. Wood; pages 49-63, copyright year 2017 by IGI Publishing (an imprint of IGI Global).

Section 3
Repurposing Wasted Food

Chapter 27
Food Waste Reduction Towards Food Sector Sustainability

Giovanni Lagioia
University of Bari Aldo Moro, Italy

Vera Amicarelli
University of Bari Aldo Moro, Italy

Teodoro Gallucci
University of Bari Aldo Moro, Italy

Christian Bux
University of Bari Aldo Moro, Italy

ABSTRACT

FAO estimates on average more than 1.3 billion tons of food loss and waste (FLW) along the whole food supply chain (equivalent to one-third of total food production) of which more than 670 million tons in developed countries and approximately 630 million tons in developing ones, showing wide differences between countries. In particular, EU data estimates an amount of more than 85 million tons of FLW, equal to approximately 20% of total food production. This research presents two main goals. First, to review the magnitude of FLW at a global and European level and its environmental, social and economic implications. Second, use Material Flow Analysis (MFA) to support and improve FLW management and its application in an Italian potato industry case study. According to the case study presented, MFA has demonstrated the advantages of tracking input and output to prevent FLW and how they provide economic, social, and environmental opportunities.

INTRODUCTION

Since each human being needs energy and chemical products to maintain his vital signs and produce cells, skin, and bones, food plays a fundamental role in human life becoming an essential commodity for human feeding (Nebbia, 1995). However, since a huge percentage of food is wasted daily, a critical question comes to mind: is food available for all people on Earth?

DOI: 10.4018/978-1-7998-5354-1.ch027

According to Food and Agriculture Organization of the United Nations [FAO] (2018), nowadays the world population amounts to approximately over 7.5 billion people, divided between rural (45%) and urban (55%) population. Moreover, a huge percentage is employed in agriculture, even with a sharp decrease between 1995 (more than 40%) and 2016 (under 27%).

Worldwide, the food production value exceeds $2.3 trillion with no homogeneous distribution (Table 1). More than 10% of the global population is undernourished because of severe food insecurity. Moreover, more than 22% of children under five suffer from stunting and more than 7% from wasting. Lastly, safely managed drinking water is used by approximately 70% of population. Thus, more than 30% people cannot access drinking water (FAO, 2018; FAO, International Fund for Agricultural Development [IFAD], United Nations International Children's Emergency Fund [UNICEF], World Food Programme [WFP], & World Health Organization [WHO], 2018).

Table 1. Worldwide food insecurity overview

Phenomena	Percentage	Million people
Undernourished people	10	750
Food insecure people	10	750
Obese people	13	975
Children under five years affected by wasting	7	50
Children under five years stunted	22	150
Children overweight under five years	5	40

Source: Authors' development based on FAO (2018)

Food insecurity presents different insecurity degrees. According to its meaning, the first indicator is uncertainty about obtaining food, followed by food quality and quantity reduction and meal skipping. In this phase of moderate food insecurity, people cannot afford a healthy diet because of insufficient money or resources. However, severe food insecurity means no food for one day or more (FAO, 2018).

These indicators focus the attention on food security and require several national and international policies to be adopted. According to the 1996 World Food Summit, food security represents a situation that exists when all people, at all times, have physical, social and economic access to sufficient, safe and nutritious food that meets their dietary needs and food preferences for an active and healthy life. In order to better understand this problem, some definitions should be taken into account. Hunger represents a physical discomfort caused by luck of food and can be measured at the individual level. Underweight means individual anthropometric variables and regards two standard deviations below the global reference values. Undernutrition concerns insufficient caloric intake according to international standards. Malnutrition is related to undernutrition, obesity, and micronutrient deficiencies (Barrett, 2010).

Trying to answer the abovementioned question (Is food available to all people on Earth?), some key factors should be considered. As stated by FAO, IFAD, UNICEF, WFP, & WHO (2018), food security is a multi-layer concept based on four key pillars of equal importance, strictly linked and affected by different variables: food availability, food access, food utilization, and food stability.

The first pillar regards food availability, considering both locally produced and imported food and existing food stock. However, food availability itself cannot ensure food security. For this reason, it is necessary to take into account food access regarding both physical and economic access to food (e.g. countries purchasing power, level of income, local infrastructures or financial means) and other practical circumstances. Food utilization, the third pillar of food security, concerns the way food is handled from hygiene perspectives along the whole supply chain. Last but not least, food stability as a macroeconomic indicator for food security considers prices, political stability, local economy but also weather issues or natural catastrophes (McCarthy et al., 2018).

Related to the factors affecting food security, they can be grouped and summarized on social, economic, and environmental grounds.

In terms of social reasons, culture affects food security. First, it regards food production, processing, and storage techniques and determines food eating models. Cultures worldwide shape food quantity and quality according to social food prescriptions, historical events or political context (Alonso, Cockx, & Swinnen, 2017).

In terms of economic issues, population growth and urbanization, it is estimated that global population growth will follow an annual rate increase of approximately 1% till 2030 and a yearly increase of more than 0.5% till 2050. It means that the population will increase from 7.5 billion people to over 9 billion people in 2050 of whom more than 65% will occupy urban areas with exaggerated urbanization trends and land losses (McCarthy et al., 2018).

Lastly, food security poses environmental issues, in particular in terms of limited natural resources and negative externalities, such as greenhouse gas (GHG) emission and water pollution. Moreover, the amount of food produced each year in each country contributes to soil exploitation and agricultural production decrease. Approximately 20 million hectare of land (for instance, equal to more than 65% of Italian total area) each year are lost through soil erosion and irrigation issues. Climate shifts have catastrophic effects on economic prosperity and agricultural production entailing population displacement and resource depletion (McCarthy et al., 2018). Based on these general considerations, food insecurity seems to be mainly due to loss and distribution problems.

This research presents two main goals. First, to review the magnitude food loss and waste (FLW) at a global and European level and its environmental, social and economic implications. Second, use Material Flow Analysis (MFA) to support and improve food loss and waste management and its application in an Italian potato industry case study. According to the case study presented, MFA has demonstrated the advantages of tracking input and output to prevent FLW and how they provide economic, social, and environmental opportunities.

The chapter is organized in two different sections. In the first one, the authors provide an overview of the main differences between food loss (FL) and food waste (FW), especially in quantity and quality at different stages of the Food Supply Chain (FSC). In the second one, the main results of MFA of Italian potato industry are presented, showing the importance of FLW adding to efficiency and sustainability.

After discussing the results, the final section concludes with some indications and recommendations to pursue food sector sustainability.

BACKGROUND

Food Supply Chain and Food Loss and Waste

As stated by FAO (2018), the food available for human consumption is measured by a dietary energy supply which is on average over 2,900 kcal/day per capita. However, there is a wide difference between the countries all around the world (Table 2).

Table 2. Worldwide dietary energy supply, crops production, and harvested area

Region	Dietary energy supply, kcal/day/ capita	Production, million tons					Harvested area, million ha
		Sugar cane	Maize	Wheat	Rice	Potatoes	
Europe	3,365	5,918	118.0	252.4	4.2	117.6	186.7
America	3,265	1,032.3	548.8	121.2	36.4	44.1	298.1
Oceania	3,002	36.2	0.6	22.7	0.3	1.6	24.7
Asia	2,824	701.3	359.6	329.4	677.3	187.4	619.5
Africa	2,593	91.4	73.5	23.3	38.0	23.5	255.8
World		1,861.2	1,100.2	749.0	756.2	374.3	1384.8

Source: Authors' development based on FAO (2018)

In descending order, Europe's average dietary energy supply is the highest (approximately 3,400 kcal/day per capita) followed by the Americas (more than 3,200 kcal/day), Oceania (about 3,000 kcal/day), Asia (more than 2,800 kcal/day), and Africa (less than 2,600 kcal/day). The highest percentage of food produced and consumed worldwide regards crops with relevance to harvest areas, yields, and quantities produced. The worldwide production shows commodities such as sugar cane (more than 1.8 billion tons in 2016), maize (more than 1.0 billion tons), wheat (approximately 750 million tons), rice (more than 740 million tons), and potatoes (approximately 370 million tons) as the top five items produced. However, cereals represent the biggest part of crop production (FAO, 2018).

Livestock covers a huge percentage of global food production. The highest amount of bred animals is represented by chickens (more than 22.7 billion heads in 2016), followed by cattle (approximately 1.5 million), ducks (more than 1.2 million), sheep (approximately 1.1 million) and goats (around 1.0 million). Moreover, fish provides over 20% of global average intake of animal protein.

With regard to the environment, on average agriculture exploits more than one-third of the total land area with its highest percentage in Asia (approximately 50% of total land in Asia) and lowest one in Europe (less than 25%). Furthermore, water represents a fundamental input for food production and its global demand (agriculture, municipalities, and industries) has increased over the past decade reaching a volume of over than 3,900 km^3 per year, of which approximately 70% (more than 2,700 km^3) in agriculture. Moreover, this sector contributes to GHG emissions with about 5 billion metric tons of CO_2 eq. per year and represents over one-fourth of global emissions (FAO, 2018).

These numbers provide an idea of environmental costs and economic and social implications associated with FSC and agricultural development. Thus, FLW entails not only social issues but also economic and environmental consequences.

Before attempting to give a definition of FLW, it is important to remark what food is. According to Food Loss and Waste Accounting and Reporting Standard, food is any substance, whether processed, semi-processed or raw, that is intended for human consumption including drinks and any other substances used for manufacture, preparation or food treatment. Subsequently, FLW can be defined as a decrease in the quantity and quality of edible food intended for human consumption, with particular difference between FL and FW (Food Loss + Waste Protocol [FLW], 2016; Pinstrup-Andersen, 2009).

FL regards essentially food production and supply system malfunctioning. It occurs along the whole supply chain between producer and market, resulting in pre-harvest problems or harvesting, handling, storage, packaging or transportation issues. Moreover, it can be determined by policy or institutional frameworks according to different national and international waste definitions and is mainly caused by managerial and technical limitations, such as lack of efficient storage technologies, improper food handling practices or inefficient packaging.

FW refers to still edible food removal from FSC for different reasons. Generally, it refers to discarding or alternative uses of still safe and nutritious food for human consumption and mainly occurs at retail or consumer levels (FAO, 2013, 2015; Rezaei & Liu, 2017) (Figure 1).

Figure 1. FLW scheme
Source: Authors' development based in Pellegrini, Sillani, Gregori, and Spada (2019)

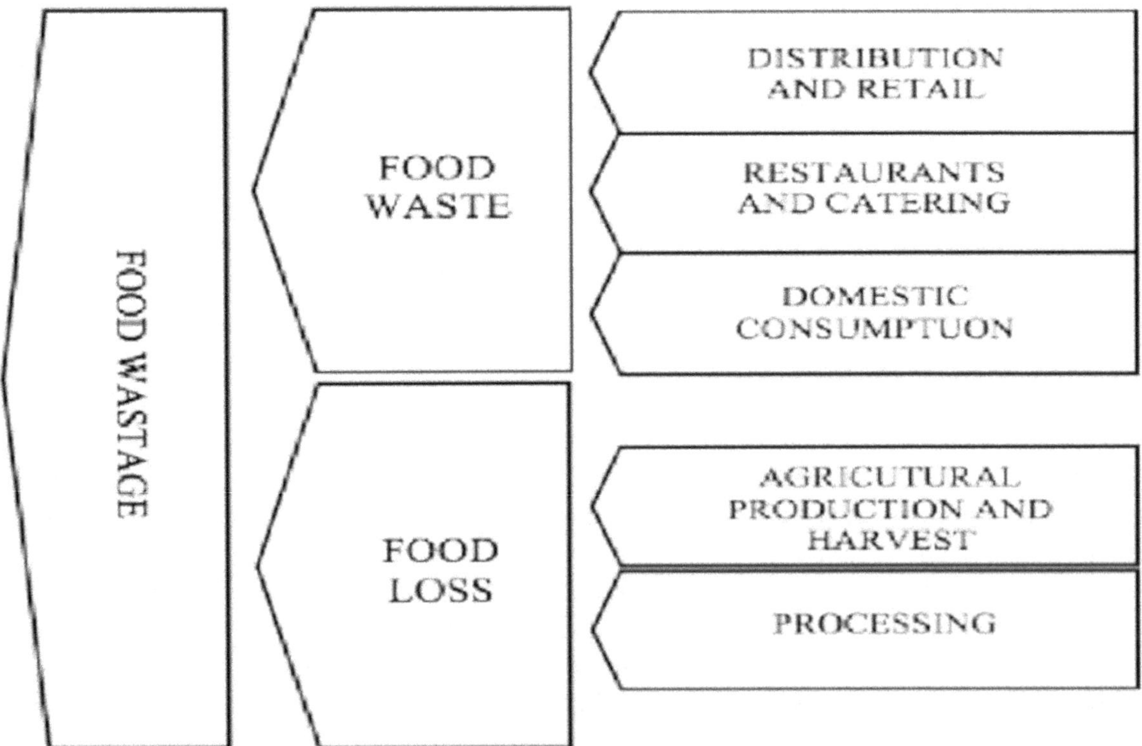

In particular, FLW occurring at different FSC stages depends essentially on its definition. However, average values can be estimated according to FAO (2015, 2019), Moller et al. (2014), and Stenmarck, Jensen, Quested, and Moates (2016). It is stated that along FSC approximately 11-23% occurs at the agricultural production and harvest stage, 17-19% at processing, 8-17% at distribution (wholesale, retail, and food service), and 52-53% at the consumption stage (households). These little differences depend on FLW definition and analysis breakdown (Corrado et al., 2019).

Food Loss and Waste: Quantity and Costs

A shared definition of FLW is not enough to minimize this phenomenon; it must be determined in quantity and quality so as to better manage it.

In the last decades, FLW has increased on a rate of more than 50%. FAO estimates on average more than 1.3 billion tons of FWL along the whole FSC (equivalent to one-third of total food production) of which more than 670 million tons in developed countries and approximately 630 million tons in developing ones, showing wide differences between countries. In particular, EU data estimates an amount of more than 85 million tons of FLW, equal to approximately 20% of total food production (more than 170 kg of FLW out of 860 kg of food produced per capita). In descending order, domestic consumption accounts for more than 45 million tons of FLW, followed by processing (approximately 17 million tons), food service, such as restaurants and catering (more than 10 million tons), agricultural production and harvesting (more than 9 million tons), and distribution and retail (about 4 million tons). Thus, EU domestic consumption and food service account for more than 60% of FLW, while agricultural production and harvest for less than 10%. (Stenmarck et al., 2016; McCarthy et al., 2018; Boiteau, 2016).

On a global level, the average FLW associated cost is equal to approximately 1.65 Euro/kg, accounting for more than $700 billion in developed countries and less than $300 billion in developing ones. Therefore, the USA wastes more than $210 billion per year, equaling 1.3% of the U.S. GDP. In the EU, this cost goes over €140 billion, of which approximately €100 billion are generated at the household level (Stenmarck et al., 2016; Boiteau, 2016; McCarthy et al., 2018; FAO, 2019).

Figure 2 shows FLW quantity and costs divided per regions and occurring between production and retail and at the consumer stage each year.

FLW differences around the world depend on the technical, economic and social development of each country. On average, more than 160 kg/year per capita is the estimated amount of FLW occurring from the production to retailing stages, ranging from the highest value in Latin America (approximately 200 kg/year per capita) to the lowest value in South and Southeast Asia (more than 100 kg/year per capita). However, although developed countries show the highest percentage at the retail level, while developing ones at the harvest and post-harvest stage, both show on average similar FLW values at the pre-consumption stages (FAO, 2019; Pellegrini et al., 2019; Philippidis, Sartori, Ferrari, & M'Barek, 2019).

Wide difference in FLW is registered at consumer level with an average value of approximately 50 kg/year per capita. According to global data, the highest value is recorded in North America and Oceania (approximately 120 kg/year per capita) and the lowest one in Sub-Saharan Africa (less than 10 kg/year per capita) (Boiteau, 2016).

FLW generally causes change worldwide, with big differences between developed and developing economies. In developed ones, the main causes for FLW relate to over-production, high consumer appearance and quality standards, higher costs for recovery and re-using than for discarding and sell-by date reached in general organized distribution. An Italian multiple-choice answer survey shows several

Figure 2. FLW quantity (kg per capita) and costs (€ per capita) per regions at different FSC stages
Source: Authors' development based in Pellegrini et al. (2019)

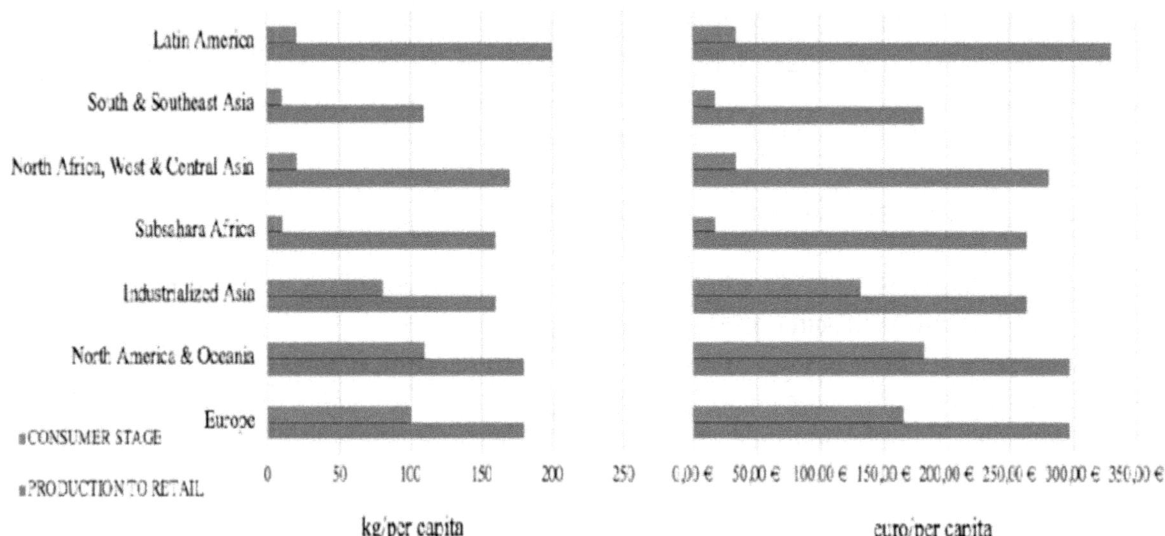

reasons for household FLW. The highest percentage of them depends on out of date food (approximately 55% of given answers) followed by moldy food (less than 40%), badly smelling or tasting food (more than 30%), wrong planning of meals (more than 25%), too much served food (approximately 20%), unintelligible data labeling (approximately 5%), incorrect storage (less than 5%) or insufficient cooking skills (less than 5%) (Jorissen, Priefer, & Brautigam, 2015).

In developing countries, the main causes for FLW concern production phases, such as agricultural ones (too early harvesting of crops), poor storage, processing, and market facilities, and lack of infra-structure (Boiteau, 2016).

Food Loss and Waste: Quality and Composition

FLW composition differs around the world, recording deep differences between regions and FLW groups. On average and based on the total production of a single food group, roots and tubers show the highest percentage (52%) and dairy products the lowest one (15%). For various reasons and in different FSG stages, more than half of the total roots and tubers and less than 50% of fruit and vegetables produced lose their value as a human diet component.

Based on 2018 production data, Figure 3 shows the worldwide FLW composition and percentage of lost or wasted food at different FSC stages. FLW is calculated as total production of a single food group (Figure 3).

Food Loss and Waste: Accounting and Reporting

FLW minimization aims at food security, economic benefits, and environmental gains. However, its management faces several challenges according to complex FLW measurement along the FSC.

Figure 3. Worldwide FLW composition at different FSC stage
Source: Authors' development based on FAO (2019)

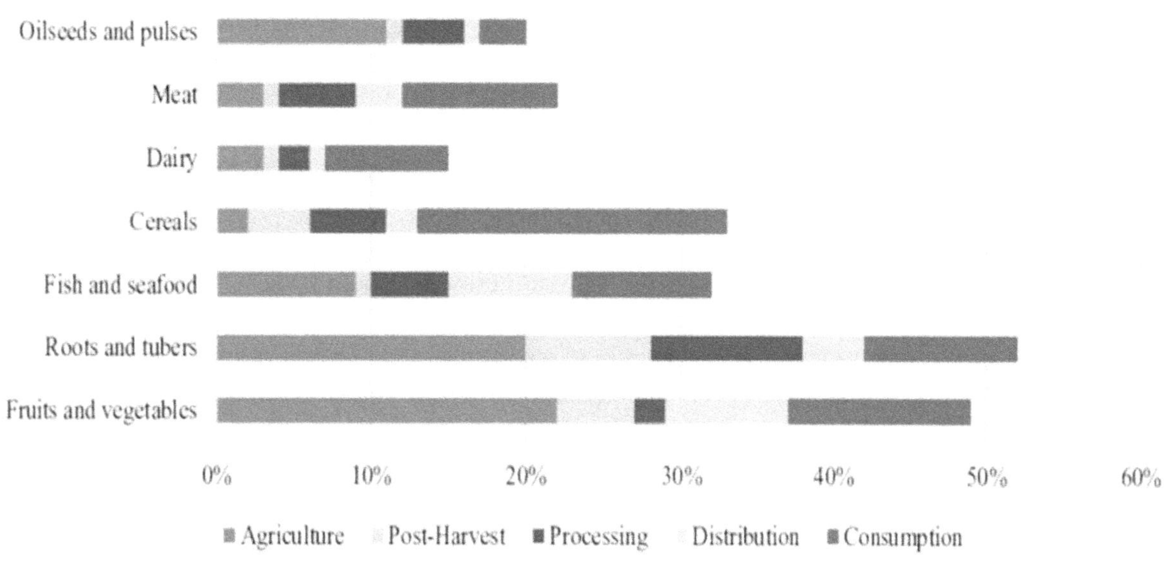

The inverted pyramid for solid waste FW management based on prevention, re-use, recycling, recovery, and disposal can be applied also to FLW (Figure 4). Generally, FLW can be used for and/or transformed in animal feed, bio-based materials, bioenergy recovery, composting or landfilling.

Figure 4. FLW management hierarchy
Source: Authors' development based on FLW (2016a, 2016b)

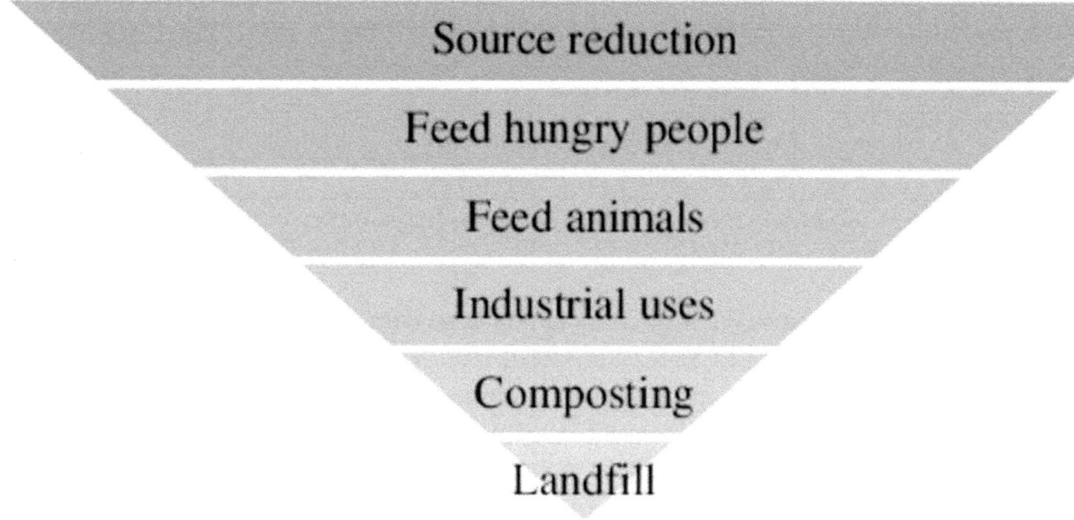

The first solution requires surplus food generation avoidance and prevention along the whole FSC, while re-use presupposes redeployment for human consumption through food redistribution and food banks. Recycling requires FLW usage as animal feed or composting, recovery means energy, solid or liquid material production (e.g. conversion into useable heat, electricity, biofuel, or fertilizers) and the last and residual option means that it has to be landfilled (Papargyropoulou, Lozano, Steinberger, Wright, & Bin Ujang, 2014; FLW, 2016a, 2016b).

However, FLW hierarchy implementation requires accurate accounting and reporting tools along the whole FSC.

At the production stage, farming and husbandry should be considered. Moreover, processing and manufacturing on the primary (e.g. drying, sieving, and milling) and secondary stages (e.g. mixing, cooking, and molding) as well as on the retail stage need particular attention. And finally, consumption distinguishing between household use, catering (e.g. restaurants), and institutions such as educational and medical treatment ones should be taken into account (Papargyropoulou et al., 2014). Table 3 details FLW causes along the FSC.

Table 3. Causes for FLW along the FSC from production to distribution

FSC stage	FLW causes
Agricultural stage (harvesting, threshing, breeding)	• Crops left in field (e.g. esthetical reasons, out of retail standard products, handling costs higher than market prices) • Crops damaged during harvesting due to poor harvesting and threshing techniques
Transport Distribution	• Poor transport infrastructure • Transport accidents and damages • Out of date products due to poor or insufficient supply programming
Primary processing Secondary processing	• Contamination and losses occurring during cleaning, classification, packaging, mixing, cooking, frying at industrial stage
Quality control	• Discharging due to out of retail standards products (e.g. esthetical or weight standards)
Storage	• Storage issues such as pests, disease, contamination due to poor storage infrastructure (e.g. lack of cooling/cold storage)
Packaging	• Packaging damages • Contaminations • Weighing, labeling, and sealing mistakes
Marketing and retail	• Publicity, selling, and distribution issues

Source: Authors' development based on Papargyropoulou et al. (2014) and Segrè and Falasconi (2011)

As stated by previous paragraphs, FLW at consumption stage deserves special mention accounting highest percentage along FSC equal to 52-53% at global level. Households FLW generation can be considered as results of food purchased, people cooking and shopping behavior and general lifestyle.

For instance, EU surveys show average households FLW accounting for more than €450 per family in 2010, however that is less if compared to 2008 (more than €550/family). The highest percentage of FLW concerns fresh products such as eggs, meat, cheese, and milk with over 35% of total purchase, followed by bread (less than 20%), fruit and vegetables (approximately 15%), cold cuts and salads (about 10%), pasta and quick-frozen (less than 5%) (Segrè & Falasconi, 2011).

In terms of FLW causes occurring at the consumption stage, it is possible to distinguish between external variables related to social and cultural issues, FSC variables regarding problems and malfunctioning along the supply chain and individual variables related to personal habits, attitudes, and values (Table 4).

Table 4. External, FSC, and individual variables influencing FLW at consumption stage

Influences source	FWL causes
External variables	• Food-safety campaigns • Household make-up • Income levels • Customs and traditions • Food fashion
FSC variables	• Products availability • Packaging • Storage guidance • Date labeling • Promotions
Individual variables	• Attitude and values • Motivation • Habits • Knowledge and skills • Facilities and resources

Source: Authors' development based on Moller et al. (2014)

Several impacts are associated with FLW from economic to environmental and social ones (Figure 5).

Figure 5. FLW economic, social, and environmental impacts
Source: Authors' development based on Barilla Center for Food and Nutrition [BCFN] (2012)

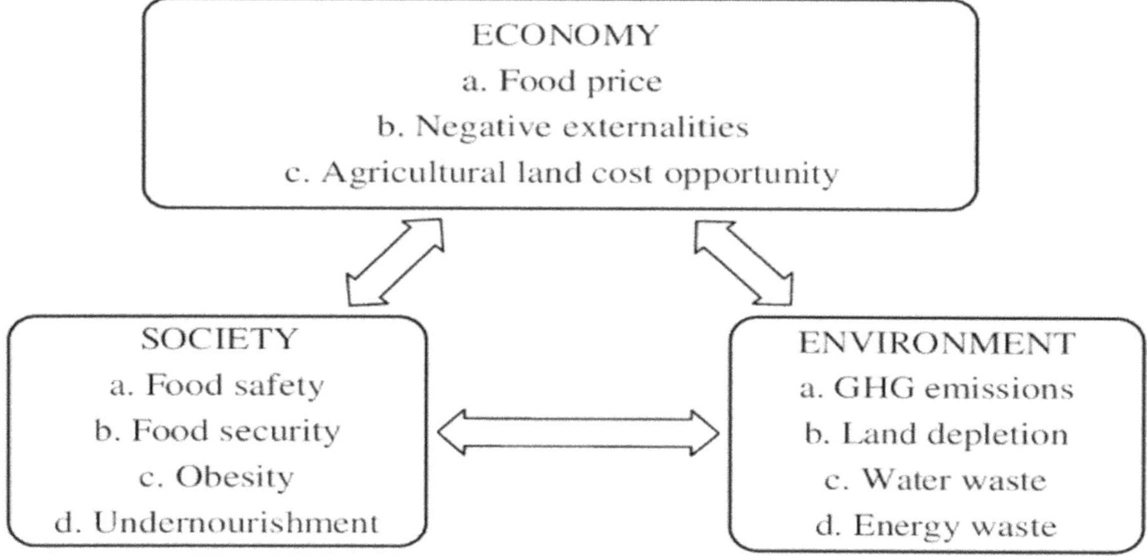

MAIN FOCUS OF THE CHAPTER

Potato FSC Case Study in Italy

As mentioned above, FLW data available are not homogenous and present several differences. Based on Italian FLW equaling on average to 150 kg/per capita per year (approximately 5% of Italian waste generation), in Italy approximately more than 9 Mt of food are wasted yearly corresponding to more than €14.5 billion loss (€1.65/kg). However, references record lower values. For instance, Segrè and Azzurro (2016), Segrè and Falasconi (2011), Segrè, Falasconi, and Politano (2016), BCFN (2012), and Pellegrini et al. (2019) estimate that Italy wastes less than 3% (approximately 2 Mt) of its national food production each year, losing approximately €3.5 billion and human feed for approximately three-quarters of its population. In particular, the highest FLW costs are associated with meat wastes for over €440 million (Bräutigam, Jörissen, & Priefer, 2014; Priefer, Jörissen, & Bräutigam, 2016).

With regard to the Italian FLW composition, drinks and dairy together account for 47%, followed by fruits and vegetables (15%), bread and sweets (13%), cereals (12%), meat (8%), oils and vegetable fats (4%), and fish (1%) (Figure 6).

Figure 6. Italian FLW composition
Source: Authors' development based on Segrè and Falasconi (2011)

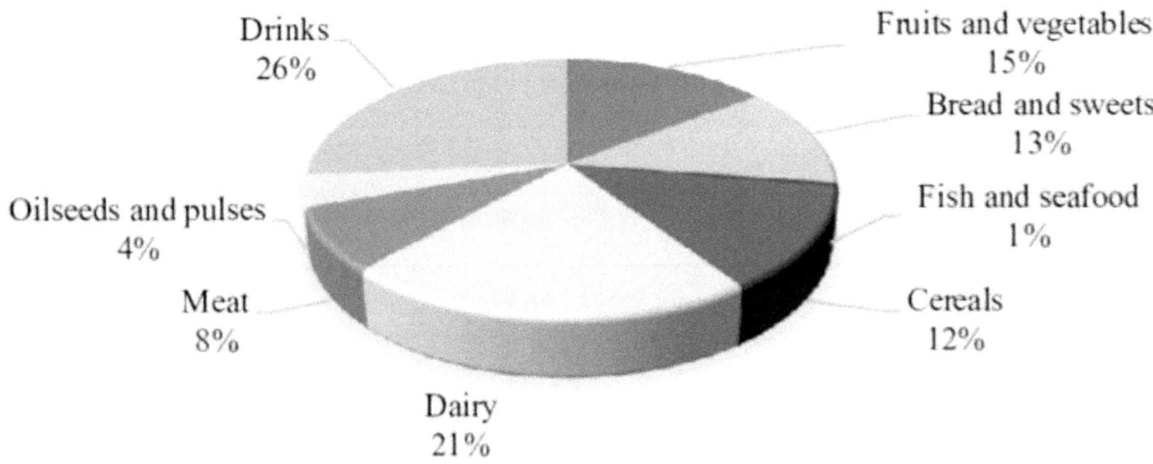

To detail: with regard to the hypothesis in which the Italian FLW follows the same trends of the global FLW (Figure 3), it is possible to calculate the Italian FLW percentages along the FSC (Figure 7).

In particular, between 2% and 12% of the FLW occurs in the agricultural stage as harvest land loss (e.g. less than 2% of citrus fruits, 5% of potatoes and legumes, and more than 12% for tomatoes) (BCFN, 2012).

The case study presented regards potato industry. The choice is based on the following considerations: potato is the fourth most important staple food worldwide after maize, wheat and rice mainly due to its starch content which is the primary energy source in the human diet. It is cultivated in about 130 countries, mostly in developing ones even if, in the last years, its production has recorded a continuously growing

Figure 7. Italian FLW composition at different FSC stages
Source: Authors' development based on FAO (2019) and Segrè and Falasconi (2011)

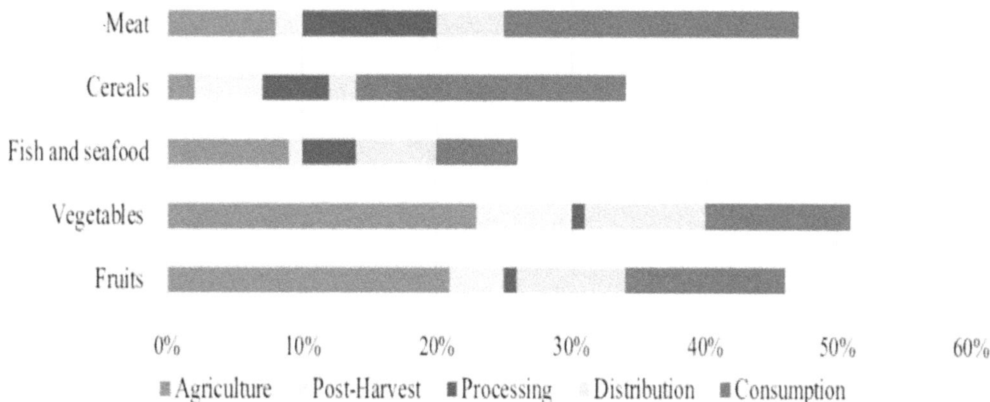

also in developing countries. It has become a crucial food both for its direct and indirect use in human diet in the European countries (Eriksson, Carlson-Nilsson, Ortíz, & Andreasson, 2016; Eurostat, 2019, FAO, n.d.). Moreover, vegetables are one of the most wasted food categories worldwide, recording high percentage of FLW along FSC. Moreover, potatoes as raw materials can be transformed in several final products, giving the chance to compare costs and wastes along different FSCs.

Worldwide, potato production (PP) is estimated to be approximately less than 390,000 kt with several changes in global markets and trades. Until the 1990s, the highest percentage was consumed in Europe, North America, and USSR countries. However, recent statistics show a sharp increase of PP in Asia, Africa, and Latin America from 30 million tons in the 1960s to more than 165 million tons in 2007. Moreover, China shows the biggest PP and approximately one-third of all potatoes is harvested between China and India (PotatoPro.com, n.d.). China accounts for about 100,000 kt, followed by India (approximately 50,000 kt) and Russia (approximately 30,000 kt). Table 5 shows PP, harvested area and yield, while Figure 8 shows PP worldwide.

Table 5. Potato production, harvested area, and yield

Phenomena	Quantity
World Potato Production (2017)	374,252,073 tons
World Potato Harvested Area (2017)	19,302,600 ha
World Potato Yield (2017)	201,108 hg/ha

Source: Authors' development based on PotatoPro.com (n.d.)

Fresh and processed potatoes global consumption is on average approximately less than 35 kg/capita each year at consumption stage. European PP accounts for more than 50,000 kt in 2018, less with more than 60,000 kt if compared to the 2017 PP. Italian PP registers more than 1,300 kt in 2018 (approximately 2.5% of European PP) (Eurostat, 2019).

Figure 8. Potato production worldwide, tons
Source: Authors' development based on FAO (2018)

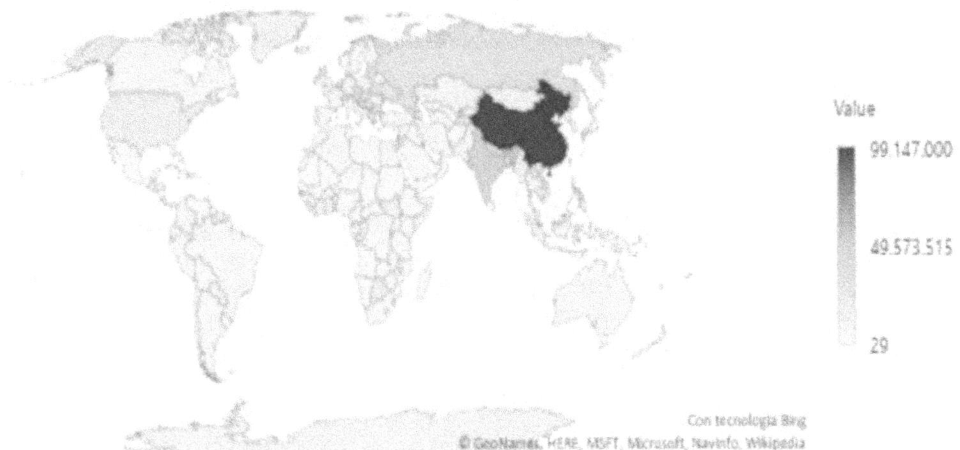

In particular, the potato FSC registers a sharp increase requiring quality standards such as dimension, shape, peel characteristics, sugar in raw content, and taste. However, the one can distinguish between potatoes for industrial use and potatoes for consumption.

Available data state that the Italian potato FSC depends approximately on 85% imported raw material, followed by 10% national produce and less than 5% is selected for planting. Moreover, Italian harvested land is approximately over 60,000 ha and PP accounts for more than 1,300 kt.

Potato consumption (PC) shows some important trends. According to an Italian consumer survey, more than 55% of consumers habitually consume them and approximately 25% is very interested in. This means that less than 2% of the population does not consume potatoes, thus becoming one of the most preferred products by consumers. Furthermore, several varieties of potatoes can be distinguished. The highest percentage of PC is registered by yellow flesh potatoes (approximately 50%), followed by new potatoes, white flesh potatoes and lastly frozen potatoes. However, their use changes according to consumer preferences. More than 60% of consumers eat baked potatoes, approximately 55% – French fries, about 50% boiled ones, and less than 30% for other preparation, showing baked and French potatoes as the preferred ones in a double-choice answer survey (Coltura & Cultura, n.d.; ISMEA, 2014; Tirelli, n.d.).

With regard to the market, Table 6 shows important details according to consumers purchase preferences.

Table 6. Consumer purchase preferences

Potato-based final product	%	kt
In jute bags	33	429
Packaged potatoes (with quality label)	25	325
Loose potatoes	24	312
Frozen potatoes	15	195
Ready for consumption (peeled, cooked)	3	39
Total	100	1,300

Source: Authors' development based on Tirelli (n.d.)

Considering that Italian PP is approximately more than 1,300 kt in 2018, it is possible to estimate and share its national transformation according to consumer purchase preferences. Applying these percentages to Italian PP, it is possible to calculate how PP is divided between industrial and consumer end-use.

After having stated PP and PC quantity and quality and remembering potatoes importance in daily diet, in consumer purchase preference and in FLW phenomena, it is possible to create a Material Flow Analysis (MFA) along the whole FSC to measure FLW. In particular, three types of industrial processing can be taken into account: frozen pre-fried potatoes, chips and dehydrated potatoes.

SOLUTIONS AND RECOMMENDATIONS

The authors have chosen to use the MFA for analyzing the potato industry. MFA is a systematic assessment of the state and change of materials flow and stocks defined in space and time. It connects sources, pathways, and intermediate and final sinks of materials. Since MFA is related to the matter of conservation law, MFA results can be controlled by mass balance comparing all inputs, stocks, and outputs (Brunner & Rechberger, 2017; Lagioia & Camaggio, 2002; Zaghdaoui, Jaegler, Gondran, & Montoya-Torres, 2017; Kytzia, Faist, & Baccini, 2004).

MFA is the main method applied in the following case study and takes into account three specific typologies of processed potatoes: pre-fried, chips, and dehydrated potatoes, which represent the highest quota of processed potatoes. According to reference literature, the main type of processed potatoes are pre-fried ones (e.g. linear sticks, zig-zag sticks, sliced potatoes), potatoes for direct consumption (e.g. chips), and dehydrated ones.

The functional unit of MFA is one ton of final product and boundaries are from the agricultural to the processing stage, without considering distribution/retail and consumption ones. However, according to different technical routes, MFA tries to summarize common sections for both pre-fried potatoes and chips and one common supply chain for dehydrated ones. MFA first deals with the agricultural stage, then the processing technologies and particular issues along the supply chain, focusing its attention to FLW along the FSC.

According to Wang et al. (2016), it is possible to calculate resources (seeds, fertilizers, and energy, without considering land and water) and waste produced along whole FSC (boundaries from agricultural stage to storage, without considering retail and consumption stages). Figure 9 illustrates in details the whole MFA from the agricultural to storage stage for pre-fried potatoes (in circles) and chips (in rectangles), showing global input-output. The agricultural stage, reception, preparation for cutting, cutting, washing, drying, burning, pre-frying and frying are common for both industrial processes. After frying, separate processes are represented (cooling-down and freezing for pre-fried potatoes and salting for chips) (Figure 9).

Starting from the agricultural stage, seeds, fertilizers, and energy are required as input. However, this stage produces land loss (5% of tubers required). To obtain a functional unit, an amount of 1.7-2.0 tons of tubers are needed in the pre-fried potatoes process, while it is 3.5-4.0 tons in the chips process. During reception and preparation for the cutting phase, approximately 1 m^3 of water are required in both processes. Moreover, about 50 kg of uncalibrated tubers are wasted while more than 0.2-0.4 tons of skins and scraps are produced. Later, during the cutting, washing, drying, and burning phases, additional water is required (5 m^3 for pre-fried potatoes and more than 15-20 m^3 for chips) with little waste. Subsequently, sticks (1.4-1.5 tons) and chips are obtained. Sticks should be about 10 cm in length and 6-12 mm in depth while chips should be 1.0-1.7 in depth.

Figure 9. MFA for pre-fried potatoes and chips (1 ton)
Source: Authors' development

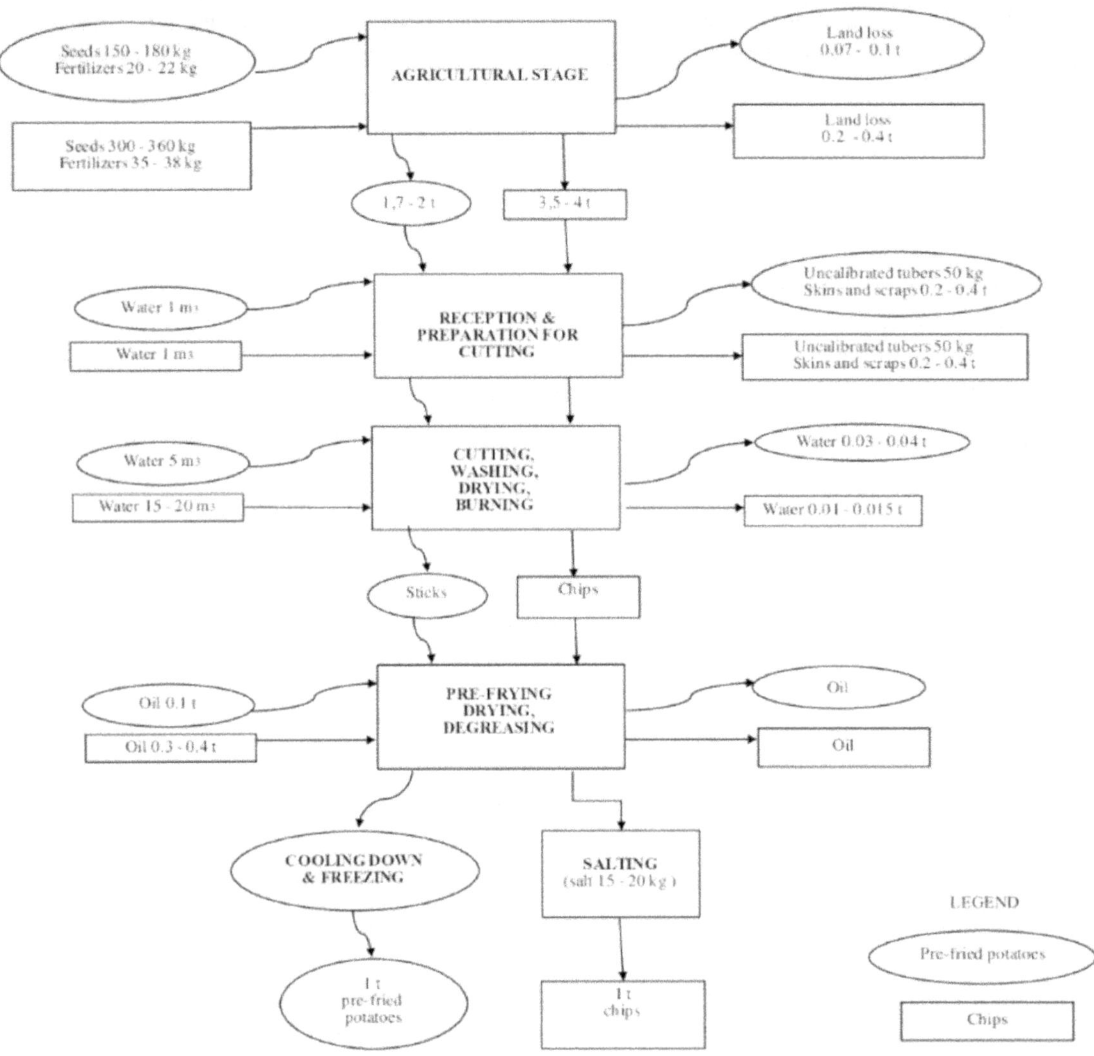

During the pre-frying, drying, and degreasing phase, oil is required in a range of 0.1-0.4 tons. After that, the process differs between pre-fried potatoes and chips. In the first case, a cooling-down and freezing phase is required, while in the second one salting (15-20 kg of salt) is needed.

Moreover, it is possible to calculate resources (seeds, fertilizers, and energy, without considering land and water) and waste produced along the whole FSC (boundaries from agricultural stage to storage, without considering retail and consumption stages) for dehydrated potatoes (Figure 10).

As stated in Figure 10, to obtain 1 ton of dehydrated potatoes (functional unit), 55-60 kg of potato seeds, 70-80 kg of fertilizers, tubers in a range of 6.3-7.3 tons, 30-35 tons of water and 40 GJ of energy, of which 3 GJ for electricity production and 37 GJ for the production of 15-20 tons of steam are required. As output, approximately 0.3-0.4 tons of land loss, 50 kg of uncalibrated tubers, 1.20-1.55 tons of skins, scraps, and waste and water, oil and steam are produced as waste and FLW.

Figure 10. MFA for dehydrated potatoes (1 ton)
Source: Authors' development

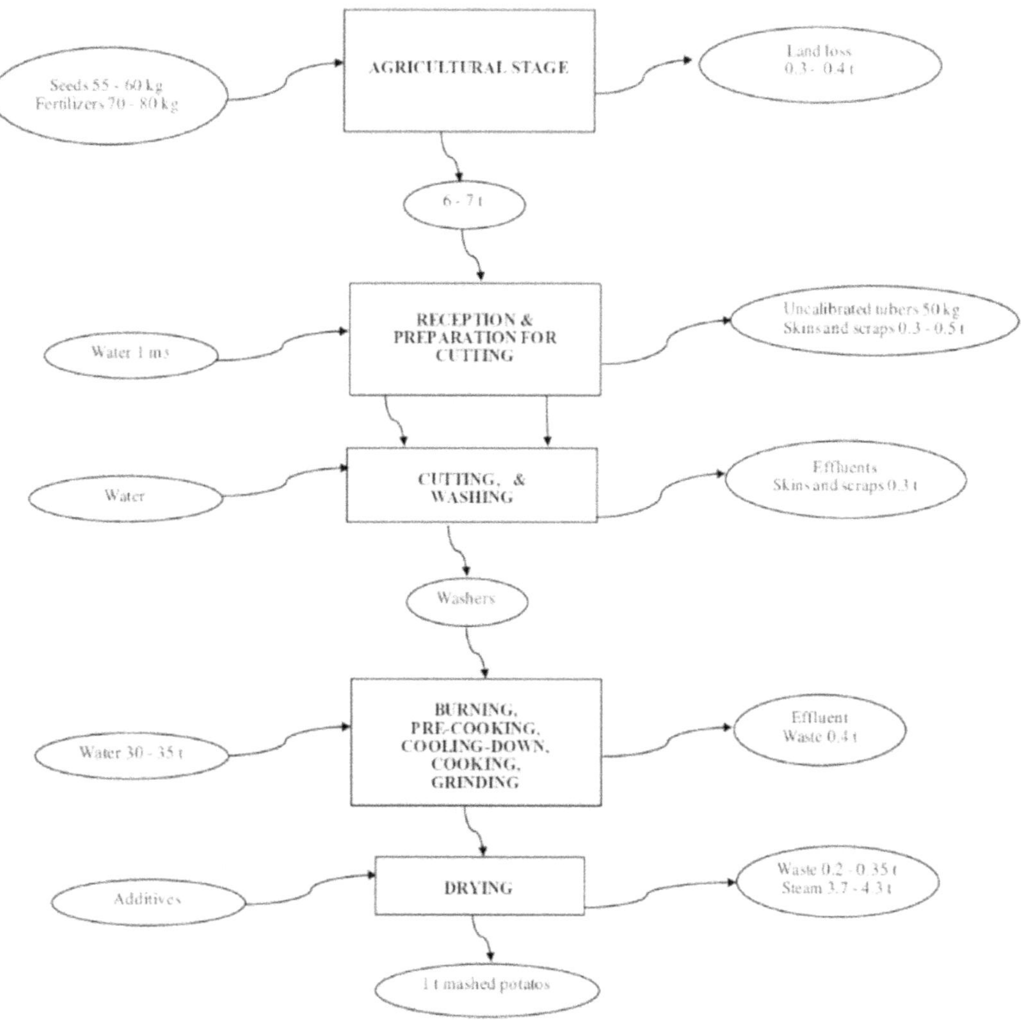

FUTURE RESEARCH DIRECTIONS

As mentioned in the previous paragraphs, the authors have chosen MFA to analyze the Italian potato industry. In particular, this tool is applied to describe and evaluate material and substance balances in a well-defined system and can be useful to define a systematic assessment of the state and change of material flows and stocks in space and time connecting sources, pathways and final sinks of materials. Moreover, since MFA is related to the matter of conservation law, its results can be controlled by mass balance comparing all inputs, stocks and outputs (Brunner & Rechberger, 2017; Zaghdaoui et al., 2017; Kytzia et al., 2004; Wang et al., 2016).

In particular, the present research uses MFA to support and improve FLW management and its application in an Italian agri-food sector towards its sustainability and main results demonstrated MFA as an important tool able to quantify and qualify natural resources utilization and economic costs associated to 1 t of final product. Moreover, MFA results are useful in FLW context to account energy and material lost or waster along FSC when food stops to be "feed" and begins to be "waste". Being MFA comparable, this tool provides useful information in order to understand if FLW associated to potato-based final products change according to new or old technologies, or to compare FLW associated to different vegetables or food FSCs.

In such context, being availability of data and FLW measurement tools European priority, authors have proposed MFA as one of the possible options for its accounting and reporting and as a basis for the construction of others environmental indicators such as carbon and water footprint or for the application of Life Cycle Assessment (LCA) methodology. Thus, its application could be improved within future studies and researches and proposed to further policy implementations, giving the chance to minimize FLW towards food safety and food security better management (Brunner & Rechberger, 2017; Caldeira, Corrado, & Sala, 2017; Zaghdaoui et al., 2017).

CONCLUSION

Table 7 shows FLW along the FSC according to the potatoes transformation quota in Table 6. FLW (kt) displays total quantity along the FSC, in a range of 585 kt and 845 kt (45-65% of global production).

Table 7. FLW (kt) along FSC for different potato-based final products

Potato-based final product	Total (kt)
In jute bags	193-279
Packaged potatoes (with quality label)	146-211
Loose potatoes	140-203
Frozen potatoes	88-127
Ready for consumption (peeled, cooked)	18-25
Total	585-845

Source: Authors' development

According to MFA methodology and Tables 6-7, potatoes FLW costs have been calculated.

With regard to pre-fried, chips, and dehydrated products, FLW occurs in a range of 585-845 kt. In terms of monetary costs and based on Istituto di Servizi per il Mercato Agricolo Alimentare (2019), FLW occurs in a range of €111.2-160.2 million (for €0.19/kg) and €274.9-€397.2 million (for €0.47/kg). Overall, FLW in PP accounts in a range of 3-12% of the Italian FLW or 0.7-2.7% considering €14.5 billion as Italian FLW associated cost.

The contribution of the MFA is a very effective tool to track input and output and in balanced mass and energy flows. As cited above, wasting food has a negative impact on many levels: ethical and social level (throwing away the food that other people could eat), economic level (people have paid for this food), environmental impacts that are underestimated (for example, CO_2 emissions derived from the improper management of organic waste). So, analyzing the factors influencing the wastage can help for better management of the whole supply chain. MFA is possible to include into the wider concept of sustainable development whose application can improve FSC management and drive the food sector towards sustainability goals. Furthermore, MFA can be integrated in the new paradigm of Circular Economy (CE). The CE concept has been introduced by Ellen MacArthur Foundation. It is an economic system where products and services are traded in closed loops or cycles. A circular economy is characterized as an economy which is regenerative by design, with the aim to retain as much value as possible of products, parts, and materials. This means that the aim should be to create a system that allows for the long life, optimal reuse, refurbishment, remanufacturing and recycling of products and materials (Ellen MacArthur Foundation, 2019).

It means that the CE paradigm can lead FLW to economic opportunities such as reuse, recycling, energy efficiency, and nutrient recovery against landfill and disposal (Garcia-Garcia, Stone, & Rahimifard, 2019; Lemaire & Limbourg, 2019; Principato, Ruini, Guidi, & Secondi, 2019; Segneanu et al., 2018). According to FLW hierarchy (Figure 4), FLW can be first reused for human consumption or secondly destined to animal feed and, if not possible, it can follow several alternative pathways such as:

- Recycling for industrial use;
- Anaerobic digestion;
- Composting;
- Combustion for energy recovery.

Several policies have adopted the CE paradigms. In particular, in Europe, European Commission (2015) proposed a transition to a more circular economy where products, materials, and resources value is maintained in the economy for as long as possible and waste generation is minimized.

This document dedicates one paragraph to FLW as an EU increasing concern. In detail, it states that FLW produces environmental impacts and financial losses for both consumers and companies and considers social implications such as limited food donation of still edible food. Moreover, it considers FLW as part of 2030 Sustainable Development Goals (SDGs), especially in terms of "Zero Hunger". Moreover, it states that FLW is still hard to quantify since there is no harmonized and reliable method to measure food waste in the EU giving public authorities the chance to assess its scale, origins, and trends. However, FLW minimization requires actions by EU Member States, regions, cities, and businesses along the whole FSC. For this reason, the EU Commission has tried to address FLW policies such as the elaboration of a common EU methodology to its measurement, the creation of an EU platform dedicated to FLW and the application of actions regarding as instance "best before" marking. The case study analyzed in Italy shows the importance of FLW accounting towards efficiency and sustainability. This is because it has become possible to develop action plans, guidelines, recommendations to address policymakers, restaurants, hotels, producers, and anyone interested in helping to reduce food waste to new managerial policy.

EU interventions against FLW can be summarized with particular attention to:

- Development of EU common methodology to measure FLW and define relevant indicators;
- Improvement of data marking use by FSC actors and its understanding by consumers (e.g. "best before" label);
- Platform involving Member States and Stakeholders to support SDGs achievement and share best practices;
- Clarification of EU legislation relating waste, food, and feed;
- Food waste facilitation and former food-stuff and by-product use.

According to EU policies and other studies and researches, and since the available amount of data on FLW is low in quality and quantity, data collection should become policy priority. Table 8 registers FLW legislative frameworks opportunities and limits according to European Parliament (2008) and Technopolis Group (2016).

Table 8. FLW legislative framework opportunities and limits

FLW hierarchy stage	Opportunities	Limits
FLW prevention	Reduction in portion sizes Tailored hygiene rules Best before practices Estimation of day-to-day customers	No legislation on portion sizes Strict hygiene rules Problems in estimation
FLW collection		Lack of collection infrastructure Expansive collection
FLW reuse	Food donations Food banks	VAT Limited liability rules
FLW recycling	Animal feed Composting	Limits in catering separation as only biotic materials can be processed Cannibalism and safeguard of animal health
FLW incineration	Biofuels generation	CO_2 emissions

Source: Authors' development based on Technopolis Group (2016)

When considering FLW prevention policies, some possible options can be taken into account, such as reduction in portion sizes, tailored hygiene rules, best before dates for products and better estimations of the number of day-to-day customers. However, several lacks can be registered: lack of rules on portion sizes, hygiene, best before dates and lack of accurate FLW definition. Moreover, in terms of FLW recovery and re-use and related separate collection, the lack of an efficient collection infrastructure determines an expansive collection process. One more option is FLW reuse through donation. However, it is limited by VAT and liability rules with negative economic incentive on food donation and competitive implications to anaerobic digestion, incineration, composting and animal feed. In terms of FLW recycling which regards food conversion into animal feed and composting, the limits are represented by lack of efficient conversion plants. Last option regards incineration, being worldwide used as a biofuel generation source. Its limit is represented by environmental impacts such as GHG and related CO2 emissions.

In conclusion, according to typologies and the FSC stage, different FLW quality can be reported with different FLW destinations, such as natural fertilizer (left in field), animal feeding, energy recovery, food banks and composting.

REFERENCES

Alonso, E. B., Cockx, L., & Swinnen, J. (2017). *Culture and Food Security*. Leuven: Centre for Institutions and Economic Performance.

Barilla Center for Food and Nutrition. (2012). *Lo sprecoalimentare: cause, impatti e proposte*. Parma: Barilla Center for Food and Nutrition.

Barrett, C. B. (2010). Measuring Food Insecurity. *Science*, *327*(5967), 825–828. doi:10.1126cience.1182768 PMID:20150491

Boiteau, J. M. (2016). *Food Loss and Waste in the United States and Worldwide*. Retrieved August 20, 2019, from https://www.worldhunger.org/food-loss-and-waste-in-the-united-states-and-worldwide/

Bräutigam, K. R., Jörissen, J., & Priefer, C. (2014). The Extent of Food Waste Generation across EU-27: Different Calculation Methods and the Reliability of their Results. *Waste Management & Research*, *32*(8), 683–694. doi:10.1177/0734242X14545374 PMID:25161274

Brunner, P. H., & Rechberger, H. (2017). *Handbook of Material Flow Analysis. For Environmental, Resource and Waste Engineers*. London: CRC Press.

Caldeira, C., Corrado, S., & Sala, S. (2017). *Food Waste Accounting – Methodologies, Challenges and Opportunities*. Brussels: Publication Office of the European Union.

Coltura & Cultura. (n.d.). *Un Volume, una Coltura*. Retrieved from https://www.colturaecultura.it/download

Corrado, S., Caldeira, C., Eriksson, M., Hanssen, O. J., Hauser, H.-E., Van Holsteijn, F., ... Sala, S. (2019). Food Waste Accounting Methodologies: Challenges, Opportunities, and Further Advancements. *Global Food Security*, *20*, 93–100. doi:10.1016/j.gfs.2019.01.002 PMID:31008044

Ellen MacArthur Foundation. (2019). *What Is the Circular Economy?* Retrieved from https://www.ellenmacarthurfoundation.org/circular-economy/what-is-the-circular-economy

Eriksson, D., Carlson-Nilsson, U., Ortíz, R., & Andreasson, E. (2016). Overview and Breeding Strategies of Table Potato Production in Sweden and the Fennoscandian Region. *Potato Research*, *59*(3), 279–294. doi:10.100711540-016-9328-6

European Commission. (2015). *Communication from the Commission to the European Parliament, the Council, the European Economic and Social Committee and the Committee of the Regions. Closing the Loop – An EU Action Plan for the Circular Economy*. Retrieved from https://eur-lex.europa.eu/legal-content/EN/TXT/?uri=CELEX:52015DC0614

European Parliament. (2008). *Directive 2008/98/EC of the European Parliament and of the Council of 19 November 2008 on Waste and Repealing Certain Directives*. Retrieved from https://eur-lex.europa.eu/legal-content/EN/TXT/?uri=celex%3A32008L0098

Eurostat. (2019). *Crop Production in EU Standard Humidity*. Retrieved from https://data.europa.eu/euodp/en/data/dataset/u33K8Gi1MFYGN7HyHUNhg

Food and Agriculture Organization of the United Nations. (2013). *Food Wastage Footprint. Impacts on Natural Resources*. Rome: Food and Agriculture Organization of the United Nations.

Food and Agriculture Organization of the United Nations. (2015). *Global Initiative on Food Loss and Waste Reduction*. Rome: Food and Agriculture Organization of the United Nations.

Food and Agriculture Organization of the United Nations. (2018). *World Food and Agriculture. Statistical Pocketbook 2018*. Rome: Food and Agriculture Organization of the United Nations.

Food and Agriculture Organization of the United Nations. International Fund for Agricultural Development, United Nations International Children's Emergency Fund, World Food Programme, & World Health Organization. (2018). The State of Food Security and Nutrition in the World 2018. Building Climate Resilience for Food Security and Nutrition. Rome: Food and Agriculture Organization of the United Nations.

Food and Agriculture Organization of the United Nations. (2019). *Save Food: Global Initiative on Food Loss and Waste Reduction*. Rome: Food and Agriculture Organization of the United Nations.

Food and Agriculture Organization of the United Nations. (n.d.). *Crops*. Retrieved from http://www.fao.org/faostat/en/#data/QC

Food Loss + Waste Protocol. (2016a). *Food Loss and Waste Accounting and Reporting Standard*. Retrieved from https://flwprotocol.org/

Food Loss + Waste Protocol. (2016b). *Guidance on FLW Quantification Methods*. Retrieved from https://flwprotocol.org/wp-content/uploads/2016/05/FLW_Protocol_Guidance_on_FLW_Quantification_Methods.pdf

Garcia-Garcia, G., Stone, J., & Rahimifard, S. (2019). Opportunities for Waste Valorisation in the Food Industry – A Case Study with Four UK Food Manufacturers. *Journal of Cleaner Production, 211*, 1339–1356. doi:10.1016/j.jclepro.2018.11.269

Istituto di Servizi per il Mercato Agricolo Alimentare. (2014). *Patate: nel 2014 la produzione italiana cresce del 20%*.

Istituto di Servizi per il Mercato Agricolo Alimentare. (2019). *Osservatorio patate. Prezzi all'origine. Trend annui*. Retrieved from http://www.ismeamercati.it/flex/cm/pages/ServeBLOB.php/L/IT/IDPagina/4845#MenuV

Jorissen, J., Priefer, C., & Brautigam, K.-R. (2015). Food Waste Generation at Household Level: Results of a Survey among Employees of Two European Research Centers in Italy and Germany. *Sustainability, 7*(3), 2695–2715. doi:10.3390u7032695

Kytzia, S., Faist, M., & Baccini, P. (2004). Economically Extended-MFA: A Material Flow Approach for a Better Understanding of Food Production Chain. *Journal of Cleaner Production, 12*(8-10), 877–889. doi:10.1016/j.jclepro.2004.02.004

Lagioia, G., & Camaggio, G. (2002). *La trasformazione industrial della patata. Dal tubero al fast food*. Bari: Progedit.

McCarthy, U., Uysal, I., Badia-Melis, R., Mercier, S., Donnell, C. O., & Ktenioudaki, A. (2018). Global Food Security – Issues, Challenges and Technological Solutions. *Trends in Food Science & Technology, 77*, 11–20. doi:10.1016/j.tifs.2018.05.002

Moller, H., Hanssen, J., Gustavsson, J., Ostergren, K., Stenmarck, A., & Dekhtyar, P. (2014). *Report on Review of (Food) Waste Reporting Methodology and Practice*. Krakeroy: Ostfold Research.

Nebbia, G. (1995). *Lezioni di Merceologia*. Rome: Laterza & Figli Spa.

Papargyropoulou, E., Lozano, R., Steinberger, J. K., Wright, N., & Bin Ujang, Z. (2014). The Food Waste Hierarchy as a Framework for the Management of Food Surplus and Food Waste. *Journal of Cleaner Production*, *76*, 106–115. doi:10.1016/j.jclepro.2014.04.020

Pellegrini, G., Sillani, S., Gregori, M., & Spada, A. (2019). Household Food Waste Reduction: Italian Consumers' Analysis for Improving Food Management. *British Food Journal*, *121*(6), 1382–1397. doi:10.1108/BFJ-07-2018-0425

Philippidis, G., Sartori, M., Ferrari, E., & M'Barek, R. (2019). Waste not, Want not: A Bio-Economic Impact Assessment of Household Food Waste Reductions in the EU. *Resources, Conservation and Recycling*, *146*, 514–522. doi:10.1016/j.resconrec.2019.04.016 PMID:31274960

Pinstrup-Andersen, P. (2009). Food Security: Definition and Measurement. *Food Security*, *1*(1), 5–7. doi:10.100712571-008-0002-y

PotatoPro.com. (n.d.). *The Potato Sector.* Retrieved from https://www.potatopro.com/world/potato-statistics

Priefer, C., Jörissen, J., & Bräutigam, K.-R. (2016). Food Waste Prevention in Europe – A Cause-Driven Approach to Identify the Most Relevant Leverage Points for Action. *Resources, Conservation and Recycling*, *109*, 155–165. doi:10.1016/j.resconrec.2016.03.004

Principato, L., Ruini, L., Guidi, M., & Secondi, L. (2019). Adopting the Circular Economy Approach on Food Loss and Waste: The Case of Italian Pasta Production. *Resources, Conservation and Recycling*, *144*, 82–89. doi:10.1016/j.resconrec.2019.01.025

Rezaei, M., & Liu, B. (2017). Food Loss and Waste in the Food Supply Chain. *Nutfruit*, 26-27.

Segneanu, A.E., Grozescu, I., Cepan, C., Cziple, F., Lazar, V., & Velciov, S. (2018). Food Security into a Circular Economy. *HSOA Journal of Food Science and Nutrition, 4*, 38.

Segrè, A., & Azzurro, P. (2016). *Spreco alimentare: dal recupero alla prevenzione. Indirizzi applicativi della legge per la limitazione degli sprechi*. Milan: Fondazione Giangiacomo Feltrinelli.

Segrè, A., & Falasconi, L. (2011). *Il libro nero dello spreco in Italia: il cibo*. Milan: Edizioni Ambiente.

Segrè, A., Falasconi, L., & Politano, A. (2016). *Crisi dei prezzi agricoli, sostenibilità e sprechi alimentari*. Retrieved from https://www.researchgate.net/publication/228837174_Crisi_dei_prezzi_agricoli_sostenibilita_e_sprechi_alimentari

Stenmarck, A., Jensen, C., Quested, T., & Moates, G. (2016). *Estimates of European Food Waste Levels*. Stockholm: IVL Swedish Environmental Research Institute.

Technopolis Group. (2016). *Regulatory Barriers for the Circular Economy. Lessons from Ten Case Studies*. Amsterdam: Technopolis Group.

Tirelli, D. (n.d.). *Richieste del consumatore*. Retrieved from https://www.colturaecultura.it/capitolo/richieste-del-consumatore

Wang, W., Jiang, D., Chen, D., Chen, Z., Zhou, W., & Zhu, B. (2016). A Material Flow Analysis (MFA)-Based Potential Analysis of Eco-Efficiency Indicators of China's Cement and Cement-Based Materials Industry. *Journal of Cleaner Production*, *112*(1), 787–796. doi:10.1016/j.jclepro.2015.06.103

Zaghdaoui, H., Jaegler, A., Gondran, N., & Montoya-Torres, J. (2017). Material Flow Analysis to Evaluate Sustainability in Supply Chains. *Proceedings of the 20th IFAC World Congress*. Toulouse: The International Federation of Automatic Control.

ADDITIONAL READING

Aramyan, L., Valeeva, N., Vittuari, M., Gaiani, S., Politano, A., & Gheoldus, M. … Hanssen, O.J. (2016). Marked-Based Instruments and Other Socio-Economic Incentives Enchancing Food Waste Prevention and Reduction. Wageningen: Wageningen UR.

Aschemann-Witzel, J., & Peschel, A. O. (2019). How Circular Will You Eat? The Sustainability Challenge in Food and Consumer Reaction to either Waste-to-Value or yet Underused Novel Ingredients in Food. *Food Quality and Preference*, *77*, 15–20. doi:10.1016/j.foodqual.2019.04.012

Boulding, K. (1996). The Economics of the Coming Spaceship Earth. In H. Jarrett (Ed.), *Environmental Quality in a Growing Economy* (pp. 3–14). Baltimore: Johns Hopkins University Press.

De Marco, O., Lagioia, G., Amicarelli, V., & Sgaramella, A. (2009). Constructing Physical Input-Output Tables with Material Flow Analysis (MFA) Data: Bottom-Up Case Studies. In S. Sangwon (Ed.), *Handbook on Input-Output Economics in Industrial Ecology* (pp. 161–187). Amsterdam: Springer Netherlands. doi:10.1007/978-1-4020-5737-3_9

European Food Banks Federation. (2016). *Circular Economy in Favour of the Most Deprived. Preventing Food Waste through Food Redistribution*. Brussels: European Food Banks Federation.

Fresco, L. O. (2009). Challenges for Food System Adaptation Today and Tomorrow. *Environmental Science & Policy*, *12*(4), 378–385. doi:10.1016/j.envsci.2008.11.001

Gustavsson, J., Cederberg, C., Sonesson, U., Van Otterdijk, R., & Meybeck, A. (2011). *Global Food Losses and Food Waste. Extent, Causes and Prevention*. Rome: Food and Agriculture Organization of the United Nations.

International Food Policy Research Institute. (2018). *2018 Global Food Policy Report*. Washington, DC: International Food Policy Research Institute.

Jeffries, N. (2018). *A Circular Economy for Food: 5 Case Studies*. Retrieved from https://medium.com/circulatenews/a-circular-economy-for-food-5-case-studies-5722728c9f1e

Kaza, S., Yao, L. C., Bhada-Tata, P., & Van Woerden, F. (2018). *What a Waste 2.0: A Global Snapshot of Solid Waste Management to 2050*. Washington, DC: World Bank. doi:10.1596/978-1-4648-1329-0

Lagioia, G., Calabrò, G., & Amicarelli, V. (2012). Empirical Study of the Environmental Management of Italy's Drinking Water Supply. *Resources, Conservation and Recycling*, *60*, 119–130. doi:10.1016/j.resconrec.2011.12.001

Renner, G. T. (1947). Geography of Industrial Localization. *Economic Geography*, *23*(3), 167–189. doi:10.2307/141510

Rood, T., Muilwijk, H., & Westhoek, H. (2017). *Food for the Circular Economy*. The Hague: PBL Netherlands Environmental Assessment Agency.

Saint Ville, A., Po, J. Y., Sen, A., & Quiñonez, H. M. (2019). Food Security and the Food Insecurity Experience Scale (FIES): Ensuring Progress by 2030. *Food Security*, *11*(3), 483–491. doi:10.100712571-019-00936-9

Tseng, M.-L., Chiu, A. S. F., Chien, C.-F., & Tan, R. R. (2019). Pathways and Barriers to Circularity in Food Systems. *Resources, Conservation and Recycling*, *143*(1), 236–237. doi:10.1016/j.resconrec.2019.01.015

KEY TERMS AND DEFINITIONS

Circular Economy: A concept that entails gradually decoupling economic activity from the consumption of finite resources, and designing waste out of the system.

Food Loss: Food that gets spilled, spoilt or otherwise lost, or incurs reduction of quality and value during its process in the food supply chain before it reaches its final product stage.

Food Sector: A collection of all activities that facilitate the consumption and supply of food products and services across the world.

Food Supply Chain: The processes that describe how food from a farm ends up on a table of a consumer, including the processes of production, processing, distribution, consumption, and disposal.

Food Waste: Food that completes the food supply chain up to a final product, of good quality and fit for consumption, but still does not get consumed because it is discarded, whether or not after it is left to spoil or expire.

Material Flow Analysis: A systematic assessment of the flows and stocks of materials within a system defined in space and time.

Sustainability: A concept focuses on meeting the needs of the present without compromising the ability of future generations to meet their needs.

This research was previously published in the Handbook of Research on Globalized Agricultural Trade and New Challenges for Food Security edited by Vasilii Erokhin and Tianming Gao; pages 147-169, copyright year 2020 by Engineering Science Reference (an imprint of IGI Global).

Chapter 28
Utilization and Management of Food Waste

Shriram M. Naikare
SNDT College of Home Science, India

ABSTRACT

The food industry generates a huge amount of waste annually around the globe from a variety of sources. Approximately one third of all food produced today goes to landfill as waste. The food waste is not only a humanitarian problem, but also a serious economic and environmental pollution problem. The global volume of food wastage has been reported to around 1.3bn tones worth to about $165 bn. In India, about 40% of the food produced is wasted, which is estimated to about Rs. 50,000 crores worth every year. The important types of food wastes generated are agricultural residue, processed food, fruit and vegetable processing, marine food, dairy processing, meat and poultry, hotel and restaurant, etc. The food industrial waste can be converted into byproducts mainly based on the processing of fruits and vegetables and allied food manufacturing, supply and distribution, livestock feed, using it as source of bioactive compounds, useful bioenergy production, artificial fertilizer and decomposed manure, a variety of chemicals, antioxidant, nutraceuticals, etc.

INTRODUCTION

Food supply and waste management are the emerging challenges for the policy makers and companies in the food supply and processing. The global population is expected to grow 9 billion and demand for food upto 77% by 2050. Over the same period, food production will be under threat from climate change, competing land uses, and erosion and diminishing supplies of clean water. The food which we consume has to undergo a series of food processing operations soon after harvesting at the farm level.

The agro-food industry generate huge amount of wastage annually around the globe from a variety of sources. Food is a basic need of human beings, while food waste has been identified a major crucial challenge faced by human community today (Gustavsson et al, 2011).

DOI: 10.4018/978-1-7998-5354-1.ch028

Over 4.2 million tons of food waste is dispersed to landfill in Australia each year. 2.7 million tons of this is from households and around 1.5 million tons of this is from commercial and industrial sector, (DEWHA, 2009) costing around $ 10.5 billion in waste disposal charges and lost product. The largest single contributor in the commercial and industrial sector is food service activities.(Example- Cafes, restaurants, fast food outlets), which generate 661,000 tons of food waste per year, followed by manufacturing (312,000 tones) and food retail (179,000 tons). Most waste in food manufacturing is unavoidable, and almost 90% is already recovered as animal feed, compost or bio-energy. (Verghese et al 2013)

Presently, around 21,000 people die every day due to hunger related causes (Vandermeersch et al, 2014) and globally one in nine people go to bed each night hungry(http.//www.fao). Nevertheless, approximately one third of all the food produced goes to landfill as waste (Memon,2010). The vast amount of food ending up as waste is not only a humanitarian problem but also serious economic, nutritional and environmental pollution problem (Sakai et al,2011, Autrey et al, 2007).

At global statistics, according to the British Institute of Mechanical Engineers (IME) half of the food produced is wasted worldwide at different stages. The global volume of the food wastage has been reported to around 1.3 billion tons. The total volume of water used each year to produce food that is lost or wasted (250 km3) i.e. equivalent to the annual flow of Russian's Volga river or three times the Lake Geneva. Similarly, 1.4 billion hectares of land 28% of the world's agriculture area is used annually to produce food that is lost or wasted (FAO, 2015). About $ 165 billion worth of food waste enters landfills each year.

In India, according to UN Development program 40% of the food produced is wasted at pre- and post-harvest stages. Ministry of Food Processing Industries, Government of India's resources about Rs. 58,000 crore worth of food is wasted every year. About 25% of fresh water used to produce food is ultimately wasted as millions of people still don't have access to drinking water. About 300 million of barrels of oil are used to produce food that is ultimately wasted. As a result, a large quantity of food is wasted and being thrown away around the world while a child dies every five seconds because of hunger. In terms of food waste- agricultural produce, meat, poultry and milk- India ranks seventh, with the Russian Federation at the top in the list. India's major land is under agriculture, hence there is highest wastage of cereals, pulses, fruits and vegetables. Meat accounts for just four percent of the food wastage but contributes 20% of the economic cost of the wastage. Wastage of fruits and vegetables is 70% of the total produce, but translated into only 40% of the economic losses. Also, rice crop emits methane, a potent global warming gas, because of the decomposition of organic matter in submerged paddy fields. Food loss and waste costs the world about $ 940 billion a year.

However, the utilization and disposal of food waste is difficult due to its inadequate biological stability, potentially pathogenic nature, high water content, potential for rapid autoxidation, microbial decomposition through high level of enzymatic activity. The world population will reach to 9.6 billion by 2050 (FAO, 2015).

WORLD ENVIRONMENTAL PROBLEMS

Population growth contributes to GHG (Green House Gas) emission through its effect on deforestation as land is grabbed for enhancing food production (Lambin and Moyfroidt, 2011). As the world's population grows and becomes more affluent, waste production rises and might double by 2025 (Hoornweg et.al, 2013). According to the US Environmental Protection Agency (EPA), food wastage currently represents the single largest type of waste entering landfills (Nishida, 2014) Wasted food leads to over utilization of water and fossil fuels and to increasing greenhouse gas emission i.e. methane and carbon di oxide arising from degradation of food in landfills (Hall et. al.,2009).

Therefore, the environmental impact of food waste is twofold (Morane, 2016)

1. It is associated with the depletion of natural resources used for its production (example soil depletion) and distribution.
2. It relates to the costs associated with waste disposal. There is a growing awareness needed to minimize the amount of food wasted at the end of the food supply chain- an issue particularly relevant in high-income countries where more than 40% of the food losses occur at retail and consumer level (FAO, 2015).

Globally per capita food waste by consumers amounts to 95-115 kg/ year in Europe and North America compared to 6-11 kg/year in South or South East Asia and Sub-saharian Africa (Gustavsson et. al., 2011). Food waste reduction at the consumption level represents indeed a large target for medium and high income countries, where evidence shows that the main source of the problem is the domestic setting (Monier et. al. 2010; Braun 2012).

Reasons for Food Losses and Food Wastage

Agricultural Production: Destruction from insects, pests, diseases, inappropriate crop cultivation practices, changing agro-climatic conditions, not meeting the quality specifications, low yielding varieties, lack of inputs, poor crop yield due to draught and natural calamities, etc.

1. **Post-Harvest Handling and Storage Practices:** Not meeting the specifications for quality and/ or poor or lack of post-harvest handling, packaging, storage facilities may lead to damage due to insect, pest, spillage, germination and degradation (lack of pack houses, packaging materials, pre-cooling facilities, storage and transport facilities (cold chain, cold storages, poor supply chain management, etc.)
2. **Lack of Primary Processing and Packaging Facilities:** Inadequate infrastructure such as godowns, ware houses, cold storages for perishable commodities, referred vans for high value commodities like grapes, strawberry, broccoli, milk and milk products, poultry, meat, fish, etc. these operations create trimmings and other food preparation waste. Inedible portions, wet or dry material, their storage and transport or proper utilization at proper stage. Wet or dry garbage may create severe problems of their proper disposal, failure may create air pollution and health hazards.
3. **Food Processing Industry Sector Waste**
4. **Distribution and Logistics (Wholesale and Retail):** Damage or loss of food in transit/ storage due to packaging failures, shelf life of processed, fresh food commodities, poor road facilities, transit storage (warehouse/ cold storage) at the port or metro cities hub. Packaging failures, product spoilage, fresh produce (perishable), may get damaged during handling, storage and distribution, short shelf life hence low sales.
5. **Food Service Sector:** Food wastage generated in the hotels, restaurants, institutional kitchens, poor management of such wet food wastages, their packaging, boxes, plastics, improper food handling, left over or stale food items.

6. **At Home:** Trimmings, cuttings, peels, stones, seeds, and other food preparation waste, damaged or spoiled food items, preparing too much food, leftover food, improper stored food and food items. The overall food loss and wastage costs the world about $ 940 billion a year. The food losses are reported to be higher in developing countries than the developed nations. However to overcome and handle the food wastage problem is a huge challenge and task all over the globe.

The overall food loss (waste) in USA alone, annually people throw away 30% of the food produced which corresponds to 40 billion liters of water. Whereas in UK, the household waste estimated to be 6.7 million MT purchased. This means that approximately 32% of all food purchased every year is not eaten. Most of this (5.9 million MT or 88%) is currently collected by local authorities. Most of the food waste (4.1 million MT or 61% is avoidable and could have been eaten if had been better managed

- The annual food losses and waste are estimated to be about 30% for cereals, 40-50% for root crops, 30% for fish and 20% for oilseeds and meat
- On globe scale, just 43% of the fruits and vegetables produced are consumed and the remaining 57% are wasted
- Food waste accounts for roughly US $680 billion in industrialized countries and US $ 310 billion in developing countries
- Roughly one-third of the food is lost or wasted that translates into 1.30 billion MT each year worth nearly one trillion US dollars and equivalent of 6-10% of human generated greenhouse gas emission (Bos and Hamelinck, 2014).

Classification of Food Waste (Based on Nature of Waste)

1. Solid Waste (Organic and Inorganic) Sources- domestic waste, factory waste, waste from oil industry, e-waste, agricultural waste, food processing waste, variety of plastic based waste, packaging material (industry and domestic waste) etc. (Mackensine et al). out of the total solid waste generated, 44% is wet (organic)
2. Wet Waste
    a. Kitchen waste (food waste, cooked and uncooked food, egg shells, meat and bones, fish, fruit and vegetable inedible portion etc.
    b. Flower, fruit and vegetable waste
    c. Garden, tree, leaves, branches, straws, trash waste
    d. Sanitary waste (drainage waste)
    e. Food industry waste (raw materials and finished goods)
    f. Food waste (left over, stale, spoiled food)
    g. Wet garbage and industry (sewage) waste
3. Dry Waste
    a. Paper, plastic (all kinds), laminates, foils
    b. Card boards, cartoons, packaging, glass bottles, metal tins and containers, strappings, foils, rags, rubber, houses, pipes, sweepings, ashes, wrappings, discarded clothes, etc.
4. Domestic Hazard Waste
    a. Compact florescent lamps, tubes, glasses
    b. Chemicals, detergents, etc.

5. Non-Hazard Waste
    a. Glass bottles, iron containers/ wares, plastic bottles/ wares and materials

Food Waste From Different Food Groups

- Cereals (grains), pulses, fruits and vegetables, meat, dairy products, marine, sugarcane, winery, plantation by-products, slaughter house, canning industry.
- Wastes are untreated and underutilized; therefore its disposal is widely adopted through burning, dumping or land filling.
- Juice industry produced a large amount of waste as peels, pulp, seeds, fiber.
- Fruit and vegetable processing industry waste.

Reasons for Food Waste Generation: Scenario

As per the FAO report, around one third of the food produced for human consumption is lost or wasted globally, which is equivalent to 1.3 billion ton each year (Gustavsson et al, 2011; WRAP, 2011). In the United States, the figure is likely to be closer to 40% (Hall et al, 2009). The per capita food loss for North America and Oceania combined is estimated to be around 280-300 kg/year, which is equivalent to around6.5 million tons of food waste in Australia (ABS, 2013).

Around 4.2 million tons of food waste is disposed to landfill in Australia each year with almost half of the commercial and industrial waste coming from the food service sector. Source: (DEWHA, 2009).

While considering the food losses/ wastes at different stages of processing, in less developed economies, foods tend to be lost at the agricultural cultivation and post-harvest stages (Kummu et al, 2012) due to the inefficient harvesting, storage, transport and processing. Waste tends to move up the distribution to the retail and consumer levels as the standard of development improves (IME, 2013, Kummu et al, 2012). This is where food is much more likely to be thrown away when it is still edible (Gustavsson, 2011). Verghese et al, 2013 reported that the largest single contributor to food waste in Australia is the food service sector (Food and beverage services) such as hotels, pubs, restaurants, cafes and commercial caterers, which recycles only 2% of the food waste they generate and send approximately 645,000 tons of landfill each year.

The second largest contributor is the food retail sector which also recycles very little (5%) and sends around 170,000 tons to landfill each year. The areas of high loss are the perishable products such as fruits, vegetables, meat, bread and cut flowers. Another 75,000 tons is sent to landfill from wholesale trade sector.

Further they observed that the food manufacturing sector generates a significant amount of food waste but with a recycling rate of 88% sends very little to landfill. A large proportion of this waste is unavoidable, for example skin, bones and other inedible food components. One of the reasons for the high recovery rate for food waste is that manufacturers produce relatively consistent and uncontaminated wastes that can be used for animal feed or as feed stock for composting.

Finally, the team reported that the remaining food waste is generated in the manufacturing and service organizations that are largely outside the food supply. Most of this waste is related to employee consumption, i.e. generated in canteens and kitchens.

Low recovery rates for commercial and industry waste sector can be attributed to inadequate infrastructure for recovery, difficulties in on-site handling, storage and collection and low value of this material compared to other recyclables (US Report, 2012). This waste represents a significant cost to business. In addition to the costs of waste disposal and recycling, the value of the food inputs that are ultimately thrown away or recycled by the commercial and industrial sector in Australia is estimated to be around $ 10.5 billion (E CSRU, 2012).

The edible components of food wasted at each stage of the supply chain in North America and Oceania. For example, wastage rates for fruits and vegetables in the supply chain are 4% in post-harvest handling and storage, 12% in distribution including retail. Overall wastage rates are highest in consumption 35% followed by agricultural production sector 20% (Gustavsson et al, 2011). Perishable products (high moisture) have a short shelf life such as fresh fruits and vegetables, baked goods, meat and seafood have a higher tendency to become waste (Mera, 2011).

Food waste is the food not suitable for human consumption, no longer fit for sale, which is subjected to livestock feed or fertilizer through decomposition. Major food waste generates during distribution or storage processes at warehousing or in-store display.

In food service operations, more food is been consumed away from home in restaurants, cafes or 'take-away' (home delivery) food (IME, 2013).

The Sustainable Restaurants Association (SRA) in UK identified three main sources of food waste and estimated that if an average restaurant reduced its waste by 20%, it could save more than 2,000 pound from avoided food costs and up to 1700 on avoided waste collection costs, 65% from preparation, 30% from customers' plates and 5% spoilage (out of date). (SRA, 2010)

In industrial countries, the large amount of food wasted is generated by households, Australians waste about $ 5.2 billion worth of food every year (Baker et al, 2009). The research on other countries has revealed some interesting insights, that perishable foods such as fruits, vegetables, dairy products and pre-prepared meals are the largest contributors to food waste. (Ventour, 2008, Williams et al, 2012)

Solutions for Reduction of Food Industry Waste

- Effective supply chain management practices to fresh agro produce (fruits and vegetables, dairy products)
- Reduction in food wastage (at processing, storage, distribution)
- Improvement in post-harvest handling practices, transport, storage and distribution of food through appropriate technologies (cold chain, improved packaging etc.)
- Value addition of the by-products generated in the food industry
- Quick and appropriate disposal of food industry wastage, garbage, effluents, sewage, etc.
- Food lost or wasted should be discarded to avoid environmental pollution (each year it accounts for 3.3 billion tons of carbon di oxide emission globally) (FAO, 2015)
- Government and Community must work collaboratively to achieve policy of zero waste or policy "No to food waste".
- The agro-industrial residue have high nutritional potential, therefore it can be utilized for production of a variety of by-products, chemicals (Grawinha et al, 2008) or any suitable disposal.
- Conversion of waste into valuable product through biodegradation/ decomposting.
- Fermentation of the solids/ semi-solid waste.
- Formation of 'Food Banks' and its timely distribution to the needy/ hungry population

- Bio gas (fuel gas) production
- Composting through earthworms/ microbes into manure

Utilization and Management of Food Waste

The food waste can be categorized as solid (organic and inorganic), semi-solid waste, dry waste and liquid (wet waste). The food processing industry generates vast, hazardous either by-product waste or material ready for discard causing harmful effect to human beings and animals, creating severe environmental pollution (solid, liquid, gas pollution)

The present scenario of overall waste management in India indicates that the waste used for biogas production 5%, composting 18% and vermicomposting 32% (Matkar and Singh, 2007)

Classification of waste according to their properties is shown in Figure 1.

Figure 1.Classification of waste

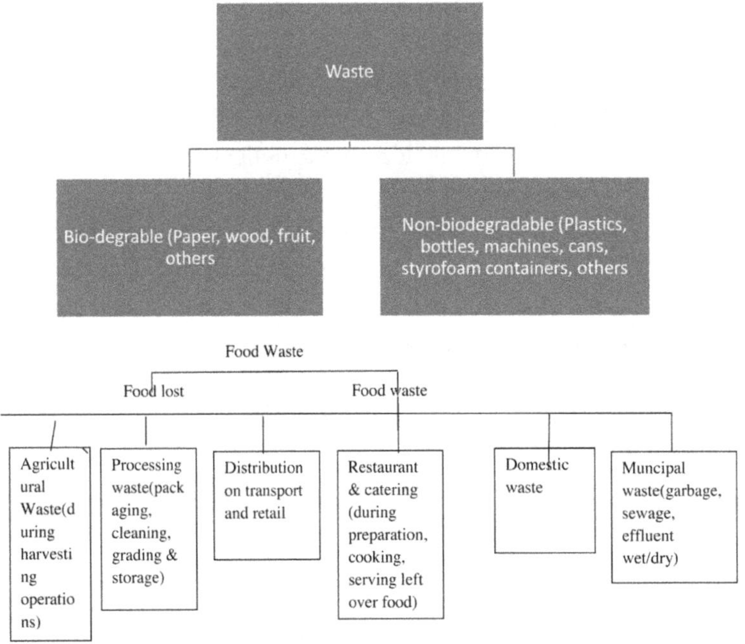

Worldwide the food waste, garbage processing has become a crucial problem.
Garbage processing countries (%)

- Austria – 63%
- Germany – 62%
- Taiwan – 60%
- Singapore – 59%
- South Korea – 49%
- Britain – 39%

- Italy – 36%
- France – 35%

Source: Strategy paper on Solid Waste management (Nitri, Nagpur)

Table 1. Different types of Garbage generated in India

TYPE OF GARBAGE	**%**
Organic	50%
Plastic	33%
Metal	1%
Paper	4%
Glass	6%
Others	6%

Source: World Bank Report on 'What a Waste', 2012

The agro industrial waste produced by food industries is mainly based on the processing of fruits and vegetables. It is estimated that the food industry in Europe generates about 250 million tons/year of byproducts, waste and effluents and 6% of them represented by fruits and vegetables (De Los Fuenters et al, 2004). Waste and byproducts include damaged fruits, leaves, unripe, immature, peels, stones, stalks, etc. A huge amount of waste are also generated during food processing of juices, canned foods, sauces, liquors, dehydration as solid and liquid residue that are usually disposed into landfills or used as compost or animal feed.

All the wastes pose increasing problems of disposal and potentially severe pollution problems. In Italy, total production of tomato accounts to nearly 9,000,000 tons/year and about 1.8% to 2.3% of them (i.e., 162,000 to 207000 tons) is discarded as waste (unripe, damaged, peels and seeds). Agro Industrial wastes represents a cheap, chemical, feed stock for extraction of useful chemicals, byproducts, since they are rich in high value components like lipids, fibers, natural pigment, carotenoids and oxidants, nutraceuticals, phenolic compounds (Velentia et al, 2014)

and reservoir of complex carbohydrates, proteins which can be utilized for the production of commercially important metabolites. Agro-Industrial wastes are useful for manufacturing of bio-fuels, enzymes, vitamins, antioxidants, animal feed, antibiotics and other chemical through solid state fermentation (SSF). A variety of micro-organisms are used for the production of these valuable products through SSF processes.

Types of Agri-Industrial Waste

It includes leaves, stalk, seed, pods, stem, peels, stubbles, plant, branches, husks, seed coat, stones, cores, etc. while the process residue include husks, immature seeds, roots, molasses, etc. the industrial waste contains peels, fruits, seeds, stones, pod shells, coconut shells and fibers, soya bean pod shells, cake, etc.

Sugar cane, rice straw, corn stalks, saw dust, sugar beet waste, pomace, barley straw, cotton stalk, oat straw, soya stalks, sunflower heads, stalks, wheat straw, <u>food industry waste</u> – potato, sweet potato, mango, orange peels, pineapple peels, coffee skins (hulls).

Table 2. Food and agricultural commodity waste world production (Million)

Sr.no	Commodity	Production yield	Waste
1	Apple	61.9	4.9
2	Banana	71.3	8.4
3	Cassava	202.6	26.8
4	Coconut	54.7	2.5
5	Citrus fruit	108.8	8.6
6	Coffee	7.8	0.1
7	Corn	221.4	26.1
8	Grape	66.6	2.2
9	Olive	16.0	0.2
10	Onion	55.1	4.7
11	Pineapple	15.3	1.6
12	Potato	327.6	22.4
13	Soybean	204.20	4.2
14	Sugar beet	249.2	0.5
15	Sugar cane	1324.0	117.5
16	Tea	3.3	0.07
17	Tomato	120.4	9.7
18	Wheat	627.1	20.0
19	Total cereals	2264.0	78.2
20	Total fruits	503.3	42.4
21	Total oil crop	132.7	10.4
22	Total vegetables	865.8	70.2

Source: FAO, 2004

Global Food Waste by Commodity

1.   Fish and sea food : 2%
2.   Oil seed and pulses : 3%
3.   Meat : 4%
4.   Milk : 8%
5.   Cereals : 20%
6.   Fruits and vegetables : 45%

Table 3. Major processed food and types of waste generated

Sr. no	Food crop	Food product	Waste
1	Rice, wheat, corn	Grain, flour, bread, biscuits, roti, cake, starch, flakes, bakery products	Straw, stem, leaves, husk, comb, hulls, fibers, brans, germ, gluten, todder
2	Fruits and vegetables	Juice, pulp, preserved products, vegetable oil, potato products, fruits, roots, tubers, bulbs, sugar dehydrated, pickles, fermented products	Rotten fruits, vegetables and their parts, pomace, skin, seeds, stones, fibers.
3	Fish and sea food	Canned, salted fish, smoked fish, processed form, dehydrated, frozen	Scales, fins, shells, bones, guts, fish oil, skeleton.
4	Meat and poultry	Processed meat(beef, pork, poultry, eggs and their products)	Blood, hairs, head, skin, horn, bones, carcass, fat, feet, guts, wide intestinal parts.
5	Dairy products	Milk, butter, cheese, milk powder, cream, ghee, paneer, ice cream,	Whey, processed water, solids, waste material, effluents etc.
6	Beverages	Cocoa, coffee, tea, fruits, alcohol(wine), molasses, grain based alcohol	Shells, seed coat, molasses, sewage water.
7	Oils	Oil, hydrogenated fat, fatty acids	Cake, solid impurities, water effluents, rancid spoiled seeds oil
8	Sugar	Sugar. jaggery, confectionary,	Solid wastage, sugar industry effluents, waste.

Source: FAO ,2015

EPA Has Given Food Recovery Hierarchy

1. **Source of Reduction:** Reduce the huge volume of food generated
2. **Feed Hungry People:** - Donate extra food to food banks, kitchens, shelters
3. **Feed Animals:** Divert food surplus to animal feed.
4. **Industrial Uses:** Extraction oils, chemicals, valuable nutrients and industrial aids from waste, conversion into fuels, drying and improving storage through powders, use in pharmaceuticals, allied uses.
5. **Composting:** Use for bio fermentation, biogas, fertilizers, composting through bacteria, earthworms, solid waste fermentation
6. **Landfill:** Incineration

The percent wastage reported along the food supply chain at different stages is

1. Pre harvest – 25% (food cost at pre harvest)
2. Post-harvest stage – 20- 40% (post-harvest losses)
3. Processing losses – 30% (grain and others – cleaning, grading, packaging)
4. Transportation – 20% (during transport spoilage, storage, poor packaging, over loading, lack of cold storages and chain transport for perishables F & V)
5. Retailing - 10% (handling, food cost, number of handlers, middle man are increased, short distance and local movement),
6. Consumption – 40% (produced, prepared food wasted during eating, kitchen storage, quality loss due to excessive purchasing).

Consequences of Food Loss

1. Wastage of valuable bulk
2. Loss of bulk nutrients
3. Loss of functional nutraceuticals nutrients (natural ingredients/ nutrients)
4. Severe problem of their disposal, transport, movement
5. Being wet/ perishable likely to undergo fermentation on quickly; need to provide additional attention.
6. Emission of toxic gases (CO_2, CO, methane), microbes, when wasted food is kept open as such or buried in landfills.
7. Air, water, atmosphere get severely polluted due to improper disposal.
8. Loss of energy, manpower, water, land, etc. for growing of the food being lost.
9. Heavy financial loss to the community/ government on disposal.
10. Loss of soil fertility (that soil remain as waste land)
11. Emission of greenhouse gases (methane, CO_2, CO, SO_2, H_2S, etc.)
12. Food industry causes health hazards and air pollution to human beings.

Measures for Reducing Food Losses

Harvesting the agricultural commodities at optimum maturity stage by adopting suitable harvesting aids.

- Proper handling and threshing, grading, drying and bagging of the produce at proper storage conditions.
- For packaging reusable plastic crates (woven bags with plastic liners) be introduced as primary or secondary packaging in supply chain operation to improve efficiencies and extend shelf life, particularly for fresh perishable produce, (Chonhenchob and Singh, 2003) and it can produce the environmental benefits of reusable, more robust structure for food supplies in the food supply chain. (Lee and Xu, 2004, Singh et.al, 2006.)
- Supply of surplus and unsalable processed food, commodities to food rescue organization from farm / food industry / food storages to food recovery organization. (Varghese et.al, 2013.)
- Pre-processing and packaging of food produce can reduce food waste in supply chain and in the home by extending the shelf life.
- Application of the improved packaging technology to fresh processed food products extended their shelf life significantly through multi-layer barrier packaging, modified atmosphere packaging (MAP), edible coatings, ethylene scavengers, oxygen and carbon dioxide scavengers, moisture absorbers, aseptic packaging, tetra pack packaging, retortable pouch packaging, vacuum packaging, N2 gas flushing packaging, grape guard pad in package etc.(Varghese et.al, 2013)
- Adoption of cold chain supply and cold storage will help to reduce the losses of perishable food commodities significantly.

Utilization of Fruits and Vegetables Waste

- Fresh wet waste utilization is worldwide concern to dictating the improvement of alternative cleaner and renewable bioenergy resources (Okonko et.al, 2009) these waste causes serious disposal problem.(Rodrigoue 2008).
- Over the last decade the annual production of fruits and vegetable have been increased by 70%. However, the economy is suffering the loss of about $ 750 billion (i.e. Rs. 47 lakh crore), as 1/3rd of the food produced goes wasted.
- The juice industries produce huge amount of waste as peels, coffee pulp waste, pomace, fruit seeds, stones, etc. All over the world the fiber sources are found to the tune of 147.2 million metric tons in 1990. (Belewu and Babalola, 2009)
- As per the composition of these agro industry waste / residue are concerned, they constitute high nutritional profile and hence being used for agro industry by products. (Grawinhna et.al, 2008)
- Various studies reported that different kinds of wastes such as pomegranate peels, lemon peels and green walnut husks can be used as natural antimicrobials (Adame et.al.)
- Same food industry by products / wastes contain high amount of proteins (soya cake ground cake), sugars (molasses) and minerals (rice bran, wheat bran). Due to high nutritional composition these residues not described as wastes but considered as raw material/ by product for other product formation and development. (Nguyen et.al, 2010).
- Fruit and vegetable processing industry has accounted 25% losses and wastes in the form of organic waste such as peel, stem, core, stones, seeds and pomace generated either from fruit discarded into the sorting operation or pomace from juice extraction.
- Waste is the potential source of functional dietary fiber for food applications some of the waste goes to animal feed for e.g. 10,000 tons of apple pomace out of total production 1 million tons is being utilized for by product processing. This by products can be utilized as a valuable source of natural food additives of high nutritional value (Husain et.al, 2015)
- The statistical figures of fruit and vegetable waste produced reported by NHB (2014-15) and Djillas (2009) were apple peel, pomace, seed- 25%, mango peels stones -45%, banana peel- 35%, citrus peel, rag, seeds – 50%, pineapple-skin, core-33%, grapes- stem, skin, seeds – 20%, guava-peel, core, seeds 10%, tomato – peel, core, seeds – 20% potato- peel- 15% and peas- shells – 40%.

By-products resulting from processing of papaya, pineapple and mango represent approx. 10 – 16% of fruit weight. In case of citrus fruits, amount residues accounts for about 50% of the original fruit weight, seeds constitute considerable proportion of grape ranging from 38 -52% on dry mater bases. (Kaur et.al, 2017).

NUTRITIONAL COMPOSITION OF FRUIT AND VEGETABLE POMACE

The nutritional value of fruits and vegetable are reported to be rich in dietary fiber, vitamins A and C, minerals (Ca, Fe, Zn, K, Cu, Ph, Mg and Mn they are good source of phytochemicals, antioxidants, L alpha tocopherol, carotenoids, beta carotene, lycopene, cryptoxanthin, zeaxanthin and lutein). (Gopalan et.al, 2016). The nutritional value apple pomace assessed by Sudha et.al. (2007) and revealed that it contains 51.1% dietary fibers, 7.31 -8.53% of fruit protein, 3.85 – 4.7% total ash, high amounts poly phenols

(7000 mg / kg), flavon-3-ols (1850-2550 mg/ kg) hydroxycinnmates and hydroxylchalcones and pectin (10-15%).apple peels were found to contain up to 33,00 mg / 100gm of phenolic compounds. Majority of total fibers was located in the peel of apple (0.91%).

Guava pomace was reported to contain high amount of total dietary fiber (63.949 / 100gm), reduced calorie content (182kcal /100gm), iron (13.8 mg /100gm), zinc (3.31mg/ 100gm) and considerable amount of ascorbic acid (Vitamin. C 87.44 mg /100gm), total carotenoids (1.25 mg/100gm), an insoluble dietary fiber (63.55mg/100gm).

In case of citrus fruits, citrus pulp obtain after juice extraction contains 41-42% dietary fiber, 6% crude protein, 6.3% ash, minerals like Calcium (7.7 gm./ kg), phosphorus(1.6 gm./ Kg) (Silva et.al, 1992). It was also found that total phenolic compounds in peels of oranges and lemon were 15% higher than that of pulp of these fruits (Gopalan et al, 2014).

Pineapple pomace has good nutritive value, rich in dietary fibers, contains calcium, phosphorus and iron. About 25% of fresh fruit is lost as pomace. Pomace contains about 1.8% ash, 21.5mg / 100gm ascorbic acid and 0.41% crude fiber (Husain et.al, 2015).

Pomegranate peels contain 249.4mg/gm. of phenolic compounds as compare to only 24.4 mg/gm of phenolic compounds found in the pulp of pomegranate.

Banana peels constituting about 40% of total weight of fresh banana as a major waste. It is rich source of starch (3%), crude protein (6-9%) total dietary fiber (43.2-49.7%) and crude fat (3.8-11.0%). Banana peels is a good source of micronutrients (K, P Ca, Mg) PUFA (linolenic acid and alpha linolenic acid) and essential amino acids (leucin, valine, phenylalanine, threonine). Moreover significant amount of lignin (6-12%) pectin (10-11%), cellulose (7.6-9.6%).

Hemi cellulose (6.4- 9.4%) and galacturonic acid is found in banana peel as dietary fiber. Moreover, Shyamala and Jamuna (2011) stated that peel had good antioxidant components and activity where the free radical scavenging activity of tannic acid (90-62%) and polyphenols (200-850mg equivalent to tannic acid /100gm) were found.

Grapes (Vitis vinifera) constitute seeds 38-52%. The seed oil is rich in unsaturated fatty acids (particularly linoleic acid) and phenolic compounds. (80% grapes used for wine world wide). During tomato processing, about 3-7% of the raw material is lost as waste. Tomato pomace generally consists of the crushed are dried skin and seeds of the fruit. Appropriately, the seeds account for 10% of fruit and 60% of the total waste. The seeds are reported to be good source of protein (35%) and fat (25%). Tomato seed oil is found to be rich in unsaturated fatty acids such as linolenic acid that has largely attracted the interest of researchers (Eller et al, 2010). As compared to seeds and pulp, the tomato peel contains higher levels of total flavonoids, total phenolic compounds, lycopene and ascorbic acid exhibiting higher antioxidant activity.

Carrot pomace, generated during processing, contains 14.75% soluble fiber, 30% insoluble fiber, 6.50 proteins, 5.12% ash, 5456 µg total carotenes and 607 µg β-carotene.

Chemically, the agricultural wastes contain 31-60% cellulose, 11-38% pentosane and 12-28% lignin. This product has been reported to be used in the alcohol production (Aappaiah, 2017). Fruits are very rich in carbohydrate and sugar content which can be a very good source of alcohol production.

Grape and wine making industry generate a number of waste and by products. These material include wine pruning, grape stalks, grape pomace, grape seeds, yeasts, tartrate, carbon dioxide and waste matter, every by- product will become fertilizers, animal feed or fuel. (Nerantzis and Tetaridis, 2006). The grape seed extracts have gained ground as nutritional supplement in view of its antioxidant activity (Arvanitoyannis et al, 2006).

Enzyme Production

Grape pomace, main polluting waste from the wine industry, is a good natural medium for solid state fermentation that is used for production of hydrolytic enzymes such as cellulases, xylanses, and pectinases using Aspergillus awamori (Botella et al, 2007). Proteolytic enzymes such as bromelain is recovered from pineapple pomace and papain from papaya latex. Moreover, orange peel and orange finished pulp, sugar beet pulping and peas waste are good substrates for polygalacturonase production. Apple pomace, a waste from the apple processing industry is also used as a substrate for pectinase production by aspergillus spp. in solid state fermentation.

Pectin Production

Pectin a heteropolysaccharide having properties like capacity to make gels, emulsify and stabilize. The major waste during processing is peel (citrus) which is widely used for the producing pectin powder; other sources of pectin are mango peels, residue of sunflower and guava (Kaur et al, 2017). Lal et al, (1988) have given the detail information about utilizing waste of fruits and vegetables. Apple peel, pomace for pectin, guava peels for preparation of guava cheese, water melon rind for pickle making, jackfruit for pectin, pineapple for vinegar production, limes for citric acid, seeds and for oil, orange, lime peel can be used for extraction of essential oil, Citrus oil/ orange oil. Banana pseudostem, leaves for preparation of paper pulp and banana fiber (for clothes) and ecofriendly containers, green papaya for latex and tutti fruiti preparation, other waste and garbage can be used in feed or decomposition of compost manuring.

1. Salad dressing- orange peels and orange waste pulp.
2. Yoghurt- added with grape pomace extract for enrichment of bioactive compound (Tseng and Zhao, 2013).
3. Grape seed oil rich in polyphenols, antioxidants and vitamins used in cooking oil.
4. Mango seed kernel oil/ fat to be used as cocoa butter equivalent.
5. Pulpy waste in ethanol production by fermentation.
6. Tomato pomace can be used in extruded products.
7. Others for recovery of fiber, vitamins, β-carotene.
8. Natural colouring pigments - beetroot (red), leaves (green), paprika red (chilli powder), turmeric (yellow), carrot (orange red), kesar (pink-yellow), radish (anthocyanin).
9. Brewery and wine industry waste- the brewery industry waste are the spent grain, the trub, and the residual yeast. Brewer spent grain (BSG) is the main by-product of brewing industry representing approximately 85% of the total by product generated. It is rich in cellulose and non-cellulosic polysaccharides (Aliyu and Bala, 2011).

Marine Industry Waste

Sea food by-products could serve as important value added nutraceuticals and functional food ingredients (Gormley, 2013). By-products from sea food processing may account for up to 80% of the harvest depending on the species. These include w-3 PFA from the livers of white lean fish waste flesh parts of fatty fish, blubber of marine animals, hydrolysates from fish guts, cleaning, peptides and products from crustaceans such as chitosan, chitosan oligomers and glucosamines. Hence, by-products from sea foods could serve as important value added nutraceuticals and functional food ingredients (Gormley, 2013). Gelatin, a thickening polysaccharide, is obtained from sea animal carcasses. Like wise the moss, agar are also obtained from sea weeds, cod liver oil from cod fish liver (Kadam and Prabha Sankar, 2010).

Meat Industry Waste

According to the European Commission (EC) the animal by-products may be defined as whole bodies or parts of creatures, products of animal origin or other products obtained from animals as carcasses, skin, bones, meat, trimmings, blood, fatty tissues, horns, feet, hoofs or intestinal organs. Meat by-products are reported to be rich in lipids, polysaccharides, proteins, and the bioactive peptides which are known to have antimicrobial, antioxidative, antithrombic, anti-hypertensive properties (Lafarga and Teagase, 2014).

Grain Processing Industry Waste

Rice bran,10 percent of the weight of rice grain, in rice milling yields the by-products20% husk, 8% bran and 2% germ. Rice bran is rich in antioxidant (polyphenols, Vit. E (alfa tocopherol) and carotenoids). Rice bran is presently used for extraction of edible rice bran oil after refining. Rice bran used in other products are bread, biscuits, pasta, noodles a n ice-creams having more functional and textural properties (Gul et al, 2015). Rice husk is a major protective covering of paddy grain which accounts to about 14% - 28% of the grain, estimated to 80 million tones (average 20% of paddy) must disposed of annually worldwide. The major application of the husk are in the production of husk ash, silicon (husk contains about 90% silica), fuel, briquettes, poultry litter, traditionally used in cattle feed, composite press boards, furfural, silicon tetrachloride, activated carbon, cement concrete, husk as fuel, electricity generation, etc. (Pillaiyar, 1988; Juliano, 1985). B- glucan extracted from grain flour which progress lipid metabolism, reduce the glycemic index and lower plasma cholesterol, lignan concentrate from flax seed which act as anticancer, antioxidant, antibacterial, antiviral and anti-inflammatory agent and phenolic compounds extracted from cereal bran which provide antioxidants resistance against free radical damage, cancer and cardiovascular diseases. Flax seed super rich in lignans can be added to different cereal based formulations like bread, muffins and other bakery products (Bainao, 2014). Maize germ obtained during grain milling is used for extraction of maize oil and it is further used for edible purposes after refining as 'Mazola oil' (Helkar. 2016)

Dairy Processing Industry Waste

Whey is a liquid by-product of dairy industry obtained during the preparation of chhana, paneer, cheese and contain casein. World whey production is estimated to about 180 to 190 X 106 tons per year with an annual increment of 1 to 2% and only 50% and only 50% of whey is utilized or processed (Roman et al, 2012). Whey contains 45 to 50% total milk solids, 70% milk sugar (lactose and galactose), 20% milk proteins (casein) and 70 – 90% milk minerals and almost all the water soluble vitamins originally present in the milk (Horton 1995). Whey disposal becomes a serious environmental pollutant being loaded with high amount of organic matter. Whey posses preventive and curative elements responsible for treatment of ailments such as arthritis, anemia and liver complaints (Cruz et al, 2009).Fruit and dairy waste based on products are attaining considerable attention due to delicious taste and market for such food products has incredible potential (Ismail et al,2011). Whey based fruit beverages are more suitable for health as compared to other drinks because of probiotic effect (Kumar 2005). Production of nourishing pleasant whey based on fruit RTS (ready- to- serve) beverages is one of the most promising trend in utilization of dairy waste whey. Whey powders are rich source of protein of high biological value (Ramos et al, 2016).

Ur is one of the by-products of milk industry having high probiotic functional, medicinal and nutritional properties (Homayouni, et al, 2012).

Summary

In general, the food industry waste could be utilized by various ways such as—

- Reduction in pre- and post- harvest losses,
- Efficient storage, packaging and distribution of food products,
- Supply chain management, cold chain management, cold storages,
- Proper modern packaging technologies be adopted widely,
- Efficient and proper collection and disposal of waste after proper segregation.
- Ultrafiltration and recovery of food waste,
- Recovery of fruit and vegetable waste (semi solid),
- Recovery of protein and other fermentable value added chemicals,
- Extraction of fat and other ingredients for manufacturing valuable items,
- Utilization of waste in animal feed after proper processing,
- Utilization in fuel, electricity energy, bio- gas generation projects,
- Decomposition of waste through microorganisms, earth worms, (composting), bio- gas production for domestic use.
- Recycling of the food waste, sewage water, effluents after proper treatment, or can be send into landfills (very little share, but care must be taken to avoid environmental pollution).
- Reduction, reuse and recycling of food waste must be mandatory enforced by the governments of the countries to their society so as to improve and protect their people's life.
- **Benefits of the recycling of waste:**
    - It reduces the amount/ expenditure required for disposal,
    - It saves natural resources,
    - It reduces the amount of energy needed for manufacturing New Products,
    - It reduces pollution and destruction,
    - It provides employment opportunities,
    - It helps to National Economy
    - It helps to maintain Zero Food Wastage

REFERENCES

Adame, Samino, & Sanchez, , & Gonzalez. (2012). In vitro estimation of the antibacterial activity and antioxidant capacity of aqueous extracts from grape seeds. *Food Control, 24,* 136 – 141.

Aliyu, S., & Bela, M. (2011). Brewer's spent grain: A review of its potential and applications. *African Journal of Biotechnology, 10,* 324–331.

Appaiah Anu, K. A. (2017). Fruit and vegetable wastes: An alternative feed stock for alcohol production. *Indian Food Industry, 36*(6), 30–41.

Arvanitoyannis, S., Ladas, D., & Mavromattes, A. (2006). Potential Uses and application of treated wine waste: A Review. *International Journal of Food Science & Technology, 41*(5), 475–487. doi:10.1111/j.1365-2621.2005.01111.x

Autrel, E., Betrhier, F., Lutze Zajac, A., & Nicolas, F. (2007). Inceneration of municipal and material recovery performances. *Journal of Hazardous Materials, 139*, 569. doi:10.1016/j.jhazmat.2006.02.065 PMID:16707217

Baker, D., Fear, J., & Denniss, R. (2009). *What a waste: An analysis of house hold expenditure on food, in policy Brief no. 6*. Canberra: The Australia Institute.

Belewu, M. A., & Babalola, F. T. (2009). Nutrient enrichment of some waste agriculture residue after solid state fermentation: Application to animal nutrition. *Animal Feed Science and Technology, 14*(4), 122.

Bos, A., & Hamelinck, C. (2014). *Green House Impact of marginal fossil fuel use*. Project no. BIEN 14973.

Butella, C., Diaz, A., Ory, I. W., Webb, C., & Blandino, A. (2007). Xylanase and pectinase production by Aspergillus awamori on grape pomace in solid state fermentation. *Process Biochem., 42*, 98-101.

Chandrasekaran. (2012). *Valorization of food processing by-products*. CRC Press.

Chonhenchob, V., & Singh, S. P. (2003). A comparison of corrugated boxes and reusable plastic containers for mango distribution. *Packaging Technology & Science, 16*(6), 231–237. doi:10.1002/pts.630

Chonhenchob, V., & Singh, S. P. (2005). Packaging performance comparison for distribution and export of papaya fruit. *Packaging Technology & Science, 18*(3), 125–131. doi:10.1002/pts.681

Cruz, A. G., Ana, A. S. J., Marchione, M. M., Teixeira, A. M., & Schmaltz, F. I. (2009). Milk drink using whey butter, cheese and acerola juice as a potential source of Vit C. *Food and Bioprocess Technology, 28*, 368–373. doi:10.100711947-008-0059-9

De Las Fuentes, L. B., Sanders, B., Lorenzo, A., & Aber, S. (2004). Awareness Agrofood wastes minimization and reduction network. Total Food Proceedings, 233 – 244.

DEWHA, National Waste Policy. (2009). Less waste more resources. Department of Environment, Heritage and the Arts, Editor, Common Wealth of Australia.

Djilas, S., Canadanovic-Brunet, J., & Cetkovic, G. (2009). By products of fruit processing as source of phytochemicals. *Chem Ind.Chem. Eng., 15*(4), 191–202. doi:10.2298/CICEQ0904191D

Eller, F. J., Mosser, J. K., Kenar, J. A., & Taylor, S. L. (2010). Extraction and analysis of tomato seed oil. *Journal of the American Oil Chemists' Society, 87*(7), 755–762. doi:10.100711746-010-1563-4

FAO. (2011). *Global food losses and waste, extent, causes and prevention*. Rome: FAO.

FAO. (2015). *The state of food insecurity in the world*. Rome: FAO.

Ganders, D. (2012). *Wasted: How America is losing up to 40 percent of its food from farm to fork to landfill*. New York: Natural Resources Defense Council.

Gopalan, C., Rama Sastri, B. V., & Balasubramanian, S. C. (2014). *Nutritive value of Indian Foods* (p. 161). Hyderabad: NIN.

Gormley, R. (2013). *Fish as a functional food: some issues and outcomes, Sea Health*. UCD.

Graminha, Goncalves, Pirota, Balsalobre, Silva, & Gomes. (2008). Enzyme production by solid feed. *Sci. Technol, 144*, 1–22.

Gul, K., Yousuf, B., Singh, A. K., Sing, P., & Wane, A. (2015). Rice Bran, Nutritional value and its emerging potential for development of functional food: A review. *J of Bioactive Carbohydrates and Dietary Fibers, 6*(1), 24–30. doi:10.1016/j.bcdf.2015.06.002

Gustavsson, J., Cederberge, Sonesson, U., Van O Hedrick, R., & Me beck, A. (2011). *Global Food issues and food waste: Extent causes and prevention*. Rome: FAO, UNO.

Hall, K. D., Quo, J., Dore, M., & Chow, C. (2009). The progressive increase of food waste in America and its environmental impact. National Institute of Diabetes and Digestive and Kidney Diseases.

Helkar, P. B., Sahoo, A. K., & Patil, N. J. (2016). Review: Food industry by-products used as a functional food ingredients. *J. of Waste Resource, 6*(3), 1-6.

Homayouni, A., Alizadeh, M., Alikhan, H., & Zijah, V. (2012). *Functional dairy probiotic development trends, concepts and products*. Intech. doi:10.5772/48797

Hoornweg, D., Bhada-Ta-ta, P., & Kennedy, C. (2013). Environment: waste production must peak this century. *Nature, 502*, 615 – 617.

Horton, B. S. (1995). Whey processing and utilization. *IDF Bulletin, 308*, 2–6.

Hossain, M. F., Akhtar, S., & Anwar, M. (2015). Nutritional value and medicinal benefits of pineapple. *Int. J. Nutri. Food Sci., 4*(1), 84–88. doi:10.11648/j.ijnfs.20150401.22

Hussein, A. M. S., Kamil, M. M., Hegazy, N. A., Mahmoud, K. F., & Ibrahim, M. A. (2015). Utilization of some fruits and vegetables by-products to produce high dietary fibre jam. *Food Sci. Quality and Mgmt, 37*, 39–45.

Institution of Mechanical Engineers (IME). (2013). *Global food waste not want not*. Author.

Ismali,, A. E., & Abdellader,, M. O., & Ali, A. (2011). Microbial and chemical evolution of whey based mango beverage, Advances. *Journal of Food Science and Technology, 38*, 250–253.

Juliano, B. O. (1985). *Rice Chemistry and Technology*. American Association of Cereal Chemistry.

Kadam, S., & Prabha Sankar, P. (2010). Marine foods as functional ingredients in bakery and pasta products. *Food Research International, 3*(8), 1975–1980. doi:10.1016/j.foodres.2010.06.007

Kaur, R., Kapoor, S., & Sharma, S. (2017). Utilization potential of fruit and vegetable pomace. *Indian Food Industry, 36*(2), 24 – 30.

Kumar, R. S. (2005). Whey beverage: A review. *Beverage and Food World*, 58-60.

Kummu, M., de Moel, H., Porkka, M., Siebert, S., Varis, O., & Ward, P. (2012). Lost food, wasted resources: Global food supply chain losses and their impact on freshwater, cropland and fertilizer use. *The Science of the Total Environment*, *43*, 477–489. doi:10.1016/j.scitotenv.2012.08.092 PMID:23032564

Lafarga, T., & Teagase, M. H. (2014). Bioactive peptides from meat muscle and by products: Generation functionality and application as functional ingredients. *Meat Science*, *98*(2), 227–239. doi:10.1016/j.meatsci.2014.05.036 PMID:24971811

Lal, G., Siddappa, G. S., & Tandon, G. L. (1988). *Preservation of Fruits and Vegetables*. New Delhi: ICAR Pub.

Lambing, E. F., & May Froidt, P. (2011). Global land use change, deglobalization and booming land scarcity. *Proceedings of the National Academy of Sciences of the United States of America*, *108*(9), 3465–3472. doi:10.1073/pnas.1100480108 PMID:21321211

Lee, S. G., & Xu, X. (2004). A simplified life cycle assessment of reusable and single -use bulk transit packaging. *Packaging Technology & Science*, *17*(2), 67–83. doi:10.1002/pts.643

Mena, C. B., Adenso-Diaz, B., & Yurt, O. (2011). The causes of food waste in the supplier – retail interface: Evidence from the UK and Spain. *Resources, Conservation and Recycling*, *55*(6), 648–654. doi:10.1016/j.resconrec.2010.09.006

Menon, M. A. (2010). Integrated solid waste management based on the '3R'approach. *J. Motor Cycles Waste*, *12*(1), 30–40. doi:10.100710163-009-0274-0

Monier, V., Shailendra, M., Escalon, V. O., Connor, C., Gibbon, T., Anderson, G., . . . Reisinger, H. (2010). Preparatory study on food waste across EU 27. European Commission (DGENV) Directorate Industry, Final Report.

Moroney, P. (2016). Recycling, recovering and preventing food waste competing solutions for food systems substantially in the United States and France. Academic Press.

Nerantzis, E. T., & Tetaridis, P. (2006). *Integrated enology: utilization of winery by-products into high value added products.* Academic Press.

Nguyen, T. A. D., Kim, K. R., Han, S. J., Cho, H., Kim, J. W., Park, S. M., & Sim, S. J. (2010). Pretreatment of rice straw with ammonia and ionic liquid for lingo cellulose conversion to fermentable sugars. *Bioresource Technology*, *101*(19), 7432–7438. doi:10.1016/j.biortech.2010.04.053 PMID:20466540

Nishida, J. (2014). Reducing food waste and promoting two recovery, globally, EPA c connect. *The Official Blog of the EPA Leadership*. Retrieved from https:/blog.epa.gov/blog/2014/reducingfood-waste-and-promotingfood-recovery-gglobally

Pillaiyar, P. (1988). *Rice post production Manual*. New Delhi: Willey Eastern Ltd.

Ramos, O. L., Rodrigues, R. M., Texeira, J. A., & Vicentre, A. A. (2016). Whey and whey powders: Production and uses. Food Science Encyclopedia of Food and Health, 498-505.

Rodríguez Couto, S. (2008). Exploitation of biological waste for the production of value added products under solid state fermentation conditions. *Biotechnology Journal*, *3*(7), 859–870. doi:10.1002/biot.200800031 PMID:18543242

Roman, A., Vetal, G., Illzes, A., Kovacs, Z., & Czermak, P. (2012). Modeling of dia filteration process for determination of acid whey: an empirical approach. *J. of food Process Engg, 35*(5), 708-714.

Sakai, S. J., Yoshida, H., Hirai, Y., & Ansari, M. (2011). International comparative study of '3R's and waste management policy developments. *Master Cycles Waste, 13*(2), 86–102. doi:10.100710163-011-0009-x

Shyamala, B. N., & Jamuna, P. (2010). Nutritional content and antinutritional properties of pulp waste from *Daucus carota* and *Beta vulgaris. Mal, 16*(3), 397-408.

Silva, A. G., Wanderley, R. C., Pedroso, A. F., & Ashbell, G. (1997). Ruminal digestion kinetics of citrus peel. *Animal Feed Science and Technology, 68*(3-4), 247–257. doi:10.1016/S0377-8401(97)00056-4

Singh, Chonhenchob, & Singh. (2006). Life cycle inventory and analysis of reusable plastic containers and display-ready corrugated containers used for packaging fresh fruits and vegetables. *Packaging Technology and Science, 19*, 279-293.

Stuart, T. (2009). *Waste: Uncovering the global food scandal.* New York: Penguin.

Sudha, M. L., Baskaran, V., & Leelavathi, K. (2007). Apple pomace as source of dietary fibre and Polyphenols and its effect on the rheological characteristics and cake m making. *Food Chemistry, 104*(2), 689–692. doi:10.1016/j.foodchem.2006.12.016

Sustainable Restaurant Association. (2010). Too good to waste; Restaurant food waste survey Report 2010, UK. Author.

Taurisano, Gianluca, Nicolas, & Di Donato. (2014). Reuse of April waste, recovery of valuable compounds by Eco-friendly techniques. *International J. of performation to Engg., 10*(4), 419-425.

Tseng, A., & Zhao, Y. (2003). wine grape pomace as antioxidant dietary fibre for enhancing nutritional value and improving stability of yoghurt and salad dressing. *Food Chemistry, 138*(1), 356–365. doi:10.1016/j.foodchem.2012.09.148 PMID:23265499

Vandermeerch, T., Alvarenga, R.A.F., Ragart, P., & Dewalf, J. (2014). Environmental sustainability assessment of food waste valorization, options, resource conserve. *Recy, 87*, 57.

Varghese, K., Lewis, H., Lockroy, S., & Williams, H. (2013). *The role of packaging in minimizing food waste in the supply chain of the future, Final report, Centre for design RMIT University.* CHEP.

Ventour, L. (2008). Food waste report v2, in the food we waste wrap and exodus market research. Weston – Super-Mare.

Williams, H., Wikstrom, F., Otterbring, T., Lofgren, M., & Gustafsson, A. (2012). Reasons for household food waste with special attention to packaging, *J. of Cleaner Production, 24*, 148.

WRAP. (2011). Fruit and Vegetable resource maps, Final Report 201., Waste and Resources Action Program (WRAP).

This research was previously published in Global Initiatives for Waste Reduction and Cutting Food Loss edited by Aparna B. Gunjal, Meghmala S. Waghmode, Neha N. Patil, and Pankaj Bhatt; pages 165-190, copyright year 2019 by Engineering Science Reference (an imprint of IGI Global).

Chapter 29
Various Approaches for Food Waste Processing and Its Management

Anupam Pandey
Kumaun University Nainital, India

Ankita Harishchandra Tripathi
Kumaun University Nainital, India

Priyanka Harishchandra Tripathi
National Institute of Pathology (ICMR), India

Satish Chandra Pandey
Kumaun University Nainital, India

Ashutosh Paliwal
Kumaun University Nainital, India

Tushar Joshi
Kumaun University Nainital, India

Veena Pande
Kumaun University Nainital, India

ABSTRACT

Food wastage is a huge crisis arising in today's world. An extensive amount of waste generation has become a serious concern of our society in the past years that affects developing and developed countries equally, and according to the Food and Agriculture Organization (FAO), as much as one-third of the food intentionally grown for human consumption is never consumed and is therefore wasted, with significant environmental, social, and economic ramifications. By wasting food, we also waste the time and energy that we have used to produce the food and as well our natural resources and the limited available agricultural land will be used up which could be handled in a much better and sustainable way. Additionally, waste has a strong financial impact and affects the environment including the overall greenhouse gas emission. In an increasingly resource-constrained world, it is imperative to reduce the high environmental, social, and economic impacts associated with this type of waste.

DOI: 10.4018/978-1-7998-5354-1.ch029

INTRODUCTION

Every year approximately 1.3 billion tons of food which equals one third of total food production worldwide is lost or wasted (Gustavsson *et al.*, 2011). Food waste is predominantly challenging in industrialized countries that have a major contribution to household food waste. As food production is resource intensive, food loses and wastes indirectly cost the environment and the major effect of this can be seen in the environmental burden in the form of, water and air pollution, deforestation, soil erosion as well as greenhouse gas emissions that occur during the processes of food production, stowage, conveyance, and waste-management (Mourad, 2016). Owing to these rising environmental burdens, social and economic concerns towards food waste is progressively accredited as a crucial issue between governments, academics, NGOs, businesses, and the general public (Beretta *et al.*, 2013; Edjabou *et al.*, 2016). Humans are totally depended on plants and animals for their nutritional assistances. The Global Food Report, by the Institute of Mechanical Engineers, has claimed that there could be a whopping three billion to be fed with food by the end of this century. In that period, one can expect great changes in the areas of wealth, calorific intake and dietary preferences of people in developing countries across the globe. Hence, it lies in our hands to focus in producing food in safer quantities by availing the best technologies.

Food waste is generally defined as the loss of materials planned for human ingestion that are afterwardeither discharged, which thereby get contaminated, degrade and are subsequently lost. As per the Food and Agriculture Organisation (FAO) of United Nations, food is "Any modification in the accessibility, edibility, wholesomeness or quality of eatable material that averts it from being eaten by people". This definition was stated for the period of post-harvest of food ending, when the point is of proprietorship of the final consumer (FAO, 1981). Another definition of FL provided by Gustavsson *et al.*, (2011) included description of food supply chain (FSC) production stage along with postharvest and processing stage.According to Parfitt *et al.*, (2010), "Food waste (FW) is the loss of food taking place either at the market stage or at final consumption and utilization stages and is generated due to the negligent behaviour on the part of retailer as well as consumer. European Project FUSIONS defines food waste as''any form of food, edible or inedible, aloof from (diverted or lost from) the food supply chain that is to be either disposed or improved (includes anaerobic digestion, incineration, composted crops, co-generation, bio-energy production, sewer disposal, landfill or discarded into the sea)'' (Östergren *et al.*, 2014). For proper metabolic functioning and cellular activities, cell needs energy and this energy comes from food. All human beings depend on food for both energy constraint and survival.

Research study carried by Smil, 2010 explained that when the losses and food wastage along the food supply chain was taken into account along with the transformation of food production into animal feed, it was reported that 43% out of the total food cultivated worldwide is directly consumed by humans. According to the Unites States Department of Agriculture USDA (2007), in the United States a total of 30% of the food intended for human feeding is wasted every year, mostly in the houses, restaurants and food service establishments. According to Eurostat data (2006) the quantity of food wasted annually in Europe is 89 million tons, equivalent to 180 kg per capita, but this figure is not inclusive of the losses that occur all through the food production and harvesting stages. Looking only at waste in the houses, and using various national data sources, it was found that the amount wasted per person per year is: 110 kg in Great Britain, 109 kg in the United States, 108 kg in Italy, 99 kg in France, 82 kg in Germany and 72 kg in Sweden.

According to (BIOIS, 2010), in food supply chain, the largest food-waste fraction is contributed by private households, therefore prevention of food waste over the final stages of supply chain is of extreme importance to prevent further changes in climate (Parfitt *et al.,* 2010). In emerging republics, the great losses are suffered at the initial level of the food supply chain, mainly due to limitation of techniques used for cultivation, harvesting, and preservation, or due to a lack of adequate transportation and storage infrastructures. In commercial countries, the largest share of waste in the food supply chain occurs in the final phase (household consumption, restaurants and food service establishments). However, even in these countries, the losses recorded at the agricultural level are not insignificant for instance, in Italy in 2009, 17.7 million tons of agricultural foodstuffs was left in the fields, representing 3.25% of total production (Segrè and Gaiani, 2011). In agriculture, research shows that the food losses are attributable to climatic and environmental dynamics, and also to disease and parasites. But there are discrepancies at this stage when we compare between emerging and advanced countries which can be credited to the accessible technology, agricultural skills and the techniques used for preparation of agricultural field, infrastructures, sowing, cultivation, harvesting, processing, and storage. In developed countries, and sometimes also in emerging countries, regulatory and economic factors play a part. However, there is undoubtedly still a long way to go in understanding the causes of the initial stages losses in the food supply chains. The primary identified reasons of waste produced during the initial processing stages of the agricultural product and semi-finished goods are inefficiencies and technical malfunctions in the production processes - commonly known as "production waste". There are many causes for food waste production throughout the distribution and sales of food (both wholesale as well as retail) which includes improper ordering and false estimation of consumer requirements.

According to a survey conducted in October 2011 by Coldiretti-SWG, Italians have reduced food waste by 57% because of the economic crisis. To combat waste and thus save more food, as many as three out of four Italians spend more carefully than before crisis. Among the measures taken to reduce food waste are to shop more wisely, reduce the quantity of food purchased (31%), increase use of leftover products in meals (24%) and pay more attention to expiration dates (18%).

Food Waste Management

Presently, due to ever increasing population, food systems have become very inefficient: it is projected that one half of all the food produced would get lost before reaching human mouth. In 2015 United Nations has established "The Sustainable Development Goal 12" that 'Safeguard maintainable production and consumption patterns' including a target specific for food waste reduction: at retail and consumer levels, halve per capita reduction in global food waste till 2030 (The Agenda For Sustainable Development 2030 (2015)). During prehistoric time, when techniques and knowledge were less, traditional methodology was used by people for waste management. The traditional method included three steps: 1. Reduce, 2. Reuse, 3. recycle.

- **Reduce:** Take minimum food which can be finished by an individual.
- **Reuse:** Food that has been cooked can be used more than once in a day.
- **Recycle:** Even after consumption, leftover food can further be used for production of some commercial products such as biofuel, ethanol etc.

Sustainable management of food waste is a importantexploration area that has speedily grown over recent years. Methodology of food waste management includes classification of food waste. Food waste can be categorized according to the type of food: drinks, meat, cereals, fish, fruits, etc. this classification is beneficial in order to quantify the quantity of food wasted on the basis of mass, economic cost, and energy content (Flores *et al.,* 1999).

Lin *et al.* classified food waste as organic crop residue (including fruits and vegetables), animal by-products, domestic waste packaging, mixed food waste and catering waste. Edjabou *et al.* included two new factors: vegetable/ animal-derived food waste and avoidable-processed/ avoidable-unprocessed food waste.

In the UK, WRAP identified supply chain stages, where food waste is generated (e.g. manufacturer, retailer) and had assess the edibility of the waste. Accordingly, food waste can be avoidable (food parts that are edible) and unavoidable (food parts that are inedible such as fruits skin, bones etc.). Furthermore, food waste can be divided at household level as cooked/uncooked, packaged/unpackaged or opened/ unopened packaging or leftovers and untouched food which usually is thrown and wasted (Matsuda *et al.,* 2012).

According to a published research in "The Food We Waste" (WRAP, 2007), the main reasons for food wastes in the home include:

- Buying too much: Due to the special offers such as "buy one get one free"
- Buying more perishable food
- Poor storage and management: Not eating food in date order, preparing too much.
- Sensitivity to food hygiene: Not taking a chance with food close to its "best before" date

Figure 1. Food waste management

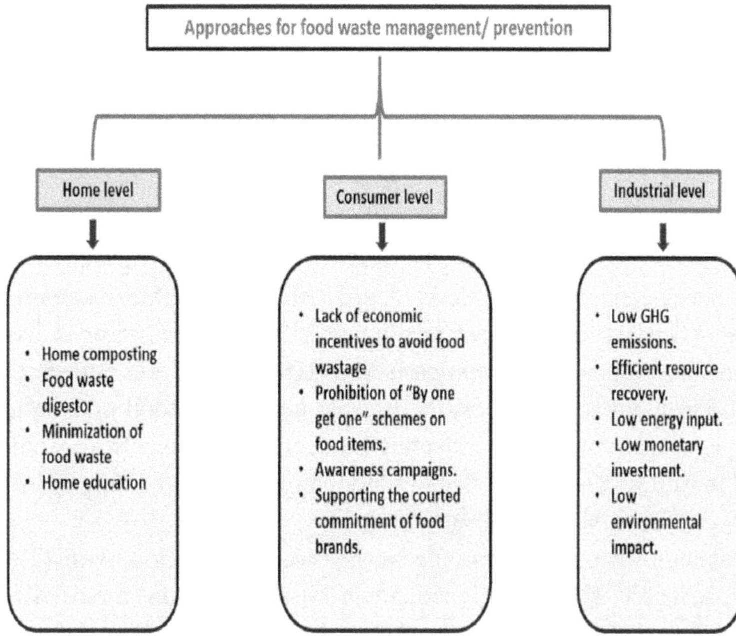

Attitudes and behaviour towards food waste are driven by a number of factors at consumer level including:

- Retail practices that encourage people to buy more than they need.
- Lack of economic incentives to avoid food waste.
- Lack of advance planning, skills and knowledge regarding food storage and preparation.

Ideas to sanitize people for management of food waste, supermarkets-initiated programs to manage food waste at consumer stage. The programs included initiatives on moving away from Buy One Get One Free promotions (these promotions are not common in other European countries) to "Buy one get one free". The buyer still benefits from the free items of food, but they can be collected at a later date when they are more likely to be consumed as the consumer will purchase smaller quantity at one time. Plans by the former government entitled "war on waste" suggested scrapping best before dates, limiting sell by labels and creating new food packaging sizes in an attempt to save $300. With "best before" dates and other labelling – The Food standards agency (FSA) found that only one-third of people correctly interpreted these terms and more than one quarter thought that food, past its best before date could be unsafe and should be thrown away (FSA, 2006). Other supermarket initiatives include "Love your leftovers" and "Great taste less waste" involving recipes cards, vouchers and website information. Many of these ideas are being introduced to reduce packaging and food waste. This is a promise signed up to by more than 40 retailers and brand owners to reduce waste and provide choices to consumers regarding the products they buy. This relates to the fact that a substantial amount of food waste is literally waste food which has not been touched by the purchaser (Hogg et al., 2007).

The second phase of the obligation was launched in March 2010 with a more focused aim to achieve a better sustainable use of resources over their entire lifecycle. The main targets of phase second are to reduce supply chain product and packaging waste by 5% and to reduce UK household food and drink waste by 4% by 2010. A report by the British Retail Consortium revealed that retailers in the UK have managed to halve waste sent to landfill from 48% to 23% since 2005. This has been achieved through re-use, using energy recovery technology and reducing consumer food waste (Barton, 2010).

Collections of Food Wastes

In UK, through the refuse stream or food waste collections (WRAP, 2009b) the local authorities have collected 5.8 tonnes of wastefood. Despite the fact, the trash stream is disposed of in landfill, in Europe the local authorities have been asked to limit the degradable waste in thrash stream. Now, though there are great differences, in Austria and Germany,near about 75% of organic waste is divided from the waste stream and collected for composting, in comparison to UK, Ireland and Greece where it is less than 10% (ACR+, 2009). For many local authorities, presenting a waste food assemblage offers a genuine solution for meeting legislative marks for collecting biodegradable waste from landfill thereby, increasing composting and recycling rates. It has been found that greater than 100kg per inhabitant of organic collection is made every year (ACR+, 2009).

In 2009, 137 local authorities in UK provided a food waste collection, with 47% offering food only collections (Brook Lyndhurst, 2009). In France, green waste collections are used widely by native authorities to capture biodegradable waste. As kerbside recycling collections now capture a broad range of dry recyclables, a large proportion of the remaining refuse stream consists of biodegradable material.

In Bournemouth, food waste makes up to 38% of the refuse stream, while green waste makes up 11% (Resource Futures, 2009). Implementing a separate food waste collection would have a significant impact on the quantity and quality of material remaining in the refuse stream and ultimately its cost of disposal.

Drivers for Collections of Food Waste

A number of strategies forsubstantialassistances to accumulating food waste separately from the waste stream. Numerous are directly related to the alteration of biodegradable waste obtained from landfill by:

- Improving recycling rates
- Reducing waste disposal costs as landfill cost increases
- Reducing the impactsassociated with landfill (toxicity in leachate, gas emissions from landfill) on environment.
- Reducing greenhouse gas emissions by eliminating putrescent content from landfill sites.

Figure 2. Food related practices and routines

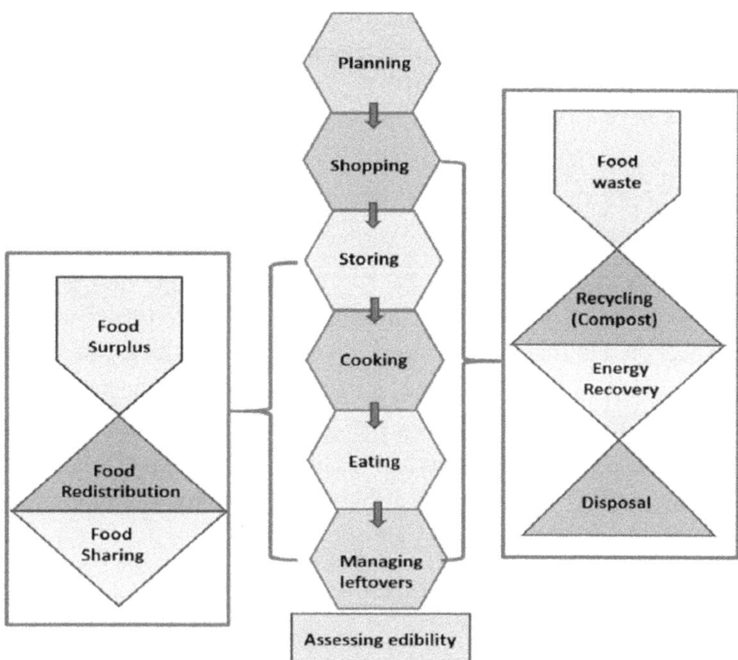

Food waste collections can also help local authorities who presently practice alternatives to landfill for the treatment of the waste stream, such as Mechanical Biological Treatment (MBT) Energy from Waste (EW) by:

- Improving recycle rates
- By producing improved quality liquid fertilizers and composts, so that they can be used for improving soil quality.

- Generating large amount of power and heat through anaerobic digestion (AD).
- Reducing annoyance created by rats, flies and vermin attracted to food in refuse stream.

The benefits will vary in different areas, depending on the local authority's current performance and collection systems already in place.

Policy Initiatives

Economic Instruments

According to Driesen, 2006; FUSIONS, 2016, economic enticements, goal is to lessen food waste through various market signals and costs. It can be in the form of taxes, subsidies, fees etc. Financial instruments are considered as an influential means to change consumption forms towards additional sustainable food practices (Reisch *et al.*, 2013). It is expected that if the actual cost of natural reserve use is replicated in charges, consumers are more expected to become active in prevention of food waste (UNEP, 2014). The volume- or weight-based fee system "Pay-As-You-Throw" (PAYT) is a mutual method that has been prompted in various countries, such as the, Sweden, Japan, Canada, United States, Taiwan, Thailand, Vietnam Korea, and China (UNEP, 2014). In these countries, implicating households for personally produced waste has been found to be an operative scheme for reduction of food waste (Chalak *et al.*, 2016; Dahlen and Lagerkvist, 2010; EEA, 2009).

Regulations

For reduction of food waste, regulatory approaches with an aim of waste reduction targets has been implemented, which includes mandatory management plans, aim to induce waste reduction, laws and standards, restrictions or covenants, penalties for those who do not obey the regulatory provisions. So far, regulations have been accepted in many countries, such as Italy, Belgium, France, and the Netherlands. The National Pact against Food Waste in France, for example, summaries eleven measures to accomplish a food waste reduction of 50% by 2025 (Mourad, 2016). One possible regulatory instrument is the evaluation and abolition of needless food-safety values that lead to high rates of food waste. In contrast to fiscal and economic incentives, well-defined principles appear to be a more operative tool to battle household food waste generation (Chalak *et al.*, 2016).

Information and Education Campaigns

Information campaigns present one of the utmost common tools used for food waste anticipation and reduction (Priefer *et al.*, 2016). Information and education movements, information stages and face-to-face door-stepping operations have been employed all over Europe to raise awareness and improve consumer's knowledge about prevention of food waste (Schanes *et al.*, 2018).

Industrial Application

Increasing efforts are currently being focused on defining effective and stable means of obtaining biofuel and bio-products from waste food materials. These opportunities could pay for benefits from an environ-

Figure 3. Approaches towards food waste management

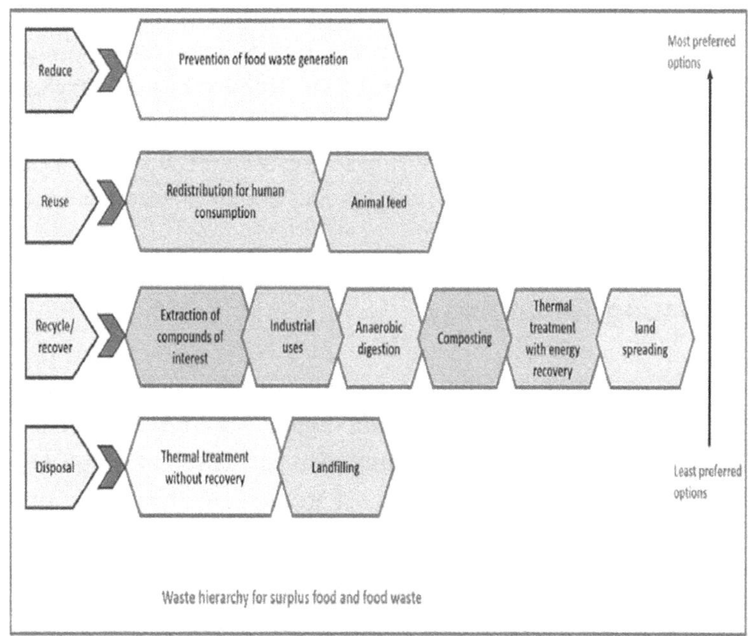

mental point of view due to the reduction of methane gas emissions from landfills and the conservation of natural resources such as coal and fossil fuels, from a social point of view since lack of food verses fuel competition, and from an economical point of view thanks to costs saving linked to surplus food production and specific investments in establishing non-food crops dedicated to biofuel or bio-plastic production. Bio-refineries are the concept underlying industrial waste food consumption. Similarly, to the transformation by oil refineries of petroleum into fuels and ingredients for use in a wide variety of consumer products, bio-refineries convert organic waste and biomasses (corn, sugar cane and other plant-based materials) into a range of ingredients for bio-based fuels or products. Waste food produced from agriculture and food processing is abundant and concentrated in specific locations. These materials could be less susceptible to deterioration if compared to food waste produced at household level at the end of the FSC (Galanakis, 2012). These characteristics highlight the potential to develop industrial utilisation processes based on symbiosis where the wastes from one sector are inputs for other sectors. Accessibility of food waste and location of potential users define the feasibility of industrial symbiosis (Mirabella *et al.*, 2014). Therefore, precise efforts will be required from the agricultural and the industrial sectors to define sustainable and inventive processes for residues use and conversion, and from governments to stimulate and support this new vision with specific legislations. The potential profitability of chemicals and biofuels produced from food waste will stimulate investments on bio-refinery chains rather than treatments of food waste in traditional waste management processes. Valorisation routes of food wastes in bio-refinery chains include both extraction of high-value components already present in the substrates to be used for nutrition or pharmaceutical applications and conversion into chemicals, materials or biofuels by the use of chemical or biological processes. Type, origin, seasonal generation and territorial distribution of food waste will affect transport logistic for its utilisation and its compatibility with the transformation process. High and concentrated volumes of food waste will be generally required to sustain large production capacities and meet economy of scale. Cost-effectiveness of conversion processes will then be ensured by security of supply at regional scale, low heterogeneity of substrates and large variety of extractable chemicals, biopolymers and biofuels. For these reasons, large fluxes of agro-industrial wastes seem to be more suitable for bio-refinery chains where stability of supply and substrate homogeneity are required for extraction or production of specific commodities while source segregated organic waste from household or restaurants would be more indicated for treatment processes where composition variability, origins and contaminations do not represent limits for the selected process (Pfaltzgraff *et al.*, 2013).

Developing Composting Technology

Sustainable food waste management system also includes development of composting technologies. Compost is generally a dark black or brown colour organic mixture formed from degradation and breakdown of organic components and is rich in humus. In agriculture, Composts are extensively used as manure/fertilizer and for soil amendments. Compost are prepared by mixing organic wastes such as leaves, food waste, garden waste with bulking agents such as wood chips. This forms an ideal environment for fungi and anaerobic bacteria to undergo the process of chemical decomposition. Maturation and curing process stabilizes the compost.

According to US EPA, composting process serve may benefits. These include:

- Decrease and exclusion of the requirement for chemical fertilizers
- Crop yields increase
- Assistance of habitat revitalization, wetland restoration, and reforestation, by modifying polluted, compressed, and marginal soils
- Capturing and destruction of 99.6 percent of industrial volatile organic chemicals (VOCs) in contaminated air;
- More cost-effective soil, water, and air remediation compared to conventional technologies;
- Extension of municipal landfill life by diverting organic materials from landfills.

Biofuel and Bioenergy Production

Food waste is characterised by a variable chemical composition depending on its source of production. Waste food materials may therefore comprise a mixture of carbohydrates, lipids and proteins, or, if generated from specific agro-industrial sectors, may be rich in one of these constituents. Different biofuels are therefore produced from food waste using bioprocesses or thermo-chemical processes, depending on their chemical composition. The use of food waste for energy production was recently reviewed by Pham *et al.*, (2015) and by Kiran *et al.*, (2014). Waste food can be converted into biofuels or energy by means of the following processes:

- Trans-esterification of oils and fats to produce biodiesel;
- Fermentation of carbohydrates to produce bioethanol or bio-butanol;
- Anaerobic digestion to produce biogas (methane rich gas);
- Dark fermentation to produce hydrogen;
- Pyrolysis and gasification;

- Hydrothermal carbonisation
- Incineration;

Not all the listed processes are currently developed at industrial level in full running mode. For example, waste food is widely studied as a substrate for the biological production of hydrogen by dark fermentation, although no full-scale applications have been realised to date (Alibardi *et al.*, 2014; De Gioannis *et al.*, 2013). Incineration is a mature technology in which waste food material directly applied to flame for decay. Incineration is applied to diminish waste volumes and produce electrical energy and heat; however, the high moisture contents of food waste limit its application together with the concerns of local communities on air emissions (Pham *et al.*, 2015). Anaerobic digestion, on the contrary, is a technology facing growing interests and large applications (Clarke and Alibardi, 2010; Levis *et al.*, 2010). The high biodegradability and moisture content of waste food are ideal characteristics for production of bio-gas and digestion residues can be used as soil conditioner or amendment or as nutrient source (e.g. ammonia or struvite). Biodiesel can be defined as short-chain alcohols and long-chain fatty acids of alkyl esters (methyl/ethyl esters) of derived from natural biological lipid sources such as vegetable oils or animal fats, which had their viscosity reduced by means of a process known as trans-esterification and are suited to use in conventional diesel engines and distributed through existing fuel infrastructure". Any fatty acid source may be used to prepare biodiesel (Refaat, 2012). Thus, any animal or plant lipid should represent a ready substrate for the production of biodiesel. However, the use of edible vegetable oils and animal fats for biodiesel production has traditionally been of high concern due to their competing with food materials. The use of non-edible vegetable oils in biodiesel production is likewise questionable, as the production of crops for fuel implies an inappropriate use of land, water, and energy resources vital for the production of food for human consumption; the use of waste oil may therefore represent a more realistic and effective element for use in the production of biodiesel (Gasparatos *et al.*, 2011; Refaat, 2012). The new technologies developed in recent years have enabled the production of biodiesel from recycled frying oils, resulting in a final quality comparable to that obtained with virgin vegetable oil biodiesel. Canakci (2007) claimed the annual production of oils, greases and animal fats from restaurants in the United States could replace more than 5 million litres of diesel fuel if collected and converted to biodiesel. Waste cooking oil requires a series of pre-treatment steps to eliminate solid impurities and reduce water contents and free fatty acids. The pre-treatment process may include washing, centrifugation, flash evaporation, and acid esterification. Final ester yield could be up to 80% (Yaakob *et al.*, 2013). These results are expected to encourage the public and private sectors to improve the collection and recycling of used cooking oil to produce biodiesel. Various microorganisms like Protists, Molds and bacteria rapidly grow on waste food from which bio-diesel can be prepared. (Ghanavati *et al.*, 2015; Kiran *et al.*, 2014). First-generation bioethanol can be derived from renewable sources of virgin feedstock; typically starch and sugar crops such as corn, wheat, or sugarcane. Indeed, most of the feed stocks used in first generation biofuel production are crops. For this reason, biofuel expansion may compete with food production both directly and indirectly (Gasparatos *et al.*, 2011). One potential advantage of cellulosic ethanol technologies is that they avoid direct competition for crops used in the food supply chain, as the materials used are non-edible; this option however should be limited to cases in which an overt sustainable surplus of crops occurs or where crop wastes and wood wastes are available as feedstock. (Pirozzi *et al.*, 2012; Refaat, 2012). Cellulosic ethanol has a number of potential benefits over corn grain ethanol, but although the cost of biomass is low, releasing fermentable sugars from these materials remains challenging. Bioethanol can be produced from FW and agricultural waste, the latter being cost-effective, renewable and abundant substrates (Kiran *et al.,* 2014).

Clostridium acetobutylicum bacteria is one of the prominent bacteria involved in the production of butanol by fermenting waste food. This bacterium poses a number of inimitable properties, including the ability to produce high yield of acetone and butanol by utilizing various starchy substances in comparison to Fernbach's original culture method of butanol and acetone production (Stoeberl *et al.,* 2011). Butanol poses greater advantages over ethanol as a fuel or merger/blending component. They require a lower vapour pressure, which enhances combustion competency, greater energy density. They even reduce viscosity of vegetable oils when mixed together in any ratio.

Thermal processes such as Pyrolysis and gasification have been used as an alternative methods in management of waste food (Pham *et al.,* 2015). The process of pyrolysis of waste food, involves heating at temperatures ranging from 400 to 800 °C, which converts the waste food materials from the solid into gas or liquid products, which can be used as raw materials or fuels proposed to consequent biochemical processes. The solid carbon thus produced is then additionally refined by adding activated charcoal. Products of pyrolysis are usually solid, liquid and gaseous, and their proportion depends upon the reaction parameters and the process of pyrolysis. Inflammable mixture of gas is obtained from the process of gasification through partial oxidation of wastefood. About 800-900°C temperature is provided during the process. The gas formed can be used directly or can be used as a fuel for engines and turbines operated through gas or even can be used as a feedstock in the production of chemicals (e.g. methanol) (Pham *et al.,* 2015).

Applicability and feasibility of these processes are strongly dependent on waste characteristics such as elemental composition, heating values, ash, moisture and volatile solids content, the presence of contaminants, bulk density. These characteristics are crucial for process performances and limit the applicability of gasification and pyrolysis. The majority of gasification technologies for example use pre-treated waste as feed stocks and no gasification/pyrolysis processes have been developed using raw food waste (Pham *et al.,* 2015). Only few researches were published on gasification or pyrolysis of food waste. Liu *et al.,* (2014) investigated the effectiveness of catalytic pyrolysis of food waste by using microwave power for heating. Opatokun *et al.,* (2015) evaluated the pyrolysis of both dry raw waste food and digested waste food after biological anaerobic treatment and concluded that both substrates demonstrated potential for fast degradation due to high volatile matter content. Energy content was for both cases mainly spread into biochar and bio-oil fractions while gases provided significantly lower energy. The use of agro-industrial residues for the extraction of high-value chemicals was recently reviewed by Mirabella *et al.,* (2014).

Biopolymers production is a panorama facing growing interest, as it is pertinent both to organic waste generated at household level and also including agro-industrial generated residues. The constituent monomers are available either through the process of fermentation of carbohydrates obtained from feedstocks by microbes, or are often genetically modified, or are obtained from chemical processing of plant oils (Fuessl *et al.,* 2012). The major focus of food waste management research is production of metabolites that can be used as biodegradable and renewable constituents of petrochemical products. Metabolites used for preparation of biopolymers include lactate which is used for the production of a plastic constituent Polylactate, Succinate used as a major precursor of detergent, plastic production, and even in pharmaceuticals. Polyhydroxyalkanotes, chiefly polyhydroxybutyrate, which are ordinary storage polymer found in many bacterial species having properties comparable to polypropylene and polyethylene (Li *et al.,* 2015). As for the biofuel production from virgin feed stocks, significant discussion surrounds the production of bio-plastics from natural materials, hovering the question as to whether they produce a harmful effect on human food supply. In this situation, the chance of using food waste in the manufacture of bio-plastics appears an extremely achievable choice. The production of pure L-lactic acid (optically active) from waste food has captivated significant attention due to its capacity to treat organic wastes with concurrent regaining of valuable by-products (Li *et al.*, 2015). A novel approach was described for operative production of optically active pure acid, L-lactic acid from waste food at moderate temperature, amending main enzyme activity by supplementation of sewage sludge and irregular basic fermentation. A production of optically pure L-lactic acid was achieved from food waste at ambient temperature with a yield of 0.52 g/g COD (Li *et al.*, 2015). Dairy industries produce large amounts of whey from processing milk for numerous industrial products. Whey is basically a by-product obtained during the process of cheese production, and its removal is presently a chief pollution problem for the dairy industry (Abdel-Rahman *et al.*, 2013). Whey is a potent and suitable raw material for lactic acid production, consisting in lactose, mineral salts, fats, proteins, water-soluble vitamins and other essential nutrients for microbial growth (Panesar *et al.*, 2007). At present, amongst the various types of starch-based biodegradable plastics such as polylactic acid (PLA) and polyvinyl acetate (PVA), the group of polyhydroxyalkanoates (PHAs) is one of the most promising. Polyhydroxyalkanoates (PHAs) are linear polyesters of hydroxyacids (hydroxyalkanoate monomers) synthesised by a wide variety of bacteria through bacterial fermentation (Reis *et al.*, 2011). The strength and toughness of PHAs are good, and they are completely resistant to moisture and feature a very low oxygen permeability. Accordingly, PHA is suitable for use in the production of bottles and water-resistant film (Van Wegen *et al.*, 1998). The simplest type of PHA is polyhydroxybutyrate (PHB). PHAs accumulate in bacteria cytoplasm as a high molecular weight polymer forming intracellular granules of 0.2– 0.7 mm in diameter. Typically, PHAs accumulate to a significant proportion of the cell dry weight when bacteria are grown in a media that is limited in a nutrient essential for growth (typically nitrogen or phosphorus), but with an abundant supply of carbon (for example glucose). Under these conditions, bacteria convert the extracellular carbon into an intracellular storage form, namely PHA. When the limiting nutrient is resupplied, intracellular PHA is degraded and the resulting carbon is used for growth (Reis *et al.*, 2011).

The main limitation in using bacterial PHAs as a source of biodegradable polymers is their production cost. In particular the average cost is by far the most significant contributor to overall PHB price, approximately two and a quarter times greater than the capital cost of equipment (Van Wegen *et al.*, 1998). Using agro-industrial food waste as substrate instead of virgin feedstock of refined sugar such as glucose, sucrose and corn steep liquor could represent a turning point. Sugarcane and beet molasses, cheese whey effluents, plant oils, swine waste liquor, vegetable and fruit wastes, effluents of palm oil mill, olive oil mill, paper mill, pull mill and hydrolysates of starch (e.g., corn and tapioca), cellulose and hemicellulose are all excellent alternatives characterised by a high organic fraction (Reis *et al.*, 2011).

CONCLUSION

Food wastage has become a major problem in today's world. In the last few years, food wastage has become a serious issue that has affected both "developed and developing countries" equally. According to Food and Agriculture Organization (FAO), about one-third or one-fifth of all the food produced remains unconsumed. Moreover, food waste has a robust financial influence and effects the environment with the total greenhouse gas emission. A number of resolutions may be applied in the suitable organization of waste food and prioritised in a parallel way to waste food management. The greatest desirable solutions are characterized by circumvention and donation of palatable portions to social services. Food waste is also employed in industrial processes for the production of biofuels or biopolymers. Further steps predict the repossession of nutrients and fixation of carbon by composting. Therefore, it is expected that there will be an increasing number of initiatives, campaigns and legislative developments in order to reach the aforementioned objectives.

REFERENCES

Abdel-Rahman, M. A., Tashiro, Y., & Sonomoto, K. (2013). Recent advances in lactic acid production by microbial fermentation processes. *Biotechnology Advances*, *31*(6), 877–902. doi:10.1016/j.biotechadv.2013.04.002 PMID:23624242

ACR+. (2009). Municipal Waste in Europe – Towards a European Recycling Society. *Victoires Editions*.

Alibardi, L., Muntoni, A., & Polettini, A. (2014). Hydrogen and waste: Illusions, challenges and perspectives. *Waste Management (New York, N.Y.)*, *34*(12), 2425–2426. doi:10.1016/j.wasman.2014.09.001 PMID:25442106

Bajón Fernández, Y., Soares, A., Villa, R., Vale, P., & Cartmell, E. (2014). Carbon capture and biogas enhancement by carbon dioxide enrichment of anaerobic digesters treating sewage sludge or food waste. *Bioresource Technology*, *159*, 1–7. doi:10.1016/j.biortech.2014.02.010 PMID:24632434

Barton, S. (2010, September 17). *Retailers halve waste to landfill since 2005*. Retrieved from https://www.letsrecycle.com/news/latest-news/retailers-halve-waste-to-landfill-since-2005/

Beretta, C., Stoessel, F., Baier, U., & Hellweg, S. (2013). Quantifying food losses and the potential for reduction in Switzerland. *Waste Management (New York, N.Y.)*, *33*(3), 764–773. doi:10.1016/j.wasman.2012.11.007 PMID:23270687

Brook Lyndhurst Blog. (2009). *Enhancing Participation in Kitchen Waste Collections*. Retrieved from http://www.brooklyndhurst.co.uk/enhancing-participation-in-kitchen-waste-collections-_119

Burkhardt, M., Koschack, T., & Busch, G. (2015). Biocatalytic methanation of hydrogen and carbon dioxide in an anaerobic three-phase system. *Bioresource Technology*, *178*, 330–333. doi:10.1016/j.biortech.2014.08.023 PMID:25193088

Canakci, M. (2007). The potential of restaurant waste lipids as biodiesel feedstocks. *Bioresource Technology*, *98*(1), 183–190. doi:10.1016/j.biortech.2005.11.022 PMID:16412631

Chalak, A., Abou-Daher, C., Chaaban, J., & Abiad, M. G. (2016). The global economic and regulatory determinants of household food waste generation: A cross-country analysis. *Waste Management (New York, N.Y.)*, *48*, 418–422. doi:10.1016/j.wasman.2015.11.040 PMID:26680687

Clarke, W. P., & Alibardi, L. (2010). Anaerobic digestion for the treatment of solid organic waste: What's hot and what's not. *Waste Management (New York, N.Y.)*, *30*(10), 1761–1762. doi:10.1016/j.wasman.2010.06.019 PMID:20638829

Dahlén, L., & Lagerkvist, A. (2010). Evaluation of recycling programmes in household waste collection systems. *Waste Management & Research, 28*(7), 577–586. doi:10.1177/0734242X09341193 PMID:19748961

De Gioannis, G., Muntoni, A., Polettini, A., & Pomi, R. (2013). A review of dark fermentative hydrogen production from biodegradable municipal waste fractions. *Waste Management (New York, N.Y.), 33*(6), 1345–1361. doi:10.1016/j.wasman.2013.02.019 PMID:23558084

Edjabou, M. E., Petersen, C., Scheutz, C., & Astrup, T. F. (2016). Food waste from Danish households: Generation and composition. *Waste Management (New York, N.Y.), 52*, 256–268. doi:10.1016/j.wasman.2016.03.032 PMID:27026492

Exodus Market Research. (2006). *A quantitative assessment of the nature, scale and origin of post consumer food waste arising in Great Britain 2006.* Author. (unpublished)

FAO. (1981). Food loss prevention in perishable crops. FAO Agricultural Services Bulletin, 43, 72.

Favaro, L., Alibardi, L., Lavagnolo, M. C., Casella, S., & Basaglia, M. (2013). Effects of inoculum and indigenous microflora on hydrogen production from the organic fraction of municipal solid waste. *International Journal of Hydrogen Energy, 38*(27), 11774–11779. doi:10.1016/j.ijhydene.2013.06.137

Flores, R. A., Shanklin, C. W., Loza-Garay, M., & Wie, S. H. (1999). Quantification and characterization of food processing wastes/ residues. *Compost Science & Utilization, 7*(1), 63–71. doi:10.1080/10 65657X.1999.10701954

Food Standards Agency. (2006). *Consumer Attitudes to Food Safety 2005.* Author.

Friends of the Earth. (2006). *Briefing: food waste collections.* Retrieved from http://www.foe.co.uk/resource/briefings/food_waste.pdf

Fuessl, A., Yamamoto, M., & Schneller, A. (2012). *Opportunities in bi-based building blocks for polycondensates and vinyl polymers. In Polymer Science: A Comprehensive Reference* (Vol. 5, pp. 49–70). Elsevier.

FUSIONS. (2016). *EU FUSIONS website.* Retrieved from www.eu-fusions.org

Galanakis, C. M. (2012). Recovery of high added-value components from food wastes: Conventional, emerging technologies and commercialized applications. *Trends in Food Science & Technology, 26*(2), 68–87. doi:10.1016/j.tifs.2012.03.003

Garcia-Garcia, G., Woolley, E., Rahimifard, S., Colwill, J., White, R., & Needham, L. (2017). A Methodology for Sustainable Management of Food Waste. *Waste and Biomass Valorization, 8*(6), 2209–2227. doi:10.100712649-016-9720-0

Gasparatos, A., Stromberg, P., & Takeuchi, K. (2011). Biofuels, ecosystem services and human wellbeing: Putting biofuels in the ecosystem services narrative. *Agriculture, Ecosystems & Environment, 142*(3-4), 111–128. doi:10.1016/j.agee.2011.04.020

Ghanavati, H., Nahvi, I., & Karimi, K. (2015). Organic fraction of municipal solid waste as a suitable feedstock for the production of lipid by oleaginous yeast Cryptococcus aerius. *Waste Management (New York, N.Y.), 38*, 141–148. doi:10.1016/j.wasman.2014.12.007 PMID:25595390

Gustavsson, J., Cederberg, C., Sonesson, U., Van Otterdijk, R., & Meybeck, A. (2011). *Global food losses and food waste: extent, causes and prevention*. Rome: FAO.

Hogg, D., Barth, J., Schleiss, K., & Favoino, E. (2007). *Dealing with food waste in the UK*. Eunomia Research and Consulting Limited. WRAP. Retrieved from http://www.wrap.org.uk/sites/files/wrap/Dealing_with_Food_Waste_-_Final_2_March_07.pdf

Kiran, E. U., Trzcinski, A. P., Ng, W. J., & Liu, Y. (2014). Bioconversion of food waste to energy: A review. *Fuel, 134*, 389–399. doi:10.1016/j.fuel.2014.05.074

Levis, J. W., Barlaz, M. A., Themelis, N. J., & Ulloa, P. (2010). Assessment of the state of food waste treatment in the United States and Canada. *Waste Management (New York, N.Y.), 30*(8-9), 1486–1494. doi:10.1016/j.wasman.2010.01.031 PMID:20171867

Li, X., Chen, Y., Zhao, S., Chen, H., Zheng, X., Luo, J., & Liu, Y. (2015). Efficient production of optically pure l-lactic acid from food waste at ambient temperature by regulating key enzyme activity. *Water Research, 70*, 148–157. doi:10.1016/j.watres.2014.11.049 PMID:25528545

Liu, H., Ma, X., Li, L., Hu, Z., Guo, P., & Jiang, Y. (2014). The catalytic pyrolysis of food waste by microwave heating. *Bioresource Technology, 166*, 45–50. doi:10.1016/j.biortech.2014.05.020 PMID:24905041

Matsuda, T., Yano, J., Hirai, Y., & Sakai, S. (2012). Life-cycle greenhouse gas inventory analysis of household waste management and food waste reduction activities in Kyoto, Japan. *The International Journal of Life Cycle Assessment, 17*(6), 743–752. doi:10.100711367-012-0400-4

Mirabella, N., Castellani, V., & Sala, S. (2014). Current options for the valorization of food manufacturing waste: A review. *Journal of Cleaner Production, 65*, 28–41. doi:10.1016/j.jclepro.2013.10.051

Mourad, M. (2016). Recycling, recovering and preventing "food waste": Competing solutions for food systems sustainability in the United States and France. *Journal of Cleaner Production, 126*, 461–477. doi:10.1016/j.jclepro.2016.03.084

Nanqi, R., Wanqian, G., Bingfeng, L., Guangli, C., & Jie, D. (2011). Biological hydrogen production by dark fermentation: Challenges and prospects towards scaled-up production. *Current Opinion in Biotechnology, 22*(3), 365–370. doi:10.1016/j.copbio.2011.04.022 PMID:21612910

Opatokun, S. A., Strezov, V., & Kan, T. (2015). Product based evaluation of pyrolysis of food waste and its digestate. *Energy, 92*, 349–354. doi:10.1016/j.energy.2015.02.098

Östergren, K., Gustavsson, J., Bos-Brouwers, H., Timmermans, T., Hansen, O.-J., Møller, H., . . . Redlingshöfer, B. (2014). FUSIONS Definitional Framework for Food Waste. Full Report.

Panesar, P. S., Kennedy, J. F., Gandhi, D. N., & Bunko, K. (2007). Bioutilisation of whey for lactic acid production. *Food Chemistry, 105*(1), 1–14. doi:10.1016/j.foodchem.2007.03.035

Parfitt, J., Barthel, M., & Macnaughton, S. (2010). Food waste within food supply chains: Quantification and potential for change to 2050. *Phil. Trans. R. Soc.*, *365*(1554), 3065–3081. doi:10.1098/rstb.2010.0126 PMID:20713403

Pfaltzgraff, L. A., De bruyn, M., Cooper, E. C., Budarin, V., & Clark, J. H. (2013). Food waste biomass: A resource for high-value chemicals. *Green Chemistry*, *15*(2), 307–3014. doi:10.1039/c2gc36978h

Pham, T. P., Kaushik, R., Parshetti, G. K., Mahmood, R., & Balasubramanian, R. (2015). Food waste-to-energy conversion technologies: Current status and future directions. *Waste Management (New York, N.Y.)*, *38*, 399–408. doi:10.1016/j.wasman.2014.12.004 PMID:25555663

Pirozzi, D., Ausiello, A., & Yousuf, A. (2012). Exploitation of Lignocellulosic Materials for the Production of II Generation Biodiesel. In *Proceeding Venice 2012, Fourth International Symposium on Energy from Biomass and Waste*. Cini Foundation.

Priefer, C., Jörissen, J., & Bräutigam, K.-R. (2016). Food waste prevention in Europe – A cause-driven approach to identify the most relevant leverage points for action. *Resources, Conservation and Recycling*, *109*, 155–165. doi:10.1016/j.resconrec.2016.03.004

Refaat, A. A. (2012). Biofuels from Waste Materials. *J. Compr. Renew. Energy*, *5*, 217–261. doi:10.1016/B978-0-08-087872-0.00518-7

Reis, M., Albuquerque, M., Villano, M., Majone, M. (2011). Mixed culture processes for Resource Futures. *Bournemouth Borough Council Waste Composition Analysis Phase 2 and Sciences*, (1), 17-26.

Reisch, L., Eberle, U., & Sylvia Lorek, S. (2013). Sustainable food consumption: an overview of contemporary issues and policies. *Sustainability: Science, Practice and Policy*, *9*(2), 7–25. doi:10.1080/1 5487733.2013.11908111

Resource Futures. (2009). *Bournemouth Borough Council Waste Composition Analysis Phase 2 and Comparative*. RF Project no.510.

Schanes, K., Dobernig, K., & Gozet, B. (2018). Food Waste Matters—A Systematic Review of Household Food Waste Practices and Their Policy Implications. *Journal of Cleaner Production*, *182*, 978–991. doi:10.1016/j.jclepro.2018.02.030

Segrè, A., & Gaiani, S. (2011). *Transforming Food Waste into Resource*. Cambridge, UK: Royal Society of Chemistry.

Smil, V. (2010). Improving efficiency and reducing waste in our food system. *Environmental Sciences*, *1*(1), 17–26. doi:10.1076/evms.1.1.17.23766

Stoeberl, M., Werkmeistera, R., Faulstichb, M., & Russa, W. (2011). Biobutanol from food wastes – fermentative production, use as biofuel and the influence on the emissions. *Procedia Food Waste*, *1*, 1868–1974.

UN General Assembly. (2015). *Resolution adopted by the General Assembly on 25 September 2015: Transforming our world: the 2030 Agenda for Sustainable Development A/RES/70/1*. Retrieved from www.un.org/ga/search/view_doc.asp? symbol=A/RES/70/1&Lang=E

UNEP. (2014). *Prevention and reduction of food and drink waste in businesses and households - Guidance for governments, local authorities, businesses and other organisations, Version 1.0*. UNEP.

Van Wegen, R. J., Ling, Y., & Middelberg, A. P. J. (1998). Industrial production of polyhydroxyalkanoates using escherichia coli: An economic analysis. *Trans. IChem, E76*(3), 417–426. doi:10.1205/026387698524848

WRAP. (2007). *Understanding Food Waste*. Research Summary. WRAP, Banbury.

WRAP. (2009a). *Household Food and Drink Waste in the UK*. WRAP, Banbury.

Yaakob, Z., Mohammad, M., Alherbawi, M., Alam, Z., & Sopian, K. (2013). Overview of the production of biodiesel from waste cooking oil. *Renewable & Sustainable Energy Reviews, 18*, 184–193. doi:10.1016/j.rser.2012.10.016

Zhang, C., Su, H., Baeyens, J., & Tan, T. (2015). Reviewing the anaerobic digestion of food waste for biogas production. *Renewable & Sustainable Energy Reviews, 38*, 383–392. doi:10.1016/j.rser.2014.05.038

This research was previously published in Global Initiatives for Waste Reduction and Cutting Food Loss edited by Aparna B. Gunjal, Meghmala S. Waghmode, Neha N. Patil, and Pankaj Bhatt; pages 191-211, copyright year 2019 by Engineering Science Reference (an imprint of IGI Global).

Chapter 30
Value–Added Products From Food Waste

Baban Baburao Gunjal
Sunrise Biotech Organisation, India

ABSTRACT

Food waste is the most challenging issue humankind is facing worldwide. Food waste, which consists of carbohydrates, proteins, lipids, and inorganic compounds, is a biodegradable waste discharged from food processing industries, households, and hospitality sectors. The management of food waste is very important. The food waste generated is usually incinerated or dumped in open areas which may cause severe health and environmental issues. The management of food waste can be done by conversion to different value-added products, for example, phytochemicals, bioactive compounds, food supplements, livestock feed, dietary fibers, biopigments and colorants, emulsifiers, edible and essential oils, biopreservatives, biofertilizers, biofuels, and single cell proteins. The value-added products from food waste will be very eco-friendly. The chapter will focus on different value-added products from food waste.

INTRODUCTION

The problem of food waste is increasing, involving all sectors of waste management from collection to disposal. Global food waste is approximately 1.3 billion tons per year (Kojima & Ishikawa, 2013). It is estimated that more food is wasted in the industrialized countries compared to the developing nations on per-capita basis (Gustavsson et al., 2011). The wastes generated from food processing industries are shown in Table 1.

Recently, there is great emphasis on the recovery, recycling and reconditioning of food waste. The efforts are made to convert food waste into value-added products (Laufenberg et al., 2003). The food waste can be converted into useful value-added products viz., phytochemicals, bioactive compounds, food supplements, livestock feed, dietary fibres, biopigments and colourants, emulsifiers, edible and essential oils, biopreservatives, biofertilizers, biofuels and single cell protein. India's share in some agricultural and horticultural produce is shown in Table 2.

DOI: 10.4018/978-1-7998-5354-1.ch030

The potential of vegetable wastes for production of value added products and for the generation of biofuels is an efficient mode of food waste management. Strategies for efficient waste management must be adopted. The best approach for the waste management is reduction of the waste at its source. Socio-economic aspect of waste generation and handling also has to be considered for adopting an efficient strategy of integrated waste management. Food waste is generated as a part of human society at small domestic level and at large industrial level. In developed countries, the waste management practices followed are viz., sanitary landfills, composting, incineration etc. Wastes are collected and mostly dumped in open or burnt in open (Sandra, 2006). This has serious impact on both environment and human health. When dumped in open or in landfills, food wastes get decomposed by the action of various microorganisms. This produces different gases like methane and carbon dioxide both of which contribute to the greenhouse effect leading to global warming (Brown & David, 1994).

The problem of food waste must be solved by converting the waste into various value-added products which will be very eco-friendly and also effective. The various value-added products from carrot, onion, pea, tomato and sugar beet are mushroom, biomethane, biohydrogen, single cell protein, biogas, bioethanol, mushroom, vinegar, α-L-arabinofuranosidase, organic acids, oligomers, fertilizers, glycoalkaloids, animal feeds, etc.

Table 1. Wastes generated from food processing industries

Food processing industry	Waste materials
Animal products	Skins, hides, blood, fats, horns, hairs, bones, liver, intestines
Poultry processing	Skin, blood, fats, hairs, feathers, bones, liver, intestines, wings, trimmed organs
Marine products processing	Shells, roes, trimmed parts, pincers
Cereals and pulse processing	Husk, hull, chaff, stalks
Fruits and vegetable processing	Skin, peels, stones, fibre, pith
Nuts	Shells, coir, pith
Spices and condiments	Hulls, stalks.

(Rao, 2010)

Table 2. India's share in some agricultural and horticultural produce

Fruit / Vegetable	Global production (%)
Mangoes	54
Cauliflower	30
Bananas	23
Green peas	36
Onions	10

Various Value-Added Products From Food Waste

The management of food waste can be done by converting into value-added products. There are many uses of exotic fruits, olives and tomatoes for the production of antioxidants, fibers, phenols, polyphenols and carotenoids. Dairy by-products and slaughter house waste can be potential source for lactic acid and protein extraction (Mirabella et al., 2014).

Fruit processing produce large amount of waste products viz., seeds, kernels, flesh and peels; which contain valuable compounds in higher quantities (Mirabella et al., 2014). Recovery of value-added products from passion fruit processing waste (Mirabella et al., 2014); and pineapple stem (Canteri et al., 2010); amino acids and phenolic compounds from mango seeds (Upadhyay et al., 2012); polyphenols, carotenoids, vitamins, enzymes and dietary fibres from mango peels (Abdalla et al., 2007); coconut protein powder from coconut processing industry waste (Ajila et al., 2010) etc. have been reported.

About 50% of the cheese-whey, the by-product of cheese manufacturing, is converted into value added products viz., whey powder, whey protein, whey permeate, bioethanol, biopolymers, hydrogen, methane, single cell protein (Siso, 1996; Yadav et al., 2015). Cheese-whey is known to consist of mostly lactose (4.5-5% w/v), soluble proteins (0.6-0.8% w/v), lipids (0.4-0.5% w/v) and mineral salts (8-10% of dried extract); less quantities of lactic acid, citric acid, non-protein nitrogen compounds and B vitamins are also reported (Prazeres et al., 2012).

Ethanol Production From the Food Waste

There is a report where food waste with a composition of 23.3% w/w total reducing sugars, 34.8% w/w starch, and 1.6% w/w fibres has been converted for the ethanol production (Zhang & Richard, 2011). Similarly, Moon et al. (2009) also studied ethanol production from food waste with high starch (30.1% w/w) and fibre (14.9% w/w) contents, with a total of 17.6% w/w reducing sugars. Matsakas et al. (2014) reported ethanol yield of 108 g/kg dry material from household food waste. The bioethanol yield from various food residues and wastes is shown in Table 3.

Table 3. Bioethanol yield from various food residues and wastes

Food residue/wastes	Country	Bioethanol yield (%)	Reference
Switch grass	USA	72	(Asli et al., 2008)
Corn steep liquor	USA and Brazil	No yield	(Ruanglek et al., 2006)
Brewer's yeast autolysate	Thailand	88	(Ruanglek et al., 2006)
Waste potato	Finland	87	(Liimatainen et al., 2004)
Oil palm empty fruit	Malaysia	Not specified	(Ibrahim et al., 2012; Razak et al., 2013)

Food Waste to Biogas

Food wastes are good source of biogas that can be used in plants. Due to high moisture content of food wastes, bioconversion technologies such as anaerobic digestion are more suitable compared to thermo-chemical conversion technologies. Many researchers have studied the potential of food waste for biogas production. Recently, Chinese researchers studied the anaerobic digestion of food waste resulting in final total solids and volatile solids. Due to this, the quantity of wasted food decreases and also produces clean biogas (Yang et al., 2015; Zhang et al., 2014).

Glycoalkaloids From Potato Waste

In countries like Ireland, the potato production in 2010 was 450,000 tonnes. Industrial processing of potatoes generates large quantities of peel which creates disposal, sanitation, and environmental problems. The potato peels are rich in glycoalkaloids such as α-solanine and α-chaconine; carbohydrates; starch; and proteins.

Marine Food Waste for Production of Oligomers

The fish waste is a potential source of high-value biochemicals, such as biopolymers (chitin, chitosan), pigments (carotenoid, astaxanthin), minerals, and proteins. The different value-added products from the marine food wastes are viz., chitin and chitosan oligomers.

Fruit Wastes for Single Cell Protein Production

Fruit wastes have been used as substrates for the production of Single Cell Protein (SCP) by many researchers. Sweet orange residues have been used for SCP production (Nwabueze & Oguntimein, 1987). Rahmat et al. (1995) used apple pomace for the production of single cell protein from *Kloechera apiculata* and *Candida utilis* so as to improve stock feed. Pineapple cannery effluent has been utilized for SCP production by Nigam (1998). Essien et al. (2005) utilized banana peel as a substrate for mould growth and biomass production.

Food Wastes as Substrates for the Production of Organic Fertilizers

After food wastes are degraded by aerobic microorganism, the secondary pollution is avoided, and has good environmental benefits. The degradation products can be divided into organic fertilizer, bio-organic fertilizer and soil conditioner, which contain plant growth promoting substances. This will reduce the use of chemical fertilizers and therefore pollution also will be reduced.

Food Processing Wastes as Substrates for the Production of Animal Feeds

The food processing wastes can be used in the production of animal feed. Soya bean cake obtained after extraction of the soya bean milk and groundnut cake obtained from the groundnut processing industry have been used for the production of animal feeds.

Vegetable Oil and Its By-Products

The vegetable oil industry generates number of waste products. India produces about 70 lakh tons of vegetable oil. The phytosterols can be obtained from vegetable oils during refining process, which has nutraceutical value. The value-added products from vegetable oil industry is shown in Table 4.

Table 4. Value-added products from vegetable oil industry

Oil seeds	Primary product	Secondary product	Value-added products
Soybean	Soyabean oil	Gum sludge, deodorizer distillate, soap stock, deoiled cake	Soy protein, isoflavones, lecithin, tocopherol, fatty acids
Cotton seed	Cotton seed oil	Gum sludge, deodourizer distillate, soap stock, deoiled cake	Protein, gossypol, fatty acids, lecithin
Sunflower	Sunflower oil	Gum sludge, deodourizer distillate, soap stock, deoiled cake	Sunflower seed protein, lecithin, tocopherol concentrate, wax, fatty acids
Rape-mustard seed	Mustard oil	Gum sludge, deodourizer distillate, soap stock, deoiled cake	Mustard seed protein, glucosinolate concentrate, lecithin, tocopherols
Palm fruit	Palm oil, palm kernel oil	Gum sludge, deodourizer distillate, soap stock, deoiled cake	Beta-carotene, tocotrienol, palm stearin, palmitic and oleic acids, lecithin, carotenoids
Rice	Rice bran oil and chemically refined oils	Gum sludge, wax sludge, deodorizer distillate, fatty acids, soap stock, deoiled cake	Rice bran protein, coenzyme Q10, rice bran fibre for food purposes, lecithin, oryzanol, tocotrienols, squalene, phytosterols, wax, fatty acids

High Value By-Products From Fruits and Vegetables

Peel is the major waste generated from fruits. The peel after fruit processing undergoes rapid changes in quality for the generation of secondary value-added products. They can be used for the production of secondary products viz., pectin, mucilage, gum, anthocyanin, carotenoids, antioxidants, antimicrobials and fermented products. Fruit peels are the best source for compounds such as polyphenols, flavonoids, tannins, catechins and vitamins. The potential anthocyanin sources are blackcurrant, chokeberry, egg-plant, orange, blackberry, vaccinium, raspberry, cherry, redcurrent, red grape, etc.

There are also many by-products which can be obtained from grape processing from seeds (grape seed oil) and skin (resveratrol, polyphenols). The use of grape skin colour powder includes beverages, sauces, baking and red wine. The extract after being processed with beverages, milk, chocolates, candy, etc. produces food products which are good for health. The grape waste can also be processed to get the value-added product polyphenolics which can be used as phytoceuticals.

Organic Acids From Food Waste

Lactic acid, acetic acid, oxalic acids are important because of their various applications existing from food industry to pharmaceuticals. They can be produced by fermentation process by the activity of different microorganisms. Various organic acids are produced by the microbial fermentation. Some of the examples are citric acid, lactic acid and acetic acid by *Aspergillus niger, Lactobacillus delbrueckii* and *Acetobacter aceti,* respectively (Sethi and Maini, 1999). Various substrates have been used for the citric acid production by fermentation process, but recently agricultural wastes have been used on high demand due to their abundant availability (Soccol et al., 2006). Among them, citric acid is an important chemical having worldwide demand due to its high usage and low toxicity. Beet molasses have been used for citric acid production. Zhang and Jin (2009) studied lactic acid production using potato starch waste where the lactic acid production obtained was 103.8 g/l in 48 h fermentation. Sugar beet molasses have been used as low-cost substrate for oxalic acid production using different reactors. High production was obtained in the reactor having nitrogen oxide (Guru et al., 2001). Acetic acid, another organic acid can be produced by carrots and white radish leafage. Carrots have been used as the substrate in the hydrothermal two stage production of acetic acid which resulted in high yield (Jin et al., 2005).

Natural Food Colours and Dyes

Natural colour has advantage over synthetic colours. These natural food colours are obtained from vegetable, animal or mineral. The natural colours come from sources viz., seeds, fruits, vegetables, leaves, algae and insects. The examples of commonly used natural colours are Annatto (seed), turmeric, beet juice (root), red cabbage (vegetable), spinach (leaf), anthocyanins, β-carotene, carmine, curcumin, canthaxanthin, etc.

Polyhydroxybutyrate Production From the Food Waste

Polyhydroxybutyrate (PHB) is a biopolymer used as a biodegradable thermoplastic material for waste management strategies and biocompatibility in medical devices (Gouda et al., 2001). It has wide applications viz., packaging, pharmaceuticals, chemical and cosmetic industries. Vegetable and food wastes have now been used as substrates for production of PHB in a cost effective way (Carucci et al., 2001; Koller et al., 2008). Rusendi and Sheppard (1995) reported the use of potato processing waste from the potato-chip plant for the production of PHB. Hafuka et al. (2011) reported 87% PHB yield from food wastes after 259 h of incubation.

CONCLUSION

Different value-added products viz., single cell protein; biogas; polymers; feed; organic fertilizers; organic acids; colours and dyes; PHB; etc. will be obtained from food waste. The value-added products from food waste will be very eco-friendly. This will help the management of food waste which is very important. The different value-added products from food waste have many applications.

Future Possibilities

Food waste recycling will help mitigate greenhouse gas emissions. Food waste management also play important role to control environmental pollutants.

REFERENCES

Abdalla, A. M., Darwish, S. M., Ayad, E. E., & El-Hamahmy, R. M. (2007). Egyptian mango by-product 1. Compositional quality of mango seed kernel. *Food Chemistry, 103*(4), 1134–1140. doi:10.1016/j.foodchem.2006.10.017

Ajila, C. M., Aalami, M., Leelavathi, K., & Rao, U. P. (2010). Mango peel powder: A potential source of antioxidant and dietary fibre in macaroni preparations. *Innovative Food Science & Emerging Technologies, 11*(1), 219–224. doi:10.1016/j.ifset.2009.10.004

Asli, I., Jennifer, N. H., & Anthony, L. (2008). Aqueous ammonia soaking of switchgrass followed by simultaneous saccharification and fermentation. *Applied Biochemistry and Biotechnology, 144*(1), 69–77. doi:10.100712010-007-8008-z PMID:18415988

Brown, K. A., & David, M. H. (1994). Using landfill gas: A UK perspective. *Renewable Energy, 5*(5-8), 774–781. doi:10.1016/0960-1481(94)90086-8

Canteri, M. G., Scheer, A., Wosiacki, G., Ginies, C., Reich, M., & Renard, C. G. (2010). A comparative study of pectin extracted from passion fruit rind flours. *Journal of Polymers and the Environment, 18*(4), 593–599. doi:10.100710924-010-0206-z

Carucci, A., Dionisi, D., Majone, M., Rolle, E., & Smurra, P. (2001). Aerobic storage by activated sludge on real wastewater. *Water Research, 35*(16), 3833–3844. doi:10.1016/S0043-1354(01)00108-7 PMID:12230166

Essien, J. P., Akpan, E. J., & Essien, E. P. (2005). Studies on mould growth and biomass production using waste banana peel. *Bioresource Technology, 96*(13), 1451–1456. doi:10.1016/j.biortech.2004.12.004 PMID:15939272

Gouda, M. K., Swellam, A. E., & Omar, S. H. (2001). Production of PHB by a *Bacillus megaterium* strain using sugarcane molasses and corn steep liquor as sole carbon and nitrogen source. *Microbiological Research Journal, 156*(3), 201–204. doi:10.1078/0944-5013-00104 PMID:11716209

Guru, M., Bilgesu, A. Y., & Pamuk, V. (2001). Production of oxalic acid from sugar beet molasses by formed nitrogen oxides. *Bioresource Technology, 77*(1), 81–86. doi:10.1016/S0960-8524(00)00122-X PMID:11211079

Gustavsson, J., Cederberg, C., Sonesson, U., van Otterdijk, R., & Meybeck, A. (2011). Global food losses and food waste. Extent, causes and prevention. Rome: Academic Press.

Hafuka, A., Sakaida, K., Satoh, H., Takahashi, M., Watanabe, Y., & Okabe, S. (2011). Effect of feeding regimens on polyhydroxybutyrate production from food wastes by *Cupriavidus necator*. *Bioresource Technology, 102*(3), 3551–3553. doi:10.1016/j.biortech.2010.09.018 PMID:20870404

Ibrahim, M. F., Abd-Azizi, S., Razak, M. A., Phang, L. Y., & Hassan, M. A. (2012). Oil palm empty fruit bunch as alternative substrate for acetone-butanol-ethanol production by *Clostridium butyricum* EB6. *Applied Biochemistry and Biotechnology, 166*(7), 1615–1625. doi:10.100712010-012-9538-6 PMID:22391689

Jin, F., Zhou, Z., Moriya, T., Kishida, H., Higashijima, H., & Enomoto, H. (2005). Controlling hydrothermal reaction pathways to improve acetic acid production from carbohydrate biomass. *Environmental Science & Technology*, *39*(6), 1893–1902. doi:10.1021/es048867a PMID:15819253

Kojima, R., & Ishikawa, M. (2013). Prevention and recycling of food wastes in Japan: Policies and achievements. Kobe University.

Koller, R., Chiellini, B. E., Fernandes, E. G., Horvat, P., Kutschera, C., Hesse, P., & Braunegg, G. (2008). Polyhydroxy alkanoate production from whey by *Pseudomonas hydrogenovora*. *Bioresource Technology*, *99*(11), 4854–4863. doi:10.1016/j.biortech.2007.09.049 PMID:18053709

Laufenberg, G., Kunz, B., & Nystroem, M. (2003). Transformation of vegetable waste into value-added products: (A) the upgrading concept; (B) practical implementations. *Bioresource Technology*, *87*(2), 167–198. doi:10.1016/S0960-8524(02)00167-0 PMID:12765356

Liimatainen, H., Kuokkanen, T. K., & Ariainen, J. (2004). Development of bioethanol production from waste potatoes. In *Proceedings of the Waste Minimization and Resources Use Optimization Conference*. University of Oulu.

Matsakas, L., Kekos, D., Loizidou, M., & Christakopoulos, P. (2014). Utilization of household food waste for the production of ethanol at high dry material content. *Biotechnology for Biofuels*, *7*(1), 1–9. doi:10.1186/1754-6834-7-4 PMID:24401142

Mirabella, N., Castellani, V., & Sala, S. (2014). Current options for the valorization of food manufacturing waste: A review. *Journal of Cleaner Production*, *65*, 28–41. doi:10.1016/j.jclepro.2013.10.051

Moon, H. C., Song, I. S., Kim, J. C., Shirai, Y., Lee, D. H., Kim, J. K., ... Cho, Y. S. (2009). Enzymatic hydrolysis of food waste and ethanol fermentation. *International Journal of Energy Research*, *33*(2), 164–172. doi:10.1002/er.1432

Nigam, J. N. (1998). Single cell protein from pineapple cannery effluent. *World Journal of Microbiology & Biotechnology*, *14*(5), 693–696. doi:10.1023/A:1008853303596

Nwabueze, T. U., & Ogumtimein, G. B. (1987). Sweet orange (*Citrus sinensis*) residue as a substrate for single cell protein production. *Biological Wastes*, *20*(1), 71–75. doi:10.1016/0269-7483(87)90085-1

Prazeres, A. R., Carvalho, F., & Rivas, J. (2012). Cheese whey management: A review. *Journal of Environmental Management*, *110*, 48–68. doi:10.1016/j.jenvman.2012.05.018 PMID:22721610

Rahmat, H., Hodge, R., Manderson, G., & Yu, P. (1995). Solid substrate fermentation of *Kloechera apiculata* and *Candida utilis* on apple pomace to produce an improved stock-feed. *World Journal of Microbiology & Biotechnology*, *11*(2), 168–170. doi:10.1007/BF00704641 PMID:24414495

Rao, D. G. (2010). *Fundamentals of food engineering*. New Delhi: PHI Learning Private Ltd.

Razak, M. A., Ibrahim, M. F., Yee, P. L., Hassan, M. A., & Abd-Azizi, S. (2013). Statistical optimization of butanol Production from oil palm decantater cake hydrolysate by *Clostridium acetobutylicum* ATCC 824. *BioResources*, *8*, 1758–1770.

Ruanglek, V., Maneewatthana, D., & Tripetchkul, S. (2006). Evaluation of thai agroindustrial wastes for bio-ethanol production by *Zymomonas mobilis*. *Process Biochemistry*, *41*(6), 1432–1437. doi:10.1016/j.procbio.2006.01.010

Rusendi, D., & Sheppard, J. D. (1995). Hydrolysis of potato processing waste for the production of poly-ß hydroxybutyrate. *Bioresource Technology*, *54*(2), 191–196. doi:10.1016/0960-8524(95)00124-7

Sandra, C. (2006). Occupational and environmental health issues of solid waste management. The World Bank Group.

Sethi, V., & Maini, S. B. (1999). Production of organic acids. In V. K. Joshi & A. Pandey (Eds.), *Biotechnology: Food Fermentation, Microbiology, Biochemistry and Technology* (pp. 1259–1290). New Delhi: Educational Publishers and Distributors.

Siso, M. G. (1996). The biotechnological utilization of cheese whey: A review. *Bioresource Technology*, *57*(1), 1–11. doi:10.1016/0960-8524(96)00036-3

Soccol, C. R., Vandenberghe, L. S., Rodrigues, C., & Pandey, A. (2006). New perspectives for citric acid production and application. *Food Technology and Biotechnology*, *44*, 141–149.

Upadhyay, A., Chompoo, J., Araki, N., & Tawata, S. (2012). Antioxidant, antimicrobial, 15-LOX, and AGEs inhibitions by pineapple stem waste. *Journal of Food Science*, *77*(1), H9–H15. doi:10.1111/j.1750-3841.2011.02437.x PMID:22260109

Yang, L., Huang, Y., Zhao, M., Huang, Z., Miao, H., Xu, Z., & Ruan, W. (2015). Enhancing biogas generation performance from food wastes by high-solids thermophilic anaerobic digestion: Effect of pH adjustment. *International Biodeterioration & Biodegradation*, *105*, 153–159. doi:10.1016/j.ibiod.2015.09.005

Zhang, C., Su, H., Baeyens, J., & Tan, T. (2014). Reviewing the anaerobic digestion of food waste for biogas production. *Renewable & Sustainable Energy Reviews*, *38*, 383–392. doi:10.1016/j.rser.2014.05.038

Zhang, X., & Richard, T. (2011). Dual enzymatic saccharification of food waste for ethanol fermentation. *Proceedings of international conference on electrical and control engineering*. 10.1109/ICECENG.2011.6058308

This research was previously published in Global Initiatives for Waste Reduction and Cutting Food Loss edited by Aparna B. Gunjal, Meghmala S. Waghmode, Neha N. Patil, and Pankaj Bhatt; pages 20-30, copyright year 2019 by Engineering Science Reference (an imprint of IGI Global).

Chapter 31
Microbe Mediated Bioconversion of Fruit Waste Into Value Added Products:
Microbes in Fruit Waste Management

Mridul Umesh
Bharathiar University, India

Thazeem Basheer
Bharathiar University, India

ABSTRACT

Biosynthetic capabilities of microbes have solved several hurdles in the human welfare. Microbes have served and continue to serve as imperial candidates in both production and management strategies. Microbe mediated techniques has emerged as ecofriendly and sustainable alternative to their synthetic counterparts. Fruit based industries produces large volumes of solid and liquid wastes contributing to increase in pollution load. Disposal of these waste not only represent loss of valuable biomass but also leads to substantial increase in Biological Oxygen Demand (BOD) and Chemical Oxygen Demand (COD). However, in spite of their pollution and hazard aspects, in many cases, fruit processing wastes have a promising potential for being chief raw materials for secondary industries. This chapter summarizes microbe mediated fermentative utilization of fruit waste, for the production of value added products like organic acid, single cell protein, bioplastics, enzymes and biogas.

INTRODUCTION

The exponential growth of the human population has led to the accumulation of huge amounts of biodegradable and non-biodegradable waste materials across the world (Rivard et al., 1995). Living conditions in the biosphere are therefore changing dramatically, in such a way that the presence of waste residues is affecting the potential survival of many species. Fruit peels are a class of agro wastes that may be

DOI: 10.4018/978-1-7998-5354-1.ch031

regarded as a non-product flow of raw materials having economic values less than the cost of collection and recovery for reuse. Fruit based industries produces large volumes of wastes, both solid and liquid; these wastes pose increased disposal and pollution (High BOD or COD) problems and represents a loss of valuable biomass and nutrients. In spite of their hazardous effects contributing to environmental pollution, fruit peels have a good potential for conversion into useful products of higher value as by-product, or even as raw materials for other industries. Fruit waste contain an appreciable amount of carbohydrates which could be utilized by microorganisms producing economically important Biopolymers, Single Cell Proteins, Organic acids, Enzymes, Biogas etc. with potential application in food, fuel, agriculture, packaging, and pharmaceutical industries.

Bioplastics especially polyhydroxyalkanoates (PHA's) are exclusively synthesized as intracellular carbon and energy storage compounds by wide range of microorganisms and are reported to be completely degraded in to benign compounds both aerobically and anaerobically (Lemoigne, 1926). Their material properties closely resemble synesthetic plastics and thus are emerging to be the best alternatives to their synthetic counterparts. The ability to be synthesized from a wide variety of waste substrates along with their fully degradable nature is an added advantage to this kind of biopolymers.

SCPs are protein rich microbial biomass or total proteins extracted from microbial cell that could be used as protein supplements in food and feed (Gour et al., 2015). Their nutritious value and growth promoting essential amino acids content makes them ideal for tackling the global issues associated with Protein Calorific Malnutrition (PCM). Production of organic acids from fruits and fruit wastes dates back to several centuries. It is still an important industry that sustains the economy of many developed, developing and under developed countries. Acetic acid, butyric acid, lactic acid, citric acid and tartaric acid are the well-known examples of microbe mediated 'organic acids'. Enzyme production from fruit wastes using microbes could pave as a sustainable method for reducing cost of production. Fruit peels are used for the commercial production of enzymes like amylase, protease, and laccase. Microbes could also be exploited as tools for production of bioethanol and biogas from fruit peels. This serves as a promising alternative for increasing energy crisis all over the world.

Fruit peel wastes could be thus considered as valuable by-product if appropriate technical means are used to increase the value of the subsequent products to exceed the cost of reprocessing. This chapter highlights easily adoptable microbiological methodologies for recycling, reprocessing and eventual utilization of fruit peel wastes for the production of value added products rather than their discharge to the environment.

Background of the Study

Fruit wastes represent an important class of food processing waste that has been turned to be a menace for all the countries due to problems associated with their disposal and treatment. Majorly it consists of large fractions of solid or semi-solid waste generated during the separation of desired products from undesired ones in early stages of processing. Undesirable constituents discharged from fruit-based industries include fruit peels, seeds, extracted pulp and pits. Usages of these wastes either as feed ingredient for livestock or application on land are two conventional methods of fruit waste management. Major characteristic of fruit processing industries are wide range of waste water and organic load. Biological Oxygen Demand (BOD) and Total Suspended Solids (TSS) accounts for the chief pollutants in the fruit-based waste. Fruit based industries are conservative and reluctant to invest capital in waste management principles. The fruit processing industry produces 12 million tons of fruit annually. This in turn generates approximately 39 billion gal of waste water and 4.7 million tons of solid residuals. Fruit processing waste majorly contain mostly biodegradable organic matter in both soluble and insoluble forms (Omoregie et al., 2013). Due to the presence of high volume of suspended solids and BOD, fruit wastes can lead to serious environmental concerns when discharged in to the main streams. Microorganisms metabolize the organic matter present in the waste water thereby reducing the oxygen concentration that leading to the death of aquatic organisms. Continuous oxygen depletion triggers the anaerobic decomposition of organic matter and producing foul odor and stream discoloration.

MAJOR FOCUS OF THE CHAPTER

The thrust for development of integrated production strategies in food industries along with substantial byproduct utilization has paved way for valorization of fruit waste rather than their usage as feed or composting materials. Microbial mediated bioconversion has always been excelled as an important tool in waste management and product development (Bayer et al., 2007).

Organic Acid

Microbes have been exploited as the important biological agents for the production of organic acid from a wide variety of substrates. This trend continues even during the 21st century due to their robust nature to support fermentation and ability to utilize even the very cheap agricultural waste serves as feed stock for organic acid production. Microbial fermentation has advantages over chemical synthesis of organic acid which includes their ability to use waste as substrate for acid production, ease in recovery process, cost of production is low and problems associated with disposal of waste chemicals is nullified. These factors make them ideal and affordable even for developing and under developed countries. The major organic acids produced from fruit waste along with their applications in various sectors are illustrated in Figure 1.

Figure 1. Important organic acid and their uses

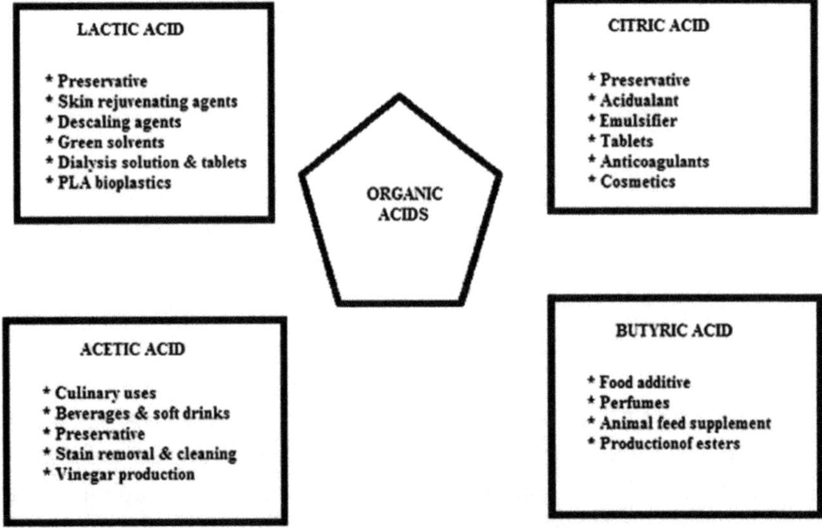

Lactic Acid

Lactic acid classified as GRAS (generally regarded as safe) for use as a food additive by the US FDA (Food and Drug Administration), can be produced by either microbial fermentation or chemical synthesis. There are two optical isomers of lactic acid: L (+) -lactic acid and D (-) –lactic acid. Depending upon organism, metabolic pathways differ when glucose is the main carbon source: homofermentative bacteria yield two lactic acid molecules from a glucose molecule whereas the heterofermentative bacteria transform a glucose molecule in to lactate, ethanol and carbon dioxide. Lactic Acid Bacteria (LAB) consist of a number of bacterial genera within the phylum *Firmicutes*. The genera *Coronobacterium, Enterococcus, Lactobacillus, Lactococcus, Lactosphaera, Leuconostoc, Melissococcus, Oenococcus, Pediococcus, Streptococcus, Tetragenococcus, Vagococcus and Weissella* are recognized as the Lactic Acid Bacteria (Ercolini et al., 2001). Lactic acid production from fruit waste was reported in many literatures (Mridul & Preethi, 2014; Pushparani et al., 2012) Production of lactic acid from fruit waste through microbial fermentation can be depicted through the flow diagram:

Fruit Waste → Acid hydrolysis/ Enzymatic treatment →Fermentable Carbohydrates → Microbial Fermentation → Recovery and Purification

Lactic acid is also used in pharmaceutical industry as an electrolyte in many parenteral and intra venal solutions that are intended to replenish the body fluids or electrolytes. Example includes Lactated Ringer's or Hartmann's solutions, CAPD (continuous ambulatory peritoneal dialysis) solution, and dialysis solution for conventional artificial kidney machines. Moreover, lactic acid is used in preparation of tablets, prostheses, surgical sutures and controlled drug delivery systems (Pushparani et al., 2012).

Lactic acid offers natural ingredients for cosmetic applications. Although primarily used as moisturizers and pH regulators, they possess multiple other properties such as antimicrobial activity, skin lightening and skin hydration. The moisturizing effect is related directly to lactate's water retaining capacity and the skin lightening action of lactic acid is produced by the suppression of the formation of tyrosinase. Since they are naturally ingredients of the human body, lactic acid and its salt fit perfectly in to the modern trend towards natural and safer formulations, and they produce such effect as skin lightening and rejuvenation which makes them very useful as active ingredients in cosmetics.

Lactic acid and its salts are used increasingly in various types of chemical products and processes. In this category of application, lactic acid function as a descaling agent, pH regulator, neutralizer, chiral intermediate, solvent, cleaning agent, metal complexing agent, antimicrobial agent, and humectants. Natural lactic acid serves as an excellent and clean solvent as compared to their synthetic counterparts for cleansing application. Due to the high solvency power and solubility of lactic acid, it is an excellent remover of polymer and resins. It is available with an isomeric purity of 98%, and is suitable as a starting material in the production of herbicides or pharmaceuticals. Since lactic acid offers better descaling properties than conventional organic descalers do, it is often used in many decalcification products, such as bathroom cleaners, coffee machines, and toilets. Ethyl lactate is used in many anti-acne preparations, because it combines excellent solvency power against oils and polymeric stains, with no environmental impact and toxicological effects.

Lactic acid is considered the most potential monomer for chemical conversion, because it contains two reactive functional groups, a carboxylic group and a hydroxyl group. Lactic acid can undergo a variety of chemical conversions into potentially useful chemicals, such as propylene oxide (via hydrogenation), acetaldehyde (via decarboxylation), acrylic acid (via dehydration), propanoic acid (via reduction), and dilactide (via self –esterification). Lactic acid has recently received a great deal of attention as a feedstock monomer for the production of Poly Lactic Acid (PLA), which serves as a biodegradable commodity plastic. The optically pure lactic acid can be polymerized in to a high molecular mass PLA through serial reactions of polydecondensation, depolymerization, and ring-opening polymerization. The resultant polymer, PLA, has numerous uses in a wide range of application, such as protective clothing, food packaging, mulch film, trash bags, rigid containers, shrink wrap and short life trays. The huge growth of the PLA market will stimulate future demands on lactic acid considerably.

Success of fermentative production of lactic acid relies on the availability of cheap raw materials, because polymer producers and other industrial users usually require large quantities of lactic acid at a relatively low cost. Raw materials for lactic acid production should have the following characteristics: cheap, low levels of contaminating microbes, rapid production rate, high yield, little or no by-product formation, ability to be fermented with little or no pretreatment and year-round availability. When refined materials are used for production the costs for production and the costs for product purification should be significantly reduced. However still it is not economically favorable as refined carbohydrates are so expensive that they eventually result in higher production costs. Therefore, there have been many attempts to screen for cheap raw material for economical production of lactic acid (John et al., 2007).

Cheap raw materials, such as starch and cellulosic materials, whey, and molasses have been used for lactic acid production. Among these, starch and cellulosic materials are currently receiving a great deal of attention, because they are cheap and abundant renewable source. The starch material used for lactic acid production includes sweet sorghum, wheat, corn, cassava, potato, rice, rye and barley. These materials have to be hydrolyzed in to fermentable sugars before fermentation, because they consist of mainly α (1, 4) and α (1, 6) linkage between glucose molecules. This hydrolysis can be simultaneously with fermentation (Ligouri et al., 2013).

Cellulosic materials have been used for lactic acid production in similar ways as starch materials. These materials consist mainly of (1, 4) – glucan and often contain xylan, arabinan, galactan and lignin. The utilization of corncob, waste paper and wood has been reported as well. Sreenath et al., (2001) investigated the production of lactic acid from agricultural residues such as alfalfa fiber, wheat bran, corn stover and wheat straw. They suggested that, during SSF of alfalfa fiber, lactic acid production was enhanced by adding pectinase and cellulase together. Garde et al., (2002), used hemicellulose hydrolyzate from wheat straw for lactic acid production by co-culture of *L. brevis* and *L. pentosus*. Fermentation of lignocellulosic hydrolyzate is inhibited usually by inhibitory compounds, such as furfural, 5-hydroxy-methyl furfural and acetic acid, which are generated during pre-treatment of lignocellulose. Most studies on methods to decrease this inhibition have been focused on the chemical and physical detoxification of the hydrolyzate. Wee et al., (2005) however, reported that the inhibition of fermentation caused by wood hydrolyzate was reduced to a slight degree by direct adaptation of LAB to the wood hydrolyzate-based medium.

Some industrial waste products, such as whey and molasses are of interest for common substrates for lactic acid production. Whey is a major by-product of the dairy industry and it contains lactose, protein, fat and mineral salts. For complete utilization of whey lactose, it is necessary to supplement whey with an additional nitrogen source. Amrane and Prigent (1998), Kulozik and Wilde (1999), and Schepers et al., (2002) supplemented whey with yeast extract for rapid production of lactic acid with *L. helveticus*. According to Fitzpatrick and O'Keeffe (2001) the addition of whey protein hydrolyzate to whey medium would make the fermentation more economically viable and would also reduce the amount of unused nutrients left during fermentation. There were several attempts to produce lactic acid from whey by batch culture of *L. casei*. Molasses is a waste product from the sugar manufacturing process and it usually contains a large amount of sucrose. *L. delbrueckii* and *E. faecalis* have recently been used for lactic acid production from molasses. Shukla et al., (2004) also reported D (–)-lactic acid production from molasses with recombinant strains of *E. coli*.

It is necessary to supplement the fermentation media with sufficient nutrients for rapid lactic acid production. The most common nutrient for lactic acid production is yeast extract, but this may contribute significantly to an increase in production costs. As an alternative to yeast extract, corn steep liquor, a by-product from the corn steeping process, has been used successfully for lactic acid production. Since it is derived from corn, 85% of its total nitrogen content is composed of proteins, peptides and amino acids. Yun et al., (2004) suggested that rice bran and wheat bran play important roles as effective nutrients for lactic acid production, because they usually contain several nutritional factors as well as fermentable carbohydrates. Kurbanoglu (2003) demonstrated that ram horn waste was an effective supplement for lactic acid production. Similarly, Bustos et al., (2004) proposed that vinification lees could be used for the formulation of low-cost media for lactic acid production. According to Wee et al., (2004) wastewater from electrodialyzed fermentation broth still contained some nutrients that could be available to LAB. Their result indicated that, if small amounts of other nutrients were supplemented to electro dialysis wastewater, then the efficiencies of fermentation would be improved significantly (Yun et al., 2004).

Agro wastes may be regarded non product flows of raw materials whose economic values are less than the cost of collection and recovery for reuse; and are therefore discarded.These wastes could be considered valuable by-product if appropriate technical means are used to increase the value of the subsequent products to exceed the cost of reprocessing. Recycling, reprocessing and eventual utilization of food processing residues offer potential of returning these by-product to beneficial uses rather than their discharge to the environment which might cause detrimental environmental effects. Food industries produces large volumes of wastes both solids and liquids; these wastes pose increasing disposal and pollution (High BOD or COD) problem and represent a loss of valuable biomass and nutrients. However, in spite of their pollution and hazard aspects, in many cases, food processing wastes have a good potential for conversion into useful products of higher value as by-product, or even as raw materials for other industries. Organic acids are example of such valuable by-product of the fermentation of high carbohydrate containing industrial substrates. Fruit peels contain an appreciable amount of carbohydrates which could be utilized by microorganisms producing intermediate volume of high value organic acid like lactic acid.

Lactic acid, an intermediate – volume specialty chemical is under increasing demand in food, pharmaceutical and chemical industries and for the production of Poly lactic acid polymers, which possess excellent biomedical applications. The global production of this organic acid is estimated to be 100 million pounds/year and is expected to grow by 8.6% annually. In India, the annual production capacity of Lactic acid is 6000t and estimated gaps of 2300t in supply by the year 2015 have been predicted, if the present level of production is not increased. Starch rich waste substrates could be used for meeting this growing demand for lactic acid, if appropriate biotechnological interventions are used and specific sectors amongst the Indian food processing industry are targeted.

The biotechnological processes for the production of lactic acid from cheap raw materials should be improved further to make them competitive with the chemically derived one.

Acetic Acid

Acetic acid is formed through multistep process involving conversion of starch to sugar by amylases, anaerobic conversion of sugars to ethanol by yeast fermentation, conversion of ethanol to hydrated acetaldehyde and dehydrogenation to acetic acid by aldehyde dehydrogenase. The last two steps are performed aerobically with the aid of acetic acid forming bacteria. Vinegar bacteria also called acetic acid bacteria, are members of the genus *Acetobacter* characterized by their ability to convert ethyl alcohol into acetic acid, by oxidation as shown below:

Fruit waste → Acetic acid bacteria/ Yeast → Anaerobic fermentation

Ethanol → Acetic acid bacteria → Oxidation → Acetic acid

Earlier processes used for making acetic acid were the Orleans process (which is also known as the slow process), the quick process (which is also called the generator process) and the submerged culture process. The quick process and submerged culture process were developed and are used for commercial acetic production today. Acetic acid can be produced from fruit peel waste containing appreciable amount of carbohydrates through fermentation process (Vikas & Mridul, 2014).

- **Citric Acid:** Citric acid is an intermediate in Tri Carboxylic Acid cycle and is a commercially valuable product with wide spread applications. It is produced through submerged fermentation in commercial scale from sucrose rich media. In small scale citric acid can be produced through solid state fermentation. In recent years, citric acid is produced from fruit wastes like grape pomace, kiwi fruit peel, carob pod, pineapple peels, orange peels and mosami peels. The microbial strains used in commercial production of citric acid from carbohydrate rich waste include *Aspergillus niger, Candida sp.* and *Bacillus licheniformis* (Kumar et al., 2003; Imandi et al., 2008).

Butyric Acid

Butyric acid belongs to the class of short chain fatty acids widely used in the manufacture of textile fibers, heat and temperature resistant films. Salts of butyric acid are used as flavoring agents in food. It is used extensively in the production of drugs used for treatment of gastrointestinal disorders and cancer (Bouallagui et al., 2004). Butyric acid is commercially produced through chemical synthesis using crude oil or through microbial fermentation approach. Despite of its high cost of production, microbial fermentation of butyric acid is unavoidable for some specific application. Butyric acid is produced by anaerobic microorganism belonging to the genera – *Clostridium, Fusobacterium* and *Sarcina*. Microbial production of butyric acid from fruit waste could be out lined in Figure 2.

Single Cell Proteins

Single cell proteins are dried microbial biomass or total proteins extracted from microbes that could be used as protein supplement in both food and feed. It is also called as bioprotein or microbial protein. Apart from high protein content (about 60-82% of dry cell weight) SCP also contains fats, carbohydrates, nucleic acids, vitamins and minerals. Another advantage with SCP is that it is rich in certain essential

Figure 2. Butyric acid production pathway

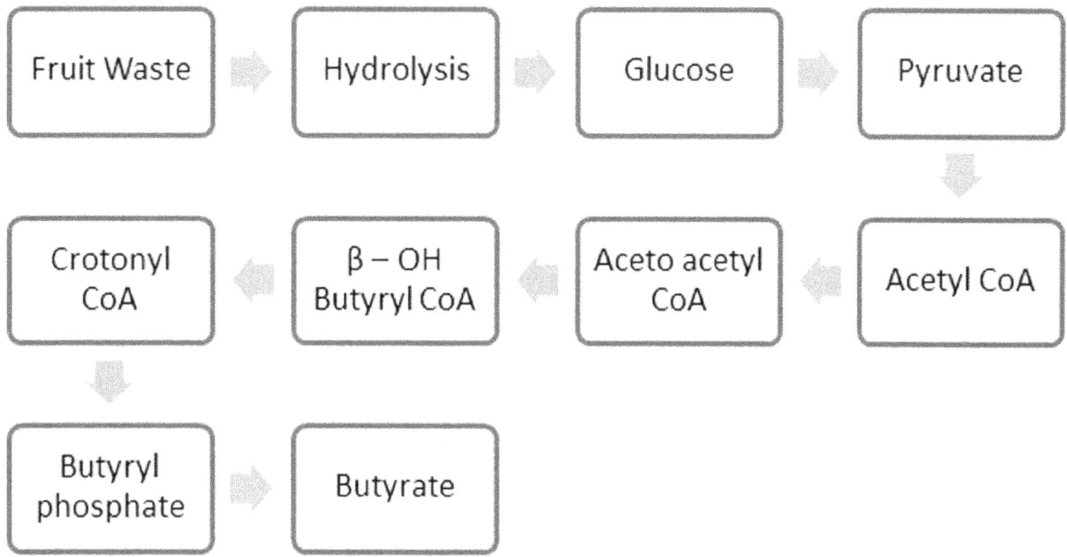

amino acids like lysine and methionine which are limiting in most plant and animal foods (Gour et al., 2015). Microbes like yeast, fungi, bacteria and algae have been used for SCP production. Yeast is another source of Single Cell Protein, and has been produced since a long time ago. Algae had drawn the attention of scientist to bridge the protein gap. Some of the algae like *Chloralla, Soenedesmus, Coelastrum* and *Spirulina* have been found to suitable for mass cultivation and utilization. The advantages in using algae include high protein and nutrient content, simple cultivation, effective utilization of solar energy and faster growth.

Many species of bacteria have been investigated for use in single cell protein production. *Methylophilus methylotrophus* with a generation time of about 2 hours and is usually and mainly used in animal feed as bacteria, in general produce a more favorable protein composition than yeast or fungi. Therefore, the large quantities of SCP animal feed can be produced using bacteria. The major factors that make bacteria ideal candidate for SCP production: their rapid growth and short generation times most can double their cell mass in 20 minutes to 2 hours. Capable of growing on a variety of raw materials, ranging from carbohydrates such as starch and sugar, hydrocarbons as methane, ethane and petrochemicals (Solomons et al., 1985; Nigam et al.,2000).

Importance of Microbial Protein

Microbial protein or SCP has various benefits over animal and plant proteins in that its requirement for growth are neither seasonal or climate dependent; it can be produced all around the year. It does not require a large expanse of land and it has high protein content with wide amino acid spectrum, low fat content and higher protein - carbohydrate ratio than forages. It can be grown on waste and it is environmental friendly as it helps in recycling waste (Gour et al., 2004). Beside nutritional value a protein should have desirable functional properties for its incorporation as food. Microbial protein has found to meet all the requirements for its inclusion as diet supplement for both human and livestock especially in the developing countries of Africa (Adedayo et al., 2011). Genetic manipulation of microbes may improve chemical composition and nutritional value and also production of microbial protein requires less labour than does agriculture production.

Benefits of Production of SCP From Microorganisms

1. Microorganisms have a high rate of multiplication and hence rapid succession of generations (algae: 2–6 hours, yeast: 1–3 hours, bacteria: 0.5–2 hours)
2. They can be easily genetically modified for varying the amino acid composition.
3. Protein content accounts for 43–85% in the dry mass.
4. They can utilize a broad spectrum of raw materials as carbon sources, which include waste products. Thus, they help in the removal of pollutants also.
5. Strains with high yield and good composition can be selected or produce relatively easily.
6. SCP production is independent of seasonal variation and usually consistent.
7. Land requirement is low and is ecologically beneficial.
8. A high solar-energy-conversion efficiency per unit area.
9. Solar energy conversion efficiency can be maximized and yield can be enhanced by easy regulation of physical and nutritional factors.
10. Algal culture can be done in space that is normally unused and so there is no need to compete for land (Rashad et al., 1990; Mateles et al., 1968; Miller et al., 1976; Parajo et al., 1995).

Limitations of SCP

Limitations of microbial proteins are enlisted below:

1. Production of non-targeted toxic end product can occur that may seriously affect health of the livestock when used as feed or may be toxic to human health.
2. Problem with digestion may occur sometimes.
3. Occurrence of allergic response in humans upon consumption of SCP may occur rarely.
4. Presence of high nucleic acid content may make SCP undesirable for human consumption and may often lead to the formation of gout and kidney stones.
5. The high nucleic acid content of many types of microbial biomass may lead to poor digestibility, gastrointestinal problem and also some skin reactions in humans.
6. Single cell protein production is a very expensive procedure as it needs high level of sterility control in the production unit or in the laboratory.

Fruit Waste as Substrate for SCP Production

Fruit waste containing an appreciable amount of complex carbohydrates need to be subjected to chemical or physical pretreatments to release the monomeric sugars that are easily fermentable (Figure 3). Apart from the carbon source, SCP production requires nitrogen and mineral supplementation depending on the targeted microorganism. Aseptic conditions need to be maintained throughout the process to prevent contamination. The starter culture is inoculated in its pure state and fermentation is carried out in aerobic conditions. Provisions for ensuring minimizing the heat generation during SCP produc-

Figure 3. SCP production from fruit waste

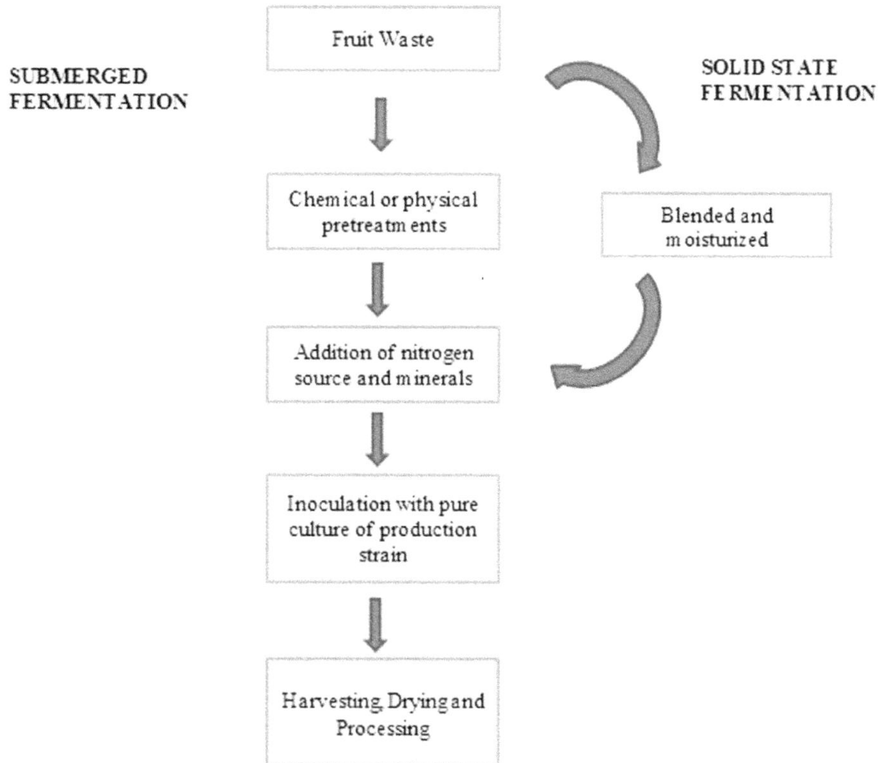

tion should be monitored precisely for maximizing the yield. The microbial biomass is harvested from the medium, dried and processed. Commercial production of SCP basically occurs through submerged fermentation using *Saccharomyces cerevisiae, Aspergillus oryzae, Rhizopus oligosporus* and *Candida utilis* (Nasseri et al., 2011).

Enzymes

Enzymes are important class of bioactive compounds that has a great industrial significance in day to day life. Using of synthetic media for enzyme production results in the overall increase in the cost of production of enzymes. Global demand for increased production of enzymes paved way for the utilization of cheap agro waste substrates like fruit waste as commercially valuable substrates for enzyme production. Fruit wastes are primarily composed of complex polysaccharide that enhances the microbial growth for the production of industrial enzymes. The important enzymes produced from fruit waste along with their potential application are enlisted below:

Pectinases

Pectinases are pectin degrading enzyme produced majorly from *Aspergillus niger, Penicillium sp., Rhizobium sp.* especially using citrus peel waste. Pectinases are broadly divided in to two:

1. Depolymerizing enzyme – breaks α 1, 4 linkage between pectin.
2. Demethoxylating enzyme – converts pectin to pectic acid.

Production of pectinase from fruit waste is outlined in Figure 4

Figure 4. Pectinase production from fruit waste

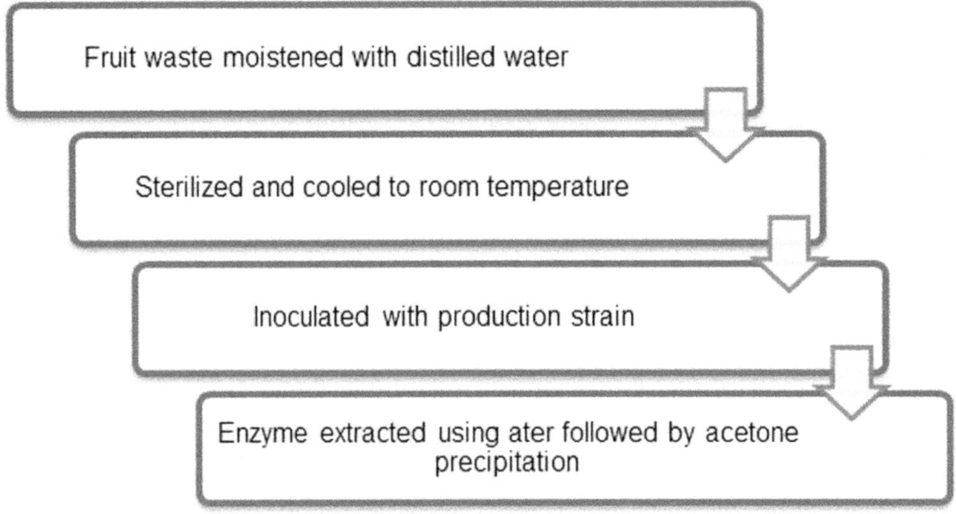

Amylase

It is a class of starch degrading enzyme basically produced from fungi, plants and animals. Bacterial amylases are commercially produced using *Bacillus sp.* and are highly compatible due to thermal stability. Important steps in amylase production is outlined in Figure 5.

Figure 5. Amylase production from fruit waste

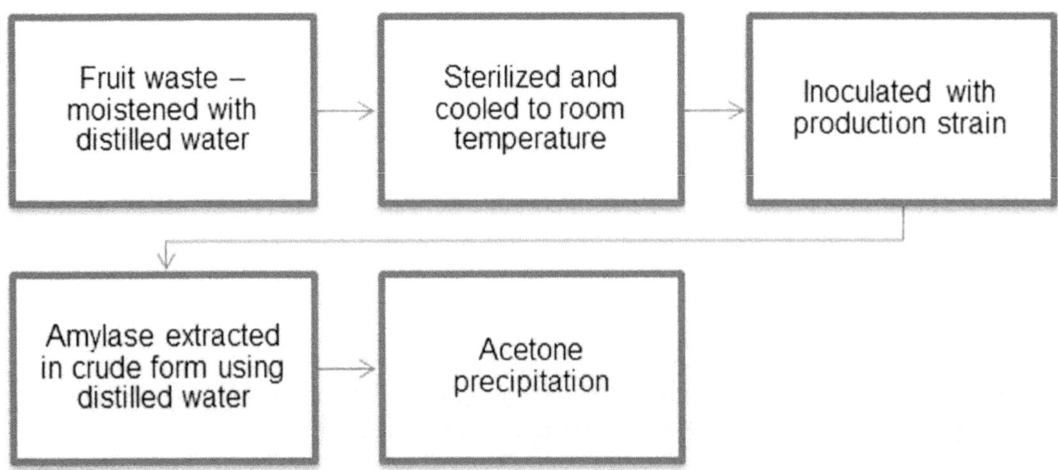

Biogas Production From Fruit Waste

The technique of using organic materials for biogas production dates back to several decades. Methane accounts for the major portion of the biogas produced by anaerobic digestion of organic matter. Biogas is basically a flammable gas produced when organic materials are fermented under anaerobic condition. It contains methane and carbon dioxide along with traces of hydrogen sulfide and water vapour. It usually burns with a pale blue flame and has a calorific value between 25.9 – 30 J/m^3 (Weiland, 2010).

The formation of biogas from fruit waste basically occurs through three major steps:

1. Complex organic molecules present in the fruit waste are decomposed by microorganisms in to simple molecules.

$$n\ (C_6H_{10}O_5) + nH_2O\ n(C_6H_{12}O_6)$$

2. These simple organic molecules are then converted in to organic acids by acid forming bacteria.

$$n(C_6H_{12}O_6)\ \xrightarrow{\text{Acid forming bacteria}}\ CH_3COOH\ \xrightarrow{\text{Amylolytic bacteria}}$$

3. These organic acids are then converted in to methane by methanogenic bacteria.

$$CH_3COOH\ \xrightarrow{\text{Methanogenic bacteria}}\ CH_4 + CO_2$$

Methanogens further carry out reduction of CO_2 formed to increase methane yield.

$$CO_2 + 4H2\ \xrightarrow{\text{Methanogenic bacteria}}\ CH_4 + 2H_2O$$

Factors affecting biogas formation are (Paul et al., 2014):

- **Nature of the Substrate:** This determines the need of any pretreatment step to release fermentable sugars.
- Temperature
- **pH:** Optimum pH range between 6.8 – 7.3
- **Agitation:** Intermediate mixing of the organic matter aids in accelerating biogas production.
- **Nutrient Supply:** Addition of nutrient sources to accelerate microbial growth can inturn increase biogas production.
- Slurry Concentration
- Digester Configuration
- **C/N Ratio:** Optimum concentration between 15-25
- **Retention Time:** At least 10 days
- Intitial feeding
- Total volatile acids
- COD

- Total Solid

The basic methodology involved in production of biogas from fruit waste is outlined below. Preparation of biogas from fruit waste preliminary involves drying of the waste followed by preparation of slurry for inoculation in to the digester of varying concentration. It is followed by inoculating the slurry with inoculum from previous batch or using cow dung containing substantial amount of methanogens.

BIOPLASTIC PRODUCTION

Plastics material is one of the most popular materials and indispensable in the present world. The word plastic comes from the Greek word "plastikos", which means 'able to be molded into different shapes' (Joel, 1995). Plastics are manmade long chain polymeric molecules (Scott, 1999). Plastics have become technologically significant since the 1940s and since then they have come to replace glass, wood, masonry and other constructional materials, and even metals in many industrial, domestic, commercial and environmental applications (Cain, 1992). Synthetic plastics are made from inorganic and organic raw materials, such as carbon, silicon, hydrogen, nitrogen, oxygen and chloride. The basic materials used for making plastics are extracted from oil, coal and natural gas (Seymour, 1989). They have versatile qualities of strength, lightness, durability and resistance to degradation. They have become an important commodity to enhance the comfort and quality of life. Accumulation of recalcitrant plastics in the environment has become a world-wide problem. During the combustion of plastic waste, hydrogen cyanide can be formed from acrylonitrile-based plastics and may cause potential health hazards are also causing other serious environmental problems due to their non-biodegradability. The sorting of wide variety of discarded plastic material is also a very time-consuming process. In such a scenario, biodegradable plastics offer the best solution to the environmental hazard posed by conventional plastics.

Synthetic Polymers and Their Impact on the Environment

The properties of plastics such as low cost, durability, lightweight, ease in processing and high resistance to chemical and biological degradation have made them an integral part of everyday life. Their chemical structure can be easily manipulated so that they can be molded into almost any desired shape and therefore are used in the manufacture of many durable, disposal goods and as packaging materials (Rivard et al., 1995; Yu, 2007). The four major commodity thermoplastic resins are, polyethylene, polypropylene, polystyrene and polyvinyl chloride. The major features of plastics that have contributed immensely towards their popularity are causing grave environmental and societal concerns. Plastics being xenobiotic in nature and are recalcitrant to microbial degradation (Flechter, 1993). Their large molecular size is responsible for the resistance of plastics to biodegradation (Reddy et al., 2003). Since their presence in nature is increased enormously during the recent years, new enzyme structures capable of degrading synthetic polymers are yet to be evolved and nature's in-built mechanisms are unable to degrade these novel unfamiliar pollutants (Reddy et al., 2003; Mueller, 2006). Approximately, 140 million tonnes per year of synthetic petroleum-based plastics are produced and several thousand tonnes of it is discarded into the environment as industrial waste products (Shimao, 2001). The accumulation of these discarded plastics in the environment is reducing the aesthetic qualities of cities, forests, water bodies as well as endangering the flora and fauna especially in the marine ecosystem (Moore, 2008; Ojumu et al., 2004). This dramatic increase in production and recalcitrant property of the synthetic polymers is imposing a strain on nature due to their persistence in the environment for centuries (Albertsson et al., 1987). Disposal of these xenobiotics is currently achieved through landfilling, incineration or recycling. Unfortunately, only a small fraction of the discarded plastic wastes reach the disposal sites while the rest litters the landscape or is blown off into the sea posing severe threat to the marine life (Moore, 2008). Incineration of plastic waste results in the generation of large amounts of carbonaceous material and undesirable pollutants such as carbon dioxide, carbon monoxide, furans, dioxins, hydrogen chloride, hydrogen cyanide, nitrogen oxides and benzopyrene which are highly corrosive and disease inducing (Jayasekara et al., 2005; Johnston, 1995; Reddy *et al.,* 2003). Recycling of synthetic plastics is disadvantageous due to alteration in the material properties, limiting its further application range and thereby inevitably increasing the cost of the recycled plastics as compared to the original form of plastics. The persistence of the discarded plastics is a global threat due to their potential adverse impacts on the environment (Mohanty et al., 2002).

Bioplastics

A fully biodegradable polymer is defined as a polymer that is completely converted by living organisms (usually microorganisms) to carbon dioxide, water and humic material. They can be completely degraded in landfills, composters or sewage treatment plants by action of naturally occurring microorganisms. Fully degradable plastics leave no toxic, visible or distinguishable residues following degradation. Bioplastics are a special type of biomaterial. They are polyesters produced by a range of microbes cultured under different nutrient and environmental conditions. These polymers are storage granules rich in lipids, are accumulated as storage materials (in the form of mobile, amorphous, liquid granules) allowing microbial survival under stress conditions. The rate of bioplastic formation, material and physicochemical properties vary depending on the production strain. They can be observed intracellularly as light-refracting granules or as electronlucent bodies that, in overproducing mutants, cause a striking alteration of the bacterial shape.

Types of Bioplastics

Biodegradable plastics can be divided into three categories:

1. **Chemically Synthesised Polymers:** Polyglycollic acid, polylactic acid, poly (ε-caprolactone), polyvinyl alcohol, poly (ethylene oxide) fall into this category. These are susceptible to enzymic or microbial attack.
2. **Starch-Based Biodegradable Plastics:** In this type, starch is added as filler and cross-linking agent to produce a blend of starch and plastic (for example, starch– polyethylene). Soil micro-organisms degrade the starch easily, thus breaking down the polymer matrix. This results in significant reduction of degradation time. But such plastics are only partially degradable. The fragments left after starch removal are recalcitrant and remain in the environment for a long time.
3. **Polyhydroxyalkanoates (PHAs):** These are the only 100% biodegradable polymers. They are polyesters of various hydroxyalkanoic acids which are synthesised by numerous micro-organisms as energy reserve materials when an essential nutrient such as nitrogen or phosphorus is available only in limiting concentrations in the presence of excess carbon source. Polyhydroxyalkanoates

(PHAs) are a family of biopolyesters synthesized and accumulated by a wide range of microorganisms as reserve food material. These are the only plastics produced exclusively by microorganisms and hence are completely degraded to benign compounds (Anderson and Dawes, 1990). They are non-polluting as they do not need catalysts or additives to promote their degradation. Plastics produced from PHAs have been reported to be truly biodegradable in both aerobic and anaerobic environments, unlike many of the "so-called" biodegradable plastics made synthetically. PHAs are composed mainly of poly-betahydroxybutyric acid (PHB) and poly-beta hydroxyvaleric acid (PHV). More than 80 different forms of PHAs have been detected in bacteria (Lee, 1996). These copolymers have better film forming and mechanical properties quite similar to low-density polyethylene. PHB was first discovered in bacteria (Lemoigne, 1926). It is a unique intracellular polymer accumulated under stress conditions but with excess carbon source.

a. **Occurrence and Biosynthesis of PHA:** There is widespread occurrence of PHA-producing organisms in the environment. The main candidates for commercial-scale PHA production are bacteria and transgenic plants. Bacterial cells are capable of accumulating PHA to levels as high as 90% (w/w) of the dry cell weight (DCW) (Steinbuchel & Lutke-Eversloh, 2003) thus emphasizing its importance as a potential candidate for PHA production. A wide variety of bacteria are able to synthesize PHA. Unbalanced nutrient supply triggers the bacteria to store the excess carbon and energy in the form of PHA. The PHA polymer is deposited in the cell cytoplasm as discrete insoluble granules which vary in number depending on the bacterial strain (Anderson & Dawes, 1990). Polyhydroxybutyrate (PHB), the first PHA to be discovered, is produced via the classical PHB biosynthetic pathway in three steps catalyzed by the PHA biosynthetic enzymes. These are polyesters containing monomers of medium chain length (mcl PHAs, C5–C14) or long-chain length (lcl PHAs, >C14). Although PHAs are structurally related to PHBs (short-chain length, scl PHAs), the microbes that synthesise PHBs usually fail to make PHAs. However, recombinant organisms containing mixed catabolic pathways are able to synthesise either polymers (or co-polymers) containing scl, mcl monomers, or both. PHA production starts in response to stress imposed on cells, usually by nitrogen or phosphorus limitation, although in the presence of abundant carbon source. Under these conditions (PHA accumulation phase), the cells do not grow or divide but instead divert their metabolites towards the biosynthesis of hydoxyalkyl-CoA (HA-coA). HA-CoA is polymerized by the enzymatic action of PHA synthase to form PHA polymer (Figure 6). Being insoluble in water, PHA begins to form amorphous and nearly spherical granules that gradually fill the cells and force them to expand (Lee et al., 1999).

b. **Chemical Structure of Polyhydroxyalkanoates:** Polyhydroxyalkanotes are hydroxyalkanoic acids linked to each other by an ester linkage. Polyhydroxybutyrate (PHB) is the most commonly occurring and hence most studied PHA. The composition of the synthesized polymer is influenced by the bacterial strain as well as type and relative quantity and quality of carbon sources supplied to the growth medium (Steinbuchel et al., 1993).

c. **General Structure of PHA:** The polyhydroxyalkanoates can be divided into three groups depending on the carbon chain length of the monomeric units (Figure 7):
   i. Short-Chain-Length (scl-PHA), which consist of 3 to 5 carbon atoms
   ii. Medium-Chain-Length (mcl-PHA), which consist of 6 to 14 carbon atoms
   iii. Long-Chain-Length (lcl-PHA), which consist of 17 to 18 carbon atoms (Volova, 2004). Biosynthetic pathway for the synthesis of PHA is illustrated in Figure 5

Figure 6. PHA production from fruit waste

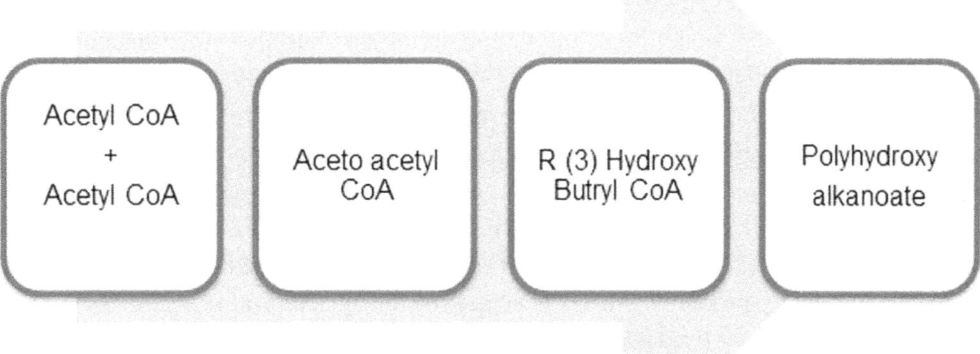

Figure 7. General structure of PHA

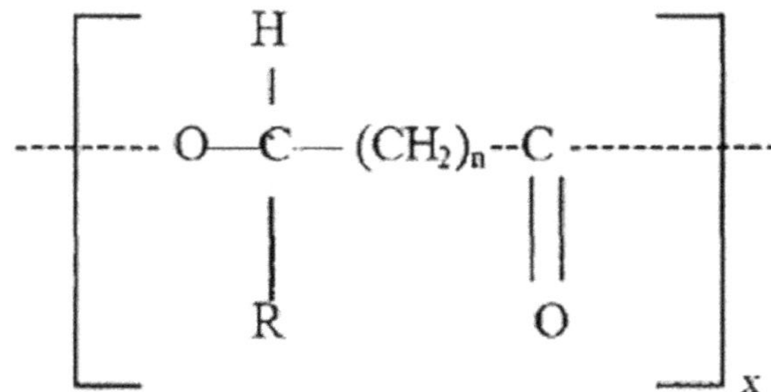

$n = 1$ R = methyl: polymer = poly(3-hydroxybutyrate)

$\quad$ R = ethyl: polymer = poly(3-hydroxyvalerate)

$n = 2$ R = hydrogen: polymer = poly(4-hydroxybutyrate)

$n = 3$ R = hydrogen: polymer = poly(5-hydroxybutyrate)

$x = 100\text{-}30000$

Bioplastic Production From Waste Substrate

The use of plastics has grown rapidly over the past few decades. An interesting alternative to decrease the environmental impacts of plastics is to replace conventional petroleum-derived polymers with bio-degradable ones. The most important factors affecting the overall economics of PHA production are PHA productivity, PHA content and PHA yield which depend mainly upon the carbon source used, the raw material cost and the recovery methods. In the manufacturing process the raw material cost, especially the carbon source greatly influences the overall cost of the final product. Synthesis of PHA using expensive carbon sources such as glucose renders the process economically non-viable. Alternatively, inexpensive and easily available raw materials such as wastes generated during agricultural and industrial processes are now being considered as potential carbon substrates (Castilho et al., 2009). These wastes contain large amounts of organic matter which can be utilized as carbon feedstock for PHA production. This will not only ensure the reduction in the raw material cost but also simultaneously save energy and decrease the costs associated with its disposal. The synthesis of value-added products such as PHA from waste carbon sources coupled with their biodegradability makes them increasingly attractive in the pursuit of sustainable development. The biological polyesters known as polyhydroxyalkanoates (PHAs) are mainly produced by microbial fermentation processes, and there is a major challenge to reduce their production costs (Nath et al., 2008). Since the traditional approach for PHA production has been based on submerged fermentation (SMF) processes, most studies reported in the literature are limited either to liquid wastes or to liquid by-products. Wastes generated in the agricultural sector are being reviewed as potential feedstock for polymer production. In a wheat-based biorefinery strategy for PHB production, accumulation of PHB occurred when wheat hydrolysate and fungal extract were provided as carbon and nitrogen sources (Koutinas et al., 2013). A large number of industrial processes generate organic wastes such as molasses and corn steep liquor which are rich in carbon. These wastes are being used for the synthesis of value-added products namely; lactic acid, ethanol, enzymes and antibiotics. Wastes generated by the fast food manufacturing units can also serve as ideal feedstock due to their organic content.

FUTURE RESEARCH DIRECTIONS

The immense fermentative potential of fruit waste along with its global availability throughout the year makes it a versatile for important fermentation process involving microbes. Microbe mediated bioconversion continues to be the most effective tool for waste management due to the inherent ability of microbial enzymes to break the most complex organic molecules. Development of integrated process for simultaneous production of more than one microbial metabolite utilizing fruit waste will be the major focus for research in the upcoming years. Research aimed at utilization of carbohydrate rich waste like fruit peels can spread light on the concept of 'Reduce, Reuse and Recycle'. Development in genetic engineering and microbial fermentation process in the upcoming years could act as promising milestones in the development of novel compounds of commercial interest from cheap raw material like fruit wastes.

CONCLUSION

Increasing concern about environment pollution due to careless discharge of waste called for development of sustainable waste management strategies for production of value added products. Fruit waste with high content of carbohydrates are easily available cheap raw material for the production of a wide range of products like organic acids, single cell protein, bioplastics, enzymes and biogas. Utilization of biomass through microbial fermentation serves as sustainable alternative for chemical synthesis process for the manufacture of products of commercial interest. Proper planning, execution, financial assistance from public and private sector for both research and product development can take this initiative in to promising domains in the future emphasizing the concept of 'Wealth from Waste'.

REFERENCES

Adedayo, M. R., Ajiboye, E. A., Akintunde, J. K., & Odaibo, A. (2011). Single cell proteins: As nutritional enhancer. *Advances in Applied Science Research*, *2*(5), 396–409.

Albertsson, A. C., Andersson, S. O., & Karlsson, S. (1987). The mechanism of biodegradation of polyethylene. *Polymer Degradation & Stability*, *18*(1), 73–87. doi:10.1016/0141-3910(87)90084-X

Amrane, A., & Prigent, Y. (1998). Lactic acid production rates during the different growth phases of *Lactobacillus helveticus* cultivated on whey supplemented with yeast extract. *Biotechnology Letters*, *20*(4), 379–383. doi:10.1023/A:1005331430943

Anderson, A. J., & Dawes, E. A. (1990). Occurrence, metabolism, metabolic role, and industrial uses of bacterial polyhydroxyalkanoates. *Microbiological Reviews*, *54*(4), 450–472. PMID:2087222

Bayer, E. A., Lamed, R., & Himmel, M. E. (2007). The potential of cellulases and cellulosomes for cellulosic waste management. *Current Opinion in Biotechnology*, *18*(3), 237–245. doi:10.1016/j.copbio.2007.04.004 PMID:17462879

Berezinaa, N., Nysb, J., & Yadaa, B. (2013). Method for the Analysis of Grafted Cellulosic Materials. *Chemical Engineering (Albany, N.Y.)*, 32.

Bouallagui, H., Torrijos, M., Godon, J. J., Moletta, R., Cheikh, R. B., Touhami, Y., & Hamdi, M. (2004). Two-phases anaerobic digestion of fruit and vegetable wastes: Bioreactors performance. *Biochemical Engineering Journal*, *21*(2), 193–197. doi:10.1016/j.bej.2004.05.001

Buss, S. E., Butler, A. P., Sollars, C. J., Perry, R., & Johnston, P. M. (1995). Mechanisms of leakage through synthetic landfill liner materials. *Water and Environment Journal: the Journal / the Chartered Institution of Water and Environmental Management*, *9*(4), 353–359. doi:10.1111/j.1747-6593.1995.tb00952.x

Bustos, G., Moldes, A. B., Alonso, J. L., & Vázquez, M. (2004). Optimization of D-lactic acid production by *Lactobacillus coryniformis* using response surface methodology. *Food Microbiology*, *21*(2), 143–148. doi:10.1016/S0740-0020(03)00061-3

Cain, R. B. (1992). Microbial degradation of synthetic polymers. *Journal of Microbial control of pollution*.

Carmo, I. M. T. D. D. (2013). *Food waste valorization through the production of polyhydroxyalkanoates by mixed microbial cultures* [Doctoral dissertation]. Faculdade de Ciências e Tecnologia.

Castilho, L. R., Mitchell, D. A., & Freire, D. M. (2009). Production of polyhydroxyalkanoates (PHAs) from waste materials and by-products by submerged and solid-state fermentation. *Bioresource Technology*, *100*(23), 5996–6009. doi:10.1016/j.biortech.2009.03.088 PMID:19581084

Chirila, T. V., Constable, I. J., Crawford, G. J., Vijayasekaran, S., Thompson, D. E., Chen, Y. C., & Griffin, B. J. (1993). Poly (2-hydroxyethyl methacrylate) sponges as implant materials: In vivo and in vitro evaluation of cellular invasion. *Biomaterials*, *14*(1), 26–38. doi:10.1016/0142-9612(93)90072-A PMID:7678755

Daramwal, N., & Gaur, R. (2004). Single cell protein. *Environmental microbiology and biotechnology, 218.*

Fitzpatrick, J. J., & O'keeffe, U. (2001). Influence of whey protein hydrolysate addition to whey permeate batch fermentations for producing lactic acid. *Process Biochemistry, 37*(2), 183–186. doi:10.1016/S0032-9592(01)00203-5

García, I. L., Lopez, J. A., Dorado, M. P., Kopsahelis, N., Alexandri, M., Papanikolaou, S., & Koutinas, A. A. (2013). Evaluation of by-products from the biodiesel industry as fermentation feedstock for poly (3-hydroxybutyrate-co-3-hydroxyvalerate) production by *Cupriavidus necator*. *Bioresource Technology, 130*, 16–22. doi:10.1016/j.biortech.2012.11.088 PMID:23280181

Garde, A., Jonsson, G., Schmidt, A. S., & Ahring, B. K. (2002). Lactic acid production from wheat straw hemicellulose hydrolysate by *Lactobacillus pentosus* and *Lactobacillus brevis*. *Bioresource Technology, 81*(3), 217–223. doi:10.1016/S0960-8524(01)00135-3 PMID:11800488

Goldberg, S. Z., Eisenberg, R., Miller, J. S., & Epstein, A. J. (1976). Tetrakis (methyl isocyanide) palladium (II) tetrakis (7, 7, 8, 8-tetracyano-p-quinodimethane), [Pd (CNMe) 4](TCNQ) 4.2 MeCN: Synthesis, structure, and physical properties. *Journal of the American Chemical Society, 98*(17), 5173–5182. doi:10.1021/ja00433a020

Imandi, S. B., Bandaru, V. V. R., Somalanka, S. R., Bandaru, S. R., & Garapati, H. R. (2008). Application of statistical experimental designs for the optimization of medium constituents for the production of citric acid from pineapple waste. *Bioresource Technology, 99*(10), 4445–4450. doi:10.1016/j.biortech.2007.08.071 PMID:17936623

Jayasekara, R., Harding, I., Bowater, I., & Lonergan, G. (2005). Biodegradability of a selected range of polymers and polymer blends and standard methods for assessment of biodegradation. *Journal of Polymers and the Environment, 13*(3), 231–251. doi:10.100710924-005-4758-2

Jendrossek, D., Knoke, I., Habibian, R. B., Steinbüchel, A., & Schlegel, H. G. (1993). Degradation of poly (3-hydroxybutyrate), PHB, by bacteria and purification of a novel PHB depolymerase from *Comamonas sp. Journal of Polymers and the Environment, 1*(1), 53–63.

John, R. P., Sukumaran, R. K., Nampoothiri, K. M., & Pandey, A. (2007). Statistical optimization of simultaneous saccharification and L (+)-lactic acid fermentation from cassava bagasse using mixed culture of lactobacilli by response surface methodology. *Biochemical Engineering Journal, 36*(3), 262–267. doi:10.1016/j.bej.2007.02.028

Ko, P. C., & Yu, Y. (1968). Production of SCP from hydrocarbons: Taiwan. *Single Cell Protein*, 225.

Kulozik, U., & Wilde, J. (1999). Rapid lactic acid production at high cell concentrations in whey ultrafiltrate by *Lactobacillus helveticus*. *Enzyme and Microbial Technology, 24*(5), 297–302. doi:10.1016/S0141-0229(98)00122-7

Kumar, D., Jain, V. K., Shanker, G., & Srivastava, A. (2003). Utilisation of fruits waste for citric acid production by solid state fermentation. *Process Biochemistry, 38*(12), 1725–1729. doi:10.1016/S0032-9592(02)00253-4

Kurbanoglu, E. B., & Kurbanoglu, N. I. (2003). Utilization for lactic acid production with a new acid hydrolysis of ram horn waste. *FEMS Microbiology Letters, 225*(1), 29–34. doi:10.1016/S0378-1097(03)00472-5 PMID:12900017

Lee, S. Y. (1996). Bacterial polyhydroxyalkanoates. *Biotechnology and Bioengineering, 49*(1), 1–14. doi:10.1002/(SICI)1097-0290(19960105)49:1<1::AID-BIT1>3.0.CO;2-P PMID:18623547

Lee, S. Y., Choi, J. I., & Wong, H. H. (1999). Recent advances in polyhydroxyalkanoate production by bacterial fermentation: Mini-review. *International Journal of Biological Macromolecules, 25*(1), 31–36. doi:10.1016/S0141-8130(99)00012-4 PMID:10416647

Lemoigne, M. (1926). Produits de deshydration et de polymerisation de l'acide boxybutyrique. *Biological science, 8,* 770-782.

Liguori, R., Amore, A., & Faraco, V. (2013). Waste valorization by biotechnological conversion into added value products. *Applied Microbiology and Biotechnology, 97*(14), 6129–6147. doi:10.100700253-013-5014-7 PMID:23749120

Mohanty, A. K., Misra, M., & Drzal, L. T. (2002). Sustainable bio-composites from renewable resources: Opportunities and challenges in the green materials world. *Journal of Polymers and the Environment, 10*(1), 19–26. doi:10.1023/A:1021013921916

Moore, C. J. (2008). Synthetic polymers in the marine environment: A rapidly increasing, long-term threat. *Environmental Research, 108*(2), 131–139. doi:10.1016/j.envres.2008.07.025 PMID:18949831

Umesh, M., & Preethi, K. (2014). Fermentative Utilization of fruit peel waste for Lactic Acid production by *Lactobacillus plantarum. Indian Journal of Applied Research, 4*(9), 449–451.

Mudaliyar, P., Sharma, L., & Kulkarni, C. (2012). Food waste management-lactic acid production by *Lactobacillus species. International Journal of Advanced Biological Research, 2*(1), 34–38.

Mueller, R. J. (2006). Biological degradation of synthetic polyesters—enzymes as potential catalysts for polyester recycling. *Process Biochemistry, 41*(10), 2124–2128. doi:10.1016/j.procbio.2006.05.018

Nasseri, A. T., Rasoul-Amini, S., Morowvat, M. H., & Ghasemi, Y. (2011). Single cell protein: Production and process. *American. Journal of Food Technology, 6*(2), 103–116. doi:10.3923/ajft.2011.103.116

Nath, A., Dixit, M., Bandiya, A., Chavda, S., & Desai, A. J. (2008). Enhanced PHB production and scale up studies using cheese whey in fed batch culture of Methylobacterium sp. ZP24. *Bioresource Technology, 99*(13), 5749–5755. doi:10.1016/j.biortech.2007.10.017 PMID:18032031

Nigam, J. N. (2000). Cultivation of Candida langeronii in sugar cane bagasse hemicellulosic hydrolyzate for the production of single cell protein. *World Journal of Microbiology & Biotechnology, 16*(4), 367–372. doi:10.1023/A:1008922806215

Oh, H., Wee, Y. J., Yun, J. S., Han, S. H., Jung, S., & Ryu, H. W. (2005). Lactic acid production from agricultural resources as cheap raw materials. *Bioresource Technology, 96*(13), 1492–1498. doi:10.1016/j.biortech.2004.11.020 PMID:15939277

Oikeh, E. I., Oriakhi, K., & Omoregie, E. S. (2013). Proximate analysis and phytochemical screening of *Citrus sinensis* fruit wastes. *The Bioscientist, 1*(2), 164–170.

Ojumu, T. V., Yu, J., & Solomon, B. O. (2004). Production of polyhydroxyalkanoates, a bacterial biodegradable polymers. *African Journal of Biotechnology, 3*(1), 18–24. doi:10.5897/AJB2004.000-2004

Pandey, A., Soccol, C. R., Nigam, P., & Soccol, V. T. (2000). Biotechnological potential of agro-industrial residues. I: Sugarcane bagasse. *Bioresource Technology, 74*(1), 69–80. doi:10.1016/S0960-8524(99)00142-X

Parajó, J. C., Santos, V., Domínguez, H., & Vázquez, M. (1995). NH 4 OH-Based pretreatment for improving the nutritional quality of single-cell protein (SCP). *Applied Biochemistry and Biotechnology, 55*(2), 133–149. doi:10.1007/BF02783554

Preethi, K., & Maha Lakshmi, G., Mridul Umesh, Priyanka, K., & Thazeem, B. (2017). Fruit peels: A potential substrate for acetic acid production using *Acetobacter aceti. International Journal of Applied Research, 2*(4), 286–291.

Rashad, M. M., Moharib, S. A., & Jwanny, E. W. (1990). Yeast conversion of mango waste or methanol to single cell protein and other metabolites. *Biological Wastes, 32*(4), 277–284. doi:10.1016/0269-7483(90)90059-2

Reddy, C. S. K., Ghai, R., & Kalia, V. (2003). Polyhydroxyalkanoates: An overview. *Bioresource Technology, 87*(2), 137–146. doi:10.1016/S0960-8524(02)00212-2 PMID:12765352

Rivard, C., Moens, L., Brigham, K. R., & Kelley, S. (1995). Starch esters as biodegradable plastics: Effects of ester group chain length and degree of substitution on anaerobic biodegradation. *Enzyme and Microbial Technology, 17*(9), 848–852. doi:10.1016/0141-0229(94)00120-G

Schepers, A. W., Thibault, J., & Lacroix, C. (2002). *Lactobacillus helveticus* growth and lactic acid production during pH-controlled batch cultures in whey permeate/yeast extract medium. Part I. multiple factor kinetic analysis. *Enzyme and Microbial Technology, 30*(2), 176–186. doi:10.1016/S0141-0229(01)00465-3

Scott, D. S., & Legge, R. L. (1999). Bioplastics. CIGR handbook of agricultural engineering, 5, 305-310.

Seymour, R. B. (1989). Polymer science before & after 1899: Notable developments during the lifetime of Maurtis Dekker. *Journal of Macromolecular Science. Chemistry, 26*(8), 1023–1032. doi:10.1080/00222338908052032

Shimao, M. (2001). Biodegradation of plastics. *Current Opinion in Biotechnology, 12*(3), 242–247. doi:10.1016/S0958-1669(00)00206-8 PMID:11404101

Shukla, V. B., Zhou, S., Yomano, L. P., Shanmugam, K. T., Preston, J. F., & Ingram, L. O. (2004). Production of d (−)-lactate from sucrose and molasses. *Biotechnology Letters, 26*(9), 689–693. doi:10.1023/B:BILE.0000024088.36803.4e PMID:15195965

Solomons, G. L. (1985). Production of biomass by filamentous fungi. *Comprehensive biotechnology: the principles, applications, and regulations of biotechnology in industry, agriculture, and medicine.*

Sreenath, H. K., Moldes, A. B., Koegel, R. G., & Straub, R. J. (2001). Lactic acid production from agriculture residues. *Biotechnology Letters, 23*(3), 179–184. doi:10.1023/A:1005651117831

Steinbüchel, A., & Lütke-Eversloh, T. (2003). Metabolic engineering and pathway construction for biotechnological production of relevant polyhydroxyalkanoates in microorganisms. *Biochemical Engineering Journal, 16*(2), 81–96. doi:10.1016/S1369-703X(03)00036-6

Vikas, O.V., & Mridul, U. (2014). Bioconversion of papaya peel waste in to vinegar by *Acetobacter aceti*. *International Journal of Scientific Research*, *3*(11), 409–411.

Volova, T. G. (2004). *Polyhydroxyalkanoates--plastic materials of the 21st century: production, properties, applications*. Nova publishers.

Wee, Y. J., Kim, J. N., Yun, J. S., & Ryu, H. W. (2004). Utilization of sugar molasses for economical L (+)-lactic acid production by batch fermentation of Enterococcus faecalis. *Enzyme and Microbial Technology*, *35*(6), 568–573. doi:10.1016/j.enzmictec.2004.08.008

Weiland, P. (2010). Biogas production: Current state and perspectives. *Applied Microbiology and Biotechnology*, *85*(4), 849–860. doi:10.100700253-009-2246-7 PMID:19777226

Wong, R. C., & Solomon, A. R. (1985). Acquired dermal smooth-muscle hamartoma. *Cutis*, *35*(4), 369–370. PMID:3996041

Yu, W. W., Chang, E., Falkner, J. C., Zhang, J., Al-Somali, A. M., Sayes, C. M., & Colvin, V. L. (2007). Forming biocompatible and nonaggregated nanocrystals in water using amphiphilic polymers. *Journal of the American Chemical Society*, *129*(10), 2871–2879. doi:10.1021/ja067184n PMID:17309256

KEY TERMS AND DEFINITIONS

Amylase: Starch degrading enzyme produced by wide variety of microbes.

Biogas: Biogas is basically a flammable gas produced when organic materials are fermented under anaerobic condition.

Bioplastics: A fully biodegradable polymer is defined as a polymer that is completely converted by living organisms, usually microorganisms, to carbon dioxide, water and humic material.

Fermentation: Metabolic process mediated by microbes that involves conversion of organic matter in to value added products.

Organic Acid: Acids derived from organic source preferably plant or animals.

Polyhydroxyalkanoates: Polyhydroxyalkanotes are hydroxyalkanoic acids linked to each other by an ester linkage

Single Cell Protein: Live or dried protein supplement produced from microbes.

This research was previously published in the Handbook of Research on Microbial Tools for Environmental Waste Management edited by Vinay Mohan Pathak and Navneet; pages 57-78, copyright year 2018 by Engineering Science Reference (an imprint of IGI Global).

Chapter 32
Industrially Important Enzymes Production From Food Waste:
An Alternative Approach to Land Filling

Madhuri Santosh Bhandwalkar
S. B. B. Alias Appasaheb Jedhe College, India

ABSTRACT

To link food demand and reduction in food waste, proactive approaches should be taken. Perishable food is mainly fruits and vegetables, waste from different processing industries like pulses, meat products, oil products, dairy products, and fishery byproducts. Conventional food waste management solution is land filling which is not sustainable as it generates global warming gases like methane and carbon dioxide. To reduce food waste, the process known as "food valorization" has become another solution to landfilling, the concept which is given by European Commission in 2012, meaning food processing waste conversion to value-added products. In this chapter the study focuses on production of industrially important enzymes from food waste which could be one of the reactive solutions. Different enzymes like pectinase, peroxidase, lipase, glucoamylase, and protease can be produced from food waste.

INTRODUCTION

Food Demand is rising globally in the proportion to rapid population growth. This leads to increase in Food production and ultimately in food waste or loss in food supply chain from initiation to final consumption. For sustainable food waste management, the waste hierarchy concept (1975) given by European Waste Policy can be useful to categorize the food waste and treat them accordingly. Some of the indicators used in food waste classification are edibility (edible/nonedible), State (Eatable/uneatable), Origin (Animal/plant) and complexity (single product/complex product). Water activity is the main factor assisting to predict the presence of microorganisms spoiling the food. Among them bacteria need water activity 0.85 and molds (0.7-0.8) for growth. It is important to treat solid food waste and liquid food waste eco-friendly.

DOI: 10.4018/978-1-7998-5354-1.ch032

Liquid waste generally contains proteins, sugars, starches, and fats. The researchers focused on the study of different problems faced by developing and developed countries regarding food waste generation and management.

Out of total industrially important enzymes production food industry useful enzymes are 45%, detergent industry 35%, textile 10%, and leather 3%. For the production, fungi and bacteria are mainly used and others involve higher plants, higher animals, yeasts and *Streptomyces*. Chapter covers the information from food waste generation, classification, different strategies used to manage food waste, microbial sources used in different enzyme production, different food waste types with examples, future aspects and conclusion.

FOOD WASTE GENERATION

According to many researchers hospitality industries and households which are the end of the food supply chain are contributing food waste generation. Developed and developing countries are defined by the Gross National Income (GNI) index. This study reveals that though the developing countries have less food demand as compared to developed countries, the food waste generation contributed by both of them is equal in quantity. Many researchers have shown that most food is wasted at the end of the food supply chain. Before considering Food Waste (FW) it is important to distinguish between food loss and food waste. (As classified in Table 1)

Food loss is the one which occurs before completing food supply chain and transformed into a final product. Before that point only food spills, lost or reduce in nutritional value and volume also. Food waste is the one which occurs after completing food supply chain. It may occur before consumption or before spoiling it is left to spoil. Table 1 explains the food loss and food waste.

Table 1. Food loss and waste along the value chain

Production	Handling and storage	Processing and packaging	Distribution and Market	Consumption
During or immediately after harvesting on the farm	After produce leaves the farm for handling, storage and transport	During industrial or domestic processing and/ or packaging	During distribution to markets, including losses and wholesale and retail markets	Losses in the home or business of the consumer, including restaurants/ caterers
Fruits bruised during picking or threshing	Edible food eaten by pests	Milk spoiled during pasteurization and processing	Edible produce sorted out due to quality	Edible produce sorted out due to quality
Crops sorted out post- harvest for not meeting quality standards	Edible produce degraded by fungus or disease	Edible fruits or grains sorted out as not suitable for processing	Edible products expired before being purchased	Food purchased but not eaten
Crops left behind in fields due to poor mechanical harvesting or sharp drop in prices	Livestock death during transport to slaughter or not accepted for slaughter	Livestock trimming during slaughtering and industrial processing	Edible products spoiled or damaged in market	Food cooked but not eaten

Source: Bagherzadeh et.al, 2014 OECD, France

FOOD WASTE CLASSIFICATION

To carry optimal food waste management, classification of food waste using their types viz., fruits, cereals, drinks, fish, meat is necessary. Activities to be treated on FW and manage them food classification is essential prerequisite. Also it decides a methodical procedure. Garcia-Garcia et al (2017) has explained these nine indicators. They are as Edibility, State, Origin, Complexity, Animal product presence, Treatment, Packaging. Food waste categorization also helps to monitor purposes like business or else so that assessing progress in the management and sustainability can easily be done. (Guillermo Garcia-Garcia et al., 2017). Figure1 describes Food Waste Management Decision Tree (FWMDT).

Best waste management option available after categorizing food waste are: Anaerobic digestion, composting or thermal treatment with energy recovery.

VARIOUS STRATEGIES FOR FOOD WASTE MANAGEMENT

According to many researchers hospitality industries and households which are the end of the food supply chain are contributing food waste generation. The best solution for handling food waste is to avoid the onset of food waste generation. As it is impossible to do so, there are various strategies which can be applied are described below.

1. **Animal Feeding:** FW generated from animal products like meat and bone meal, edible tallow, restaurant grease, feather meal, fish meal, dairy whey, dry milk are used as animal feed. FW has high coefficient variations which causes increase in digestibility coefficient and if it contains primary nutrients around 3/4th part of total FW, can be recognized as feed additive. Also there are chances of causing diseases to animals, so less preferable solution for considering FW treatment.
2. **Anaerobic Digestion:** Anaerobic digestion is considered as one of the effective method to treat FW and getting biogas like methane. For enhancing anaerobic digestion of FW, pretreatment like physical methods with measures of mechanical grinding, ultrasound, microwave, thermal, pressure –depressure or chemical method with the use of acid and biological method using biological solubilization is done followed by co-digestion. Co-digestion is done to overcome inhibition of anaerobic digestion due to high lipid content. It is done by addition of organic substances like cattle manure (CM), green waste, and sewage sludge.

Balancing the nutrient imbalance and reducing energy expenses required for anaerobic digestion are the challenges for this treatment.

3. **Composting:** C:N ratio is significant (25:1 to 35:1 suitable for microbial activity)in the successful composting process as less ratio means excess nitrogen leads to ammonia production causing odor problems and high ratio means high carbon content leading to complete utilization of Nitrogen before carbon containing material decomposition. (Rynk. R., ed. 11992).Proper composting can give us sufficient temperature rise destructing pathogen, weeding seeds along with 40% volume reduction.(S.M. Schaub and J.J. Leonard)

4. **Incineration:** Previous studies suggest that incineration is used to produce thermal energy and can be used to reduce the volume of waste.(AnqiGao et al.).It is energy consuming as moisture content is high and incineration causes air pollution.

MICROBIAL SOURCES USED IN DIFFERENT FOOD WASTE FOR THE ENZYME PRODUCTION

As Microbial Growth is short, the requirements of industries for enzyme production using microbial source is fulfilled. The food waste is nutrient and organic rich source for production of valuable products like organic acids, methane, chemical, ethanol and most importantly enzymes using various technical processes.

There is tremendous potential in glucoamylase and protease enzymes for applying in pharmaceutical; food industrial processes. It has been demonstrated that glucoamylase and protease can be effectively produced from waste bread using solid state fermentation.

Scientists have produced the laccase production by fungus *Trametes hirsute* of family Polyporaceae using potato, orange, and apple peelings (Jasminailerdži). Laccase is lignin modifying enzyme. To remove phenolic compounds in the recovery process of enzymes laccase and peroxidase enzymes have been effective. It has been shown that by solid state fermentation three fungal enzymes (invertase, pectinase, and tannase) produced by *Aspergillus niger* produced higher yield compared to submerged fermentation. Physiological studies explain the reason behind this result. Such comparison studies are also helpful to get maximum enzyme production using fungus. Glucose oxidase enzyme production using the waste mycelium of *A.niger* is the other example. If *A. niger* waste mycelium is present in food waste containing sodium gluconate, potassium gluconate can be used for Glucose oxidase enzyme production. The study revealed that maintaining metal ions accelerates Glucose oxidase activity.

Scientists have been proposed an idea to valorize the molecules like amino acids and sugars recovered from bakery waste to feedstocks in bioconversion process. In this study they have given an innovative approach by using Bakery waste for valorization, biocolorant and enzyme production. Nutrient rich hydrolysate containing free amino nitrogen, sugars and phosphates was generated using bakery waste by *Aspergillus awamori* and *Aspergillus oryzae*. This hydrolysate was used for bio-colorant production and solid state fermentation for glucoamylase and protease enzyme production using filamentous fungus *Monascuspurpureus*.

Another interesting approach of linking discovery of renewable fuel and focus to use food waste as raw material for biofuels production has been done. Leonidas Matsakas and Paul Christakopoulos have been successful in ethanol production from enzymatically treated dried food waste using enzymes produced on-site. The ethanol production from source House hold food waste had been evaluated and also produced hydrolytic enzymes for cellulose hydrolysis in- house using thermophilic fungus *Myceliophthora thermophila*. After studying enzyme production it was optimized for an enzymatic activity up to 0.28 FPU/ml in the cell free broth. The enzymes produced in this way with 30% (w/w) were used to hydrolyze cellulose in obtaining sugars for ethanol production. A considerable amount of ethanol production was found to be produced when enzymes were added as compare to the control where no saccharification by enzymes was done.

TYPES OF VARIOUS FOOD WASTE USED FOR DIFFERENT ENZYMES

Food Waste Containing Bread, Savory, Waste Cakes, Cafeteria Waste, Fruits, Vegetables and Potatoes

Number of Enzyme recovery steps needed is proportional to degree of purity and safety needed for that enzyme. Saccharification of FW is the important step in bioconversion of polymers to their monomers. Glucoamylase is the industrially important enzyme. In situ enzyme production without downstream processing is a less expensive, productive method.(Merino and Cherry,2007,Wangetet..al.2010).This strategy has been used by many researchers.

EsraUckunKiran et.al, studied glucoamylase production using *Aspergillus awamori*by solid state fermentation. FW was bread, savory, waste cakes, cafeteria waste, fruits, vegetables, and potatoes. This study proved that cake waste was best substrate for glucoamylase production (Source: Biofuel Research Journal 3 (2014) 98-105).

For Glucoamylase production, food waste is sterilized and fermented after inoculating A.awarmori . Once fermentation is completed, enzyme is extracted with the addition of enzyme carrier and enzyme is stored.

In second step food waste in hydrolytic reactor,enzyme in proportion to food waste volume is added to give glucose rich bioliuid.

Thus initial pH of 7.9, initial moisture content of 69.6% was found to be optimum for glucoamylase production using *Aspergillus awamori*. The enzyme solution produced was used for Saccharifiation of starch present in FW.

FOOD PROCESSING WASTES

Protease Production

Industrial Protease production is contributing 65% of the global market. They are useful in food industry, detergent industry and pharmaceutical industry. The production of enzymes like proteases, lipases, chitinolytic enzymes, ligninolytic enzymes from Fish wastes (heads, viscera, chitinous material, wastewater, etc.) was studied in details by Faouzi Ben Rebah . *Bacillus cereus* Strain grown in fish processing waste based media was mostly used in protease production.

Fish raw materials used in growth media were heads and viscera of *Sardinella*, viscera from rainbow trout, swordfish, Acid hydrolyzed tuna waste, defatted tuna waste. Among these heads and viscera of *Sardinella* waste when used to grow *Pseudomonas aeruginosa showed* protease activity maximum that is 7,800 U/ml (Table 2).

Lipases Enzymes

Lipases the next industrially important enzyme class can be produced in significant quantity using *Staphylococcus xylosus* growth in fish processing waste based media as mentioned in Table 2.

Table 3 gives the details about production of lipases.

Table 2. Protease production by various microbial strains grown in fish processing waste based media

Fish raw materials	Preparation of the growth media	Microbial strains	Activity (U/ml)	References
Heads and viscera of *Sardinella*	Raw materials cooked, pressed, minced and dried (80 °C, 24–48 h)	*Pseudomonas aeruginosa MN7*	7,800	Triki-Ellouz et al. (2003)
Heads and viscera of *Sardinella*	Raw materials cooked, pressed, minced and dried (80 °C, 24–48 h)	*Bacillus subtilis*	720	Ellouz et al. (2001)
Viscera from rainbow trout, swordfish, squid and yellowfin tuna	For peptone preparation, raw materials were ground with water and supernatant recovered after centrifugation was processed	*Vibrio anguillarum*	35–68	Vazquez et al. (2006)
Viscera from rainbow trout, swordfish, squid and yellowfin tuna	For peptone preparation, raw materials were ground with water and supernatant recovered after centrifugation was processed	*Vibrio splendidus*	9–30	Vazquez et al. (2006)
Raw tuna waste	Raw materials cooked, bones removed, pressed to remove water and fat, pressed, minced and dried (80 °C, 24–48 h)	*Bacillus cereus*	74.77	Esakkiraj et al. (2009)
Defatted tuna waste	Extraction with chloroform/methanol	*Bacillus cereus*	134.57	Esakkiraj et al. (2009)
Acid-hydrolyzed tuna waste	Method described by Gao et al. (2006)	*Bacillus cereus*	60.37	Esakkiraj et al. (2009)
Alkali-hydrolyzed tuna waste	Method described by Batista (1999)	Bacillus cereus	65.96	Esakkiraj et al. (2009)

Source: Biotech (2013) 3:255–265

Table 3. Production of lipase by different microbial species grown in fish processing by-products

Fish raw materials	Preparation of the growth media	Microbial strains	Lipase activity (U/ml)	References
Defatted tuna by-products	Extraction with chloroform/methanol[a]	*Staphylococcus epidermidis*CMST Pi 2	12.63	Esakkiraj et al. (2010a)
Defatted tuna by-products	Extractionwith chloroform/methanol[a]	*Staphylococcus epidermidis*CMST Pi 2	14.20	Esakkiraj et al. (2010a)
Tuna by-products	Raw materials were cooked, bones were removed, pressed to remove water and fat, pressed, minced and dried(80 °C, 24–48 h)[a]	*Staphylococcus epidermidis*CMST Pi 2	8.17	Esakkiraj et al. (2010a)
Shrimp by-products	Raw materials were boiled (100 °C for 20 min) in water and supernatants were recuperated by centrifugation[b]	*Staphylococcus xylosus*	19–28	Ben Rebah et al. (2008)
Cuttlefish by-products	Raw materials were boiled (100 °C for 20 min) in water and supernatants were recuperated by centrifugation[b]	*Staphylococcus xylosus*	5–9.50	Ben Rebah et al. (2008)
Tuna by-products	Raw materials were boiled (100 °C for 20 min) in water and supernatants were recuperated by centrifugation[b]	*Staphylococcus xylosus*	0–4	Ben Rebah et al. (2008)

a To the basal medium, fish powder obtained after processing was added at different proportions
b The supernatant was used as a nutrient source for lipase production
Source: 3 Biotech (2013) 3:255–265

Staphylococcus xylosus showed 19-28 U/ml lipase activity using Shrimp by-products, which is in considerable amount as compared to other raw materials. (Table 3).

Chitinolytic enzymes, Ligninolytic enzymes are equally important. It has been known that chitinases are useful in Single cell Protein production and isolating protoplast from yeast and fungi. (Dahiya et al. 2006). Shrimp waste from sea food can be a substrate for fermentative production of chitinase enzyme by solid state fermentation after mild treatment. (Y.L.Ramchandra et.al 2008) .They isolated *Oerskovia* Sp., *Sporolactobacillus* Sp.2, and *Sporolactobacillus* Sp.2 giving maximum of 56.8, 34.0, and 17.2 U/g, IDS chitinase production.

Ligninolytic enzymes are effective in xenobiotic substance removal and hence more study is needed to focus on this as xenobiotic is toxic to human and animal health.

FUTURE ASPECTS

As compare to chemical and physical degradation of food waste biological decomposing is effective and better for economic and ecological reason. To reduce food loss there is need to implement different policies like enabling export, reducing transport regulations, supporting food processing.

Enzymes, the high value added compounds have different challenges bound to its recovery from food waste. Considering all the parameters discussed in the chapter it interprets that more innovative techniques are needed to apply for recovery of enzymes. Nanotechnology is a promising technique to use in enzyme production using Food waste. Hydroxy nanoparticles can act as a chaperon; this property can be applied in the future.

CONCLUSION

All the enzymes aforementioned have been produced and they have high market potential. General techniques that are used in the recovery of enzymes can be applied to enzyme production using food waste. Isolation, Fractionation, precipitation, centrifugation, ultrafiltration, chromatography, electrophoresis and liquid - liquid extraction are the available methods for enzyme purification. It is not sufficient to use single method for isolating and purifying enzymes. Precipitation (salt precipitation, Solvent precipitation and isoelectric precipitation) is the initial step used for isolating enzyme. Later on chromatography techniques (Gel filtration chromatography, Ion exchange chromatography, Adsorption chromatography and Affinity chromatography) are used. Recombinant DNA technology has wide application in production of industrially important enzymes with desired characteristics, using food waste, resulting in cost effective manner.

REFERENCES

Ahamed, A., Yin, K., Ng, B. J. H., Ren, F., Chang, V. W.-C., & Wang, J.-Y. (2016). Life cycle assessment of the present and proposed food waste management technologies from environmental and economic impact perspectives. *Journal of Cleaner Production*, *131*, 607–614. doi:10.1016/j.jclepro.2016.04.127

Anto, H., Trivedi, U. B., & Patel, K. C. (2006). Glucoamylase production by solid- state fermentation using rice flake manufacturing waste products as substrate. *Bioresource Technology, 97*(10), 1161–1166. doi:10.1016/j.biortech.2005.05.007 PMID:16006122

Ben Rebah, F., Frikha, F., Kammoun, W., Belbahri, L., Gargouri, Y., & Miled, N. (2008). Culture of Staphylococcus xylosus in fish processing by-product-based media for lipase production. Lett. *Applied Microbiology, 47*(6), 549–554. doi:10.1111/j.1472-765X.2008.02465.x PMID:19120924

Ben Rebah & Miled. (2013). Fish processing wastes for microbial enzyme production: A review. *Biotech, 3*, 255–265.

Ćilerdžić, Stajić, Vukojević, Duletić-Laušević, & Knežević. (2011). Potential of *Tramete Hirsuta* to Produce Ligninolytic Enzymes during Degradation Of Agricultural Residues. *BioResources, 6*(3), 2885–2895.

Dahiya, N., Tewari, R., & Hoondal, G. S. (2006). Biotechnological aspects of chitinolytic enzymes: A review. *Applied Microbiology and Biotechnology, 71*(6), 773–782. doi:10.100700253-005-0183-7 PMID:16249876

DeWitt, C. A. M., & Morrissey, M. T. (2002). Pilot plant recovery of catheptic proteases from surimi wash water. *Bioresource Technology, 82*(3), 295–301. doi:10.1016/S0960-8524(01)00178-X PMID:11991080

Esakkiraj, P., Austin Jeba Dhas, G., Palavesam, A., & Immanuel, G. (2010a). Media preparation using tuna-processing wastes for improved lipase production by shrimp gut isolate *Staphylococcus epidermidis* CMST Pi2. *Applied Biochemistry and Biotechnology, 160*(4), 1254–1265. doi:10.100712010-009-8632-x PMID:19430738

Esakkiraj, P., Rajkumarbharathi, M., Palavesam, A., & Immanuel, G. (2010b). Lipase production by *Staphylococcus epidermidis* CMST-Pi 1 isolated from the gut of shrimp *Penaeusindicus. Annals of Microbiology, 60*(1), 37–42. doi:10.100713213-009-0003-x

Gaoa, A. (2017). Comparison between the technologies for food waste treatment. *Energy Procedia, 105*, 3915–3921. doi:10.1016/j.egypro.2017.03.811

Garcia-Garcia, Woolley, & Rahimifard, Colwill, White, & Needham. (2017). A Methodology for Sustainable Management of Food Waste. *Waste and Biomass Valorization, 8*, 2209–2227.

Kiran, Trzcinski, & Liu. (2014). Glucoamylase production from food waste by solid state fermentation and its evaluation in the hydrolysis of domestic food waste. *Biofuel Research Journal, 3*, 98–105.

Moldes, D., Gallego, P. P., Rodriguez Couto, S., & Sanroman, M. A. (2003). Grape seeds: The best lignocellulosic waste to produce laccase by solid state cultures of Trameteshirsuta. *Biotechnology Letters, 25*(6), 491–495. doi:10.1023/A:1022660230653 PMID:12882277

Ramchandra, Y. L., Padmalatha Rai, S., Sujan Ganapathy, P. S., Sudeep, H. V., & Krushnamurthy, N. B. (2008). Chitinase Production by Solid State Fermentation using Shrimp waste. *Asian Journal Of Microbiol.Biotech.Env.Sc., 10*(3), 615–620.

Rasit & Kuan. (2018). Investigation on the Influence of Bio-catalytic Enzyme Produced from Fruit and Vegetable Waste on Palm Oil Mill Effluent. *IOP Conf. Series: Earth and Environmental Science, 140.*

Rosales, E., Rodriguez Couto, S., & Sanhromán, M. A. (2007). Increased laccase production by *Tramete shirsuta* grown on ground orange peelings. *Enzyme and Microbial Technology*, *40*(5), 1286–1290. doi:10.1016/j.enzmictec.2006.09.015

Rosales, S., Rodríguez Couto, S., & Sanromán, A. (2002). New uses of food waste: Application to laccase production by *Tramete shirsuta*. *Biotechnology Letters*, *24*(9), 701–704. doi:10.1023/A:1015234100459

Schaub, S. M., & Leonard, J. J. (1996). Composting: An alternative waste management option for food processing industries. *Trends in Food Science & Technology*, *7*(8), 263–268. doi:10.1016/0924-2244(96)10029-7

Sharma, R., Chisti, Y., & Banerjee, U. C. (2001). Production, purification, characterization and applications of lipases. *Biotechnology Advances*, *19*(8), 627–662. doi:10.1016/S0734-9750(01)00086-6 PMID:14550014

Uçkun, E. (2014). Glucoamylase production from food waste by solid state fermentation and its evaluation in the hydrolysis of domestic food waste. *Biofuel Research Journal*, *3*, 98–105.

Unakal. (2012). Production of α-amylase using banana waste by *Bacillus subtilis* under solid state fermentation. *European Journal of Experimental Biology*, *2*(4), 1044–1052.

Wang, Q. H., Liu, Y. Y., & Ma, H. Z. (2010). On-site production of crude glucoamylase for kitchen waste hydrolysis. *Waste Management & Research*, *28*(6), 539–544. doi:10.1177/0734242X09354353 PMID:20015936

Wohlgemuth, Sigma-Aldrich, Buchs, & Switzerland. (2011). Product Recovery. Comprehensive Biotechnology, 2, 591-601.

This research was previously published in Global Initiatives for Waste Reduction and Cutting Food Loss edited by Aparna B. Gunjal, Meghmala S. Waghmode, Neha N. Patil, and Pankaj Bhatt; pages 31-42, copyright year 2019 by Engineering Science Reference (an imprint of IGI Global).

Chapter 33

Recent Advances in Waste Cooking Oil Management and Applications for Sustainable Environment

Ching Thian Tye
Universiti Sains Malaysia, Malaysia

ABSTRACT

This chapter discusses the management of waste cooking oil (WCO) in a sustainable manner in order to protect the environmental pollution. Increasing consumption of edible oils worldwide leads to generation of substantial amount of waste cooking oil (WCO). While WCO is not considered toxic, large amount of WCO can contribute to environment pollution if not being handled properly. The huge generation of WCO in the world creates problem of collection, treatment and disposal. Due to its chemical features, the recycling of WCO not only provides a renewable feedstock for producing biofuels and bio-based products, but also alleviates environmental pollution arising from its improper handling. This chapter also provides an overview of some recent approaches in WCO recycling and applications.

INTRODUCTION

The increase of population and living standards has led to higher demand of edible oils worldwide. This can be seen from the growth in global production of vegetable oils of 90.5 million metric tons in year 2000/2001 to 197.23 million metric tons in year 2017/2018 (Statista, 2019a). Edible oils are oils mainly extracted from plants or vegetables such as, oil palm fruit, soybean, rapeseed, sunflower seed, peanut, coconut and etc. Palm oil is the most common type of edible oil (Statista, 2019b). Edible oils consist mostly of triacylglycerides (96%) that composed of different fatty acids and some other compounds such as free fatty acids, phospholipids, phytosterols, tocopherols, other antioxidants or waxes (Matthäus, 2010).

DOI: 10.4018/978-1-7998-5354-1.ch033

All over the world, edible oil is essential in food preparation and substantial quantity of edible oils are used for food frying either in home, restaurants or in food industry. Waste cooking oils (WCO) are bio-based oils that have been used for the same purpose. During the frying process, cooking oil undergoes various physical and chemical changes due to chemical reactions including hydrolysis, thermal degradation, oxidation, and polymerization (Panadare & Rathod, 2015). Repeated frying and usage of edible oil alters its physiochemical and nutrition properties, and leads to the formation of Total Polar Compounds (TPCs), which in high rates have been found to have a negative effect on a person's health. At certain point after reused multiple times, the oil becomes unfit for human consumption and may pose serious health risks such as hypertension, liver disease, increased cholesterol and atherosclerosis by consuming such oil (The news minute, 2019).

High amount of cooking oil consumption leads to significant wastage. WCO and fat generated from kitchens and food preparation have created serious problems for their disposal, due to its slow degradation. Proper waste management is thus necessary for WCO in order to preserve a sustainable environment.

WCO implies an economic loss in edible oils. Due to its chemical composition and physical nature, WCO can be considered as a potential waste which can be utilized as energy source and raw material for chemical or biological processes. It has been getting more attention as a low-cost feedstock for producing biodiesel or other biofuels and nonfuel products comparing to the use of edible oils as a food resource for human beings. The present article provides an overview regarding recent advancement in WCOs management and applications for recycled WCO.

DETRIMENTAL EFFECTS OF FOOD DERIVED USED OIL AND FAT

Fat and oil consumption per capita in developed countries was estimated at over 50 kg/annum compared to less than 20 kg/annum in less developed countries (Williams, Clarkson, Mant, Drinkwater, & May, 2012). It is estimated that 2.5 L of WCO are produced per person per month domestically (European Biomass Industry Association, 2015). In Japan, it is presumed that 100–140 ktonne WCO from household sector are discarded every year (Ministry of Environment, 2006). Oil cannot be removed from cooking operations as it is inveterate in many culinary customs. Used cooking oil is considered a waste upon being discharged into the sewer systems. The waste oil from multiple sites can accumulate in the sewer with other non-flushable waste to cause sewage blockage and overflow, leading to odor, nuisance and creating the corrosion of sewer lines under anaerobic conditions. It has been estimated that 50-75% of approximately 24,750 inline blockages per year in the UK (Arthur et al., 2008) are due to fat, oil and grease (FOG) deposits (Keener et al., 2008). In 2000, the Drainage Services Department of Hong Kong claimed that more than 60% of sewer blockages were due to excessive grease build-ups (Chan, 2010). These deposits can impact human health and the environment.

In addition, oil and fat that pass through the sewer system and enter wastewater treatment plants will increase the difficulties to treat. Additional techniques such as dissolved air flotation, centrifugation, filtration, biological removal and ultrafiltration are needed, in order to treat the oil contaminated water, which leading to increase operational and maintenance costs (Wallace et al., 2017).

Another concern is gutter oil, which is illicit cooking oil that has been recycled from waste oil collected from restaurant fryers, drains, grease traps, and slaughterhouse waste has emerged as a serious food-safety issue in China. Taking food prepared from oxidation and hydrogenation of this 'gutter oil' can cause health problems in humans (Lu & Wu, 2014). In September 2014, an incident of "food safety scandal" was reported in Taiwan (Wee, Budiman, Su, Chang, & Chen, 2016). It was related to the usage of gutter/tainted oil by several oil suppliers, in which the series of food safety incidents affected 1,256 businesses.

WASTE OIL MANAGEMENT

WCO does not contain toxic components or heavy metals commonly found in the used petroleum derived oil products. Nevertheless, used cooking oils should not be simply disposed and need to be handled properly. Appropriate waste oil management is important for sustainable development. European countries utilize the waste hierarchy, as depicted in Figure 1, to manage WCO (European Parliament Council, 2008). The waste hierarchy refers to prevention as the preferred method when tackling waste but when this is not feasible, the 3Rs (reduce, reuse or recycle) are the next option (Wallace, Gibbons, O'Dwyer, & Curran, 2017). Disposal of the used oil is to be totally avoided if possible.

Figure 1. Waste Hierarchy in relation to waste cooking oil management, adapted from European Parliament Council (2008)
Source: (Wallace et al., 2017)

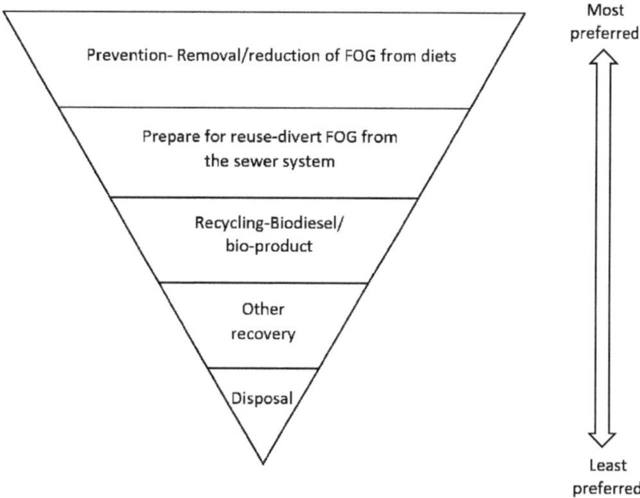

The aim for any effective waste management is to minimize the production of waste and reuse waste produced. Education and awareness campaigns with the stakeholders are the foundation for all waste oil management initiatives. There are policies and regulations for how used cooking oils are to be collected, stored, transported and processed in different countries in order to ensure a sustainable living environment in long run. The following sections are some recent trends of international waste oil management approaches.

Public Awareness and Prevention

Public awareness is the key to successful waste oil management. With waste the result of human activities, a proper understanding of waste management issues is paramount, without which the success of even the best-conceived waste management plan becomes doubtful. A high level of public awareness regarding the issue can reduce the waste oil production at the top of the waste hierarchy. This can prevent and reduce the detrimental effects resulted from the waste oil generated. Public awareness can be achieved via public educational campaigns to mitigate domestic sewer deposits and inappropriate waste oil disposal. The public must be made aware of waste management issues to understand the consequences of improper management of waste and how it may ultimately pose a serious threat to their lives and well-being (Hasan, 2004).

In the meantime, attempts to increase public awareness and some regulatory preventive measurement have been carried out. All facilities with a trade effluent discharge are potential fat, oil and grease (FOG) producers. Many authorities around the world get to reduce FOG waste entering the sewerage system by requiring or enforcing the installation of grease trapping systems (GTSs) (He et al., 2013). Since the year 2000, the UK Building Regulations have required all new and converted premises to install grease management systems. Before the year 2000, food service outlets generally only had a GTSs if they had been identified as problematic. Even when GTSs were installed, maintenance was often poor, which resulted in FOG entering the sewer systems (Williams et al., 2012).

Waste Cooking Oil Recovery

When WCO generation is unavoidable, affords to recover the WCO are necessary in order to minimize the detrimental consequences. In terms of WCO recovery, it is found that an effective domestic WCO collection systems will reduce the WCO discharging down into the sewer system. Many countries' local authorities have started the system to collect the WCO from residential areas in addition to industry sector. For instance, in the United Kingdom, local authority has a legal duty under the Environmental Protection Act 1990 to collect household waste such as WCO (UK Environmental Law Association). The estimated WCO collected in Europe annually is 100,000-700,000 tonnes (Iglesias, Laca, Herrero, & Díaz, 2012).

In Asia, commencing from October 2014, the government of Republic of China (Taiwan) has made the recycling of WCO from residential and commercial sectors in Taiwan mandatory. The WCO produced by households and institutions can be collected by local environmental protection bureaus or sanitation teams, which are legally obliged to manage it. The WCOs that are produced by small-scale commercial stores (e.g., restaurant, snack bar, vendor, night market) can also be collected by municipal collection teams. In the meantime, in order to maintain effective WCO collection and to track its flow, applications for permits are henceforth to be reviewed and issued by local governments. The collected amounts of WCO was reported increased significantly from 1599 tonnes in 2015 to 12,591 tonnes in 2017, reflecting on the WCO recycling regulation effective since 2015 (Tsai, 2019).

A study using life cycle sustainability assessment (LCSA) methodology showed that domestic WCO collection systems through urban collection centers (UCC) has better environmental and economic performance compared to those collection systems through schools and door-to-door cities in Mediterranean countries (Vinyes, Oliver-Solà, Ugaya, Rieradevall, & Gasol, 2013). LCSA is the combination of life cycle assessment, life cycle costing, and social life cycle assessment.

European Biomass Industry Association carried out a multi country initiative RecOil project that involved Spain, Greece, Italy, Portugal, Belgium and Denmark. The RecOil project found that it was possible to collect 2.5 liters of WCO per household per month (European Biomass Industry Association, 2015). 60% of used cooking oil is found improperly disposed of. Information among 44 different WCO collection systems implemented was analyzed. 180 tonnes and 80 tonnes of WCO was collected from restaurants and private households, respectively, approximately 45% of the estimated potential of 400 tonnes per year from restaurants and 16% of the estimated potential of 500 tonnes from private households. Nearly €30,000 was saved from the cost of maintaining the wastewater treatment plants. The project highlighted the benefits of utilizing the waste stream and the potential saving available.

Apart from direct WCO collection, it is equally important to create an eco-system that encompasses the complete life cycle of the WCO recovery, in this case, from public education, to establishing effective oil collection to the producing of value-added end product, such as bio-diesel. With this in mind, on 1st of July 2018, the Food Safety and Standards Authority of India (FSSAI) announced the new regulations for monitoring WCO. The implementation of the regulations will require focus on consumer education, enforcement as well as creation of an eco-system for collection of WCO to produce biodiesel. FSSAI is in discussion with the Indian Biodiesel Association to establish a nation-wide eco-system for collection of used cooking oil and its conversion to bio-diesel (The Hindu Business line, 2018).

WASTE COOKING OIL RECYCLING AND APPLICATIONS

Concerns of world crude oil reserve depleting and impact of fossil fuels to the environment has led to searching for alternative renewable replacement. Use of WCO into the fuel mix has been an attractive one. Motivated by the aforementioned needs, the WCO recycling industry has grown over the past five years as both upstream and downstream markets have fared well (IBIS world, 2018). There are companies who offer services for WCO collection, grease trap maintenance, meat byproduct collection and deadstock pickup to the customers. This has directly promoting in WCO reused and recycling process. This is a good example of waste management not only solves the derived pollution problem, but also can become a resourceful feedstock for fuel production and a series of other applications. The following section states the various applications of WCO.

Conversion of Waste Cooking Oil Into Fuel

At least 8.9 million tons of WCO is produced worldwide annually. Many countries encourage the conversion of WCO to liquid fuel such as biodiesel, bio gasoline and green aviation fuel. China has been promoting this since 2006 and first implemented the Renewable Energy Law in 2006. Then, it is followed by the various medium- and long-term Renewable Energy Development Plans in later years. Liquid biofuels are important components in these legal initiatives to promote renewable energy (Liang, Liu, Xu, & Zhang, 2013).

WCO is one of the most prudent sources of energy because of its restrictions for food use, cheap, availability and appropriateness for fuel production. WCO can be converted into biofuel via different pathways or reactions. The most commons include transesterification, hydrocracking, catalytic cracking and pyrolysis (Table 1). With the different process, the properties and applications of the derived biofuel is also different. Some recent advances in WCO recycling via these processes are also discussed.

Table 1. Common processes used in WCO recycling and treating

Process	Operating Conditions	Major Product
Transesterification	React with alcohol at 60°C with the presence of base catalyst.	FAME (biodiesel), glycerol
Catalytic cracking	At 300-500 °C with selective catalyst.	Gasoline
Hydrodeoxygenation	With H_2 at 290-400 °C with metal catalyst.	C15-C18 hydrocarbons
Pyrolysis	At 550-800 °C in an inert atmosphere.	Bio-oil

Transesterification

Transesterification is the most widely used industrial process to produce biodiesel from vegetable or plant oil because the process is simple and cost effective. In this process, the fat or oil is first purified and then reacted with an alcohol, usually methanol (CH_3OH) or ethanol (CH_3CH_2OH), in the presence of a catalyst such as potassium hydroxide (KOH) or sodium hydroxide (NaOH) (Figure 2). When this process occurs, the triglycerides (oil or fat) is transformed to form esters and glycerol. The esters that remain are called biodiesel. In case of methanol used, a more common term used for biodiesel is fatty acid methyl ester (FAME). During the transesterification process, the reactant that reacts with methanol is triglyceride molecules (major component) in the plant or vegetable derived oil. Therefore, WCO with triglyceride as the major compound has been a very good candidate. In addition, there is another by–product, glycerol form in this process which can help in production economic. In the process, after the reaction, FAME is separated from glycerol.

Figure 2. Transesterification of triglyceride (vegetable oil) into FAME and glycerol
R is the mixture of hydrocarbon parts of different fatty acids present in the triglyceride

$$
\begin{array}{ccccc}
\begin{matrix} O \\ \| \\ CH_2\text{-}O\text{-}C\text{-}R_1 \\ | \quad O \\ \quad \| \\ CH\text{-}O\text{-}C\text{-}R_2 \\ | \quad O \\ \quad \| \\ CH_2\text{-}O\text{-}C\text{-}R_3 \end{matrix}
& + \; 3CH_3\text{-}OH
& \xrightarrow[\text{catalyst}]{\substack{60\text{-}90°C \\ \text{Alkaline}}}
& \begin{matrix} O \\ \| \\ CH_3\text{-}O\text{-}C\text{-}R_1 \\ O \\ \| \\ CH_3\text{-}O\text{-}C\text{-}R_2 \\ O \\ \| \\ CH_3\text{-}O\text{-}C\text{-}R_3 \end{matrix}
& + \; \begin{matrix} CH_2\text{-}OH \\ | \\ CH\text{-}OH \\ | \\ CH_2\text{-}OH \end{matrix}
\\
\text{Triglyceride} & \text{Methanol} & & \text{FAME} & \text{Glycerol} \\
& & & \text{(biodiesel)} &
\end{array}
$$

Biodiesel have similar physical characteristics as those of fossil diesel fuels. The high viscosity of vegetable oils is reduced by the transesterification process. Biodiesel blend is the blend of fossil diesel and FAME (Khalid & Khalid, 2011). A different set of additives is required for biodiesel blend than fossil diesel which is for correcting low temperature behaviour and slowing down of the oxidation processes of biodiesel in storage (ETIP Bioenergy, 2019). Biodiesel is non-toxic and biodegradable. Using WCO as the feedstock in transesterification process is also found to have lower greenhouse gases compare to fresh cooking oil in life cycle assessment.

Over the year, effort is still going on to improve the process in order to optimize the yield from transesterification of WCO. This includes improvement from operating condition, catalysts used as well as using WCO from different sources as feedstock. Mohadesi et al. (2019) investigated the transesterification of WCO with methanol in the presence of potassium hydroxide as the catalyst using a semi-industrial pilot of microreactor with 50 tubes to produce 5 L/h biodiesel. The authors claimed the highest level of biodiesel purity or FAMEs obtained at 98.26%.

In Indonesia, effects of alcohol type and base catalyst used during transesterification were investigated using chicken fat and WCO to produce methyl esters. The reaction process was run for 90 minutes at 60°C and 2000 rpm stirring rate. Maximum methyl esters yield of 91% was reported. The fuel properties of methyl esters produced with methanol and sugarcane spirits were close to each other. The production cost of biodiesels from chicken fat and WCO were reported cheaper than market biodiesel selling price (Soegiantoro, Chang, Rahmawati, Christiani, & Mufrodi, 2019).

Kataria et al. (2019) studied a heterogeneous base catalyzed transesterification under different reactant proportions: the molar ratio of alcohol to oil and mass ratio of catalyst to oil, for the optimum production of biodiesel. The optimum condition for base catalyzed transesterification of WCO was determined as 12:1 and 5 wt.% of zinc doped calcium oxide. The fuel properties of the produced biodiesel and their blend for different ratios were comparable with properties of fossil diesel and ASTM biodiesel standards. Tests have been conducted on a CI engine and the biodiesel produced using heterogeneous catalyst was found suitable to be used as diesel oil blends, having lesser emissions as compared to fossil diesel.

Esterification

Some WCOs have high free fatty acid (FFA) content, (>1%). In such cases, saponification hinders separation of the ester from glycerin and reduces the yield and formation rate of FAME during transesterification (Lucena, Silva, & Fernandes, 2008). Therefore, WCO with FFA contains higher than 1% needs to go through a pretreatment process before transesterification. Esterification is another process that converts component in WCO into biodiesel or FAME. The process is similar to transesterification as WCO is reacted with methanol to produce FAME. However, the component involve in the reaction is the free fatty acid in the WCO. FFA in WCO react with methanol to produce FAME and water. Figure 3 represents the reaction.

Figure 3. Esterification of free fatty acid into FAME (biodiesel) and water

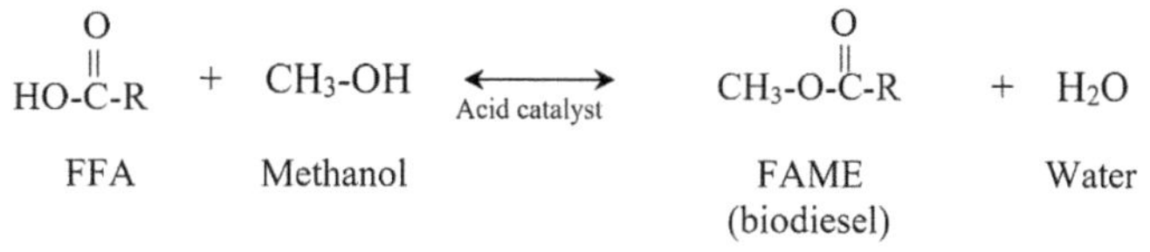

$$\underset{\text{FFA}}{\text{HO-C-R}} \;+\; \underset{\text{Methanol}}{\text{CH}_3\text{-OH}} \;\underset{\text{Acid catalyst}}{\rightleftharpoons}\; \underset{\substack{\text{FAME}\\ \text{(biodiesel)}}}{\text{CH}_3\text{-O-C-R}} \;+\; \underset{\text{Water}}{\text{H}_2\text{O}}$$

Pretreatment of WCO with esterification was found to be the most efficient using acidic catalyst. The FFA was reported to reduce up to 88.8% at 60 °C with 1:2.5 methanol to oil molar ratio (Sahar, Sadaf, Iqbal, Ullah, & Iqbal, 2018). In general, the process for biodiesel or FAME production is as shown in Figure 4.

Figure 4. Transesterification process to produce FAME

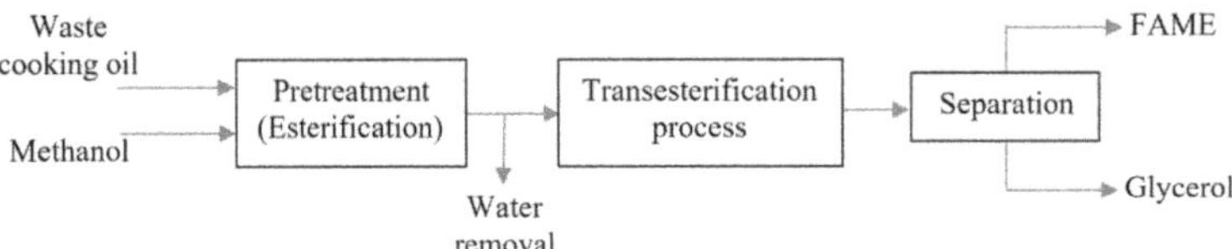

Catalytic Cracking

Catalytic cracking has been a conventional process used to treat waste oil. It is considered to be inexpensive in terms of energy consumption to convert petroleum feedstocks to lighter fractions of gasoline boiling range. Catalytic cracking process is carried out with selective catalyst at temperature within 300-500°C. Conversion of WCO into green fuel via catalytic cracking has also been carried out. The product obtained from catalytic cracking of vegetable oils includes organic liquid product, gas, coke and water. The distributions of products yield were influenced by various factors such as composition of feedstock, reaction temperature, residence/reaction time, nature and the type of catalyst used (Wakoc, Reshadb, Bhaleraoa, & Goud, 2018). During the conversion of vegetable oils under catalytic cracking conditions, the gasoline fraction can be produced in an amount of up to 40% (of feedstock mass), as well as 10–15 wt. % propane–propylene (PPF) and butane–butylene (BBF) fractions (Doronin, Potapenko, Lipin, Sorokina, & Buluchevskaya, 2012).

The major difference in catalytic cracking of WCO compare to the conventional petroleum catalytic cracking process is the feedstock. Therefore, studies of various potential catalysts such as composite zeolite, functionalized ZSM-5, metals etc. have been carried out (Chang & Tye, 2013; Chiam & Tye, 2013; Abdul Majed & Tye, 2018). The liquid fuel obtained from catalytic cracking process after water removal is mainly hydrocarbon, which has very similar properties as the fossil fuel with much lower oxygen content. This has made it a favorable process to convert WCO to fuel.

Hydrodeoxygenation

In order to improve the yield of liquid fuel in the cracking process, hydrogen is added during reaction. The process is called hydrodeoxygenation. There has been commercial production of renewable aviation fuel from plant/vegetable oil via hydrodeoxygenation. Successful green fuel production from vegetable has also leading to using WCO with similar properties as the feedstock. Li et al. (2018) claims a nearly complete conversion and 90% selectivity to C15-C18 hydrocarbons was achieved at 350 °C.

Pyrolysis

Pyrolysis is another process used to convert biomass into bio-oil or fuel. Pyrolysis is a thermal decomposition process that carried out at elevated temperatures (550-800 °C) in an inert atmosphere. Pyrolysis of WCO can produce bio-oil (main product) of high caloric value (high heating value ~ 8843 kg/Kcal) which can be further processed into liquid fuel.

The gas and solid byproducts of pyrolysis of waste oil are also have their respective applications as seen in Figure 5. The gases product (syngas) with heating value up to 8 MJ/kg is suitable as an energy source and the biochar which is rich in iron and organic carbon is suitable (Trabelsi, Zaafouri, Baghdadi, Naoui, & Ouerghi, 2018).

Figure 5. Pyrolysis of waste cooking oil

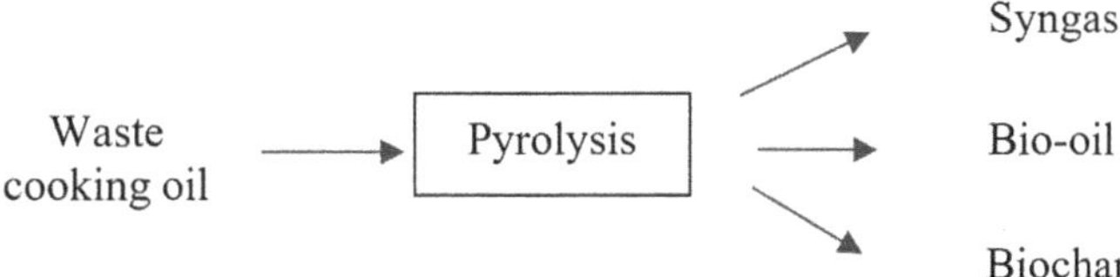

Waste Cooking Oil as Building Material

Other than fuel, WCO has also been used and tested for other applications such as construction and building material. It was added in the synthesis of lime mortars for restorative materials. Application of ordinary Portland cement (OPC) binders for repair and rehabilitation of old buildings is proven to be unsuitable, due to incompatibility problems frequently associated with the pathology origin in the restoration of historical buildings. The low affinity of OPC binders/mortars with historical substrates has been an issue (Grilo et al., 2014).

New lime mortars with addition of WCO was synthesized for restorative rendering applications. Air-, formulated- and hydraulic-lime mortars were synthesized with inclusion of used sunflower cooking oils and, brick waste powder as pozzolanic addition, when necessary. The results of WCOs addition in the mortars exhibited promising hydrophobic effects, such as sorptivity reduction up to 60 times and improvement of superficial durability. Addition of high-oleic acid cooking oil in 13 wt.% in the formulated and hydraulic lime mortars was reported to increase their hydrophobicity without worsening their mechanical strengths. All the investigated mortars exhibited appropriate indexes as restorative materials (Pahlavan, Manzi, Rodriguez-Estrada, Bignozzi, 2017). Later, another test: air and formulated lime mortars with pulverized brick waste were synthesized with addition of used cooking oil and albumen. Parallel additions of oil and albumen in lime mortars was found increased their hydrophobicity and superficial durability without retarding their setting time due to the role of fatty acids and unfolded proteins under alkaline conditions. Though there are still issues to which, (decreased in permeability values and setting kinetics), the parallel valorization showed high potentials in synthesis of restorative mortars design (Pahlavan, Manzi, Sansonetti, & Bignozzi, 2018).

On the other hand, the possibility of WCO as grinding aid in the production of Portland cement was also assessed. Cement clinker and gypsum were interground with various WCOs. In overall, WCO favorably improves cement grinding. Additionally, certain WCO increased the cement strength (Li, Zhao, Huang, Jiang, & Chen, 2016). All of these studies showed that WCO has its values as construction material.

Waste Cooking Oil in Pavement

Asphalt binder or bitumen plays an important role in the composition of bituminous pavements. Hot mix asphalt (HMA) is the most widely used binder for pavement. Application of recycled pavement materials to produce new pavement materials results in considerable savings of material, and energy. The main problem pertaining to the use of the recycled asphalt pavement (RAP) material in HMA is the ageing of bitumen, which limits the percentage of applied RAP in HMA.

In 2012, waste residential cooking oil was used to rejuvenate the used bituminous binder. The physical properties of the original bitumen, aged bitumen and rejuvenated bitumen were measured and compared by the conventional bitumen binder tests such as softening point, penetration and Brookfield viscosity. The results showed that the aged bitumen was rejuvenated by the WCO due to a change in its physical properties, which resemble the physical properties of original bitumen (80/100). The optimum percentage of WCO for the rejuvenated aged bitumen group of 50/60, 40/50, and 30/40 was reported by adding 1%, 3–4%, and 4–5% of WCO, respectively. The statistical analyses also confirms that there was no significant difference between the original asphalt binder and rejuvenated asphalt binder (Asli, Ahmadinia, Zargar, & Karim, 2012).

Later, similar tests were carried out, Sun et al. (2016) analyzed the properties of asphalt binder modified by bio-oil derived from WCO. The bio-oil, black oily liquid, used was the by-product of WCO refining for biodiesel. The bio-oil derived from WCO is found mainly composed of aromatics, resins and saturates. It was also reported that almost no chemical reactions between bio-oil and control asphalt was observed. The addition of bio-oil decreases the softening point and viscosity, increases the penetration and ductility of control asphalt binder. Furthermore, the addition of bio-oil was found could reduce the deformation resistance and elastic recovery performance of control asphalt and improve the stress relaxation property and thermal cracking resistance of control asphalt (Sun et al., 2016). Again, WCO residue was used in the preparation of HMA using recycled pavement material recently and encouraging results obtained (Ma et al., 2019). Therefore, WCO especially the residue actually is a cheap and widely available potential component, which can be applied in asphalt aggregate preparation for pavement.

Waste Cooking Oil as Cooling Medium

Vegetable oils, due to their attractive properties like renewability, low toxicity, biodegradability, high fire point and availability are considered as a reliable substitute for petroleum-based oils in transformer cooling system (Qiu et al., 2011). Hence, WCOs, with similar properties, instead of the fresh vegetable oil is considered a potential alternative cooling medium source for electrical transformer as well. The performance of WCO after transesterification process (mainly with fatty acid methyl ester) for application in electrical transformers as cooling medium was evaluated and compared to the mineral oil. Based on the study by Raeisian et al. (2019), the breakdown voltage and thermal conductivity (the two main indexes) of transformer that using WCO derived oil as cooling medium are, respectively, 48% and 33%, higher than those of the mineral oil. Furthermore, the transformer hotspot temperature with WCO derived oil is 3°C lower than the mineral oil and the transformer experiences lower temperature in the thermally critical region. Therefore, WCO derived oil was found to be an effective alternative cooling medium for liquid-filled transformers.

Waste Cooking Oil as Chemical Sources

Vegetable oils are made up predominantly of triesters of glycerol with fatty acids and commonly are called triglycerides. The many derivatives of fatty acids manufactures are used in surface coatings, plastics, detergents, lubricants, etc, where the long hydrocarbon chain confer needed plasticity, surface activity, or lubricity (Abdullah & Salimon, 2010). Therefore, large amount of WCOs that is generated daily widely can be considered a rich resource of fatty acid. This has leading to the eco-development of various WCO materials.

WCOs have the potential to be an economic alternative for synthesizing different biomaterials. WCO methyl esters were used as starting material and being structurally modified via epoxidation reaction to epoxide WCO esters. Epoxides are produced by reaction of double bonds with peracids. An example of epoxidation reaction is shown in Figure 6.

Figure 6. Epoxidation of palmitoleic acid

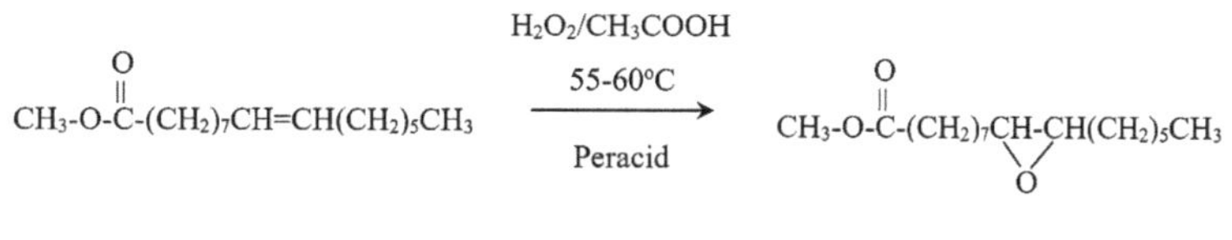

$$CH_3\text{-}O\text{-}\overset{\overset{O}{\|}}{C}\text{-}(CH_2)_7CH=CH(CH_2)_5CH_3 \quad \xrightarrow[\text{Peracid}]{\overset{H_2O_2/CH_3COOH}{55\text{-}60°C}} \quad CH_3\text{-}O\text{-}\overset{\overset{O}{\|}}{C}\text{-}(CH_2)_7\underset{\underset{O}{\diagdown\diagup}}{CH\text{-}CH}(CH_2)_5CH_3$$

Zheng et al. (2018) tested the waste epoxide cooking oil 2-ethylhexyl esters as bio-plasticizer to substitute toxic plasticizer dioctyl phthalate used during poly(vinyl chloride) or PVC processing. Most of the plasticizers used during PVC processing are typically toxic petroleum-based phthalates. The epoxide WCO 2-ethylhexyl esters was found to have superior low temperature property, oxidation stability, and remarkably reduced the glass transition temperature of PVC, comparing to the conventional epoxy compound. It was proven to be an effective alternative to dioctyl phthalate, replacing about 40% of the total plasticizer (Zheng et al., 2018).

Another plasticizer (acetylated-fatty acid methyl ester-citric acid ester, ACFAME-CAE) for PVC was synthesized by using WCO and citric acid as raw materials. The mechanical properties of PVC films with AC-FAME-CAE plasticizer were found better than those of PVC films plasticized by ESO (epoxidized soybean oil) and as good as those of PVC films plasticized by dioctyl phthalate, the conventional plasticizer (Feng et al., 2018).

Waste cooking oil (WCO) has also been used as feedstock for different processes such as to produce aromatics from catalytic fast pyrolysis reaction (Wang, Zhong, Ding, Zhang, & Ruan, 2017). All these efforts have led to a more environmentally friendly process and product.

Waste Cooking Oil as Lubricant

WCO has been using as lubricant for some general work. It can also be used as a feedstock to produce specific lubricant formulation. An organic medium dispersible Cu nanoparticle was directly prepared in a WCO via a "wet chemistry" approach. Blending of nano-copper based additive and PAO6 base oil results in a stable formulation without segregation phenomena. The role of the copper nanoadditives as friction modifier was found to improve oxidative stability of a mixture (Sarno, Spina, & Senatore, 2019).

Waste Cooking Oil as Detergent

WCO can be used to make soap or detergent which can be further used as dish washing, laundry washing, house cleaning, animal or vehicle cleaning use. Low grade soaps can be directly obtained by having WCO reacts with alkali metal hydroxide (approximately 1-5%), via saponification method (Panadare, & Rathod, 2015). There is patented method to produce liquid soap or detergent from WCO in which amine derivatives is used to produce a mild liquid soaps which are safe to handle and without unpleasant odorous substances (Kazuo, 1989).

Recently, Junior et al. (2019) used WCO to synthesize an environmentally friendly detergent: anionic surfactant methyl ester sulfonate (MES). MES was combined with ZnO nanoparticles, producing nanofluidic detergent. WCO was filtered, neutralized and bleached before it underwent transesterification with methanol. The as-produced methyl ester was then undergone sulfonation process to become MES surfactant. The product was then further purified with methanol and neutralized by sodium hydroxide. Liquid detergent comprising of 15% MES concentration and 0.1% ZnO nanoparticles exhibits notable stability, while retaining 64.97% stain removal as well as 82.36% stain degradation.

Waste Cooking Oil as Solvents for Pollutants

WCO with its organic property is also explored for its tendency to solubilize small organic molecules. Tarnpradab et al. (2016) employed WCOs to treat the emission produced during the rice husk pyrolysis. In particular, WCO was found able to reduce the content of organic hydrocarbon contaminants with a molecular weight higher than that of benzene (which are generally referred to as tar). In the study, heavy tar was reported absorbed by WCO through a dissolution mechanism and several data about the saturation levels were reported (Mannu et al. 2019).

Waste Cooking Oil as a Component of Animal Feed

Oils and fats are essential components of animal diet as they serve high energy diets as well as some essential fatty acids are needed and are not synthesised by animals. Very economical WCOs that bind the other ingredients of animal feed together fulfilled this requirement (Panadare, & Rathod, 2015). Food provided to the animals like poultry farms and pigs, indirectly come to human beings via food chain. It should be free from any toxic and unsafe components. Due to food safety, UK government only allow WCO which is collected by a licensed waste carrier, treated well and certified to be used in animal feeds (Panadare, & Rathod, 2015).

Harmful chemicals, especially malondialdehyde and other peroxidation products, such as 2-thiobarbituric acid are generated due to thermal reaction during cooking or frying. This makes it unfit as a component for animal feed. Hence, necessary treating process is needed for WCO prior to be used in animal feed. However, conventional techniques like filtration, degumming, bleaching, and deodorizing processes failed in the removal of those harmful materials. Wei et al. (2011) developed a simple and reliable method to measure the content of malondialdehyde in WCO and studied the removal of malondialdehyde and other 2-thiobarbituric acid reactive substances via three methods: water extraction, physical adsorption, and chemical adsorption. Chemical adsorption using lysine or monosodium glutamate as chemical adsorbent was reported to be the most effective. The authors claimed that removal of 80% of those substances from WCO was achieved.

CONCLUSION

With proper management strategies, WCO can be converted into useful bio base material and helps in alleviating the environmental pollution. More noticeably, WCO represents a renewable resource to produce fuels or can be used as alternative feedstocks in replacements of petroleum-based chemicals. In some cases, it is utilized as a high energy feed additive in various livestock feeding products. WCO is normally a repeatedly used cooking oil. It is vital to understand that oil becomes too acidic when reused multiple times, and after a certain point, the oil becomes unsafe for consumption. This will cause health hazards when people consume it or its processing products. Noting that *repeated frying of oil leads to changes in physiochemical, nutritional, and sensory properties of edible oil,* the FSSAI has announced that restaurants will no longer be able to reuse cooking oil more than three times (The news minute, 2019). Therefore, the reuse of WCO as a feed additive without proper treatment should be banned to prevent it from re-entering the food chain. By the way, recycling of WCO is a sustainable way of using the waste resources that can decrease environmental pollution and promote social and economic benefits.

ACKNOWLEDGMENT

This work was conducted under FRGS 2019-1 by Ministry of Education Malaysia.

REFERENCES

Abdul Majed, M. A.,, & Tye, C. T. (2018). Catalytic cracking of used vegetable oil to green fuel with metal functionalized zsm-5 catalysts. *The Malaysian Journal of Analytical Sciences, 22*(1), 8–16.

Abdullah, B. M., & Salimon, J. (2010). Epoxidation of vegetable oils and fatty acids: catalysts, methods and advantages. *Journal of Applied Sciences (Faisalabad), 10*(15), 1545–1553. doi:10.3923/jas.2010.1545.1553

Asli, H., Ahmadinia, E., Zargar, M., & Karim, M. R. (2012). Investigation on physical properties of waste cooking oil – Rejuvenated bitumen binder. *Construction & Building Materials, 37*, 398–405. doi:10.1016/j.conbuildmat.2012.07.042

BioenergyE. T. I. P. (2019). *Transesterification to biodiesel.* Retrieved from http://www.etipbioenergy.eu/value-chains/conversion-technologies/conventional-technologies/transesterification-to-biodiesel

Chang, W. H.,, & Tye, C. T. (2013). Catalytic cracking of used palm oil using composite zeolite. *The Malaysian Journal of Analytical Sciences, 17*(1), 176–184.

Chen, R.-X.,, & Wang, W.-C. (2019). The production of renewable aviation fuel from waste cooking oil. Part I: Bio-alkane conversion through hydroprocessing of oil. *Renewable Energy, 135*, 819–835. doi:10.1016/j.renene.2018.12.048

Chiam, L. T.,, & Tye, C. T. (2013). Deoxygenation of plant fatty acid using NiSnK/SiO$_2$ as catalyst. *The Malaysian Journal of Analytical Sciences, 17*(1), 129–138.

Doronin, V. P., Potapenko, O. V., Lipin, P. V., Sorokina, T. P., & Buluchevskaya, L. A. (2012). Catalytic cracking of vegetable oils for production of high octane gasoline and petrochemical feedstock. *Petroleum Chemistry*, *52*(6), 392–400. doi:10.1134/S0965544112060059

European Biomass Industry Association. (2015). Transformation of used cooking oil into biodiesel: from waste to resource. Promotion of used cooking oil recycling for sustainable biodiesel production (RecOil). Retrieved from http://www.eubren.com/UCO_to_Biodiesel_2030 _01.pdf

Feng, G., Hu, L., Ma, Y., Jia, P., Hu, Y., Zhang, M., ... Zhou, Y. (2018). An efficient bio-based plasticizer for poly (vinyl chloride) from waste cooking oil and citric acid: Synthesis and evaluation in PVC films. *Journal of Cleaner Production*, *189*, 334–343. doi:10.1016/j.jclepro.2018.04.085

Grilo, J., Faria, P., Veiga, R., Silva, A. S., Silva, V., & Velosa, A. (2014). New natural hydraulic lime mortars – physical and microstructural properties in different curing conditions. *Construction & Building Materials*, *54*, 378–384. doi:10.1016/j.conbuildmat.2013.12.078

Hasan, S. E. (2004). Public awareness is key to successful waste management. *Journal of Environmental Science and Health. Part A, Toxic/Hazardous Substances & Environmental Engineering*, *39*(2), 483–492. doi:10.1081/ESE-120027539 PMID:15027831

IBIS world. (2018). *Cooking oil recycling industry in the US*. Industry Market Research Report. September, 2018.

Iglesias, L., Laca, A., Herrero, M., & Díaz, M. (2012). A life cycle assessment comparison between centralized and decentralized biodiesel production from raw sunflower oil and waste cooking oils. *Journal of Cleaner Production*, *37*, 162–171. doi:10.1016/j.jclepro.2012.07.002

Junior, G. D., Ibadurrohman, M., & Slamet. (2019). Synthesis of eco-friendly liquid detergent from waste cooking oil and ZnO nanoparticles. In *AIP Conference Proceedings* (vol. 2085(1), 020075). doi:. doi:10.1063/1.5095053

Kataria, J., Mohapatra, S. K., & Kundu, K. (2019). Biodiesel production from waste cooking oil using heterogeneous catalysts and its operational characteristics on variable compression ratio CI engine. *Journal of the Energy Institute*, *92*(2), 275–287. doi:10.1016/j.joei.2018.01.008

Kazuo, S. US Pat. 4839089, Mimasu Oil Chemical Co., Ltd., (1989).

Khalid, K., & Khalid, K. (2011). Transesterification of palm oil for the production of biodiesel. *American Journal of Applied Sciences*, *8*(8), 804–809. doi:10.3844/ajassp.2011.804.809

Li, H., Zhao, J., Huang, Y., Jiang, Z., & Chen, Q. (2016). Investigation on the potential of waste cooking oil as a grinding aid in Portland cement. *Journal of Environmental Management*, *184*(3), 545–551. doi:10.1016/j.jenvman.2016.10.027 PMID:27793479

Li, Z., Huang, Z., Ding, S., Li, F., & Chen, C. (2018). Catalytic conversion of waste cooking oil to fuel oil: Catalyst design and effect of solvent. *Energy*, *157*, 270–277. doi:10.1016/j.energy.2018.05.156

Liang, S., Liu, Z., Xu, M., & Zhang, T. (2013). Waste oil derived biofuels in China bring brightness for global GHG mitigation. *Bioresource Technology*, *131*, 139–145. doi:10.1016/j.biortech.2012.12.008 PMID:23340111

Lucena, I. L., Silva, G. F., & Fernandes, F. A. N. (2008). Biodiesel production by esterification of oleic acid with methanol using a water adsorption apparatus. *Industrial & Engineering Chemistry Research*, *47*(18), 6885–6889. doi:10.1021/ie800547h

Ma, J., Sun, D., Pang, Q., Sun, G., Hu, M., & Lu, T. (2019). Potential of recycled concrete aggregate pretreated with waste cooking oil residue for hot mix asphalt. *Journal of Cleaner Production*, *221*, 469–479. doi:10.1016/j.jclepro.2019.02.256

Mannu, A., Ferro, M., Pietro, M. E. D., & Mele, A. (2019). Innovative applications of waste cooking oil as raw material. *Science Progress*, *102*(2), 153–160. doi:10.1177/0036850419854252

Matthäus, B. (2010). Oxidation in foods and beverages and antioxidant applications: management in different industry sectors. Chapter 6 - Oxidation of edible oils. Woodhead Publishing Series in Food Science, Technology and Nutrition, 183-238.

Ministry of Environment (2006). Report on promotion of eco-fuel for transportation.

Mohadesi, M., Aghel, B., Maleki, M., & Ansari, A. (2019). Production of biodiesel from waste cooking oil using a homogeneous catalyst: Study of semi-industrial pilot of microreactor. *Renewable Energy*, *136*, 677–682. doi:10.1016/j.renene.2019.01.039

Pahlavan, P., Manzi, S., Rodriguez-Estrada, M. T., & Bignozzi, M. C. (2017). Valorization of spent cooking oils in hydrophobic waste-based lime mortars for restorative rendering applications. *Construction & Building Materials*, *146*, 199–209. doi:10.1016/j.conbuildmat.2017.04.001

Pahlavan, P., Manzi, S., Sansonetti, A., & Bignozzi, M. C. (2018). Valorization of organic additions in restorative lime mortars: Spent cooking oil and albumen. *Construction & Building Materials*, *181*, 650–658. doi:10.1016/j.conbuildmat.2018.06.089

Panadare, D. C., & Rathod, V. K. (2015). Applications of waste cooking oil other than biodiesel: A review. *Iranian Journal of Chemical Engineering*, *12*, 55–76.

Qiu, F., Li, Y., Yang, D., Li, X., & Sun, P. (2011). Biodiesel production from mixed soybean oil and rapeseed oil. *Applied Energy*, *88*(6), 2050–2055. doi:10.1016/j.apenergy.2010.12.070

Raeisian, L., Niazmand, H., Ebrahimnia-Bajestan, E., & Werle, P. (2019). Feasibility study of waste vegetable oil as an alternative cooling medium in transformers. *Applied Thermal Engineering*, *151*, 308–317. doi:10.1016/j.applthermaleng.2019.02.010

Sahar, S., Sadaf, S., Iqbal, J., Ullah, I., Bhatti, H. N., Nouren, S., ... Iqbal, M. (2018). Biodiesel production from waste cooking oil: An efficient technique to convert waste into biodiesel. *Sustainable Cities and Society*, *41*, 220–226. doi:10.1016/j.scs.2018.05.037

Sarno, M., Spina, D., & Senatore, A. (2019). One-step nanohybrid synthesis in waste cooking oil, for direct lower environmental impact and stable lubricant formulation. *Tribology International*, *135*, 355–367. doi:10.1016/j.triboint.2019.03.025

Soegiantoro, G. H., Chang, J., Rahmawati, P., Christiani, M. F., & Mufrodi, Z. (2019). Home-made eco green biodiesel from chicken fat (CIAT) and waste cooking oil (PAIL). *Energy Procedia*, *158*, 1105–1109. doi:10.1016/j.egypro.2019.01.267

Solway Recycling Ltd. (2019). Some legal requirements for consideration when arranging a cooking oil collection. Retrieved from https://www.solwayrecycling.co.uk/recycling-services/oil-collection/legal-requirements-of-cooking-oil-collection

Statista. (2019a). *Global production of vegetable oils from 2000/01 to 2018/19 (in million metric tons)*. Retrieved from https://www.statista.com/statistics/263978/global-vegetable-oil-production-since-2000-2001/

Statista. (2019b). *Consumption of vegetable oils worldwide from 2013/14 to 2018/2019, by oil type (in million metric tons)*. Retrieved from https://www.statista.com/statistics/263937/vegetable-oils-global-consumption/

Sun, Z., Yi, J., Huang, Y., Feng, D., & Guo, C. (2016). Properties of asphalt binder modified by bio-oil derived from waste cooking oil. *Construction & Building Materials*, *102*, 496–504. doi:10.1016/j.conbuildmat.2015.10.173

Tarnpradab, T., Unyaphan, S., Takahashi, F., & Yoshikawa, K. (2016). Tar removal capacity of waste cooking oil absorption and waste char adsorption for rice husk gasification. *Biofuels*, *7*(4), 401–412. doi:10.1080/17597269.2016.1147919

The Hindu Business line. (2018). *New regulations for 'used cooking oil' come into effect*. Retrieved from https://www.thehindubusinessline.com/economy/policy/new-regulations-for-used-cooking-oil-come-into-effect/article24314377.ece

The news minute. (2019). *Restaurants can no longer reuse cooking oils as per new food safety regulations*. Retrieved from https://www.thenewsminute.com/article/restaurants-can-no-longer-reuse-cooking-oils-new-food-safety-regulations-96723

Trabelsi, A. B. H., Zaafouri, K., Baghdadi, W., Naoui, S., & Ouerghi, A. (2018). Second generation biofuels production from waste cooking oil via pyrolysis process. *Renewable Energy*, *126*, 888–896. doi:10.1016/j.renene.2018.04.002

Tsai, W.-T. (2019). Mandatory recycling of waste cooking oil from residential and commercial sectors in Taiwan. *Resources*, *8*(1), 38. doi:10.3390/resources8010038

UK Environmental Law Association. (2017). *The plain guide to environmental law*. Retrieved from http://www.environmentlaw.org.uk/rte.asp?id=85

Vinyes, E., Oliver-Solà, J., Ugaya, C., Rieradevall, J., & Gasol, C. M. (2013). Application of LCSA to used cooking oil waste management. *The International Journal of Life Cycle Assessment*, *18*(2), 445–455. doi:10.100711367-012-0482-z

Wakoc, F. M., Reshadb, A. S., Bhaleraoa, M. S., & Goud, V. V. (2018). Catalytic cracking of waste cooking oil for biofuel production using zirconium oxide catalyst. *Industrial Crops and Products*, *118*, 282–289. doi:10.1016/j.indcrop.2018.03.057

Wallace, T., Gibbons, D., O'Dwyer, M., & Curran, T. P. (2017). International evolution of fat, oil and grease (FOG) waste management - A review. *Journal of Environmental Management*, *187*, 424–435. doi:10.1016/j.jenvman.2016.11.003 PMID:27838205

Wang, J., Zhong, Z., Ding, K., Zhang, B., & Ruan, R. (2017). Successive desilication and dealumination of HZSM-5 in catalytic conversion of waste cooking oil to produce aromatics. *Energy Conversion and Management, 147*, 100–107. doi:10.1016/j.enconman.2017.05.050

Wee, H. M., Budiman, S. D., Su, L. C., Chang, M., & Chen, R. (2016). Responsible supply chain management-An analysis of Taiwanese gutter oil scandal using the theory of constraint. *International Journal of Logistics Research and Applications, 19*(5), 380–394. doi:10.1080/13675567.2015.1090964

Wei, Z., Li, X., Thushara, D., & Liu, Y. (2011). Determinations and removal of malodialdehyde and other 2-thiobarbituric acid reactive substances in waste cooking oil. *Journal of Food Engineering, 107*(3-4), 379–384. doi:10.1016/j.jfoodeng.2011.06.032

Williams, J. B., Clarkson, C., Mant, C., Drinkwater, A., & May, E. (2012). Fat, oil and grease deposits in sewers: Characterisation of deposits and formation mechanisms. *Water Research, 46*(19), 6319–6328. doi:10.1016/j.watres.2012.09.002 PMID:23039918

Zheng, T., Wu, Z., Xie, Q., Fang, J., Hu, Y., Lu, M., ... Ji, J. (2018). Structural modification of waste cooking oil methyl esters as cleaner plasticizer to substitute toxic dioctyl phthalate. *Journal of Cleaner Production, 186*, 1021–1030. doi:10.1016/j.jclepro.2018.03.175

KEY TERMS AND DEFINITIONS

Biodiesel: Long chain alkyl esters that is made by catalytic reaction of triglycerides and alcohol.
Hydrodeoxygenation: A process for removing oxygen from oxygen containing compound by reacting with hydrogen.
Prevention: Action to stop something to happen.
Pyrolysis: A thermal decomposition process of materials at elevated temperatures in an inert atmosphere.
Recycling: A process to convert waste materials into new materials and objects.
Transesterification: A chemical reaction involves ester and alcohol.
Waste Cooking Oil: Used vegetable oils and animal fats derived from cooking.

This research was previously published in the Handbook of Research on Resource Management for Pollution and Waste Treatment edited by Augustine Chioma Affam and Ezerie Henry Ezechi; pages 47-63, copyright year 2020 by Engineering Science Reference (an imprint of IGI Global).

Index

A

Active 22, 25-30, 34, 39-40, 54, 83, 90, 94, 96, 130-133, 135, 141, 144-145, 148-149, 151-154, 156-162, 171, 182-184, 186-189, 191-197, 202-203, 206, 218, 230, 251, 306, 357, 363, 381, 446, 535, 584, 589, 607, 711-712, 748, 788, 815-816, 821, 832, 902, 905, 914-915, 924, 926, 929-930, 947, 954, 961-962, 965, 1045, 1119-1120, 1194, 1246, 1248, 1250-1251, 1255

active packaging 131, 148, 151-154, 157, 159, 161-162, 182-183, 186-189, 192-194, 196-197

agbiotech 813-814, 817-819, 821-827, 829, 832

Agbiotech/Transgenic Science 813

Agricultural Composting 662, 669

Agricultural Cooperative 834, 837-838, 842, 844-845, 848-849

agricultural crop value 948, 956-957, 959, 961-962, 968

Agricultural Engineering 624, 725-726, 728, 731-732, 742-744, 748

Agricultural Inputs 148, 183, 948, 952, 965, 968

agricultural outputs 948-949, 951, 968, 1083

Agricultural Production 217-218, 235, 287, 407, 536, 539, 560, 563, 685, 687, 690, 694, 698, 704, 725-727, 729-731, 740, 745-746, 753, 778, 790, 818, 822, 826, 832, 834, 836, 841-843, 846, 851, 884-887, 889, 891-894, 896, 898-899, 902-904, 906-907, 909, 918-919, 926-928, 930-932, 936, 939-941, 948-949, 951, 953-954, 963, 965, 972, 974, 1001, 1006, 1039, 1174, 1189, 1233, 1254

Agriculture 3-11, 16, 18, 21-22, 26, 29, 35, 37, 54, 64, 94, 98-99, 114, 141, 144, 159-160, 179, 193, 195, 211, 217, 244, 247, 256, 258, 277, 281, 288, 290, 300, 302-306, 314, 341, 350, 382, 392, 405-407, 421, 425-426, 460, 477, 481-482, 494, 498-502, 506, 508, 517-518, 529, 531, 535, 537, 553-554, 556, 559, 574, 578-580, 585-586, 589, 591, 605, 612, 624, 656, 664, 667-668, 671, 685, 687, 691, 694-697, 699-702, 704, 716, 719, 725-726, 730-732, 740, 743-746, 748-751, 753-756, 758, 762-769, 771-774, 776-779, 783-806, 814-815, 817, 819-820, 822-824, 827-831, 833-834, 837-843, 846-848, 850-851, 856, 858-859, 861-862, 866, 872, 880-889, 891-894, 896-905, 908, 910, 919, 921-923, 926-928, 932-934, 938, 940-957, 959, 963, 965-968, 973-977, 982, 984-987, 989-990, 993, 995-998, 1003, 1006-1009, 1012-1014, 1019, 1021, 1025, 1031-1032, 1034-1038, 1041, 1043, 1046, 1051, 1054, 1056, 1059, 1063-1064, 1066-1067, 1072-1077, 1081, 1083, 1085, 1087-1090, 1093, 1106, 1108, 1119, 1123, 1125-1126, 1128, 1136-1138, 1147, 1152-1154, 1169, 1173-1174, 1177-1178, 1180, 1182-1186, 1203-1204, 1206-1207, 1209, 1230, 1252-1253, 1259-1260, 1269-1271, 1273, 1277, 1279, 1295-1300, 1308-1313, 1315

Agri-Industrial Waste 565

Agroecology 800, 822, 827, 832

Agrofood Supply Chain 239

agro-industrial complex 725-727, 740, 742-743, 747-748, 903, 924

agro-materials 652

Ai 26, 361, 401-402, 734, 738, 771-779, 783-789, 791, 797, 800, 803, 805, 807, 1252

air curtain 99, 104-106, 108, 112-113, 119-121

air infiltration 99-100, 104, 108, 113, 121

air velocity 99, 104, 113

alien genes 1168

allergic reactions 1168, 1175-1176, 1200

Alleviation 1007

Amelioration 854, 862-863

Amylase 605, 614, 625, 664

anaemia 1000, 1175, 1210, 1218-1219, 1231

anaerobic digestion 406, 409, 412, 421-424, 426, 551-552, 579, 584, 586-587, 590, 594, 597-598, 603, 615, 621, 628

analytic hierarchy process (AHP) 265, 395-396, 476

Analytics 340, 348, 351, 382, 447, 457, 682, 745, 753,

F

M

T

U

V

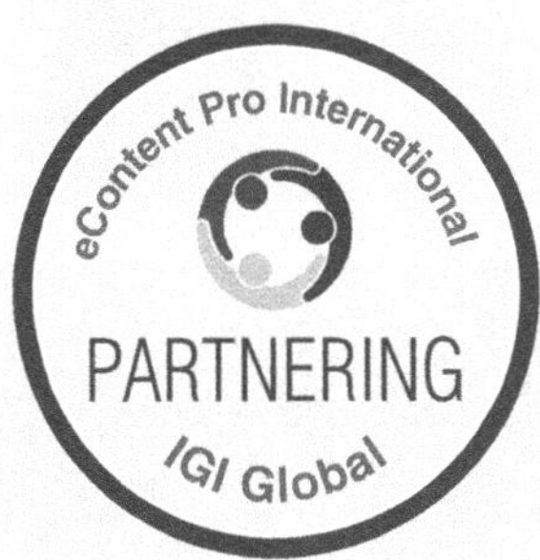

IGI Global Proudly Partners With eContent Pro International

Receive a 25% Discount on all Editorial Services

Editorial Services

IGI Global expects all final manuscripts submitted for publication to be in their final form. This means they must be reviewed, revised, and professionally copy edited prior to their final submission. Not only does this support with accelerating the publication process, but it also ensures that the highest quality scholarly work can be disseminated.

English Language Copy Editing

Let eContent Pro International's expert copy editors perform edits on your manuscript to resolve spelling, punctuaion, grammar, syntax, flow, formatting issues and more.

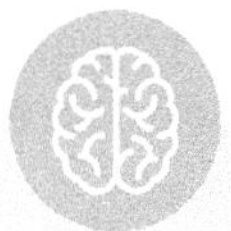

Scientific and Scholarly Editing

Allow colleagues in your research area to examine the content of your manuscript and provide you with valuable feedback and suggestions before submission.

Figure, Table, Chart & Equation Conversions

Do you have poor quality figures? Do you need visual elements in your manuscript created or converted? A design expert can help!

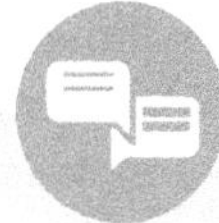

Translation

Need your documjent translated into English? eContent Pro International's expert translators are fluent in English and more than 40 different languages.

Hear What Your Colleagues are Saying About Editorial Services Supported by IGI Global

"The service was very fast, very thorough, and very helpful in ensuring our chapter meets the criteria and requirements of the book's editors. I was quite impressed and happy with your service."

– Prof. Tom Brinthaupt,
Middle Tennessee State University, USA

"I found the work actually spectacular. The editing, formatting, and other checks were very thorough. The turnaround time was great as well. I will definitely use eContent Pro in the future."

– Nickanor Amwata, Lecturer,
University of Kurdistan Hawler, Iraq

"I was impressed that it was done timely, and wherever the content was not clear for the reader, the paper was improved with better readability for the audience."

– Prof. James Chilembwe,
Mzuzu University, Malawi

Email: customerservice@econtentpro.com   **www.igi-global.com/editorial-service-partners**

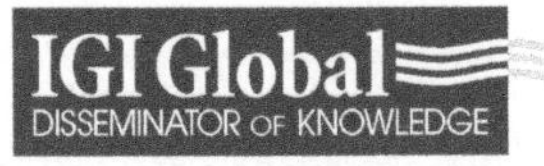

Celebrating Over 30 Years of Scholarly Knowledge Creation & Dissemination

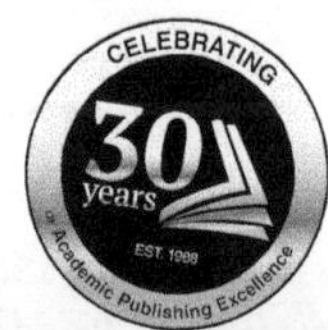

InfoSci®-Books

A Database of Over 5,300+ Reference Books Containing Over 100,000+ Chapters Focusing on Emerging Research

GAIN ACCESS TO **THOUSANDS** OF REFERENCE BOOKS AT **A FRACTION** OF THEIR INDIVIDUAL LIST **PRICE**.

InfoSci®-Books Database

The **InfoSci®-Books** database is a collection of over 5,300+ IGI Global single and multi-volume reference books, handbooks of research, and encyclopedias, encompassing groundbreaking research from prominent experts worldwide that span over 350+ topics in 11 core subject areas including business, computer science, education, science and engineering, social sciences and more.

Open Access Fee Waiver (Offset Model) Initiative

For any library that invests in IGI Global's InfoSci-Journals and/ or InfoSci-Books databases, IGI Global will match the library's investment with a fund of equal value to go toward **subsidizing the OA article processing charges (APCs) for their students, faculty, and staff** at that institution when their work is submitted and accepted under OA into an IGI Global journal.*

INFOSCI® PLATFORM FEATURES

- No DRM
- No Set-Up or Maintenance Fees
- A Guarantee of No More Than a 5% Annual Increase
- Full-Text HTML and PDF Viewing Options
- Downloadable MARC Records
- Unlimited Simultaneous Access
- COUNTER 5 Compliant Reports
- Formatted Citations With Ability to Export to RefWorks and EasyBib
- No Embargo of Content (Research is Available Months in Advance of the Print Release)

*The fund will be offered on an annual basis and expire at the end of the subscription period. The fund would renew as the subscription is renewed for each year thereafter. The open access fees will be waived after the student, faculty, or staff's paper has been vetted and accepted into an IGI Global journal and the fund can only be used toward publishing OA in an IGI Global journal. Libraries in developing countries will have the match on their investment doubled.

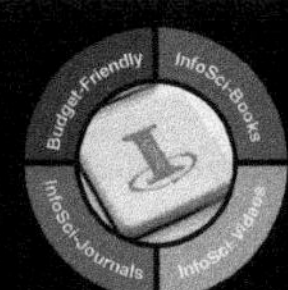

To Learn More or To Purchase This Database:

www.igi-global.com/infosci-books

eresources@igi-global.com • Toll Free: 1-866-342-6657 ext. 100 • Phone: 717-533-8845 x100

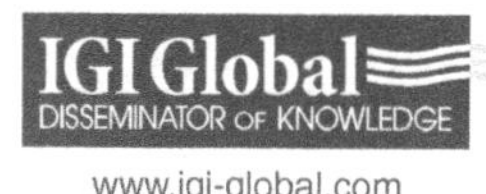

Publisher of Peer-Reviewed, Timely, and Innovative Academic Research Since 1988

IGI Global's Transformative Open Access (OA) Model:
How to Turn Your University Library's Database Acquisitions Into a Source of OA Funding

In response to the OA movement and well in advance of Plan S, IGI Global, early last year, unveiled their OA Fee Waiver (Read & Publish) Initiative.

Under this initiative, librarians who invest in IGI Global's InfoSci-Books (5,300+ reference books) and/or InfoSci-Journals (185+ scholarly journals) databases will be able to subsidize their patron's OA article processing charges (APC) when their work is submitted and accepted (after the peer review process) into an IGI Global journal. *See website for details.

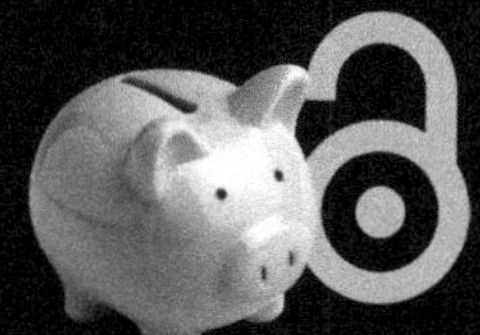

How Does it Work?

1. When a library subscribes or perpetually purchases IGI Global's InfoSci-Databases and/or their discipline/subject-focused subsets, IGI Global will match the library's investment with a fund of equal value to go toward subsidizing the OA article processing charges (APCs) for their patrons.

   Researchers: **Be sure to recommend the InfoSci-Books and InfoSci-Journals to take advantage of this initiative.**

2. When a student, faculty, or staff member submits a paper and it is accepted (following the peer review) into one of IGI Global's 185+ scholarly journals, the author will have the option to have their paper published under a traditional publishing model or as OA.

3. When the author chooses to have their paper published under OA, IGI Global will notify them of the OA Fee Waiver (Read and Publish) Initiative. If the author decides they would like to take advantage of this initiative, IGI Global will deduct the US$ 2,000 APC from the created fund.

4. This fund will be offered on an annual basis and will renew as the subscription is renewed for each year thereafter. IGI Global will manage the fund and award the APC waivers unless the librarian has a preference as to how the funds should be managed.

Hear From the Experts on This Initiative:

"I'm very happy to have been able to make one of my recent research contributions, "Visualizing the Social Media Conversations of a National Information Technology Professional Association" featured in the *International Journal of Human Capital and Information Technology Professionals*, freely available along with having access to the valuable resources found within IGI Global's InfoSci-Journals database."

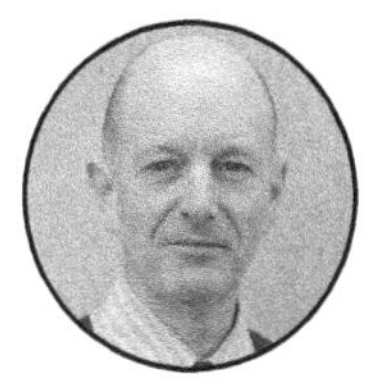

– **Prof. Stuart Palmer**,
Deakin University, Australia

Research Anthology on Food Waste Reduction and Alternative Diets for Food and Nutrition Security

Information Resources Management Association
USA

Volume II

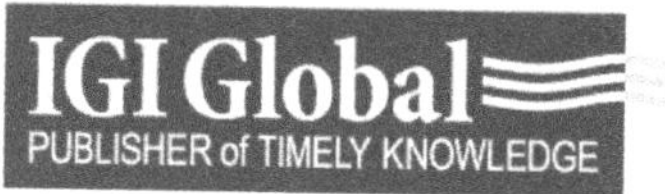

Published in the United States of America by
IGI Global
Engineering Science Reference (an imprint of IGI Global)
701 E. Chocolate Avenue
Hershey PA, USA 17033
Tel: 717-533-8845
Fax: 717-533-8661
E-mail: cust@igi-global.com
Web site: http://www.igi-global.com

Library of Congress Cataloging-in-Publication Data

Names: Information Resources Management Association, editor.
Title: Research anthology on food waste reduction and alternative diets for
    food and nutrition security / Information Resources Management
    Association, editor.
Description: Hershey, PA : Engineering Science Reference, an imprint of IGI
    Global, [2021] | Includes bibliographical references and index. |
    Summary: "This book explores methods for reducing waste and cutting food
    loss in order to help the environment and support local communities as
    well as solve issues including that of land space. It also provides
    vital research on the development of plant-based foods, meat-alternative
    diets, and nutritional outcomes"-- Provided by publisher.
Identifiers: LCCN 2020009128 (print) | LCCN 2020009129 (ebook) | ISBN
    9781799853541 (hardcover) | ISBN 9781799853558 (ebook)
Subjects: LCSH: Food industry and trade--Waste disposal.
Classification: LCC TD899.F585 R47 2020 (print) | LCC TD899.F585 (ebook)
    | DDC 363.72/88--dc23
LC record available at https://lccn.loc.gov/2020009128
LC ebook record available at https://lccn.loc.gov/2020009129

British Cataloguing in Publication Data
A Cataloguing in Publication record for this book is available from the British Library.

The views expressed in this book are those of the authors, but not necessarily of the publisher.

For electronic access to this publication, please contact: eresources@igi-global.com.

List of Contributors

Table of Contents

Dheeraj Kumar, National Institute of Technology, Durgapur, India
Md. Farrukh, Echelon Institute of Technology, India
Nadeem Faisal, ITM University, Gwalior, India

Basak Gokce Col, Istanbul Gelisim University, Turkey
Sergen Tuggum, Tekirdag Namik Kemal University, Turkey
Seydi Yıkmış, Tekirdağ Namık Kemal University, Turkey

Alperen Koker, Middle East Technical University, Turkey
İlhami Okur, Middle East Technical University, Turkey
Sebnem Ozturkoglu-Budak, Ankara University, Turkey
Hami Alpas, Middle East Technical University, Turkey

Nazli Turkmen, Ankara University, Turkey
Sebnem Ozturkoglu-Budak, Ankara University, Turkey

Tejinder Pal Singh, College of Dairy Science and Food Technology, India
Sarang Dilip Pophaly, College of Dairy Science and Food Technology, India
Ruby Siwach, College of Dairy Science and Food Technology, India

Inna Simakova, Saratov State Vavilov Agrarian University, Russia
Victoria Strizhevskaya, Saratov State Vavilov Agrarian University, Russia
Igor Vorotnikov, Saratov State Vavilov Agrarian University, Russia
Fedor Pertsevyi, Sumy National Agrarian University, Ukraine

Section 3
Repurposing Wasted Food

Volume II

Section 4
Sustainable Agricultural Production

Section 5
Sustainable Consumption and Alternative Diets

Preface

Of the utmost importance in every country are the accessibility, availability, and stability of food. As increasing populations, reduction in farmland, climate change, improper transportation of food, unbalanced dieting habits, increased cases of foodborne illness, and other factors have put a strain on resources, issues with food waste, food scarcity, and food safety have increased. It has become imperative for sustainable agriculture to be discussed and transformed through the use of technologies that can increase efficiency and crop output. Similarly, food supply chains and food preservation must be reexamined to procure solutions that mitigate the amount of food that is wasted due to such factors as improper refrigeration or handling methods that render the products unsafe for consumption.

Alternatively, this distinctive reference source also looks past the technological and sustainable methods that can be applied to the production and distribution of food and incorporates applications for repurposing food that is wasted. This innovative research examines the conversion of waste byproduct into livestock feed, value-added products, and more. Additionally, the content includes a unique perspective on eating habits and the ways in which society can transform to include more sustainable and environmentally-friendly food products into their diets. Such research includes the analysis of plant-based proteins, soybeans, insects, and new meat alternatives that present sustainable food consumption options without sacrificing nutrition security as well. The book serves to incorporate case studies and applications in these areas in order to assist in reducing food waste, increasing consumer awareness of their food choices, and improving the quality of the farming industry and agricultural technologies of the future.

Thus, the *Research Anthology on Food Waste Reduction and Alternative Diets* seeks to fill the void for an all-encompassing and comprehensive reference book covering the latest and emerging research, concepts, and theories for the better understanding of food waste reduction and management and the technologies being implemented for both. This two-volume reference collection of reprinted IGI Global book chapters and journal articles that have been handpicked by the editor and editorial team of this research anthology on this topic will empower farmers, experts in the agricultural industry, nutritionists, supply chain managers, food safety experts, technologists, policymakers, professionals, students, researchers, and academicians with a strong understanding of critical issues within food waste reduction by exploring preservation technologies, food safety, food supply chain management and improvement, along with the conversion of waste into useful byproducts and the ethical production and consumption of food.

The *Research Anthology on Food Waste Reduction and Alternative Diets* is organized into five sections that provide comprehensive coverage of important topics. The sections are:

1. Food Safety and Preservation Technologies;
2. Food Supply Chain Management;

3.   Repurposing Wasted Food;
4.   Sustainable Agricultural Production;
5.   Sustainable Consumption and Alternative Diets.

The following paragraphs provide a summary of what to expect from this invaluable reference tool.

Section 1, "Food Safety and Preservation Technologies," opens this comprehensive reference work with research on the latest tools and technologies being used to safely preserve various types of food products. Opening this book is "Food Quality and Safety Regulation Systems at a Glance," by Profs. Arvind Kumar Singh and Dixit V. Bhalani of Central Salt and Marine Chemicals Research Institute, India and Prof. Poonam Singh Thakur from Rashtrasant Tukadoji Maharaj Nagpur University, India, which explains the role of various assessment agencies and their rights and workflows in ensuring the quality and safety of food products. The next chapter, "Ecological Chemistry Aspects of Food Safety," written by Prof. Rodica Sturza of the Technical University of Moldova, Moldova, reflects on the studies carried out over the last decade, with the subject being soil, water, vegetal raw materials, and wines from the Republic of Moldova. Following this is the chapter "Food Safety and Climate Change: Case of Mycotoxins," by Prof. Abdellah Zinedine of Chouaib Doukkali University, Morocco and Prof. Samira El Akhdari from the Ministry of National Education, Morocco, which gives an overview about the major mycotoxins, masked mycotoxins, and emerging mycotoxins found on various grains and agricultural commodities and their negative impacts. The chapter "Investigation Into Fermentation: A Journey Into Cultural Relevance and Mindful Eating," by Prof. Kris Krautkremer of Kingsport City Schools, USA and Prof. Cerrone Renee Foster of East Tennessee State University, USA, focuses on fermentation, its role in cellular respiration, and practical uses of fermentation for food preservation and nutrient bioavailability. The next chapter, "Technologies for Monitoring the Safety of Perishable Food Products," authored by Prof. Pedro Dinis from Gaspar University of Beira Interior, Portugal; Prof. Pedro Dinho da Silva of the University of Beira Interior, Portugal; Profs. Luís Pinto Andrade and José Nunes from the Polytechnic Institute of Castelo Branco, Portugal; and Prof. Christophe Espírito Santo from the Agrofood Technological Center, Portugal, addresses food safety issues, namely factors related to microbial growth responsible for food deterioration, and modern monitoring technologies. The chapter "Closed Refrigerated Display Cabinets: Is It Worth It for Food Quality?" by Prof. Onrawee Laguerre of the National Research Institute of Science and Technology for Environment and Agriculture IRSTEA, France and Prof. Nattawut Chaomuang from King Mongkut's Institute of Technology Ladkrabang, Thailand, presents state-of-the-art studies on refrigerated display cabinets with further information on the airflow and temperature profile in the closed display cabinet, the influence of the presence of doors, and the frequency of door openings and the room temperature. The following chapter, "Nanocomposites in the Food Packaging Industry: Recent Trends and Applications," by Prof. Dheeraj Kumar of the National Institute of Technology, Durgapur, India and Prof. Md. Farrukh from the Echelon Institute of Technology, India, focuses on nano-composite materials that enhance the antimicrobial, mechanical, thermal, as well as barrier properties against the migrating element in the food packaging system. "Non-Thermal Food Preservation Methods in the Meat Industry," by Prof. Basak Gokce Col of Istanbul Gelisim University, Turkey and Profs. Sergen Tuggum and Seydi Yıkmış of Tekirdağ Namık Kemal University, Turkey, focuses on two novel approaches to meat preservation: non-thermal Pulsed Electric Field and Atmospheric Pressure Cold Plasma APCP Technologies. Next is "Non-Thermal Preservation of Dairy Products: Principles, Recent Advances, and Future Prospects," written by Profs. Alperen Koker and İlhami Okur from Middle East Technical University, Turkey; Prof. Sebnem Ozturkoglu-Budak of Ankara University, Turkey; and Prof. Hami

Alpas from Middle East Technical University, Turkey, which gives general principles of non-thermal techniques, current applications with dairy products, and recent advances in the dairy industry. The following chapter, "Novel Packaging Technologies in Dairy Products: Principles and Recent Advances," by Profs. Sebnem Ozturkoglu-Budak and Nazli Turkmen from Ankara University, Turkey informs about the general principles of the novel packaging techniques, such as nanotechnology, active packaging, and intelligent/smart packaging, and their current applications in dairy technology. "Biopreservatives for Improved Shelf-Life and Safety of Dairy Products: Biopreservatives for Dairy Products," by Profs. Sarang Dilip Pophaly, Tejinder Pal Singh, and Ruby Siwach of the College of Dairy Science and Food Technology, India provides a scientific background on bio preservation, a detailed look at its functionality, as well as giving food applications and further commercial aspects of bio preservatives derived from microbial sources. Concluding this section is the chapter "Resource-Saving Technology of Dehydration of Fruit and Vegetable Raw Materials: Scientific Rationale and Cost Efficiency," by Profs. Inna Simakova, Victoria Strizhevskaya, and Igor Vorotnikov of Saratov State Vavilov Agrarian University, Russia and Prof. Fedor Pertsevyi of Sumy National Agrarian University, Ukraine. It presents a solution to the insufficient consumption of fruits and vegetables in the diet of modern people with the development of technology for the dehydration of fruit and vegetables applicable directly at the harvesting site.

Section 2, "Food Supply Chain Management," presents extensive coverage on the latest findings in identifying and managing risks in food supply chain management as well as providing coverage on the technological advancements for managing food loss and waste. Starting off this section is the chapter "Managing Risk in Global Food Supply Chains: Improving Food Security and Sustainability" by Prof. Marco A. Miranda-Ackerman from the Universidad Autónoma de Baja Callifornia, Mexico; Profs. Betzabé Ruiz-Morales and Irma Cristina Espitia-Moreno from the Universidad Michoacana de San Nicolás de Hidalgo, Mexico; Prof. Citlali Colin-Chávez of CONACYT, Centro de Investigación en Alimentación y Desarrollo, Mexico & Centro de Innovación y Desarrollo Agroalimentario de Michoacán, Mexico; and Prof. Karina Cecilia Arredondo-Soto from the Universidad Autónoma de Baja Callifornia, Mexico, which presents an overview of the main risks involved in global food supply chains, as well as some techniques for risk management. The next chapter, "Risks in Sustainable Food Supply Chain Management," written by Prof. Yogesh Kumar Sharma of Graphic Era University, India; Prof. Sachin Kumar Mangla from the University of Plymouth, UK; and Prof. Pravin P. Patil of Graphic Era University, India, discusses the risks in the adoption of sustainable food supply chain management SFSCM and ranks the risks by using the Fuzzy Analytic Hierarchy Process FAHP technique. "Building a Sustainable Food Supply Chain and Managing Food Losses," by Profs. A D Nuwan Gunarathne, D. G. Navaratne, M. L. S. Gunaratne, Amanda Erasha, and Yasasi Tharindra Perera of the University of Sri Jayewardenepura, Sri Lanka, provides a conceptual model, incorporating stakeholder management and other behavioral aspects, to build a sustainable food supply chain while minimizing the food waste that occurs at different stages. The following chapter, "Logistic Strategies to Minimize Losses and Waste in Food Supply Chains," authored by Prof. Betzabé Ruiz-Morales from the Universidad Michoacana de San Nicolás de Hidalgo, Mexico; Prof. Marco A. Miranda-Ackerman of Universidad Autónoma de Baja Callifornia, Mexico; and Prof. Irma Cristina Espitia-Moreno from Universidad Michoacana de San Nicolás de Hidalgo, Mexico, proposes sustainable supply chains in agrifoods, achieved through logistical strategies to minimize food waste and losses. "From Information Sharing to Information Utilization in Food Supply Chains," by Prof. Kasper Kiil from Norwegian University of Science and Technology, Trondheim, Norway & Aalborg University, Aalborg, Denmark; Prof. Hans-Henrik Hvolby from Aalborg University, Aalborg, Denmark & Norwegian University of Science and Technology, Trondheim, Norway; Profs. Jacques

Trienekens and Behzad Behdani from Wageningen University, Wageningen, The Netherlands; and Prof. Jan Ola Strandhagen of Norwegian University of Science and Technology, Trondheim, Norway, uses a case study methodology and literature review to identify the characteristics of information sharing, and conceptualize how to move from information sharing to information utilization in food supply chains. The next chapter, "IoT-Based Cold Chain Logistics Monitoring," written by Profs. Afreen Mohsin and Siva S. Yellampalli of UTL Technologies, India aims to reduce the extent of human presence along the cold chain and fill existing gaps through the use a powerful tool in the form of the IoT. "An Exploratory Study on Blockchain Application in a Food Processing Supply Chain to Reduce Waste," by Ms. Emily Anne Carey from Samsung Electronics, UK and Dr. Nachiappan Subramanian an Independent Researcher, UK, uses a case study approach to explore the feasibility of using blockchain in the beef supply chain to reduce waste. Next is "Performance Evaluation of Food Cold Chain Logistics Enterprise Based on the AHP and Entropy," by Profs. Yazhou Xiong, Jie Zhao, and Jie Lan from Hubei Polytechnic University, Huangshi, China, evaluates the system of food cold chain logistics from four aspects, including the financial management, cold chain logistics process, development ability and customer service, based on the analytic hierarchy process. The chapter "A Circular Economy Perspective for Dairy Supply Chains," by Profs. Dimitrios Vlachos and Christina Paraskevopoulou of Aristotle University of Thessaloniki, Greece, provides a CE perspective for the dairy supply chain by identifying and analyzing the associated technologies and strategies through a literature review taxonomy based on the related stage of the supply chain. The following chapter, "Consumer Purchase Preference for the Perception of Quality of Perishable Products in a Smart City," by Profs. Iván Alonso Rebollar-Xochicale and Fernando Maldonado-Azpeitia from the Universidad Autónoma de Querétaro, Mexico, discusses the consumers role in determining food waste along the supply chain and how companies can correctly implement supply chains in smart cities for perishable products. "Methodology for the Design of Traceability System in Food Assistance Supply Chains: Case Bienestarina, Colombia," by Prof. Feizar Javier Rueda-Velasco of Universidad Distrital "Francisco José de Caldas", Colombia; Prof. Angie Monsalve-Salamanca from Universidad Nacional de Colombia, Colombia; and Prof. Wilson Adarme-Jaimes from Universidad Nacional de Colombia, Colombia, proposes a methodology for the design of traceability systems in FAP which allows increasing supply chain visibility, coordination between deliveries and social conditions, and therefore, possible impacts on public policy implications. Next is "Analyzing Sustainable Food Supply Chain Management Challenges in India," written by Profs. Pravin P. Patil, Sachin Kumar Mangla, Yogesh Kumar Sharma, and Surbhi Uniyal from Graphic Era University, India. It identifies 11 challenges in sustainable food supply chain management and uses the integration of fuzzy with DEMATEL to analyze the challenges in SFSCM. "Wastage and Cold Chain Infrastructure Relationship in Indian Food Supply Chain: A Study From Farm to Retail," by Profs. Saurav Negi and Neeraj Anand from the University of Petroleum and Energy Studies, India, outlines the extent of fruits and vegetables waste in India (at various stages from farm to retail) and its ramifications on food production and safety in the cold chain sector. The chapter "Perishable Goods Supply Cold Chain Management in India," authored by Prof. Anju Bharti from Maharaja Agrasen Institute of Management Studies, India and Prof. Arun Mittal of Birla Institute of Technology, India, explores the cold chain potential in India that still remains untapped and the challenges the country faces in becoming a part of the global trade in perishable products and quality produce. This section ends with the chapter "Factors That impact Quality during the Transportation of Tomatoes: Evidence From India," by Profs. Saurav Negi, Neeraj Anand, and Shantanu Trivedi from the University of Petroleum and Energy Studies, Dehradun, India. It provides information on the current status of tomato transportation and related issues and challenges in India and the ways in which stakeholders can improve efficiency in the transportation stage of the supply chain.

Section 3, "Repurposing Wasted Food," reveals the latest research on the history, process, technologies, and conversion of food waste into value added byproducts. The opening chapter, "Food Waste Reduction Towards Food Sector Sustainability," by Profs. Giovanni Lagioia, Vera Amicarelli,, Teodoro Gallucci, and Christian Bux from the University of Bari Aldo Moro, Italy, reviews the magnitude of FLW at a global and European level and its environmental, social, and economic implications as well as using Material Flow Analysis to support and improve FLW management and application. The following chapter, "Utilization and Management of Food Waste," by Prof. Shriram M. Naikare of SNDT College of Home Science, India, explores how the different types of food industrial waste can be converted into byproducts for livestock feed, bioenergy production, artificial fertilizer and more. Next is "Various Approaches for Food Waste Processing and Its Management," by Prof. Priyanka Harishchandra Tripathi from National Institute of Pathology ICMR, India and Profs. Anupam Pandey, Ashutosh Paliwal, Ankita Harishchandra Tripathi, Satish Chandra Pandey, Tushar Joshi, and Veena Pande from Kumaun University Nainital, India, looks into global food wastage and the approaches to manage and reduce the high environmental, social, and economic impacts associated with this type of waste. "Value-Added Products From Food Waste," written by Dr. Baban Baburao Gunjal of Sunrise Biotech Organisation, India, explains how the management of food waste can be done by conversion to different value-added products. The chapter "Microbe Mediated Bioconversion of Fruit Waste Into Value Added Products: Microbes in Fruit Waste Management," by Profs. and Thazeem Basheer from Bharathiar University, India, summarizes microbe mediated fermentative utilization of fruit waste for the production of value-added products like organic acid, single cell protein, bioplastics, enzymes, and biogas. The next chapter, "Industrially Important Enzymes Production From Food Waste: An Alternative Approach to Land Filling," by Prof. Madhuri Santosh Bhandwalkar of S. B. B. Alias Appasaheb Jedhe College, India, focuses on the production of industrially important enzymes from food waste such as pectinase, peroxidase, lipase, glucoamylase, and protease. "Recent Advances in Waste Cooking Oil Management and Applications for Sustainable Environment," by Prof. Ching Thian Tye from Universiti Sains Malaysia, Malaysia, discusses the management of waste cooking oil WCO in a sustainable manner and provides an overview of the most recent approaches in WCO recycling and applications. "Impacts of Food Industrial Wastes on Soil and Its Utilization as Novel Approach for Value Addition," by Prof. Ifra Ashraf from SKUAST-K, India; Prof. Shazia Ramzan of University of Kashmir, India; and Prof. Nowsheeba Rashid from Amity University, India, describes the new, innate, and monetary sources of colorants, protein, dietary fiber, flavoring, antimicrobials, and antioxidants, which can be utilized in the food industry as a basis of natural food additives. The next chapter, "Allocation Optimization Problem for Peruvian Food Bank," by Prof. Ricardo Campos-Caycho, Renzo A. Benavente-Sotelo, Yasser A. Hidalgo-Gómez, Christian A. Blas-Bazán, Pamela Ivonne Borja-Ramos, Stephanie M. Dueñas-Calderón, Patricia Elkfury-Cominges, Pamela Arista-Yampi, and Jorge Luis Yupanqui-Chacón from Pontificia Universidad Católica del Perú, Peru, uses the tools of operations research to determine a solution to the problem of maximizing the combination of food orders to be distributed based on their total nutritional value to the beneficiaries, seeking maximum coverage and minimum logistic costs. The final chapter in this section, "Economic and Environmental Costs of Meat Waste in the US," by Profs. Nicholas Hardersen and Jadwiga R. Ziolkowska of University of Oklahoma, USA, monetizes the annual costs of natural resources including water, land, and energy, as well as emissions of methane and nitrous oxide embedded in wasted meat in the United States.

Section 4, "Sustainable Agricultural Production," discusses leading research on the issues, challenges, and benefits in smart farming and the tools, techniques, and technologies that have been studied in a variety of regions to improve agricultural production. Opening this chapter is "Tropospheric Ozone Pollution, Agriculture, and Food Security," by Prof. Pooja Singh from Banaras Hindu University, India; Prof. Abhijit Sarkar of the University of Gour Banga, India; and Prof. Sambit Datta from the University of Calcutta, India, reviews the available literature and discusses the impact of tropospheric ozone 03 gas on modern day agricultural production worldwide. The next chapter, "Technical Equipment of Agricultural Production: The Effects for Food Security," written by Prof. Mikail Khudzhatov from Peoples' Friendship University of Russia RUDN University, Russia and Prof. Alexander Arskiy of Russian Academy of Personnel Support for the Agroindustrial Complex, Russia, analyzes the current state of the world market of agricultural machinery, develops the methodology of assessment of the competitiveness of agricultural machinery in the domestic market, and elaborates the definition of effective methods of management of logistics costs at the operation of agricultural machinery. The chapter "Issues and Challenges in Smart Farming for Sustainable Agriculture," by Profs. Immanuel Zion Ramdinthara and Shanthi Bala P. of Pondicherry University, India, focuses on sustainable agriculture and covers the benefits, where it can be used, and common practices. Next is "Disrupting Agriculture: The Status and Prospects for AI and Big Data in Smart Agriculture," by Profs. Omar F. El-Gayar and Martinson Q. Ofori from Dakota State University, USA. It conducts a systematic review focusing on big data and artificial intelligence in agriculture and emphasis the potential, key drivers, and challenges of its use. "Agbiotech, Sustainability, and Food Security Connection to Public Health," by Prof. Ike Valentine Iyioke from Michigan State University, USA, includes an integrative model of food security linking sociocultural, public policy, and ecological aspects to public health and analyzes both sides of the argument for and against agricultural biotechnology. The following chapter, "Agricultural Cooperatives for Sustainable Development of Rural Territories and Food Security: Morocco's Experience," by Prof. Maria Fedorova from Omsk State Technical University, Russia and Prof. Ismail Taaricht of Cadi Ayyad University, Morocco, uses the Moroccan agriculture cooperatives as a case of cooperative longevity and survival in order to observe the evolution and processes of adaptation to the distinct economic, social, and environmental demands of a broad range of member-owners. The next chapter, "Towards the Development of Salt-Tolerant Potato," written by Prof. John Okoth Omondi from Ben Gurion University of the Negev, Israel, explores the salinity management of potatoes and breeding and genetic engineering towards the development of salt-tolerant potatoes. "Local Production-Based Dietary Supplement Distribution in Emerging Countries: Bienestarina Distribution in Colombia," by Prof. Jesus Gonzalez-Feliu from Mines Saint-Etienne, France; Prof. Carlos Osorio-Ramírez of National University of Colombia, Colombia; Prof. Laura Palacios-Arguello from Mines Saint-Etienne, France; and Prof. Carlos Alberto Talamantes from Autonomous University of Ciudad Juarez, Mexico, presents an analysis of the Bienestarina supply chain based on the four elements: steering, organization, development, and financial issues. The chapter "State Support of Agricultural Production in Emerging Countries as a Tool to Ensure Food Security," by Profs. Anna Ivolga and Marina Lescheva from Stavropol State Agrarian University, Russian Federation and Prof. Oleksandr Labenko from National University of Life and Environmental Sciences of Ukraine, Ukraine, explores how agricultural protectionism and support of domestic farmers affect the level of food security on the emerging markets in the conditions of expanding globalization and liberalization of trade in food. The following chapter, "New Approaches to Agricultural Production Management in the Arctic: Organic Farming and Food Security," by Prof. Mykhailo Guz from the National University of Life and Environmental Sciences of Ukraine, Ukraine, discusses the potential of organic farming as a solution to the food insecurity problem and sustainable development in the rural northern areas in the Arctic. Next is "Produce Internationally, Consume Locally: Changing Paradigm of China's Food Security Policy," by Prof. Vasilii Erokhin of Harbin Engineering University, China. It discusses how China's Belt and Road Initiative may serve improving food security of the country by establishing of a predictable system of agricultural production and trade across Eurasia, particularly with the involvement of land-abundant Russia and the countries of Central Asia. The chapter "Financing and Training Imperatives for Resilient Agriculture in Nigeria," by Augustine Odinakachukwu Ejiogu from Imo State University, Nigeria, focuses on the financing and training imperatives for resilient agriculture in Nigeria and proposes a twin-track approach to addressing the challenge of agriculture as a development issue by both encouraging agri-business and supporting the large population of smallholders. The next chapter, "Determinants of Agricultural Production in Romania: A Panel Data Approach," by Profs. Alina Zaharia and Simona Roxana Pătărlăgeanu of The Bucharest University of Economic Studies, Romania, examines a panel data approach to determine the contribution of several factors on the agricultural output in terms of value and of yield in Romania. Closing this section is "Farm Security for Food Security: Dealing With Farm Theft in the Caribbean Region," by Profs. Wendy-Ann Isaac, Wayne Ganpat, and Michael Joseph, The University of Trinidad and Tobago, Trinidad and Tobago, examines the current status of farm theft in the Caribbean region, explores some of the main factors influencing farm theft, reviews some of the strategies attempted in the Caribbean and other places around the world, and makes several suggestions to create a more secure food region.

Section 5, "Sustainable Consumption and Alternative Diets," concludes this reference work with research on the way consumers choose their food and diets, the alternative diet types and foods that can be consumed to increase sustainability and the effects of consumption choices in climate change and possible solutions for the future. Opening the last section of this reference book is "A Review on Impact of Changing Climate on Sustainable Food Consumption," by Prof. Tosin Kolajo Gbadegesin from the University of Ibadan, Nigeria. It examines the impact of the changing climate on sustainable food consumption by identifying the effects of this changing climate on nutrition, food production, and food consumption, and also provides recommendations on sustainable food consumption measures. The next chapter, "Comparing the Effects of Unsustainable Production and Consumption of Food on Health and Policy Across Developed and Less Developed Countries," by Prof. Josue Mbonigaba of the University of KwaZulu-Natal, South Africa, aims to document the evidence of the difference in nature and extent of unsustainable food consumption across high-income countries HICs and low-income countries LICs. Following this chapter is "Sustainable Food Consumption in the Neoliberal Order: Challenges and Policy Implications," by Profs. Luke A. Amadi and Henry E. Alapiki from the University of Port Harcourt, Nigeria, which turns to the original impetus of sustainable food consumption and the question of how neoliberal order can be reconciled with the need to save the ecology. Next is "Food and Environment: A Review on the Sustainability of Six Different Dietary Patterns," by Prof. Pedro Pinheiro Gomes of National Statistics Institute, Portugal. It assesses the impacts of six dietary patterns while emphasizing protein overconsumption and sustainability of food systems and the nutritional disparities existent within these different patterns and the potential to make changes. "Re-Thinking Meat: How Climate Change Is Disrupting the Food Industry," by Dr. Jeff Anhang from The World Bank Group, USA, describes the ideal that sacrificing meat will benefit the climate; however, these efforts have not been linked to reduced meat consumption and instead this chapter offers alternative modes to disrupting meat production and consumption. The chapter "Normality, Naturalness, Necessity, and Nutritiousness of the New Meat Alternatives," by Prof. Diana Bogueva from Curtin University, Australia and Prof. Kurt Schmidinger of

Vienna University, Austria, examines the social readiness and acceptability of new meat alternatives as normal, natural, necessary, and nutritious amongst Gen Y and Gen Z consumers. The following chapter, "New Meat Without Livestock," by Profs. Dora Marinova and Diana Bogueva of Curtin University, Australia and Prof. Kurt Schmidinger from the University of Vienna, Austria, summarizes the global problems associated with livestock production and meat consumption and shows solution strategies through replacing animal products with plant-based alternatives. "Application of the Dietary Processed Sulfur Supplementation for Enhancing Nutritional and Functional Properties of Meat Products," by Prof. Chi-Ho Lee from Konkuk University, South Korea, focuses on strategies to investigate the changes in physical, physicochemical, and microbial properties of meat and meat products in dietary processed sulfur fed animals. Another chapter, "Nutritional Benefits of Selected Plant-Based Proteins as Meat Alternatives," written by Prof. Seydi Yıkmış from Tekirdağ Namık Kemal University, Turkey; Prof. Ramazan Mert Atan of Bandırma Onyedi Eylül University, Turkey; Prof. Nursena Kağan from Tekirdağ Namık Kemal University, Turkey; Prof. Levent Gülüm of Abant İzzet Baysal University, Turkey; Prof. Harun Aksu from Istanbul University – Cerrahpaşa, Turkey; and Prof. Mehmet Alpaslan from Tekirdağ Namık Kemal University, Turkey, describes the nutritional benefits and current uses of nine non-animal protein sources and the health benefits arising from replacing animal protein. The chapter "Understanding Gender Identities and Food Preferences to Increase the Consumption of a Plant-Based Diet With Heuristics," by Prof. Estela Seabra from The New School, USA, discerns existent food preferences and their correlation with women and men, and gender biases, in America and accounts for gender norms, cultural roles, and subconscious behavior in these decisions. The following chapter, "Lifelong Consumption of Plant-Based GM Foods: Is It Safe?" authored by Prof. Matthew Chidozie Ogwu of Seoul National University, South Korea, seeks to highlight general concerns and potential lifelong effects of consuming GM plant-based food including socioeconomic effects, development of new diseases, and potential effects on the environment and biodiversity. The chapter "Nutritional Properties of Edible Insects," by Prof. Anna K. Żołnierczyk from Wrocław University of Environmental and Life Sciences, Poland, explores how the consumption of edible insects can build a well-balanced diet, the nutrients within insects, and the benefits of insect production as compared to livestock production. Another chapter, "The Nutritional and Health Potential of Blackjack Bidens pilosa l.: A Review – Promoting the Use of Blackjack for Food," by Dr. Rose Mujila Mboya an Independent Researcher, Pietermaritzburg, South Africa, reviews the advantages and disadvantages of blackjack and argues for the deliberation of promoting its use for food. "Special Legume-Based Food as a Solution to Food and Nutrition Insecurity Problem in the Arctic," by Prof. Liudmila Nadtochii of ITMO University, Russia; Prof. Anna Veber from Omsk State Agrarian University, Russia; Prof. Svetlana Leonova of Bashkir State Agrarian University, Russia; Prof. Nina Kazydub from Omsk State Agrarian University, Russia; and Prof. Inna Simakova from Saratov State Agrarian University, Russia, discusses the potential of legume-based food products to contribute to the improvement of food and nutrition security in northern communities. Another chapter, "Soybeans Consumption and Production in China: Sustainability Perspective," by Profs. Dora Marinova and Xiumei Guo from Curtin University, Australia; Prof. Amzad Hossain of Curtin University, Australia & Rajshahi University, Bangladesh; Prof. Xiaoling Shao from Nanjing Audit University, China; and Prof. Shagufta M. Trishna from Curtin University, Australia, examines the trends in soy consumption and production in China and explores people's dietary preferences for soybeans, including concerns about the import of genetically modified soybeans. The next chapter, "The Potential of Traditional Leafy Vegetables for Improving Food Security in Africa," by Profs. Praxedis Dube, Wim J. M. Heijman, and Rico Ihle from Wageningen University, The Netherlands and Prof. Justus Ochieng from World Vegetable Center, Eastern and Southern Africa, Tanzania, assesses the potential of traditional leafy vegetables in improving food security in Africa by proposing research on the seeds, seed systems, processing methods, and increasing of consumption. Concluding this reference book is "Veganism in the Bhagwad Gita," by Prof. Pratyush Ranjan of G. M. University, India, which seeks directions from the Gita (the Song of the Spirit) on the appropriate principled responses to the animal agriculture industry, including that of changing dietary habits towards plant-based sources, before finally exploring whether the Gita would promote veganism.

Although the primary organization of the contents in this work is based on its five sections, offering a progression of coverage of the important concepts, methodologies, technologies, applications, social issues, and emerging trends, the reader can also identify specific contents by utilizing the extensive indexing system listed at the end. As a comprehensive collection of research on the latest findings related to reducing food waste and managing food waste, the *Research Anthology on Food Waste Reduction and Alternative Diets* provides farmers, experts in the agricultural industry, nutritionists, policymakers, researchers, academicians, students, and all audiences with a complete understanding of sustainable agriculture, food waste, food consumption, and food security through the lens of upcoming technologies, case studies, current methodologies, and theories. Given the vast number of issues concerning food waste and agricultural sustainability throughout countries around the world, this extensive book addresses the demand for a resource that encompasses the most pertinent research in methods being employed to globally bolster sustainability when it comes to food and agriculture.

Chapter 34
Impacts of Food Industrial Wastes on Soil and Its Utilization as Novel Approach for Value Addition

Nowsheeba Rashid
Amity University, India

Ifra Ashraf
SKUAST-K, India

Shazia Ramzan
University of Kashmir, India

ABSTRACT

Among the various agro-industries, food processing industries are the second prime generator of wastes after domestic sewage. In the current epoch of the rapid budding world, the wastes are mounting, which robustly sway the health of ecosystems and eventually the human population. For that reason, each agro-industrial sector has critical stipulation toward the secure utilization of agro-materials all the way through recycling of wastes. A crude disposal and littering of these waste materials frequently signifies a problem that is additionally provoked by different legal restrictions. Inadequate management of these solid waste constituents could lead to drastic change in physico-chemical properties of soils. The waste product, which is discarded into the environment, is loaded with valuable compounds. They are new, innate, and monetary sources of colorants, protein, dietary fiber, flavoring, antimicrobials, and antioxidants, which can be utilized in the food industry as a basis of natural food additives.

DOI: 10.4018/978-1-7998-5354-1.ch034

INTRODUCTION

India is a largely populated country which exists as the major reason for massive waste generation created frequently out of domestic & industrial actions which includes removal of peel followed by cutting of raw fruits and vegetables former to processing, eating and cooking (William, 2005). FAO revealed that every year, about one-third of all the food produced for the purpose of human consumption globally is lost or wasted. Large amounts of food processing by-product wastes are generated all over the world. It is estimated that about 5 million tons of sugar beet pulp and 3.5 million tons of brewers grain and almost half a million tons of onion peeling waste are created annually (Awarenet, 2004).This food wastage generation predicts a huge missed opportunity to enhance global food security, but also to alleviate environmental impacts and exhaustive resource use from food chains. According to the various quantitative food losses and waste estimations globally per year are roughly 40-50% for root crops, fruits and vegetables, 20% for oil seeds, meat and dairy plus 35% for fish and 30% for cereals (Gowe, 2015).

At the present epoch, ample quantity of waste generated marks food industry. As per the latest research carried out by FAO, almost 1.3 billion tons of food has been exhausted globally per year, which symbolizes nearly one third of the overall production of food industry (Gustafssonet al., 2013). Referring to the individual supplement fruit processing industries contribute more than 0.5 billion tons of waste. Thus, providing globally the accessibility of feed stock and encouraging the researchers, scientists and other authorities to exercise comprehensive studies on the various value added potential of fruit processing waste (FPW). On the other hand, vegetables are essential but uneconomical i.e. they produce ample waste concentration about 25%- 30% of inedible products (Ajila et al., 2010). Around twenty peculiar kinds of plants are generally developed for vegetables in the United States (US). Including this in each State these plants are grown on commercial basis out of which maximum population resides in New York, Texas, California, and Wisconsin. The profits from them to cultivars approach approximately to 300 million dollars annually despite of the fact not more than 20 to 30% of the crop is consumed. In this perspective, the utilization of the whole plant tissue could have cost-effective benefits to cultivars and a positive brunt on the environment, leading to a superior multiplicity of products (Cerezal & Duarte, 2005). Out of the total wastes 4 million tons of them are generally leaves. Several wastes are left as such on the soil to be plowed underneath. Few of them are fed, some are discarded in dumps and some are a simple nuisance a small portion is synthetically dehydrated for feed. The most prominent component of the wastes is water which accounts nearly about 75 to 90% (Willaman & Eskew, 1943). On a comparison fruit processing waste are originated to be selective and concentrated in nature as compared to other biomass derived waste. Besides, the greatest contribution provided is the utilization of peels, pomace and seed fractions as an excellent feedstock for recovery of bioactive compounds which include flavonoids, lipids, dietary fibers, pectin, etc (Kowalska et al., 2017; Banerjee et al., 2017).

A novel bio-refinery method would aim to manufacture a wider variety of important chemicals from fruit and vegetable processing waste. The wastes from bulk of the withdrawal processes may supplementary be used as recycle sources for creation of bio-fuels. These all benefits will open up as a scope for future utilization of fruit and vegetable waste for therapeutic and nutraceutical purpose as well as a great source for value addition of the end products.

According to the data acquired on global trend of fruit and vegetable production, the total of residues with prospective consumption after processing has been anticipated in millions tons every year. This demands the use of different forms of energy, water and other factors providing a by-product potential as the cardinal significance. This comes into being due to the presence of biocomponents, which may

Table 1. Percentage of food wastes and by-products in fruit and vegetable production

Production process	%age of wastes and by-products
White wine production Crow	20-30
Red wine production	20-30
Fruit and vegetable juice production	30-50
Fruit and vegetable processing and preservation	5-30
Vegetable oil production	40-70
Corn starch production	41-43
Potato starch production	80
Wheat starch production	50
Sugar production from sugar beet	85

Source: (Sadh et al. 2018)

be utilized for novel food production. This demands an appropriate measure to convert by-products into value added products for the reason of their calculus natural components.

To conquer the existing environmental condition, scientific communities have been exploiting industrial as well as agricultural wastes and effluents via process of recycling and clean technology, by modified and integrated utilization of waste or merely returning to the place of their origin and nature. Over the years pollution and organization of huge quantities of wastes generated by diverse industrial activities have been main problems practiced by developing countries. More demanding is the precarious disposal of these wastes into the ambient surroundings and biodegradation tribulations linked with it. These have resulted to substitution means of reclaiming the surroundings through bioremediation, phyto-remediation and air contamination control. Bioremediation involves the employment of microorganisms to break complex materials into simpler end products. These micro-organisms have advanced a host of enzymes that support in biodegradation of natural products contained by the ecosystem. This microbial clean-up (Bioremediation) method removes a number of supplementary destructive pollutants and conceivably is the most environmentally safe process used nowadays (Adriaens & Hickey, 1993; Beg et al, 2003; Van Hamme et al, 2003).

An additional source of industrial solid wastes is produced from pulp and paper mechanized plants. Pulp and paper are feigned from lignocellulosic raw materials from wood, recycled paper and agricultural residues. These wastes are typically disposed via landfill and incineration processes (Karthikeyan & Balasubramanian, 2010). These methods of dumping could be destructive to ecosystem and cause diseases to man. Many studies have been reported on the management of pulp and paper mill effluents via biological method like conventional aerobic, anaerobic action and use of white-rot fungi in the conduct (Wong et al, 2006; Wu et al, 2005; Dalentoft & Thulin, 1997). Recently, mushrooms are considered as the most advantageous and environment-friendly technique for recycling of the vast lignocellulosic waste substrates (Gume et al, 2013; Rai & Ahlawat, 2002) Figure1 depicts the illustration of recycled value-added applications of agro-industrial wastes. This chapter reviews numerous kinds of agro-industrial wastes and their principle recycled products which can be utilized in the factual world (Yusuf, 2017)

Figure 1. Schematic representation of recycled value-added applications of agro-industrial wastes

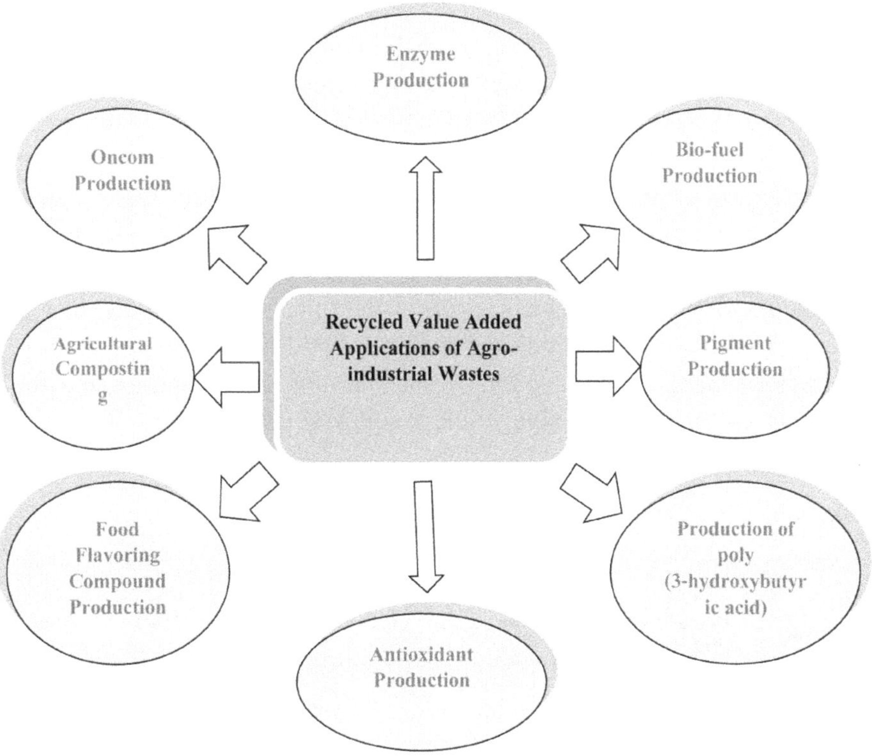

Figure 2. Representation of agro industrial wastes (Yusuf, 2017)

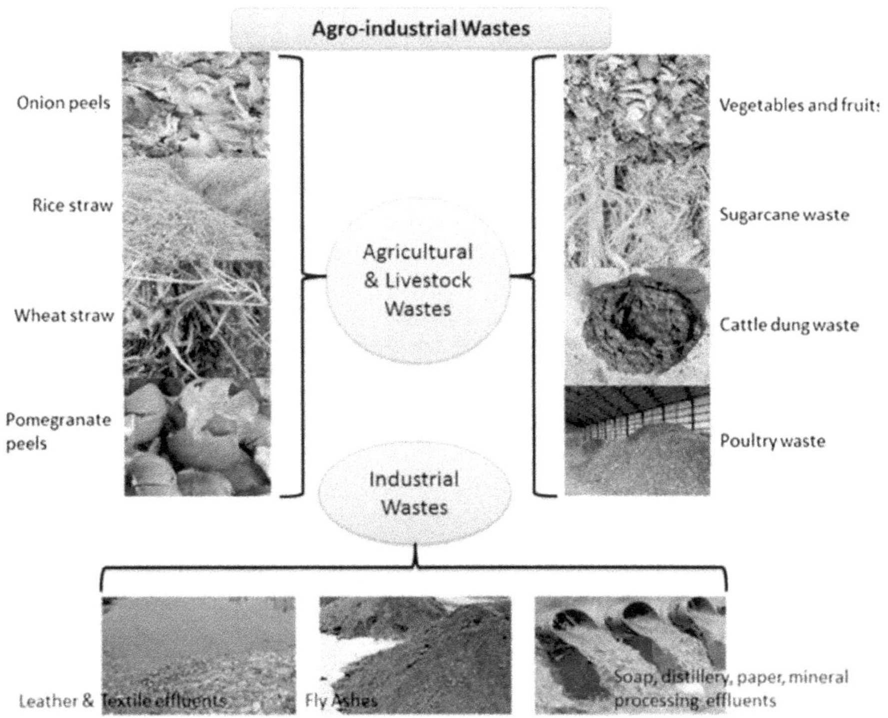

AGRO-INDUSTRIAL WASTE MATERIALS

Nowadays, one of the major sources of pollution is mostly organic waste from agro-industries. As a known fact regarding wastes mainly originating out of food industries comprise waste from pruning, manure, livestock slurry, and crop remains (Figure 2). Also, industries produce organic wastes, which constitute the by-products from agri-food industry (Table 2) like sludge from wool, coffee dregs, degummed fruits and legumes, bagasse, milk serum, cellulose, etc (Figure 3). These organic wastes goes on multiplying day by day and well thought-out to have damaging impacts on the overall environment. In this view, a number of countries prepared certain laws and rules to prevent on description of ecological concerns. Therefore, norm implies to the waste and includes the main explanations and ethics that administer waste management, highlight that waste appraisal and exclusion must be executed without generating risks for soil, water, air, or the fauna and flora to reduce such harmful effects and legalize the use of natural wastes as fertilizers in agriculture (Directive, 2008; Venglovsky et al.,2006).

Table 2. Composition of fruit industrial waste

Fruit industrial waste	Chemical Composition (%w/w)								References
	Cellulose	Hemi-cellulose	Lignin	Ash	Total solids	Moisture	Total carbon	Total nitrogen	
Potato peel waste	2.2%	-	-	7.7%	-	9.89	1.3%	-	Al-Weshahy and Rao (2012)
Orange Peel	9.21%	10.5%	0.84%	3.5%	-	11.86	-	-	Rivas et al. (2008)
Coffee skin	23.77 (gg/100g)	16.68%	28.58 (g/100g)	5.36 (g/100g)	-	-	C/N 14.41	-	Ballesteros et al.(2014)
Pineapple Peel	18.11	-	1.37	-	93.6	91	40.8	0.99	Paepatung et al. (2009)

In order to decrease the industrial pollution, a novel and clean technology can be executed to curtail organic waste via recycling. The clean technology assessment is a successful and efficient procedure that comprises five steps given below:

- Planning and organization
- Pre-assessment
- Assessment
- Feasibility study and
- Implementation

Figure 3. Agro-industrial wastes and their types

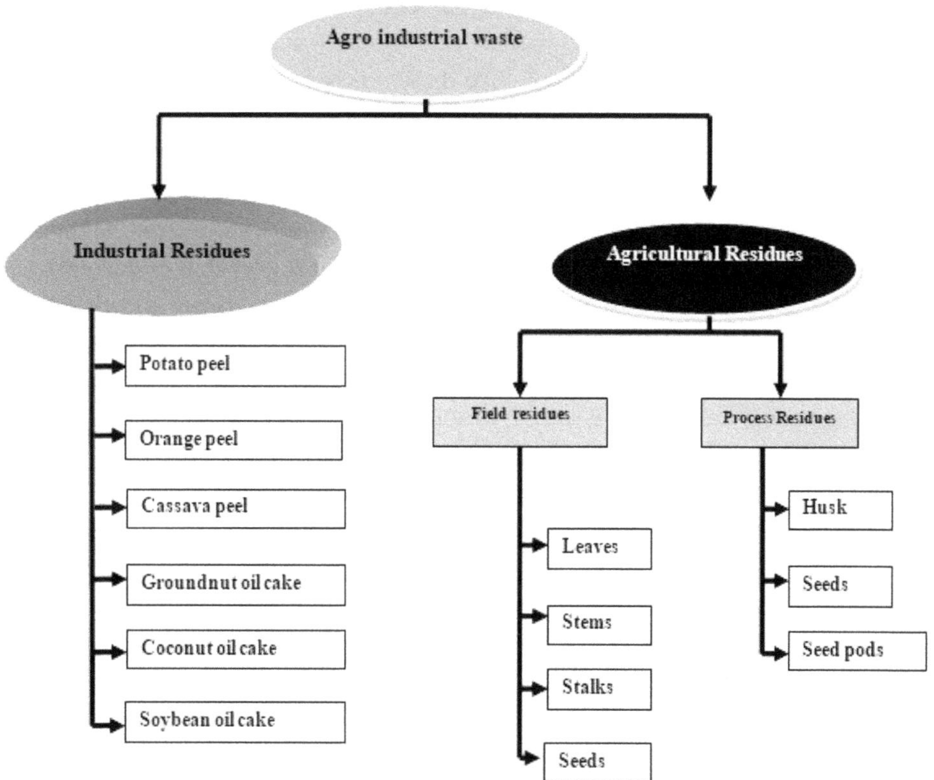

VALUE-ADDED APPLICATIONS OF RECYCLED AGRO-INDUSTRIAL WASTES

Production of Bio Fuels

Bio-fuels continue to be important because of the fact that they are used as an alternative for fossil fuels. It is revealed from the previous studies that the bio-fuels are fabricated from affirmative agro-industrial left over's like sugar beet waste, rice straw, corn stalks,(Figure 4) sweet potato waste, potato waste, sawdust, sugarcane and bagasse (Duhan et al., 2013; Kumar et al., 2014). It is found that in the year 2011, bio-ethanol production increased all over the world as much as 85 billion liters of bio-ethanol are reported to be produced (Avci et al., 2013; Saini et al., 2014). As the main concern nowadays is to reduce industrial waste and at the same time preserving our soil and environment from these pollution calamities. Hence, it is elucidated that with the help of agricultural residues, the deforestation can be decreased thus resulting in less dependence on forest woody biomass. Despite the fact that agro-industrial residues have short harvest time thus, reduce the extra consistently presented to bio-ethanol production (Limayema & Ricke, 2012). Several researchers have accomplished the production of ethanol from materials withlingo-cellulosic composition (Cadoche & López, 1989; Bjerre et al., 1996). Najafi et al. (2009) furthermore, premeditated the manufacture of bio-ethanol from a variety of agricultural residues attained from diverse agricultural crops. A range of agro-industrial wastes utilized for the production of bio-ethanol for next generation are discussed by Saini et al. (2014). They paid attention to the use of lingo-cellulosic composition of diverse agro-industrial wastes and accomplished the fact that the bio-fuels are valuable substitutes of different fossil fuels like diesel and petrol. On the basis of their debate and analysis of various approaches for bio-fuel creation, it is undoubtedly revealed that the lingo-cellulosic consequential bio-fuels are cost effective and also eco-friendly as well as substituent source of energy for upcoming generations. One more study for making of biogas by means of a variety of food industrial residues from diverse sources as well as two weeds namely *Eichornia crassipes* solms and *Typha angustifolia* L. were conceded out by Paepatung et al. (2009). A fast growth in population in most of the developing countries and also their fast expansion in industrialization creates the elevated demand for cheap sources of energy by means of cost-effective food industrial and other agricultural residues (Figure 4). An ample amount of vital waste is obtainable in these countries for the fabrication of bio-fuels. In a way Mushimiyimana and Tallapragada (2016) formed bio-ethanol by using wastes out of vegetable's via fermentation technique with the aid of baker's yeast *Saccharomyces cerevisiae*. In the study they made use of common vegetables residues such as carrot peel, potato peel, and onion peel. Bio-ethanol manufacture could be best substitute for the utilization of agricultural residues. Utilization of the stems of banana as a substrate for the production of bio-ethanol is an excellent alternative in India because of enormous availability of pseudo banana stem as a squander. Ingale et al. (2014) fashioned bio-ethanol by means of pseudo banana stem as a substrate with pre-treatment using microbes such as *Aspergillus fumigatus and Aspergillus ellipticus*. Furthermore, Maiti et al. (2016) utilizedfood industrial residues for the fabrication of butanol by making use of *Clostridium beijerinckii*. The highest amount of butanol (11.04 g/l) was produced subsequent to 96 hours of fermentation from the food industrial residue like SIW (starch industry wastewater). Hence, the utilization of economical and biologically agricultural waste for the creation of priceless bio-fuels is a healthier pathway for the accomplishment of necessity of energy through restricted resources and also eliminating the threat to the soil environment.

Production of Enzyme

One of the most important phenomena for the transformation of agricultural wastes into valuable products is enzymatic hydrolysis which is a valuable and significant technique. Consumption of food industrial wastes proposes enormous prospective for decreasing the production costs and mounting the usage of enzymes for industrial functions. As a known fact that agro-industrial wastes include sugarcane bagasse, wheat bran, wheat straw, corncob, rice bran, etc. are low price and have abundantly obtainable natural carbon sources which can be effectively utilized for the creation of scientifically essential enzymes (Jecu, 2000). A technique known as microbial culture-based solid state fermentation (Salim et al., 2017) is presently used to ferment various agro-industrial residual substrates and by-products for the successful production of cellulases (Salim et al., 2017), consequently, in a supplementary study explained the fabrication of enzymes by a recently secluded *Bacillus* sp. TMF-1 in solid-state fermentation on food industrial by-products. In this research, they achieved α-amylases, cellulases, pectinases and proteases (Krishna, 2005)

Figure 4. Positive impacts of using wastes

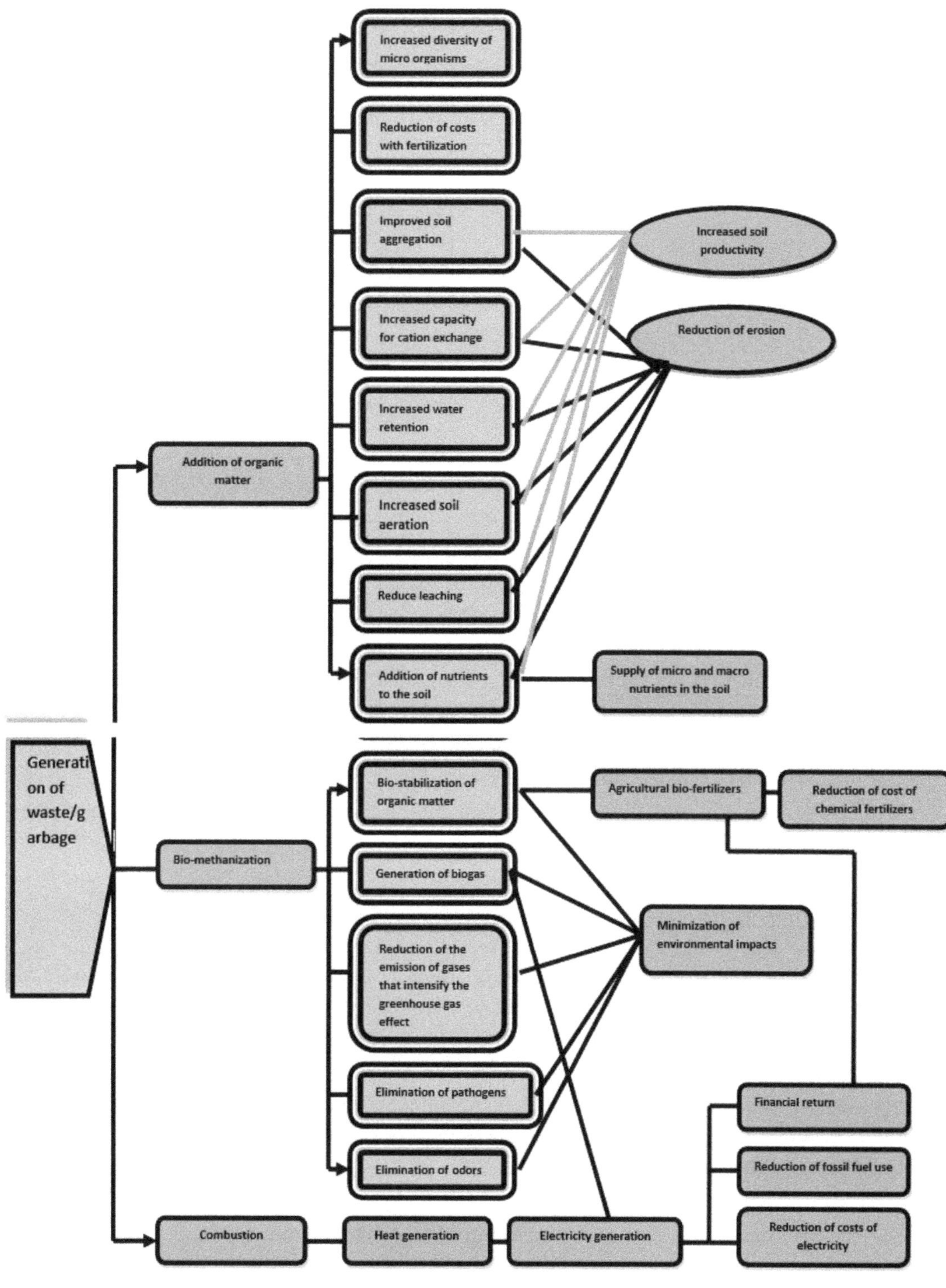

Table 3. Studies on production of enzymes by microorganisms using agro-industrial wastes

Substrates	Enzymes	Microorganisms	References
Papaya waste Groundnut oil cake(GOC) Wheat bran and orange peel Linseed oil cake(LOC) Orange peel Coconut oil cake(COC) Rice bran Corn bran (Rice, Wheat, Blackgram) bran and soyabean Fruit peel waste	α-Amylase Lipase Pectin methyl esterase Lipase α-Amylase α-Amylase α-Amylase α-Amylase α-Amylase Invertase	*A. niger* *C. rugosa* *P. notatum* *P. aeruginosa* *A. niger* *A. oryzae* *Bacillus* sp. *Bacillus* sp. *A. niger* *A. niger*	Sharanappa et al. (2011) Rekha et al. (2012) Gayen and Ghosh (2011) Parihar (2012) Sindiri et al. (2013) Ramachandran et al. (2004) Sodhi et al. (2005) Sodhi et al. (2005) Akpan et al. (1999) Mehta and Duhan (2014)

Antioxidant Production

Fruit peels such as skins are loaded with nutrients and include many phytochemicals that may be competently used as drugs or as food supplements or replacers (Bobinaitė et al., 2016). Antioxidants are excellent compounds as they act as additives in foodstuffs in order to enhance their nutritional value or in manufacture of fruit puree (Chacko & Estherlydia, 2014). In addition their sensory properties act as a raw material for the creation of food dyes. Very essential is the prospect of preserved and improved quality as a consequence of avoiding food oxidation (Ayala-Zavala & González-Aguilar, 2011). The probable antioxidative position and bioavailability of byproducts from creation of nectar of the pomegranate fruit were examined under a study (Surek & Nilufer-Erdil, 2016). Pomegranate seeds and the impulsive obtained by sedimentation of nectar comprise a good supply of anthocyanins. Filter cake, sediment peel contained extra phenolic compounds and were characterized by elevated antioxidant action than those extracted from the pomegranate nectar. In the certain studies the antioxidant activity and overall content of polyphenols of tomato skin were found to be 38.2 and 66.5% elevated, correspondingly, in comparison to the seeds of tomatoes (Sarkar & Kaul, 2014).

Production of Oncom

Oncom is a native fermented product of Indonesia which is prepared from a number of agricultural wastes. Basically, there are three categories of oncom. Out of these three categories, the most eminent is that prepared from peanut press-cake, waste merchandise from peanut oil processing industries. This is known as oncomkacang, it is accepted in West Java (VanVeen et al., 1968; Beuchat, 1986). Another type is oncomtahoo, it is admired in Jakarta. It is manufactured from the solid wastes out of tahoo, which is a curd of soya bean. Its preparation is analogous to that for oncomkacang. The third type is prepared from the solid wastes of starch flour (Hunkwe) and mungbean (*Phaseolus radiata*) and is popularly known by the name of oncomampashunkwe (Steinkraus, 1983).

The High-quality oncom (Figure 5), conventional Indonesian fermented food, was primed by the inoculation of pure culture of numerous Neurospora, Rhizopus, and Mucor strains. Even though the role of Mucor in oncom making was not recognized, many Mucor strains could create high-quality oncom. Solid inoculum includes each of 4 Mucor, 4 Rhizopus, and 3 Neurospora strains with utilization of cooked rice as a transporter were primed to manufacture high-quality oncom. All inoculum apart from one contained a sufficient amount of living cells to make oncom after storage for 180 days at room temperature. Bandung red oncom and bogor red oncom formed by the local manufacturer using the solid inoculum had very good eminence. They were brought to the neighboring market and well acknowledged by the consumers. The raw materials of oncom are chiefly the waste of agricultural goods and there are many types of oncom by the mixture of several molds and raw materials. The temperature of the solid substrate fermentation used for fermented foods in Southeast Asia is well thought-out to be mesophilic as the incubation is usually conceded out at room temperature in a very consistent steamy environment of 25° to 32°C. Oncom is the cheapest product because the raw materials for oncom are mostly the waste of agricultural products that still hold high quantity of protein appropriate for consumers with low-incomes. Thus, the enhancement of the quality of oncom ought to result not only in a deliverance of good and cheap food with high protein content, but also in the competent use of agricultural products. On the other hand, no attempt has been made to advance the quality of oncom and to deal out the enhanced products (Sastraatmadja et al,2001)

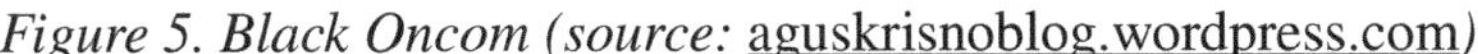

Figure 5. Black Oncom (source: aguskrisnoblog.wordpress.com*)*

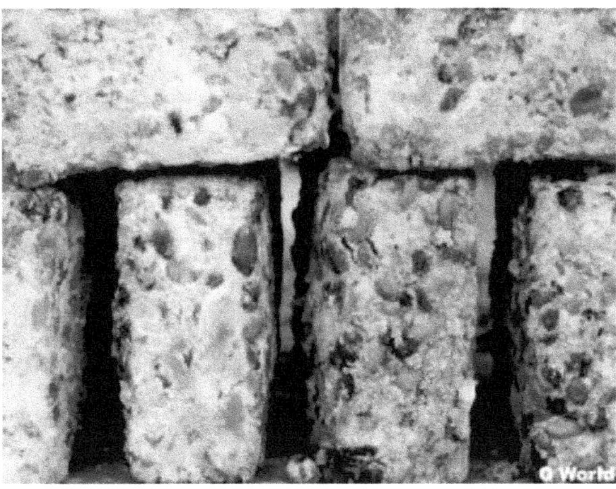

PRODUCTION OF FOOD FLAVORING COMPOUNDS

The wastes out of agro-industries are cheap and sustainable resources for the fabrication of renewable technique for value-added products. A lot of natural flavoring agents can be formed out of these wastes via microbial conversions. Because of the importance gained by potential flavorings they are being widely used. They are extensively used in various dishes as seasoning. Besides, most of them are utilized by traditional medicine, e.g. certain essential oils that are rich in terpene compounds are acknowledged for supporting in the treatment and curability of enormous health problems. An important purpose of some of them leads to various activities such as antifungal, anti viral, anti inflammatory, anti mutagenic, antibacterial, vermicide and anticancer activities (Raut & Karuppayil, 2014; Felipe et al., 2017).At the present epoch flavor companies are concerned with the aromas and flavors which are more stable and don't escape openly besides under specifically defined conditions i.e. they are mostly microscopically encapsulated (Arvanitoyannis & Varzakas, 2008).

Sometimes various factors affect the existence or availability of specific flavoring extracts such as their existence being uneconomical due to high cost or its unavailability. This leads to a great switch towards the commercial flavoring adoption. These trendy flavorings are nothing but an equal or adjacent chemical substitutes or equivalents of the existing natural flavours commonly known as the 'nature-identical (Mantzouridou et al., 2015). The production of the specific enzymatic as well as the whole-cell biocatalysis has gained a cardinal attention as well as a novelty. Their approach has been greatly observed as a substitute for the better development of several esters when compared to any naturally or chemically synthesized enzymes (Zhuang et al., 2015). These extractions of the enzymes from the particular organisms serve various vital benefits which mainly include superior productivity with respect to the elevated catalyst concentration, as well as the simpler product refinement. Some researches provide three main methods exercised for the process of aroma compounds production (Felipe et al., 2017). These processes include the method of chemical synthesis, extraction from natural sources and some of the biotechnological production processes resulting in the development of the bio-aromas.

However, among all the above-mentioned techniques majority advantages are contributed by the biotechnological process. The importance can be approved or confirmed by its natural product development as a versatile resultant. Furthermore, the most novel advantage offered is the development of the better, suitable and sustainable preservation approach towards the environment. Bioaroma production extends its approach towards the most unique renewable processing characteristic. This imparts requirement of very simple operation conditions responsible for non-toxic waste generation thus, sometimes availing the agro-industrial residues. The vital substitute is a by-product of fruit and vegetable waste which is a prospective resource of flavor production (Sadh et al., 2018).

Production of Poly (3-Hydroxybutyric Acid)

Citrus fruits are devoured throughout the world for diverse industrial purposes such as fruit juice, jams and jelly manufacture. So these categories of industries also produces an enormous quantity of waste in the form of peel residue or in supplementary form but these citrus wastes if used in fermentation process yield novel products as they contain huge quantity of carbohydrates. Various researchers obtained useful by-products by utilizing these residues besides Sukan et al. (2014) utilized orange peel waste for the creation of Poly (3-HB). Their outcome showed that orange peel is a rich and unutilized food industrial waste which can be utilized for novel approaches (Figure 6). In their research they reported first time the production of Poly (3-HB) utilizing orange peel as a solitary carbon source followed by a very simple pre-treatment method thus, preserving the soil environment and at the same time proving to be a sustainable novel product (Sadh et al., 2018).

Recycled Agricultural Composting

In recent epoch, composting techniques have been reevaluated in most countries around the globe and incorporated into the novel 4-R strategy, together with countries of America, Asia, Africa and Europe. The progresses made in composting techniques in India all through the early fraction of the preceding century have led to the novel composting operations. Composting as we know is a controlled process which uses innate and natural microorganisms existing in organic matter as well as soil to decay organic wastes (Sadh et al., 2018). These microorganisms necessitate adequate vital nutrients, oxygen as well as water in order to decompose the organic matter at an accelerated speed. The raw materials which de-

Figure 6. Putative metabolic pathway of PHA synthesis from γ- butyrolactone in H.pseudoflava (Ahn et al., 2000)

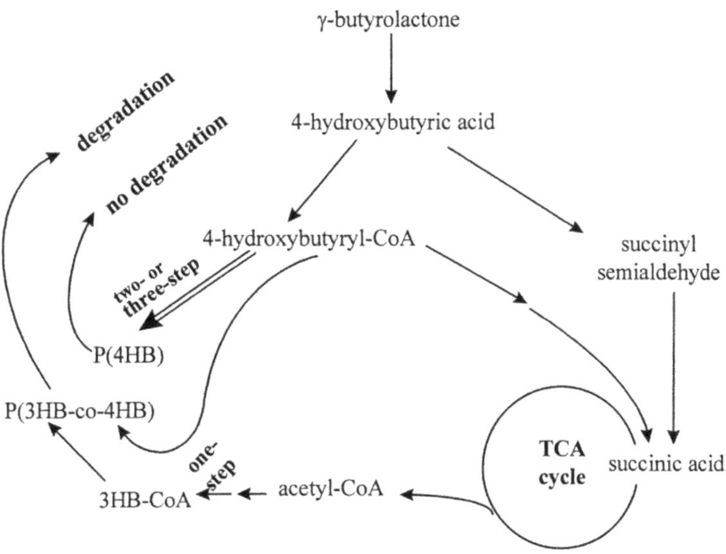

compose after going into the compost are habitually referred as feedstock. The end product i.e. compost, has a dark brown, humus-like appearance and can be easily hence safely stored, handled, and applied to land as a priceless soil conditioner (Lopez-Real, 1996).

FUTURE PROSPECTS

Agro-industrial wastes or residues are loaded with nutrients as well as bioactive compounds. These wastes encompass inconsistency in their composition such as proteins, sugars, and minerals; therefore, they should be well thought-out to be "raw material" instead of "wastes" for several other industrial purposes. The amount of such nutrients in these wastes proposes appropriate circumstances for the productive expansion of microorganisms. The microorganisms have prospective to reprocess the waste as raw materials for their development through fermentation processes. The food industrial wastes can be used as solid support i.e. substrate in solid state fermentation technique for the manufacture of a variety of important valuable compounds. The utilization of agricultural as well as agro-based industry wastes as raw materials can facilitate to decrease the manufacturing cost and contribute in recycling of residues as well as to construct the eco-friendly environment. Currently, several studies have been performed to use solid wastes from human activities as soil conditioners and/or fertilizers for increasing crop productivity. Therefore, studies that monitor organic waste effects on agricultural soils deserve the attention of the international scientific community, as it enables increases in the productivity of agricultural crops, fiber, and biomass energy combined to reduce risks to human, plant, and animal health and environment.

CONCLUSION

There have been growing remarks and evidences of various value added food products developed from the food industrial residues. Among which the majority have been significantly implemented for the various cardinal purposes in such a way that there value is unhampered and not being adversely affected. However, their production can itself be a challenge to the manufacturer for the reason of imparting additional cost to the processing value and adding to the economical values or the overall cost. However, in the mean time value addition of products may also lead to a remarkable growth in terms of the profit, but the identification, selection, manufacturing itself pertains to a major challenge. This depends on the manufacturing practices, consumption on the agro-economic level and the slightest threats imparted to the global environment. There is a extensive dialogue regarding the suitable forms of dumping and use of the solid wastes, and their reuse on agricultural soil has been measured the most remarkable option, both from the environmental standpoint and the economic one. However, their use in agriculture should be headed by a scrutiny of environmental and economic impact and the indiscriminate utilization of wastes may lead to contamination.

REFERENCES

Adriaens, P., & Hickey, W. J. (1993). Article. In D. L. Stone (Ed.), Biotechnology for the Treatment of Hazardous Waste (pp. 97–120). Ann Arbor, MI: Lewis Publishers.

Ahn, W. S., Park, S. J., & Lee, S. Y. (2000). Production of Poly(3-Hydroxybutyrate) by Fed-Batch Culture of Recombinant Escherichia coli with a Highly Concentrated Whey Solution. *Applied and Environmental Microbiology*, *66*(8), 3624–3627. doi:10.1128/AEM.66.8.3624-3627.2000 PMID:10919830

Ajila, C. M., Aalami, M., Leelavathi, K., & Rao, U. P. (2010). Mango peel powder: A potential source of antioxidant and dietary fiber in macaroni preparations. *Innovative Food Science & Emerging Technologies*, *11*(1), 219–224. doi:10.1016/j.ifset.2009.10.004

Akpan, I., Bankole, M. O., Adesemowo, A. M., & Latunde, D. G. (1999). Production of amylase by *A. niger*in a cheap solid medium using rice bran and agricultural materials. *Tropical Science*, *39*, 77–79.

Al-Weshahy, A., & Rao, V. A. (2012). Potato peel as a source of important phytochemical antioxidant nutraceuticals and their role in human health-A review. In *Phytochemicals as Nutraceuticals-Global Approaches to Their Role in Nutrition and Health*. InTech. doi:10.5772/30459

Arvanitoyannis, I. S., & Varzakas, T. H. (2008). Vegetable waste management: Treatment methods and potential uses of treated waste. Waste Management for the Food Industries, 703-752.

Avci, A., Saha, B. C., Dien, B. S., Kennedy, G. J., & Cotta, M. A. (2013). Response surface optimization of corn stover pretreatment using dilute phosphoric acid for enzymatic hydrolysis and ethanol production. *Bioresource Technology*, *130*, 603–612. doi:10.1016/j.biortech.2012.12.104 PMID:23334017

Awarenet. (2004). *Hand book of waste management and co-products recovery in food processing*. Academic Press.

Ayala-Zavala, J. F., & González-Aguilar, G. A. (2010). Use of additives to preserve the quality of fresh-cut fruits and vegetables. In *Advances in fresh-cut fruits and vegetables processing* (pp. 233–256). CRC Press. doi:10.1201/b10263-10

Ballesteros, L. F., Teixeira, J. A., & Mussatto, S. I. (2014). Chemical, functional, and structural properties of spent coffee grounds and coffee silverskin. *Food and Bioprocess Technology, 7*(12), 3493–3503. doi:10.100711947-014-1349-z

Banerjee, J., Singh, R., Vijayaraghavan, R., MacFarlane, D., Patti, A. F., & Arora, A. (2017). Bioactives from fruit processing wastes: Green approaches to valuable chemicals. *Food Chemistry, 225*, 10–22. doi:10.1016/j.foodchem.2016.12.093 PMID:28193402

Beg, M. U., Saeed, T., Al-Muzaini, S., Beg, K. R., & Al-Bahloul, M. (2003). Distribution of petroleum hydrocarbon in sediment from coastal area receiving industrial effluents in Kuwait. *Ecotoxicology and Environmental Safety, 54*(1), 47–55. doi:10.1016/S0147-6513(02)00019-2 PMID:12547635

Beuchat, L. R. (1986). Oncom (fermented peanut presscake). In N. R. Reddy, M. D. Pierson, & D. K. Salunkhe (Eds.), *Legume-based fermented foods* (pp. 135–144). Boca Raton, FL: CRC Press.

Bjerre, A. B., Olesen, A. B., Fernqvist, T., Plöger, A., & Schmidt, A. S. (1996). Pretreatment of wheat straw using combined wet oxidation and alkaline hydrolysis resulting in convertible cellulose and hemicellulose. *Biotechnology and Bioengineering, 49*(5), 568–577. doi:10.1002/(SICI)1097-0290(19960305)49:5<568::AID-BIT10>3.0.CO;2-6 PMID:18623619

Bobinaitė, R., Viskelis, P., Bobinas, Č., Mieželienė, A., Alenčikienė, G., & Venskutonis, P. R. (2016). Raspberry marc extracts increase antioxidative potential, ellagic acid, ellagitannin and anthocyanin concentrations in fruit purees. *Lebensmittel-Wissenschaft + Technologie, 66*, 460–467. doi:10.1016/j.lwt.2015.10.069

Cadoche, L., & López, G. D. (1989). Assessment of size reduction as a preliminary step in the production of ethanol from lignocellulosic wastes. *Biological Wastes, 30*(2), 153–157. doi:10.1016/0269-7483(89)90069-4

Cerezal, P., & Duarte, G. (2005). Utilización de cáscaras en la elaboración de productosconcentrados de tuna (Opuntiaficus-índica (L.)Miller). *Journal of the Professional Association for Cactus Development*, 61-83.

Chacko, C. M., & Estherlydia, D. (2014). Antimicrobial evaluation of jams made from indigenous fruit peels. *International Journal of Advanced Research, 2*(1), 202–207.

Dalentoft, E., & Thulin, P. (1997). The use of aerobic selectors in activated sludge systems for treatment of wastewater from the pulp and paper industry. *Water Science and Technology, 35*(2-3), 181–188. doi:10.2166/wst.1997.0513

Directive, E. C. (2008). 105/EC of the European Parliament and of the Council of 16 December 2008 on environmental quality standards in the field of water policy, amending and subsequently repealing Council Directives 82/176. *EEC, 83*(513), 84–97.

Duhan, J. S., Kumar, A., & Tanwar, S. K. (2013). Bioethanol production from starchy part of tuberous plant (potato) using Saccharomyces cerevisiae MTCC-170. *African Journal of Microbiological Research, 7*(46), 5253–5260. doi:10.5897/AJMR2013.6122

Felipe, L., de Oliveira, A. M., & Bicas, J. L. (2017). Bioaromas–Perspectives for sustainable development. *Trends in Food Science & Technology, 62*, 141–153. doi:10.1016/j.tifs.2017.02.005

Gayen, S., & Ghosh, U. (2011). Pectinmethylesterase Production from mixed agro- wastes by Penicilliumnotatum NCIM. 923 in Solid-State fermentation. *Journal of Bioremediation & Biodegradation, 2*(02), 119. doi:10.4172/2155-6199.1000119

Gowe, C. (2015). Review on potential use of fruit and vegetables by-products as a valuable source of natural food additives. *Food Science and Quality Management, 45*, 47–61.

Gume, B., Muleta, D., & Abate, D. (2013). Evaluation of locally available substrates for cultivation of oyster mushroom (Pleurotus ostreatus) in Jimma, Ethiopia. *African Journal of Microbiological Research, 7*(20), 2228–2237. doi:10.5897/AJMR12.895

Gustafsson, J., Cederberg, C., Sonesson, U., & Emanuelsson, A. (2013). *The methodology of the FAO study: Global Food Losses and Food Waste-extent, causes and prevention.* SIK Institutetförlivsmedelochbioteknik.

Ingale, S., Joshi, S. J., & Gupte, A. (2014). Production of bioethanol using agricultural waste: Banana pseudo stem. *Brazilian Journal of Microbiology, 45*(3), 885–892. doi:10.1590/S1517-83822014000300018 PMID:25477922

Jecu, L. (2000). Solid state fermentation of agricultural wastes for endoglucanase production. *Industrial Crops and Products, 11*(1), 1–5. doi:10.1016/S0926-6690(99)00022-9

Karthikeyan, K., & Balasubramanian, S. (2010). Studies on the characterization and possibilities of reutilization of solid wastes from a waste paper based paper industry. *Global Journal of Environmental Research, 4*(1), 18–22.

Kowalska, H., Czajkowska, K., Cichowska, J., & Lenart, A. (2017). What's new in biopotential of fruit and vegetable by-products applied in the food processing industry. *Trends in Food Science & Technology, 67*, 150–159. doi:10.1016/j.tifs.2017.06.016

Krishna, C. (2005). Solid-state fermentation systems—An overview. *Critical Reviews in Biotechnology, 25*(1-2), 1–30. doi:10.1080/07388550590925383 PMID:15999850

Kumar, A., Duhan, J. S., Gahlawat, S., & Gahlawat, S. K. (2014). Production of ethanol from tuberous plant (sweet potato) using *Saccharomyces cerevisiae* MTCC-170. *African Journal of Biotechnology, 13*(28).

Limayem, A., & Ricke, S. C. (2012). Lignocellulosic biomass for bioethanol production: Current perspectives, potential issues and future prospects. *Progress in Energy and Combustion Science, 38*(4), 449–467. doi:10.1016/j.pecs.2012.03.002

Lopez-Real, J. M. (1996). Composting of Agricultural Wastes. In M. de Bertoldi, P. Sequi, B. Lemmes, & T. Papi (Eds.), *The Science of Composting* (pp. 542–550). Dordrecht, The Netherlands: Springer. doi:10.1007/978-94-009-1569-5_51

Maiti, S., Sarma, S. J., Brar, S. K., Le Bihan, Y., Drogui, P., Buelna, G., & Verma, M. (2016). Agro-industrial wastes as feedstock for sustainable bio-production of butanol by *Clostridium beijerinckii*. *Food and Bioproducts Processing*, *98*, 217–226. doi:10.1016/j.fbp.2016.01.002

Mantzouridou, F. T., Paraskevopoulou, A., & Lalou, S. (2015). Yeast flavour production by solid state fermentation of orange peel waste. *Biochemical Engineering Journal*, *101*, 1–8. doi:10.1016/j.bej.2015.04.013

Mehta, K., & Duhan, J. S. (2014). Production of invertase from Aspergillusniger using fruit peel waste as a substrate. *International Journal of Pharma and Bio Sciences*, *5*(2), 353–360.

Mushimiyimana, I., &Tallapragada, P. (2016). *Bioethanol production from agro wastes by acid hydrolysis and fermentation process*. Academic Press.

Najafi, G., Ghobadian, B., Tavakoli, T., & Yusaf, T. (2009). Potential of bioethanol production from agricultural wastes in Iran. *Renewable & Sustainable Energy Reviews*, *13*(6-7), 1418–1427. doi:10.1016/j.rser.2008.08.010

Paepatung, N., Nopharatana, A., & Songkasiri, W. (2009). Bio-methane potential of biological solid materials and agricultural wastes. *Asian Journal on Energy and Environment*, *10*(1), 19–27.

Parihar, D. K. (2012). Production of lipase utilizing linseed oilcake as fermentation substrate. *Int. J. Sci. Environ. Technol*, *1*(3), 135–143.

Rai, R. D., & Ahlawat, O. P. (2002). Edible fungi: Biotechnological approaches. In *Applied Mycology and Biotechnology* (Vol. 2, pp. 87–121). Elsevier.

Ramachandran, S., Patel, A. K., Nampoothiri, K. M., Francis, F., Nagy, V., Szakacs, G., & Pandey, A. (2004). Coconut oil cake—a potential raw material for the production of α-amylase. *Bioresource Technology*, *93*(2), 169–174. doi:10.1016/j.biortech.2003.10.021 PMID:15051078

Raut, J. S., & Karuppayil, S. M. (2014). A status review on the medicinal properties of essential oils. *Industrial Crops and Products*, *62*, 250–264. doi:10.1016/j.indcrop.2014.05.055

Rekha, K. S. S., Lakshmi, M. V. C., Devi, V. S., & Siddartha Kumar, M. (2012). Production and optimization of lipase from *Candida rugosa* using groundnut oilcake under solid state fermentation. *Biosensors*, *27*, 31.

Rivas, B., Torrado, A., Torre, P., Converti, A., & Domínguez, J. M. (2008). Submerged citric acid fermentation on orange peel autohydrolysate. *Journal of Agricultural and Food Chemistry*, *56*(7), 2380–2387. doi:10.1021/jf073388r PMID:18321055

Sadh, P. K., Duhan, S., & Duhan, J. S. (2018). Agro-industrial wastes and their utilization using solid state fermentation: A review. *Bioresources and Bioprocessing*, *5*(1), 1. doi:10.118640643-017-0187-z

Saini, J. K., Saini, R., & Tewari, L. (2014). Lignocellulosic agriculture wastes as biomass feedstocks for second-generation bioethanol production: Concepts and recent developments. 3. *Biotechnology (Faisalabad)*, *5*(4), 337–353. doi:10.100713205-014-0246-5 PMID:28324547

Salim, A. A., Grbavčić, S., Šekuljica, N., Stefanović, A., Tanasković, S. J., Luković, N., & Knežević-Jugović, Z. (2017). Production of enzymes by a newly isolated Bacillus sp. TMF-1 in solid state fermentation on agricultural by-products: The evaluation of substrate pretreatment methods. *Bioresource Technology*, *228*, 193–200. doi:10.1016/j.biortech.2016.12.081 PMID:28063362

Sarkar, A., & Kaul, P. (2014). Evaluation of Tomato Processing By-Products: A Comparative Study in a Pilot Scale Setup. *Journal of Food Process Engineering*, *37*(3), 299–307. doi:10.1111/jfpe.12086

Sastraatmadja, D. D., Tomita, F., & Ksai, T. (2001). Production of high-quality oncom, a traditional Indonesian fermented food, by the inoculation with selected mold strains in the form of pure culture and solid inoculum. *Journal-Graduate School of Agriculture Hokkaido University*, *70*(2), 111–128.

Sindiri, M. K., Machavarapu, M., & Vangalapati, M. (2013). Alfa-amylase production and purification using fermented orange peel in solid state fermentation by *Aspergillusniger. Ind J Appl Res*, *3*(8), 49–5. doi:10.15373/2249555X/AUG2013/16

Sodhi, H. K., Sharma, K., Gupta, J. K., & Soni, S. K. (2005). Production of a thermostable α-amylase from Bacillus sp. PS-7 by solid state fermentation and its synergistic use in the hydrolysis of malt starch for alcohol production. *Process Biochemistry*, *40*(2), 525–534. doi:10.1016/j.procbio.2003.10.008

Steinkraus, K. H. (1983). *Handbook of indigenous fermented foods*. New York: M Dekker Inc.

Sukan, A., Roy, I., & Keshavarz, T. (2014). Agro-industrial waste materials as substrates for the production of poly (3-hydroxybutyric acid). *Journal of Biomaterials and Nanobiotechnology*, *5*(4), 229–240. doi:10.4236/jbnb.2014.54027

Surek, E., & Nilufer-Erdil, D. (2016). Phenolic contents, antioxidant activities and potential bioaccessibilities of industrial pomegranate nectar processing wastes. *International Journal of Food Science & Technology*, *51*(1), 231–239. doi:10.1111/ijfs.13000

Van Hamme, J. D., Singh, A., & Ward, O. P. (2003). Recent advances in petroleum microbiology. *Microbiology and Molecular Biology Reviews*, *67*(4), 503–549. doi:10.1128/MMBR.67.4.503-549.2003 PMID:14665675

VanVeen, A. G., Graham, D. C. W., & Steinkraus, K. H. (1968). Fermented peanut press cake. *Cereal Sci Today*, *13*, 96–99.

Venglovsky, J., Martinez, J., & Placha, I. (2006). Hygienic and ecological risks connected with utilization of animal manures and biosolids in agriculture. *Livestock Science*, *102*(3), 197–203. doi:10.1016/j.livsci.2006.03.017

Willaman, J., & Eskew, R. (1943). *Uses for vegetable wastes*. Academic Press.

William, P. T. (2005). Water treatment and disposal. John Wiley.

Wong, S. S., Teng, T. T., Ahmad, A. L., Zuhairi, A., & Najafpour, G. (2006). Treatment of pulp and paper mill wastewater by polyacrylamide (PAM) in polymer induced flocculation. *Journal of Hazardous Materials*, *135*(1-3), 378–388. doi:10.1016/j.jhazmat.2005.11.076 PMID:16431022

Wu, J., Xiao, Y. Z., & Yu, H. Q. (2005). Degradation of lignin in pulp mill wastewaters by white-rot fungi on biofilm. *Bioresource Technology*, 96(12), 1357–1363. doi:10.1016/j.biortech.2004.11.019 PMID:15792583

Yusuf, M. (2017). Agro-Industrial Waste Materials and their Recycled Value-Added Applications. Handbook of Ecomaterials, 1-11.

Zhuang, S., Fu, J., Powell, C., Huang, J., Xia, Y., & Yan, R. (2015). Production of medium-chain volatile flavour esters in Pichiapastoris whole-cell biocatalysts with extracellular expression of Saccharomyces cerevisiae acyl-CoA: Ethanol O-acyltransferase Eht1 or Eeb1. *SpringerPlus*, 4(1), 467. doi:10.118640064-015-1195-0 PMID:26357598

KEY TERMS AND DEFINITIONS

Agricultural Composting: Composting is the biological decomposition of organic materials by microorganisms under controlled, aerobic conditions to a relatively stable humus-like material called compost. Composting can happen in many different ways using a variety of materials, methods, equipment, and scales of operation. For agricultural operations the common materials or feedstocks that are composted are livestock manures and bedding and various residual plant materials (straw, culls, on-farm processing wastes, etc.).

Bagasse: Bagasse is the dry pulpy fibrous residue that remains after sugarcane or sorghum stalks are crushed to extract their juice. It is used as a biofuel for the production of heat, energy, and electricity, and in the manufacture of pulp and building materials.

Biofuel: Biofuel is any fuel that is derived from biomass—that is, plant or algae material or animal waste. Since such feedstock material can be replenished readily, biofuel is considered to be a source of renewable energy, unlike fossil fuels such as petroleum, coal, and natural gas.

Biomass: Biomass is organic matter, such as leaves, stems, wood. All plants collectively produce biomass that can be converted into usable energy.

Nutraceuticals: Neutraceuticals are defined as ingredients that have health benefits beyond basic nutrition. They are also defined as parts of a food or a whole food that have a medical or health benefit, including the prevention and treatment of disease.

This research was previously published in Innovative Waste Management Technologies for Sustainable Development edited by Rouf Ahmad Bhat, Humaira Qadri, Khursheed Ahmad Wani, Gowhar Hamid Dar, and Mohammad Aneesul Mehmood; pages 226-243, copyright year 2020 by Engineering Science Reference (an imprint of IGI Global).

Chapter 35
Allocation Optimization Problem for Peruvian Food Bank

Ricardo Campos-Caycho
Pontificia Universidad Católica, Peru

Pamela Ivonne Borja-Ramos
Pontificia Universidad Católica del Perú, Peru

Renzo A. Benavente-Sotelo
Ponticia Universidad Católica del Perú, Peru

Stephanie M. Dueñas-Calderón
Pontificia Universidad Católica del Perú, Peru

Yasser A. Hidalgo-Gómez
Pontificia Universidad Católica del Perú, Peru

Patricia Elkfury-Cominges
Pontificia Universidad Católica del Perú, Peru

Christian A. Blas-Bazán
Pontificia Universidad Católica del Perú, Peru

Pamela Arista-Yampi
Pontificia Universidad Católica del Perú, Peru

Jorge Luis Yupanqui-Chacón
Pontificia Universidad Católica del Perú, Peru

ABSTRACT

Food insecurity is a recurrent condition in which members of a household do not have enough food to cover their nutritional needs; this condition contributes to increasing social vulnerability of those affected. In Peru, there are more than 9 million people who suffer this condition, which generates malnutrition and anemia, mostly in children. On the other hand, the waste of food is associated with production the large amounts of greenhouse gas emissions that affect global warming. According to reports in Peru, 20% of what is food produced becomes waste. This scenario in terms of food for Peruvians represents 3 billion calories in wasted food that could feed 2 million people. The Peruvian Food Bank manages food donations, ensuring this food can reach people in need through humanitarian aid entities. This applied research work uses the tools of operations research to determine a solution to the problem of maximizing the combination of food orders to be distributed based on their total nutritional value to the beneficiaries, seeking maximum coverage and minimum logistic costs.

DOI: 10.4018/978-1-7998-5354-1.ch035

INTRODUCTION

Social vulnerability is expressed by the risk of households to suffer a deterioration in the conditions of quality of life, i.e. to fall into a state of poverty that does not allow the individual to cover their basic needs, including housing, education, work and food. In Peru, although there is an increase in the GDP, the percentage of citizens living in extreme poverty reaches 24.4% (INEI, 2017: INEI; National Institute of Statistics and Informatics).

In Peru malnutrition was reduced from 25.4% to 15.2% (PAN, 2012); despite this, child malnutrition in our country continues to be an important reason for death according to UNICEF data, with nearly half a million children under of 5 years, those affected. This is one of the reasons why projects such as food banks seek to recover food that is in the period limit and conditions of consumption do not turn into waste, to benefit less favored people, involving participation and solidarity of NGO's and companies, who participate voluntarily with their donations.

Food banks are non-profit institutions that have the function of acquiring food from different entities or suppliers (national and international), so that they can then be distributed to people to cover their basic nutritional needs of a specific population. Therefore, these institutions not only contribute to the health and welfare of society, but also contribute to preventing the generation of food waste and the preservation of the environment. According to the FAO (Food and Agriculture Organization of the United Nations), around a third of the foods in the whole world are wasted before people consume them and this becomes, therefore, garbage. The contribution of the food bank for this case is that foods that have already reached their life cycle or that are obsolete so that other organizations are redistributed optimally, and solid waste management is improved (FAO, 2013). Food banks seek to promote the social development of vulnerable communities, through the management of donations of goods, under a quality control system; that is, to serve as a link between donors and the vulnerable population that suffers from poverty, hunger and malnutrition, improving nutritional levels and sensitizing the community through volunteering (McCrindle. 2017; Delpish et al., 2018; Gonzales-Feliu et al., 2018).

Another important aspect to consider is the environment, since the production of food affects this with the waste that is generated every day and these foods could be used by food banks. Using these resources in vain would be a very bad decision. The waste will be in the form of solids, liquids, oils and more, which will then have to go through a process of biodegradation. In addition, we must consider the carbon footprint of wasted food that increases the emission of greenhouse gases and the effect it has on water, which we will drink later; as well as nitrogen emissions that directly affect the air we breathe. (Wang et al., 2006).

This work is presented following next order: first, a literature review about main theory frame is presented, after main issues related to Peruvian food bank supply chain is analyzed, an optimization model is proposed, and finally main results are discussed. The results show that the food loads to be sent can be maximized, increasing the coverage to the institutions from the current 24 to 69 at a lower transportation cost.

BACKGROUND

Because of seeking a solution for problems such as malnutrition caused by hunger and social vulnerability (Phil et al., 2017), Food Banks all over the world have occupied a very important place in different societies, since they are responsible for the distribution of donated products to communities that do not have the possibility of acquiring food (FAO, 2012). The following lines show examples of these organizations and their effects in different countries.

In Australia, Foodbank has a presence in every state in the country and is responsible for distributing food to hungry people with the help of approximately 100 employees and more than 3,000 volunteers. They work with the entire Australian food and grocery industry (farmers, wholesalers, manufacturers and retailers, as well as companies that donate as social responsibility). Many Australians (45%) who experience food insecurity have skipped a meal and 28% have spent a whole day without eating (Foodbank Australia, 2017). Australians with food insecurity report more frequently lethargy or fatigue (42%), a decrease in mental health (38%) and a loss of confidence (35%) due to lack of food (Foodbank Australia, 2017). In 2017 alone, Foodbank provided enough food for more than 67 million meals to charities and schools in the country, being the main source of food for them and improving the quality of their lives.

In Brazil, the urban harvest, the name for the food collection process in good condition for consumption and distribution to institutions, is restricted only to the city of São Paulo and the metropolitan region. The synthesis of the 2017 Social Indicators reveals that more than 52 million Brazilians, the equivalent of 25.4% of the population, live on the poverty line, so they benefit from this program. According to the Activity Report presented by BA Brasil, 2017 was the year in which it was possible to collect the largest amount of food, reaching 610,886.12 kg, being able to serve 45 institutions and benefit 20,726 people served, being 69.64% adults, 26.04% Children and teenagers and 4.32% elderly.

Les Restaurants de Coeur, is a French association as other European initiatives (Booth and Whelan, 2014)., whose objectives is to help and provide voluntary assistance to the poor, especially in the food sector. There are currently 1,651 people with housing difficulties, of which 1,628 are in emergency with only 243 beds of emergency accommodation. For this, since its creation in 1990, there are 71,000 volunteers, 102 workshops, 84 local gardens and integration sites open all year. They have managed to distribute 135.8 million meals, of which 87.7 million are donations, bequests and events.

In the United States there is the Feeding America charity, which has offices in all states and feeds more than 46 million people. They not only have pantries, but also dining rooms. This country realized that in the United States 72 billion pounds of safe and edible food are wasted each year and this can help feed the entire country. That's why the Feeding America organization is focused on working with the help of farms, manufacturers and consumer-oriented businesses (Allen, 2015: 2018). For example, there are three innovative solutions to avoid food waste. The first is that trucks pick up unsold Starbucks food every night. The second idea comes from Second Harvest Food Bank of Middle Tennessee, which rescues not standard beans from culture. Finally, Meal Connect, helps to link food banks with restaurants or any place where food is sold, so when food is available, it is collected and sent directly to the food bank. The application of these three ideas has made it possible, during the last year, that 3,300 million pounds of food have been saved (Feeding America, 2018).

MAIN FOCUS OF THE CHAPTER

Theoretical and Methodological Framework

Diet problem is defined by the search for a correct allocation of food by minimizing the cost of the food consumed during the day without neglecting the nutrients that a person should consume (Czyzyk and

Wisniewski, 1996). The problem of diets was proposed by George Stigler in 1945 under the name of "Cost of subsistence" and is to meet the minimum nutritional needs of a person considering raw material cost. This problem was solved by Dantzig (1990) using the simplex method. While Garille and Gass (2001) updated it with nutrition information and food cost data. Joseph Balintfly proposes in 1979 a modification to the problem raised by Stigler and names it the "The cost of a decent subsistence", in this case the problem is defined as the level of the minimum budget to satisfy the nutritional needs of an average person within a certain society considering their food preferences. Bas (2014) introduces a mixed-integer programming model for the dietary problem of glycemic load values of foods into objective function, it is well-known the relation between high glycemic load diets and chronic diseases such as obesity, diabetes mellitus, cardiovascular diseases, and various types of cancer. On the other hand, in a paper presented by Metecan and Egemen (2017) a genetic algorithm was used to simultaneously optimize two goals; Minimize the total cost of the supply chain and the variety of military battalion dishes. van Dooren (2018) presents a work that consolidates the diet problem by consolidating various proposals in the literature and the methods used.

The problem of the diet presented in the context of organizations such as food banks, has important considerations not considered in the original problem, such as the responsibility of food distribution by NGOs that try to reduce beneficiaries' food insecurity. Three goals are proposals for this food models; objectives of equity, effectiveness and efficiency are common in models that consider public services (Savas 1978). However, (Orgut et al., 2016) mention that these objectives may conflict with one another resulting in trade-offs for decision making, furthermore they propose food banks daily performs its activity seeking balance cost, access and quality. Equity implies serving the needs of the customer fairly. The definition of the term "equity" is subjective and can have different implications for different systems (Stone 1997). Savas (1978) defines equity in the public sector broadly as the fairness, impartiality, or equality of service.

Food Insecurity in Peru

According to INEI, chronic malnutrition in children decreased 5.2% in the last 5 years in Peru. It also indicates that the prevalence of chronic malnutrition, according to the WHO (World Health Organization), is higher in the rural area (25.3%) than in the urban area (8.2%). The highest rates were registered in Huancavelica (31.2%), Cajamarca (26.6%), Loreto (23.8%), Pasco (22.8%), Apurímac (20.9%) and Ayacucho (20%). Regarding anemia, in children from 6 to 35 months it was 43.6% in 2017, and in the last 5 years it decreased by 0.9%. In the rural area it was 53.3% and in the urban area it was 40%. The INEI reported that anemia affected more than half of the lowest quintile (55.3%), as well as children whose mothers did not have an education level or only had a primary education. The highest rates are found in Puno (75.9%), Loreto (61.5%) and Ucayali (59.1%). The Peruvian government has proposed reducing anemia from 43.6% to 19% in 2021, the year of the Bicentennial of Independence. The National Plan for the Reduction of Chronic Infantile Anemia and Malnutrition, which has been in force for more than 2 decades and is updated every 4 years, is now available. It is a policy aimed at addressing the problems of nutritional deficiency in the country. Currently, it is planned to cover anemia with new approaches, this means not only implementing micronutrients, but also promoting the consumption of iron-rich foods.

The Law for the Promotion of Healthy Eating for Children and Adolescents (Law No. 30021) is a law based on overweight and obesity that has increased in recent years in these groups. The law can include an improvement in many aspects, such as promoting the consumption of foods that are rich in nutrients and can fight school anemia, as well as having children that grow better because their protein intake is higher. What this law does is protect the most vulnerable groups, for adults, the decision to consume a food is more independent. What is sought is to provide information for these groups to make decisions and anticipate the change of attitude towards a healthy diet to prevent excess weight and thus prevent the onset of diseases such as high blood pressure, diabetes, etc.

Characterization of Lima-Callao Food Bank

On August 8, 2016, Peruvian national law N ° 30498 "Law that promotes the donation of food and facilitates the transport of donations in situations of natural disasters" is published in the official newspaper "El Peruano". The law was an important initiative of the Peruvian State in trying to reduce the amount of food destroyed due to its non-commercialization (Siesquén and Orbegoso, 2015). The objective of the law is not only to increase donations for the most vulnerable population, but also to reduce and subsequently prohibit the destruction of food by the food industry, since it is estimated that 20% of food that are produced are discarded (FAO, 2013) and still 30% of the population suffers from food insecurity (INS, 2013). Likewise, it seeks to improve the quality of life of communities in which the state has little or no presence due to its limited management capacity. For the law to be adequately enforced and the number of people suffering from food insecurity to be reduced, companies will be required to make the donated food fit for human consumption and they will be liable for any damage caused to the person that consumes food in poor condition. If it is proven that due to bad practices the organizations that receive the donated food damaged the food, they will be the legal responsible for the damages caused. In this way, the state ensures that the health of the people who receive the donations is not violated. To promote this measure, the state will deduct up to 10% of the income tax for donated food and will not consider the general sales tax for these items. For this the company must coordinate their donations with charitable institutions and social assistance or beneficiary to certify the amount donated and their condition. The donation will be made to receiving entities that will oversee the distribution in favour of the people in need. The food that is received cannot be marketed for any reason. Currently, in Peru there are initiatives whose main objective is the reduction of food insecurity in the poorest people, among which the most outstanding are the following:

- **National Program of Food Assistance (PRONAA)**: Its purpose is to help raise the food and nutrition level of the population living in extreme poverty through child feeding programs, dining programs, promotion of food security and food assistance to the affected population for a phenomenon or natural damage.
- **Qali Warma**: National School Feeding Program that aims to guarantee food service during every day of the school-year in public schools in vulnerable areas. This service aids with breakfasts and lunches aimed at the school population between 3 and 12 years. (Qali Warma, 2016).
- **Glass of Milk Program**: According to the Ministry of Development and Social Inclusion (MIDIS), it is a program that provides a daily food ration to a beneficiary population living in poverty and extreme poverty. Its main objective is to improve the nutritional level in these sectors, taking care of children, pregnant and breastfeeding mothers, the elderly and people affected by the illness TBC. Although this is a national program, each municipality is responsible for this initiative in their localities.

The Food Bank of Peru (BAP) is a non-profit organization whose purpose is to reduce the food insecurity of the people in need by donating food. This entity receives food from its main donors such as supermarkets, food production companies, food business and logistics operators. Subsequently, these foods are distributed in the shortest time possible to community support centres belonging to their network for the distribution of food to the vulnerable population. This work is remarkable because in Peru there are more than 1 million people living in extreme poverty and do not have resources to feed themselves (INEI, 2017), in addition to 9 million people who suffer from food insecurity, which, it generates diseases such as anemia (INS, 2013). This organization considers of vital importance the reduction of hunger because this problem is linked to undernourishment, intellectual development, fewer opportunities and therefore, poverty, which generates a difficult cycle to break when faced with these realities.

BAP was founded in Peru in 2014, at the initiative of professionals and entrepreneurs in the food sector interested in an organization like this operating in the country. The food bank has built a strong network of contacts with donors and charities in these years of operation, however there are still many entities that need donations and for limitations in its logistics, the bank cannot supply them. Also, this organization is part of the Global Food Banking Network, so it is essential that it meets the quality standards that this organization demands of its members, for instance guarantee that the food donated will be distributed among the people who need it the most, ensuring the safety of food. The BAP distributes different products of first necessity that are apt for the consumption or human use. Table 1 will show the products received by this institution from the beginning of its operations. The diversity of the products will depend on the entities that make voluntary contributions to this organization

Table 1. Products distribute by BAP

	Product Category	**Product**
1	Meats and Derivatives	Meat of chicken, beef, pork, eggs, fish, etc.
2	Beverages	Mineral water, soft drinks, malt drinks, etc.
3	Cereals and Derivatives	Bulk wheat, cookies, pastry dough, brownies, etc.
4	Milk and derivatives	Milk, yogurt
5	Groceries	Oil, sugar, rice, condiments, mayonnaise, noodles, flour, spices etc.
6	Food supplements	Similac, PVO, Ensure, etc.
7	Fruits	Mango, tangerine, yacon, blueberries, grapes, apples, etc.
8	Vegetables	Lettuce, tomatoes, beets, etc.
9	Hygiene and Personal Use	Shampoo, soaps, detergents, etc.

This institution has suppliers of manufacturing items, distributors and logistics companies that favor the viability of their projects. Table 2 shows the main companies that support the BAP as well as the description of their collaboration and the products they donate.

There are two types of donations, which follow two different flows; The first flow represents a cross-docking model – Type 1 (Figure 1) and in the second group the model is presented in which donations are received directly to the warehouse and an allocation of the received products is made (Figure 2).

Type 1 process in details consist in:

Table 2. Donating companies with support BAP activities

	Donating Companies	Type of Assistance Provided
1	Supermercados Peruanos	Fruits, vegetables, groceries, cereals
2	Plaza Vea	Fruits, vegetables, groceries, cereals
3	Backus	Beverages
4	Vivanda	Fruits, vegetables, groceries, cereals
5	P&G	Hygiene items and personal use
6	Agrícola Norsur	Meats and derivatives
7	Ransa	Logistical support (buses, trucks)

Figure 1. BAP cross docking process: Type 1

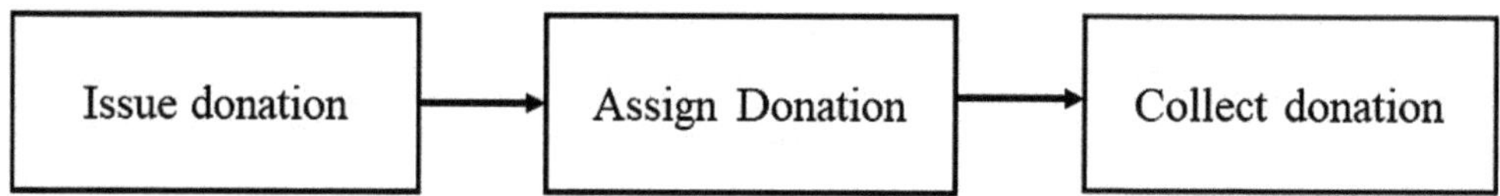

- Issue donation: The company communicates with the food bank and informs that in its stores there are products that can be donated to charities.
- Assign Donation: This allocation depends on the route established for each charity according to its distance to the donors' warehouses. In this process the bank communicates with these centres to inform them that there are products in certain stores and that they can be picked up at a certain time, in addition, informs of the capacity of the trucks for their pick-up.
- Collect donation: The beneficiaries, together with a voluntary representative of the food bank, receive the donation and verify that it is in good condition and suitable for human consumption. Subsequently, the beneficiary collects the products and returns to the point of departure.

Figure 2. BAP storage process: Type 2

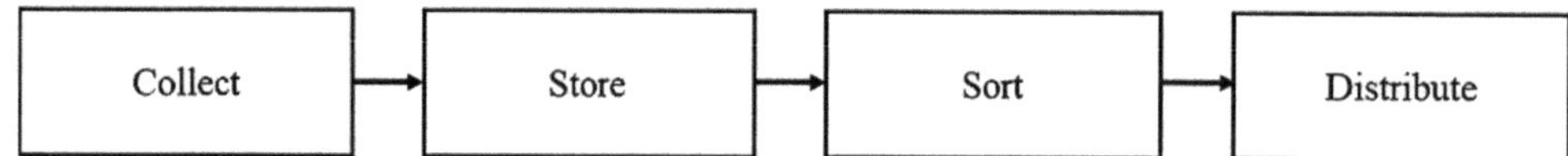

Type 2 process in details consist in:

- Collect: This is the process in which all products donated by industrial companies are collected. In general, donations are transported by a logistics operator that provides the service at zero cost.
- Store: In this process we proceed to assign a space to donations in your warehouse waiting for their classification.

- Sort: The donated products are analysed and assigned to the favoured beneficiaries according to their needs of use. Currently the company does not have a prioritization process in this operation, in such a way that the donations are distributed according to the intuition of the manager and the logistics capacity of the charities.
- Distribute: In this process, transport management is carried out from the bank's warehouse to the beneficiaries' warehouse. This process can be carried out through the mobility of the beneficiary organizations or by logistics operators at zero cost.

The following Tables specify the activities of the BAP that they carry out to manage the donations to the beneficiary centres.

Table 3. BAP cross docking activities in detail

	Process	Responsable	Activities
1	BAP receives a request to collect donations	Customer service	The donor company communicates with the BAP by mail or phone call consulting if there is a charitable institution that can collect food for that day.
2	Donor sends information on quantity, format, weight and time window to BAP	Customer service	This information is communicated without any established format. According to these data, the necessary transports will be required. Inventory levels are reviewed.
3	BAP reviews list of sponsor carriers	Transport	The BAP analyzes the list of institutions that can provide the transport service and that meet the quality standards required by the products (eg, control of the cold chain).
4	BAP confirms pick-up between transporters and donors.	Customer service	Through continuous communications between donors and transporters, time windows are established for the collection of donations according to the capacities of the vehicles.
5	Donations are received in BAP warehouse	Warehouse	The transport company delivers the donations to the warehouse and delivers quality certification of the food provided by the donors.
6	BAP Volunteer validates inventory entry	Warehouse	The certifications and the discharge are validated by voluntary personnel to ensure the condition of the food upon entering the BAP.
7	Monitoring inventory levels to assemble donation packages	Warehouse	Depending on the type of donations received, the donation packages are assembled according to the maximum date of consumption.

Table 4. BAP storage activities in detail

	Process	Responsable	Activities
1	BAP receives request for donations	Customer service	The donor company communicates with BAP by mail or phone call informing the amount of food that is available for delivery.
2	The pick-up route is identified and assigned to the beneficiary	Customer service	Through a routing scheme, the route that each beneficiary institution must follow to collect the maximum amount of food is determined.
3	Beneficiary goes to the donor's headquarters	Transport	This transport is carried out by a unit belonging to the beneficiary institution.
4	Volunteer BAP validates donations to the beneficiary	Warehouse	Through a validation format, the amount and status of donated food is certified.
5	Beneficiary goes to his warehouse with the certified donation	Transport	The route should not be extended for a long time due to the transportation of perishable food.

The process, as well as for cross docking and storage, begins in the same way, when a donor contacts the BAP and specifies the quantity of products that will be provided to them so that they can contact the beneficiaries and ensure the transportation service. From this moment both processes differ. Cross docking has the particularity that the beneficiary, to have the possibility of belonging to this system, must have its own transport to collect the donations. Once the beneficiary has been defined, a route already established by the BAP is assigned to them to have a route in which they can collect donations from different stores in the same route.

To validate the information provided by the donor and to comply with the quality requirements, the BAP assigns a volunteer to meet the beneficiary from the beginning of the route until the end of the route. Once the route is done and the donated products have been collected, the beneficiary proceeds to retire to their facilities. In this model it is complicated to establish food allocation criteria since it depends on the availability of the beneficiary's mobility and the donor's precision in describing their products. Donations that go through a storage process require more precise information management because an adequate space must be designated in the BAP temporary warehouse according to specifications such as type of product, quantity, weight and time-window or life time of the BAP. Likewise, the BAP must take charge of transporting the products to their warehouses and therefore must manage with various logistics operators so that they can perform this service at zero cost. In the BAP's warehouse, they can establish a food allocation criterion since the resources they have, are known exactly. Currently BAP serves 24 beneficiaries' institution.

Logistics Decisions and Optimization Problem

In this sense, a food bank model optimization is proposed seeking allocation of food in an equitable and effective way (Sengul et al., 2013; Martins et al., 2016, Delpish et al., 2018; Reihaneh and Ghoniem, 2018). The authors defined that they will achieve equity by reducing the absolute deviation between the proportion of food sent to an institution and their relative needs. Likewise, efficiency will be achieved by maximizing the amount of food distributed. It is important to emphasize that the costs will not be analysed because transportation costs between warehouses would favour easily accessible institutions and priority would not be given to the most distant and most needy charities. The objective function (1) minimizes the total of undistributed food, that is, the surplus. The restriction (2) ensures that the proportion of food distributed in each institution j does not vary by more than the limit K with their food needs. Restriction (3) ensures that the amount of food available is equal to the amount distributed along with the surplus. The restriction (4) represents the capacity of each institution to receive donations and the restriction (5) is the condition of non-negativity.

To maximize the amount distributed in the network, following a prioritization and respecting the limitations of the system, the following optimization model was designed by linear programming.

The objective function is available:

$$Max \sum_{i=1}^{n} \sum_{j=1}^{m} X_{ij} * P_i \tag{1}$$

Subject to the following restrictions:

$$\sum_{i=1}^{n} X_{ij} * NC_{ik} + \sum_{h=1}^{s} W_{hj} * NB_{ik} \leq M_{jk} \, \forall j \in Institutions, k \in Nutrients \tag{2}$$

$$\sum_{i=1}^{n} X_{ij} * NC_{ik} + \sum_{h=1}^{s} W_{hj} * NB_{ik} \geq m_{jk} \, \forall j \in Institutions, k \in Nutrients \tag{3}$$

$$\sum_{i=1}^{n} \sum_{j=1}^{m} X_{ij} \leq A_{i} \forall i \in Food \tag{4}$$

$$\sum_{h=1}^{s} W_{hj} \geq a_{j} \forall j \in Institutions \tag{5}$$

$$\sum_{i=1}^{n} X_{i} + \sum_{h=1}^{s} W_{hj} \leq C_{j} \forall j \in Institutions \tag{6}$$

$$X_{ij} \geq 0 \forall i \in Food, j \in Institutions \tag{7}$$

$$W_{hj} \geq 0 \forall h \in Drinks, j \in Institutions \tag{8}$$

The objective function is shown in equation (1) and represents that the total amount distributed is maximized respecting the given prioritization. The constraints (2) and (3) indicate the limits within which the amount of nutrients distributed to each institution must be found. Constraint (4) limits the total amount of food that can be distributed from donations for each type of food. The constraint (5) indicates the minimum amount of water that must be transported to the institutions. The constraint (6) represents the maximum amount that can be transported to each institution due to the capacity of the vehicles. The constraints (7) and (8) show the range of existence of the variables X and W, respectively.

This linear programming model was translated into the AMPL language and was run in the full student version using version 12.6.3.0 of the CPLEX solver. It ran on a core i5 laptop with 8 GB of RAM. Next, the model is shown in the interface within the AMPL IDE optimizer software.

```
maximize Coverage:
        sum{i in Food, j in Institution} QFood[i,j]*Priority[i];
subject to CotaMax {j in Institution,k in Nutrients}:
        sum{i in Food} QFood[i,j]*CompositionF[i,k] +
sum{h in Drinks} QDrinks[h,j]*CompositionD[h,k]
<= MaxNutrients[j,k];
subject to CotaMin {j in Institution,k in Nutrients}:
```

```
        sum{i in Food} QFood[i,j]*CompositionF[i,k] +
sum{h in Drinks} QDrinks[h,j]*CompositionD[h,k]
>= MinNutrients[j,k];
subject to Availability {i in Food}:
        sum{j in Institution} QFood[i,j] <= FoodAvailable[i];
subject to DistDrink {j in Institution}:
        sum{h in Drinks} QDrinks[h,j] >= DrinkReq [j];
subject to Reception {j in Institution}:
        sum{i in Food} QFood[i,j] +
sum{h in Drinks} QDrinks[h,j] <= Capacity[j];
```

After executing the linear programming model, it was possible to distribute each food and drink following optimizations criteria's previously defined. The following table shows how much was distributed for each type of food and drink:

Table 5. Results after executing linear programming model

Kind	Quantity
Food 1	1,084
Food 2	1,071
Food 3	1,364
Food 4	833
Food 5	731
Food 6	1,151
Food 7	800
Food 8	1,387
Food 9	773
Food 10	855
Drink 1	12,198
Drink 2	14,345
Drink 3	13,846

It should be noted that these results respected the limits of nutrition limits per institution and operational in terms of transport capacity.

RESULTS DISCUSSION AND PRACTICAL IMPLICATIONS

After executing the linear programming model, it was possible to distribute each food and drink appropriately to 69 institutions, that is mean 45 institutions more. Beneficiaries' institutions receive all kinds of food from different donors' institutions, but there is no control or efficient distribution of food. In addition, it should be considered that beneficiaries do not work in the same conditions, since they serve different types of people and some institutions serve more people than others.

Other issues to be resolve, at present, is the donations are assigned to beneficiaries associations without any type of allocation criteria and there is no prioritization among the institutions that are part of the network. Then, according to the topic described above, it is proposed to model the greatest amount of food that is given to an institution with a high priority index. This will allow the Food Bank of Peru to meet its objective of reducing food insecurity under the criteria of equity, efficiency and effectiveness.

FUTURE RESEARCH DIRECTIONS

In the case of Peru, we must consider the percentage of citizens who consider themselves in poverty, which is 21.7% of the population, which means that all people survive with less than 338 soles per month, a figure that responds to basic needs, but not to food. (INEI, 2017). In addition, it should be noted that in 2017 poverty increased to 44% of the population in rural areas (INEI, 2017) and it must be considered that these data will never be accurate due to the centralization of the country and other factors.

On the contrary, the GDP would continue to grow although slowing down. For the year 2017, a growth of 2.5% is verified. This indicator contradicts the levels of poverty in the country and is also a research opportunity, as well as the factors that can be added to the model in this document to obtain a more precise result when it comes to prioritizing areas and quantities to deliver donations, that will be reflected in a more efficient supply chain and more distributed aid throughout the country.

CONCLUSION

The proposal integrates the development of different aspects, including the issue of nutrition, which is affected in the most vulnerable population of society, which is part of the main objective of the work. We identified different organized entities that integrate the constant feeding service within the social support provided to 24 direct beneficiaries, who belong to the population of Lima in a situation of malnutrition. Each organization that benefits will receive a specific amount of a specific food and water, according to the number of children and the necessary nutrients.

Through linear programming, we can take advantage of the data obtained by the zones, as well as the statistical studies, to maximize the aid in a more efficient way to people who are in situations of poverty. It must be borne in mind that in order to have an adequate distribution it is not only necessary to have an accurate planning, or with the food to distribute, but also an infrastructure that allows such distribution. Without distribution warehouses, enough and adequate means of transport, and without adequate communication channels, optimal distribution of food is also not possible.

It should also be considered that if what is desired is to combat malnutrition in the country, the problem does not end when all areas of Peru have the capacity to provide caloric protein needs to their population, either because they are self-sufficient or because They have received from other places, but it is also necessary that these foods are distributed properly among the population and that there is a control of the effects produced in the improvement of the nutritional problem until the complete elimination of child malnutrition in Peru.

ACKNOWLEDGMENT

We would like to thank Dr. Jorge Vargas-Florez for their assistance in the creation of this chapter.

REFERENCES

Allen, J. (2015). *Food Banks Embrace the Power of Logistics Drawn from E-Commerce*. Retrieved from https://nonprofitquarterly.org/2015/12/04/food-banks-embrace-the-power-of-logistics-drawn-from-e-commerce/

Allen, J. (2018). *Food Bank of Delaware to Offer Warehouse and Logistics Training This Fall*. Retrieved from https://www.fbd.org/food-bank-of-delaware-to-offer-warehouse-and-logistics-training-this-fall/

Banco de Alimentos Brasil. (2018). *Key figures*. Retrieved from https://www.bancodealimentos.org.br/o-que-fazemos/

Banco de Alimentos del Peru. (2018). *Key figures*. Retrieved from http://bancodealimentosperu.org/

Bas, E. (2014). A robust optimization approach to diet problem with overall glycemic load as objective function. *Applied Mathematical Modelling, 38*(1), 4926–4940. doi:10.1016/j.apm.2014.03.049

Booth, S., & Whelan, J. (2014). Hungry for change: The food banking industry in Australia. *British Food Journal, 116*(9), 1392–1404. doi:10.1108/BFJ-01-2014-0037

Czyzyk, J., & Wisniewski, T. (1996). *The Diet Problem: a Www-based Interactive Case Study in Linear Programming*. Retrieve from http://ftp.mcs.anl.gov/pub/tech_reports/reports/P602.pdf

Dantzig, G. B. (1990, July - August). The Practice of Mathematical Programming. *Interfaces, 20*(4), 43–47. doi:10.1287/inte.20.4.43

Delpish, R., Jiang, S., Davis, L., & Odubela, K. (2019). A Visual Analytics Approach to Combat Confirmation Bias for a Local Food Bank. In R. Boring (Ed.), *Advances in Human Error, Reliability, Resilience, and Performance. AHFE 2018. Advances in Intelligent Systems and Computing* (Vol. 778). Cham: Springer. doi:10.1007/978-3-319-94391-6_2

FAO. (2012). *Mesa Redonda sobre políticas: protección social en favor de la seguridad alimentaria y la nutrición 2012*. Retrieve from http://www.fao.org/docrep/meeting/026/me589S.pdf

FAO. (2013). *Food wastage footprint: Impacts on natural resources*. Advanced online publication http://www.fao.org/docrep/018/i3347e/i3347e.pdf

Feeding America. (2018). *Fighting Food Waste With Food Rescue*. Retrieved from http://www.feedingamerica.org/our-work/our-approach/reduce-food-waste.html

Foodbank. (2018). *Data base*. Retrieved from https://www.foodbank.org.au/

Garille, S. G., & Gass, S. I. (2001). *Stigler's Diet Problem*. Revisited. *Operations Research, 49*(1), 1–13. doi:10.1287/opre.49.1.1.11187

Gonzalez-Feliu, J., Osorio-Ramirez, C., Palacios-Arguello, L., & Talamantes, C. A. (2018). Local production-based dietary supplement distribution in emerging countries: Bienestarina Distribution in Colombia. In Establishing Food Security and Alternatives to International Trade in Emerging Economies (pp. 297-315). IGI Global. doi:10.4018/978-1-5225-2733-6.ch014

INEI. (2017). *Evolución de la Pobreza Monetaria 2007-2016*. Retrieve from https://www.inei.gob.pe/media/cifras_de_pobreza/pobreza2016.pdf

INS. (2013). *Estado nutricional en el Perú por etapas de vida; 2012-2013*. Retrieve from https://web.ins.gob.pe/sites/default/files/Archivos/cenan/van/vigilacia_poblacion/VIN_ENAHO_etapas_de_vida_2012-2013.pdf

Les Restaurants de Coeur. (2018). *Key figures*. Retrieved from https://www.restosducoeur.org/chiffres-cles/

Martins, C. L., Melo, I. M. T., & Pato, I. M. V. (2016). *Redesigning a food bank supply chain network, Part I: Background and mathematical formulation*. Retrieved from https://pdfs.semanticscholar.org/c9cc/702e43a87213a11c6fd94e6a1311d64293c4.pdf

McCrindle. (2017). *Foodbank hunger report 2017*. Retrieved from https://www.foodbank.org.au/wp-content/uploads/2017/10/Foodbank-Hunger-Report-2017.pdf

Metecan, C., & Egemen, B. C. (2017). A Novel Approach for Stigler'S Diet Problem in Genetic Algorithm. *Proceedings of the 9th International Conference on Information Management and Engineering*.

Orgut, I. S., Brock, L. G., III, Davis, L. B., Ivy, J. S., Jiang, S., Morgan, S. D., . . . Middleton, E. (2016). Achieving Equity, Effectiveness, and Efficiency in Food Bank Operations: Strategies for Feeding America with Implications for Global Hunger Relief. In Advances in Managing Humanitarian Operations in International Series in Operations Research & Management Science (vol. 235, pp. 229-256). Springer International Publishing Switzerland.

Orgut, I. S., Ivy, J., Uzsoy, R., & Wilson, J. R. (2016). Modeling for the equitable and effective distribution of donated food under capacity constraints. *IIE Transactions*, *48*(3), 252–266. doi:10.1080/0740817X.2015.1063792

Phil, A., Fangzhou, L., Augis, F., Patama, M., & Mouhdi, O. (2017). *The food wastage phenomena: An overview of the current situation in three countries: France, Finland and Taiwan*. Retrieved from http://www.helsinki.fi/henvi/teaching/Reports_15/03_Food_wastage.pdf

Qali Warma. (2016). *Evaluación Anual del Plan Operativo Institucional 2016*. Retrieve from http://www.qw.gob.pe/wp-content/uploads/2017/03/Evaluacion-Anual-POI-2016.pdf

Reihaneh, M., & Ghoniem, A. (2018). *A multi-start optimization-based heuristic for a food bank distribution problem*. Retrieved from https://www-scopus com.ezproxybib.pucp.edu.pe/record/display.uri?eid=2-s2.085018280373&origin=resultslist&sort=plf-f&src=s&st1

Relatório de Atividades. (2017). *Key figures*. Retrieved from http://www.bancodealmentos.org.br/relatorios/relatorio-a4ebook2017-0523.pdf

Savas, E. S. (1978). On equity in providing public services. *Management Science*, *24*(8), 800–808. doi:10.1287/mnsc.24.8.800

Siesquén, D., & Orbegoso, M. (2015). *Proyecto de inversión para la creación de un banco de alimentos en la ciudad de Chiclayo*. Tesis para optar el título de Licenciado en Administración de Empresas. Chiclayo: Universidad Católica Santo Toribio de Mogrovejo, Escuela de Administración de Empresas. Retrieved from http://tesis.usat.edu.pe/bitstream/usat/889/1/TL_SiesquenBallenaDiana_OrbegosoZelvaggioMaria.pdf

Stone, D. A. (1997). *Policy paradox: the art of political decision making*. New York: WW Norton.

van Dooren, C. (2018). A Review of the Use of Linear Programming to Optimize Diets, *Nutritiously*, Economically and Environmentally. *Frontiers in Nutrition.*, *5*(48), 1–15. PMID:29977894

KEY TERMS AND DEFINITIONS

Food Insecurity: Refers to the lack of access to sufficient good, healthy and culturally appropriate food. Food safety is when a person is able to obtain a sufficient amount of healthy food daily. People who do not consume enough food every day suffer from food insecurity.

GDP: Gross domestic product. It is the monetary value of all finished goods and services produced in a country, which is generally measured every year.

Malnutrition: This term addresses three major groups of conditions: malnutrition, which includes weight loss (low weight for height), stunting (low height for age) and low weight (low weight for age); Malnutrition related to micronutrients, which includes deficiencies of micronutrients (lack of important vitamins and minerals) or excess of micronutrients; and overweight, obesity and non-communicable diseases related to diet (such as heart disease, stroke, diabetes and some types of cancer).

Poverty: Occurs when people cannot meet the basic physical and mental needs of a decent life, due to lack of resources (such as food).

Reverse Logistics: Means, for all operations, reuse, or products and materials.

Social Group: Any group of human beings who are, have been recently or anticipate being in some kind of interrelation or having certain things in common.

Utility: In the context of this document, it is worthwhile for some purposes, the goods provided by a certain process.

This research was previously published in the Handbook of Research on Urban and Humanitarian Logistics edited by Jesus Gonzalez-Feliu, Mario Chong, Jorge Vargas Florez, and Julio Padilla Solis; pages 201-215, copyright year 2019 by Information Science Reference (an imprint of IGI Global).

Chapter 36
Economic and Environmental Costs of Meat Waste in the US

Nicholas Hardersen
University of Oklahoma, USA

Jadwiga R. Ziolkowska
University of Oklahoma, USA

ABSTRACT

Food waste is a major issue around the globe impacting food security, resource use, economic operations, and the environment. Meat waste, constituting approximately half of total annual meat production in the United States, is particularly relevant to address due to significant resource inputs used in livestock breeding and the meat production process. In this chapter, the authors monetize annual costs of natural resources including water, land, and energy, as well as emissions of methane and nitrous oxide embedded in wasted meat in the United States. Results indicate the total annual cost of $32-32.5 billion. The outcomes substantiate the need to reduce current levels of wasted meat in order to minimize economic, social, and environmental impacts on natural resources and make food and meat production more sustainable.

INTRODUCTION

One-quarter to one-half of total agricultural production is wasted at different points along the global food supply chain each year, amounting to approximately 1.3 billion tons (Gustavsson et al., 2011; Kummu et al., 2012; Lipinski et al., 2013; Lundqvist et al., 2008). Regardless of the varying estimates in the literature, the amount of wasted food is substantial and directly translates into quantities of natural resources used for food production that are also wasted when food is discarded. The food waste problem and its impacts are discussed below followed by a closer exploration of animal husbandry and meat waste.

DOI: 10.4018/978-1-7998-5354-1.ch036

Food Waste Problem and Impacts on Natural Resources

Global food surplus, and particularly the surplus in high-income developed countries, has increased dramatically in the last few decades and is a root cause of food waste (Papargyropoulou et al., 2014). Agronomists recommend a food supply of 130 percent (2600 kcal/capita/day) to protect against unexpected environmental disasters as a result of resource overuse that may cause famine (Papargyropoulou et al., 2014). High-income developed countries regularly produce on average at least 1000 kcal/capita/day above the recommended food supply (1500 kcal/capita/day extra in the US), which could feed nearly 700 million people with an adequate vegetarian diet (Smil, 2004).

Both developed and developing countries generate large quantities of food waste, though they differ substantially in terms of where it occurs in the supply chain. Poor infrastructure for post-harvest storage, handling and distribution are the primary reasons why food is wasted in developing countries. On the contrary, in developed countries, while significant amounts of food are lost early in the supply chain due to out-grading from superficial appearance standards or unfavorable market conditions, negligent consumer behavior is responsible for the largest share of waste (Figure 1). According to Gustavsson et al. (2011), consumers in developed countries waste approximately 95-115 kg/capita/year, whereas consumers in developing countries waste only 6-11 kg/capita/year.

Figure 1. Food lost or wasted by region and stage in value chain, 2009 (percent of kcal lost and wasted)
Source: Lipinski et al. (2013) based on FAO (2011)

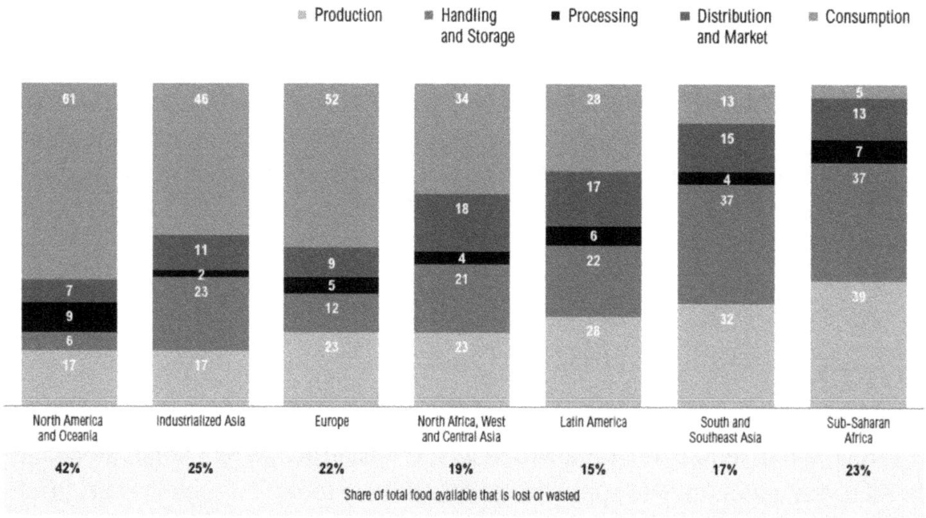

In the United States (US), since 1974 waste has increased by 50 percent along the food supply chain and amounted to losses of 1400 kcal/capita/day, or 150 trillion kcal/year in 2009 (Hall et al., 2009). In 2012, the US produced 518 billion pounds (or 235 billion kg) of food, of which 45 percent was lost or wasted (Toth & Dou, 2016). Consumers were responsible for 47 percent (i.e., 110 billion pounds) of wasted food, while retail was responsible for 19 percent (i.e., 45 billion pounds) (Toth & Dou, 2016). The total economic value of food waste at the retail and consumer level in the United States is worth a staggering $165.6 billion, or $390/capita/year (Buzby & Hyman, 2012). Over half of the total consumer generated economic losses ($197/capita/year) was from meat waste. Wasting meat and meat products can have the most serious environmental impacts out of all food categories due to the resource-intensive nature of animal husbandry, which is the focus of this chapter and is discussed in the following sections.

Another major problem related to food waste regards the numerous implications for resource loss and environmental degradation. Food production covers 38 percent of global ice-free land area, of which 12 percent (1.53 billion ha) is devoted to crops and 26 percent (3.38 billion ha) is devoted to pastures (Foley et al., 2011). The total land area used to grow food that is eventually wasted equals 1.4 billion ha, or 30 percent of the global agricultural land (FAO, 2013). Toth and Dou (2016) estimated that 65 million acres of US cropland is embedded in food waste, while 40 million of these acres are used to grow crops for animal feed.

Other environmental impacts related to food waste regard application of artificial fertilizers, which can be beneficial for increasing crop yields initially, but over time its excessive use contributes to soil, water and air pollution (Sage, 2012). Uptake rates of fertilizers by plants are inefficient at approximately 40-50 percent, meaning that at least half of applied fertilizers are dispersed into the environment (Sage, 2012). Moreover, chemical runoff from fertilizers contributes to freshwater pollution in aquifers and surface bodies and is also the major cause of hypoxic zones found on coastlines around the world, and in the Gulf of Mexico in the US (Diaz & Rosenberg, 2008). Fertilizer use is also the major cause of nitrous oxide (N_2O) emissions, a greenhouse gas (GHG) 256 times more potent than carbon dioxide (CO_2). The US agriculture emits 318.4 million metric tons of N_2O each year from soil management (EPA, 2016). Considering that 45 percent of food in the US is wasted, 143.28 million metric tons of N_2O emissions result from waste each year (Toth & Dou, 2016).

In addition, one quarter of freshwater usage globally and in the US is embedded in food waste (Hall et al., 2009; Kummu et al., 2012; Toth & Dou, 2016). According to Toth & Dou (2016), 18 trillion gallons (or 68 trillion litres) of irrigation water in the US was used to grow wasted food in 2012, mostly in central and western regions where aquifers and surface water bodies are already used at unsustainable rates.

Moreover, greenhouse gas emissions occur at every stage of the food supply chain, from farm to fork and at disposal. Global annual emissions from food waste equal 3.3 Gt of CO_2 emission equivalent (FAO, 2013). One mitigation option to significantly decrease food waste emissions is to eliminate the practice of landfilling organic waste. Currently, 97 percent of food waste in the US is sent to landfill where it decomposes in anaerobic conditions to emit methane, a greenhouse gas 21-25 times more powerful than carbon dioxide (Papargryopoulou et al., 2014).

There is a range of other environmental impacts that food waste can cause indirectly as a result of agricultural production methods. Biodiversity and ecosystem services are two of the most important measures of ecological health that are negatively affected by industrialized agriculture. These impacts are occurring mainly from excessive chemical fertilizer and pesticide inputs that cause pollution, land-use change, habitat loss, large-scale monocultures, overexploitation, and generate invasive species (Steinfeld et al., 2006). Issues related to ecosystem functioning may potentially have serious implications in the future that could impact societies over extended spatio-temporal scales.

Monetizing ecological health however is difficult (Ziolkowska, 2017). Integrating its true costs into economic valuations needs to be prioritized in order to achieve long-term sustainability. Substantial reduction of food waste could theoretically minimize pressures exerted on biodiversity and ecosystem services. While recognizing the difficulty of quantifying economic and environmental impacts of food waste, following a study by Ziolkowska (2017), this research aims at monetizing food waste and resource losses related to animal and meat production in the US.

Impacts of Animal Husbandry and Meat Waste

By 2050, the world population is expected to reach 9 billion people, which will result in a 70-100 percent increase in food demand (Godfray et al., 2010). Global Gross Domestic Product (GDP) per capita is also expected to increase steadily at 2 percent/annum (Kearney, 2010). Rising incomes have been correlated with increasing meat consumption and decreasing consumption of staple crops at the same time (Bouwman et al., 2013; Kearney, 2010; McMichael et al., 2007; Steinfeld et al., 2006). China is a prime example of this transformation. Between 1963 and 2003 the GDP/capita increased from $74.3 to $1,288.6, while meat consumption increased by 349 percent in the same time frame (Kearney, 2010; World Bank, 2017). The average global increase in meat consumption during this time period has been much less drastic at 63 percent (Kearney, 2010), however, meat production is projected to more than double from 229 million tons in 1999/2001 to 465 million tons in 2050 (Steinfeld et al., 2006). The rapidly growing demand for meat will be met almost entirely through industrial livestock production systems, including concentrated animal feed operations (CAFOs), intensification of existing grazing systems, and spatial expansion of managed grazing systems largely in tropical forests (McAlpine et al., 2009; Naylor et al., 2005). Considering that one-third of global crop production is already fed to livestock, it should be expected that this pattern may intensify substantially in the future. Consequently, insuring food security for 9 billion people might prove to be very challenging due to limited resource availability.

Raising livestock for human consumption is a very resource-intensive process. This is true for both industrial and pasture systems, though pasture systems generally pose lower environmental impacts as they do not rely on growing crops for feed. Livestock production has been described as the "single largest anthropogenic user of land" and it occupies 3.73 billion hectares, or around 75 percent of global agricultural land (Steinfeld et al., 2006, p. xxi). Water requirements for livestock vary considerably among animals, though each animal has extremely high consumptive water use. In comparison to the water requirements for production of 1 kg of wheat (500-4 000 liters), producing 1 kg meat requires 5000-20000 liters (Lundqvist et al., 2008). Most of the water requirements to produce meat stem from the feed conversion efficiency of an animal, feed composition and origin of the feed (Mekonnen & Hoekstra, 2010). Around 18 percent of anthropogenic GHG emissions are attributable to livestock, of which most are methane and nitrous oxide emissions (McAlpine et al., 2009). Livestock contributes significantly to acidification and eutrophication of ecosystems from manure and soil management (Figure 2). They can also degrade soil through compaction and from overgrazing which eventually causes erosion. Producing meat is inherently inefficient due to poor feed conversion efficiencies, particularly in ruminants (Pimentel & Pimentel, 2008). Poor feed conversion efficiency means that more crops must be grown to produce the desired amount of protein, which translates to higher inputs of water, energy, and land. Beef is the most inefficient and resource-intensive animal to raise among all livestock categories and contributes the most to GHG emissions (de Vries & de Boer, 2010). According to Smil (2002), 89-97 percent of the gross energy content and 80-96 percent of total protein content in feed crops are not converted to edible protein and fat. Moreover, there is enough energy content in the 700 million tons of cereal and legumes fed to livestock each year to feed more than three billion people on a diet of corn, barley, sorghum and soy (de Vries & de Boer, 2010).

Also, the resource intensity and environmentally damaging aspects of livestock production raise important ethical questions about livestock breeding, meat consumption, living conditions and animal treatment. Questions are being raised about the legitimacy of animal production in the face of one billion people lacking food security as of today, while this number is anticipated to increase drastically by

Figure 2. Percentage of the overall national environmental burdens exerted by the individual animal categories
Source: Eshel et al. (2014)
Legend: Nr – reactive nitrogen fertilizer

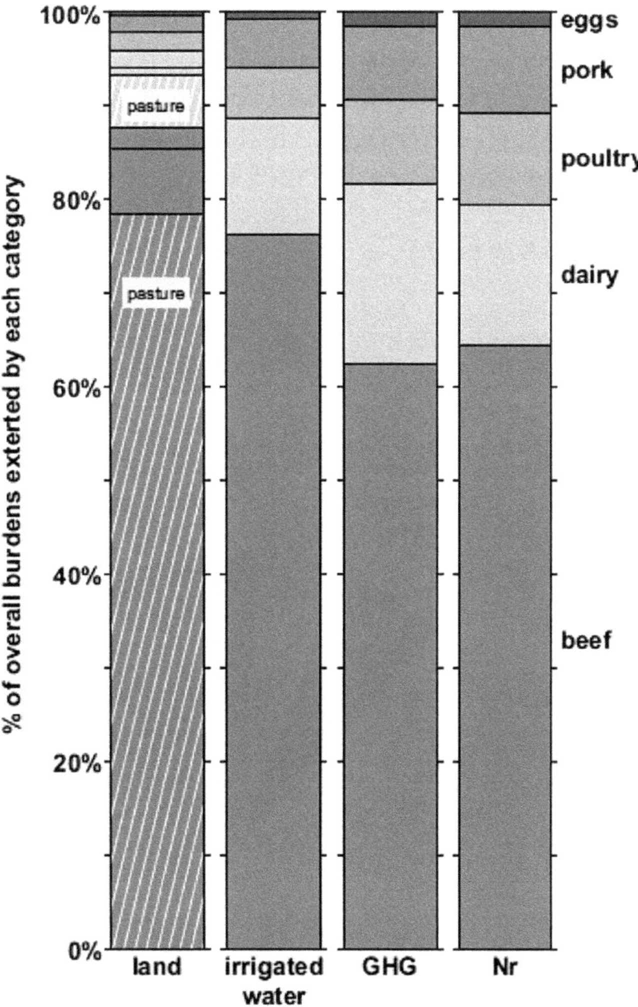

2050 due to increasing population (Pimentel & Pimentel, 2008; Smil, 2002). An additional 2.5 billion hectares would be required if the entire world population consumed 80 kg of meat/capita/year, which is the average intake of meat in a Western diet (Naylor et al., 2005). Although this scenario is unlikely to happen, a significant increase in meat consumption is expected (Keyzer et al., 2005), which will put substantially more pressure on resources and the environment.

A consequent question refers to ethical and moral aspects of wasting meat. According to Lipinski et al. (2013), of the 1.3 billion tons or 1.5 quadrillion kcal of food wasted each year, meat waste comprises 4% of total weight and 7% of total calories wasted. This means that 52 million tons or 105 trillion kcal of meat are wasted each year, which is equivalent to 16.8 percent of the total livestock production of 308.5 million tons in 2013 (FAO, 2014). Further, this equals 19 percent of total kcal available from meat (Lipinski et al., 2013). Although the proportion of meat waste is small compared to other food categories, meat requires significantly more resources to produce and causes significantly more environmental impacts than typical grains, fruit or vegetable crops (Pimentel & Pimentel, 2008). In developing countries meat is often lost or wasted in agricultural production due to high animal mortality rates from diseases and also due to poor infrastructure and distribution networks that fail to keep meat from spoiling (Gustavsson et al., 2011). In developed countries, consumption and retail stages of the food supply chain comprise approximately 50 percent of the total meat waste (Gustavsson et al., 2011). In the US, meat waste makes up 17.7 percent of the total food waste stream (Toth & Dou, 2016). As a percentage of total meat production, 41.5 billion pounds out of 83 billion pounds, i.e., 49.8 percent, were wasted in 2012 (Toth & Dou, 2016). In monetary values, in 2008, food loss of meat, poultry, and fish combined amounted to $66 231 million (41% of the total value of food loss in that year), while dairy product waste contributed by the additional 14% (Figure 3).

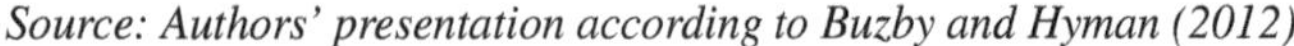

Figure 3. Different food groups' contribution to the total value of food loss ($165,579 million) in US in 2008
Source: Authors' presentation according to Buzby and Hyman (2012)

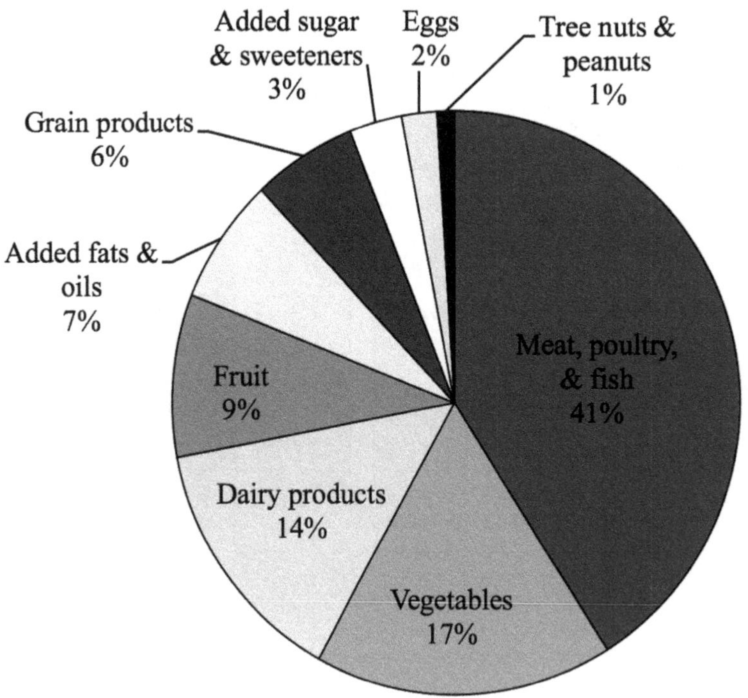

RESEARCH PURPOSE AND RELEVANCE

This chapter presents an economic cost analysis related to meat waste in the US. Wasted meat makes up 49.8 percent of the total meat production in the US (Toth & Dou, 2016). Meat waste surrounds two main issues: 1) resource use, environmental impacts and costs of raising livestock, and 2) economic and environmental impacts of wasting meat and meat products.

Livestock production is very resource intensive, particularly in terms of land, water and energy use (Eshel et al., 2014; Pimentel & Pimentel, 2008; Steinfeld et al., 2006). It is also the largest anthropogenic contributor to methane and nitrous oxide emissions, which are much more powerful GHGs than carbon dioxide. Wasting meat has high opportunity costs as these resources and money applied to meat production could be used in alternative ways to cope with other social issues, e.g. health problems caused by industrial agriculture.

While there is a common understanding about tremendous resource inputs for meat production, research quantifying those inputs and economic losses is still limited, as it is challenging at the same time due to data paucity. However, monetizing resource costs and GHG emissions associated with food waste that causes economic losses, environmental degradation and food insecurity may be a powerful tool for raising awareness, educating and incentivizing individuals, corporations, and governments to undertake actions towards reducing food waste (Ziolkowska, 2017).

Building on a study by Ziolkowska (2017) who quantified economic costs of the total food waste in the US, this chapter provides new insights into an economic analysis of resource and monetary losses caused specifically by meat waste.

METHODOLOGY AND DATA

For the presented analysis, a literature review on statistical specifications of meat waste and resource waste for meat production, has been conducted based on peer-reviewed journal articles, book chapters, and numerous reports from US Department of Agriculture (USDA), Environmental Protection Agency (EPA), and nonprofit organizations. Further, quantitative estimation of monetary costs related to meat waste and resource use for meat production was calculated, focused specifically on costs of energy, water and land use as well as methane and nitrous oxide emissions. While N_2O is not necessarily a relevant gas emitter from the total food waste perspective, it is particularly relevant to consider in calculations of meat waste as around two-thirds of global N_2O emissions are generated from livestock production (McMichael et al., 2007; Steinfeld et al., 2006).

As research in this field is still limited, data and statistics required for the analysis presented in this chapter have been scarce at times or they represent different years due to missing temporal analyses on this topic in the literature. The calculated values are approximate and are based on the amount of resources used/emissions generated, their respective prices and the percent of wasted meat within the US. These results do not represent total costs over the entire life cycle of meat production, consumption, and disposal which are much higher.

The analysis of monetary resource losses and costs associated with meat waste is based on the methodology presented by Ziolkowska (2017), while this study expands this methodological application by including nitrous oxide assessment and methane emissions in the meat pre-disposal stage. A series of equations presented below are used to calculate the impacts of meat waste on natural resources.

Water

The cost of wasted water was calculated as follows:

$$Cost\ of\ water\ for\ meat\ production(\$) = price\ of\ water\ per\ acre(\$/ac)$$
$$* irrigated\ acres\ for\ feed\ crops\ and\ animal\ husbandry(ac)$$

(1)

$$Cost\ of\ wasted\ water\ in\ meat\ production(\$) = \%\ of\ wasted\ meat\ products$$
$$* cost\ of\ water\ for\ meat\ production$$

(2)

Only direct water costs were considered in this analysis, while water costs related to production factors were omitted here, as it would go beyond the scope of this study.

The total land area used for cropland in the US in 2013 was 408 million acres, of which 55.3 million acres were irrigated (USDA, 2014). Of the 55.3 million irrigated acres, 27 percent were used to grow feed crops, which equals 14.9 million acres (Eshel et al., 2014). For non-feed crop purposes, additional irrigation is required to raise livestock. In 2013, non-feed crop irrigation requirements equaled 7 480 247 acres and were as follows: 5 966 127 acres for beef cattle ranching and farming, 698 465 acres for cattle feedlots and 815 655 acres for all other animal specialties (USDA, 2014). Thus, the total irrigation requirements to raise livestock in 2013 were 22 380 247 acres. The price of water in 2008 was \$26–\$71 per acre (Ziolkowska, 2017), while the 'shadow price' of water was not considered (Ziolkowska, 2015), which would otherwise elevate the cost of water applied in this analysis. Two calculations were conducted to estimate the cost of wasted water, based on the minimum and maximum costs for water per acre in 2008 (rather than averaging the data) to provide a more detailed picture of the cost estimates.

Land

The cost of land use embedded in meat waste was calculated based on the following three equations to account for the different agricultural land uses and their differing prices per acre:

$$Cost\ of\ land\ use\ (\$)\left[irrigated\ cropland\right] = land\ rent\ (\$) * \%\ of\ wasted\ meat\ products \tag{3}$$

$$Cost\ of\ land\ use\ (\$)\left[non\text{-}irrigated\ cropland\right] = land\ rent\ (\$) * \%\ of\ wasted\ meat\ products \tag{4}$$

$$Cost\ of\ land\ use\ (\$)\left[pastureland\right] = land\ rent\ pastureland * \%\ of\ wasted\ meat\ products \tag{5}$$

For equation 3, the total irrigated acres for feed crops (14.9 million acres) (Eshel et al., 2014) and acres for animal husbandry (7.5 million acres) (USDA, 2014) were summed up to a total of 22.4 million acres. The land rent for irrigated cropland in 2014 ranged from \$64 to \$405 per acre (USDA, 2015). To derive the total land rent for irrigated acres, the minimum and maximum land rent values were each multiplied by the total irrigated acres for livestock, and finally averaged.

In equation 4, non-irrigated acres for livestock production embedded in meat waste, the total irrigated acres for feed crops we subtracted from the total acreage used for crops and processed roughage that amounted to 0.6 million km² (148.2 million acres) annually from 2000 to 2010 (Eshel et al., 2014).

Subtracting 14.9 million irrigated acres for feed crops from the total acreage used for crops and processed roughage (148.3 million acres) resulted in the total of 133.4 million non-irrigated acres. In 2014, the land rent for non-irrigated acres ranged from $14 to $206 per acre (USDA, 2015). Irrigated acres were calculated with the same methodological procedure as above, where the minimum and maximum land rent cost for non-irrigated acres were each multiplied by the total non-irrigated acres. Ultimately the values were averaged for clarity of the presented calculations and results and due to the fact that each equation relied on different land rent costs.

The annual land rent for pastureland in the US was $7.4 billion in 2014 (Ziolkowska, 2017). This calculation is based on an assumption that the majority of pastureland is used to raise livestock, though there might be slight deviations in terms of differing pastureland uses. This could arise from the emerging trend of agro-ecological farming methods that combine livestock and crop production. However, these types of land uses still remain marginal at this point in time. The annual land rent for pastureland, $7.4 billion, was multiplied by the percent of wasted meat in 2012, namely 49.8% (Toth & Dou, 2016).

Energy

The cost of lost energy from meat waste was calculated with the following equation:

$$\text{Cost of lost energy from wasted meat}(\$) = \sum \begin{bmatrix} energy\, lost\left(BTU\right) * \% \text{ of energy source used} \\ *\text{price for energy source}\left(\$\,/\text{ million BTU}\right) \end{bmatrix}$$

$$(6)$$

Both direct and indirect energy costs from wasted meat were considered. Direct energy sources on farms in 2011 made up 66 percent of total energy use, while indirect sources represented 34 percent (Ziolkowska, 2017). The energy source estimates were derived from Miranowski (2002). Direct energy sources account for: 27 percent from diesel; 9 percent from gasoline; 5 percent from LP gas/propane; 4 percent from natural gas; and 21 percent from electricity. Indirect energy sources include: 28 percent for fertilizers production and 6 percent for pesticide production. The prices for energy sources were derived from Rapier (2010) and are as follows (in $/million BTU[1]): $15.49 for diesel; $17.81 for gasoline; $13.28 for LP gas/propane; $5.69 for natural gas; $26.31 for electricity; and $1.32 for coal. The amount of energy lost from wasted meat in the US in 2007 amounted to 972.1 trillion BTU (Cuéllar & Webber, 2010). This estimate includes energy used in production, transportation, handling and processing of meat. To calculate the cost of direct energy losses from meat waste, the percentage of energy from each source was multiplied by its corresponding price/million BTU and by the amount of energy lost due to meat waste. The estimates for the respective energy sources were further summed up to one final value.

Calculating the cost of energy loss from indirect energy sources involved the knowledge that a ton of artificial fertilizer requires 73 percent of natural gas and 27 percent of coal to produce (Kelischek, 2011). Accordingly, each of these values was multiplied by their corresponding prices/million BTU and by the amount of energy loss due to meat waste. Also in this case the estimates for the respective indirect energy sources were summed up to one final value.

Methane

The cost of methane from meat waste was calculated with the following two equations:

$$Cost\ of\ methane\ from\ wasted\ meat(\$)\big[pre-disposal\big] = carbon\ tax(\$/ton)$$
$$*livestock\ CH_4\ emissions\big(MMT\ CO_2\ eq.\big)$$
$$*\%\ of\ wasted\ meat\ products$$

$$(7)$$

$$Cost\ of\ methane\ from\ wasted\ meat(\$)\big[landfill\big] = carbon\ tax(\$/ton)$$
$$*total\ US\ methane\ emissions\big(MMT\ CO_2\ eq.\big)$$
$$*\ \%\ of\ methane\ from\ landfill\big(20\%\big)$$
$$*\ \%\ of\ meat\ in\ total\ food\ waste\ in\ landfill\big(7.08\%\big)$$

$$(8)$$

In this analysis, a calculation of pre-disposal methane emissions was included due to the fact that almost all methane generated during agricultural production is attributable to livestock. However, landfill methane emissions are still important and necessary to consider in the analysis of food waste emissions. For both, equation 7 and 8, the carbon tax estimate implemented in British Columbia, Canada was included at $23/ton (CAN $30/ton) of CO_2 emission equivalent. As of 2012, this tax was the most stringent carbon tax in the western hemisphere (World Bank, 2016). In 2014, the US emitted 6870 million metric tons (MMT) of CO_2 equivalent (EPA, 2016). Methane emissions made up 11 percent of total emissions, which equals 775.7 MMT. Agriculture is responsible for 237.7 MMT, of which 225.5 MMT is generated during livestock production (164.3 MMT from enteric fermentation and 61.2 MMT from manure management) (EPA, 2016).

For equation 7, pre-disposal methane emissions, the hypothetical carbon tax was multiplied by total livestock methane emissions and the percent of wasted meat. Landfills are responsible for 20 percent of US methane emissions (EPA, 2016). Considering that 40 percent of landfill methane emissions are attributable to anaerobically decomposing food waste (Ziolkowska, 2017), and that meat makes up 17.7 percent of total food waste (Toth & Dou, 2016), meat waste is theoretically responsible for 7.08 percent of landfill methane emissions. This calculation does not consider the different carbon intensities of organic waste, which could theoretically slightly alter the estimates. To calculate the total cost of landfill methane emissions from wasted meat, the assumed carbon tax was multiplied by the total US methane emissions, the percent of methane from landfills, and the percent of landfill emissions from wasted meat.

Nitrous Oxide

The cost of N_2O emissions from meat waste was calculated with the following equation:

$$\begin{array}{l} Cost\,of\,nitrous\,oxide\,emissions \\ from\,wasted\,meat\,(\$) \end{array} = carbon\,tax\,(\$\,/\,ton)$$

$$*total\,N_2O\,emissions\,from\,livestock\,(MMT\,CO_2\,eq.) \tag{9}$$
$$*\%\,of\,wasted\,meat\,products$$

The US agriculture is responsible for 336 MMT of nitrous oxide emissions each year, of which 318.4 MMT come from soil management and 17.5 MMT from manure management (EPA, 2016). At the same time, 40 percent of US cropland is used for feed crops (Eshel et al., 2014), which translates to 127.36 MMT of N_2O from feed crops. Adding the N_2O estimates attributable to manure management and to cropland for feed crop production, the total of 144.86 MMT of N_2O was estimated that is attributable to livestock production. To calculate the cost of N_2O emissions from meat waste, the assumed carbon tax was multiplied by the total N_2O emissions from livestock and the percent of meat waste in the US.

RESULTS

The results of this analysis show that the total costs of meat waste in the US, under the assumption of this study, amount to a total of \$32-32.5 billion per year (Table 1). Costs related to land use (including both cropland and pastureland costs) embedded in meat waste make up the biggest portion of economic losses and equal to \$13.6 billion per year (Figure 4). Energy losses also represent an enormous cost of \$13.1 billion per year.

The methane costs for pre-disposal livestock emissions amount to \$3.1 billion per year, while landfill emissions cost \$0.2 billion per year. Water was found to be the least costly resource, at \$0.3-\$0.8 billion per year. Ziolkowska (2017) found that water costs for all food waste were similarly the lowest in her study among different resources. However, she emphasized that water costs would be substantially higher if the true value of water as a resource was incorporated into valuations. The same could apply to all resources, particularly those used for food production. Lastly, nitrous oxide emissions from meat waste would cost approximately \$1.7 billion per year based on the British Columbia carbon tax calculation of CO_2 equivalent emissions.

Table 1. Costs related to meat waste by resource category

Resource	Cost of Meat Waste (Billion US$)
Water	0.3 – 0.8
Land Use (Cropland)	9.9
Land Use (Pastureland)	3.7
Energy	13.1
Methane Emissions (pre-disposal)	3.1
Methane Emissions (landfill)	0.2
Nitrous Oxide Emissions	1.7
Sum	**32 – 32.5**

Figure 4. Percent of costs related to meat waste by resource category

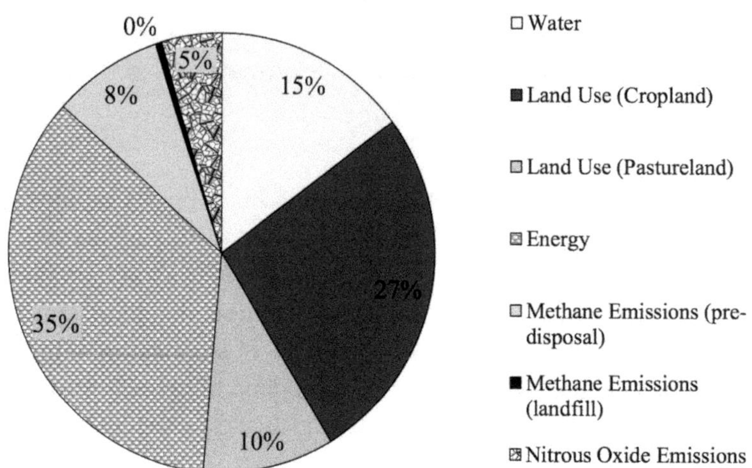

DISCUSSION

Based on the presented analysis, the US is losing substantial amounts of money (~$32 billion) annually due to meat waste. This estimated amount could be utilized to improve sustainability at different social, environmental or economic levels in the food production process. In addition, if resources and environmental impacts were valued for their true worth and costs to society, the presented results would fall much higher.

The vast amount of land being used to grow feed crops for livestock that is eventually wasted and the resulting costs have significant implications for several reasons. First, almost all land used to grow feed crops in the US is farmed industrially, which leads to harmful implications for the environment. Industrial agriculture negatively impacts ecosystems through overuse of fertilizers and pesticides, which consequently leads to water, air and soil pollution and degradation. Additionally, it fosters monocultures that impair biodiversity and deplete natural resources. Soil loss is one of the most pressing concerns for society's ability to produce sufficient amounts of food. Each year in the US, around 90 percent of cropland is losing soil at an average rate of 13 times faster than the estimated sustainable rate of 1 ton/ha/year (Pimentel & Pimentel, 2008). This development may lead to intensified land conversion into cropland in the future to compensate for the currently occurring losses, with amplified habitat and biodiversity declines. Cropland used to produce feed crops may lose even more topsoil each year than the average loss rates due to monocultures, abandonment of crop rotations, removal of tree shelter belts, leaving soil fallow without protective biomass cover and the use of heavy farm machinery (Pimentel & Pimentel, 2008).

Second, land used for feed crop production has very high opportunity costs, meaning that it has a very high alternative-use value and could be applied to grow crops for food production (including specialty crops like fruits and vegetables). Using land to grow food crops rather than feed crops would help provide calories to many more people. To put this in perspective, 45 million tons of plant protein is fed to livestock in the US each year, which produces only 7.5 million tons of animal protein for human consumption (Pimentel & Pimentel, 2008). In other words, it takes around 6 kg of plant protein to produce

1 kg of animal protein, while this plant protein could be utilized more efficiently to satisfy increasing food demands of the growing population.

Furthermore, unsustainable soil management, which often results from excessive fertilization of industrialized feed crops, is responsible for the majority of N_2O emissions from livestock production. Nitrous oxide emissions are miniscule in comparison to anthropogenic carbon dioxide emissions, but their global warming potential is 256 times as powerful, and thus needs to be seriously considered as efforts to mitigate GHG emissions across the world begin after the 2016 Paris Climate Agreement.

Demand for meat products is expected to increase rapidly by 2050 and consequently N_2O emissions will rise as well (Pelletier & Tyedmers, 2010). A carbon tax on polluters could be an effective measure to reduce N_2O emissions, while also raising revenues for the government. The hypothetical cost of N_2O emissions from meat waste, at \$1.7 billion per year, is significant in itself. Wasted meat makes up almost half of all meat produced and thus the income from a carbon tax on N_2O emissions from all meat production would amount to around \$3.4 billion per year. Considering that N_2O emissions are much more harmful than CO_2 emissions, the question about the appropriate carbon tax level might be a topic for scientific and political discussions.

It also needs to be emphasized that over-fertilization is more harmful to the environment than N_2O emissions alone. Plants only take up around half of the applied nitrogen fertilizers, while the remaining is dispersed into the environment (Sage, 2012). Bouwman et al. (2013) estimated that a surplus of 138 trillion grams of nitrogen is inputted into the environment every single year, far exceeding natural levels in the nitrogen cycle. The severe environmental consequences and potential economic costs of N_2O emissions underline the need to reduce feed crop cultivation and usage for livestock breeding and meat production.

Furthermore, water is becoming an increasingly scarce resource around the world and will only become scarcer as unsustainable water management practices continue (Lundqvist et al., 2008; Mekonnen & Hoekstra, 2010). As mentioned above, water is not priced for its true economic value as a resource and in many cases it is used without any regard for future stocks. When meat waste is combined with already unsustainable water management practices in food production, the unfolding picture becomes even more troubling in terms of sustainable resource allocation. Meat requires much more water than any other food produced, besides dairy, and approximately two-thirds (14.9 of 22.4 million acres) of the irrigation water requirements come from feed crop production (Eshel et al., 2014; USDA, 2014). Livestock conversion efficiencies from feed to protein are different for each animal but each species requires significant quantities. For example, feed and forage crops require 500-2000 l of water per kg of plant biomass produced, while producing 1 kg beef requires ~43 000 l of water, 43 times more water than 1 kg of grain (Pimentel & Pimentel, 2008).

In terms of energy use, industrial agriculture is a heavy user of fossil energy and a large portion of energy demand on farms comes from meat production. In fact, the agricultural stage of meat production requires 778 trillion BTU out of 1 270 trillion BTU from all food categories (Cuéllar & Webber, 2010). On average, 25 kcals of fossil energy are required to produce 1 kcal of animal protein, which is 10 times greater than the average energy requirements for grain protein (Pimentel & Pimentel, 2008). Other supply chain energy users, such as transportation, processing and handling, are similar in terms of overall energy use, but meat production is still a heavy energy user in all stages. It is implicit that lost energy from meat waste, at 49.8 percent of total production, is responsible for significant costs of \$13.1 billion per year. Compared to the cost of lost energy from total food waste in Ziolkowska (2017), the lost energy from meat waste makes up slightly less than half of total economic losses ($13.1 billion out of $29.4 billion).

In regard to environmental impacts, landfill methane emissions from meat waste are insignificant compared to methane emissions generated during agricultural production that can be attributed to meat waste. Reducing meat waste (and in fact food waste in general) from landfills should be a primary goal of sustainable societies. Globally, ruminants are responsible for around 77 percent of livestock methane emissions from enteric fermentation (Herrero et al., 2013), while in the US they account for approximately 73 percent (EPA, 2016). Similarly, to nitrous oxide emissions, a higher pricing scheme for methane emissions than current carbon taxes could be considered.

The remainder of livestock methane emissions occurs mainly from manure management. Moreover, improper manure management also contributes to eutrophication, leaching of nitrates into groundwater, and excessively high nutrient levels in the soil that can volatize into nitrous oxides, nitrogen oxides, and ammonia which can ultimately cause acidification of ecosystems (Steinfeld et al., 2006). Switching from industrial livestock systems to pasture-based livestock systems, while simultaneously reducing meat production, could help mitigate this issue. Also, reducing consumption of ruminant meat from cows, goats, and sheep could significantly suppress methane emissions. Currently, the average American diet, including large quantities of meat, produces 1485 kg more of CO_2 emission equivalent than an average vegan or plant-based diet (Eshel & Martin, 2006). Educating societies about impacts of meat consumption on the environment could serve as a social marketing tool to influence people's behavior.

CONCLUSION

In this study, economic costs of meat waste in the US were quantified. The results show that meat waste generates substantial annual costs of $32-32.5 billion in regard to land, water, energy applied to produce meat as well as in methane and N_2O emissions. The estimates would most likely increase substantially if existing economic approaches of resources valuation and environmental impacts better represented resource values and were more accurately embedded in resource and product prices. It can be argued that this undervaluation is a root cause of modern environmental tragedies occurring across the world. The same can be stated about food waste and societal disconnect from food production. Considering food security as a granted right, missing understanding of food production and cultural/behavioral consumption habits lead to food waste as the ultimate result.

The solution to the food waste problem may rely on improving awareness specifically about monetary losses related to meat/food waste for consumers, businesses and governments, as they are the major decision-makers in implementing change on either household level or by means of legislative measures. Policies incentivizing or dis-incentivizing certain food waste behaviors or else mandatory initiatives, e.g. citywide compost collection with penalties for non-compliance (as currently applied in Seattle, WA) could be one of possible actions in this direction. Also, educational programs, especially in schools, need to be enacted to create a notion about the need to reduce food/meat waste to limit unnecessary financial losses and to conserve natural resources at the same time.

ACKNOWLEDGMENT

This research was supported by the German Academy of Sciences Leopoldina.

REFERENCES

Bouwman, L., Goldewijk, K. K., Van Der Hoek, K. W., Beusen, A. H., Van Vuuren, D. P., Willems, J., & Stehfest, E. (2013). Exploring global changes in nitrogen and phosphorus cycles in agriculture induced by livestock production over the 1900-2050 period. *Proceedings of the National Academy of Sciences of the United States of America, 110*(52), 20882–20887. doi:10.1073/pnas.1012878108 PMID:21576477

Buzby, J. C., & Hyman, J. (2012). Total and per capita value of food loss in the United States. *Food Policy, 37*(5), 561–570. doi:10.1016/j.foodpol.2012.06.002

Cuéllar, A. D., & Webber, M. E. (2010). Wasted food, wasted energy: The embedded energy in food waste in the United States. *Environmental Science & Technology, 44*(16), 6464–6469. doi:10.1021/es100310d PMID:20704248

de Vries, M., & de Boer, I. J. M. (2010). Comparing environmental impacts for livestock products: A review of life cycle assessments. *Livestock Science, 128*(1–3), 1–11. doi:10.1016/j.livsci.2009.11.007

Diaz, R. J., & Rosenberg, R. (2008). Spreading dead zones and consequences for marine ecosystems. *Science, 321*(5891), 926–929. doi:10.1126cience.1156401 PMID:18703733

Environmental Protection Agency (EPA). (2016). Inventory of US greenhouse gas emissions and sinks: 1990-2014. Washington, DC: EPA. Retrieved from https://www.epa.gov/sites/production/files/2016-04/documents/us-ghg-inventory-2016-main-text.pdf

Eshel, G., & Martin, P. A. (2006). Diet, energy, and global warming. *Earth Interactions, 10*(9), 1–17. doi:10.1175/EI167.1

Eshel, G., Shepon, A., Makov, T., & Milo, R. (2014). Land, irrigation water, greenhouse gas, and reactive nitrogen burdens of meat, eggs, and dairy production in the United States. *Proceedings of the National Academy of Sciences of the United States of America, 111*(33), 11996–12001. doi:10.1073/pnas.1402183111 PMID:25049416

Foley, J. A., Ramankutty, N., Brauman, K. A., Cassidy, E. S., Gerber, J. S., Johnston, M., ... Zaks, D. P. M. (2011). Solutions for a cultivated planet. *Nature, 478*(7369), 337–342. doi:10.1038/nature10452 PMID:21993620

Food and Agriculture Organization of the United Nations (FAO). (2011). *Global food losses and food waste—extent, causes and prevention.* Rome, Italy: FAO.

Food and Agriculture Organization of the United Nations (FAO). (2013). *Food wastage footprint: Impacts on natural resources.* Summary Report. Retrieved from http://www.fao.org/docrep/018/i3347e/i3347e.pdf

Food and Agriculture Organization of the United Nations (FAO). (2014). *Animal Production and Health: Meat Consumption*. Agriculture and Consumer Protection Department. Retrieved from http://www.fao.org/ag/againfo/themes/en/meat/background.html

Godfray, H. C. J., Beddington, J. R., Crute, I. R., Haddad, L., Lawrence, D., Muir, J. F., & Toulmin, C. (2010). Food security: The challenge of feeding 9 billion people. *Science, 327*(5967), 812–818. doi:10.1126cience.1185383 PMID:20110467

Gustavsson, J., Cederberg, C., Sonesson, U., van Otterdijk, R., & Meybeck, A. (2011). Global food losses and food waste: Extent, causes and prevention. *Food and Agriculture Organization of the United Nations, 38.* doi:10.1098/rstb.2010.0126

Hall, K. D., Guo, J., Dore, M., & Chow, C. C. (2009). The progressive increase of food waste in America and its environmental impact. *PLoS One, 4*(11), e7940. doi:10.1371/journal.pone.0007940 PMID:19946359

Herrero, M., Havlík, P., Valin, H., Notenbaert, A., Rufino, M. C., & Thornton, P. K., … Obersteiner, M. (2013). Biomass use, production, feed efficiencies, and greenhouse gas emissions from global livestock systems. *Proceedings of the National Academy of Sciences of the United States of America, 110,* 20888–20893. 10.1073/pnas.1308149110

Kearney, J. (2010). Food consumption trends and drivers. *Philosophical Transactions of the Royal Society of London. Series B, Biological Sciences, 365*(1554), 2793–2807. doi:10.1098/rstb.2010.0149 PMID:20713385

Kelischek, N. (2011). Energy budget of nitrogen use in the United States. *Journal of Student Research in Environmental Science at Appalachian, 1*(1), 32–35. Retrieved from http://pimlico.phys.appstate.edu/JSRESA/kelischek.1-1.pdf

Keyzer, M. A., Merbis, M. D., Pavel, I. F. P. W., & van Wesenbeeck, C. F. A. (2005). Diet shifts towards meat and the effects on cereal use: Can we feed the animals in 2030. *Ecological Economics, 55*(2), 187–202. doi:10.1016/j.ecolecon.2004.12.002

Kummu, M., de Moel, H., Porkka, M., Siebert, S., Varis, O., & Ward, P. J. (2012). Lost food, wasted resources: Global food supply chain losses and their impacts on freshwater, cropland, and fertiliser use. *The Science of the Total Environment, 438,* 477–489. doi:10.1016/j.scitotenv.2012.08.092 PMID:23032564

Lipinski, B., Hanson, C., Lomax, J., Kitinoja, L., Waite, R., & Searchinger, T. (2013). *Reducing food loss and waste* (Working Paper). World Resource Institute. Retrieved from http://pdf.wri.org/reducing_food_loss_and_waste.pdf

Lundqvist, J., De Fraiture, C., & Molden, D. (2008). *Saving water: From field to fork – curbing losses and wastage in the food chain. SIWI Policy Brief.* Stockholm, Sweden: Stockholm International Water Institute.

McAlpine, C. A., Etter, A., Fearnside, P. M., Seabrook, L., & Laurance, W. F. (2009). Increasing world consumption of beef as a driver of regional and global change: A call for policy action based on evidence from Queensland (Australia), Colombia and Brazil. *Global Environmental Change, 19*(1), 21–33. doi:10.1016/j.gloenvcha.2008.10.008

McMichael, A. J., Powles, J. W., Butler, C. D., & Uauy, R. (2007). Food, livestock production, energy, climate change, and health. *Lancet, 370*(9594), 1253–1263. doi:10.1016/S0140-6736(07)61256-2 PMID:17868818

Mekonnen, M. M., & Hoekstra, A. Y. (2010). The green, blue and grey water footprint of farm animals and animal products.: Vol. 1. *Main report*. Delft, the Netherlands: UNESCO. Retrieved from http://waterfootprint.org/media/downloads/Report-48-WaterFootprint-AnimalProducts-Vol1.pdf

Miranowski, J. (2002) Energy Consumption in U.S. Agriculture. Presentation for Farm Foundation. Retrieved from https://www.farmfoundation.org/projects/documents/miranowski.ppt

Naylor, R., Steinfeld, H., Falcon, Q., Galloway, J., Smil, V., Bradford, E., ... Mooney, H. (2005). Agriculture: Losing the links between livestock and land. *Science, 310*(5754), 1621–162. doi:10.1126cience.1117856 PMID:16339432

Papargyropoulou, E., Lozano, R., & Steinberger, K., J., Wright, N., & bin Ujang, Z. (. (2014). The food waste hierarchy as a framework for the management of food surplus and food waste. *Journal of Cleaner Production, 76*, 106–115. doi:10.1016/j.jclepro.2014.04.020

Pelletier, N., & Tyedmers, P. (2010). Forecasting potential global environmental costs of livestock production 2000-2050. *Proceedings of the National Academy of Sciences of the United States of America, 107*(43), 18371–18374. doi:10.1073/pnas.1004659107 PMID:20921375

Pimentel, D., & Pimentel, M. H. (2008). *Food, energy, and society* (3rd ed.). Boca Raton, FL: CRC Press.

Rapier. (2010, January 26). The price of energy. *Forbes*. Retrieved from https://www.forbes.com/sites/energysource/2010/01/26/the-price-of-energy/#25cf888f67b1

Sage, C. (2012). *Environment and food*. London, UK: Routledge.

Smil, V. (2002). Worldwide transformation of diets, burdens of meat production and opportunities for novel food proteins. *Enzyme and Microbial Technology, 30*(3), 305–311. doi:10.1016/S0141-0229(01)00504-X

Smil, V. (2004). Improving efficiency and reducing waste in our food system. *Environmental Sciences, 1*(1), 17–26. doi:10.1076/evms.1.1.17.23766

Spooner, B. (2016). Food Waste and Food Security in a Globalizing World. In *Food Waste Across the Supply Chain: A US Perspective on a Global Problem* (pp. 73–85). University of Pennsylvania.

Steinfeld, H., Gerber, P., Wassenaar, T., Castel, V., Rosales, M., & De Haan, C. (2006). *Livestock's long shadow: Environmental issues and options*. Rome, Italy: FAO.

Toth, J. D., & Dou, Z. (2016). Wasted food, wasted resources: Land, irrigation water, and nutrients associated with food wastage in the U.S. In Z. Dou, J. D. Ferguson, D. T. Galligan, A. M. Kelly, S. M. Finn, & R. Giegengack (Eds.), *Food waste across the supply chain: A US perspective on a global problem* (pp. 57–71). Ames, IO: Council for Agricultural Science and Technology.

United States Department of Agriculture (USDA). (2014). 2012 Census of Agriculture: Farm and Ranch Irrigation Survey 2013. USDA Census of Agriculture. Retrieved from https://www.agcensus.usda.gov/Publications/2012/Online_Resources/Farm_and_Ranch_Irrigation_Survey/

United States Department of Agriculture (USDA). (2015). 2014 Land values and cash rents: Cropland and pasture. National Agriculture Statistics Service (NASS) Highlights. Retrieved from https://www. nass.usda.gov/Publications/Highlights/2014_LandValues_CashRents/LVCR.pdf

World Bank. (2016). State and trends of carbon pricing. Washington, DC: World Bank Group. Retrieved from http://documents.worldbank.org/curated/en/598811476464765822/State-and-trends-of-carbon-pricing

World Bank. (2017). *GDP per capita (current US$)*. Retrieved from http://data.worldbank.org/indicator/NY.GDP.PCAP.CD

Ziolkowska, J. R. (2015). Shadow price of water for irrigation – a case of the High Plains. *Agricultural Water Management, 153*, 20–31. doi:10.1016/j.agwat.2015.01.024

Ziolkowska, J. R. (2017). Economic and environmental costs of agricultural food losses and waste in the US. *International Journal of Food Engineering, 3*(2), 140–145.

KEY TERMS AND DEFINITIONS

Agriculture: Science or practice of farming (soil cultivation for growing crops and grazing animals) to provide food, wool, and other products.

Animal Husbandry: The raising of any animal species to consume and/or utilize for various purposes.

Food Security: The state (of an individual or societies) of having a sufficient quantity of affordable and nutritious food.

Food Waste: The loss or wastage of edible food at any point in a food supply chain.

Livestock: Any living animal or group of animals used in animal husbandry to consume and/or use for various purposes.

Monetary Valuation: Assigning economic value and/or cost to a specific resource or product.

Natural Resources: Naturally occurring materials or substances that can be used for various purposes to gain specific benefits.

Sustainability: The ability to maintain environmental, social, and economic systems and capital indefinitely for the present generation to meet its needs without compromising the ability of future generations to meet their own needs.

ENDNOTE

[1]   BTU – British thermal unit; 1 BTU = 1055 joules.

Sustainable Agricultural Production

Chapter 37
Tropospheric Ozone Pollution, Agriculture, and Food Security

Abhijit Sarkar
University of Gour Banga, India

Sambit Datta
University of Calcutta, India

Pooja Singh
Banaras Hindu University, India

ABSTRACT

Increasing population and unsustainable exploitation of nature and natural resources have made "food security" a burning issue in the 21ˢᵗ century. During the last 50 years, the global population has more than doubled, from 3 billion in 1959 to 6.7 billion in 2009. It is predicted that the human population will reach 8.7 - 11.3 billion by the year 2050. Growth in the global livestock industry has also been continuous over the last two decades. An almost 82% increase in future livestock is expected in developing countries within 2020, due to an expanding requirement for food of animal origin. Hence, the future demand of this increased human and livestock population will put enormous pressure on the agricultural sectors for providing sufficient food and fodder as well as income, employment and other essential ecosystem services. Therefore, a normal approach for any nation / region is to strengthen its agricultural production for meeting future demands and provide food security. Tropospheric ozone (O_3), a secondary air pollutant and a major greenhouse gas, has already been recognized as a major component of predicted global climate change. Numerous studies have confirmed the negative impact of O_3 on agricultural productivity throughout the world. The present chapter reviews the available literature, and catalogue the impact of this important gas pollutant on modern day agricultural production worldwide.

DOI: 10.4018/978-1-7998-5354-1.ch037

INTRODUCTION

Ozone (O_3) whether in stratosphere or troposphere has been a major talking issue for scientists, policy makers, and even the common man since last couple of decades. In stratosphere this tri-oxygen provides a crucial barrier against incoming solar ultraviolet radiation and protects life on earth; so depletion of O_3 layer in stratosphere is a problem. However, in troposphere it is a gaseous pollutant with negative impact on human and animal respiration as well as causing severe damage to both natural and cultivated plant populations (Cho et al, 2011); so, rising of O_3 level in troposphere is again a major crisis. Now, which one is more serious problem – might be a million-dollar question; but, this present section mainly focuses to review the available scientific literatures which specifically deal with the O_3 formed in the troposphere and its further consequences mainly on plant's health and productivity. Although, some O_3 is believed to be transferred from the stratosphere to the troposphere too; but the amount is debatable (Jaffe, 2003).

THE ATMOSPHERIC O_3: GOOD UP HIGH, BAD NEARBY

Ozone is generally present as a trace gas in our atmosphere, averaging about three molecules for every 10 million air molecules. In spite of this very small quantity, O_3 plays a vital function in controlling the atmospheric chemistry. This trace gas is mainly found in two different regions of Earth's atmosphere. The major amount of the total atmospheric O_3 (approximately 90%) exist in a layer that begins between 10 and 17 kilometers above the Earth's surface and extends up to about 50 kilometers. This region of the atmosphere is called 'stratosphere' and the stratospheric O_3 is commonly known as the 'ozone layer'. The remaining O_3 is present in the lower region of the atmosphere, which is commonly called 'troposphere'. Though the O_3 molecules at upper atmosphere, i.e. stratosphere, and lower atmosphere, i.e. troposphere, are chemically identical but they perform very different roles in atmosphere as well as show very different effects on the living world too. The stratospheric O_3 (sometimes referred as 'good ozone') plays a valuable role for living world by absorbing most of the biologically damaging ultraviolet sunlight (UV-B), allowing only a small amount to reach the Earth's surface. The absorption of ultraviolet radiation by O_3 creates a source of heat, which actually forms the stratosphere itself (a region in which the temperature rises as one goes to higher altitudes). Ozone thus plays a key role in the temperature structure of the Earth's atmosphere. Without the filtering action of the O_3 layer, more of the Sun's UV – B radiation would penetrate the atmosphere and would reach the Earth's surface. Many experimental studies of plants and animals and clinical studies of humans have shown the harmful effects of excessive exposure to UV-B radiation. However, in the troposphere, O_3 acts as a harmful gaseous pollutant which itself affects the health and productivity of all the living forms.

TROPOSPHERIC OZONE CYCLE: FORMATION, DEPOSITION AND TRANSPORT OF OZONE IN TROPOSPHERE

Being a secondary pollutant in nature tropospheric O_3 is generally formed by the photo-chemical reactions between oxides of nitrogen (NO_x) and volatile organic compounds (VOCs) in the presence of bright sunlight. Even, O_3 also formed from the methane emitted from swamps and wetlands and some other primary pollutants through similar reactions; and through long range transport O_3 travels huge distances and spreads over larger areas (Kondratyev & Varotsos, 2001; Varotsos et al., 2004). VOCs emission has not contributed significantly to increasing tropospheric O_3 concentrations (Fiore et al., 2002).

The chemical reactions involved in tropospheric O_3 formation are a series of complex cycles in which carbon-monoxide and VOCs are oxidized to water vapor and carbon dioxide. The oxidation occurs in carbon monoxide due to hydroxyl radical ($OH^.$). The resultant hydrogen atom reacts rapidly with oxygen to give a per-oxy radical ($HO_2^.$).

$$OH^. + CO \rightarrow H + CO_2$$
$$H + O_2 \rightarrow HO_2^.$$

Peroxy radicals react with NO to give NO_2, which is photolyzed to give atomic oxygen and by reacting with oxygen, a molecule of O_3 is formed.

$$HO_2^. + NO \rightarrow OH^. + NO_2$$
$$NO_x + radiations\ (>380\ nm) \rightarrow NO + O$$
$$O + O_2 \rightarrow O_3$$

Besides, O_3 formation also depends upon reaction of methane (CH_4), carbon monoxide (CO) and non-methane hydrocarbons (NMHCs) with O_2.

Formation of O_3 from carbon monoxide

$$CO + 2O_2 + hv \rightarrow CO_2 + O_3$$

Formation of O_3 from methane

$$CH_4 + 4O_2 + 2hv \rightarrow HCHO + H_2O + 2O_3$$
$$HCHO + hv \rightarrow H + HCO\ (\lambda < 330nm)$$
$$HCO + hv \rightarrow H + CO\ (\lambda < 360nm)$$
$$CO + 2O_2 + hv \rightarrow CO_2 + O_3$$

Formation of O_3 from non-methane hydrocarbons

$$RH + 4O_2 + 2hv \rightarrow RCHO + H_2O + 2O_3.$$

So, it is quite clear that formation of O_3 in troposphere is long process which involves a number of primary pollutants. Ozone in upper layer of troposphere can have a lifetime of many days or even a week or two. This is because the major loss processes, scavenging by nitric oxide and dry deposition occur at or very close to the surface of the Earth. This means that O_3 produced in one region can, if lifted to higher levels, travel to another region, increasing the background O_3 concentrations of that region, even if the sources of O_3 precursors are absent (Reid, 2007). A number of studies in U.K., Europe and U.S.A., have examined surface O_3 concentrations in relation to other regional air movements (Van Dop et al., 1987; Comrie & Yarnal, 1992).

Ozone concentrations also varied due to different atmospheric physical factors like simple air circulation index involving anticyclonic and cyclonic air movement has been demonstrated at Sibton, U. K.

(Davies et al., 1987). Davies et al. (1992) indicated a positive surface ozone/wind speed relationship in winter and a negative relationship in summer at Bottesford, U.K. and other European stations, which are strongly influenced by westerly winds. It has been shown by Fiore et al. (2002) and Jaffe et al. (2003) that western North America receives a background O_3 contribution from Asia and Europe, Europe receives O_3 transported from both North America and Asia (Auvray & Bey, 2005). High levels of O_3 are recorded from remote rural areas hundreds or thousands of miles away from the original sources (Prather et al., 2003). Ozone along with the precursors are found to be transported over the Pacific Ocean and occasionally reaching North America from East Asian countries (Hoell et al., 1997; Mauzerall et al., 2000; Derwent et al., 2004).

TRENDS IN TROPOSPHERIC O_3 CONCENTRATIONS: PAST, PRESENT AND FUTURE

As a secondary air pollutant, the regional mapping of O_3 concentration throughout the globe is a quite critical thing. However, researchers found that the amount of tropspheric O_3 is constantly increasing worldwide (Mittal et al., 2007; Cho et al., 2011; Rai et al, 2012). Ozone occurs naturally at low concentrations ranging from 5 to 15 ppb (Marenco et al., 1994). The earliest O_3 measurements began in mid-1800s when more than 300 stations recorded O_3 concentrations in different parts of Europe and USA. However, the continuity of O_3 monitoring was maintained only at a few stations and hence long term data are limited. These data indicated towards a general indication of what the natural background levels of O_3 would be in the absence of significant anthropogenic influences.

Ozone Concentration Around the Globe

Ozone concentrations around the globe showed a diverse picture. Evaluation of daily O_3 concentrations over Athens over a period of 1901- 1940 gives a range of about 20 ppb (Varotsos & Cartalis, 1991). Measurements from Great Lakes area of North America yielded an average daily maximum of approximately 19 ppb in the late 19th century (Bojkov, 1986). European measurements between 1850s and 1900 were found to be in the range of 17 -23 ppb approximately (Bojkov, 1986). Using O_3 data collected at Montsouris, France, between 1876 and 1910, Volz and Kley (1988) reported an annual average range between 5- 16 ppb over a period of 11 ppb. Background O_3 concentrations have more than doubled in the last century (Meehl et al., 2007) and there are also evidences of increase in annual mean values ranging from 0.1 to 1 ppb per year (Coyle et al., 2003). In UK, O_3 concentrations are predicted to reach 30- 40 ppb in rural areas resulting in doubling of AOT40 values by 2030 (Coyle et al., 2003). Clean Air Status and Trends Network (CASTNet, 2004) recorded O_3 concentrations from 11 National Parks in USA (designated as protected areas) and showed that annual medians at US parks ranged from 13 to 47 ppb, while maxima ranged from 49 to 109 ppb (CASTNet, 2004). In Canada, Canadian Air and Precipitation Network (CAPMoN) has recorded annual median O_3 concentrations at Canadian background sites ranging between 23 to 34 ppb, while annual maxima ranged from 63 to 108 ppb (Vingarzan, 2004). A Community Multiscale Air Quality Model has calculated highest O_3 concentrations ranging from 55 to 70 ppb during May and June in the boundary layer over East China and Japan (Yamaji et al., 2006). Rate of increase of tropospheric O_3 concentrations over East Asia is larger than in any other area of Northern mid latitudes (Akimoto et al., 1994; Kaneyasu et al., 2000). This unusual increase can be attributed to increased anthropogenic emissions of O_3 precursors released from rapidly emerging industrialized Asian continent (Hoell et al., 1997). O_3, along with the precursors are transported over the Pacific Ocean and occasionally reaching North America (Hoell et al., 1997; Mauzerall et al., 2000; Derwent et al., 2004).

India: A Future O_3 Hot Spot

Very few systematic data of O_3 monitoring are available in spite of the favourable climatic conditions for O_3 formation in the country. At Varanasi, situated in northern India, mean O_3 concentrations were 34.68 ppb during 1989 - 1991 (Pandey et al., 1992), 45 to 48 ppb during 1999 - 2001 (Agrawal et al., 2003), 45.18 to 62.35 ppb during summer and 28.55 to 44.25 ppb during winter from 2002 to 2006 (Tiwari et al., 2008), and 41.65 to 54.2 ppb during 2006 - 2007 (Singh et al., 2009). Daytime O_3 concentration at an urban site in Delhi varied between 9.4 to 128.3 ppb in 1991 (Varshney & Aggarwal, 1992) and between 34 to 126 ppb during winter in 1993 (Singh et al., 1997). An annual average daytime O_3 concentration of 27 ppb was reported at Pune, an urban site situated in western India between August 1991 to July 1992 (Khemani et al., 1995). Lal et al. (2000) reported that daytime mean O_3 concentration rarely exceeded 80 ppb at an urban site at Ahemedabad situated in western India from 1991 to 1995. Ozone concentrations varying from 40 - 50 ppb were recorded from an urban and rural site in Maharashtra, India during 2001- 2005 (Debaye & Kakade, 2009). Using chemical transport model named HANK, Mittal et al. (2007) calculated that 8 h daily average O_3 concentration varied between 33 - 40 ppb in Varanasi during February to April, 2000. Roy et al. (2009) used a REMO - CTM model to study the distribution of AOT40 (accumulated exposure to ozone above a threshold of 40 ppb) over the Indian region and observed high AOT40 values, exceeding the threshold set by WHO (3 ppm.h for 3 months) for agricultural crops over most of the fertile Indo Gangetic Plains. Elevated monthly AOT40 values for O_3 were found between November and May, while highest value was recorded in March over Pune (Roy et al., 2009). Regular measurements over a period of 6 months (November to April, 2003) have also shown that AOT40 values for O_3 exceeded up to 36 ppm.h, which is almost 3.6 times the critical level set for the protection of forests (Roy et al., 2009). In India, the number of measurement centers performing valid and long term representative measurements of surface O_3 and their precursors is too small. Recently a new grided emission inventory of O_3 precursors over Indian geographical region has been prepared by Roy et al. (2008).

TROPOSPHERIC OZONE AND PLANT LIFE

Since O_3 entry through the leaf cuticle is negligible, stomata play a fundamental role in determining the flux of O_3 in to the apoplastic region of the plants (Kerstein & Lendzian, 1989; Leitao et al., 2003). The flux of O_3 from troposphere into the plants depends on different resistances at various levels, i.e.- aerodynamic resistance depending on atmospheric resistance boundary layer resistance caused by a layer of laminar air adjacent to the leaves, the stomatal resistance exerted by the stomatal pores and an internal resistance of the plants (Guderian, 1985). The sensitivity of plants to O_3 depends upon their stomatal response. Since O_3 exposure generally results in decline in stomatal aperture, plants that show more rapid stomatal closure are reported to be more resistant in population level studies (Winner et al., 1997). However, O_3 induced declines in stomatal apertures may be of limited protective value, since stomatal closure is generally a consequence of damage to photosynthetic apparatus (Farage & Long, 1995). Martin et al.

(2000) modelled the data from earlier literature and showed that in most of the cases, stomatal aperture caused by acute O_3 exposure can be predicted by changes occurring in the mesophyll photosynthesis. After entering through stomata, O_3 can directly react with the plasma membrane through 'ozonolysis' or it can be converted into reactive oxygen species (ROS) and hydrogen peroxide (H_2O_2), which can alter cellular functions causing cell death, premature senescence, and the up- or down-regulation of specific genes (Long et al., 2002; Fiscus et al., 2005). In the chloroplast, O_3-induced responses could directly or indirectly impair the light and dark reactions of photosynthesis (Fiscus et al., 2005). Different studies indicate that O_3 damages the photosynthetic machinery leading to a progressive loss in the amount as well as activity of ribulose-1,5-bisphosphate carboxylase/oxygenase (RuBisCO) (Agrawal et al., 2002; Cho et al., 2008). Miller et al. (1999) reported that O_3 specifically induced 12 senescence-related genes in *Arabidopsis thaliana* (ecotype Lansberg *erecta*) leading to premature senescence. It should be noted that the O_3-induced early senescence involves many genes associated with natural senescence in *Arabidopsis*. Therefore, the harmful effects of O_3 on the plant have normally been attributed to foliar injuries leading to early senescence; decreases in light interception and photosynthesis, consequent reductions in assimilate availability and alterations at the gene and protein levels.

Effect of O_3 on Lower Group of Plants

Most of the studies in present days were mainly concerned with the higher plants. Though, O_3 can cause severe harm to lower group of plants also. Frederick and Heath (1970), exposed photosynthetic green algae *Chlorella sorokiniana* var pacificensis to a controlled O_3 exposure (2.6 μ moles min^{-1} O_3 was supplied to the medium) and observed an exponential decline in its viability. They also observed that, this decline in cell viability was highly correlated with the production of malondialdehyde, arising from the oxidative break down of unsaturated fatty acid material. Paralkar and Edzwald (1996), observed that, lower dose of O_3 generally increased the release of extra-cellular organic matter (EOM) in algae but the same O_3 in higher concentration affects the structure of EOM (by lowering the molecular size) which may hinder in subsequent coagulation. Plummer and Edzwald (2001), in their experiment with two different algae (*Scenedesmus* sp. and *Cyclotella* sp.), found that ozone exposure in the culture of respective algae increased the production of chloroform and chlorinated haloacetic acid (HAA). According to them, a pre-ozonation with 1mgL^{-1} O_3 has increased chloroform formation from *Scenedesmus* sp. by $17 - 44\%$ and from *Cyclotella* sp. by $5 - 26\%$. Chlorinated HAA also increased by $38 - 78\%$ for *Cyclotella* sp. 3mg L^{-1} pre-ozonation. In their study, they also reported that SEM studies revealed severe cell alterations in *Scenedesmus* sp. after O_3 exposure. Plummer and Edzwald (2002), in another report, showed that O_3 improved the coagulation of *Scenedesmus* sp. Chen et al. (2009) also found the same type of results in their study and concluded that, O_3 not only improved the coagulation but it also increased the cell lyses in algae.

Effect of O_3 on Higher Group of Plants: Mainly Agricultural Crops

Physiological Responses

Tropospheric O_3 and their generated ROS are known to alter membrane properties and membrane bound organelles like chloroplast, which may lead to destruction of photosynthetic pigments, and thus ultimately affect photosynthetic activity. Accelerated chlorophyll destruction is reported due to induced metabolic changes within the plant cells caused by oxidative force of O_3 (Rai et al., 2011). Several studies have suggested chlorophyll content of leaves as an indicator of stress under O_3 exposure (Sarkar & Agrawal, 2010; Leitao et al., 2007). Total chlorophyll content decreased significantly by 14, 32, 52 and 47% at elevated levels of O_3 i.e 74, 86, 100 and 124 ppb, respectively in maize plants (Leitao et al., 2007). In a study with 20 cultivars of wheat, Biswas et al. (2008) found 24-35% reductions in total chlorophyll content in recent cultivars and 3- 12% in older cultivars of wheat exposed to 82 ppb O_3 for 7 h day^{-1} over 21 days in OTCs suggesting that recent cultivars are more sensitive than older ones. Similar finding was also reported by Pleijel et al. (2006) with two wheat cultivars, one modern cultivar "Dragon" and another 100-year-old "Lantvete" when exposed to 57 ppb of O_3 (non-filtered chamber receiving elevated O_3) compared to 9 ppb O_3 (filtered chamber). It was found that O_3 induced decline in flag leaf chlorophyll content tended to proceed at a faster rate in "Dragon" compared with Lantvete. Reduction in chlorophyll content is known to reflect the activation of leaf senescence. The degradation of chloroplastic absorbing pigments might be an adaptive response to limit the production of ROS mainly driven in chloroplasts by excess absorption in photosynthetic apparatus (Herbinger et al., 2002).

Carotenoids are vital photoprotective agents, which prevent photoxidative chlorophyll destruction (Singh et al., 2009). Carotenoid content also reduced due to oxidative destruction under O_3 stress, leading to a decreased capacity to protect photosystems against photo oxidation (Singh et al., 2009). Hence, the loss of chlorophyll and carotenoids can produce a decrease in the light absorbing capacity to develop thermal dissipation energy under O_3 exposures (Singh et al., 2009).

Several studies have indicated that an early or primary response to O_3 in leaves is an interference with photosynthesis, carbohydrate metabolism, partitioning of photosynthetic products between mobile and stored pools in the leaf, and/or the translocation of photosynthate within the plants. Reductions in Ps have been widely reported under ambient field conditions at higher concentrations of air pollutants (Feng et al., 2011; Akhtar et al., 2011; Rai et al., 2011) Meta data analyses of heat, soybean and rice varieties (Feng & Kobayashi, 2009) showed varying degrees of negative response of photosynthesis under O_3 exposure. Tropospheric ozone also reduces assimilation by decreasing leaf longevity and increasing senescence in wheat plants grown in NFCs compared to FCs (Rai et al., 2011). Loss of assimilation capacity was attributed to reduced carboxylation efficiency, which can be directly related to loss of Rubisco activity. Ozone affects the synthesis as well as leads to the degradation of Rubisco due to its oxidation (Agrawal et al., 2002). Non denatured Rubisco has a large number of free- sulphydryl (-SH) residues and these groups are responsible for maintaining the correct structural conformation of Rubisco. Ozone induced oxidation of SH groups in Rubisco could alter the structural conformation of this enzyme, resulting in reduced catalytic activity and increased vulnerability (Agrawal et al., 2002).

Ozone caused reduction in the level of RNA transcript for the small subunit (rbcS) of Rubisco and also decreased the expression of photosynthetic genes for Rubisco and Rubisco activase (Feng et al., 2008). Ozone led to reductions in m RNA levels of both small (rbcS) and large (rbcL) subunits of Rubisco in wheat (Sarkar et al., 2010). In a proteomic analysis conducted under in- vivo condition on rice seedlings exposed to O_3 (40, 80, 120 ppb for 6 h d^{-1} for 9 d), reductions in expression of Rubisco large subunit (LSU) and small subunit (SSU) were reported (Feng et al., 2008). Agrawal et al. (2002) found that O_3 imposes a negative effect on energy metabolism by altering gene expression of enzymes involved in energy metabolism i.e. fructose bisphosphate aldolasechloroplast P and ATP synthase beta subunit. This leads to reduction in ATP production through photophosphorylation and thus affects the Calvin cycle in photosynthesis. Similar findings of reductions in expression of large subunit (LSU) and small subunit (SSU) of Rubisco were observed in rice cultivars Shivani and Malviya dhan 36 grown in

NFCs at a rural site of Varanasi at 20 ppb above ambient O_3 level (51ppb) under natural field conditions (Sarkar and Agrawal, 2010).

Sarkar et al. (2010) reported more reductions in Ps in sensitive cultivar of wheat than tolerant cultivar, which also showed higher reduction in g_s suggesting more stomatal closure to avoid O_3 uptake. Response of rice cultivars showed a contrasting trend as sensitive cultivar NDR 97 showed higher Ps rate and more reductions in g_s compared to Saurabh 950, a tolerant cultivar (Rai and Agrawal, 2008).

Biswas et al. (2008) and Pleijel et al. (2006) found that modern or cultivated species demonstrated higher O_3 flux as shown by increased g_s resulting in higher relative reduction in Ps than wild/old species of wheat. Two cultivars of clover exposed to 150 ppb for 3 h showed 37% reduction in Ps and 38% in g_s in *Trifolium repens*, a sensitive cultivar while tolerant cultivar *T. pretense* did not show any change in Ps and g_s suggesting that tolerant cultivar performed better due to better ability of photosynthetically active mesophyll cells to cope up with photo oxidative stress (Degl' Innocenti et al., 2003). Similar findings were also recorded in two tomato genotypes 93.1033/1 and Cuor di Bue exposed to O_3 (150 ppb for 3.5 h) (Degl'Innocenti et al., 2007). Among bush bean cultivars, exposed with 160 ppb O_3 for 3 h, higher reduction in Ps was recorded in sensitive cultivar (36%) while no change was recorded in tolerant cultivar (Guidi et al., 2009). Rice cultivars (Sufi and Bijoy) of Bangladesh ozone at 60 and 100 ppb concentrations reduced Ps rate by 27.6- 39.9% in Sufi and Bijoy cultivar suggesting no variation in sensitivity. Feng et al. (2011) exposed wheat cultivars at 27% higher ambient O_3 (52.1 ppb for 7 h) on wheat cultivars Yanmai 16 (Y 16) and Yangfumai 2 (Y 2) after flag leaf development and found significant reductions in Ps rate and stomatal conductance in Y2.

The reduction in photosynthesis may also occur due to structural damage of thylakoids, which affects the photosynthetic transport of electron, indicated as reduction in Fv/Fm ratio. Reduction of Fv/Fm ratio indicates an alteration of PS II photochemistry associated with a sign of photoinhibition, making plants more sensitive to light. Lowering of Fv/Fm ratio is observed in lettuce cv Vallaolid (2.5%) and Morella (2.6%) at mean O_3 concentration of 60 ppb (Calatayud and Barreno, 2004). Fv/Fm ratio reduced by:

- 12% in white clover sensitive clone (NC-S) at 200 ppb O_3 for 5 h d^{-1} (Francini et al., 2007),
- by 9.3% in snap bean cv S 156 at 60 ppb O_3 (Flowers et al., 2009), and
- by 5.4% in wheat cv M 234 at mean O_3 concentration of 42.4 ppb (Rai et al., 2007).

Ishii et al. (2005) also found lowering of Fv/Fm ratio in rice cv. MR 84 and MR 185, at low, medium and high O_3 doses of 27, 55 and 87 ppb.

The reduction in Fm under ambient O_3 levels is ascribed to decline in the ability to reduce the primary acceptor Q_A and associated increase in non- photochemical quenching. Reductions recorded in variable fluorescence (Fv) are more strongly correlated with lowering of Fm, suggesting impairment of an electron transport, which involves a recombination reaction between P 680 and reduced phaeophytin (Phaeo$^-$) within photosystem II (PS II) or directly affecting a PS II antenna system (Ishii et al., 2005). Degl Innocenti et al. (2003) exposed *T. repens* and *T. pretense* to 150 ppb O_3 for 3 h and maximum reductions in Fm and Fo was recorded in sensitive cultivar *T. pretense* (28 and 13.2%). But, after post fumigation recovery in Fv/Fm ratio was observed in *T. repense* and no recovery in *T. pretense*. Under O_3 exposure, there are several reports for increase in Fo and a parallel decrease in Fm on wheat (Rai et al., 2007) and rice (Rai and Agrawal, 2008) suggesting impairment of PS II activity due to the inability of the reduced plastoquinone acceptor Q_A to oxidize completely because of retardation of the electron flow through PS II or to the separation of light harvesting chl a/b protein complexes. This effect may be due to the inhibition of Calvin cycle activity as indicated by the reduction in CO_2 assimilation rates, signifying that O_3 increased excitation pressure on PS II reaction centres and thus decreased the possibility of e⁻ transport from PS II to PS I (Sarkar et al., 2010).

Biochemical Response

After O_3 exposure there is a need to tune the level of ROS produced to achieve a positive cell reaction through the signaling cascade without inducing uncontrolled cell death. As ROS are physiologically generated from various sources during cell metabolism, plants have evolved very efficient enzymatic and non- enzymatic antioxidant defense system, capable of detoxifying substantial amount of these reactive oxygen species. The antioxidant defence system plays a fundamental role in determining the cell fate, not only by keeping ROS level under control, but also acting as a central component of the cell redox balance and of the signaling modulation.

The first line of defence against O_3 derived ROS is the apoplast, where ascorbate (ASC) is believed to provide important protection from the oxidative injury. The O_3 induced changes in apoplast ascorbate and redox state was first reported in 1996 (Ranieri et al., 2000). Ranieri et al. (1996) showed that enhanced apoplast ascorbate level, while intracellular concentration did not vary markedly, supporting the hypothesis of an O_3 induced stimulation of ASC synthesis followed by active export to the apoplast in young asymptomatic and mature symptomatic leaves of pumpkin exposed to 150 ppb O_3 (5 h d⁻¹, 5 days). The protective role of ASC as ROS scavenger is also supported by the enhanced O_3^- sensitivity shown by mutant deficient in ASC (Conklin et al., 1996). The importance of ascorbic acid is demonstrated in the VTC 1 mutant of *Arabidopsis* where low ascorbic acid (AA) content in leaf tissue was associated with increased O_3 sensitivity. There is also evidence that O_3 tolerant genotypes have elevated AA content (Burkey et al., 2000, Robinson and Britz, 2000). Burkey and Eason (2002) exposed three cultivars i.e. Tendrette and Provider (O_3 tolerant) and Oregon-91 (O_3 sensitive) and four experimental lines R 123, R 142, S 144 and S 156 of snap bean (*Phaseolus vulgaris* L.) to 75 ppb O_3 for 12 h and found higher levels of leaf apoplast ASC in O_3 tolerant genotypes relative to sensitive lines. Higher apoplast AA/ASC_T ratio was found in O_3 tolerant cultivars than sensitive lines suggesting greater capacity for transport of DHA (dehydroascorbate) from the apoplast into the cytoplasm.

Leaf ascorbic acid content and redox status were compared in O_3 tolerant (Provider) and O_3 sensitive (S 156) genotypes of snap bean exposed to 71 ppb O_3 in open top chambers (OTCs) for 10 days in mature leaves early in the morning (06:00- 08:00 h) or in the afternoon (13:00- 15:00 h) (Burkey et al., 2003). Results showed that total ascorbate content [AA+ DHA] of leaf tissue was 28% higher in tolerant genotype compared to sensitive ones, exhibiting that tolerant cultivar (Provider) maintains total ascorbate content under O3 stress and level of apoplastic ascorbate were significantly higher in the afternoon than early morning for both genotypes. Rai and Agrawal (2008) found higher ascorbic acid content in sensitive cultivar of rice NDR- 97 compared to tolerant cultivar Saurabh 950 exposed to ambient O_3 concentration of 35.5 ppb grown in OTCs. Higher ascorbic acid content was observed in tolerant soybean cultivar PK 472 compared to sensitive cultivar Bragg at 70 and 100 ppb O_3 for 4 h from germination to maturity. Feng et al. (2010) showed that leaf apoplastic ascorbate content was 33.5% higher in tolerant wheat cultivar Y2 exposed to elevated O_3 concentration (83.8 ppb) which was 27% higher than the ambient O_3 concentration (66 ppb). Since, ASC is synthesized inside the cells and the oxidized form must be transported back into symplast to be re- reduced, the transport rate across the plasma membrane must be taken into account when discussing the antioxidative capacity of apoplastic ASC in the detoxification of

O_3. Burkey and Eason (2002) showed that transport of DHA from the apoplast into the cytoplasm was higher in tolerant genotypes of snapbean than sensitive lines.

The antioxidant role played by ASC depends mainly on the cell ability to maintain it in a reduced state and it occurs at the cost of reduced glutathione (GSH) by monodehydroascorbate reductase (MDHAR) or dehydroascorbate reductase (DHAR). Glutathione is generated by glutathione reductase (GR) at the expense of NADPH oxidation in Halliwell- Asada cycle. Among the tobacco cvs Bel B and Bel W3 known for their differential sensitivity to O_3, reductions in the chloroplastic GR mRNA was recorded in Bel W3 at exposure of 150 ppb to O_3 for 5 h (Pasqualini et al., 2001). Ascorbate may act as reducing substrate for ascorbate peroxidase (APX), which is one of the most efficient ROS scavenging systems. In sunflower, increased level of extracellular APX activity may contribute to avoid the buildup of toxic H_2O_2 concentrations (Ranieri et al., 2003). The higher constitutive APX activity measured in a resistant white clover clone with respect to a sensitive clone was further enhanced following long term exposure to O_3 (60 ppb for 5 h d^{-1} for 56 days). Sarkar et al. (2010) reported increase in APX and GR activities in wheat cultivars exposed to elevated O_3

Genome and Proteome Response

Over the years, many integrated and individual studies on O_3 stress responses have been reported in several plant species, and such studies have used typical research approaches. Although the demonstration of complicated mechanisms of O_3 response in plants has been attempted, much work still remains to be done in this area. In recent years, analyses have been performed to obtain information on O_3-triggered responses in plants; to this end, many high-throughput 'omics' approaches were performed in:

- *Arabidopsis* (Mahalingam et al. 2006; Tamaoki et al. 2003),
- Bean (Torres et al. 2007),
- Maize (Torres et al. 2007),
- Pepper (Lee and Yun 2006),
- Rice (Agrawal et al. 2002; Cho et al. 2008), and
- Wheat (Sarkar et al., 2010).

However, as the present chapter mainly deals with the agricultural crops; in following section we will discuss about the '-*omics*' responses of some important crops under O_3 stress.

Among all the major crops, rice (*Oryza sativa* L.) has been studied most for its response to O_3-stress (Agrawal et al., 2002; Cho et al., 2008, Feng et al., 2008; Frei et al., 2010). Agrawal et al. (2002) first reported a detailed combined trancriptomics and proteiomics response of rice plants under elevated O_3-exposure. Two weeks old rice (*cv.* Nipponbare) seedlings were exposed to 200 ppb of O_3 for three days in a controlled fumigation chambers. A drastic visible necrotic damage in O_3-exposed leaves and consequent increase in ascorbate peroxidase protein(s) accompanied by rapid changes in the immune-blotting analysis and 2-DE protein profiles were observed. They also reported nearly 52 differentially expressed proteins; among which, O_3 caused drastic reductions in the major leaf photosynthetic proteins, including the abundantly present ribulose-1, 5-bisphosphate carboxylase/oxygenase (Rubisco) and induction of various defense/stress related proteins. Most prominent change in the rice leaves, within 24 h post-treatment with O_3, was:

- The induced accumulation of a pathogenesis related (PR) class 5 protein,
- Three PR 10 class proteins, ascorbate peroxidase(s),
- Superoxide dismutase,
- Calcium-binding protein,
- Calreticulin, a novel ATP-dependent CLP protease, and
- An unknown protein.

Feng et al. (2008) also followed similar experimental model with two weeks old rice seedlings exposed at 0, 40, 80 and 120 ppb O_3 for nine days. A drastic damage in the photosynthetic proteins, mainly – large and small sub units of RuBisCO, and primary metabolism related proteins; but an induced expression of some major antioxidant, like - glutathione S transferase and Mn superoxide dismutase, and defense / stress related proteins, like - pathogenesis-related (PR) class 5 protein (PR5) and two PR10 proteins OsPR10/PBZ1 and RSOsPR10 were reported. Feng et al. (2008) also confirmed that the damage in rice proteome is strictly O_3-dose dependent. In another independent study, Cho et al (2008) also checked the expression profiles of genes in leaves of two weeks old rice seedlings exposed to 200 ppb O_3 for 1, 12 and 24 h using a 22K rice DNA microarray chip. A total of 1535 genes were differentially expressed more than fivefold over the control. Their functional categories suggested that genes involved in transcription, pentose phosphate pathway and signal transduction at 1h, and genes related to antioxidant enzymes, ribosomal protein, post-translational modification (PTM), signal transduction, jasmonate, ethylene and secondary metabolism at 12 and 24h play a crucial role in O_3- response (Cho et al., 2008). Recently, Frei et al. (2010) have tried to identify the possible mechanism of O_3-response in rice seedlings by characterizing two important quantitative trait loci (QTL), in two different chromosome segment substitution lines (SL15 and SL41); and demonstrated that the activity of some major antioxidant genes might contribute significantly in the response strategy of rice plant under higher O_3-stress.

In contrast with the above laboratory based experimental models, Sarkar and Agrawal (2010b) had applied '*field based integrated –omics*' approach to understand the background of O_3 response in two high yielding cultivars (*Malviya dhan 36* and *Shivani*) of mature rice plants under natural conditions; and, found dependable phenotypical response, in the form of foliar injury, followed by definite changes in leaf proteome. Major damage in the photosynthetic, like – large and small sub units of Rubisco, and primary metabolism related proteins; but an induced expression of some antioxidant and defense / stress related proteins in rice leaf proteome were reported.

Wheat (*Triticum aestivum* L.) is the third most important crop around the globe, and nearly two third of the world population depends on this crop for their primary nutrition supplement. Sarkar et al. (2010) recently employed '*field based integrated –omics*' approach to understand the background of O_3 response in two wheat cultivars (cvs Sonalika and HUW 510) against elevated O_3 concentrations (ambient + 10 and 20 ppb) under near natural conditions using OTCs. Results of their study showed drastic reductions in the abundantly present Rubisco large and small subunits. Western blot analysis confirmed induced accumulation of antioxidative enzymes like superoxide dismutase and ascorbate peroxidase protein(s) and common defense/stress-related thaumatin-like protein(s). 2-DGE analysis revealed a total of 38 differentially expressed protein spots, common in both the wheat cultivars. Among those, some major leaf photosynthetic proteins (including Rubisco and Rubisco activase) and important energy metabolism proteins (including ATP synthase, aldolase, and phosphoglycerate kinase) were drastically reduced, whereas some stress/defense-related proteins (such as harpin-binding protein and germin-like protein) were induced.

Maize (*Zea mays* L.) is another important crop at global context. Being a C$_4$ crop, its response to climate change has been always bit different from the others. Torres et al. (2007) have done detailed investigation of O$_3$ response in maize (cv. Guarare 8128) plants through gel based 'omics' approaches. In that experiment, 16-day-old maize plants (grown in controlled environment at green house) were exposed to 200 ppb O$_3$ for 72 h., and then the response was compared with a controlled plant (grown under filtered pollutant-free air). Results showed that nearly 12 protein spots were differentially expressed under O$_3$ exposure, and can be exploited as marker proteins. Expression levels of catalase (increased), SOD (decreased), and APX (increased) were drastically changed by O$_3$ depending on the leaf stage, whereas cross-reacting heat-shock proteins (HSPs; 24 and 30 kDa) and naringenin-7-*O*-methyltransferase (NOMT; 41 kDa) proteins were strongly increased in O$_3$-stressed younger leaves. The study also enumerated leaf injury as bio-marker under O$_3$ stress in maize leaves.

Torres et al. (2007) also conducted a study on response of cultivated bean (*Phaseolus vulgaris* L. cv. IDIAP R-3) against O$_3$ stress using the same experimental protocol, and the effects were evaluated through integrated 'omics' approach using gel-based proteomics followed by MS and immunoblotting. Results showed that in bean leaves two SOD proteins (19 and 20 kDa) were dramatically decreased, while APX (25 kDa), small HSP (33 kDa) and a NOMT (41 kDa) were increased after O$_3$ fumigation.

Lee and Yun (2006) applied cDNA microarrays to monitor the transcriptome of ozone stress-regulated genes (ORGs) in two pepper cultivars [*Capsicum annuum* cv. Dabotop (O$_3$-sensitive) and cv. Buchon (O$_3$-tolerant)]. Ozone stress up- or down-regulated 180 genes more than three-fold with respect to their controls. Transcripts of 84 ORGs increased, transcripts of 88 others diminished, and those of eight either accumulated or diminished at different time points in the two cultivars or changed in only one of the cultivars. 67% (120) of the ORGs were regulated differently in O$_3$-sensitive and ozone-tolerant pepper cultivars, most being specifically up-regulated in the O$_3$-sensitive cultivar.

Tripathi et al. (2010) analyzed the response of linseed plants under elevated O$_3$-stress through combined genomics and proteomics approaches. The results showed that 10 ppb elevation over ambient O$_3$ concentration can cause 50% damage in the genome stability of linseed plants. In line to the genome response, leaf proteome also got severely affected under O$_3$-stress, and the damages were mainly found on the photosynthetic and primary metabolism related proteins.

Growth and Yield Response

Tropospheric O$_3$ was found to adversely affect the growth and yield of a variety of agricultural plants. Tropospheric O$_3$ reduced the marketable yield of a range of crop species even in the absence of visible injury, primarily through its effects in reducing photosynthetic rates and accelerating leaf senescence (Ashmore, 2005). Cultivar sensitivity was evaluated on the basis of experiments conducted in open top chambers (Sarkar et al., 2010) and FACE experiments (Zhu et al., 2011).

In Pakistan, 29- 47% yield reductions were reported for 6 varieties of wheat (Maggs et al., 1995; Wahid et al., 1995), 28- 42% for two varieties of rice (Wahid et al., 1995) and 37- 46% for 2 varieties of soybean (Wahid, 2006) due to different pollutants in the ambient air. Exposure of O$_3$ at 80 ppb concentration for 1.5 h daily for 30 days showed yield reductions of:

- 29.5% in *Vicia faba*, 20.6% in *Oryza sativa*,
- 13% in *Panicum miliaceum,* and
- 9.7% in *Cicer arietinum* (Agrawal, 2005).

Differential responses were recorded among different crops and their cultivars. Maximum reductions were found in soybean (40- 60%) followed by wheat (20- 40%), rice (10- 20%) and minimum in barley (Feng & Kobayashi, 2009). Studies by Emberson et al. (2009), Feng and Kobayashi (2009) and Mills et al. (2007) found same trend of sensitivity, reporting legumes to be most sensitive and barley to be most resistant under O_3 exposure.

In open top chamber studies, wheat and soybean cultivars were studied extensively. Ozone exposure 70 and 100 ppb for 4 h d^{-1} for 70 days led to reductions in yield by 13.9 and 10% and 33.5 and 25% in soybean cv PK 472 and Bragg (Singh et al., 2010). The yield reductions in wheat cv HP 1209 and M 234 at O_3 concentration of 70 and 100 ppb for 4 h daily for 70 days were 8 and 4.7 and 17 and 15.5%, respectively (Agrawal, 2005). Rai et al. (2007) found 20.7% reductions in yield of wheat cv M 234 grown in chambers ventilated with ambient air (40.6 ppb) as compared to filtered chamber. Analysing the cultivar sensitivity response, Sarkar and Agrawal (2010) found reductions of 7, 16.7 and 22% in wheat cv. Sonalika and 8.4, 18.5 and 25% in cultivar HUW 510 grown in NFCs (45.3 ppb), NFCLOs (50.4 ppb) and NFCHOs (55.6 ppb) compared to FCs. Rai and Agrawal (2008) reported yield reductions of 10 and 14% in rice cultivars Saurabh 950 and NDR 97 at ambient O_3 concentration of 35.5 ppb grown in open top chambers. Among soybean cultivars, highest reduction in yield was recorded in Forrest under O_3 exposure as compared to Essex (Robinson and Britz, 2000). In SoyFACE experiment, 10 soybean cultivars were exposed to ambient (46.3 and 37.9 ppb) and elevated (46.3 and 37.9) O_3 concentrations in 2007- 2008. Yield reductions varied from 11.3- 36.8% in 2007 and 7.5- 16% in 2008 in ambient and elevated O_3 levels and the yield response relationships also indicated that Loda and Pana were tolerant and IA 3010 was sensitive (Betzbergler). Zhu *et al.* (2011) exposed four winter wheat cultivars (Yannog 19, Yangmai 16, Yangmain 15 and Yangfumai 2) under elevated O_3 with a FACE system from 2007 to 2009 with mean O_3 levels of 56.9 ppb for 7 h in 2006- 2007, 57.6 ppb in 2007- 2008 and 57.3 ppb for 2008- 2009. The grain yield reductions recorded were 18.7, 34.7 and10.1% in Y 19 in three consecutive years of O_3 exposure from 2006 to 2009.

Morgan et al. (2003) showed that a 23% increase in O_3 from an average daytime ambient level of 56 ppb to 69 ppb, will lead to 20% more reduction in soybean yield. Feng and Kobayashi (2009) calculated that at projected O_3 concentration (51- 75 ppb), the yield losses would be 10% more for soybean, wheat and rice and 20% more for bean than at present ambient level of O_3 (41- 40 ppb), thus predicting that future rise in O_3 is a significant threat to food production in the world.

CONCLUSION

On the basis of different studies conducted worldwide using different study approaches such as open top chambers (OTCs) and FACE experiments showed economic losses varies from Rs.1972- 77,055 in major crops. Rai et al. (2011) reported economic loss of Rs 1,208- 30,550 ha^{-1} for major agricultural crops wheat, rice, mustard, urd, soybean, pea and mungbean grown at ambient O_3 using different studies approach like and field transect study (FTS) in India. Even, globally Van Dingenen (2009) using a global chemistry transport model a global economic loss of approximately US $ 14- 26 billion has been calculated at world market prices for the year 2000. Emberson et al. (2009) conducted modeling based studies to assess the extent and magnitude of O3 risk to agriculture suggest that yield losses of 5- 20% for important crops may be common in areas experiencing elevated O_3 concentrations and also concluded Asian grown wheat and rice cultivars are more sensitive to O3 than the North American cultivars. The economic loss for 23 horticultural and agricultural crops due to O_3 was estimated to be 3% (€ 6.7 billion) for the base year 2000 (Holland et al., 2006). But with the scenario of implementation of current legislation, the overall loss of all crop species is estimated to be 2% (€ 4.5 billion) for 2020 (Holland et al., 2006). The scenario is however, entirely different for Asia due to tremendous increase in anthropogenic activities and rapid expansion of economy, leading an increased emission of O_3 precursors.

ACKNOWLEDGMENT

AS acknowledges the financial assistance from University Grant Commission, New Delhi, GoI, and University of Gour Banga, Malda, India.

REFERENCES

Auvray, M., & Bey, I. (2005). Long-range transport to Europe: Seasonal variations and implications for the European ozone budget. *Journal of Geophysical Research, 110*.

Avol, E. L., Linn, W. S., Venet, T. G., Shamoo, D. A., & Hackney, J. D. (1984). Comparative respiratory effects of ozone and ambient oxidant pollution exposure during heavy exercise. *Journal of the Air Pollution Control Association, 31*, 666–668. PMID:6481003

Bates, L. S., Waldren, R. P., & Teare, I. D. (1973). Rapid determination of free proline for water stress studies. *Plant and Soil, 39*(1), 205–207. doi:10.1007/BF00018060

Beauchamp, C., & Fridovich, I. (1971). Superoxide dismutase: Improved assays and an assay applicable to acrylamide gels. *Annals of Biochemistry, 44*(1), 276–287. doi:10.1016/0003-2697(71)90370-8 PMID:4943714

Bell, J. N. B., & Ashmore, M. R. (1986). Design and construction of open top chambers and methods of filteration (equipment and cost). In *Proceedings of II European open top chambers workshop*.

Biswas, D. K., Xu, H., Li, Y. G., Liu, M. Z., Chen, Y. H., Sun, J. Z., & Jiang, G. M. (2008b). Assessing the genetic relatedness of higher ozone sensitivity of modern wheat to its wild and cultivated progenitors/relatives. *Journal of Experimental Botany, 59*(4), 951–963. doi:10.1093/jxb/ern022 PMID:18310606

Biswas, D. K., Xu, H., Li, Y. G., Sun, J. Z., Wang, X. Z., Han, X. G., & Jiang, G. M. (2008a). Genotypic differences in leaf biochemical, physiological and growth responses to ozone in 20 winter wheat cultivars released over the past 60 years. *Global Change Biology, 14*, 46–59.

Black, V. J., Black, C. R., Roberts, J. A., & Stewart, C. A. (2000). Impact of ozone on the reproductive development of plants. *The New Phytologist, 147*, 421–447. doi:10.1046/j.1469-8137.2000.00721.x

Bojkov, R. D. (1986). Surface ozone during the second half of the nineteenth century. *Journal of Climate and Applied Meteorology, 25*(3), 343–352. doi:10.1175/1520-0450(1986)025<0343:SODTSH>2.0.CO;2

Bray, H. G., & Thorpe, W. Y. (1954). Analysis of phenolic compounds of interest in metabolism. In D. Click (Ed.), *Methods of Biochemical Analysis*. New York: Interscience Publications Inc. doi:10.1002/9780470110171.ch2

Britton, C., & Mehley, A. C. (1955). Assay of catalase and peroxidase. In S. P. Colowick & N. O. Kalpan (Eds.), *Method in enzymology* (Vol. 2, pp. 764–775). New York: Academic Press.

Calatayud, A., & Barreno, E. (2001). Chlorophyll fluorescence, antioxidant enzymes and lipid peroxidation in tomato in response to ozone and benomyl. *Environmental Pollution*, *115*(2), 283–289. doi:10.1016/S0269-7491(01)00101-4 PMID:11706801

CASTNet (Clean Air Status and Trends Network). (2004). Retrieved from http://www.epa.gov/castnet/

Chan, L. Y., & Helen Wu, W. Y. (1993). Study of bus commuter and pedestrian exposure to traffic air pollution in Hong Kong. *Environment International*, *19*, 121–132. doi:10.1016/0160-4120(93)90363-M

Chan, L. Y., Qin, Y., & Chan, C. Y. (1996). Vehicular emission exposures of public transport commuters and pedestrians in commercial districts, Hong Kong. In B. Caussade, H. Power, & C. A. Brebbiav (Eds.), Air pollution IV, Monitoring, simulation and control. Computation mechanism publication (pp. 593–600). Academic Press.

Cho, K., Shibato, J., Agrawal, G. K., Jung, Y., Kubo, A., Jwa, N.-S., & … (2008). Integrated Transcriptomics, Proteomics, and Metabolomics Analyses to Survey Ozone Responses in the Leaves of Rice Seedling. *Journal of Proteome Research*, *7*(7), 2980–2998. doi:10.1021/pr800128q PMID:18517257

Cho, K., Tiwari, S., Agrawal, S. B., Torres, N. L., Agrawal, M., Sarkar, A., & … (2011). Tropospheric ozone and plants: Absorption, responses, and consequences. *Reviews of Environmental Contamination and Toxicology*, *212*, 61–111. doi:10.1007/978-1-4419-8453-1_3 PMID:21432055

Comrie, A. C., & Yarnal, B. (1992). Relationships Between Synoptic-Scale Atmospheric Circulation and Ozone Concentrations in Metropolitan Pittsburgh, Pennsylvania. *Atmospheric Environment*, *26B*, 301–312.

Coyle, M., Flower, D., & Ashmore, M. (2003). New directions: Implications of increasing tropospheric background ozone concentrations for vegetation. *Atmospheric Environment*, *37*(1), 153–154. doi:10.1016/S1352-2310(02)00861-0

Darrall, N. M. (1989). The effect of air pollutants on physiological processes in plants. *Plant, Cell & Environment*, *12*(1), 1–30. doi:10.1111/j.1365-3040.1989.tb01913.x

Davies, T. D., Kelly, P. H., Brimblecombe, P., & Gair, A. J. (1987). Surface ozone concentrations and climate: preliminary analysis. *Prec. WMO Conference on air pollution modeling and its application* (Vol. 2). Geneva: World Meteorological Organisation.

Davies, T. D., Kelly, P. M., Low, P. S., & Pierce, C. E. (1992). Surface ozone concentrations in Europe: Link with the regional scale atmospheric circulation. *Journal of Geophysical Research*, *97*(D9), 9819–9832. doi:10.1029/92JD00419

Debaje, S. B., & Kakade, A. D. (2009). Surface ozone variability over western Maharashtra, India. *Journal of Hazardous Materials*, *161*(2-3), 686–700. doi:10.1016/j.jhazmat.2008.04.010 PMID:18486330

Degl'Innocenti, E., Guidi, L., & Soldatini, G. F. (2002). Characterization of the photosynthetic response of tobacco leaves to ozone: Carbon dioxide assimilation and chlorophyll fluorescence. *Journal of Plant Physiology*, *159*(8), 845–853. doi:10.1078/0176-1617-00519

Degl'Innocenti, E., Guidi, L., & Soldatini, G. F. (2007). Effects of elevated ozone on chlorophyll a fluorescence in symptomatic and asymptomatic leaves of two tomato genotypes. *Biologia Plantarum*, *51*(2), 313–321. doi:10.100710535-007-0061-5

Derwent, R. G., Stevenson, D. S., Collins, W. J., & Johnson, C. E. (2004). Intercontinental transport and the origins of the ozone observed at surface sites in Europe. *Atmospheric Environment*, *38*(13), 1891–1901. doi:10.1016/j.atmosenv.2004.01.008

Dubois, M., Gilles, K. A., Hamilton, J. K., Roberts, P. A., & Smith, F. (1956). Colorimetric method for determination of sugars and related substances. *Analytical Chemistry*, *28*(3), 350–356. doi:10.1021/ac60111a017

Duxbury, A. C., & Yentsch, C. S. (1956). Plankton pigment monographs. *Journal of Marine Research*, *15*, 91–101.

Emberson, L. D., Buker, P., Ashmore, M. R., Mills, G., Jackson, L. S., Agrawal, M., & ... (2009). A comparison of North- America and Asian exposure- response data for ozone effects on crop yields. *Atmospheric Environment*, *43*(12), 1945–1953. doi:10.1016/j.atmosenv.2009.01.005

FAOSTAT. (2007). *Food and Agriculture Organisation of the United Nations*. Retrieved from http://faostat.fao.org

Farage, P. K., & Long, S. P. (1995). An in vivo analusis of photosynthesis during short term ozone exposure in three contrasting species. *Photosynthesis Research*, *43*(1), 11–21. doi:10.1007/BF00029457 PMID:24306634

Feng, Z., & Kobayashi, K. (2009). Assessing the impacts of current and future concentrations of surface ozone on crop yield with meta-analysis. *Atmospheric Environment*, *43*(8), 1510–1519. doi:10.1016/j.atmosenv.2008.11.033

Feng, Z., Kobayashi, K., Wang, X., & Feng, Z. (2009). A meta-analysis of responses of wheat yield formation to elevated ozone concentration. *Chinese Science Bulletin*, *54*, 249–255.

Feng, Z. Z., Kobayashi, K., & Ainsworth, E. A. (2008). Impact of elevated ozone concentration on growth, physiology and yield of wheat (*Triticum aestivum* L.): A meta- analysis. *Global Change Biology*, *14*, 2696–2708.

Fiore, A.M., Jacob, D.J., Bey, I., Yantosca, R.M., Field, B.D., & Wilkinson, J.G. (2002). Background ozone over the United States in summer: origin and contribution to pollution episodes. *Journal of Geophysical Research*, *107*(15), ACH11-1–ACH 11-25.

Flowers, M. D., Fiscus, E. L., Burkey, K. O., Booker, F. L., & Dubois, J. J. B. (2007). Photosynthesis, chlorophyll fluorescence, and yield of snap bean (*Phaseolus vulgaris* L.) genotypes differing in sensitivity to ozone. *Environmental and Experimental Botany*, *61*(2), 190–198. doi:10.1016/j.envexpbot.2007.05.009

Fridovich, I. (1974). Superoxide Dismutase. *Advances in Enzymology*, *41*, 35–97. PMID:4371571

Heath, R. L. (2008). Modification of the biochemical pathways of plants induced by ozone: What are the varied routes to changes? *Environmental Pollution*, *155*(3), 453–463. doi:10.1016/j.envpol.2008.03.010 PMID:18456378

Heath, R. L., & Packer, L. (1968). Photoperoxidation in isolated chloroplasts. *Archives of Biochemistry and Biophysics*, *125*(1), 189–198. doi:10.1016/0003-9861(68)90654-1 PMID:5655425

HEI. (1988). *(Health Effect Institute) Air pollution. The automobile and public health*. Washington, DC: National Academic Press.

Heidenreich, B., Bieber, E., Sandermann, H., & Ernst, D. (2006). Identification of a new member of the WRKY family in tobacco. involved in ozone-induced gene regulation? *Acta Physiologiae Plantarum*, *28*(2), 117–125. doi:10.100711738-006-0038-6

Herbart, D., Philipps, P. J., & Strange, R. E. (1971). Estimation of reducing sugars. In J. R. Norries & D. W. Robbins (Eds.), *Methods in microbiology* (pp. 209–344). New York: Academic Press, London.

Hoell, J. M., Davis, D. D., Liu, S. C., Newell, R. E., Akimoto, H., McNeal, R. J., & Bendura, R. J. (1997). The Pacific Exploratory Mission- West B (PEM-West B). *Journal of Geophysical Research*, *102*(28), 223–228, 239.

Holland, M., Kinghorn, S., Emberson, L., Cinderby, S., Ashmoe, M., Mills, G., & Harmens, H. (2006). *Development of a framework for probabilistic assessment of the economic losses caused by ozone damage to crops in Europe*. CEH Project No. C02309NEW. Report to U.K. Department of Environment, Food and Rural affairs under contract 1/2/170 1/3/205.

Hunt, R. (1982). *Growth Curves*. London: Edward Arnold Publishers Ltd.

IPCC. (2007). *Climate change 2007: The Scientific Basis. Contribution of Working Group I to the Fourth Assessment Report of the Intergovernmental Panel on Climate Change*. Cambridge, UK: Cambridge University Press.

Ishii, S., Marshall, F.M., & Bell, J.N.B. (n.d.). Physiological and morphological responses of locally grown Malaysian rice cultivars (*Oryza sativa* L.) to different ozone concentrations. *Water, Air and Soil Pollution, 155*, 205-221.

Ishii, S., Marshall, F. M., Bell, J. N. B., & Abdullah, A. M. (2004). Impact of ambient air pollution on locally grown rice cultivars (*Oryza sativa* L.) in Malaysia. *Water, Air, and Soil Pollution*, *154*(1-4), 187–201. doi:10.1023/B:WATE.0000022964.55434.05

Jackson, M. L. (1958). *Soil Chemical Analysis*. New Delhi: Prentice- Hall of India Pvt. Ltd.

Jaffe, D., Price, H., Parrish, D., Goldstein, A., & Harris, J. (2003). Increasing background ozone during spring on the west coast of North America. *Geophysical Research Letters*, 30.

Jain, S. L., Arya, B. C., Kumar, A., Ghude, S. D., & Kulkarni, P. S. (2005). Observational study of surface ozone at New Delhi, India. *International Journal of Remote Sensing, 26*(16), 3515–3524. doi:10.1080/01431160500076616

Joo, J. H., Wang, S., Chen, J. G., Jones, A. M., & Fedoroff, N. V. (2005). Different signaling and cell death roles of heterotrimeric G protein a and b subunits in the *Arabidopsis* oxidative stress response to ozone. *The Plant Cell, 17*(3), 957–970. doi:10.1105/tpc.104.029603 PMID:15705948

Jorge, S. A. C., Menck, C. F. M., Sies, H., Osborne, M. R., Phillips, D. H., Sarasin, A., & Stary, A. (2002). Mutagenic fingerprint of ozone in human cells. *DNA Repair, 1*(5), 369–378. doi:10.1016/S1568-7864(02)00011-3 PMID:12509241

Kampa, M., & Castanas, E. (2008). Human health effects of air pollution. *Environmental Pollution, 151*(2), 362–367. doi:10.1016/j.envpol.2007.06.012 PMID:17646040

Kaneyasu, N., Takeuchi, K., Hayashi, M., Fujita, S. I., Uno, I., & Sasaki, H. (2000). Outflow patterns of pollutants from east Asia to the north Pacific in the winter monsoon. *Journal of Geophysical Research, 105*(D13), 17361–17377. doi:10.1029/2000JD900138

Kangasjarvi, J., Jaspers, P., & Kollist, H. (2005). Signalling and cell death in ozone-exposed plants. *Plant, Cell & Environment, 28*(8), 1021–1036. doi:10.1111/j.1365-3040.2005.01325.x

Keller, Th., & Schwager, H. (1977). Air pollution and ascorbic acid. *European Journal of Forest Pathology, 7*(6), 338–350. doi:10.1111/j.1439-0329.1977.tb00603.x

Kersteins, G., & Lendzian, K. J. (1989). Interactions between ozone and plant cuticles. 1. Ozone deposition and permeability. *The New Phytologist, 112*(1), 13–19. doi:10.1111/j.1469-8137.1989.tb00303.x

Khemani, L. T., Momin, G. A., Rao, P. S. P., Vijaykumar, R., & Safai, P. D. (1995). Study of surface ozone behaviour at urban and forested sites in India. *Atmospheric Environment, 29*(16), 2021–2024. doi:10.1016/1352-2310(94)00293-T

Khemani, L. T., Momin, G. A., Rao, P. S. P., Vijaykumar, R., & Safai, P. D. (1995). Study of ozone behaviour at urban and forested sites in India. *Atmospheric Environment, 29*(16), 2021–2024. doi:10.1016/1352-2310(94)00293-T

Kondratyev, K. Y., & Varotsos, C. A. (2001). Global tropospheric ozone dynamics-part II: numerical modeling of tropospheric ozone variability-part I: tropospheric ozone precursors. *Environment Science Pollution Research, 8*(2), 113–119. doi:10.1007/BF02987304

Krupa, S. V., & Manning, W. J. (1988). Atmospheric ozone: Formation and effects on vegetation. *Environmental Pollution, 50*(1-2), 101–137. doi:10.1016/0269-7491(88)90187-X PMID:15092655

Laemmli, U. K. (1970). Cleavage of Structural Proteins during the Assembly of the Head of. Bacteriophage T4. *Nature, 227*(5259), 680–685. doi:10.1038/227680a0 PMID:5432063

Lal, S., Naja, M., & Subbaraya, B. H. (2000). Seasonal variations in surface ozone and its precursors over an urban site in India. *Atmospheric Environment, 34*(17), 2713–2724. doi:10.1016/S1352-2310(99)00510-5

Lee, S., & Yun, S. C. (2006). The ozone stress transcriptome of pepper (Capsicum annuum L.). *Molecules and Cells, 21*, 197–205. PMID:16682813

Leitao, L., Dizengremel, P., & Biolley, J.-P. (2008). Foliar CO_2 fixation in bean (Phaseolus vulgaris L.) submitted to elevated ozone: Distinct changes in Rubisco and PEPc activities in relation to pigment content. *Ecotoxicology and Environmental Safety, 69*(3), 531–540. doi:10.1016/j.ecoenv.2006.10.010 PMID:17141868

Leitao, L., Goulas, P., & Biolley, J. P. (2003). Time-course of Rubisco oxidation in beans (*Phaseolus vulgaris* L) subjected to a long-term ozone stress. *Plant Science, 165*(3), 613–620. doi:10.1016/S0168-9452(03)00230-9

Levy, J. I., Chemerynski, S. M., & Sarnat, J. A. (2005). Ozone exposure and mortality: An empiric Bayes metaregression analysis. *Epidemiology (Cambridge, Mass.), 16*(4), 458–468. doi:10.1097/01. ede.0000165820.08301.b3 PMID:15951663

Linn, W. S., Avol, E. L., Shamoo, D. A., Spier, C. E., Valencia, L. M., Venet, T. G., & ... (1986). A dose-response study of healthy, heavily exercising men exposed to ozone at concentrations near the ambient air quality standard. *Toxicology and Industrial Health, 2*(1), 99–112. doi:10.1177/074823378600200105 PMID:3787644

Lippmann, M. (1989). Effects of ozone on respiratory function and structure. *Annual Review of Public Health, 10*(1), 49–67. doi:10.1146/annurev.pu.10.050189.000405 PMID:2655642

Long, S. P., Ainsworth, E. A., Leakey, A. D. B., & Morgan, P. B. (2005). Global food insecurity. Treatment of major food crops with elevated carbon dioxide or ozone under large-scale fully open-air conditions suggests recent models may have overestimated future yields. *Philos. T.R. Soc. B., 360*(1463), 2011–2020. doi:10.1098/rstb.2005.1749 PMID:16433090

Long, S. P., & Naidu, S. L. (2002). Effects of oxidants at biochemical, cell and physiological levels with particular reference to ozone. In J. N. B. Bell & M. Treshow (Eds.), *Air Pollution and Plant Life* (p. 69). West Sussex, UK: John Wiley & Sons Ltd.

Lowry, O. H., Rosebrough, N. J., Farr, A. L., & Randall, R. J. (1951). Protein measurement with the foliar phenol reagent. *The Journal of Biological Chemistry, 193*, 265–275. PMID:14907713

Maclachlan, S., & Zalik, S. (1963). Plastid structure, chlorophyll concentration and free amino acid composition of a chlorophyll mutant of barley. *Canadian Journal of Botany, 41*(7), 1053–1062. doi:10.1139/b63-088

Maggs, R., Wahid, A., Shamsi, S. R. A., & Ashmore, M. R. (1995). Effects of ambient air pollution on wheat and rice yield in Pakistan. *Water, Air, and Soil Pollution, 85*(3), 1311–1316. doi:10.1007/BF00477163

Mahalingam, R., Jambunathan, N., Gunjan, S. K., Faustin, E., Weng, H., & Ayoubi, P. (2006). Analysis of oxidative signaling induced by ozone in Arabidopsis thaliana. *Plant, Cell & Environment, 29*(7), 1357–1371. doi:10.1111/j.1365-3040.2006.01516.x PMID:17080957

Marenco, A. H., Gouget, P. N., & Pages, J. P. (1994). Evidence of a long term increase in tropospheric ozone from Pic Du Midi data series, consequences, positive radiative forcing. *Journal of Geophysical Research, 99*(D8), 166–177. doi:10.1029/94JD00021

Martin, M. J., Farage, P. K., Humphries, S. W., & Long, S. P. (2000). Can the stomatal changes caused by acute ozone exposure be predicted by changes occurring in the mesophyll? A simplification for models of vegetation response in tropospheric elevated ozone episodes. *Australian Journal of Plant Physiology, 27*, 211–219.

Mauzerall, D. L., Narita, D., Akimoto, H., Horowitz, L., & Waters, S. (2000). Seasonal characteristics of tropospheric ozone production and mixing ratios of East Asia: A global three-dimensional chemical transport model analysis. *Journal of Geophysical Research, 105*.

McCready, R. M., Guggolz, J., Silveira, V., & Owens, A. (1950). Determination of starch and amylose in vegetables. *Analytical Chemistry, 22*(9), 1156–1158. doi:10.1021/ac60045a016

McDonnell, W. F., Chapman, R. S., & Leigh, M. W. (1985). Respiratory responses of vigorously exercising children to 0.12 ppm ozone exposure. *The American Review of Respiratory Disease, 132*(4), 875–879. PMID:4051323

Meehl, G. A., Stocker, T. F., Collins, W. D., Friedlingstein, P., Gaye, A. T., … Zhao, Z.C. (2007). Global climate projections. In Climate Change: The Physical Science Basis. Contribution of Working Group I to the Fourth Assessment Report of the Intergovernmental Panel on Climate Change. Cambridge University Press.

Mills, G., Buse, A., Gimeno, B., Bermejo, V., Holland, M., Emberson, L., & Pleijel, H. (2007). A synthesis of AOT40-based response functions and critical levels of ozone for agricultural and horticultural crops. *Atmospheric Environment, 41*(12), 2630–2643. doi:10.1016/j.atmosenv.2006.11.016

Mittal, M. L., Hess, P. G., Jain, S. L., Arya, B. C., & Sharma, C. (2007). Surface ozone in the Indian region. *Atmospheric Environment, 41*(31), 6572–6578. doi:10.1016/j.atmosenv.2007.04.035

Rai, R., Rajput, M., Agrawal, M., et al. (n. d.). Gaseous Air Pollutants: A review on current and future trends of emissions and impact of agricultue. *Journal of Scientific Research, 55*, 72-110.

Schönbein, C. F. (1843). Ueber die Natur des eigenthümlichen Geruches, welcher sich sowohl am positiven Pole eine Säule während der Wasserelektrolyse, wie auch beim Ausströmen der gewöhnlichen Elektricität aus Spitzen entwickelt. *Ann. Phys. Chem., 1843*(59), 240-55.

Varotsos, C., & Cartalis, C. (1991). Re-evaluation of surface ozone over Athens, Greece, for the period 1901–1940. *Atmospheric Research, 26*(4), 303–310. doi:10.1016/0169-8095(91)90024-Q

Varotsos, C., Cartalis, C., Vlamakis, A., Tzanis, C., & Keramitsoglou, I. (2004). The long term coupling between column ozone and tropopause properties. *Journal of Climate, 17*(19), 3843–3854. doi:10.1175/1520-0442(2004)017<3843:TLCBCO>2.0.CO;2

Varshney, C. K., & Aggarwal, M. (1992). Ozone pollution in the urban atmosphere of Delhi. *Atmospheric Environment, 26*, 291–294.

Velissariou, D. (1999). Toxic effects and losses of commercial value of lettuce and other vegetables due to photochemical air pollution in agricultural areas of Attica, Greece. In J. Fuhrer & B. Achermann (Eds.), *Critical Levels for Ozone – Level II* (p. 253). Bern, Switzerland: Swiss Agency for Environment, Forest and Landscape.

Vingarzan, R. (2004). A review of surface ozone background levels and trends. *Atmospheric Environment, 38*(21), 3431–3442. doi:10.1016/j.atmosenv.2004.03.030

Vollenweider, P., Woodcock, H., Kelbty, M. J., & Hofer, R. M. (2003). Reduction of stem growth and site dependency of leaf injury in Massachusetts black cherries exhibiting ozone symptoms. *Environmental Pollution, 125*(3), 467–480. doi:10.1016/S0269-7491(03)00079-4 PMID:12826424

Volz, A., & Kley, D. (1988). Evaluation of the montsouris series of ozone measurements made in the 19th-century. *Nature, 332*(6161), 240–242. doi:10.1038/332240a0

Chapter 38
Technical Equipment of Agricultural Production:
The Effects for Food Security

Mikail Khudzhatov

https://orcid.org/0000-0001-6683-3206

Peoples' Friendship University of Russia (RUDN University), Russia

Alexander Arskiy

https://orcid.org/0000-0001-7417-6795

Russian Academy of Personnel Support for the Agroindustrial Complex, Russia

ABSTRACT

The guarantee of a sufficient food supply is one of the challenges in both international and national economic security. Development of world agriculture is impossible without using advanced technologies. Their application in agriculture depends on the security of agricultural producers with highly effective agricultural machinery for which agricultural engineering serves. Agricultural engineering is an important element of the agro-industrial complex of any state providing it with necessary machinery and equipment. One of the important directions of the establishment of food security is the development of agricultural engineering. In this regard, the chapter analyses the current state of the world market of agricultural machinery; develops the methodology of assessment of the competitiveness of agricultural machinery in the domestic market; and elaborates the definition of effective methods of management of logistics costs at the operation of agricultural machinery.

INTRODUCTION

Ensuring a sufficient food supply is one of the most critical challenges in establishing both international and national economic security. In this context, it is important to make a differentiation between food security and food self-sufficiency.

DOI: 10.4018/978-1-7998-5354-1.ch038

Food self-sufficiency is defined as the ability of a state to meet domestic food needs. The level of food self-sufficiency, calculated as the ratio of its national production to domestic consumption, varies for different countries. It is determined by the effective public demand for food, development of the agro-industrial complex, size of its commodity resources, degree of profitability, and reliability of international food relations (Ibragimov & Dokholyan, 2010).

The concept of food security is not limited to direct provision of food to the population, although this task is its ultimate goal. The food security system also includes the establishment of strategic food stocks; formation of the optimal ratio of food for the country by means of domestic production and import; development of food base of agriculture and the network of enterprises for the processing of raw materials, as well as trade in these raw materials and foodstuffs; expansion of transport networks for the supply of raw materials to food industry and food to consumers (Shapkina, 2012).

The term "food security" is widely used in the literature. In a general sense, it includes various aspects of activities related to the development of agricultural and agro-industrial production, food supply, and provision of targeted social food aid to population. Narrowly defined, food security of a country is the level of dependence on imports of basic types of food. Anisimov, Gapov, Rodionova, and Saurenko (2019) generalized an approach to understanding food security as a state of the global economy which provided physical access to food and economic opportunity to purchase it in the required quantity for all social groups.

Food security is provided by a set of economic and social conditions associated with the development of food production and general state of the national and global economy. Food security level is ensured both by domestic food products and the availability of financial resources to import the required volume of food. Every government in the pursuance of national security interests strives minimizing the degree of potential vulnerability of food security parameters (Khudzhatov, 2018a) and stabilizing food supply amid any external fluctuations (inflation, currency deficit, violations of food imports, embargo on supplies, etc.).

Establishment of food security includes the stability of both internal (preferably) and external food sources, as well as the availability of reserve funds.

The rational level of food security involves optimal use of the agricultural potential of a country for the needs of the domestic market and intensification of foreign economic activity in the terms of import of food and raw materials (in the volume required to close food supply gaps taking into account international division of labor and situation on the global market).

One of the key challenges in establishing food security is the development of domestic agro-industrial complex, which includes production of food and agricultural products and agricultural engineering (Figure 1).

Globally, development of agricultural production is hardly possible without using advanced technologies. Their application depends on the provision of agricultural producers with high-efficient agricultural machinery which is a major goal of agricultural mechanical engineering. It is also important to note that the global trade in agricultural machinery allows ensuring food security in the countries where domestic agricultural mechanical engineering is not capable to saturate domestic market with agricultural machinery. The above provisions determined the relevance of this chapter in the context of ensuring food security at a national level.

Figure 1. Structure of the agro-industrial complex
Source: Authors' development based on Khudzhatov (2018b)

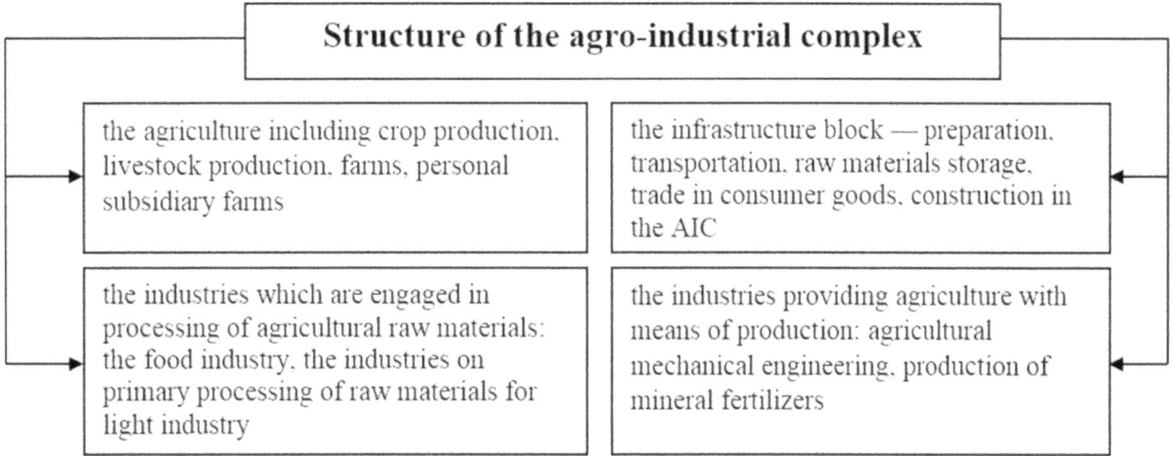

BACKGROUND

Agricultural mechanical engineering is an important element of agro-industrial complex of any state, providing it with necessary machinery and equipment. High mechanization of work is the key for growth of volumes and qualities of the produced agricultural products and, as a result, it has a positive impact on food security of a country.

According to food security programs of many countries, major food products have to be produced domestically. Particularly, Russia sets the following security thresholds: grain – 95%; sugar – 80%; vegetable oil – 80%; meat and meat products – 85%; milk and dairy products – 90%; potatoes – 95% (President of the Russian Federation, 2010). To be able to achieve the established levels of domestic agricultural production and in such a way ensure food security, agricultural sector has to implement advanced agricultural mechanical engineering.

Economic mechanisms, preconditions, and methodological aspects of business development in the agricultural machinery market have been studied internationally by many scholars (Bortolini, Cascini, Gamberi, Mora, & Regattieri, 2014; Huang, Yun, You, & Wu, 2011; Liu, Hu, Jette-Nantel, & Tian, 2014; Staus & Becker, 2012; Yakymenko, 2013; Yu, Leng, & Zhang, 2012; Zhovnovach, 2014).

Muzlera (2014) defined agricultural machinery market as an exchange of machinery and agricultural equipment. Among the major segments of agricultural machinery market are agricultural goods, combine harvesters, cultivators, walking tractors, plows, drill machines, and mowing machines (Bortolini, Mora, Cascini, & Gamberi, 2014). Agricultural machinery market is central for establishing national food security as it creates infrastructure required for the development of agricultural production (Morozova, Litvinova, Rodina, & Prosvirkin, 2015).

Peculiarities of business activities under the conditions of international trade integration and global competition for the enterprises operating in various countries have been examined by Antonakakis and Tondl (2014), Ganushchak-Yefimenko (2013a, 2013b), and Gong and Kim (2013). In such conditions, entrepreneurs may benefit from entering new markets of foreign countries (Bull, 2014). At the same time, globalization brings international competition to domestic markets (Wirtz, Tuzovic, & Ehret,

2015). Increasing competition is an inseparable element of integration processes in the global economy (Goncalves & Madi, 2013).

Among other scholars, Clapp and Helleiner (2012), Khafizova, Galimardanova, and Salmina (2014), Mulatu and Wossink (2014), Vosta (2014), and Yushkevych (2013) investigated major challenges and problems related to the functioning of agricultural machinery market in the conditions of international trade integration and elaborated state regulations needed to support domestic producers. In the conditions of international trade integration, national markets of agricultural machinery face intensifying competition (Solovchuk, 2015). Often, foreign competitors win the struggle and in such a way threaten national food security (Gnedenko & Kazmin, 2015). To support and protect national producers, governments implement various regulations in the sphere of agricultural machinery markets by providing tax subsidies and more favorable conditions to domestic actors (Morozova & Litvinova, 2014).

Studying and assessing competitiveness on the agricultural machinery market in relation to its influence on food security is of particular relevance today. Economic literature provides a variety of approaches to understanding competitiveness. In the most general sense, it is defined as an ability to be ahead of the others using the advantages in the achievement of the goals (Chaynikova, 2007). According to Mazilkina and Panichkina (2009), the variety of approaches to defining competitiveness may be explained by the following issues:

- Features of problem definition and research objective that require an author to focus on particular aspect of competitiveness
- Characteristics of an object under study (item, service), subject of competition (enterprise, industries, regions, national economy, state), subject to competition (demand, market, production factors), scale of activity (commodity, branch, regional, interregional, world markets)

When competitiveness is considered as a property of a product or service, its quantitative characteristic may be reflected by various parameters, quality being the most widespread one.

Similar approaches to the determination of the level of competitiveness have been elaborated by Tikhonov (1985), Fatkhutdinov (2005), Okrenilov (1998), and Rybakov (1995), who all have measured the level of competitiveness by a ratio of integrated indicators of competitiveness of the products consumed by a standard customer during a standard lifetime. There are alternative approaches to the assessment of competitiveness of technical products. According to Ferapontov (1994), competitiveness may be measured as a relation of complex indicator of quality to the actual price of its implementation.

The relationships between the impact of the production and trade of agricultural equipment on food security were studied by Gebbers and Adamchuk (2010), Auat Cheein and Carelli (2013), and Ncube, French, and Mupangwa (2018). However, in general, in the academic literature, trade in agricultural machinery remains one of the understudied aspects of food security.

Thus, at the national level, food security should be considered as a component of the aggregated concept of national economic security. One of the important directions of ensuring food security is the creation and development of agricultural engineering. In this regard, this chapter attempts analyzing current state of the global market of agricultural machinery, developing of a methodology of assessment of competitiveness of agricultural machinery in domestic market; defining effective methods of management of logistic costs associated with the operation of agricultural machinery. These research directions are one of the most relevant in terms of ensuring food security of a country by means of advanced agricultural engineering.

MAIN FOCUS OF THE CHAPTER

International Trade in Agricultural Machinery

At present stage, main development characteristics of the global economy are transnationalization and globalization which together cause the emergence of interdependence of national economies. Economic relations between the countries are beyond bilateral, and the center of gravity is displaced towards multilateral economic cooperation. In such patterns, agricultural machinery industry is being increasingly integrated to the global market and is characterized by high extent of globalization. Mechanization influences on the quantitative and qualitative growth of agricultural production. Currently, most of large producers of agricultural machinery are multinational corporations which have manufacturing and assembly enterprises around the world (Mechanical Engineering Portal, n.d.).

Agricultural machinery market is segmented based on the type of a product, function, and regions (Figure 2).

Figure 2. Segments of the global market of agricultural machinery
Source: Authors' development based on Grand View Research (2018)

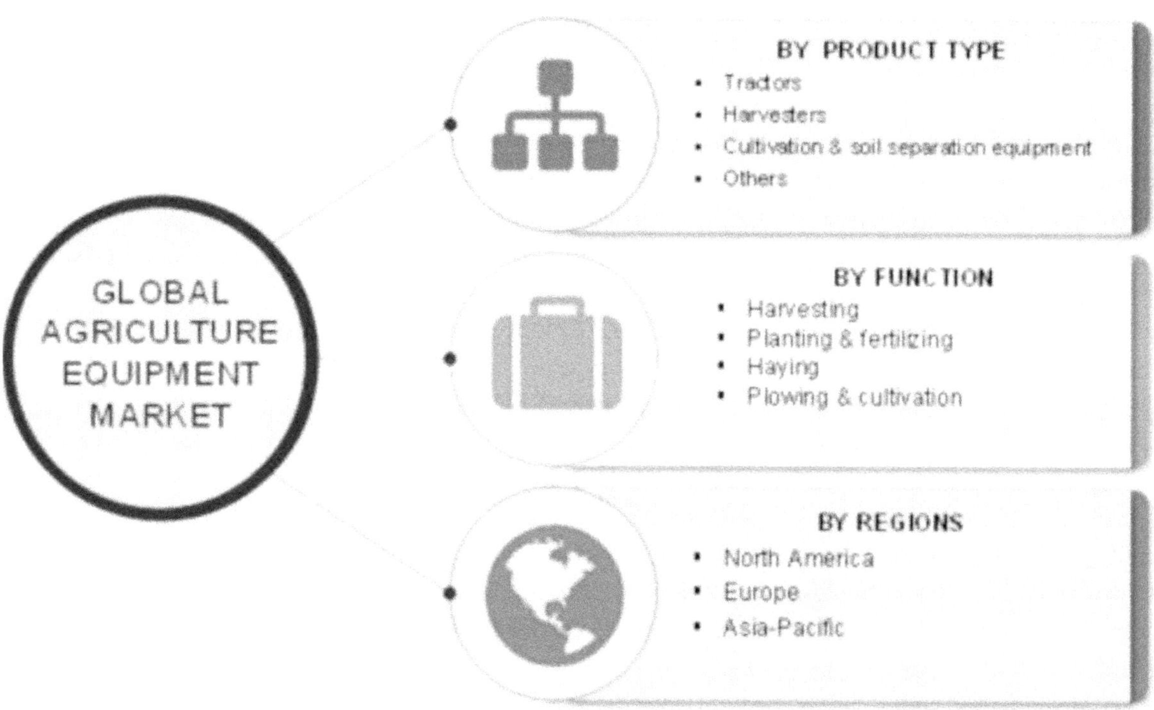

Types include tractors, harvesters, cultivation and soil separation equipment (Research and Markets, 2018). The segment of agricultural tractors is the biggest one. The share of tractors in total sales of agricultural machinery increased from 30% in 2011 up to 44% in 2018. The growth due to the increase in demand for food products, shortage of labor, and expanded government subsidies towards mechanization. The world market of tractors declined from 1.8 million machines in 2014 down to 1.68 million machines in 2015, but it is expected to grow up to 2.15 million machines in 2020 (Agriculture Equipment Market, 2019). Tractors are widely used in various spheres of agricultural production for soil cultivation, plowing, and landing.

In previous years, sales volume of equipment for plowing and cultivation has been increasing by 9%. This sector is now the fastest growing one among other types of agricultural machinery sectors. The volume has already reached $10 billion as farmers in developing countries purchase larger and more difficult equipment for soil cultivation in their attempts to increase efficiency of agricultural production. Demand for spare parts and attachable equipment grows by 5.5%. In this segment, the sales volume was $27.8 billion in 2018 (Research and Markets, 2018).

In relation to the functions of agricultural machinery, the market is segmented across harvesting, planting, fertilizing, haying, plowing, and cultivation. Harvesting machinery reduces dependence on labor, helps meeting growing demands of urban dwellers, and help breaking up soil efficiently. These factors accelerate the need for agricultural equipment for harvesting by farmers.

By regions, global agricultural machinery market spans across North America, Europe, Asia Pacific, and other regions. Global market of agricultural machinery is high fragmented due many producers and other actors, most of which are technologically advanced transnational companies which widely apply innovations to develop their production and distribution chains. As a result, smaller local suppliers experience difficulties when competing with larger actors, related particularly to quality, technology, and price. Global market of agricultural machinery is dominated by four largest companies which aggregated share of the market is over 40%. The biggest actor John Deere (USA) –18% of the global market of agricultural machinery. The other three are Case New-Holland (Italy) – 11%, AGCO (USA) – 7%, and Claas (Germany) – 4%. At the same time, there are many niche companies which focus on particular narrow segments of the market. German producers Fella, Krone, and Welger specialize in production of fodder harvesting machines. Kverneland (Norway), Kuhn (France), and Pottinger (Austria) – on soil-cultivating and fodder harvesting equipment. The USA, Germany, France, and Italy are major producers of agricultural machinery in the world (Medvedeva, 2018).

According to VDMA Agricultural Machinery Producers, the leading association of agricultural machinery producers which includes over 160 companies in Germany and worldwide, in 2108, global aggregated output of agricultural machinery reached $175 billion (Gotz, 2017). During previous eight years, the output has been increasing rapidly. Compared to 2010, in 2018, the output increased by 60% (average annual growth by 8%) (Figure 3).

The output has been driven by population growth, urbanization, and higher productivity demand amid the decrease in the acreage of agricultural land. Taken together, those factors have led to the growth in demand for agricultural machinery. Technological advancement for developing more efficient products, while keeping in mind the country-specific requirements, will provide opportunities for future growth of the sector. The key factors influencing the sale of agricultural equipment are the level of net farm income and, to a lesser extent, interest rates, and general economic conditions, availability of financing and related subsidy programs, farmland prices, and farm debt levels. Net farm income is primarily impacted by the volume of acreage planted, commodity and livestock prices, stock levels, the impacts of ethanol demand, farm operating expenses (which includes fertilizer and fuel costs), crop yields, fluctuations in currency exchange rates, tax incentives, and government subsidies. Farmers tend to postpone the purchase of equipment when the farm economy declines and increase their purchases when economic conditions improve.

Figure 3. Global production of agricultural machinery, $ billion
Source: Authors' development based on Gotz (2017)

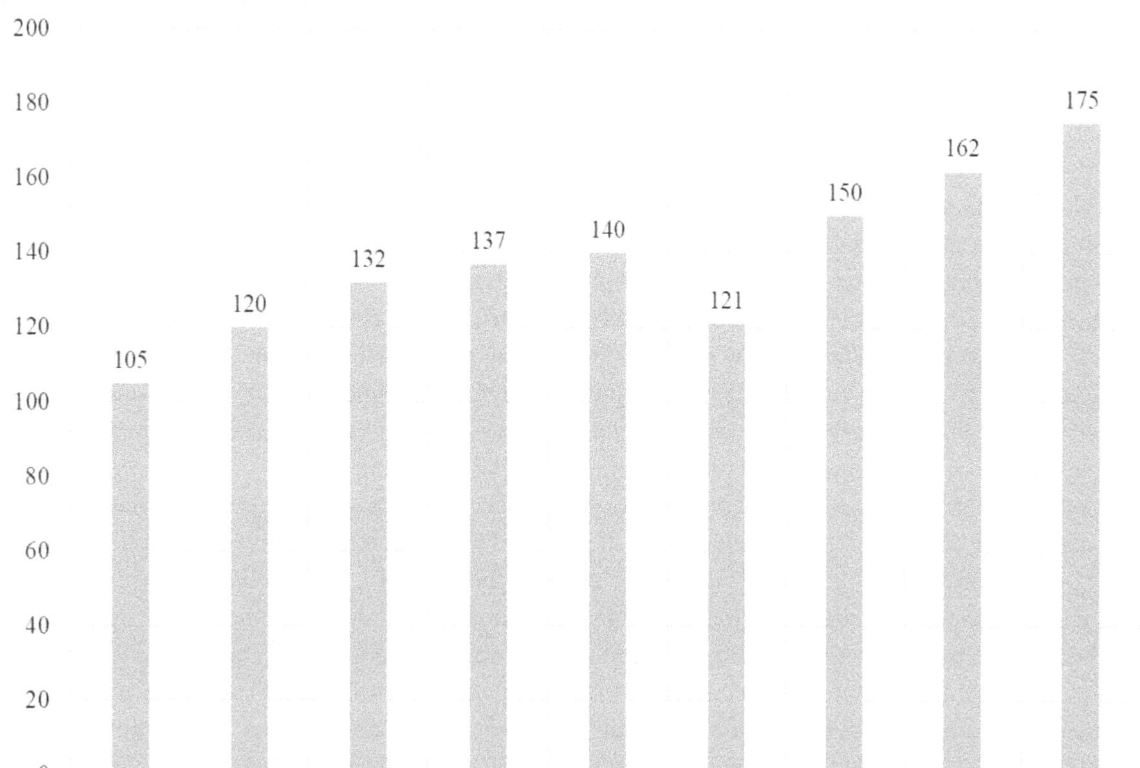

Growth happened due to the increase in sales in emerging economies, primarily, China and India. By 2022, the Asia Pacific region will lead the agriculture machinery market by reaching nearly $74 billion due to growing demand for food. This may skyrocket a demand for agricultural machinery. There will be an inevitable need for agricultural equipment in the region due to these factors. Continuous adoption of technologically advanced devices due to supportive initiatives by the governments coupled with farmers' awareness programs can drive agricultural equipment market in Asia Pacific. In India, there has been noted an emergence of startups in the sphere of agricultural engineering. For instance, Agribolo located in Rajasthan is a farming services platform which provides such services as information dissemination, quality input procurement, market linkages, irrigation facilities, and farming equipment (Mordor Intelligence, 2017).

Apart from China and India, the agricultural machinery markets in Thailand and Indonesia are expanding too. In the region of Central and Latin America, the sales increased in 2011-2012 due to the economic boom in Brazil and development of mechanization in agricultural production in Argentina. However, in 2014-2018, the economic decline in both Brazil and Argentina caused the decrease in the sales of agricultural machinery in the region. North America and Western Europe recorded growth below average till 2018. In both regions, demand is conditioned by technical achievements, such as increase in efficiency provided by new advanced equipment which allows farmers replacing outdated machinery in an economically effective manner. However, in the developed countries, many farmers postponed replacement of outdated equipment during economic crisis of 2008-2010, avoiding large purchases of new equipment because of uncertain economic situation. After the crisis, in 2011, the demand for new agricultural machinery emerged. Since a replacement cycle usually takes eight-nine years, the spike demand in 2011 resulted in a fact that many farmers did not seek replacement of agricultural machinery until 2018 and demand for agricultural machinery thus decreased.

With rapid technological development coupled with growing population, agricultural equipment market in North America is set to grow steadily. Moreover, there has been increase in the use of advanced agricultural equipment for more effective, reliable and time-saving production in the USA and Canada. Rapid introduction of advanced agricultural equipment in Europe can bolster the market growth in this region. Introduction of advanced equipment, such as multi-purpose tractors, will fuel the demand for agricultural equipment in Europe, thus positively impacting the growth of the market. For instance, in June 2018, SIWI Agriculture Ltd. Europe developed an automated hitch system to boost agricultural productivity and promote safety. This system enables a tractor driver to stay in a cabin instead of manually coupling and uncoupling between the implement, carriage, and the tractor.

Growth of the world population and increase in income per capita in emerging economies have resulted in the increase of demand for food products. By 2050, world population is forecasted to reach 9.5 billion people (7.4 billion in 2016). Farmers will need to increase the level of mechanization to be able to meet the growing demand. Global agricultural machinery market will grow amid the shortage of agricultural work because of mechanization and concentration of government support programs on promotion of agricultural machinery. In most of the countries worldwide, the governments will subsidize agricultural machinery production and agricultural engineering to increase production of food. The loans have been already intensively granted by banks and non-bank finance corporations to farmers to buy cars on tick. For example, in 2015, India allocated \$127.9 billion for crediting of farmers, and \$3.76 billion for the development of infrastructure of rural development (Ereport, n.d.).

It is supposed that the global market of agricultural machinery will experience a moderate growth by 7.3% (average) in 2018-2022. By 2022, the size of the market will reach \$200 billion. Considering the growing investment opportunities in the agricultural sector, it is expected that the market of agricultural machinery will have a positive trend in 2020.

Among the agricultural machinery markets of Brazil, the USA, France, Germany, and Russia, Russian market is the one most dependent on imports. When Russia accessed the World Trade Organization (WTO), import duties on agricultural machinery were reduced by 5-10% which resulted in the increase of the openness of domestic market to foreign producers (Alekseyeva, 2018). The markets of Brazil and the USA, on the contrary, are those the most protected. Both countries are self-sufficient in the production of tractors and other agricultural machinery (Government of the Russian Federation, 2017).

It is important to note that in terms of food security it is necessary to have a methodology for assessing the competitiveness of agricultural machinery in the domestic market.

Measuring Competitiveness of Agricultural Machinery in the Domestic Market

An analysis of the existing approaches to the assessment of competitiveness of agricultural machinery allows allocating two methodologies. The first one reflects subjective preferences of consumers, while the second one reveals a position of agricultural machinery producers.

First approach is to calculate the integrated measure of competitiveness of agricultural machinery J_K:

$$JK = \frac{An}{Ac}\gamma 1 + \frac{Bn}{Bc}\gamma 2 + \frac{Cn}{Cc}\gamma 3 + \frac{Dn}{Dc}\gamma 4 + \frac{En}{Ec}\gamma 5 \tag{1}$$

A_n, A_c – cost of performance of work of this type (direct costs of funds for operation of the equipment) on new equipment and the one by a competitor, respectively;

B_n, B_c – labor productivity (activities carried out by an operator by means of a technical unit) on new equipment and the one by a competitor, respectively;

C_n, C_c – payback period of full costs of acquisition and operation on new equipment and the one by a competitor, respectively;

D_n, D_c – decrease in a loss of agricultural products on new equipment and the one by a competitor, respectively;

E_n, E_c – fuel costs related to the use of new equipment and the one by a competitor, respectively;

γ_1, γ_2, γ_3, γ_4, γ_5 – specific weight (importance) of the parameters.

According to this approach, a client chooses one or several indicators, a specific weight of the chosen indicators is accepted to a unit, and the specific weight of other indicators – to zero. If money is a major factor, then the cost index of works or a payback period are the most significant. When a cost of fuel is high and technical parameters are relatively equal to each other, a client may select the machinery with the highest efficiency in terms of fuel consumption. The main shortcoming of this approach is its subjective character as it considers only preferences of certain consumers and therefore does not provide an adequate assessment of competitiveness of agricultural machinery.

Second approach assumes an establishment of parameters which are the subjects of comparison and assessment with their quantitative expression and establishment of "ponderability" for characteristic of degree of satisfaction of a client's specific need. The specified list includes three groups of parameters: standard and legal, technical, and economic.

Standard and legal parameters establish compliance of a product to the legal standards and norms regulating the actual level and required thresholds of these parameters. Accounting of standard parameters can be provided by introduction of special indicator with two values of 1 or 0. If a machinery meets legal standards, the indicator is 1, otherwise, it is 0.

General standard and legal parameter J_{LP} represents the work of individual parameters:

$$JLP = \prod_{i=1}^{n} q_i \tag{2}$$

q_i – individual parameter
n – number of standard parameters in the sample

If at least one of individual parameters is equal to 0 (technical tool on any indicator does not meet legal standard), then general indicator is equal to 0 too. That means a machine is not competitive in the market.

Technical parameters reflect the relation of physical volume of the products to the expenses of resources in natural measuring instruments. To find the general technical parameter J_{TP}, the importance (specific weight) of each individual parameter included the general set should be considered:

$$JTP = \sum_{i=1}^{n} \frac{bin}{bin}\, ai \tag{3}$$

b_{io} – individual technical parameter of a machine (domestic production)
$b_{i\kappa}$ – individual technical parameter of a machine (foreign competitor)
a_i – specific weight of individual technical parameter
n – number of technical parameters in the sample

Economic parameters are based on actual costs and do not depend on expert assessment. The price of agricultural machinery P_C is calculated as follows:

$$PC = Pn + Po \tag{4}$$

P_M – price of a machinery
P_0 – operation price of a machinery
P_M price is determined as follows:

$$Pn = \frac{P}{n} \tag{5}$$

P – selling price of a machinery
n – depreciation term
P_0 operation price is calculated as follows:

$$Po = Et + Es + Ef + Er + Em \tag{6}$$

E_t – transportation costs
E_s – annual charges on compensation of service staff
E_f – annual charges on fuels and lubricants
E_r – annual charges on repair
E_m – annual charges on maintenance

The aggregated economic measure E_{EP} is calculated as follows:

$$EEP = \frac{Pcd}{Pcc} \tag{7}$$

P_{cd} – price of consumption of domestic equipment
P_{cc} – price of consumption of foreign equipment

The lower the consumption price, the higher the competitiveness of a machinery, as it means that a client has an opportunity to get a unit of quality cheaper compared to a competitor.

On the basis of the aggregated measures of standard, technical, and economic parameters, the integrated measure of competitiveness *(IC)* is determined:

$$IC = PC \times \frac{JTP}{EEP} \tag{8}$$

Consequently, agricultural machinery of domestic production is more competitive compared to the imports if $IC \geq 1$. This approach, however, has several shortcomings:

- Aggregated measure of standard and legal parameters amounts to either 0 or 1. It has significant effect on the integrated measure of competitiveness, however, it does not make much sense measuring the competitiveness of agricultural machinery scored 0 as it does not meet required standards and legal regulations.
- Aggregated measure of technical parameters provides a weight basis for individual indicators. Measuring aggregated parameter on a basis of similar technical indicator may result in different weights for various objects.
- Specified approach ignores investment parameters as it does not consider the interests of investors, creditors, and other actors in agricultural machinery market.

Consequently, the existing approaches to the measurement of competitiveness of agricultural machinery require improvement. The specified shortcomings cause a need in the more substantiated choice by a client of particular type of equipment. The authors offer a combination of technical, economic, and investment parameters of the compared agricultural machinery options as a basis for new approach. The key technical parameters are capacity, engine capacity, reliability (time between failures), and productivity. Economic parameters include price of agricultural machinery and operation price. Among investment parameters of competitiveness, the most important ones are fuel consumption at maximum power, cost of power unit of an engine, cost of unit of mass (Zhudro, 2009).

The specified characteristics can be estimated on the basis of micro indexes of technical, economic, and investment parameters. MI_T micro index of technical parameters is determined as follows:

$$MIt = \sum_{i=1}^{n} SiPi \tag{9}$$

$S_i = b_{io}/b_{ik}$, i = 1, 2, ..., n;

b_{io}, b_{ik} – individual technical indicator of agricultural machinery (domestic vs foreign, respectively);
P_i – weight of *i* in relation to total *n*.

When calculating the general indicator for technical parameters, there is a problem with the determination of a weight base for individual indicators and discovering general parameter on its basis. To solve this problem, the authors carry out a comparison of technical parameters of agricultural machinery on the basis of convolutions of quantitative indices (Anisimov, 2009).

Formally, a convolution of technical characteristics of the two items is possible in a form of the following task. There are J items of agricultural machinery under comparison. Each of J items is characterized by a set of technical indicators. Generally, I types of indicators are established. For each parameter, a value is set: x_{ij}, $i = 1, 2, ..., I, j = 1, 2, ..., J$ where i – index of an indicator type, j – index of agricultural machinery.

At the first stage, it is necessary to define the coefficients B_j, $j = 1, 2, ..., J$ commensurabilities of the compared items of machinery. To find the coefficients, it is necessary to choose the reference agricultural machinery. As a standard, it is accepted a conditional machinery which has the maximum values of technical characteristics out of the machinery units under study, that is:

$$x_{i\mathfrak{m}} = \max x_{ij}, i = 1, 2, ..., I, j = 1, 2, ..., J \tag{10}$$

At the second stage, each of the agricultural machinery units taken as a standard one is characterized by the sizes:

$$S_{ij} = x_{ij} / x_{i\mathfrak{m}}, i = 1, 2, ..., I, j = 1, 2, ..., J \tag{11}$$

Enter parameters d_{ij} such, that:

$$d_{ij} = \begin{cases} 1, & \text{if increase } x_{ij} \text{ leads to an increase inefficiency of the machines} \\ 0, & \text{otherwise} \end{cases}$$

Then, the efficiency of each of the agricultural machinery units can be characterized by the sizes:

$$S'_{ij} = d_{ij} S_{ij}, i = 1, 2, ..., I, j = 1, 2, ..., J \tag{12}$$

Taking into account the values of the coefficients B_j, $j = 1, 2, ..., J$ commensurabilities of the agricultural machinery units under study are defined by a ratio:

$$Bj = \sum_{i=1}^{I} S'ij \times Pi \tag{13}$$

P_i – weight of i indicator in relation to total I.

In a basis of definition of P_i, $i = 1, 2, ..., I$ can be put the principle of a maximum of entropy. The essence of the principle is that at the measurement of competitiveness of agricultural machinery, the available information does not allow determining the efficiency of a machinery precisely by technical indicators and distribution of probabilities. Therefore, it is necessary to choose the steadiest one from all possible distributions. It is the distribution providing maximum of uncertainty (entropy), and, therefore, a minimum of conjectures in the developing information situation.

Practical opportunities according to the analysis of possible values of the considered weight coefficients of P_i, $i = 1, 2, ..., I$ are limited to pair comparison and establishment of some linear relations of an order on a set:

$$P = \{P_i\}, i = 1, 2, ..., I \tag{14}$$

In this regard, the problem of determination of sizes P, $i = 1, 2, ..., I$ comes down to the choice of a method of transformation of the preferences set in the form of the system of the relations of an order in dot estimates.

Convenient method of such transformation for the benefit of a problem of determination of weight coefficients of technical characteristics of the alternative agricultural machinery is use of the models offered by Fishbern for a priori receiving the linear restrictions of dot estimates of probabilities of events which do not contradict a system.

Information and theoretical justification of objectivity of Fishbern's estimates relies on the principle of maximum uncertainty:

$$E\left(p\right) = \prod_{i=1}^{I} p_i^{I-k+1} \tag{15}$$

p_i – probability of approach of i of an event from full group of I events reaches a maximum on Fishbern's estimates.

Taking into account that various technical characteristics of agricultural machinery units may be equal, the steadiest one (the possessing maximum of entropy of E(p)) is the uniform distribution. Then Pi . $i = 1, 2, ..., I$ are determined by a formula:

$$Pi = \frac{\sum_{j=1}^{J} S'ij}{\sum_{i=1}^{I}\sum_{j=1}^{J} S'ij} \tag{16}$$

Thus, in such technique of weight of P_i, $i = 1, 2, ..., I$ technical indicators and coefficients of B_j, $j = 1, 2, ..., J$ commensurabilities of the agricultural machinery are appointed not randomly, and are at a minimum of conjectures, on the basis of real characteristics of agricultural machinery units under consideration. It provides a certain objectivity to the results of comparison of agricultural machinery on their technical parameters received at its application (Khudzhatov, 2017).

MI_E micro index of economic parameters is defined as follows:

$$MIe = \frac{Pcd}{Pcc} \tag{17}$$

P_{cd} – price of domestic equipment
P_{cc} – price of competing foreign equipment

MI_I micro index of investment parameters is defined as follows:

$$MIi = \sum_{i=1}^{n} \frac{n\ in}{n\ in}\ ai \qquad (18)$$

c_{io} – individual investment parameter of a machine (domestic production)
c_{jk} – individual investment parameter of a machine (foreign competitor)
a_i – weight of i-individual investment parameter

On the basis of micro indexes of technical, economic, and investment parameters, integrated index of competitiveness (*IIC*) of agricultural machinery is defined:

$$IIC = \frac{MIt}{MIi \times MIe} \qquad (19)$$

If $IIC \geq 1$, then technical disadvantages of domestic machinery are compensated by lower costs of acquisition and operation and more favorable conditions for investors, or the high price of consumption of this equipment and big investment expenses are compensated by its technical advantages. In both cases, domestic equipment is more competitive compared to the foreign one.

The application of the methodology is demonstrated on the cases of combine harvesters of Acros 585 (Rostselmash, Russia) and W650 (John Deere, USA). At the first stage, micro index of technical parameters is defined (Table 1).

Table 1. Key technical parameters of combine harvesters

Combine harvester	Speed of unloading, l/sec	Engine capacity, hp	Capacity of the fuel tank, l	Productivity, ha/h
Acros 585	90	300	540	4.1
John Deere W650	88	324	800	6.9

Source: Authors' development

Having taken W650 John Deere combine as a standard, the authors then define weight indicators of technical parameters (Table 2).

Table 2. Weight indicators of technical parameters

Speed of unloading, P_1	Engine capacity, P_2	Capacity of the fuel tank, P_3	Productivity, P_4
0.29	0.28	0.17	0.26

Source: Authors' development

Further, micro index of technical parameters is calculated: $MI_T = 0.83$.

At the next stage, micro index of economic parameters is defined. It is necessary to define a price of each machinery item under study. This price consists of the price of a machine and operation price (Table 3, Table 4).

Table 3. Price of combines per year

Combine harvester	Average market price in domestic market, $	Depreciation term, years	Price per year, $
Acros 585	138,462	10	13,846
John Deere W650	200,000	15	13,338

Source: Authors' development

Table 4. Operation price of combines per year, $

Combine harvester	Transportation costs	Annual charges on compensation of personnel	Annual charges on fuel and lubricants	Annual charges on repair	Annual charges on servicing	Operation price per year
Acros 585	569.5	453.1	890.2	1,304.6	1,659.5	4,876.9
John Deere W650	668.9	509.4	1,146.3	624.6	738.5	3,687.7

Source: Authors' development

At the next stage, the price is calculated for each combine: Acros 585 – $18,723, John Deere W650 – $17,026. Micro index of economic parameters: $MI_E = 1.1$. Finally, micro index of investment parameters is defined. For this purpose, individual investment parameters of the combines are determined (Table 5).

Table 5. Individual investment parameters of combine harvesters

Combine harvester	Specific fuel consumption at the maximum power, kg/t	Specific cost of engine power unit, $/hp	Specific cost of mass unit, $/kg
Acros 585	4.2	461.5	8.8
John Deere W650	3.9	617.3	12.8

Source: Authors' development

Micro index of investment parameters in the condition of equality of specific weights of individual parameters: $MI_I = 0.84$.

Based on the calculation above, integrated index of competitiveness is determined for a domestic agricultural machinery unit in comparison with a foreign analog in domestic market:

$$IIC = \frac{0,83}{1,1 \times 0,84} = 0,9$$

As *IIC* < 1, Russian Acros 585 is considered as not competitive in comparison with W650 John Deere. At the same time, higher technological level of W650 John Deere provides lower price of consumption in comparison with Acros 585 and also compensates higher investment expenses. Therefore, at the expense of more considerable investment investments, John Deere is more competitive. Thus, the developed methodology for measuring competitiveness of agricultural machinery in domestic market allows considering a wide range of parameters and indicators and also revealing key problems when using agricultural machinery of different producers. At the same time, this methodology is simple in practical application as it does not require complex calculations.

Management of Logistics Costs in the Operation of Agricultural Machinery

Logistics costs is one of the main factors which affects the economic efficiency of agricultural enterprise. A relevant task is to measure the impact of the dynamics of logistics costs on the cost of agricultural products. One of the objectives of this chapter is to assess the impact of the dynamics of logistics costs on the cost of agricultural products, namely the study of the variable costs of diesel fuel during transportation of agricultural products.

The logistics costs associated with transportation of agricultural products are divided into fixed and variable ones. Variable costs include those resulting from the material costs of the motor fuel consumed by a vehicle, as well as ensuring the operation of the auxiliary units (refrigerator compartment compressor and cargo compartment climate control).

In order to measure the impact of the dynamics of logistics costs on the cost of agricultural products, the authors considered a specific type of a vehicle – grain carrier on the basis of KAMAZ 65115 (carrying capacity – 14 tons, cargo hold – 26 m^3). Consumption of motor fuel per 100 km is 27.4 liters (empty) and 32.0 liters (loaded) at air temperature above +10°C. This type of grain carrier is selected due to its average performance parameters among the trucks used in cargo transportation in agriculture. Serving the agro-industrial complex, therefore, its performance parameters provide sufficient accuracy of modeling. The average distance of transportation from agricultural enterprise to grain storage is 50 km (Arskiy, 2018a).

There is a need to assess the impact of the dynamics of the cost of motor fuel on the value of logistics costs due to their stable positive dynamics in recent years. The rise in the cost of motor fuel has a certain effect on the increase in logistics costs. A study is carried out to measure the influence of logistics costs on the cost of agricultural production and economic performance of an agricultural enterprise (Arskiy, 2018b). The authors study the cost of motor fuel in the countries of the Eurasian Economic Union (EAEU) actively engaged in farming: Russia, Kazakhstan, and Belarus. KAMAZ 65115 is the most commonly used agricultural cargo vehicle across all three countries (Table 6).

Table 6. Diesel fuel costs in the selected EAEU countries in January-May 2018

Country	Diesel fuel costs in January 2018, $/l	Diesel fuel costs in May 2018, $/l	Change
Russia	0.63	0.65	+3.2%
Kazakhstan	0.48	0.51	+5.9%
Belarus	0.65	0.68	+4.5%

Source: Authors' development on Eurasian Economic Commission (2019)

Based on the data of Table 6, the following findings are revealed:

- The dynamics of diesel fuel costs in Russia in the first half of 2018 is positive and amounts to +3.2%. The growth is due to the decline in world oil prices, which conditioned lower attractiveness of domestic market for diesel fuel producers.
- The dynamics of diesel fuel costs in Kazakhstan in the first half of 2018 is positive and amounts to +5.9%. The growth is due to the lack of sufficient refining capacity (oil refineries). Kazakhstan currently imports fuel from Russia, but there are plans to develop domestic refinery industry (there are three refining factories in the country, the fourth one will be launched in the near future).
- The dynamics of diesel fuel costs in Belarus in the first half of 2018 is positive and amount at +4.5%. Belarus imports fuel from Russia, prices in the two markets correlate closely.

There is a steady positive dynamics of changes in retail consumer prices for diesel fuel used by agricultural enterprises in their logistics. The on-going increase of logistics costs requires the assessment of their impact on the economic performance of agricultural enterprises. In this study, the authors calculate motor fuel costs associated with the transportation of grain from agricultural enterprise (field, storage) to grain elevator. The algorithm of the model (V) is as follows (Arskiy, 2016):

$$V = d_1 \times \frac{n_1}{100} + d_2 \times \frac{n_2}{100} \tag{20}$$

d_1 – distance from agricultural enterprise (warehouse, field) to the distribution point (elevator)
n_1 – liters of motor fuel per 100 km (loaded)
d_2 – distance from agricultural enterprise (warehouse, field) to the elevator
n_2 – liters of motor fuel per 100 km (empty)

Using the parameters of KAMAZ 65115, the calculations are made based on the average cost of the volume of motor fuel spent in January 2018 ($18.76) and May 2018 ($19.38). The difference between May 2018 and January 2018 is $0.62. Based on the data presented, it is possible to determine the increase in transportation costs per one ton of grain at the rate of fourteen tons of grain transported at a time: 0.62 / 14 = $0.044. Having taken $138.5 for the cost of one ton of wheat (class 3, ex-warehouse delivery terms), the authors calculate the increase in logistics costs of motor fuel in comparison with the relative period of 2017: 0.044 / 138.5 = 0.03%. The algorithm of the model for measuring the impact of the dynamics of motor fuel costs on logistics costs (E) is as follows:

$$E = \frac{\left(\left(d_1 \times \frac{n_1}{100} + d_2 \times \frac{n_2}{100}\right) \times C_1\right) - \left(\left(d_1 \times \frac{n_1}{100} + d_2 \times \frac{n_2}{100}\right) \times C_2\right)}{V} \times 100 \tag{21}$$

C_1 – motor fuel costs in the period under study
C_2 – motor fuel costs in the previous period

V – volume of transported cargo (tons)

P – contract value per ton of transported cargo

When $E < 1$, the influence of the actual positive dynamics of logistics costs on production costs of agricultural enterprise is insignificant.

In case of the selected EAEU countries, it is found that the dynamics of diesel fuel costs is positive. This factor determines a need to take into account the increasing costs in the logistics process of agricultural enterprise. In general, it can be concluded that there is no actual influence of motor fuel costs on the structure and volume of the corresponding logistic costs due to the meager amount of the increase in logistic costs in terms of value relative to the cost of the transported cargo. This study is based on the simplest methods of calculation when dynamics has a direct impact on the level of logistics costs. At the same time, it is necessary to practice a rational approach in forming assessments of the influence of these factors on the economic efficiency of agricultural enterprise. These estimates should also be formed taking into account government subsidies and subsidies enjoyed by some market actors while affecting the competitive market environment.

SOLUTIONS AND RECOMMENDATIONS

In general, the study of current challenges of agro-industrial complex is essential in terms of ensuring food security. Each country has to develop domestic system of agricultural engineering to obtain high performance of agricultural industry. Global market of agricultural machinery tends to grow at the expense of significant contribution of developing states which realized an importance of agricultural engineering for ensuring food security. Agricultural machinery produced in a country has to be competitive in domestic market in terms of not only technical characteristics but also economic and investment parameters. Otherwise, domestic producers may lose competition to international agro-engineering companies. Besides, measuring logistic costs associated with the operation of agricultural machinery is important. In this context, a country has to react to the world prices for oil adequately. The implementation of some of the findings of this study may allow increasing food security of a country in terms of improving technical capacity of agro-industrial sector.

FUTURE RESEARCH DIRECTIONS

Practical recommendations elaborated in this study contain some provisions which have universal character and can be implemented across various industries. The findings obtained and discussed in this chapter can become a basis for further investigations in the sphere of development of agro-industrial complex. The task for further research is the elaboration of scientific and methodical device for providing an integration of state mechanisms of stimulation of investments into agricultural sector.

CONCLUSION

The study of food security issues is essential for any country. Food security is a part of national security of a country providing its population with food products. Complex food security is impossible without development of various elements of agro-industrial complex, agricultural engineering being one of them. The scientific and methodical device of assessment of competitiveness of agricultural machinery in domestic market and calculation of logistic costs at its functioning allows defining shortcomings of agricultural engineering and ways of their correction. Implementation of the findings provides a solution of a practical problem of ensuring food security of a country by means of improvement of technical capacity of agro-industrial complex.

Thus, the study conducted in the chapter makes it possible to distinguish the link between trade in agricultural machinery and food security. Developed agricultural machinery allows ensuring food security of a country, while global production of agricultural machinery allows ensuring food security in a global scale.

REFERENCES

Agriculture Equipment Market. (2019). *Report*. Retrieved from https://www.farmmachinerysales.com.au/

Alekseyeva, Y. (2018). *Russia – Agricultural Equipment*. Retrieved from https://www.export.gov/article?id=Russia-Agricultural-Equipment

Anisimov, E., Gapov, M., Rodionova, E., & Saurenko, T. (2019). The Model for Determining Rational Inventory in Occasional Demand Supply Chains. *International Journal of Supply Chain Management*, *8*(1), 86–89.

Anisimov, V. (2009). *Optimization: An Adaptive Approach to Investment Management under Uncertainty*. Moscow: Publishing House of the Russian Customs Academy.

Antonakakis, N., & Tondl, G. (2014). Does Integration and Economic Policy Coordination Promote Business Cycle Synchronization in the EU? *Empirica*, *41*(3), 541–575. doi:10.100710663-014-9254-2

Arskiy, A. (2016). Peculiarities of Calculation of Logistics Costs. Motor Fuel. *World of Modern Science*, *35*(1), 34–37.

Arskiy, A. (2018a). Management of Logistics Costs of Enterprises of Agro-Industrial Complex. *Bulletin of the Moscow University of Finance and Law*, *1*, 98–102.

Arskiy, A. (2018b). Assessment of Efficiency of Management Decisions in Crisis Management of Agricultural Enterprise. *Marketing and Logistics*, *16*(2), 6–11.

Auat Cheein, F. A., & Carelli, R. (2013). Agricultural Robotics: Unmanned Robotic Service Units in Agricultural Tasks. *IEEE Industrial Electronics Magazine*, *7*(3), 48–58. doi:10.1109/MIE.2013.2252957

Bortolini, M., Cascini, A., Gamberi, M., Mora, C., & Regattieri, A. (2014). Sustainable Design and Life Cycle Assessment of an Innovative Multi-Functional Haymaking Agricultural Machinery. *Journal of Cleaner Production*, *82*, 23–36. doi:10.1016/j.jclepro.2014.06.054

Bortolini, M., Mora, C., Cascini, A., & Gamberi, M. (2014). Environmental Assessment of an Innovative Agricultural Machinery. *International Journal of Operations and Quantitative Management*, *20*(3), 243–258.

Bull, B. (2014). The Development of Business Associations in Central America: The Role of International Actors and Economic Integration. *Journal of Public Affairs*, *14*(3-4), 331–345. doi:10.1002/pa.1420

Chaynikova, L. (2007). *Competitiveness of an Enterprise: Scientific and Practical Study*. Tambov: Tambov State Technical University.

Clapp, J., & Helleiner, E. (2012). Troubled Futures? The Global Food Crisis and the Politics of Agricultural Derivatives Regulation. *Review of International Political Economy*, *19*(2), 181–207. doi:10.1 080/09692290.2010.514528

Ereport.ru. (n.d.). *World Market of Agricultural Machinery and Equipment*. Retrieved from http://www. ereport.ru/articles/commod/mirovoj-rynok-selskohozjajstvennoj-tehniki.htm

Eurasian Economic Commission. (2019). *Statistics of the EAEU*. Retrieved from http://www.eurasian-commission.org/ru/act/integr_i_makroec/dep_stat/union_stat/Pages/default.aspx

Fatkhutdinov, R. (2005). *Strategic Competitiveness*. Moscow: Economy.

Ferapontov, A. (1994). One of Variants of Mathematical Model of Indicators of Competitiveness of Technical Production. *Standards and Quality*, *4*, 44–45.

Ganushchak-Yefimenko, L. (2013a). Economic Integration as a Basis for Small and Medium Enterprises Business. *Actual Problems of Economics*, *141*(3), 70–77.

Ganushchak-Yefimenko, L. (2013b). Management of Innovation Potential Development of Small and Medium Business Based on Economic Integration. *Actual Problems of Economics*, *144*(6), 72–79.

Gebbers, R., & Adamchuk, V. (2010). Precision Agriculture and Food Security. *Science*, *327*(5967), 828–831. doi:10.1126cience.1183899 PMID:20150492

Gnedenko, E., & Kazmin, M. (2015). Agricultural Land and Regulation in the Transition Economy of Russia. *International Advances in Economic Research*, *21*(3), 347–348. doi:10.100711294-015-9535-y

Goncalves, J. R. B., & Madi, M. A. C. (2013). Global Economic Integration, Business Expansion and Consumer Credit in Brazil, 1994-2010. *International Journal of Green Economics*, *7*(3), 213–225. doi:10.1504/IJGE.2013.058164

Gong, C., & Kim, S. (2013). Economic Integration and Business Cycle Synchronization in Asia. *Asian Economic Papers*, *12*(1), 76–99. doi:10.1162/ASEP_a_00188

Gotz, C. (2017). *Upswing in Agricultural Machinery Industry*. Retrieved from https://lt.vdma.org/en/viewer/-/v2article/render/19870108

Government of the Russian Federation. (2017). *Order #1455-r from July 7, 2017, "Strategy of Development of Agricultural Engineering in Russia"*. Retrieved from http://government.ru/docs/28393/

Grand View Research. (2018). *Agricultural Machinery Market Analysis, Market Size, Application Analysis, Regional Outlook, Competitive Strategies, and Segment Forecasts, 2016 to 2024*. Retrieved from https://www.grandviewresearch.com/industry-analysis/agricultural-machinery-market/methodology

Huang, H., Yun, Z., You, L., & Wu, J. (2011). Forecast of Subsidy for Purchasing Agricultural Machinery Based on Life Cycle Theory in China. *Paper presented at the International Conference on Management and Service Science*, Wuhan. Academic Press. 10.1109/ICMSS.2011.5998516

Ibragimov, M.-T., & Dokholyan, S. (2010). Methodological Approaches to the Assessment of Food Security of the Region. *Regional Problems of Economic Transformation, 26*(4), 172–193.

Khafizova, A., Galimardanova, Y., & Salmina, S. (2014). Tax Regulation of Activity of Agricultural Commodity Producers. *Mediterranean Journal of Social Sciences, 24*(5), 421–425.

Khudzhatov, M. (2017). The Study of Differentiation of Foreign Trade Prices by Using of Dispersion Analysis. *RUDN Journal of Economics, 25*(1), 91–101. doi:10.22363/2313-2329-2017-25-1-91-101

Khudzhatov, M. (2018a). *Enhancement of Customs Instruments of Promotion of Foreign Investments in Agricultural Mechanical Engineering in Russia*. Moscow: DPK Press.

Khudzhatov, M. (2018b). The Use of Customs Instruments for Stimulation of Foreign Investment in Agricultural Machinery in Russia. *Marketing and Logistics, 15*(1), 58–70.

Liu, Y., Hu, W., Jette-Nantel, S., & Tian, Z. (2014). The Influence of Labor Price Change on Agricultural Machinery Usage in Chinese Agriculture. *Canadian Journal of Agricultural Economics, 62*(2), 219–243. doi:10.1111/cjag.12024

Mazilkina, E., & Panichkina, G. (2009). *Competitiveness Management*. Moscow: Omega-L.

Mechanical Engineering Portal. (n.d.). *Analytics*. Retrieved from http://www.mashportal.ru/analytics.aspx

Medvedeva, A. (2018). *World Market of Agricultural Machinery – Stability and Need for Innovations*. Retrieved from https://www.agroxxi.ru/selhoztehnika/novosti/mirovoi-rynok-selskohozjaistvennoi-tehniki-stabilnost-i-potrebnost-v-innovacijah.html

Mordor Intelligence. (2017). *Agricultural Machinery Market – Segmented by Type (Tractors, Plowing and Cultivating Machinery, Planting Machinery, Harvesting Machinery, Haying and Forage Machinery, Irrigation Machinery), by Geography – Analysis of Growth, Trends and Progress (2019-2024)*. Retrieved from https://www.mordorintelligence.com/industry-reports/agricultural-machinery-market?gclid=Cjw KCAiAiJPkBRAuEiwAEDXZZW41MxYmd5jvxtxaw-6prmgjEvU3F_UY1hMAd9lfiZtwtE8rLKLc-MxoCqwwQAvD_BwE

Morozova, I., & Litvinova, T. (2014). Russian Market of Agricultural Equipment: Challenges and Opportunities. *Asian Social Science, 23*(10), 68–77.

Morozova, I., Litvinova, T., Rodina, E., & Prosvirkin, N. (2015). Marketing Mix in the Market of Agricultural Machinery: Problems and Prospects. *Mediterranean Journal of Social Sciences, 36*(6), 19–26.

Mulatu, A., & Wossink, A. (2014). Environmental Regulation and Location of Industrialized Agricultural Production in Europe. *Land Economics, 90*(3), 509–537. doi:10.3368/le.90.3.509

Muzlera, J. (2014). Capitalization Strategies and Labor in Agricultural Machinery Contractors in Argentina. *Research in Rural Sociology and Development, 20*, 57–74. doi:10.1108/S1057-192220140000020002

Ncube, B., French, A., & Mupangwa, W. (2018). Precision Agriculture and Food Security in Africa. In P. Mensah, D. Katerere, S. Hachigonta, & A. Roodt (Eds.), *Systems Analysis Approach for Complex Global Challenges* (pp. 159–178). Heidelberg: Springer. doi:10.1007/978-3-319-71486-8_9

Okrenilov, V. (1998). *Quality Management: Scientific and Practical Study*. Moscow: Economics.

President of the Russian Federation. (2010). *Decree #120 from January 30, 2010, "Food Security Doctrine of the Russian Federation"*. Retrieved from http://www.garant.ru/hotlaw/federal/228793/

Research and Markets. (2018). *Global Agricultural Machinery Market – Industry Trends, Opportunities and Forecasts to 2023*. Retrieved from https://www.researchandmarkets.com/research/b6lzkj/global?w=5

Rybakov, I. (1995). Quality and Competitiveness in Market Relations. *Standards and Quality, 12*, 43–47.

Shapkina, L. (2012). Regional Aspects of Management of Food Security. *Terra Economicus, 1-2*, 128–131.

Solovchuk, K. (2015). Regulation and Support for Innovations in the Agricultural Sector of the European Union. *Actual Problems of Economics, 165*(3), 62–68.

Staus, A., & Becker, T. (2012). Attributes of Overall Satisfaction of Agricultural Machinery Dealers Using a Three-Factor Model. *Journal of Business and Industrial Marketing, 27*(8), 635–643. doi:10.1108/08858621211273583

Tikhonov, P. (1985). *Competitiveness of Industrial Products*. Moscow: Publishing House of Standards.

Vosta, M. (2014). The Foodstuffs Market in the CR and Its Regulation within the Framework of the EU Agricultural Policy. *Agricultural Economics – Czech, 60*, 279-286.

Wirtz, J., Tuzovic, S., & Ehret, M. (2015). Global Business Services: Increasing Specialization and Integration of the World Economy as Drivers of Economic Growth. *Journal of Service Management, 26*(4), 565–587. doi:10.1108/JOSM-01-2015-0024

Yakymenko, O. (2013). Peculiarities in Strategic Management of Enterprise Development in Agricultural Machinery Sector. *Actual Problems of Economics, 147*(9), 138–144.

Yu, X., Leng, Z., & Zhang, H. (2012). Optimal Models for Impact of Agricultural Machinery System on Agricultural Production in Heilongjiang Agricultural Reclamation Area. *Paper presented at the 24th Chinese Control and Decision Conference*, Taiyuan. Academic Press. 10.1109/CCDC.2012.6244128

Yushkevych, O. (2013). Regulation Mechanisms in the Development of Agricultural Enterprises. *Actual Problems of Economics, 147*(9), 132–137.

Zhovnovach, R. (2014). Satisfaction of Consumers' Demand as the Basis for Planning Competitiveness of Agricultural Machinery Enterprises. *Actual Problems of Economics, 155*(5), 171–180.

Zhudro, M. (2009). *Development of Economic Instruments of Increase of Competitiveness of the Use of Agricultural Technology*. Gorki: Belsha.

ADDITIONAL READING

Arskiy, A. (2017). Factor of the Economic Potential of the Customs Territory in the Anti-Crisis Management of a Trucking Enterprise. *Marketing and Logistics*, *13*(5), 6–12.

Bruck, T., & d'Errico, M. (2019). Food Security and Violent Conflict: Introduction to the Special Issue. *World Development*, *117*, 167–171. doi:10.1016/j.worlddev.2019.01.007

Choi, T., Chiu, C., & Chan, H. (2016). Risk Management of Logistics Systems. *Transportation Research Part E, Logistics and Transportation Review*, *90*, 1–6. doi:10.1016/j.tre.2016.03.007

Colin, E. C. (2009). Mathematical Programming Accelerates Implementation of Agro-Industrial Sugarcane Complex. *European Journal of Operational Research*, *199*(1), 232–235. doi:10.1016/j.ejor.2008.11.016

Erokhin, V. (2016). Development of Rural Territories in the Russian Far East and in Heilongjiang Province of China. *Agricultural Bulletin of Stavropol region, 23*(3), 256-260.

Hossain, M., Mullally, C., & Niaz Asadullah, M. (2019). Alternatives to Calorie-Based Indicators of Food Security: An Application of Machine Learning Methods. *Food Policy*, *84*, 77–91. doi:10.1016/j.foodpol.2019.03.001

Kain, R., & Verma, A. (2018). Logistics Management in Supply Chain – An Overview. *Materials Today: Proceedings*, *5*(2), 3811–3816.

Kou, Z., & Wu, C. (2018). Smartphone Based Operating Behavior Modelling of Agricultural Machinery. *IFAC-PapersOnLine*, *17*(51), 521–525. doi:10.1016/j.ifacol.2018.08.156

Kwesi-Buor, J., Menachof, D., & Talas, R. (2019). Scenario Analysis and Disaster Preparedness for Port and Maritime Logistics Risk Management. *Accident; Analysis and Prevention*, *123*, 433–447. doi:10.1016/j.aap.2016.07.013 PMID:27491716

Peng, W., & Berry, E. (2019). The Concept of Food Security. In Encyclopedia of Food Security and Sustainability (Vol. 2, pp. 1-7). Elsevier.

Perez-Moreno, S., Rodriguez, B., & Luque, M. (2016). Assessing Global Competitiveness under Multi-Criteria Perspective. *Economic Modelling*, *53*, 398–408. doi:10.1016/j.econmod.2015.10.030

Prosekov, A., & Ivanova, S. (2018). Food Security: The Challenge of the Present. *Geoforum*, *91*, 73–77. doi:10.1016/j.geoforum.2018.02.030

Sahnoun, H., Serbaji, M., Karray, B., & Medhioub, K. (2012). GIS and Multi-Criteria Analysis to Select Potential Sites of Agro-Industrial Complex. *Environmental Earth Sciences*, *66*(8), 2477–2489. doi:10.100712665-011-1471-4

Soltan, M., Elsamadony, M., & Tawfik, A. (2017). Biological Hydrogen Promotion via Integrated Fermentation of Complex Agro-Industrial Wastes. *Applied Energy*, *185*, 929–938. doi:10.1016/j.apenergy.2016.10.002

KEY TERMS AND DEFINITIONS

Agricultural Engineering: An area of industry engaged in the production and maintenance of equipment designed to work in agriculture.

Agro-Industrial Complex: A combination of several sectors of the economy aimed at the production and processing of agricultural raw materials and obtaining products from it, brought to the end consumer.

Competitiveness: An ability of a particular object or entity to surpass competitors in a given environment.

Entropy: A measure of the chaotic, disordered nature of a system.

Eurasian Economic Union: The union of Armenia, Belarus, Kazakhstan, Kyrgyzstan, and Russia established in 2014 for the effective promotion of free movement of goods, services, capital, and labor between participating countries.

Fishburne's Rule: An optimal distribution of the weights of the indicators from the point of view of informational entropy.

Food Security: A situation in which all people have physical and economic access to sufficient, quantitatively safe food to lead an active and healthy life at all times.

Logistics Costs: Relate to the charges for various transportation methods, including train travel, trucks, air travel, and ocean transport. Additional logistics costs include fuel, warehousing space, packaging, security, materials handling, tariffs, and duties.

Principle of Maximum Entropy: A probability distribution which best represents the current state of knowledge is the one with largest entropy, in the context of precisely stated prior data (such as a proposition that expresses testable information).

World Trade Organization: International organization established on 1 January 1995 to liberalize international trade and regulate the trade and political relations of member.

This research was previously published in the Handbook of Research on Globalized Agricultural Trade and New Challenges for Food Security edited by Vasilii Erokhin and Tianming Gao; pages 105-128, copyright year 2020 by Engineering Science Reference (an imprint of IGI Global).

Chapter 39
Issues and Challenges in Smart Farming for Sustainable Agriculture

Immanuel Zion Ramdinthara
Pondicherry University, India

Shanthi Bala P.
Pondicherry University, India

ABSTRACT

Sustainable agriculture helps to promote farming practices and methods in order to sustain farmers and resources. It is economically viable, socially supportive, and economically sound. It assists to maintain soil quality, reduce soil erosion and degradation, and also save water resources. Sustainable agriculture improves the biodiversity of the land and thus leads to the healthy and natural environment. The sustainable agriculture is very essential to ordinate with the increasing demand for the food, climate change, and degradation of the ecosystem in future. It plays a major role for preserving natural resources, reducing greenhouse gas emissions, halting biodiversity loss, and caring for valued landscapes. Sustainable agriculture is applied to farming in order to preserve the nature without compromising the quality of the future generation basic needs and thus enable to make smartness in farming. The common practices included in smart farming for sustainable agriculture are crop rotations that mitigate weeds, disease, insect, and other pest problems.

INTRODUCTION

The word "sustainable" is the process of maintaining changes in the environment. Sustainable agriculture is a measure in which it should emphasize long-term support in producing food and beverages and also at the same time in an eco-friendly mannered (Srisruthi, Swarna, Ros, & Elizabeth, 2016). Sustainable agriculture helps to balance the needs for food with ecological preservation. It helps to promote farming practices and methods in order to sustain farmers and resources. It is economically viable, socially sup-

DOI: 10.4018/978-1-7998-5354-1.ch039

portive and economically sound. It assists to maintain soil quality, reduce soil erosion and degradation and also save water resources. Sustainable agriculture improves the biodiversity of the land and thus leads to a healthy and natural environment. Sustainable agriculture is important ordinate with the increasing demand for the food and control climate change and degradation of the ecosystem in the future. It plays a major role in preserving natural resources, reducing greenhouse gas emissions, halting biodiversity loss and caring valued landscapes.

Sustainable Agriculture

Sustainable agriculture is applied to farming in order to preserve nature without compromising the quality of the future generation basic needs and thus enable to make smartness in farming. The common practices included in smart farming for sustainable agriculture are crop rotations that mitigate weeds, disease, insect and other pest problems. Thus it leads a way to make the hazardless environment. Sustainable agriculture comprises of sustainability of farmers, the productivity of agricultural resources and environment-friendly. Recycling and harvesting of water is the milestone to form sustainable agriculture. Moreover, as the need for food rises every day, it has to be preserved in order to meet the need sufficiently.

The living organisms are dependent on the nature of biodiversity. This has been contaminated slowly by emitting wastes, degraded dead plants, use of fertilizers and pesticides, dilution of water, etc. Moreover, because of this desecration of an environment and emission of greenhouse gases actually affects the plants, animals as well as human beings. So, it is very important to sustain and make a better environment for plants and for human beings. Thus, smart farming is a primary key to meet better agricultural systems and make better sustainable agriculture for the future.

Figure 1. Three factors for sustainable agriculture

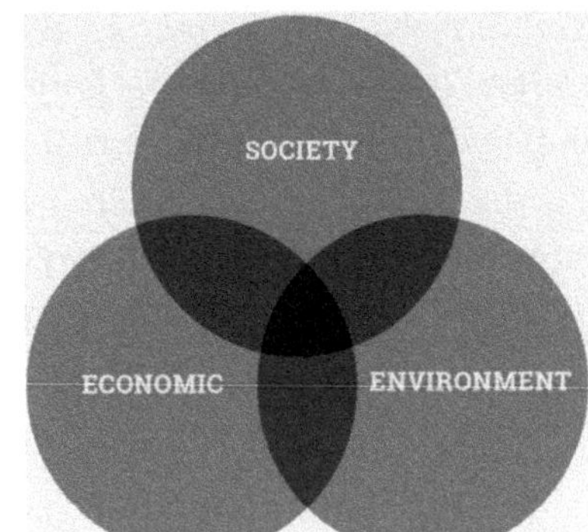

Smart Farming

The sustainability of agriculture can be carried up with a technique called smart farming. Smart farming is basically a concept of promoting precision agriculture and create eco-friendliness to increase the quantity and quality of the nourishment with modern sophisticated technology (O'Grady & O'Hare, 2017). Smart farming enables the farmers to monitor and control over the plants remotely and satisfy their necessary requirements of the plants and animals. Internet of Things (IoT) is a new technology that enables the devices to connect remotely in order to achieve smart farming (Patil & Kale, 2016). Smart farming delivers simplicity for the farmers to harvest and yield crops as automation of sensors and machines that replaces the early typical workforce of farming and it is much faster and reliable than ever before. The technologies transform the typical way of farming to automated devices which brings revolution in the history of agriculture.

Farming was completely dependent on labor force until it meets new technology in recent years. With the advancement in technologies, farmers could possibly make higher production and it has a great impact on the agricultural economy. It also helps in bridging the gap between the small and large-scale businessman. The technologies brought an ability to communicate with all over the world and explore what is going on on the other side of the world. This way methods and techniques can be shared by farmers across the globe.

Before the technologies come into existence, farmers and labors face a lot of problems in selling out the products that had been harvested as they hardly get the secondary buyers. Fortunately, even if there are buyers for the products, the farmers could not sell it off at a reasonable price. However, the emergence of technology had swiped away the nightmare that has held the farmers in misery. Agriculture has met a new technology which actually changed the typical way of farming and conventional techniques were transformed into a technique called the Internet of Things. This technology has drastically changed the way of farming and has much more potential of establishing better precision agriculture.

Internet of Things

The Internet of things is the interconnection of different devices over the internet through the cloud server. IoT is implemented and deployed in different platforms like Hospital, Traffic, Government Offices, vehicle, and agriculture, etc. (Asghari, Rahmani, & Javadi, 2019). There is a tremendous impact on agriculture and has assisted human labors and promotes simplicity (Khanna & Kaur, 2019). The technology has the ability to monitor the plants and animals and also can retrieve information remotely in the device like handheld and mobile phones. Moreover, the primary obstacles that the farmers faced to get a productive agriculture product are unpredictable weather, water scarcity, pests, and diseases. Unpredictable weather is apparently caused due to the pollution emitted by the human from industrial wastes and smoke from vehicles etc. Agriculture is completely dependant on the weather condition as it requires rainwater and light for photosynthesis. However, because of the pollution and wastes from industries and individuals, the weather of the season became uncertain and farmers faced problems because of unpredictable weather which affect the crops and falling of productivity.

Devices and sensors enable the farmers to predict weather and anticipate the amount of production. Secondly, Water scarcity is also the most common problem faced by farmers. This could also be more or less resulted by pollution and global warming. Water had been tremendously contaminated by industrial wastes and human daily wastes. Moreover, most of the inhabitants simply waste water and dump the waste in the sea. However, the people came to realize that the earth is in critical as summer became hotter and hotter and winter becomes extremely cold. This is a big sign of the consequences of human action. So, awareness had been given in educational institution and society to save rainwater and maintain waste properly. This is where technologies are highly important as they can be made in such a way it would assist human in any means. In many developed countries like USA, Israel and some of the European Countries, IoT plays a vital role in everyday living as even garbage trucks are automated to identify and differentiate degradable and nondegradable substances and wastes.

IoT has significantly played a very important role in the harvesting of water as it monitors the amount and controls the flow, it evaluated the amount of water required by the plants and supply them an adequate amount which saves a huge amount of water than ever before(Yong et al., 2018). Conventional water sprinkler was used in lawns and gardens which also saves a fair amount of water as compared to the manual methods of watering plants. Moreover, technologies become even better and smarter. Water sprinkler could not only supply water but also controls with different parameters prior to the humidity of the soil, grass, and plants. Sensors are connected to the cloud through the gateway and could be able to monitor the status and supply water exactly what the soil and plant need remotely through handheld devices and computers (Mekala & Viswanathan, 2017). Moreover, other means of harvesting water is drip irrigation. This has been widely used in many parts of the world. Drip irrigation is the method of dropping water directly to the root of the plants to an adequate amount (Joshi & Ali, 2017). This technology is used a wide and huge piping method which would supply many plants in large scale.

One of the problems that farmers encountered other than water scarcity is the disease and pests which destroy their crops and plants which keeps the farmers in devastation. It is difficult for the farmers to anticipate the invasions of the diseases as these are small and tiny substances which cannot be seen especially plants in a wide area of land. The farm production apparently deteriorated as the diseases had invaded many plants in the farms and the farmers could barely monitor every plant. It was problematic for the farmers to monitor and observe each and every plant manually whether it had suffered from disease or not. However, IoT technology fortunate farmers and lead them to a new milestone in the agricultural field. This technology has transformed the conventional way of farming to a new era of farming (Mittal & Singh, 2007).

Figure 2. User's mostly browsed IoT on the internet
(Source: www.i-scoop.eu)

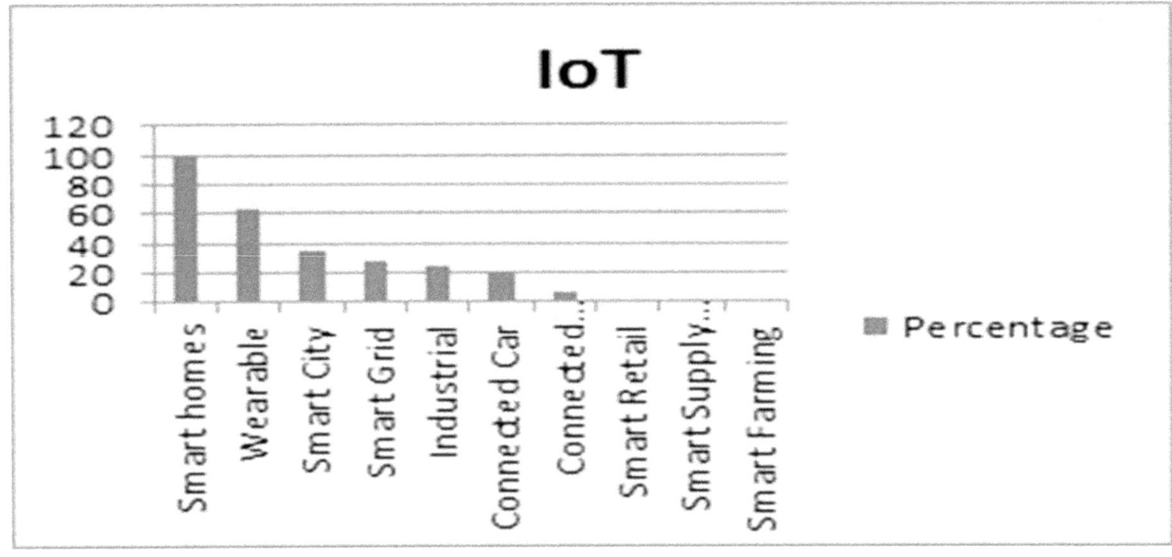

Machine Learning

A machine Learning algorithm is basically a subset of Artificial Intelligence which helps to train and to learn automatically and improve the experience without any human consent and without explicitly programmed. This technology is thriving in the agriculture sector as it could perform a task automatically and also improved the technology of IoT. Machine Learning has become very powerful, accurate and efficient because it can make the best feasible solution for many situations. The term "Machine Learning" was coined by Arthur Samuel in the year 1959. It was used in several problems solving. Improvement takes place over time, it became a very powerful algorithm or system where the machine can learn and act accordingly and smartly. Machine Learning can be broken down in three subgroups called Supervised Learning, Unsupervised Learning and Reinforcement Learning. Supervised Learning is basically a machine learning algorithm that deals with labeled datasets. Whereas in unsupervised learning, the datasets are scattered, unknown, unclassified and it can be any group of different variables. In Reinforcement learning, the software has to take action in the environment and acquire the most feasible solution. It is like a trial and error approach.

The weather has a huge dependency for farming so it is necessary for the farmers to monitor and predict for the upcoming season which would ideally significant for the plants (A. Toreti, A. Maiorano, G. De Sanctis, H. Webber, A.C. Ruane, D. Fumagalli, A. Ceglar,S. Niemeyer, M. Zampieri, 2019). Fortunately, Machine Learning has the capability to predict the weather from previous records or datasets using regression techniques. This is quite powerful for prediction but unfortunately human has emitted pollution which makes the weather hard to predict as it is unbalanced.

Farmers are opportune with the ability to classify plants variations, diseases, and pest which is aid by the machine learning algorithm called classification. Nowadays, many species are classified using the sensor which helps the farmers to identify the plants and supply fertilizers and water accordingly. It also can classify diseases and pest within the leaves which helps the farmers to save the plants or trees at the early stages.

The incorporation of Machine Learning and the Internet of Things had made a revolutionary in the agriculture domain and thriven the technology to the next generation. Farmers are able to monitor and control the devices and sensors accurately and make a hike on agricultural production. However, there are some limitations of these two techniques which are basically in the analysis of data and records. These technologies are powerful for the smaller datasets and a small group of parameters, however, when the data becomes extremely large, it does not work quite well and often leads to redundancy and inaccurate of data manipulation. Data Analytics is the process of organizing and modeling a set of data in order to be able to manipulate these data accordingly. This technology has improved the dataset generated by the sensors and stored in a proper format. With this data, a problem can be solved and the decision could be made from the data stored.

RELATED WORK

Sustainable agriculture is a measure in which farming would be taken in a smarter manner and eco-friendly. Many research is carried out in the agricultural domain and it is drastically evolving as compared with the earlier conventional type of farming. A focus is on the Internet of Things and Machine Learning algorithm as these two technologies are the most powerful and most feasible algorithm for solving a problem. As agriculture is important for livelihood, it is necessary to take a challenge for the researcher, students, and enthusiasts in order to develop the farming system, irrigation system, and marketing system, etc.

Water is a primary need for the plant's growth. So, it is necessary to aware of the preservation of water with the new technologies like automatic water sprinkling systems, irrigation system and desalination of sea water. Some countries like Israel and the US have adopted and practices water preservation by implementing drip irrigation and desalination. Drip irrigation is basically a watering system used in agriculture for watering plants economically and also sufficiently. It saves water as it drips within a fraction of time and does not waste. It is a big challenge to improve the conventional drip irrigation technique and to perform it in a smarter way in which it can actually monitor the soil moisture and plants humidity (Pandithurai, Aishwarya, Aparna, & Kavitha, 2017). Over the year, water had been wasted due to improper water systems and preservations. In many countries, water scarcity is a major problem for the development of agriculture. Now, a sensor technology helps to monitor the pH of the soil, soil moisture and nitrogen content of the soil for the plants to consume the exact required amount of water and mineral.

Water sprinkler is another way of conserving water and watering plants economically for the adequate use of water. In recent decades, a conventional water sprinkler was used where it supplies water to the plants by sprinkling over the plants under the control of the operator. It is a semi-automatic in which the operator controls the switch where it could be turned on and off with operator acknowledgment.

IoT and Machine Learning are used in many agricultural platforms for smarter and better systems for upcoming experiences. So, these technologies can assist the farmers in monitoring the humidity of the soil, the pH level of the soil, and minerals, etc. The characteristics of all plants differ from one another, for instance, the amount of water required to grow and kinds of soil mineral and soil pH to have proper growth. So, in order to grow plants and yield crops faster, it is very important to implement a system where each plant gets its requirements. Sensors like Arduino, RasberryPi, and Zigbee are the most common devices used by many authors for monitoring the soil. These sensors are actually electronic components which can generate data from the sensor in the form of magnetic waves and current (Kalaivani, Allirani, & Priya, 2011). Data and information can be accessed and processed through the cloud server from anywhere on handheld devices for monitor and control. In this way, specific plant requirement can be measured and supply an adequate amount of minerals and herbicide.

During the late twentieth century, trackers and animals like horse, buffaloes, and cows are the main sources of energy for farming. Especially tractor and machines run by steam is apparently, afforded only by some of the countries from the American continent and Europeans. In other parts of the world like the African continent and South East Asian continent, workforce and animals are the primary sources of energy for farming. When the technological revolution in agriculture began, the American continent and Europeans are the countries to lead and it was growing exponentially. Since the 21st century, technology thrived rapidly and the Internet of Things was introduced which becomes a very important technology for many domains. Machine Learning has also improved soon after the introduction of IoT. These two technologies completely change the way of conventional farming to digital farming.

So, in this modern age of technology, diseases and pests could be easily detected using sensors and image processing which is an application of IoT and Machine Learning. Machines are trained to identify which plants are growing well and healthy. Image processing is used for visual identification in classification, detection of diseases. It is basically the process of comparing the images that have been captured by the visual camera or Aerial drones with several sample pictures (Dimitriadis & Goumopoulos, 2008).

Image processing is generally used for the plant disease detection that helps farmers to prevent the deterioration of plants and crops due to the pests and diseases (Gandhi, Nimbalkar, Yelamanchili, &

Ponkshe, 2018). Plant disease is one of the most destructive measures in the agricultural sector which often brought the farmer in misery. An image-based classification system for plants diseases (Athani, Tejeshwar, Patil, Patil, & Kulkarni, 2017). Datasets are taken manually from the input device and to augment the input dataset, Generative Adversarial Network is used and further classified using Convolutional Network (CNN). In agriculture, water preservation is one of the vital measures that must be taken in order to sustain the life of plants and trees. They have introduced a system that measures the soil moisture and humidity using sensor and IoT technology. The main objective is to utilize the water for irrigation. The plant would be watered adequately without wasting any of the water in order to meet the needs of plants as well as to save the water. The Arduino sensor is deployed in the soil and fetches information in the form of data. Soil moisture and soil pH level is measured and processed further using the Neural network algorithm.

Data Analytics is also a significant topic in modern technology as data is generated at every moment. Every enterprises, company, and machine significantly generated information or data to process and records all the transaction. Data Analytics is a science of analyzing a large group of unlabeled data and manage the trends, groups, and types to form a uniform database. Data Analytics and Big data are already implemented in many domains like offices, hospitals, and airport, etc (Lim, Kim, & Maglio, 2018). Big Data is a new approach used for managing and manipulating a massive group of raw data and store for future reference and for a better future experience. It could collect information from a different platform and organize them for comparison and survey (Wolfert, Ge, Verdouw, & Bogaardt, 2017).

TECHNOLOGIES FOR SUSTAINABLE AGRICULTURE

Technologies for Smart Farming

The labor force is the primary source of power and energy engaged in agriculture in the late 20th century although some conventional machines and animals are still in use. The farmers were often frustrated and devastated because of the unpredictable situation like weather change, water shortage, pests, diseases and calamities, etc. Season of the year was the only thing that could be anticipated by the farmers but, now even time of the season gradually changes because of global warming and pollution.

However, the 21st century brought the technological revolution which gradually changes the way of farming. The animals are used for farming like horses and buffaloes were replaced with tractor and machines. In the early days, machines were operated physically by farmers or operators which is through tremendous ease as compared to the labor force farming. The technological revolution brought tremendous changes to farming and increase crop productivity. The evolution had brought machines like a tractor, truck, combine harvester, etc which is called mechanization. There are different types of technologies which together makes farming smart. They are:

- Sensing technology
- Software application
- Information and Communication technology
- Positioning technology
- Hardware and Software system that enabled IoT-based
- Data Analytics

Sensing Technology

Sensing technology is basically a device which has the ability to measure certain properties of some components or variables. Sensing technology changes the typical ways of farming in many ways such as monitoring the plants, monitoring soil moisture, minerals and pH level. Weather forecasting became much accurate. Weather conditions are also one of the primary measures to be monitored as particular crops required to be grown inadequate temperature level. There are several brands for a sensor such as Flir, UNO, Raspberry Pi and Arduino, etc.

Software Application

A software application is a group of programs that can perform specific task and functions. It is the interpreter between the users and the hardware. Many software developers and communities develop several software applications which promotes simplicity in operation of hardware devices and machines to perform tasks without much of human assistance. The software application provides a privilege to the users to touch and control over the devices and machines and helps to perform a specific task. In farming, Software Application is the module which controls and operates over all the sensor and farming devices through handheld devices and computers.

Information and Communication Technology

Information and communication technology refers to a technology that provides access to data and information through telecommunication and internet interconnection. This technology allows the user to exchange data and information through network interconnection from device to another. There are different types of interconnection and communication such as Wireless Sensor Network (WSN), Radio Frequency Identification (RFID), and Zigbee network, etc. These types of communication are used in many domains such as Airport, Traffic, hospitals and even in agriculture. Wireless Sensor Network is a type of communication that has a standard of 802.15.4 that probably covers up to 100 meters depending on the settings and devices used. This is widely used for monitoring soil moisture, soil pH level, soil minerals, disease and pests and even weather prediction which is control through the cloud server (Abhiram Singh & T. P. Sharma, 2014).

A Radio Frequency Identification (RFID) technology refer to a wireless system that allows the device to read information from a certain distance without any physical contact. It provides a method to transmit and receive data from one point to another. This is widely used as a barcode reader and ID scanner, etc. RFID is also used for identifying animals in the livestock and for labeling the animals (Ruiz-Garcia & Lunadei, 2011).

Zigbee is of 802.15.4 standard which is a high-level communication protocol and it is used to create a small personal area network with low power and low bandwidth. This communication is generally used in a small area. It is suitable for farming within a specific area which connects the sensors and the controller.

Positioning Technology

Positioning technology is a technology for determining a position and orientation of an object or a thing. It is widely used today for determining the location on a map. Global Positioning System (GPS) and Global Information System are the two prominent systems which are used by many companies like Google Map for locating positions. In smart farming, positioning system plays a vital role in which the farmers enables to locate particular crops over the wide field when required which makes it faster. It also helps in identifying areas which are suitable for cultivation, etc.

Hardware and Software System That Enables IoT-Based

In the world of computing, hardware and software always come together which connects and communicate to perform a task. Hardware comprises a physical electronic substance like Devices and sensors. Software is the group of commands or program which makes the hardware works such as Arduino software, Machine Learning, and ThinkSpeak, etc.

Data Analytics

Data Analytics is the process of organizing a group of raw data into uniform sets of information which can be referred and manipulate for a better experience. In farming, as the farmer has to record information about different types of crops and their properties, data analytics can be helpful in manipulating the data as per required.

Figure 3. Different factors making farming smart

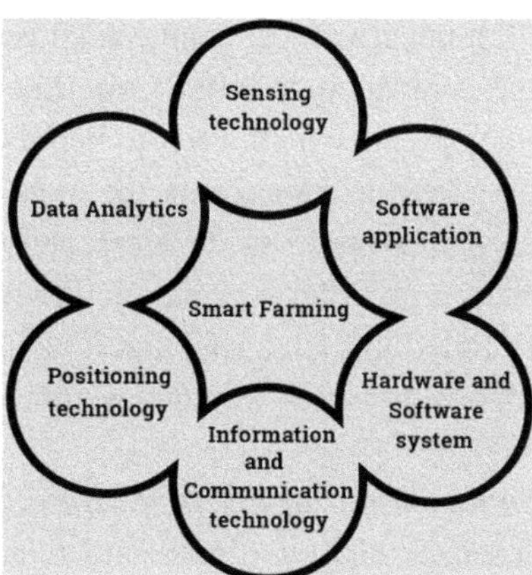

The figure above shows the important six factors that make farming smart.

With the growth of population globally, the need for food has also arisen respectively, so, it is necessary to aware of food security to meet the need. Moreover, due to the pollution and wastes, the form of season gradually changes and weather are improper as compare with the early days. The weather became unpredictable and farmers the most sufferers as plants required proper light and water for their growth. That is why smart farming is important to control all the problems much accurate.

Smart farming is the only feasible way to sustain agriculture and produce quality products at a higher quantity. It is highly efficient as compared with conventional techniques. IoT technology that provides uses sensors like sound, light, temperature, humidity and soil moisture which can be used as a measure to monitor the crop's and plant's growth and identify the requirements of fertilizers and minerals of the plants (Biradar & Shabadi, 2017).

Parameters for Smart Farming

The different parameters that are used in smart farming are as follows:

- Disease detection
- Smart water sprinkler
- Soil moisture
- Soil pH
- Soil minerals
- Soil temperature
- Water Sprinkler
- Drip Irrigation

Basically, farming is improved since recent years with the use of sophisticated technologies which for faster work and profitable. Some of the technologies are

Disease Detection

During a period of harvesting and cultivation, farmers are often disturbed by pests and diseases. Plants disease are very common among different varieties of plants and it is usually caused by fungus, bacteria, and virus. The occurrence of disease in plants may differ from time to time. There is the season when diseases are likely to spread and attack plants which leads to decrease crop production rates. The sensor technology and Machine Learning help in monitoring the plant's health and detection of diseases at the early stages when plants leaves can be cured easily. Here, sensors like Visual sensors and camera are highly used for disease detection as it provides a visual picture for any detection which is much accurate and reliable. The camera is installed in such a way that it would scan the leaves real-time further processed with Machine Learning algorithm which would classify the pest and the disease found on the leaves (Singh, Varsha, & Misra, 2015).

These diseases are also detected with various devices like an electromagnetic sensor, Optical sensor, Mechanical sensor, electrochemical sensor, airflow sensor, and an acoustic sensor.

Smart Water Sprinkler

The advancement in technology has also brought a technique for the preservation of water. In the earlier system of a sprinkling of water, the water sprinkler was controlled by the operators or farmers towards their knowledge and experiences to utilize and save water. However, in the present technology, the soil is being sensed initially using sensors which check the humidity and moisture of the soil and pass input

Figure 4. Disease detection with image processing technique
(Source: bitrefine.group)

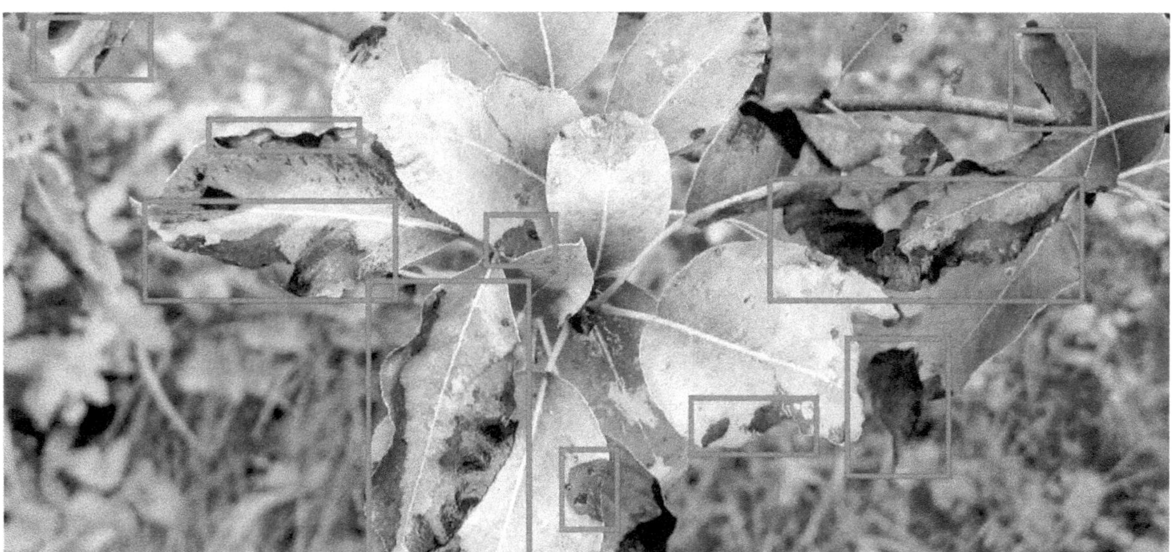

parameter for the further process to control the water sprinkler depending on the inputs requirements. This technique is much more sophisticated and more efficient as compared with recent technology.

Weather Forecasting

Crop cultivation completely dependent on the weather condition as crops certain ranges of temperature where it can live and grow. So, it is crucial to control the farmers in order to increase the food production rate and maintain high food security. As human is emitting pollution to the environment, it also has a great effect on climate weather change. This has made farmers in misery as they are not able to anticipate for the upcoming weather. However, with the help of technology, it is possible to predict for the upcoming weather for the better farming experience. Sensors for weather forecasting are used widely in agricultural systems.

Soil pH Level

Soil pH is the measure of acidity and alkalinity in the soil. It consists of level 1 to 14 where 7 is the neutral level for the plants to adapt to live and grow. However, some plant has the ability to adapt and even thrived beyond the neutral level. So, it is very important to know the kind of soil so that the farmers may seed the particular plants and trees in order to thrive. IoT technology has changed the conventional way of measuring soil pH with chemicals. Sensors technology like Arduino are widely used for monitoring the soil pH with device probe dipped in the soil which receives a signal in the form of Radiofrequency.

The sensor which looks like a pen is dipped into the soil. It is functioning like potentiometer and signal or data information would be sent to the board for further processes.

Figure 5. UNO soil pH sensor

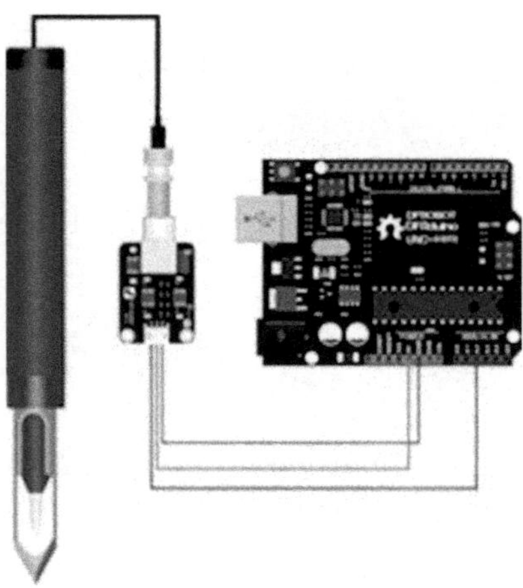

Soil Moisture

The number of water requirements for every plant could probably differ from plants to plants in order to grow. So, in order to supply a sufficient amount of water a probe sensor is used which measures the water content of the soil (Pandithurai et al., 2017). Arduino, Zigbee, and raspberry are the common sensors that are mostly used today. The soil moisture sensor has two probes which allow current to flow.

Figure 6. Soil moisture sensor

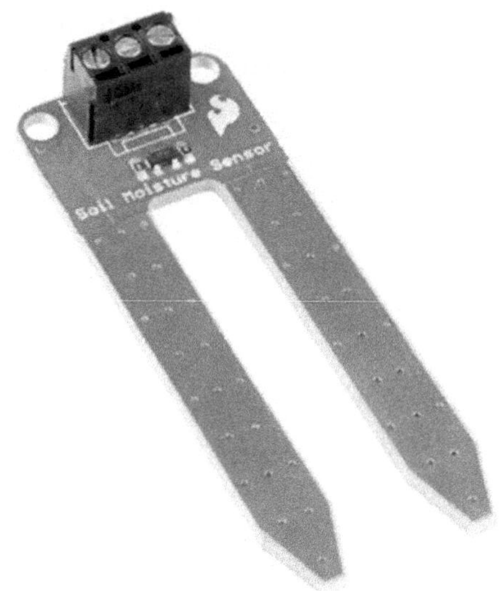

Soil Temperature

Soil temperature is the measurement of the warmth of the soil. Plants have an ideal temperature range to grow which is of 65-75 F (18-25C). However, there are several crops that have different ranges of temperature in which it can survive. In the early days, measuring the temperature of soil not possible so, it could be proof by monitoring the growth of plants. As the technologies emerged, however, the sensor technology enables the farmers to anticipate the conditions of the soil.

Soil Minerals

Soil contains a number of minerals, nutrients which are essential for the plants to grow like phosphorus denoted as (P), nitrogen denoted as (N) and potassium denoted as (K). These minerals help the plants to grow as it is the primary nutrients for the plants. On the hand, there is an excessive amount of these minerals present which actually lead to contaminate the groundwater. So, it has to be neutralized just enough for the plants and soil. Excessive use of fertilizers and herbicides is harmful to the crops and plants as well as for the consumers. So, it is important to avoid these chemicals and promote using of technologies for monitoring of soil mineral for better growth of the plants.

Figure 7. Mineral sensor

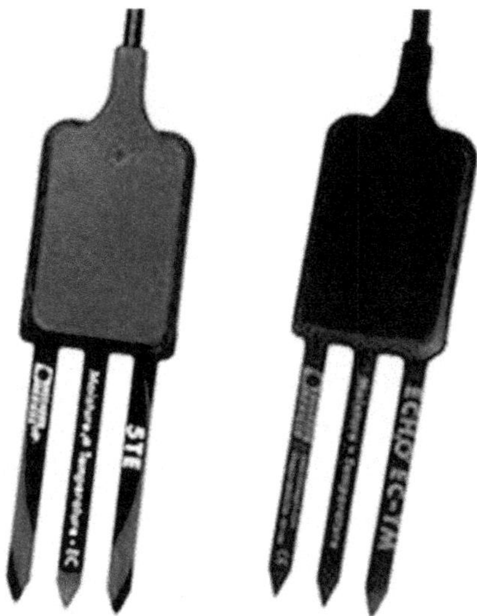

Drip Irrigation

Drip Irrigation is an irrigation system that provides the ability to save water by dripping waste slowly to the root of the plants which can be buried inside or on top of the soil surface. It has the potential to save water because the water is dropping within a certain period of time. It also helps in minimizing the evaporation of water. Drip irrigation was first introduced by Simcha Blass and his son Yeshayahu in 1959 in Israel which reduces the water consumption and increase crop yields and productivity. Drip

Irrigation is the reason behind the success in the agriculture sector. Israel is a desert where the country has only 20% of arable land. Apparently, it is because of the drip irrigation and technology that lifted the country up to this level and became on the most advanced country in agriculture. Drip irrigation has a great impact on farming and it can possibly increase crop yields and productivity (Kavianand, Nivas, Kiruthika, & Lalitha, 2016). The figure shows how drip irrigation works. The water source provides water to the pipe where the there are small knob or outlet valve where it drips the water.

Figure 8. Drip irrigation

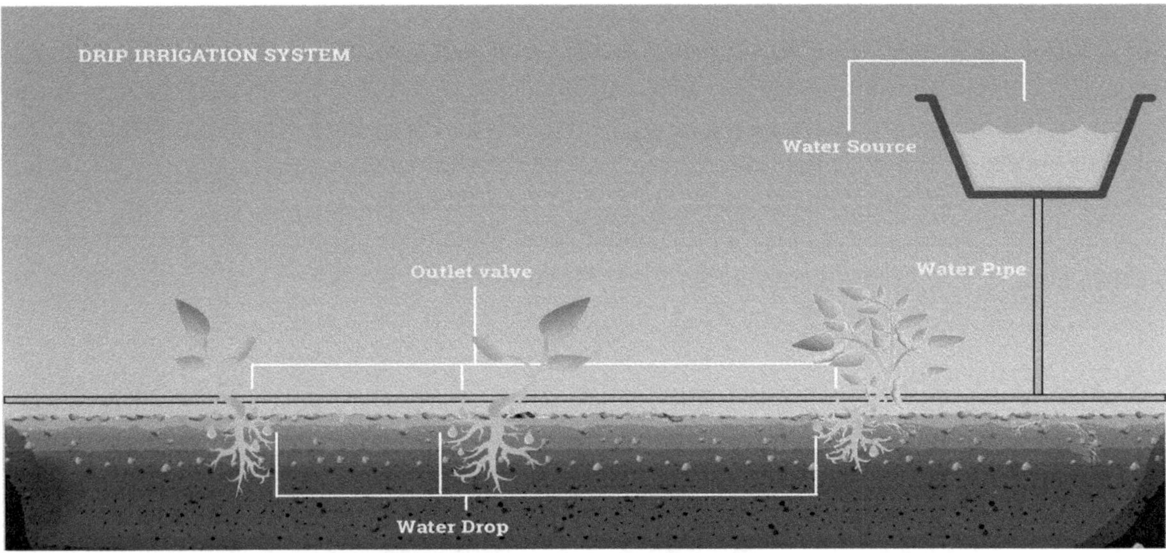

IoT AND MACHINE LEARNING FOR PRECISION AGRICULTURE

Significance of Incorporating IoT and Machine Learning

The Wireless sensor network technology has thrived in the technology world and it transforms the conventional ways of the manual system to an automatic smart system (Deepika & Rajapirian, 2016). Nowadays, station, office, home, airport, farming, and traffic interconnect with the help of IoT technology. This is one of the fastest growing technologies as it had connected 15.41 billion devices in 2015 and estimated that 75.44 billion IoT devices would be connected by 2025 (Source: www.statista.com/statistics/471264/iot-number-of-connected-devices-worldwide/). Internet of Things provides a common platform for all the devices where information and data can be shared and also provide a common language for all the devices for communication. Moreover, IoT provides accessibility from any platform and devices to all the information gathered and stored in a database. It provides authority to the users to retrieve the data as per the requirement for better experiences and it enables the users to monitor and control from any handheld device and computers. For instance, the fitness band is a new IoT technology that observes human gesture, behavior, and heartbeats which is actually a health monitoring device.

Figure 9. IoT and machine learning working mechanism
(Source: https://twitter.com/kirkdborne/status/762654729939869696)

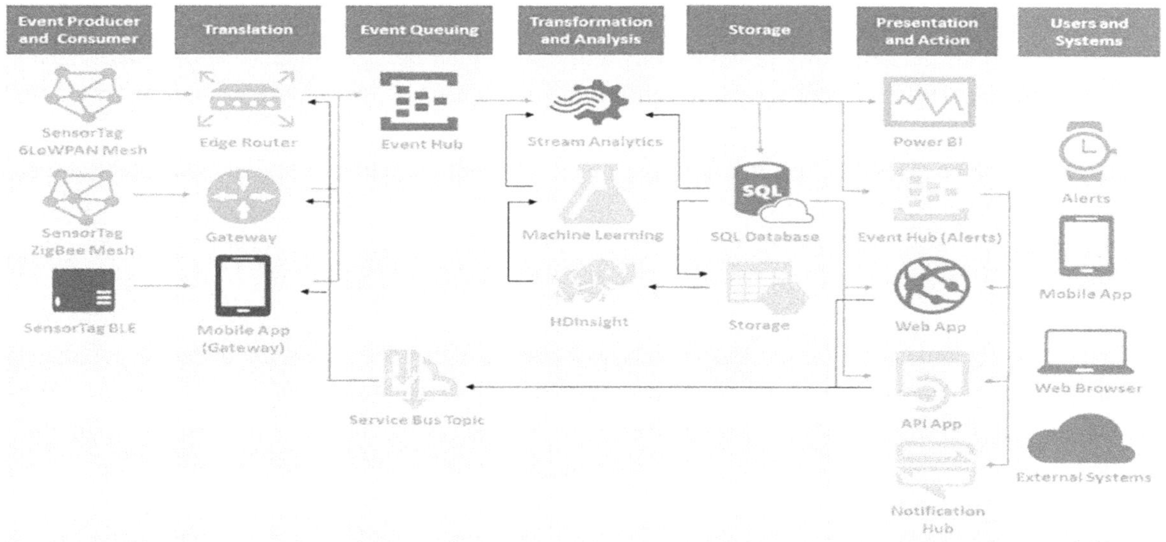

With the revolutionary in the system of farming, the Internet of Things (IoT) has been introduced which is basically the interconnection of all devices and sensors over the internet. This technology has drastically changed the life of a farmer as they can monitor and control over the farms and plants on the tips of their hand using handheld devices and laptops etc. This technology had made farming much faster and accurate and which ultimately lead to high productivity.

In this world of technology, IoT has emerges to wide ranges in almost every domain such as hospitals, traffic, vehicle, machines and even household which make technology smart. Technically, sensors are installed and are all connected all over the world through internet connectivity and data and information could be interchange and exchange from one domain to the other.

Machine Learning is an algorithm that teaches systems to work progressively for a better experience and make decisions from experience without explicitly programmed. It literally means training a computer to solve a certain level of real-time problems encountered in human life and without a human assistant. Machine Learning is a powerful system which is widely used in many domains such as a vehicle, agriculture, traffic, market and homes, etc. For instance, a self-driving car is one of the most prominent automated device built with a Machine learning algorithm. So, IoT and Machine Learning technologies have a high potential to create a revolutionary in the technology world. It is the combination of all the expert machines and intelligent system connecting together that enables to communicate and exchange information for a better experience.

Applications

Precision Farming

Precision farming is the measures that have taken to improve the system of farming with sophisticated technologies that provide efficiency and accuracy. Farming has been enriched with the technologies like sensors, automated machines, robots, autonomous vehicles and control systems. These technologies are used in different parameter and in different geographical places. These technologies could share data and information with high-speed internet connectivity. The Internet plays a vital role in the field of agriculture as it has the capability of controlling and bringing all devices together at one platform and share information. This connectivity has made farming effortless but also accurate and it has promoted control remotely.

In order to make precision farming, farming has to be smart, intelligent and also efficient and accurate at the same time.

Agricultural Drones

The drone has become a very important device in farming. It has been used for different parameters such as irrigation, disease detection, soil analysis, health assessment and so on. It has a very high time complexity and simplicity which can save a lot of time. With the drone, farmers could be able to monitor the crop, its health, yield prediction, plant height and amount of water requirement by placing camera which captures the image.

Livestock Monitoring

The animals in the livestock are large in numbers and it is very difficult for the farmers to monitor animal's health individually, behavior and diseases spread among the animals. Here, with the help of camera or sensor animal can be monitored real-time and retrieve images and data of the animal behavior and gesture anytime needed where it is very easy to identify the condition of animals. There are often spread of contagious diseases like H1N1, swine flu, fowlpox and bird flu which are easily spread amongst one another. So, monitoring of these animals would highly help to avoid the spreading of diseases amongst the animals by isolating the one with the disease.

Smart Greenhouse

The greenhouse is an enhancement of the system of farming in order to yield crops better and more productive. The main idea of implementing greenhouse is to maintain climate, weather, and humidity for the proper growth of the plants. In the greenhouse, plants and crops are growing rigorously as they are under proper environment. However, the conventional greenhouse has a limitation on automation where works are manually operated. To enhance the technology, smart greenhouse came into the picture with the help of IoT technology where it monitors the humidity, temperature, and climate specifically. IoT provides farmers with the ability to monitor and control over the internet through Wifi connections.

ISSUES AND PROBLEMS FOR IMPLEMENTING SMART FARMING

Technology has elevated the system of farming and has provided efficiency, accuracy and time complexity. Smart farming delivers an increase in productivity and yield crops. However, there are problems in adopting technologies in smart farming, these are:

High Cost of Technology

Recent technologies such as the Internet of Things and Machine Learning etc could minimize the workforce as it performs task really fast and accurate on the devices and machines etc, so, it is anticipated that the machine would probably replace the farmers in the near future. However, this is not really the case at some point as in some countries in the African continent and South East Asian continent because many countries had undergone through poverty where the workforce was the main source of energy in the agricultural fields. Therefore, deployment and implementation of devices and technologies are still not in the process. Implementation of devices practically on the field would probably require couples of sensors which would actually cost a huge amount of money. So, there are fewer chances of mechanizing the system of farming for the farmers while there are times when they only get just their daily bread. It would have been difficult for them to afford these kinds of devices while they are still having difficulties in implementing conventional tools for yielding of crops, productivity, and exports.

Unreachability of Rural Areas

Agriculture and farming take place in the countryside and isolated area where spaces are available for farming. It is because farming is more effective in a place where there the land is much arable than the land contaminated by the wastes and chemicals emits by the human. However, the implementation of technologies in these areas could be problematic as electricity and network coverage area are limited to the remote and rural area. So, people living in these areas often had a problem with electricity and power.

Immediate implementation of technology in farming would be difficult as farming needs huge acres of land and there are places in rural areas where internet connection and electricity has not reached in.

Ignorance by the Authorities

Farming typically takes place in the remote areas and mountainous regions where crops can easily adapt and soil compatibility is higher. Geographically, it has a high potential for yielding crops on a large scale with high productivity. However, the people who are actually farmers living in this area are poor. They are generally ignored by the authorities and hardly get financial support. The authorities support is probably the only way for the farmers to sustain agriculture. Farmers in these places do not have the capability of affording sophisticated farming devices and machines. Despite being mechanizing the system of farming, they could not even buy fertilizers and pesticides. Farmers from South Asian and South East Asian generally face these problems (Babar Shahbaz, Tanvir Ali1, Izhar A. Khan and Munir Ahmad, 2010).

Lack of Financial Resources

A group of financial supporters like governments and private banks and private money lenders could not give loans to the farmers because of several loans not being paid. This is because in some cases, the farmer could not get expected yield productions because of several calamities like droughts, Storms, unexpected increase in temperature and flood. Moreover, pests and diseases are also destroying the crops and it has been a nightmare for the farmers. So, many farmers eventually ended up with nothing in their hands. So, in many countries from the African continent and South East Asian continent farmers are poor and frustrated and even committed suicide.

Lack of Knowledge

Farmers in developing countries are mostly uneducated and unskilled because neither they are an urge to acquire knowledge of new technologies nor the authorities give awareness of the importance of new technologies (J. M. Kimiti, D. W. Odee & B. Vanlauwe, 2009). So, this is the main factor why farmers prefer the conventional type of farming over smart farming as it needs less money to spend (Abdul Rasheed Khan, M.K. Dubey, P.K. Bisen and K.K. Saxena, 2007).

A Development Project in Nigeria called FADAMA is an objective which will increase the incomes for farmers of rural areas and develop sustainable agriculture. It actually helps the farmers by financing them and makes them aware of the knowledge in anyways in order to develop and sustain a better way of farming, irrigation and increase food security in the country.

FUTURE RESEARCH DIRECTIONS

Internet of things is a technology that thrived on a very large scale and it enlarged its boundary in many domains, especially in the agricultural sector it has promoted simplicity for the farmers and increases yield productions. The estimation states that by 2020, over 24 billion devices would be connected with IoT. So, as the connectivity increases, security should go along the pace of new technology to protect systems from redundancy and several errors. This is also a big challenge for researchers and students to be aware of better security systems. Moreover, on the other side of the technology world, machine learning has grown so fast and is adopted in many. There are lots of researchers and enthusiasts people in many parts of the country seeking to enhance and make computer smart like a human. Incorporating of machine learning algorithms and IoT has the huge potential and feasible on the agriculture sector for making precision agriculture. So, a researcher, a student and enthusiasts must aware of these technologies and bring these technologies to its best for making a better smart farming experience.

CONCLUSION

In this chapter, different types of techniques which were used for farming and the modern sophisticated technologies are discussed and how it has an impact on farming and the overview of all the technologies. Apparently, the population growth rate is increasing exponentially which led the demand for food has risen respectively, so it is necessary for everyone to aware of the food security in order to sustain precision agriculture. Pollution and waste contaminate seawater, rivers, lakes and even the soil which actually affects human livelihood. The lakes and rivers water is the main source of water for consumption and for irrigation. Because of this contamination of these water, diseases like bacteria and viruses are often spread in human and plants, which is very dangerous for health. So, it is very important and crucial to emphasize on implementation of technologies irrigation, agriculture and drinking water in order to sustain mental well being. As agriculture is necessary for human livelihood, it is our duty to seek a better way of farming with modern technology to sustain Precision Agriculture.

ACKNOWLEDGMENT

This research received no specific grant from any funding agency in the public, commercial, or not-for-profit sectors.

REFERENCES

Asghari, P., Rahmani, A. M., & Javadi, H. H. S. (2019). Internet of Things applications: A systematic review. *Computer Networks*, *148*, 241–261. doi:10.1016/j.comnet.2018.12.008

Athani, S., Tejeshwar, C. H., Patil, M. M., Patil, P., & Kulkarni, R. (2017). Soil moisture monitoring using IoT enabled Arduino sensors with neural networks for improving soil management for farmers and predict seasonal rainfall for planning future harvest in North Karnataka — India. In *2017 International Conference on I-SMAC (IoT in Social, Mobile, Analytics and Cloud) (I-SMAC)* (pp. 43–48). Palladam, Tamilnadu, India: IEEE. 10.1109/I-SMAC.2017.8058385

Biradar, H. B., & Shabadi, L. (2017). Review on IOT based multidisciplinary models for smart farming. In *2017 2nd IEEE International Conference on Recent Trends in Electronics, Information & Communication Technology (RTEICT)* (pp. 1923–1926). Bangalore: IEEE. 10.1109/RTEICT.2017.8256932

Deepika, G., & Rajapirian, P. (2016). Wireless sensor network in precision agriculture: A survey. In *2016 International Conference on Emerging Trends in Engineering, Technology and Science (ICETETS)* (pp. 1–4). Pudukkottai, India: IEEE. 10.1109/ICETETS.2016.7603070

Dimitriadis, S., & Goumopoulos, C. (2008). Applying Machine Learning to Extract New Knowledge in Precision Agriculture Applications. In *2008 Panhellenic Conference on Informatics* (pp. 100–104). Samos, Greece: IEEE. 10.1109/PCI.2008.30

Gandhi, R., Nimbalkar, S., Yelamanchili, N., & Ponkshe, S. (2018). Plant disease detection using CNNs and GANs as an augmentative approach. In *2018 IEEE International Conference on Innovative Research and Development (ICIRD)* (pp. 1–5). Bangkok: IEEE. 10.1109/ICIRD.2018.8376321

Joshi, A., & Ali, L. (2017). A detailed survey on auto irrigation system. In *2017 Conference on Emerging Devices and Smart Systems (ICEDSS)* (pp. 90–95). Mallasamudram, Tiruchengode, India: IEEE. 10.1109/ICEDSS.2017.8073665

Kalaivani, T., Allirani, A., & Priya, P. (2011). A survey on Zigbee based wireless sensor networks in agriculture. In *3rd International Conference on Trendz in Information Sciences & Computing (TISC2011)* (pp. 85–89). Chennai, India: IEEE. 10.1109/TISC.2011.6169090

Kavianand, G., Nivas, V. M., Kiruthika, R., & Lalitha, S. (2016). *Smart drip irrigation system for sustainable agriculture. In 2016 IEEE Technological Innovations in ICT for Agriculture and Rural Development (TIAR)* (pp. 19–22). Chennai, India: IEEE; doi:10.1109/TIAR.2016.7801206

Khan, A. R., Dubey, M. K., Bisen, P. K., & Saxena, K. K. (2007). Constraints faced by farmers of Narsing Kheda village of Sihore district. *Young (up to 30 yrs.), 8,* 16.

Khanna, A., & Kaur, S. (2019). Evolution of Internet of Things (IoT) and its significant impact in the field of Precision Agriculture. *Computers and Electronics in Agriculture, 157,* 218–231. doi:10.1016/j.compag.2018.12.039

Kimiti, J. M., Odee, D. W., & Vanlauwe, B. (2009). *Area under grain legumes cultivation and problems faced by smallholder farmers in legume production in the semi-arid eastern Kenya.* Academic Press.

Lim, C., Kim, K.-J., & Maglio, P. P. (2018). Smart cities with big data: Reference models, challenges, and considerations. *Cities (London, England), 82,* 86–99. doi:10.1016/j.cities.2018.04.011

Mekala, M. S., & Viswanathan, P. (2017). A Survey: Smart agriculture IoT with cloud computing. In *2017 International conference on Microelectronic Devices, Circuits and Systems (ICMDCS)* (pp. 1–7). Vellore: IEEE. 10.1109/ICMDCS.2017.8211551

Mittal, A., & Singh, A. (2007). Microcontroller based pest management system. In *Second International Conference on Systems (ICONS'07)* (pp. 43–43). Martinique, France: IEEE. 10.1109/ICONS.2007.35

O'Grady, M. J., & O'Hare, G. M. P. (2017). Modelling the smart farm. *Information Processing in Agriculture, 4*(3), 179–187. doi:10.1016/j.inpa.2017.05.001

Pandithurai, O., Aishwarya, S., Aparna, B., & Kavitha, K. (2017). Agro-tech: A digital model for monitoring soil and crops using internet of things (IOT). In *2017 Third International Conference on Science Technology Engineering & Management (ICONSTEM)* (pp. 342–346). Chennai, India: IEEE. 10.1109/ICONSTEM.2017.8261306

Patil, K. A., & Kale, N. R. (2016). A model for smart agriculture using IoT. In *2016 International Conference on Global Trends in Signal Processing, Information Computing and Communication (ICGTSPICC)* (pp. 543–545). Jalgaon, India: IEEE. 10.1109/ICGTSPICC.2016.7955360

Shahbaz, B., Ali, T., Khan, I. A., & Ahmad, M. (2010). An analysis of the problems faced by farmers in the mountains of Northwest Pakistan: Challenges for agri. extension. *Pakistan Journal of Agricultural Sciences, 47*(4), 417–420.

Singh, A., & Sharma, T. P. (2014, July). A survey on area coverage in wireless sensor networks. In *2014 International Conference on Control, Instrumentation, Communication and Computational Technologies (ICCICCT)* (pp. 829-836). IEEE. 10.1109/ICCICCT.2014.6993073

Singh, V., Varsha, & Misra, A. K. (2015). Detection of unhealthy region of plant leaves using image processing and genetic algorithm. In *2015 International Conference on Advances in Computer Engineering and Applications* (pp. 1028–1032). Ghaziabad, India: IEEE. 10.1109/ICACEA.2015.7164858

Srisruthi, S., Swarna, N., Ros, G. M. S., & Elizabeth, E. (2016). Sustainable agriculture using eco-friendly and energy efficient sensor technology. In *2016 IEEE International Conference on Recent Trends in Electronics, Information & Communication Technology (RTEICT)* (pp. 1442–1446). Bangalore, India: IEEE. 10.1109/RTEICT.2016.7808070

Toreti, A., Maiorano, A., De Sanctis, G., Webber, H., Ruane, A. C., Fumagalli, D., ... Zampieri, M. (2019). Using reanalysis in crop monitoring and forecasting systems. *Agricultural Systems*, *168*, 144–153. doi:10.1016/j.agsy.2018.07.001 PMID:30774182

Wolfert, S., Ge, L., Verdouw, C., & Bogaardt, M.-J. (2017). Big Data in Smart Farming – A review. *Agricultural Systems*, *153*, 69–80. doi:10.1016/j.agsy.2017.01.023

Yong, W., Shuaishuai, L., Li, L., Minzan, L., Ming, L., Arvanitis, K. G., ... Sigrimis, N. (2018). Smart Sensors from Ground to Cloud and Web Intelligence. *IFAC-PapersOnLine*, *51*(17), 31–38. doi:10.1016/j.ifacol.2018.08.057

ADDITIONAL READING

Ferentinos, K. P. (2018). Deep learning models for plant disease detection and diagnosis. *Computers and Electronics in Agriculture*, *145*, 311–318. doi:10.1016/j.compag.2018.01.009

Goap et al. - 2018 - An IoT based smart irrigation management system us.pdf. (n.d.).

Ip, R. H. L., Ang, L.-M., Seng, K. P., Broster, J. C., & Pratley, J. E. (2018). Big data and machine learning for crop protection. *Computers and Electronics in Agriculture*, *151*, 376–383. doi:10.1016/j.compag.2018.06.008

Ma, C., Zhang, H. H., & Wang, X. (2014). Machine learning for Big Data analytics in plants. *Trends in Plant Science*, *19*(12), 798–808. doi:10.1016/j.tplants.2014.08.004 PMID:25223304

Mohamad Noor, M., & Hassan, W. H. (2019). Current research on Internet of Things (IoT) security: A survey. *Computer Networks*, *148*, 283–294. doi:10.1016/j.comnet.2018.11.025

Mostafa, H., El-Nady, R., Awad, M., & El-Ansary, M. (2018). Drip irrigation management for wheat under clay soil in arid conditions. *Ecological Engineering*, *121*, 35–43. doi:10.1016/j.ecoleng.2017.09.003

Rehman, T. U., Mahmud, M. S., Chang, Y. K., Jin, J., & Shin, J. (2019). Current and future applications of statistical machine learning algorithms for agricultural machine vision systems. *Computers and Electronics in Agriculture*, *156*, 585–605. doi:10.1016/j.compag.2018.12.006

Ruiz-Garcia, L., & Lunadei, L. (2011). The role of RFID in agriculture: Applications, limitations and challenges. *Computers and Electronics in Agriculture*, *79*(1), 42–50. doi:10.1016/j.compag.2011.08.010

Scheberl, L., Scharenbroch, B. C., Werner, L. P., Prater, J. R., & Fite, K. L. (2019). Evaluation of soil pH and soil moisture with different field sensors: Case study urban soil. *Urban Forestry & Urban Greening*, *38*, 267–279. doi:10.1016/j.ufug.2019.01.001

Yong, W., Shuaishuai, L., Li, L., Minzan, L., Ming, L., Arvanitis, K. G., ... Sigrimis, N. (2018). Smart Sensors from Ground to Cloud and Web Intelligence. *IFAC-PapersOnLine*, *51*(17), 31–38. doi:10.1016/j.ifacol.2018.08.057

Zamora-Izquierdo, M. A., Santa, J., Martínez, J. A., Martínez, V., & Skarmeta, A. F. (2019). Smart farming IoT platform based on edge and cloud computing. *Biosystems Engineering*, *177*, 4–17. doi:10.1016/j.biosystemseng.2018.10.014

This research was previously published in Modern Techniques for Agricultural Disease Management and Crop Yield Prediction edited by N. Pradeep, Sandeep Kautish, C.R. Nirmala, Vishal Goyal, and Sonia Abdellatif; pages 1-22, copyright year 2020 by Engineering Science Reference (an imprint of IGI Global).

Chapter 40
Disrupting Agriculture:
The Status and Prospects for AI and Big Data in Smart Agriculture

Omar F. El-Gayar
https://orcid.org/0000-0001-8657-8732
Dakota State University, USA

Martinson Q. Ofori
https://orcid.org/0000-0002-6581-8909
Dakota State University, USA

ABSTRACT

The United Nations (UN) Food and Agriculture (FAO) estimates that farmers will need to produce about 70% more food by 2050. To accommodate the growing demand, the agricultural industry has grown from labor-intensive to smart agriculture, or Agriculture 4.0, which includes farm equipment that are enhanced using autonomous unmanned decision systems (robotics), big data, and artificial intelligence. In this chapter, the authors conduct a systematic review focusing on big data and artificial intelligence in agriculture. To further guide the literature review process and organize the findings, they devise a framework based on extant literature. The framework is aimed to capture key aspects of agricultural processes, supporting supply chain, key stakeholders with a particular emphasis on the potential, drivers, and challenges of big data and artificial intelligence. They discuss how this new paradigm may be shaped differently depending on context, namely developed and developing countries.

INTRODUCTION

The Agricultural Revolution between the 17th to late 19th centuries brought about productivity through the mechanization of farm work. As the human population continues to grow, however, the demand for land, food, and resources have become more intense making it necessary to reinvent the agricultural sector. Even with the continuous advancements in agriculture, the sector is still faced with several issues such as climate change, competition for land and water resources, food waste attributed to post-harvest handling

DOI: 10.4018/978-1-7998-5354-1.ch040

and storage, and more. The 2018 Global Report on Food Crisis stated that *"out of the 51 countries that experienced food crises in 2017, conflict and insecurity were the major drivers of food insecurity in 18 countries, where almost 74 million people faced Crisis (IPC/CH Phase 3), Emergency (IPC/CH Phase 4) or Catastrophe/Famine (IPC/CH Phase 5) conditions"* (Food Security Information Network, 2018). The United Nations (UN) Food and Agriculture Organization (FAO) estimates that farmers will need to produce about 70% more food by 2050. How is the sector prepared for increased production of food despite competing with humans for land? What is the optimal use for resources despite climate change? Will agriculture meet global food needs as projected by the UN?

In this regard, an emerging trend is the use of *"smart"* technologies in farming commonly referred to as Smart Agriculture. As CEMA (2017) puts it, the main difference between Precision Agriculture and its successor, Smart Agriculture, is that while the former improves the accuracy of operations and allows the management of in-field (or in-herd) variations by providing for plants (or animals) the optimal resources needed for growth, the latter uses big data analytics and artificial intelligence (AI) to act on data collected by the farm equipment. It has been suggested that Smart Agriculture solves the problem of generalization whilst providing autonomy for farm decisions enhanced by context, situation and location awareness (Wolfert et al., 2014). In this paper, we define Smart Agriculture as the use of precision agriculture technologies aided by big data and AI to make informed autonomous farm decisions that save resources in short term and increase the quality of produce in long term.

In essence, as has been done by blockchain and cryptocurrency in the payment industry, virtual reality in the entertainment industry, and trendsetters like 3D printing and augmented reality, big data and artificial intelligence (AI) in agriculture are disruptive technologies that, as defined by Christensen (1997), are changing the entire outlook of the industry through new ideas for problem solving with the hope of eventually displacing existing practices. However, as with any disruptive innovation, the impact on the target sector and society at large can have far-reaching implications. Big data and AI are already starting to reshape the manner we handle agricultural tasks such as harvesting, crop and soil management, and accounting for environmental impact on yield using predictive analytics. Examples range from robots employing advanced machine vision for harvesting pepper (Simon, 2018), to optimizing crop yields in India (Microsoft, Inc., 2018). Further, the socio-technical, and socio-economic drivers and challenges for the development and diffusion of smart agriculture are context dependent. While developed countries may be driven by a severe shortage of labor, developing countries are driven by the sheer need to support their fast-growing populations. The development and diffusion in developing countries will have to consider factors such as the nascent supporting technology infrastructure.

Being a novelty field with so much potential and rising popularity, several researchers have tried to measure the impact of Smart Agriculture and its effect on traditional agricultural practices. Big data management and analysis especially has been a major theme for most researchers in trying to understand the opportunities inherent in its incorporation into farms (Chi et al., 2016; Coble et al., 2018; Kamilaris & Prenafeta-Boldú, 2018; Nandyala & Kim, 2016; Waga & Rabah, 2014; Woodard, 2016). Wolfert et al., (2017) went further to develop a conceptual framework to analyze big data in Smart Farming applications from a socio-economic perspective. Other reviews have been more geo-specific: as has been done to understand applications of big data in developing countries (Ali et al., 2016; Misaki et al., 2018; Olaniyi et al., 2018; Protopop & Shanoyan, 2016); or more domain-specific: such as deep learning applications (Kamilaris & Prenafeta-Boldú, 2018; Zhu et al., 2018), hyper-spectral analysis (Khan et al., 2018; Thenkabail et al., 2012), and wireless technology (Mark et al., 2016). This chapter aims to contribute to existing literature by emphasizing the AI dimension of the conversation through an examination of how the relationship between these two innovations are disrupting agriculture. Specifically, this chapter addresses the following research questions:

1. What is the current status of Big Data and AI in smart agriculture?
2. What are the drivers and challenges underlying this paradigm shift?
3. What are the prospects of Big Data and AI as disruptive technology in agriculture?

Addressing these research questions, we conduct a systematic review focusing on big data and AI in agriculture. The review spans the last decade and covers peer-reviewed scholarly publications as well as, given the emerging field, *grey* literature, example industry reports. To further guide the literature review process and organize the findings, we devise a framework based on extant literature. The framework aims to capture key aspects of agricultural processes supporting supply chain and key stakeholders with a particular emphasis on the potential, drivers, and challenges of big data and artificial intelligence. We also discuss how this new paradigm may be shaped differently depending on context, namely developed and developing countries. In this chapter, Smart Agriculture, Smart Farming and Agriculture 4.0 are used to interchangeably.

The chapter is organized as follows: The following two sections describe the background and methodology for the systematic review and introduce the proposed conceptual framework, respectively. Next, we present the results followed by a discussion of the findings with respect to the current status and prospects of big data and AI in agriculture as well as the drivers and challenges moving forward.

BACKGROUND

Industrial revolutions have always gone in tandem with agriculture, and just like the Industrial Revolution 4.0, the agricultural industry has grown from the labor-intensive Agriculture 1.0, high productivity gains of the *green* Agriculture 2.0, *precision farming* through guidance systems, sensors, and telematics of Agriculture 3.0 through to Agriculture 4.0, or Smart Agriculture, which consists of farm equipment that are enhanced using autonomous unmanned decision systems (robotics), data and artificial intelligence (Cho, 2018; Wolfert et al., 2017). To understand the relevance of this slow but gradual change towards automation based on farm data, it is necessary to examine the value chain of agriculture as well as concepts related to big data and AI.

The Agriculture Value Chain

In this review we breakdown agriculture's value chain into its components as:

Pre-Production: Any activity that occurs before actual planting takes place is classified under the pre-production phase. These activities include land preparation, seed quality control, and all other planning activities, that can be very crucial to healthy crop production and potential crop yield (Krishnan & Surya Rao, 2005; Oshunsanya, 2013).

Production: The production phase covers every on-field activity such as planting, fertilizer application, irrigation, pest and weed control. Precision Agriculture delivered a plethora of mechanization improvements in this aspect of agriculture. Herein, we identify how big data and AI have further optimized production decisions – both autonomous and human-led. Cost, time and any other resource savings are brought to the forefront by examining process improvements.

Post-Production: Robotic harvesting has been around as far back as the 1980's, and this has been popularized and applied to various types of commodities: eggplants, tomatoes, cucumber, and strawberries (Arima et al., 1994; Arima et al., 2001; Hayashi et al., 2002; Kawamura et al., 1984; Kondo et al., 1996). Smart Agriculture provides an avenue for further improving accuracy of harvest, supply chain, and marketing operations, hereby reducing yield waste and increasing profit margins.

AI and Big Data

The concept and real-world application of artificial intelligence has existed since circa 1950. The concern for AI has been developing systems that act as rational agents taking the best possible action in any given situation (Russell & Norvig, 2010). Cockburn et al. (2018) groups AI applications into three interrelated separate streams: symbolic systems such as natural language processing and image recognition: have been successfully applied at various levels but also been criticized for their inability to be scaled towards commercial solutions; robotics: used heavily for industrial automation; and the learning approach: that given some inputs can predict the presence of particular physical or logical events. As demonstrated in Figure 1., these streams are not so far from the sub-specialties proposed by Michael Mills of Neota Logic (Martin, 2016). Just like the streams proposed by Cockburn et al. (2018), he divides AI into robotics, cognition tools such as Natural Language Processing and Vision systems used to capture and synthesize text, voice and images; Machine Learning consisting of deep learning and predictive analytics through supervised and unsupervised learning used to find previously unknown relationships in data; and other concepts such as Expert Systems and Planning, and Scheduling & Optimization.

Big data, on the other hand, refers to large amounts of unstructured data produced by high-performing applications (Cuzzocrea, et al., 2011). It is characterized by the 3V model proposed by Laney (2001) consisting of *volume*, *variety*, and *velocity*. Many authors have extended these 3Vs to include *value* and *veracity* (Bello-Orgaz et al., 2016; Cuzzocrea et al., 2011). Big data methodologies, such as data mining, serve up huge datasets made up of both structured and unstructured data (Fan & Bifet, 2013; Ghosh & Nath, 2016). What is inherently clear, however, is that big data is beyond the analysis capabilities of traditional relational databases (IBM, 2018).

By employing machine learning techniques, AI provides the needed analytic capabilities that support Data-Driven Decisions (DDD) (Bengio, 2009, 2013; Najafabadi et al., 2015). As the name implies, a data-driven decision is one made by using up-to-date data to analyze the facts in data and draw conclusions. As such, we consider big data and AI's value and potential as a derivative of their combined ability to provide automated DDD which result in higher productivity and market value (Brynjolfsson et al., 2011; Provost & Fawcett, 2013).

There is a plethora of underlying technologies (Hadoop, MapReduce, Spark, Mahout, Hive, etc.) and techniques (Naive Bayes, Regression Models, K-Nearest Neighbors, Decision Trees, Boosting Algorithms, Genetic Algorithms, Neural Networks etc.) used in processing, mining and analyzing big data. Our focus, however, is on value which typically is derived from deploying AI-based analytics to big data.

Overall, there are four types of analytics – descriptive, diagnostic, predictive, and prescriptive (Markkanen, 2015; Rajeswari et al., 2017). In this chapter, we focus on the latter three progressions of deriving value from big data where AI techniques are most prevalent:

Figure 1. Fields of AI. Source: (Mills, 2015)

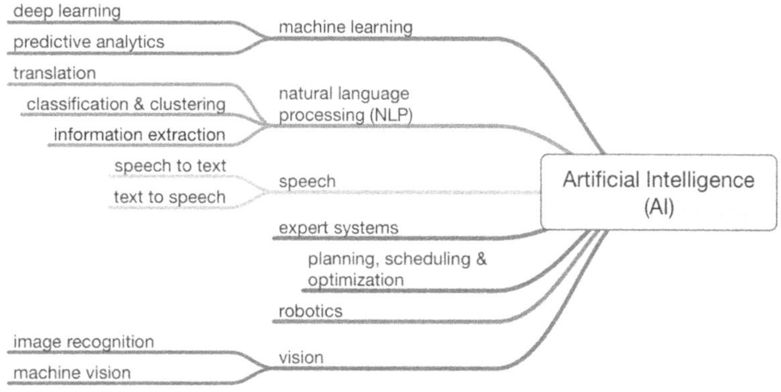

Diagnostic

This function aims at providing answers to the question: *why did it happen?* (Gartner, 2018). Diagnostic Analytics is sometimes combined with Descriptive Analytics with some researchers even calling it a step 1.5 before the next phase (Markkanen, 2015). This is because it is the most abstract of the phases: an explorative step that exists mainly to drill down on reasons behind certain trends. However, it is still key in understanding data trends, especially as machine learning models can quickly find patterns in data that human analysts might not be as quick to identify. A simple example will be where a business, before restocking due to a sudden rise in the sales of a commodity, uses this type of analytics to understand why there is an increase in sales and thereby prevent over (or under) stocking on the said commodity.

Predictive

Any analytics model that emphasizes prediction, rapid analysis, business relevance of resulting insights, and ease of use (sometimes through automated decision making) is considered Predictive Analytics. It is primarily concerned with: *what could happen* (Gartner, 2018; IBM, 2013). Some of the more common predictive models include regression analysis, decision trees, forecasting, multivariate statistics, pattern matching, and neural networks. While there are close parallels between this type of analytics and machine learning, it is important to underline that Predictive Analytics merely employs machine learning algorithms in making estimations of future outcomes however they are not the same. (Wakefield, 2018). Business uses for Predictive Analytics include risk outcomes of various business decisions, sales forecasting, deriving marketing insight for proper market segmentation, and even financial modeling aimed at forecasting business performance.

Prescriptive

Prescriptive Analytics forms part of the paradigm of advanced analytics that explores data to provide possible actions. In essence, it provides answers to the question: *what should be done?* (Gartner, 2018; IBM, 2013; Markkanen, 2015). In essence, it builds on Predictive Analytics to provide possible actions to take and the effect of such decisions. Techniques employed with this type of analytics include simulation, graph analysis, recommender systems, complex event processing, heuristics, neural networks, and machine learning. By continuously *learning* from new data, the accuracy of prescriptions improves with each iteration.

Related Work

Big data applications have been used to deal with several agricultural issues and there are many agricultural areas where big data solutions have been deployed. These include but are not limited to weather forecasting, land conservation, weed detection, biodiversity, and remote sensing (Coble et al., 2018; Kamilaris et al., 2017). Kamilaris et al., (2017) go further to state some potential areas for big data application, especially in the supply chain where there is a need for quality products and better yield and demand estimation. This view is similar to the position taken by Wolfert et al. (2017). They propose a conceptual framework to analyze big data applications in Smart Farming from a socio-economic perspective. Their findings demonstrate that big data applications in agriculture are changing the scope of the industry through push-pull mechanisms. The push factors are driven by advancements in technology, massive amounts of data generation and storage, and digital connectivity. The pull factors, on the other hand, are mainly through population and business demand: the public being interested in food sustainability, security, and nutrition; and to the farmer, smart farming being mainly about efficiency and profitability.

The recent resurgence of AI, and associated techniques like machine learning, is also pushing the limits for Smart Farming. Machine learning is often the most used technique employed by researchers for big data analysis, although other statistical models like time series analysis, and spike and regression analysis have also been used for forecasting agricultural events (Coble et al., 2018; Kamilaris et al., 2017). One branch of machine learning which has been applied, especially to computer vision and image analysis in agriculture, is deep learning. In a recent paper, Kamilaris & Prenafeta-Boldú (2018) surveyed several applications of deep learning in agriculture. Interestingly, they found that deep learning has been applied not only to imaging but sensory data and other environmental variables. Recurrent Neural Networks (RNN), a type of deep learning, were seen to offer higher performance due to their ability to capture both space and time dimension. Zhu et al. (2018) also surveyed deep learning applications in agriculture and discovered similar result. They found that RNN had been used for land cover classification, phenotype recognition, crop yield estimation, leaf area index estimation, weather prediction, soil moisture estimation, animal research, and event date estimation.

The value of big data in smart agriculture, with the right analysis, can provide a win-win situation for all stakeholders. The potential for revenue growth and increased production efficiency, however, still seem unable to drive large-scale adoption. Several challenges have been found by researchers. Wolfert et al. (2017) discussed technical and organizational challenges with the latter being the most important. One of the biggest challenges was found to be governance issues regarding privacy and security of big data leading to its underutilization in smart farming. This sentiment is echoed by several other researchers (Coble et al., 2018; Kamilaris et al., 2017; Nandyala & Kim, 2016). In developing countries, the challenge for adoption runs deeper than data security. The most glaring being the lack of adequate physical and legal infrastructure to allow collection, storage and processing of data (Kshetri, 2014; Misaki et al., 2018; Protopop & Shanoyan, 2016). Another issue raised by researchers has been the high illiteracy levels amongst farmers in these areas which has contributed to the lack of awareness and trust in smart technology. Further, Misaki et al. (2018) discuss at length issues regarding farmers' belief that integration of big data applications will result in undue advantage for their competitors and even drive up land value and seed prices.

In this chapter, we discuss the current and future prospects of smart farming, the machine learning techniques that have been most prevalent, and how the relationship between big data and AI is disrupting agriculture. This chapter aims to contribute to existing literature by emphasizing the AI dimension of the conversation through an examination of how the relationship between these two innovations are disrupting agriculture. We explore the gap inherent in current literature which have been more geo-specific (Ali et al., 2016; Misaki et al., 2018; Olaniyi et al., 2018; Protopop & Shanoyan, 2016); or domain-specific such as deep learning (Kamilaris & Prenafeta-Boldú, 2018; Zhu et al., 2018), hyper-spectral analysis (Khan et al., 2018; Thenkabail et al., 2012), and wireless technology (Mark et al., 2016).

METHODS

In this systematic review, we use guidelines in accordance with the Preferred Reporting Items for Systematic Reviews and Meta-Analyses (PRISMA) (Liberati et al., 2009). The PRISMA statement provides an evidence-based minimum set of items for reporting systematic reviews and meta-analyses with the aim of improving the quality of reporting by authors of systematic reviews.

Data Sources and Search Strategy

We systematically reviewed literature from Web of Science, IEEE Xplore Digital Library, and Science-Direct (Elsevier) using a Boolean search query consisting of three groups of keywords that is big data and AI technologies (big data, artificial intelligence, data mining, machine learning, deep learning, neural networks etc.) and associated with either the set of keywords representing smart agriculture (smart agric*, smart farm*, agriculture 4.0, digital farm*, precision farm* etc.), or agriculture in general (agric*, farm*, agronom*, cultivat* etc.). To further enrich the data retrieved, literature from ACM Digital Library, Agricola and *grey* literature from sources such as industry reports and non-peer-reviewed publications from Google Scholar are considered. Big data is a relatively new subject area; the first academic reference to big data was by Weiss & Indurkhya (1997), as such, the survey targeted literature published a decade after this first publication, that is, the period between January 2008 to September 2018. Due to language barrier, only English language publications are considered. Relevant works outside the specified timespan are considered if cited by included sources and are determined to be of importance to the chapter.

Study Selection

Papers focusing on areas other than agriculture are excluded, for example, the review excluded papers about the technologies themselves where agriculture was mentioned only as an area of application. Further, the review limits the definition of agriculture to agronomy (crop cultivation and soil management), hence livestock production and aquaculture applications are excluded as well. Other exclusion criteria included papers that are comparing technologies already covered such as reviews, surveys, and duplicates.

CONCEPTUAL FRAMEWORK

The conceptual framework (Figure 2.) serves as a background for the systematic review of big data and AI technologies in agriculture. We posit that the interaction between agriculture and smart technology, that is AI and big data, is a cross relationship between the agricultural value chain and the levels of analytics. As such, using the simple agricultural value chain and the levels of analytics described in the background, we break down agricultural production from inputs to distribution as a basis for identifying any form of disruption in the entire chain (Kaplinsky & Morris, 2001). For the purposes of this review, we emphasize the efficiencies these technologies bring to agricultural production and the magnitude of the value added, or prospects of value, as we move upstream in the agricultural value chain. Consequently, papers will be classified based on their potential value in this chain and not solely on technique alone.

Figure 2. Conceptual framework for reviewing literature

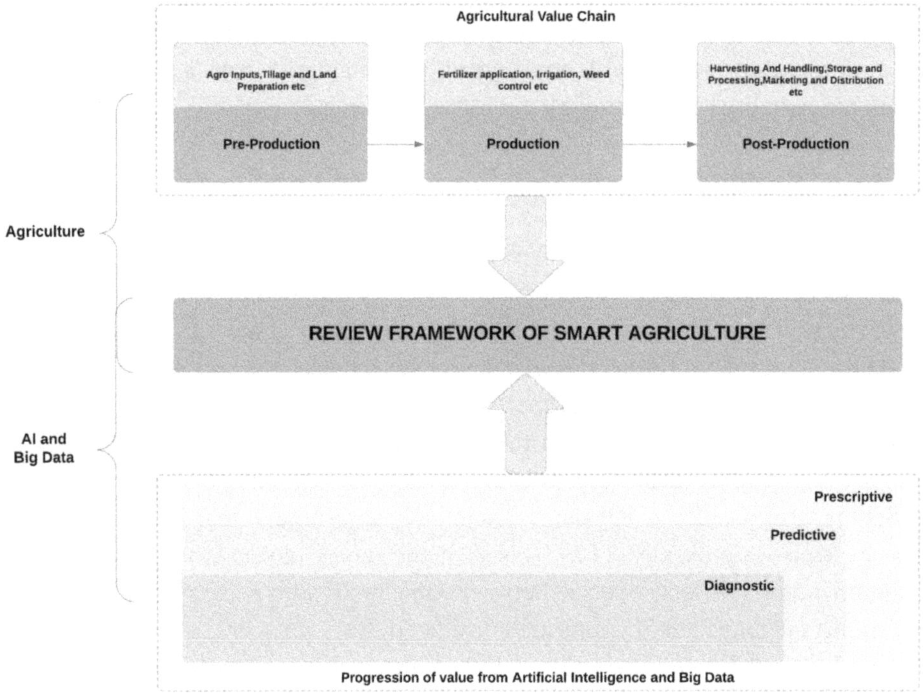

Starting from the bottom, researchers employ diagnostic analytics techniques in order to understand why an event has happened or is happening. In classifying papers as having used diagnostic analytics, we refer to papers that try to provide an interpretation of environmental or societal indices and cropping using AI and big data. We look at studies that identify anomalies, do data discovery, or determine causal relationships. The middle tier, predictive analytics, identifies mainly two categories of studies: those that forecast future events or classify the existence, or non-existence, of certain agents. In each part of the value chain, there are different types of predictions to be made: in production, for example, there are advantages to both identification of weeds and yield forecasting. At the very top is prescriptive analytics where we highlight studies that adopt AI and big data to provide recommendations. Studies that provide automated decisions and or apply business rules to prescribe actions. Some recommendations may not necessarily provide optimal solutions but rather simulate the possible effects of decision making. Simulations can be used, for example, to identify yield in different weather conditions.

RESULTS

As depicted in Figure 3., the search yielded 581 titles, of which 24 duplicates were excluded. The 557 remaining articles underwent careful title and abstract assessment; 59 were rejected on basis of being a survey, review, case study or comparative study; 94 excluded for being based purely on soil science; 125 articles based on animals, technology or precision agriculture were also excluded as well as 56 other off-topic articles. A total of 223 articles met our initial eligibility criteria and underwent full review out of which 153 articles covering the entire spectrum of AI and big data in agriculture were selected. Figure 4. depicts the trend line of papers over the analysis period.

Figure 3. Study selection process for systematic review

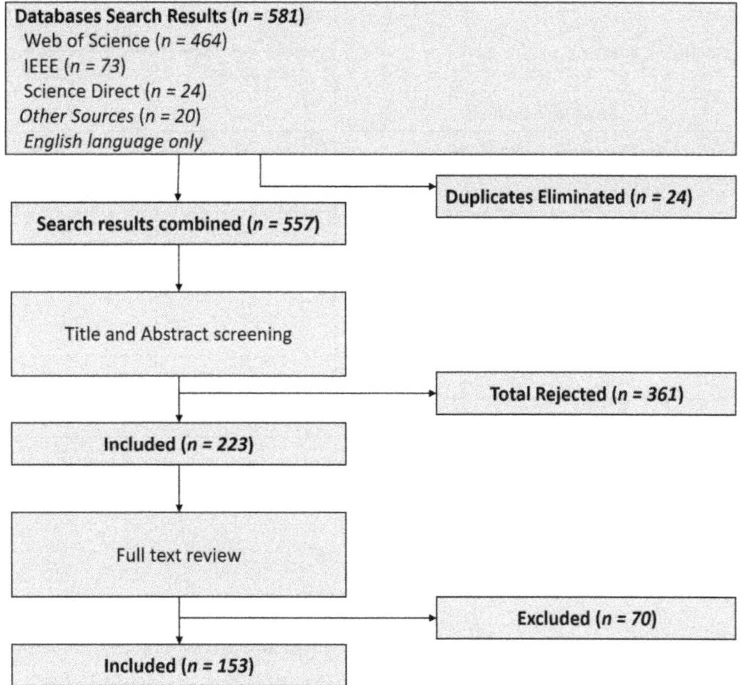

Predictive (72.54%) and Prescriptive (22.88%) were the most prevalent. The majority of the work done has been during the Production phase of agriculture (61.43%) with 78 (62.17%) of that value being Predictive, and 16 (15.01%) being Prescriptive as shown in Table 1. See the Appendix (Table 2., Table 3. and Table 4.) for summary information of each included article in our study.

Figure 4. Distribution of papers by years

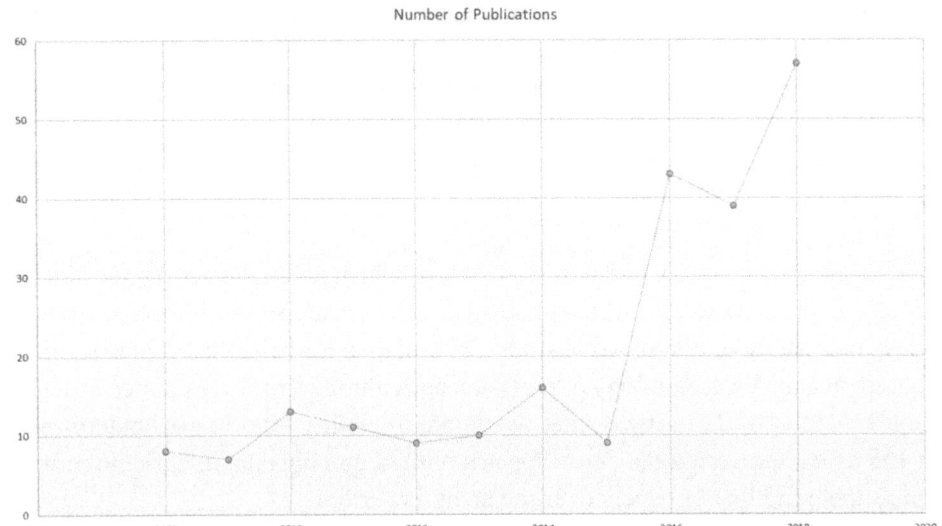

Table 1. Key findings

Agricultural Value Chain		Big Data and AI		
		Diagnostic	*Predictive*	*Prescriptive*
Pre-production	Seeds & Seedlings		4	3
	Soil, Tillage and Land Preparation	1	7	
	Other Pre-planting Activities	2	6	8
Production	Planting, Irrigation & Fertilizer Application	1	16	8
	Weed, Disease & Pest Control	2	33	7
	Yield, Weather, Energy & Other Farm Management Activities	2	29	1
Post-production	Harvest & Handling		6	7
	Storage & Processing		4	3
	Market & Consumer		10	1

Pre-Production

Seeds & Seedlings: Seven studies focused on improving the seeding process. Four studies employed the use of predictive techniques to classify infected and non-infected seedlings, sort quality of seedlings, and to predict yield (Emamgholizadeh et al., 2015; Griffel et al., 2018; Lamsal et al., 2017; Silva et al., 2013). Prescriptive methods was employed in the three remaining papers in recommending the right amount of phosphogypsum to be used when the farmer uses no-till management, optimization and seed density simulation (Caires & Guimaraes, 2018; Dornelles et al., 2018; Tesfaye et al., 2016).

Soil, Tillage and Land Preparation: Out of eight studies, one study employed diagnostic methods aimed at analyzing the effects of soil properties on traction force and traction effiency in a bid to optimize tillage (Pentos & Pieczarka, 2017). All other papers, were predictive in nature; five focused on predicting soil properties; others focused on predicting and optimizing vitro proliferation and estimating fuel consumption during tillage and soil preparation (Ajdadi et al., 2016; Arteta et al., 2018; Borges et al., 2017; Calderano et al., 2014; Pentos & Pieczarka, 2017; Pike et al., 2009; Prasad et al., 2018; Quraishi & Mouazen, 2013).

Other Pre-planting Activities: Two papers using diagnostic methods applied supervised feature selection to define traits affecting water content in maize and Spearson's rank correlation to determine association between climatic indices and maize and sorghum yields (Byakatonda et al., 2018; Shekoofa et al., 2011). Six studies used predictive methods in various aspects; for drought assessment and water planning, for forecasting seasonal variability and temperature, and for appraising mechanization on farms to predicting the success of an agricultural enterprise based on their capital (Bakhshi et al, 2016; Osman et al., 2015; Park et al., 2016; Smith et al., 2009; Zangeneh et al., 2010; Zhong et al., 2009). Prescriptive methods was the focus of the larger number of studies done in this area with the eight studies found devoted to prescribing and simulating management routes based on seeding density, land use conversion, and crop sequence (Delgado et al., 2008; Dornelles et al., 2018; Jimenez et al., 2009; Rajeswari et al., 2017; Renaud-Gentie et al., 2014; Rizzo et al., 2014; Snow & Lovattb, 2008; Zhong et al., 2009).

Production

Planting, Irrigation & Fertilizer Application

We found twenty-five papers that addressed this area of the agricultural cycle. One paper used data mining to analyze the spatial relationship between environmental and social factors and maize cultivation (Ureta et al., 2013). Sixteen papers concentrated on prediction of evapotranspiration and irrigation, chlorophyll and nitrogen estimation, and prediction of soil properties. Eight papers were prescriptive in nature and dealt mainly with water and irrigation management, and fertilizer recommendation.

Weed, Disease & Pest Control

Almost a third (29.41%) of all studies pertained to studies directed at solving issues with weeds, diseases and pests. A total of forty-five studies were found. Two papers that employed diagnostic methods saw the introduction of electronic devices designed to quantify climatic variables complemented by a mobile application for diagnosing casual agents of wilt complex disease, and data mining techniques applied to understand the relation between crop, weather, environment and leaf spot disease. Thirty-three papers dealt in various degrees with weed detection and mapping, disease detection and diagnosis, and pest classification and identification. Appendix Table B provides a breakdown of the papers, area of application and machine learning technique applied.

Yield, Weather, Energy & Other Farm Management Activities

Of the thirty-two papers found in this area; two employed diagnostic techniques for determining appropriate environmental conditions for obtaining high yields and for modeling crop sequences (Jimenez et al., 2011; Xiao et al., 2014), twenty-nine papers were predictive in nature focusing on various agricultural improvements such as yield prediction, greenhouse management, energy input and output modeling, and temperature prediction, the remaining publication used prescriptive methods to for weather prediction and autonomous robot fruit harvesting (Sennaar, 2017).

Post-Production

Harvest & Handling

Thirteen studies examined the harvesting and handling process. Six of these studies were predictive in nature and aimed at forecasting the readiness of various agricultural produce for harvest; strawberry, apple, sugarcane, kiwi fruit, coffee, and even herbs. The seven remaining studies used prescriptive methods; six studies aimed at determining ideal time for harvesting and automated robotic harvesting, and the last study focused on sorting already harvested fruit using decision trees.

Storage & Processing

A total of seven papers, four on predictive and three on prescriptive methods were chosen. One study proposed a real-time classification method for Anthurium cultivars aimed at increasing the postharvest processing process and two studies were on predicting biomass for agricultural and industrial processes. Smith et al., (2009) introduced a system for year-round temperature prediction deployed on the website of the Georgia Automated Environmental Monitoring Network which will be suitable for managing and planning storage activity. The prescriptive papers were; Babazadeh et al., (2016) proposed a classification method for potato tubers based on solanine toxicant, Wu et al., (2014) proposed a control system for tobacco flue-curing barns, and Guine et al. (2018) evaluated the influence of production conditions and other factors on the total phenolic compounds and antioxidant activity of blueberries.

Market & Consumer

Predictive techniques were used ten papers mostly for price forecasting and measuring colorimetric properties of fruit. The one prescriptive paper found was on a decision support model aimed at improving export process.

Machine Learning Techniques

As demonstrated in Figure 5., artificial neural networks (ANN) was the most used technique by researchers with a link strength of 108 and was used in 76 of our surveyed literature. This stems from the range of application of ANN algorithms. They are used in classification of remote sensing imagery to time series forecasting. The use of Support Vector Machines (SVM) algorithm was also popular amongst researchers. It was used in 22 papers with a total link strength of 43. SVM supports both classification and regression problems. We also found that statistical models like Linear and Logistic Regression are still applied especially new variants of the model like Multiple Linear Regression which is used in cases where there are more than one explanatory variables. They were used in 10 and 4 papers, respectively.

Figure 5: A network of machine learning techniques and areas of application

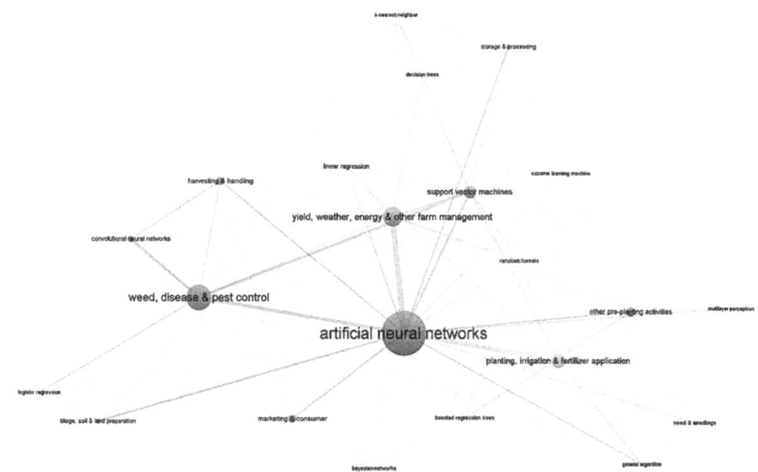

DISCUSSION

Current State of Big Data and AI in Agriculture

Big data in smart agriculture originates from farm sensors, drones, satellite stations, published industry performance, price index databases, and several other sources. In line with the characteristics of big data, the volume, variety, and velocity of agricultural data allows the use of AI to solve several agricultural issues and drive efficiency along the agriculture value chain. Our findings demonstrate that the amount of relevant studies spans the entire spectrum of agriculture value chain, although evidence points to the prominence of the production phase.

The approaches used by researchers contain a range of machine learning technique that can be applied to different problems along the value chain. Figure 5. demonstrates that ANN, which is inspired by the biological neural network of the human brain, is the most popular technique used by researchers in the surveyed studies. It has shown promise in the application of deep learning models to on-farm decision making. Other techniques like Support Vector Machines, Convolutional Neural Networks (CNN), and Genetic Algorithms (GA) have been used to various degrees. The use of GA, especially, is interesting as it is also inspired by natural selection and belongs to the larger class of evolutionary algorithms. They are often used in solutions that require bio-inspired operators such as mutation, crossover, and selection. SVM, on the other hand, are used in both classification and regression analysis. GA is often used in combination with either ANN or SVM.

As pointed out earlier in this chapter, smart agriculture is a novelty field, and this may explain the large amounts of academic research available in literature. The ideal scenario is to have more commercially usable studies that employ prescriptive techniques at scale. Some potentially disruptive applications of such studies include two in Spain: a hybrid system modeled on farmer's behavior to predict irrigation depths (Perea R et al., 2018), and the automatic translation of agricultural regulations into machine-processable rules (Espejo-Garcia et al., 2018). While commercial application of big data and AI may not be ubiquitous in agriculture yet, startups such as Trace Genomics and VineView have embraced the use of machine learning for diagnosing soil defects and for crop analysis respectively. The former has already raised $19 million in funding from 6 investors, and the latter $4.9 million from 3 investors as of December 2018 (Crunchbase, 2018; Sennaar, 2017; Trace Genomics, 2018; VineView, 2018). In a recent report, McKinsey Global Institute pointed to the fact that although AI adoption in industries outside the tech sector was still at an experimental stage, external investment into the innovation had grown three times more since 2013 (Columbus, 2016). Such investments represent a win for researchers and the agricultural industry, and as more and more research efforts continue to pour in, investors will be more willing to back commercial forays into big data and AI on the farm.

As we discuss in the ensuing section, the challenges and drivers for developed and developing countries in smart farm adoption may be motivated by slightly different circumstances. While the research also appears to originate predominantly from developed countries where the technological infrastructure, availability of capital, and supporting organizational and cultural structures are more conducive to such innovations, the research agenda from the surveyed literature is very similar. Further, there has been accounts of attempts to introduce smart agriculture in lesser developed regions of the world. Examples include: drought-tolerant maize varieties used in southern Africa to evaluate their performance (Tesfaye et al., 2016), and estimating evapotranspiration in India (Kumar et al., 2016). Price index prediction has been of special interest to researchers in Brazil and South Africa (Ayankoya et al,, 2016; Correa et al., 2016; Orge Pinheiro & de Senna, 2017; Ribeiro & Oliveira, 2011). This is one such area that can drive government policy in the developing countries and bridge the gap to developed countries.

Drivers and Challenges of AI and Big Data in Agriculture

Drivers for AI and big data in agriculture can be broadly addressed along economic, business, and technology dimensions as follows:

Economic Drivers

The UN FAO (2017) lists ten important challenges in their mission to eradicating hunger and malnutrition, and ensuring food security and agricultural productivity. These challenges include but are not limited to; improving agricultural productivity and sustainability to meet increasing demand, ensuring a sustainable natural resource base, addressing climate change and intensification of natural hazards, eradicating extreme poverty and reducing inequality, and preventing transboundary and emerging agriculture and food system threats. We envision that these same challenges will be key economic drivers for the integration of technology into not only on-farm activity but the entire agricultural value chain.

Evidence from our review also suggests that the aforementioned challenges are driving academic research. Machine vision systems backed by ANN have been used in robotizing farm work in a bid to optimize previously tedious and overly manual processes. In order to conserve natural resources such as land and water, and to battle climate change, there has been focus on soil classification, evapotranspiration, and smart irrigation. Process improvements have been made to weed, diseases and pest control to assist in fighting threats to food production and ensuring food security. Again, planning sales, export and import, and determining the price point of produce through yield prediction will be important for combating economic issues such as inflation.

Business Drivers

Businesses will rely on big data and AI for informed insights into decision making. The opportunity to preemptively grow through data-driven innovation, decision making, and discovery will drive even more businesses to move from more traditional ways (relying on farmer experience) to big data-driven artificial intelligence. AI will provide agriculture with more sustainable processes that take as input environmental factors and provide recommendations that saves business resources and increase yield. From a financial standpoint, both the farmer, investors and distributors have a lot to gain from yield, weather and energy predictions in a bid to plan business models and stock supply lines. Early detection of diseases and pest have immense cost and yield benefits to everyone involved in production.

On the other hand, as available workforce continues to dwindle in the agricultural sector, automation through predictive and prescriptive methods will decrease timelines and cost and increase quality of processes and produce. Human decisions can be mimicked and optimized through algorithms that continually self-correct based on new parameters. Tasks such as sorting of seeds and weed control, which are slow when done manually and potentially hurtful when done mechanically without any insights, have the potential of being entirely overhauled through proper classification of plants.

Technology Drivers

As has been pointed out, sensors and IoT devices from the precision agriculture are generating unprecedented amounts of data that will only continue to increase with time. Cloud computing has enabled storage and compute power to become cheaper through a "pay-for-what-you-use" model; ensuring a cost-effective avenue for retrieving value from big data. With cloud computing the agricultural sector can now afford to optimize efforts without necessarily allocating up-front capital. Technological trends like Infrastructure as a Service (IaaS), Software as a Service (SaaS), and Platform as a Service (PaaS) will drive farmers to focus on what they do best, farm, while leveraging such services to grow and advance yield. Researchers such as Alipio et al. (2017) and Rajeswari et al., (2017) have integrated cloud computing into their smart agricultural models due to their scalability over traditional systems and economical cost.

Like any innovation however, we envision several challenges, most notably are:

Data Ownership and Security

Privacy is a key concern for cybersecurity associated with data generation. Innovations like the ifarma, a cloud based farm management information system (FMIS), where farmers are provided with end-user license agreement give the farmer total ownership of data (Paraforos et al., 2016). The industry, however, needs regulations around ensuring privacy and securing data as has been done for the financial and health fields through the Gramm-Leach-Bliley Act of 1999 (GLBA), Health Insurance Portability and Accountability Act of 1996 (HIPAA) and most recently the European General Data Protection Regulation (GDRP).

Data Stream Consolidation and Interoperability

While this may be a challenging task due to the volume and variability of data, it makes for a better analysis on a regional and global level when data is consolidated and curated on global scales. Especially in the wake of proper regulations and privacy controls, it will allow proper global forecasts into food sustainability.

Data Transport and Hosting

Cloud infrastructure seems to provide evidence of readiness to take on large amounts of data, however location and retrieval of data is important for building real-time decisions.

Data Processing Power: It is undoubted that computing power has increased considerably over the years, but so has big data. It is clear that faster and more reliable algorithms need to be tested to allow for commercial applications of big data in agriculture. There is a special need for more research in the areas of automated feature engineering and dimensionality reduction.

Transparent, Explainable, and Accountable AI

Similar to other domains such as healthcare, the transparency, explainability, and accountability of AI algorithms may pose a particular challenge with respect to the credibility, trustworthiness, and ultimate adoption of these techniques in the field. The extent of impact - including possible regulations (Wachter, Mittelstadt, & Floridi, 2017) is likely to vary depending on the application on hand and represents and open area for research.

Inexpensive and Commercial AI

One of the barriers to adoption of AI is the funds needed to employ the requisite talent to deploy data solutions. Data scientist are some of the most expensive talents to hire today. While most companies believe AI is plug-and-play, it requires massive amounts of domain knowledge, proper key performance indicators, and long timelines to deploy robust solutions. Largescale adoption of AI stems from the development of agriculture-friendly commercial solutions that do not require an extensive computer or statistical knowledge.

Bridging Divide Between Developed and Developing Countries

A number of papers have presented initiatives in developing countries such as Iran, South Africa, India, Brazil and Argentina (Caires & Guimaraes, 2018; Ferraro et al., 2012; Khashei-Siuki et al., 2011; Kumar et al., 2016; Tesfaye et al., 2016), it stands to reason that the problem for the adoption and diffusion of big data and AI in these developing countries is not due to lack of research or technical capability. Misaki et al., (2018) in a recent survey pointed to lack of trust and transparency between farmers, technology providers and government organizations; inappropriate cultural context; illiteracy amongst farmers; inadequate infrastructure; low awareness; bureaucracy; and a few others as challenges facing small-scale farmers in sub-Saharan Africa. Of particular significance for most developing, and some developed countries, additional challenges include:

IT Infrastructure & Power Supply

Saidu, et al. (2017) pointed to challenges such as lack of infrastructure and erratic power supply as major barriers to adoption of on-farm information technology in developing areas.

Organizational and Cultural Practices

Despite strong evidence of government in developing countries readiness to support technology adoption, there are concerns on possible disruption of the way of doing things which may act as a barrier to Smart Agriculture (Aleke et al., 2011).

As much as these and other challenges such as the ones we discussed above exist for developing countries, we propose a backward integration of big data and AI into their processes. Starting from the 'Market and Consumer' section of the agricultural value chain, AI can be used to analyze prevailing trends. There is strong evidence of the proliferation of mobile phones, internet and social media in developing countries, and they have shown increasing effects on agricultural development (Olaniyi et al., 2018). Supply chain management and development can be enhanced through analysis of big data, especially from social media, to examine trends and user perception. Availability of price indices online can also be used to shape export and import benchmarks.

Prospects of Big Data and AI Technologies in Agriculture

Years of research have gone into developing many types of sensors for recording agronomically relevant parameters, collecting enough data via Internet of Things (IoT) and sensor networks, developing farm management systems, devising AI-driven farm machinery, and the like. By 2020, it is estimated that about 75 million agricultural IoT devices will be in use with an average farm generating up to 4.1 million data points daily by 2050 as compared to the 190,000 data points generated in 2014 (Clercq et al., 2018).

Due to the fluidity and hierarchically distributed open form of big data, capturing value requires real-time information to be dredged out of said data. It is required that analysis of the data takes as little time as possible and give a better profit margin as compared to good human-made management decisions. As a result, AI algorithms are being trained to provide this value (Özdemir & Hekim, 2018; Weltzien, 2016). Table 1. and Figure 4. points to an increase in the amount of relevant research taking on this challenge. Further, it can be said that many of the problems in agriculture are represented by over-parameterized nonlinear systems that may only be solved with the help AI. AI can recognize patterns and make predictions based on historically generated data and through automation, apply to real-time systems, as such the focus on predictive and prescriptive methods by most researchers (Özdemir & Hekim, 2018; Weltzien, 2016).

The major shortfall of ANN and most AI algorithms is the need for longer training times and the risk of either unintentional (example overfitting) or intentional (example malicious intent) bias. In such cases, a solution that might work for one problem, might not generalize well to other problems. *Cognitive Neural Networks* and *Deep Reasoning* algorithms will be most beneficial in such situations. Algorithms that go beyond recognizing and identifying attributes of objects (example perception and classification) to recognizing the causal relationships inherent and basing explainable decisions on these relationships (cognitive reasoning) (Battaglia et al., 2016; IBM, 2015; Y. Wang, 2016). We envision that they will be critical going forward. AI that is explainable will be more important especially for accountability in the wake of increasing data protection regulations that penalize companies for reasoning, or lack thereof, behind decision making. While deep reasoning is still in a very experimental phase, other methods (such as *Reinforcement Learning*; *Transfer Learning*; and *Active Learning*) can cater to current needs in terms of training times and optimal use of computing power.

A Futuristic Smart Farm Scenario

In principle, AI and machines can learn to perform any agricultural task given relevant data and parameters to learn from. The future for AI and farming lies in its very definition, that given any situation will act as a rational agent to take the best action possible. In future farming scenarios, we expect that big data and AI will disrupt the entire agriculture value chain. In this section we will paint two contrasting scenarios representing the current state of agriculture and the ideal smart farm for the future.

Typically, a farmer decides how and when to till the fields. When tilling is complete, planting of crops is done, typically with a planter attached to a tractor. In the rest of the season, the farmer manually monitors for the onset of diseases or harmful insects and should there be the need, may use an aerial applicator to fly over the farm and apply fungicides, weedicides, herbicides, and other chemicals to control any such problems. Irrigation is sometimes used but most farmers rely on rainfall for crop water supply. At harvest time, a harvester is used, and crops are sent to storing barns or silos till they can be sold off to food distributors. Although some farmers have the opportunity to sell to different markets, they are usually not in control of prices offered.

In a future smart farm, an AI system will identify optimal seed varieties and optimal planting times based on soil properties and weather data. The same system will control agro-robots that till and plant the seeds. After planting and germination, a drone is programmed to fly over the farm and collect image data which is immediately processed by the system. This allows for instant detection of crop diseases and pest infestation. In other parts of the field, seedlings suffering from late shoot or some form of damage will be marked for immediate replanting. At the end of the flight, the software then delivers population counts and yield estimates. More data will be collected from satellite imagery and a prediction is made if, for instance, a swarm of insects have infested nearby farms and are headed for that general area. This prediction can be corroborated by mining social media data. Consequently, the AI will estimate potential damage and recalibrate yield for each possible action to take should there be an infestation.

Further, the AI system shall control the nutrient and water needs of each plant and perform irrigation and spraying automatically. These calibrations will be readjusted daily based on how the crops are faring. At harvest time, the system then notifies the farmer and provides the most optimal pricing and distribution channels using pricing index databases. When the farm produce is shipped off to the food distributor, the system will upload production data to their database. This means in the end; the consumer can also immediately identify which chemicals have gone into the production and under which conditions their food was produced.

These scenarios show that not only will prescriptive analytics be key to the future farm but if done right, will disrupt the entire value chain and deliver in a manner that will benefit every stakeholder in the food production chain.

CONCLUSION

Smart Agriculture is making strides in the fight towards food security and sustainability. In this chapter, we have systematically reviewed the literature on big data and AI applications in a bid to identify the status and prospects of these technologies in disrupting agriculture. The combination of big data and AI drives value through their analytics capabilities. This chapter presents a conceptual framework that examines the agricultural value chain along the lines of the different types of business analytics. Our findings demonstrate that works dedicated to weed, disease and pest control, and yield, weather and energy predictions is of most interest to researchers. As much as these technologies are a relatively new phenomenon, there are successful commercial implementations in countries such as Canada, Iran and Spain. The trajectory of the number of works in the field has picked up pace in recent years and investors have shown commitment to backing commercially viable solutions.

We expect that economic factors such as import and export planning, and price point predictions, business factors like process optimization and dwindling agricultural workforce, and technological factors such as the increase in computing power will drive the agenda for Smart Agriculture. Challenges include data ownership, stream consolidation, transport, hosting and processing power. Developing countries especially, face an uphill battle in putting in place the right infrastructure and doing away with years of skills honed through social and cultural practices.

It should be noted that the scope of the systematic literature review is limited to articles published in the English language and is dominated by peer-review literature indexed in scholarly databases. As such, the research represents a strong academic focus capturing current research contributions and potential for future research. As the proliferation of big data and AI into agriculture continues, future reviews could increase reliance on 'grey literature' with an increased emphasis on commercialization endeavors of the technology.

REFERENCES

Aghighi, H., Azadbakht, M., Ashourloo, D., Shahrabi, H. S., & Radiom, S. (2018). Machine Learning Regression Techniques for the Silage Maize Yield Prediction Using Time-Series Images of Landsat 8 OLI. *IEEE Journal of Selected Topics in Applied Earth Observations and Remote Sensing*, 1–15. doi:10.1109/JSTARS.2018.2823361

Ahmed, F., Al-Mamun, H. A., Bari, A. S. M. H., Hossain, E., & Kwan, P. (2012). Classification of crops and weeds from digital images: A support vector machine approach. *Crop Protection*, *40*, 98–104. doi:10.1016/j.cropro.2012.04.024

Ajdadi, F. R., Gilandeh, Y. A., Mollazade, K., & Hasanzadeh, R. P. R. (2016). Application of machine vision for classification of soil aggregate size. *Soil & Tillage Research*, *162*, 8–17. doi:10.1016/j.still.2016.04.012

Akbarzadeh, S., Paap, A., Ahderom, S., Apopei, B., & Alameh, K. (2018). Plant discrimination by Support Vector Machine classifier based on spectral reflectance. *Computers and Electronics in Agriculture*, *148*, 250–258. doi:10.1016/j.compag.2018.03.026

Aleke, B., Ojiako, U., & Wainwright, D. W. (2011). ICT adoption in developing countries: Perspectives from small-scale agribusinesses. *Journal of Enterprise Information Management, 24*(1), 68–84. doi:10.1108/17410391111097438

Ali, A., Qadir, J., Rasool, R., Sathiaseelan, A., Zwitter, A., & Crowcroft, J. (2016). Big data for development: Applications and techniques. *Big Data Analytics, 1*(1), 2. doi:10.118641044-016-0002-4

Ali, M., Deo, R. C., Downs, N. J., & Maraseni, T. (2018). Multi-stage committee based extreme learning machine model incorporating the influence of climate parameters and seasonality on drought forecasting. *Computers and Electronics in Agriculture, 152*, 149–165. doi:10.1016/j.compag.2018.07.013

Alipio, M. I., Dela Cruz, A. E. M., Doria, J. D. A., & Fruto, R. M. S. (2017). A smart hydroponics farming system using exact inference in Bayesian network. *2017 IEEE 6th Global Conference on Consumer Electronics (GCCE)*, 1–5. 10.1109/GCCE.2017.8229470

Ancin-Murguzur, F. J., Barbero-Lopez, A., Kontunen-Soppela, S., & Haapala, A. (2018). Automated image analysis tool to measure microbial growth on solid cultures. *Computers and Electronics in Agriculture, 151*, 426–430. doi:10.1016/j.compag.2018.06.031

Aquino, C. F., Chamhum Salomao, L. C., & Azevedo, A. M. (2016). High-efficiency phenotyping for vitamin A in banana using artificial neural networks and colorimetric data. *Bragantia, 75*(3), 268–274. doi:10.1590/1678-4499.467

Arima, S., Kondo, N., Shibano, Y., Fujiura, T., Yamashita, J., & Nakamura, H. (1994). Studies on Cucumber Harvesting Robot (Part 2). *Journal of the Japanese Society of Agricultural Machinery, 56*(6), 69–76. doi:10.11357/jsam1937.56.6_69

Arima, S., Kondo, N., Yagi, Y., Monta, M., & Yoshida, Y. (2001). Harvesting robot for strawberry grown on table top culture, 1: Harvesting robot using 5 DOF manipulator. *Journal of Society of High Technology in Agriculture*. Retrieved from http://agris.fao.org/agris-search/search.do?recordID=JP2001006293

Arteta, T. A., Hameg, R., Landin, M., Gallego, P. P., & Barreal, M. E. (2018). Neural networks models as decision-making tool for in vitro proliferation of hardy kiwi. *European Journal of Horticultural Science, 83*(4), 259–265. doi:10.17660/eJHS.2018/83.4.6

Ayankoya, K., Calitz, A. P., & Greyling, J. H. (2016). Real-Time Grain Commodities Price Predictions In South Africa: A Big Data And Neural Networks Approach. *Agrekon, 55*(4), 483–508. doi:10.1080/03031853.2016.1243060

Babazadeh, S., Moghaddam, P. A., Sabatyan, A., & Sharifian, F. (2016). Classification of potato tubers based on solanine toxicant using laser induced light backscattering imaging. *Computers and Electronics in Agriculture, 129*, 1–8. doi:10.1016/j.compag.2016.09.009

Bakhshi, M., Pourtaheri, M., & Eftekhari, A. R. (2016). Developing a Model to Predict Success of Agricultural Production Enterprises Based on Their Capitals. *Journal of Agricultural Science and Technology, 18*(6), 1443–1454.

Bakhshipour, A., & Jafari, A. (2018). Evaluation of support vector machine and artificial neural networks in weed detection using shape features. *Computers and Electronics in Agriculture, 145*, 153–160. doi:10.1016/j.compag.2017.12.032

Bakhshipour, A., Jafari, A., Nassiri, S. M., & Zare, D. (2017). Weed segmentation using texture features extracted from wavelet sub-images. *Biosystems Engineering, 157*, 1–12. doi:10.1016/j.biosystemseng.2017.02.002

Battaglia, P. W., Pascanu, R., Lai, M., Rezende, D., & Kavukcuoglu, K. (2016). *Interaction Networks for Learning about Objects, Relations and Physics.* Retrieved from http://arxiv.org/abs/1612.00222

Bello-Orgaz, G., Jung, J. J., & Camacho, D. (2016). Social big data: Recent achievements and new challenges. *Information Fusion, 28*, 45–59. doi:10.1016/j.inffus.2015.08.005

Bengio, Y. (2009). Learning Deep Architectures for AI. *Foundations and Trends® in Machine Learning, 2*(1), 1–127. doi:10.1561/2200000006

Bengio, Y. (2013). Deep Learning of Representations: Looking Forward. In A.-H. Dediu, C. Martín-Vide, R. Mitkov, & B. Truthe (Eds.), Statistical Language and Speech Processing (Vol. 7978, pp. 1–37). Academic Press. doi:10.1007/978-3-642-39593-2_1

Borges, P. H. M., Mendoza, Z. M. S. H., Maia, J. C. S., Bianchini, A., & Fernandes, H. C. (2017). Estimation Of Fuel Consumption In Agricultural Mechanized Operations Using Artificial Neural Networks. *Engenharia Agrícola, 37*(1), 136–147. doi:10.1590/1809-4430-eng.agric.v37n1p136-147/2017

Brynjolfsson, E., Hitt, L. M., & Kim, H. H. (2011). *Strength in Numbers: How Does Data-Driven Decision-Making Affect Firm Performance?* SSRN Electronic Journal. doi:10.2139srn.1819486

Byakatonda, J., Parida, B. P., Kenabatho, P. K., & Moalafhi, D. B. (2018). Influence of climate variability and length of rainy season on crop yields in semiarid Botswana. *Agricultural and Forest Meteorology, 248*, 130–144. doi:10.1016/j.agrformet.2017.09.016

Caires, E. F., & Guimaraes, A. M. (2018). A Novel Phosphogypsum Application Recommendation Method under Continuous No-Till Management in Brazil. *Agronomy Journal, 110*(5), 1987–1995. doi:10.2134/agronj2017.11.0642

Calderano, B. F., Polivanov, H., da Silva Chagas, C., de Carvalho, W. J., Barroso, E. V., Teixeira Guerra, A. J., & Calderano, S. B. (2014). Artificial Neural Networks Applied for Soil Class Prediction in Mountainous Landscape of The Serra Do Mar. *Revista Brasileira de Ciência do Solo, 38*(6), 1681–1693. doi:10.1590/S0100-06832014000600003

Camargo, A., Molina, J. P., Cadena-Torres, J., Jimenez, N., & Kim, J. T. (2012). Intelligent systems for the assessment of crop disorders. *Computers and Electronics in Agriculture, 85*, 1–7. doi:10.1016/j.compag.2012.02.017

Cameron, M., Viviers, W., & Steenkamp, E. (2017). Breaking the "big data" barrier when selecting agricultural export markets: An innovative approach. *Agrekon, 56*(2), 139–157. doi:10.1080/03031853.2017.1298456

Castaneda-Miranda, A., & Castano, V. M. (2017). Smart frost control in greenhouses by neural networks models. *Computers and Electronics in Agriculture*, *137*, 102–114. doi:10.1016/j.compag.2017.03.024

Castro, C. A. de O., Resende, R. T., Kuki, K. N., Carneiro, V. Q., Marcatti, G. E., Cruz, C. D., & Motoike, S. Y. (2017). High-performance prediction of macauba fruit biomass for agricultural and industrial purposes using Artificial Neural Networks. *Industrial Crops and Products*, *108*, 806–813. doi:10.1016/j.indcrop.2017.07.031

CEMA - European Agricultural Machinery. (2017, February 13). *Digital Farming: what does it really mean?* Retrieved September 24, 2018, from http://www.cema-agri.org/page/digital-farming-what-does-it-really-mean

Chantre, G. R., Vigna, M. R., Renzi, J. P., & Blanco, A. M. (2018). A flexible and practical approach for real-time weed emergence prediction based on Artificial Neural Networks. *Biosystems Engineering*, *170*, 51–60. doi:10.1016/j.biosystemseng.2018.03.014

Chapman, R., Cook, S., Donough, C., Lim, Y. L., Vun Vui Ho, P., Lo, K. W., & Oberthür, T. (2018). Using Bayesian networks to predict future yield functions with data from commercial oil palm plantations: A proof of concept analysis. *Computers and Electronics in Agriculture*, *151*, 338–348. doi:10.1016/j.compag.2018.06.006

Chaudhary, A., Kolhe, S., & Kamal, R. (2016). A hybrid ensemble for classification in multiclass datasets: An application to oilseed disease dataset. *Computers and Electronics in Agriculture*, *124*, 65–72. doi:10.1016/j.compag.2016.03.026

Cheng, X., Zhang, Y., Chen, Y., Wu, Y., & Yue, Y. (2017). Pest identification via deep residual learning in complex background. *Computers and Electronics in Agriculture*, *141*, 351–356. doi:10.1016/j.compag.2017.08.005

Chi, M., Plaza, A., Benediktsson, J. A., Sun, Z., Shen, J., & Zhu, Y. (2016). Big Data for Remote Sensing: Challenges and Opportunities. *Proceedings of the IEEE*, *104*(11), 2207–2219. doi:10.1109/JPROC.2016.2598228

Cho, G. (2018). The Australian digital farmer: challenges and opportunities. *IOP Conference Series: Earth and Environmental Science*, *185*, 012036. 10.1088/1755-1315/185/1/012036

Christensen, C. (1997). *The Revolutionary Book that Will Change the Way You Do Business (Collins Business Essentials)*. New York: Harper Paperbacks.

Chung, C.-L., Huang, K.-J., Chen, S.-Y., Lai, M.-H., Chen, Y.-C., & Kuo, Y.-F. (2016). Detecting Bakanae disease in rice seedlings by machine vision. *Computers and Electronics in Agriculture*, *121*, 404–411. doi:10.1016/j.compag.2016.01.008

Clercq, M. D., Vats, A., & Biel, A. (2018). Agriculture 4.0: The Future of Farming Technology. *World Government Summit*, 30.

Coble, K. H., Mishra, A. K., Ferrell, S., & Griffin, T. (2018). Big Data in Agriculture: A Challenge for the Future. *Applied Economic Perspectives and Policy*, *40*(1), 79–96. doi:10.1093/aepp/ppx056

Cockburn, I., Henderson, R., & Stern, S. (2018). *The Impact of Artificial Intelligence on Innovation* (No. w24449). doi:10.3386/w24449

Columbus, L. (2016). *McKinsey's 2016 Analytics Study Defines The Future Of Machine Learning.* Retrieved November 14, 2018, from https://www.forbes.com/sites/louiscolumbus/2016/12/18/mckinseys-2016-analytics-study-defines-the-future-machine-learning/#3da708d214eb

Correa, F. E., Oliveira, M. D. B., Gama, J., Correa, P. L. P., & Rady, J. (2016). Analyzing the behavior dynamics of grain price indexes using Tucker tensor decomposition and spatio-temporal trajectories. *Computers and Electronics in Agriculture, 120,* 72–78. doi:10.1016/j.compag.2015.11.011

Costa, A. G., Pinto, F., Motoike, S. Y., Braga Júnior, R. A., & Gracia, L. M. N. (2018). Classification of Macaw Palm Fruits from Colorimetric Properties for Determining the Harvest Moment. *Engenharia Agrícola, 38*(4), 634–641. doi:10.1590/1809-4430-eng.agric.v38n4p634-641/2018

Crunchbase. (2018). *Crunchbase: Discover innovative companies and the people behind them.* Retrieved December 17, 2018, from Crunchbase website: https://www.crunchbase.com

Cuzzocrea, A., Song, I.-Y., & Davis, K. C. (2011). *Analytics over large-scale multidimensional data: the big data revolution!* Academic Press.

da Silva, C. A. Junior, Nanni, M. R., Teodoro, P. E., & Capristo Silva, G. F. (2017). Vegetation Indices for Discrimination of Soybean Areas: A New Approach. *Agronomy Journal, 109*(4), 1331–1343. doi:10.2134/agronj2017.01.0003

de Barros, M. M., da Silva, F. M., Costa, A. G., Ferraz, G. A. e S., & da Silva, F. C. (2018). Use of classifier to determine coffee harvest time by detachment force. *Revista Brasileira de Engenharia Agrícola e Ambiental, 22*(5), 366–370. doi:10.1590/1807-1929/agriambi.v22n5p366-370

Delgado, G., Aranda, V., Calero, J., Sanchez-Maranon, M., Serrano, J. M., Sanchez, D., & Vila, M. A. (2008). Building a fuzzy logic information network and a decision-support system for olive cultivation in Andalusia. *Spanish Journal of Agricultural Research, 6*(2), 252–263. doi:10.5424jar/2008062-316

Demir, B. (2018). Application of data mining and adaptive neuro-fuzzy structure to predict color parameters of walnuts (Juglans regia L.). *Turkish Journal of Agriculture and Forestry, 42*(3), 216–225. doi:10.3906/tar-1801-78

Demir, B., Gurbuz, F., Eski, I., Kus, Z. A., Yilmaz, K. U., & Ercisli, S. (2018). Possible Use of Data Mining for Analysis and Prediction of Apple Physical Properties. *Erwerbs-Obstbau, 60*(1), 1–7. doi:10.100710341-017-0330-1

Diaz, I., Mazza, S. M., Combarro, E. F., Gimenez, L. I., & Gaiad, J. E. (2017). Machine learning applied to the prediction of citrus production. *Spanish Journal of Agricultural Research, 15*(2), e0205. doi:10.5424jar/2017152-9090

Dimililer, K., & Zarrouk, S. (2017). ICSPI: Intelligent Classification System of Pest Insects Based on Image Processing and Neural Arbitration. *Applied Engineering in Agriculture, 33*(4), 453–460. doi:10.13031/aea.12161

Ding, W., & Taylor, G. (2016). Automatic moth detection from trap images for pest management. *Computers and Electronics in Agriculture, 123*, 17–28. doi:10.1016/j.compag.2016.02.003

Dornelles, E. F., Kraisig, A. R., da Silva, J. A. G., Sawicki, S., Roos-Frantz, F., & Carbonera, R. (2018). Artificial intelligence in seeding density optimization and yield simulation for oat. *Revista Brasileira de Engenharia Agrícola e Ambiental, 22*(3), 183–188. doi:10.1590/1807-1929/agriambi.v22n3p183-188

Dos Santos Ferreira, A., Matte Freitas, D., Gonçalves da Silva, G., Pistori, H., & Folhes, M. T. (2017). Weed detection in soybean crops using ConvNets. *Computers and Electronics in Agriculture, 143*, 314–324. doi:10.1016/j.compag.2017.10.027

Du, K., Sun, Z., Li, Y., Zheng, F., Chu, J., & Su, Y. (2016). Diagnostic Model For Wheat Leaf Conditions Using Image Features And A Support Vector Machine. *Transactions of the ASABE, 59*(5), 1041–1052. doi:10.13031/trans.59.11434

Ebrahimi, E., & Mollazade, K. (2010). Integrating fuzzy data mining and impulse acoustic techniques for almond nuts sorting. *Australian Journal of Crop Science, 4*(5), 353–358.

Emamgholizadeh, S., Parsaeian, M., & Baradaran, M. (2015). Seed yield prediction of sesame using artificial neural network. *European Journal of Agronomy, 68*, 89–96. doi:10.1016/j.eja.2015.04.010

Espejo-Garcia, B., Martinez-Guanter, J., Perez-Ruiz, M., Lopez-Pellicer, F. J., & Javier Zarazaga-Soria, F. (2018). Machine learning for automatic rule classification of agricultural regulations: A case study in Spain. *Computers and Electronics in Agriculture, 150*, 343–352. doi:10.1016/j.compag.2018.05.007

Espinoza, K., Valera, D. L., Torres, J. A., Lopez, A., & Molina-Aiz, F. D. (2016). Combination of image processing and artificial neural networks as a novel approach for the identification of Bemisia tabaci and Frankliniella occidentalis on sticky traps in greenhouse agriculture. *Computers and Electronics in Agriculture, 127*, 495–505. doi:10.1016/j.compag.2016.07.008

Everingham, Y., Sexton, J., Skocaj, D., & Inman-Bamber, G. (2016). Accurate prediction of sugarcane yield using a random forest algorithm. *Agronomy for Sustainable Development, 36*(2), 27. doi:10.100713593-016-0364-z

Everingham, Y. L., Smyth, C. W., & Inman-Bamber, N. G. (2009). Ensemble data mining approaches to forecast regional sugarcane crop production. *Agricultural and Forest Meteorology, 149*(3–4), 689–696. doi:10.1016/j.agrformet.2008.10.018

Fan, W., & Bifet, A. (2013). Mining big data: Current status and forecast to the future. *ACM SIGKDD Explorations Newsletter, 14*(2), 1. doi:10.1145/2481244.2481246

Farjam, A., Omid, M., Akram, A., & Niari, Z. F. (2014). A Neural Network Based Modeling and Sensitivity Analysis of Energy Inputs for Predicting Seed and Grain Corn Yields. *Journal of Agricultural Science and Technology, 16*(4), 767–778.

Feng, Y., Peng, Y., Cui, N., Gong, D., & Zhang, K. (2017). Modeling reference evapotranspiration using extreme learning machine and generalized regression neural network only with temperature data. *Computers and Electronics in Agriculture, 136*, 71–78. doi:10.1016/j.compag.2017.01.027

Ferentinos, K. P. (2018). Deep learning models for plant disease detection and diagnosis. *Computers and Electronics in Agriculture, 145,* 311–318. doi:10.1016/j.compag.2018.01.009

Fernandes, J. L., Rocha, J. V., & Camargo Lamparelli, R. A. (2011). Sugarcane yield estimates using time series analysis of spot vegetation images. *Scientia Agrícola, 68*(2), 139–146. doi:10.1590/S0103-90162011000200002

Fernandez, R., Montes, H., Surdilovic, J., Surdilovic, D., Gonzalez-De-Santos, P., & Armada, M. (2018). Automatic Detection of Field-Grown Cucumbers for Robotic Harvesting. *IEEE Access: Practical Innovations, Open Solutions, 6,* 35512–35527. doi:10.1109/ACCESS.2018.2851376

Ferraro, D. O., Ghersa, C. M., & Rivero, D. E. (2012). Weed Vegetation of Sugarcane Cropping Systems of Northern Argentina: Data-Mining Methods for Assessing the Environmental and Management Effects on Species Composition. *Weed Science, 60*(1), 27–33. doi:10.1614/WS-D-11-00023.1

Food and Agriculture Organization of the United Nations. (Ed.). (2017). *The future of food and agriculture: trends and challenges.* Rome: Food and Agriculture Organization of the United Nations.

Food Security Information Network. (2018). *Global Report on Food Crises 2018.* Retrieved from http://www.fsincop.net/fileadmin/user_upload/fsin/docs/global_report/2018/GRFC_2018_Full_report_EN_Low_resolution.pdf

Fortin, J. G., Anctil, F., Parent, L.-E., & Bolinder, M. A. (2011). Site-specific early season potato yield forecast by neural network in Eastern Canada. *Precision Agriculture, 12*(6), 905–923. doi:10.100711119-011-9233-6

Fukuda, S., Spreer, W., Yasunaga, E., Yuge, K., Sardsud, V., & Mueller, J. (2013). Random Forests modelling for the estimation of mango (Mangifera indica L. cv. Chok Anan) fruit yields under different irrigation regimes. *Agricultural Water Management, 116,* 142–150. doi:10.1016/j.agwat.2012.07.003

Garcia-Santillan, I. D., & Pajares, G. (2018). On-line crop/weed discrimination through the Mahalanobis distance from images in maize fields. *Biosystems Engineering, 166,* 28–43. doi:10.1016/j.biosystemseng.2017.11.003

Gartner. (2018). *Gartner IT Glossary.* Retrieved November 14, 2018, from https://www.gartner.com/it-glossary/

Ghosh, K., & Nath, A. (2016). Big Data: Security Issues, Challenges and Future Scope. *International Journal of Research Studies in Computer Science and Engineering, 3*(3). doi:10.20431/2349-4859.0303001

Goldstein, A., Fink, L., Meitin, A., Bohadana, S., Lutenberg, O., & Ravid, G. (2018). Applying machine learning on sensor data for irrigation recommendations: Revealing the agronomist's tacit knowledge. *Precision Agriculture, 19*(3), 421–444. doi:10.100711119-017-9527-4

Gómez-Casero, M. T., Castillejo-Gonzalez, I. L., Garcia-Ferrer, A., Peña-Barragán, J. M., Jurado-Expósito, M., Garcia-Torres, L., & López-Granados, F. (2010). Spectral discrimination of wild oat and canary grass in wheat fields for less herbicide application. *Agronomy for Sustainable Development, 30*(3), 689–699. doi:10.1051/agro/2009052

Gonzalez-Sanchez, A., Frausto-Solis, J., & Ojeda-Bustamante, W. (2014). Predictive ability of machine learning methods for massive crop yield prediction. *Spanish Journal of Agricultural Research, 12*(2), 313–328. doi:10.5424jar/2014122-4439

Goumopoulos, C., O'Flynn, B., & Kameas, A. (2014). Automated zone-specific irrigation with wireless sensor/actuator network and adaptable decision support. *Computers and Electronics in Agriculture, 105*, 20–33. doi:10.1016/j.compag.2014.03.012

Griffel, L. M., Delparte, D., & Edwards, J. (2018). Using Support Vector Machines classification to differentiate spectral signatures of potato plants infected with Potato Virus Y. *Computers and Electronics in Agriculture, 153*, 318–324. doi:10.1016/j.compag.2018.08.027

Guine, R. P. F., Matos, S., Goncalves, F. J., Costa, D., & Mendes, M. (2018). Evaluation of phenolic compounds and antioxidant activity of blueberries and modelization by artificial neural networks. *International Journal of Fruit Science, 18*(2), 199–214. doi:10.1080/15538362.2018.1425653

Gutierrez, M., Alegret, S., Caceres, R., Casadesus, J., Marfa, O., & del Valle, M. (2008). Nutrient solution monitoring in greenhouse cultivation employing a potentiometric electronic tongue. *Journal of Agricultural and Food Chemistry, 56*(6), 1810–1817. doi:10.1021/jf073438s PMID:18303814

Gutierrez, P. A., López-Granados, F., Peña-Barragán, J. M., Jurado-Expósito, M., Gómez-Casero, M. T., & Hervas-Martinez, C. (2008). Mapping sunflower yield as affected by Ridolfia segetum patches and elevation by applying evolutionary product unit neural networks to remote sensed data. *Computers and Electronics in Agriculture, 60*(2), 122–132. doi:10.1016/j.compag.2007.07.011

Gutierrez, P. A., López-Granados, F., Peña-Barragán, J. M., Jurado-Expósito, M., & Hervas-Martinez, C. (2008). Logistic regression product-unit neural networks for mapping Ridolfia segetum infestations in sunflower crop using multitemporal remote sensed data. *Computers and Electronics in Agriculture, 64*(2), 293–306. doi:10.1016/j.compag.2008.06.001

Hamedani, S. R., Liaqat, M., Shamshirband, S., Al-Razgan, O. S., Al-Shammari, E. T., & Petkovic, D. (2015). Comparative Study of Soft Computing Methodologies for Energy Input-Output Analysis to Predict Potato Production. *American Journal of Potato Research, 92*(3), 426–434. doi:10.100712230-015-9453-9

Harada, M., Tominaga, T., Hiramatsu, K., & Marui, A. (2013). Real-Time Prediction Of Chlorophyll-A Time Series In A Eutrophic Agricultural Reservoir In A Coastal Zone Using Recurrent Neural Networks With Periodic Chaos Neurons. *Irrigation and Drainage, 62*(1), 36–43. doi:10.1002/ird.1757

Hassanien, A. E., Gaber, T., Mokhtar, U., & Hefny, H. (2017). An improved moth flame optimization algorithm based on rough sets for tomato diseases detection. *Computers and Electronics in Agriculture, 136*, 86–96. doi:10.1016/j.compag.2017.02.026

Hayashi, S., Ganno, K., Ishii, Y., & Tanaka, I. (2002). Robotic Harvesting System for Eggplants. *Japan Agricultural Research Quarterly: JARQ, 36*(3), 163–168. doi:10.6090/jarq.36.163

Heim, R. H. J., Wright, I. J., Chang, H.-C., Carnegie, A. J., Pegg, G. S., Lancaster, E. K., ... Oldeland, J. (2018). Detecting myrtle rust (Austropuccinia psidii) on lemon myrtle trees using spectral signatures and machine learning. *Plant Pathology, 67*(5), 1114–1121. doi:10.1111/ppa.12830

Hill, B. D., Kalischuk, M., Waterer, D. R., Bizimungu, B., Howard, R., & Kawchuk, L. M. (2011). An Environmental Model Predicting Bacterial Ring Rot Symptom Expression. *American Journal of Potato Research*, *88*(3), 294–301. doi:10.100712230-011-9193-4

Husin, Z., Shakaff, A. Y. M., Aziz, A. H. A., Farook, R. S. M., Jaafar, M. N., Hashim, U., & Harun, A. (2012). Embedded portable device for herb leaves recognition using image processing techniques and neural network algorithm. *Computers and Electronics in Agriculture*, *89*, 18–29. doi:10.1016/j.compag.2012.07.009

IBM. (2013). *Descriptive, predictive, prescriptive: Transforming asset and facilities management with analytics*. IBM.

IBM. (2015, September 11). *The new AI innovation equation*. Retrieved April 16, 2019, from IBM Cognitive - What's next for AI website: http://www.ibm.com/watson/advantage-reports/future-of-artificial-intelligence/ai-innovation-equation.html

IBM. (2018, October 30). *Big Data Analytics*. Retrieved January 9, 2019, from https://www.ibm.com/analytics/hadoop/big-data-analytics

Ilic, M., Ilic, S., Jovic, S., & Panic, S. (2018). Early cherry fruit pathogen disease detection based on data mining prediction. *Computers and Electronics in Agriculture*, *150*, 418–425. doi:10.1016/j.compag.2018.05.008

Jimenez, D., Cock, J., Jarvis, A., Garcia, J., Satizabal, H. F., Van Damme, P., ... Barreto-Sanz, M. A. (2011). Interpretation of commercial production information: A case study of lulo (Solanum quitoense), an under-researched Andean fruit. *Agricultural Systems*, *104*(3), 258–270. doi:10.1016/j.agsy.2010.10.004

Jimenez, D., Cock, J., Satizabal, H. F., Barreto, M. A., Perez-Uribe, A., Jarvis, A., & Van Damme, P. (2009). Analysis of Andean blackberry (Rubus glaucus) production models obtained by means of artificial neural networks exploiting information collected by small-scale growers in Colombia and publicly available meteorological data. *Computers and Electronics in Agriculture*, *69*(2), 198–208. doi:10.1016/j.compag.2009.08.008

Jokic, A., Zavargo, Z., Gyura, J., Radivojevic, S., & Seres, Z. (2010). An Artificial Neural Network Approach to Prediction of Sugar Beet Yield and Quality in Serbia. In *Sugar Beet Crops: Growth, Fertilization & Yield* (pp. 153–166). Academic Press. Retrieved from https://www.researchgate.net/publication/281874792_An_artificial_neural_network_approach_to_prediction_of_sugar_beet_yield_and_quality_in_Serbia

Kamilaris, A., Kartakoullis, A., & Prenafeta-Boldú, F. X. (2017). A review on the practice of big data analysis in agriculture. *Computers and Electronics in Agriculture*, *143*, 23–37. doi:10.1016/j.compag.2017.09.037

Kamilaris, A., & Prenafeta-Boldú, F. X. (2018). Deep learning in agriculture: A survey. *Computers and Electronics in Agriculture*, *147*, 70–90. doi:10.1016/j.compag.2018.02.016

Kaplinsky, R., & Morris, M. (2001). *A Handbook for Value Chain Research*. 113.

Kawamura, N., Namikawa, K., Fujiura, T., & Ura, M. (1984). Study on Agricultural Robot (Part 1). *Journal of the Japanese Society of Agricultural Machinery, 46*(3), 353–358. doi:10.11357/jsam1937.46.3_353

Khan, M. J., Khan, H. S., Yousaf, A., Khurshid, K., & Abbas, A. (2018). Modern Trends in Hyperspectral Image Analysis: A Review. *IEEE Access: Practical Innovations, Open Solutions, 6*, 14118–14129. doi:10.1109/ACCESS.2018.2812999

Khanal, S., Fulton, J., Klopfenstein, A., Douridas, N., & Shearer, S. (2018). Integration of high resolution remotely sensed data and machine learning techniques for spatial prediction of soil properties and corn yield. *Computers and Electronics in Agriculture, 153*, 213–225. doi:10.1016/j.compag.2018.07.016

Khashei-Siuki, A., Kouchakzadeh, M., & Ghahraman, B. (2011). Predicting Dryland Wheat Yield from Meteorological Data Using Expert System, Khorasan Province, Iran. *Journal of Agricultural Science and Technology, 13*(4), 627–640.

Khazaei, J., Naghavi, M. R., Jahansouz, M. R., & Salimi-Khorshidi, G. (2008). Yield estimation and clustering of chickpea genotypes using soft computing techniques. *Agronomy Journal, 100*(4), 1077–1087. doi:10.2134/agronj2006.0244

Khoshnevisan, B., Rafiee, S., & Mousazadeh, H. (2013). Environmental impact assessment of open field and greenhouse strawberry production. *European Journal of Agronomy, 50*, 29–37. doi:10.1016/j.eja.2013.05.003

Khoshnevisan, B., Rafiee, S., Omid, M., Mousazadeh, H., & Rajaeifar, M. A. (2014). Application of artificial neural networks for prediction of output energy and GHG emissions in potato production in Iran. *Agricultural Systems, 123*, 120–127. doi:10.1016/j.agsy.2013.10.003

Kondo, N., Nishitsuji, Y., Ling, P. P., & Ting, K. C. (1996). Visual Feedback Guided Robotic Cherry Tomato Harvesting. *Transactions of the ASAE. American Society of Agricultural Engineers, 39*(6), 2331–2338. doi:10.13031/2013.27744

Kouadio, L., Deo, R. C., Byrareddy, V., Adamowski, J. F., Mushtaq, S., & Nguyen, V. P. (2018). Artificial intelligence approach for the prediction of Robusta coffee yield using soil fertility properties. *Computers and Electronics in Agriculture, 155*, 324–338. doi:10.1016/j.compag.2018.10.014

Krishnan, P., & Surya Rao, A. V. (2005). Effects of genotype and environment on seed yield and quality of rice. *The Journal of Agricultural Science, 143*(04), 283–292. doi:10.1017/S0021859605005496

Kshetri, N. (2014). The emerging role of Big Data in key development issues: Opportunities, challenges, and concerns. *Big Data & Society, 1*(2). doi:10.1177/2053951714564227

Kumar, D., Adamowski, J., Suresh, R., & Ozga-Zielinski, B. (2016). Estimating Evapotranspiration Using an Extreme Learning Machine Model: Case Study in North Bihar, India. *Journal of Irrigation and Drainage Engineering, 142*(9), 04016032. doi:10.1061/(ASCE)IR.1943-4774.0001044

Kus, Z. A., Demir, B., Eski, I., Gurbuz, F., & Ercisli, S. (2017). Estimation of the Colour Properties of Apples Varieties Using Neural Network. *Erwerbs-Obstbau, 59*(4), 291–299. doi:10.100710341-017-0324-z

Lamsal, A., Welch, S. M., Jones, J. W., Boote, K. J., Asebedo, A., Crain, J., ... Arachchige, P. G. (2017). Efficient crop model parameter estimation and site characterization using large breeding trial data sets. *Agricultural Systems, 157*, 170–184. doi:10.1016/j.agsy.2017.07.016

Laney, D. (2001). *3D Data Management: Controlling Data Volume, Velocity, and Variety* [Technical Report]. Retrieved from https://blogs.gartner.com/doug-laney/files/2012/01/ad949-3D-Data-Management-Controlling-Data-Volume-Velocity-and-Variety.pdf

Liao, M.-S., Chuang, C.-L., Lin, T.-S., Chen, C.-P., Zheng, X.-Y., Chen, P.-T., ... Jiang, J.-A. (2012). Development of an autonomous early warning system for Bactrocera dorsalis (Hendel) outbreaks in remote fruit orchards. *Computers and Electronics in Agriculture, 88*, 1–12. doi:10.1016/j.compag.2012.06.008

Liberati, A., Altman, D. G., Tetzlaff, J., Mulrow, C., Gøtzsche, P. C., Ioannidis, J. P., ... Moher, D. (2009). The PRISMA statement for reporting systematic reviews and meta-analyses of studies that evaluate health care interventions: Explanation and elaboration. *PLoS Medicine, 6*(7). doi:10.1371/journal.pmed.1000100 PMID:19621070

Liu, Z.-Y., Wu, H.-F., & Huang, J.-F. (2010). Application of neural networks to discriminate fungal infection levels in rice panicles using hyperspectral reflectance and principal components analysis. *Computers and Electronics in Agriculture, 72*(2), 99–106. doi:10.1016/j.compag.2010.03.003

Logan, T. M., McLeod, S., & Guikema, S. (2016). Predictive models in horticulture: A case study with Royal Gala apples. *Scientia Horticulturae, 209*, 201–213. doi:10.1016/j.scienta.2016.06.033

López-Granados, F., Gómez-Casero, M. T., Peña-Barragán, J. M., Jurado-Expósito, M., & García-Torres, L. (2010). Classifying Irrigated Crops as Affected by Phenological Stage Using Discriminant Analysis and Neural Networks. *Journal of the American Society for Horticultural Science, 135*(5), 465–473. doi:10.21273/JASHS.135.5.465

Lu, J., Hu, J., Zhao, G., Mei, F., & Zhang, C. (2017). An in-field automatic wheat disease diagnosis system. *Computers and Electronics in Agriculture, 142*(A), 369–379. doi:10.1016/j.compag.2017.09.012

Mahmoud, T., Dong, Z. Y., & Ma, J. (2018). Advanced method for short-term wind power prediction with multiple observation points using extreme learning machines. *The Journal of Engineering, 2018*(1), 29–38. doi:10.1049/joe.2017.0338

Mark, T. B., Griffin, T. W., & Whitacre, B. E. (2016). The Role of Wireless Broadband Connectivity on `Big Data' and the Agricultural Industry in the United States and Australia. *International Food and Agribusiness Management Review, 19*(A), 43–56.

Markkanen, A. (2015). IoT Analytics Today and in 2020. *ABI Research*, 10.

Martin, K. (2016, April 27). How will artificial intelligence affect legal practice? *Thomson Reuters*. Retrieved April 1, 2019, from Answers On website: https://blogs.thomsonreuters.com/answerson/artificial-intelligence-legal-practice/

Mattar, M. A., El-Marazky, M. S., & Ahmed, K. A. (2017). Modeling sprinkler irrigation infiltration based on a fuzzy-logic approach. *Spanish Journal of Agricultural Research, 15*(1), e1201. doi:10.5424jar/2017151-9179

Microsoft, Inc. (2018). *Digital Agriculture: Farmers in India are using AI to increase crop yields*. Retrieved September 25, 2018, from Microsoft News Center India website: https://news.microsoft.com/en-in/features/ai-agriculture-icrisat-upl-india/

Mills, M. (2015). *Artificial Intelligence in Law – The State of Play in 2015?* Retrieved April 29, 2019, from Legal IT Insider website: https://www.legaltechnology.com/latest-news/artificial-intelligence-in-law-the-state-of-play-in-2015/

Misaki, E., Apiola, M., Gaiani, S., & Tedre, M. (2018). Challenges facing sub-Saharan small-scale farmers in accessing farming information through mobile phones: A systematic literature review. *The Electronic Journal on Information Systems in Developing Countries*, 84(4), e12034. doi:10.1002/isd2.12034

Moller, A. B., Beucher, A., Iversen, B. V., & Greve, M. H. (2018). Predicting artificially drained areas by means of a selective model ensemble. *Geoderma*, 320, 30–42. doi:10.1016/j.geoderma.2018.01.018

Najafabadi, M. M., Villanustre, F., Khoshgoftaar, T. M., Seliya, N., Wald, R., & Muharemagic, E. (2015). Deep learning applications and challenges in big data analytics. *Journal of Big Data*, 2(1), 1. doi:10.118640537-014-0007-7

Nandyala, C. S., & Kim, H.-K. (2016). Big and Meta Data Management for U-Agriculture Mobile Services. *International Journal of Software Engineering and Its Applications*, 10(2), 257–270. doi:10.14257/ijseia.2016.10.2.21

Navarro-Hellin, H., Martinez-del-Rincon, J., Domingo-Miguel, R., Soto-Valles, F., & Torres-Sanchez, R. (2016). A decision support system for managing irrigation in agriculture. *Computers and Electronics in Agriculture*, 124, 121–131. doi:10.1016/j.compag.2016.04.003

Olaniyi, E., Оланії, Е., & Оланиии, Э. (2018). Digital Agriculture: Mobile Phones, Internet & Agricultural Development in Africa. *Actual Problems of Economics*, 16.

Oo, L. M., & Aung, N. Z. (2018). A simple and efficient method for automatic strawberry shape and size estimation and classification. *Biosystems Engineering*, 170, 96–107. doi:10.1016/j.biosystemseng.2018.04.004

Orge Pinheiro, C. A., & de Senna, V. (2017). Multivariate analysis and neural networks application to price forecasting in the Brazilian agricultural market. *Ciência Rural*, 47(1). doi:10.1590/0103-8478cr20160077

Oshunsanya, S. O. (2013). Crop Yields as Influenced by Land Preparation Methods Established Within Vetiver Grass Alleys for Sustainable Agriculture in Southwest Nigeria. *Agroecology and Sustainable Food Systems*, 37(5), 578–591. doi:10.1080/21683565.2012.762439

Osman, J., Inglada, J., & Dejoux, J.-F. (2015). Assessment of a Markov logic model of crop rotations for early crop mapping. *Computers and Electronics in Agriculture*, 113, 234–243. doi:10.1016/j.compag.2015.02.015

Özdemir, V., & Hekim, N. (2018). Birth of Industry 5.0: Making Sense of Big Data with Artificial Intelligence, "The Internet of Things" and Next-Generation Technology Policy. *OMICS: A Journal of Integrative Biology*, 22(1), 65–76. doi:10.1089/omi.2017.0194 PMID:29293405

Pallottino, F., Menesatti, P., Figorilli, S., Antonucci, F., Tomasone, R., Colantoni, A., & Costa, C. (2018). Machine Vision Retrofit System for Mechanical Weed Control in Precision Agriculture Applications. *Sustainability*, *10*(7), 2209. doi:10.3390u10072209

Pandorfi, H., Bezerra, A. C., Atarassi, R. T., Vieira, F. M. C., Barbosa Filho, J. A. D., & Guiselini, C. (2016). Artificial neural networks employment in the prediction of evapotranspiration of greenhouse-grown sweet pepper. *Revista Brasileira de Engenharia Agrícola e Ambiental*, *20*(6), 507–512. doi:10.1590/1807-1929/agriambi.v20n6p507-512

Pantazi, X. E., Tamouridou, A. A., Alexandridis, T. K., Lagopodi, A. L., Kashefi, J., & Moshou, D. (2017). Evaluation of hierarchical self-organising maps for weed mapping using UAS multispectral imagery. *Computers and Electronics in Agriculture*, *139*, 224–230. doi:10.1016/j.compag.2017.05.026

Paraforos, D. S., Vassiliadis, V., Kortenbruck, D., Stamkopoulos, K., Ziogas, V., Sapounas, A. A., & Griepentrog, H. W. (2016). A Farm Management Information System Using Future Internet Technologies. *IFAC-PapersOnLine*, *49*(16), 324–329. doi:10.1016/j.ifacol.2016.10.060

Park, S., Im, J., Jang, E., & Rhee, J. (2016). Drought assessment and monitoring through blending of multi-sensor indices using machine learning approaches for different climate regions. *Agricultural and Forest Meteorology*, *216*, 157–169. doi:10.1016/j.agrformet.2015.10.011

Peloia, P. R., & Rodrigues, L. H. A. (2016). Identification Of Commercial Blocks Of Outstanding Performance Of Sugarcane Using Data Mining. *Engenharia Agrícola*, *36*(5), 895–901. doi:10.1590/1809-4430-Eng.Agric.v36n5p895-901/2016

Pentos, K., & Pieczarka, K. (2017). Applying an artificial neural network approach to the analysis of tractive properties in changing soil conditions. *Soil & Tillage Research*, *165*, 113–120. doi:10.1016/j.still.2016.08.005

Perea, R. (2018). Prediction of applied irrigation depths at farm level using artificial intelligence techniques. *Agricultural Water Management*, *206*, 229–240. doi:10.1016/j.agwat.2018.05.019

Pike, A. C., Mueller, T. G., Schoergendorfer, A., Shearer, S. A., & Karathanasis, A. D. (2009). Erosion Index Derived from Terrain Attributes using Logistic Regression and Neural Networks. *Agronomy Journal*, *101*(5), 1068–1079. doi:10.2134/agronj2008.0207x

Pineda, M., Pérez-Bueno, M. L., & Barón, M. (2018). Detection of Bacterial Infection in Melon Plants by Classification Methods Based on Imaging Data. *Frontiers in Plant Science*, *9*, 164. doi:10.3389/fpls.2018.00164 PMID:29491881

Pour, A. S., Chegini, G., Zarafshan, P., & Massah, J. (2018). Curvature-based pattern recognition for cultivar classification of Anthurium flowers. *Postharvest Biology and Technology*, *139*, 67–74. doi:10.1016/j.postharvbio.2018.01.013

Prasad, R., Deo, R. C., Li, Y., & Maraseni, T. (2018). Soil moisture forecasting by a hybrid machine learning technique: ELM integrated with ensemble empirical mode decomposition. *Geoderma*, *330*, 136–161. doi:10.1016/j.geoderma.2018.05.035

Protopop, I., & Shanoyan, A. (2016). Big Data and Smallholder Farmers: Big Data Applications in the Agri-Food Supply Chain in Developing Countries. *International Food and Agribusiness Management Review, 19*(A, SI), 173–190.

Provost, F., & Fawcett, T. (2013). Data Science and its Relationship to Big Data and Data-Driven Decision Making. *Big Data, 1*(1), 51–59. doi:10.1089/big.2013.1508 PMID:27447038

Quraishi, M. Z., & Mouazen, A. M. (2013). Development of a methodology for in situ assessment of topsoil dry bulk density. *Soil & Tillage Research, 126*, 229–237. doi:10.1016/j.still.2012.08.009

Rajeswari, S., Suthendran, K., & Rajakumar, K. (2017). A smart agricultural model by integrating IoT, mobile and cloud-based big data analytics. *2017 International Conference on Intelligent Computing and Control (I2C2)*, 1–5. 10.1109/I2C2.2017.8321902

Ramirez-Gil, J. G., Martinez, G. O. G., & Osorio, J. G. M. (2018). Design of electronic devices for monitoring climatic variables and development of an early warning system for the avocado wilt complex disease. *Computers and Electronics in Agriculture, 153*, 134–143. doi:10.1016/j.compag.2018.08.002

Rathod, S., Singh, K. N., Patil, S. G., Naik, R. H., Ray, M., & Meena, V. S. (2018). Modeling and forecasting of oilseed production of India through artificial intelligence techniques. *Indian Journal of Agricultural Sciences, 88*(1), 22–27.

Renaud-Gentie, C., Burgos, S., & Benoit, M. (2014). Choosing the most representative technical management routes within diverse management practices: Application to vineyards in the Loire Valley for environmental and quality assessment. *European Journal of Agronomy, 56*, 19–36. doi:10.1016/j.eja.2014.03.002

Ribeiro, C. O., & Oliveira, S. M. (2011). A hybrid commodity price-forecasting model applied to the sugar-alcohol sector. *The Australian Journal of Agricultural and Resource Economics, 55*(2), 180–198. doi:10.1111/j.1467-8489.2011.00534.x

Rizzo, D., Martin, L., & Wohlfahrt, J. (2014). Miscanthus spatial location as seen by farmers: A machine learning approach to model real criteria. *Biomass and Bioenergy, 66*, 348–363. doi:10.1016/j.biombioe.2014.02.035

Romero, J. R., Roncallo, P. F., Akkiraju, P. C., Ponzoni, I., Echenique, V. C., & Carballido, J. A. (2013). Using classification algorithms for predicting durum wheat yield in the province of Buenos Aires. *Computers and Electronics in Agriculture, 96*, 173–179. doi:10.1016/j.compag.2013.05.006

Russell, S. J., & Norvig, P. (2010). *Artificial intelligence: A Modern Approach* (3rd ed.). Upper Saddle River, NJ: Prentice Hall.

Sa, I., Ge, Z., Dayoub, F., Upcroft, B., Perez, T., & McCool, C. (2016). DeepFruits: A Fruit Detection System Using Deep Neural Networks. *Sensors (Basel), 16*(8), 1222. doi:10.339016081222 PMID:27527168

Sabanci, K., & Aydin, C. (2017). Smart Robotic Weed Control System for Sugar Beet. *Journal of Agricultural Science and Technology, 19*(1), 73–83.

Safa, M., Samarasinghe, S., & Nejat, M. (2015). Prediction of Wheat Production Using Artificial Neural Networks and Investigating Indirect Factors Affecting It: Case Study in Canterbury Province, New Zealand. *Journal of Agricultural Science and Technology*, *17*(4), 791–803.

Safavi, H. R., Mehrparvar, M., & Szidarovszky, F. (2016). Conjunctive Management of Surface and Ground Water Resources Using Conflict Resolution Approach. *Journal of Irrigation and Drainage Engineering*, *142*(4), 05016001. doi:10.1061/(ASCE)IR.1943-4774.0000991

Saidu, A., Clarkson, A. M., Adamu, S. H., Mohammed, M., & Jibo, I. (2017). Application of ICT in Agriculture. *Opportunities and Challenges in Developing Countries.*, *3*, 11.

Sennaar, K. (2017, October 16). *AI in Agriculture - Present Applications and Impact*. Retrieved September 24, 2018, from TechEmergence website: https://www.techemergence.com/ai-agriculture-present-applications-impact/

Shamshiri, R. R., Weltzien, C., Hameed, I. A., Yule, I. J., Grift, T. E., Balasundram, S. K., ... Chowdhary, G. (2018). Research and development in agricultural robotics: A perspective of digital farming. *International Journal of Agricultural and Biological Engineering*, *11*(4), 1–14. doi:10.25165/j.ijabe.20181104.4278

Sharma, N., Sharma, P., Irwin, D., & Shenoy, P. (2011). Predicting solar generation from weather forecasts using machine learning. *2011 IEEE International Conference on Smart Grid Communications (SmartGridComm)*, 528–533. 10.1109/SmartGridComm.2011.6102379

Shekoofa, A., Emam, Y., Ebrahimi, M., & Ebrahimie, E. (2011). Application of supervised feature selection methods to define the most important traits affecting maximum kernel water content in maize. *Australian Journal of Crop Science*, *5*(2), 162–168.

Sideratos, G., & Hatziargyriou, N. D. (2012). Probabilistic Wind Power Forecasting Using Radial Basis Function Neural Networks. *IEEE Transactions on Power Systems*, *27*(4), 1788–1796. doi:10.1109/TPWRS.2012.2187803

Silva, L. O. L. A., Koga, M. L., Cugnasca, C. E., & Costa, A. H. R. (2013). Comparative assessment of feature selection and classification techniques for visual inspection of pot plant seedlings. *Computers and Electronics in Agriculture*, *97*, 47–55. doi:10.1016/j.compag.2013.07.001

Simon, M. (2018, September 25). The Creepy-Cute Robot that Picks Peppers With its Face. *Wired*. Retrieved from https://www.wired.com/story/the-creepy-cute-robot-that-picks-peppers/

Sirsat, M. S., Cernadas, E., Fernandez-Delgado, M., & Khan, R. (2017). Classification of agricultural soil parameters in India. *Computers and Electronics in Agriculture*, *135*, 269–279. doi:10.1016/j.compag.2017.01.019

Smith, B. A., Hoogenboom, G., & McClendon, R. W. (2009). Artificial neural networks for automated year-round temperature prediction. *Computers and Electronics in Agriculture*, *68*(1), 52–61. doi:10.1016/j.compag.2009.04.003

Snow, V. O., & Lovattb, S. J. (2008). A general planner for agro-ecosystem models. *Computers and Electronics in Agriculture*, *60*(2), 201–211. doi:10.1016/j.compag.2007.08.001

Soh, Y. W., Koo, C. H., Huang, Y. F., & Fung, K. F. (2018). Application of artificial intelligence models for the prediction of standardized precipitation evapotranspiration index (SPEI) at Langat River Basin, Malaysia. *Computers and Electronics in Agriculture, 144*, 164–173. doi:10.1016/j.compag.2017.12.002

Sonobe, R., Tani, H., Wang, X., Kojima, Y., & Kobayashi, N. (2015). Extreme Learning Machine-based Crop Classification using ALOS/PALSAR Images. *Japan Agricultural Research Quarterly, 49*(4), 377–381. doi:10.6090/jarq.49.377

Stastny, J., Konecny, V., & Trenz, O. (2011). Agricultural data prediction by means of neural network. *Agricultural Economics-Zemedelska Ekonomika, 57*(7), 356–361. doi:10.17221/108/2011-AGRICECON

Suh, H. K., Ijsselmuiden, J., Hofstee, J. W., & van Henten, E. J. (2018). Transfer learning for the classification of sugar beet and volunteer potato under field conditions. *Biosystems Engineering, 174*, 50–65. doi:10.1016/j.biosystemseng.2018.06.017

Sujaritha, M., Annadurai, S., Satheeshkumar, J., Sharan, S. K., & Mahesh, L. (2017). Weed detecting robot in sugarcane fields using fuzzy real time classifier. *Computers and Electronics in Agriculture, 134*, 160–171. doi:10.1016/j.compag.2017.01.008

Sulistyo, S. B., Woo, W. L., & Dlay, S. S. (2017). Regularized Neural Networks Fusion and Genetic Algorithm Based On-Field Nitrogen Status Estimation of Wheat Plants. *IEEE Transactions on Industrial Informatics, 13*(1), 103–114. doi:10.1109/TII.2016.2628439

Tamaddoni-Nezhad, A., Milani, G. A., Raybould, A., Muggleton, S., & Bohan, D. A. (2013). Construction and Validation of Food Webs Using Logic-Based Machine Learning and Text Mining. In G. Woodward & D. A. Bohan (Eds.), Advances in Ecological Research, Vol 49: Ecological Networks in an Agricultural World (pp. 225–289). Academic Press. doi:10.1016/B978-0-12-420002-9.00004-4

Tan, D. S., Leong, R. N., Laguna, A. F., Ngo, C. A., Lao, A., Amalin, D. M., & Alvindia, D. G. (2018). AuToDiDAC: Automated Tool for Disease Detection and Assessment for Cacao Black Pod Rot. *Crop Protection, 103*, 98–102. doi:10.1016/j.cropro.2017.09.017

Tesfaye, K., Sonder, K., Cairns, J., Magorokosho, C., Tarekegn, A., Kassie, G. T., … Erenstein, O. (2016). Targeting Drought-Tolerant Maize Varieties in Southern Africa: A Geospatial Crop Modeling Approach Using Big Data. *International Food and Agribusiness Management Review, 19*(A, SI), 75–92.

Thenkabail, P. S., Lyon, J. G., & Huete, A. (2012). Advances in Hyperspectral Remote Sensing of Vegetation and Agricultural Croplands. In P. S. Thenkabail, J. G. Lyon, & A. Huete (Eds.), Hyperspectral Remote Sensing of Vegetation (pp. 3–35). Academic Press. Retrieved from https://pubs.er.usgs.gov/publication/70098951

Torkashvand, A. M., Ahmadi, A., & Nikravesh, N. L. (2017). Prediction of kiwifruit firmness using fruit mineral nutrient concentration by artificial neural network (ANN) and multiple linear regressions (MLR). *Journal of Integrative Agriculture, 16*(7), 1634–1644. doi:10.1016/S2095-3119(16)61546-0

Torres-Sospedra, J., & Nebot, P. (2014). Two-stage procedure based on smoothed ensembles of neural networks applied to weed detection in orange groves. *Biosystems Engineering, 123*, 40–55. doi:10.1016/j.biosystemseng.2014.05.005

Trace Genomics. (2018). *Trace Genomics*. Retrieved December 17, 2018, from https://www.tracege-nomics.com/#/

Tripathy, A. K., Adinarayana, J., Vijayalakshmi, K., Merchant, S. N., Desai, U. B., Ninomiya, S., ... Kiura, T. (2014). Knowledge discovery and Leaf Spot dynamics of groundnut crop through wireless sensor network and data mining techniques. *Computers and Electronics in Agriculture, 107*, 104–114. doi:10.1016/j.compag.2014.05.009

Ureta, C., Gonzalez-Salazar, C., Gonzalez, E. J., Alvarez-Buylla, E. R., & Martinez-Meyer, E. (2013). Environmental and social factors account for Mexican maize richness and distribution: A data mining approach. *Agriculture, Ecosystems & Environment, 179*, 25–34. doi:10.1016/j.agee.2013.06.017

VineView. (2018). *Aerial Vineyard Mapping - Vigor & Grapevine Disease*. Retrieved December 17, 2018, from VineView website: https://www.vineview.ca/

Wachter, S., Mittelstadt, B., & Floridi, L. (2017). Transparent, explainable, and accountable AI for robotics. *Science Robotics, 2*(6). doi:10.1126cirobotics.aan6080

Waga, D., & Rabah, K. (2014). Environmental Conditions' Big Data Management and Cloud Computing Analytics for Sustainable Agriculture. *World Journal of Computer Application and Technology, 9*.

Wakefield, K. (2018). *Predictive analytics and machine learning*. Retrieved November 14, 2018, from https://www.sas.com/en_gb/insights/articles/analytics/a-guide-to-predictive-analytics-and-machine-learning.html

Wang, L., Niu, Z., Kisi, O., Li, C., & Yu, D. (2017). Pan evaporation modeling using four different heuristic approaches. *Computers and Electronics in Agriculture, 140*, 203–213. doi:10.1016/j.compag.2017.05.036

Wang, Y. (2016). Deep reasoning and thinking beyond deep learning by cognitive robots and brain-inspired systems. *2016 IEEE 15th International Conference on Cognitive Informatics Cognitive Computing (ICCI*CC)*, 3–3. 10.1109/ICCI-CC.2016.7862095

Wang, Z., Hu, M., & Zhai, G. (2018). Application of Deep Learning Architectures for Accurate and Rapid Detection of Internal Mechanical Damage of Blueberry Using Hyperspectral Transmittance Data. *Sensors (Basel), 18*(4), 1126. doi:10.339018041126 PMID:29642454

Wang, L., Zhou, X., Zhu, X., & Guo, W. (2017). Estimation of leaf nitrogen concentration in wheat using the MK-SVR algorithm and satellite remote sensing data. *Computers and Electronics in Agriculture, 140*, 327–337. doi:10.1016/j.compag.2017.05.023

Wang, Li'ai, Zhou, X., Zhu, X., Dong, Z., & Guo, W. (2016). Estimation of biomass in wheat using random forest regression algorithm and remote sensing data. *Crop Journal, 4*(3), 212–219. doi:10.1016/j.cj.2016.01.008

Weiss, S. M., & Indurkhya, N. (1997). *Predictive data mining: a practical guide*. Retrieved from https://www.elsevier.com/books/predictive-data-mining/weiss/978-0-08-051465-9

Weltzien, C. (2016). *Digital agriculture – or why agriculture 4.0 still offers only modest returns*. Academic Press.

Wolfert, S., Ge, L., Verdouw, C., & Bogaardt, M.-J. (2017). Big Data in Smart Farming – A review. *Agricultural Systems*, *153*, 69–80. doi:10.1016/j.agsy.2017.01.023

Wolfert, S., Goense, D., & Sorensen, C. A. G. (2014). A Future Internet Collaboration Platform for Safe and Healthy Food from Farm to Fork. *2014 Annual SRII Global Conference*, 266–273. 10.1109/SRII.2014.47

Woodard, J. (2016). Big data and Ag-Analytics An open source, open data platform for agricultural & environmental finance, insurance, and risk. *Agricultural Finance Review*, *76*(1), 15–26. doi:10.1108/AFR-03-2016-0018

Wu, J., Yang, S. X., & Tian, F. (2014). A novel intelligent control system for flue-curing barns based on real-time image features. *Biosystems Engineering*, *123*, 77–90. doi:10.1016/j.biosystemseng.2014.05.008

Xiao, Y., Mignolet, C., Mari, J.-F., & Benoit, M. (2014). Modeling the spatial distribution of crop sequences at a large regional scale using land-cover survey data: A case from France. *Computers and Electronics in Agriculture*, *102*, 51–63. doi:10.1016/j.compag.2014.01.010

Yongting, T., & Jun, Z. (2017). Automatic apple recognition based on the fusion of color and 3D feature for robotic fruit picking. *Computers and Electronics in Agriculture, 142*(A), 388–396. doi:10.1016/j.compag.2017.09.019

Zangeneh, M., Omid, M., & Akram, A. (2010). Assessment of agricultural mechanization status of potato production by means of artificial Neural Network model. *Australian Journal of Crop Science*, *4*(5), 372–377.

Zhang, X., Qiao, Y., Meng, F., Fan, C., & Zhang, M. (2018). Identification of Maize Leaf Diseases Using Improved Deep Convolutional Neural Networks. *IEEE Access: Practical Innovations, Open Solutions*, *6*, 30370–30377. doi:10.1109/ACCESS.2018.2844405

Zhang, Z., Gong, Y., & Wang, Z. (2018). Accessible remote sensing data based reference evapotranspiration estimation modelling. *Agricultural Water Management*, *210*, 59–69. doi:10.1016/j.agwat.2018.07.039

Zhong, L., Hawkins, T., Holland, K., Gong, P., & Biging, G. (2009). Satellite imagery can support water planning in the Central Valley. *California Agriculture*, *63*(4), 220–224. doi:10.3733/ca.v063n04p220

Zhong, T. Y., Zhang, X. Y., & Huang, X. J. (2009). Simulation of farmer decision on land use conversions using decision tree method in Jiangsu Province, China. *Spanish Journal of Agricultural Research*, *7*(3), 687–698. doi:10.5424jar/2009073-454

Zhu, N., Liu, X., Liu, Z., Hu, K., Wang, Y., Tan, J., ... Guo, Y. (2018). Deep learning for smart agriculture: Concepts, tools, applications, and opportunities. *International Journal of Agricultural and Biological Engineering*, *11*(4), 21–28. doi:10.25165/j.ijabe.20181104.4475

KEY TERMS AND DEFINITIONS

AI: Artificial intelligence.
ANN: Artificial neural networks.
DDD: Data-driven decisions.
ELM: Extreme learning machine.
IoT: Internet of things.
RNN: Recurrent neural networks.
SVM: Support vector machine.

This research was previously published in AI and Big Data's Potential for Disruptive Innovation edited by Moses Strydom and Sheryl Buckley; pages 174-215, copyright year 2020 by Engineering Science Reference (an imprint of IGI Global).

APPENDIX

Table 2. Breakdown of papers on Pre-Production phase

Pre-Production Category	Type	Main Study Objectives/Impact	Technique	References
Seeds & Seedlings	Predictive	Pot plant seedling classification	Feature Selection	(Silva et al., 2013)
		Seed yield prediction	Artificial Neural Networks	(Emamgholizadeh et al., 2015)
		Estimate cultivar and site-specific parameters from breeding trial data	Holographic Genetic Algorithm	(Lamsal et al., 2017)
		Classification tool for Potato Virus Y detection	Support Vector Machines	(Griffel et al., 2018)
	Prescriptive	Target drought-tolerant maize varieties	Spatial Modeling	(Tesfaye et al., 2016)
		Seeding density optimization	Artificial Neural Networks	(Dornelles et al., 2018)
		Phosphogypsum Application Recommendation	M5-Rules Algorithm, Regression Models	(Caires & Guimaraes, 2018)
Soil, Tillage and Land Preparation	Diagnostic	Analyze the effects of soil texture, moisture, compaction, horizontal deformation and vertical load on traction force and traction efficiency	Artificial Neural Networks	(Pentos & Pieczarka, 2017)
	Predictive	Erosion Index prediction to aid conservation planning	Logistic Regression, Artificial Neural Networks	(Pike et al., 2009)
		Soil classification	Artificial Neural Networks	(Ajdadi et al., 2016; Calderano et al., 2014)
		Estimation of fuel consumption in agricultural mechanized operations	Artificial Neural Networks	(Borges et al. 2017)
		Prediction of key factors for a successful kiwi micropropagation	Artificial Neural Networks: Neuro Fuzzy logic models	(Arteta et al., 2018)
		Generating soil moisture forecasts	Artificial Neural Networks	(Prasad et al., 2018)
Other Pre-planting Activities	Diagnostic	Selection of important traits contributing to maximum kernel water content of maize	Supervised Feature Selection	(Shekoofa et al., 2011)
		Determining association between climatic indices and maize and sorghum yields	Spearman's Rank Correlation, Artificial Neural Networks	(Byakatonda et al., 2018)
	Predictive	Using satellite imagery to estimate water usage	Supervised Maximum Likelihood Classification	(L. Zhong et al., 2009)
		Predicting machinery energy ratio for target farming systems	Artificial Neural Networks	(Zangeneh et al., 2010)
		Predicting crops present in a given field using crop sequence of previous years	Markov Logic Networks	(Osman et al., 2015)
		Drought assessment and monitoring	Random Forest, Boosted Regression Trees, Cubist	(Park et al., 2016)
		Year-round temperature prediction	Artificial Neural Networks	(Smith et al., 2009)
	Prescriptive	Creating rule-based information system for decision making	Fuzzy Data-Mining, Decision Trees, Simulation Models, MapReduce Algorithms	(Delgado et al., 2008; Rajeswari et al., 2017; Snow & Lovattb, 2008)
		Land use conversion simulation	Classification and Regression Tree	(Zhong et al., 2009)
		Production Models based on soil and meteorological data	Artificial Neural Networks: Multilayer Perceptron and Self-Organizing Maps	(Jimenez et al., 2009)
		Classifying technical management routes of farmers	Data Mining, Ascendant Hierarchical Clustering, K-Means Clustering	(Renaud-Gentie et al., 2014)
		Miscanthus location probabilities through farmers' criteria	Boosted Regression Trees	(Rizzo et al., 2014)
		Yield simulation	Artificial Neural Networks, Genetic Algorithm	(Dornelles et al., 2018)

Table 3. Breakdown of papers on Production phase

Production Category	Type	Main Study Objectives/Impact	Technique	References
Planting, Irrigation & Fertilizer Application	*Diagnostic*	Evaluate spatial relationships of environmental and social factors with the spatial distribution of races and that can harbor highest number of races	Data Mining	(Ureta et al., 2013)
	Predictive	Monitoring nutrient solution compositions	Artificial Neural Networks	(Gutierrez et al., 2008)
		Estimating of nutrient content of plants	Artificial Neural Networks: Recurrent Neural Networks, Multiple Linear Regression, Multiple-Kernel Support Vector Regression, Genetic Algorithm	(Harada et al., 2013; Sulistyo et al., 2017; Liai Wang et al., 2017)
		Drought forecasting, assessment and monitoring	Extreme Learning Machine, Artificial Neural Networks, Multiple Linear Regression, Random Forests, Boosted Regression Trees, Cubist	(Ali et al., 2018; Park et al., 2016)
		Prediction of evapotranspiration	Artificial Neural Networks: Generalized Regression Neural Networks, Support Vector Machines, Extreme Learning Machine, Genetic Programming, Multiple Linear Regression, Multivariate Adaptive Regression Spline, Least Square Support Vector Regression	(Feng et al., 2017; Kumar et al., 2016; Pandorfi et al., 2016; Soh et al., 2018; Wang et al, 2017; Zhang et al., 2018)
		Modeling irrigation systems	Artificial Neural Networks, Fuzzy Logic, Genetic Algorithm	(Mattar, El-Marazky, & Ahmed, 2017; Perea R et al., 2018)
		Mapping extent of artificially drained areas	Selective Ensemble	(Moller et al., 2018)
		Prediction of soil properties	Linear Regression, Random Forests, Artificial Neural Networks, Support Vector Machine, Gradient Boosting, Cubist	(Khanal et al., 2018)
	Prescriptive	Classification of irrigated crops	Artificial Neural Networks: Multilayer Perceptron and Radial Basis Function	(López-Granados et al., 2010)
		Decision support system for Automated irrigation	Partial Least Square Regression, Artificial Neural Networks: Adaptive Neuro Fuzzy Inference Systems, Gradient Boosting	(Goldstein et al., 2018; Goumopoulos et al., 2014; Navarro-Hellin et al., 2016)
		Surface and ground Water management using conflict resolution	Artificial Neural Networks, Genetic Algorithm	(Safavi et al., 2016)
		Identification of well performing crops	Regression Trees, K-Means Clustering	(Peloia & Rodrigues, 2016)
		Soil classification	Support Vector Machines, Random Forests, Extreme Learning Machine	(Sirsat et al., 2017)
		Automating the growing process of crops via smart hydroponics	Bayesian Networks	(Alipio et al., 2017)

continues on following page

Table 3. Continued

Production Category	Type	Main Study Objectives/Impact	Technique	References
Weed, Disease & Pest Control	Diagnostic	Understanding the relationship between crop, weather, environment and disease	Multivariate Regression	(Tripathy et al., 2014)
		Early warning system, diagnosis, and management practices of avocado wilt complex disease.	Correlation Models	(Ramirez-Gil et al., 2018)
	Predictive	Weed discrimination	Logistic Regression, Fuzzy Logic, Artificial Neural Networks, Convolutional Neural Networks, Support Vector Machines, Principal Component Analysis, Naïve Bayes, Ensemble Algorithm, Discriminant Analysis	(Akbarzadeh et al., 2018; Bakhshipour & Jafari, 2018; Bakhshipour et al., 2017; Chantre et al., 2018; Dos Santos et al., 2017; Gómez-Casero et al., 2010; Gutierrez et al., 2008; Pantazi et al., 2017; Sujaritha et al., 2017; Torres-Sospedra & Nebot, 2014)
		Fungal infection discrimination	Principal Component Analysis, Artificial Neural Networks: Learning Vector Quantization	(Chung et al., 2016; Heim et al., 2018; Liu et al., 2010)
		Prediction of bacterial infection	Artificial Neural Networks, Support Vector Machines	(Hill et al., 2011; Liao et al., 2012; Pineda et al., 2018)
		Information system for assessment of crop disorders	Support Vector Machines	(Camargo et al., 2012)
		Remote sensing crop classification	Extreme Machine Learning	(Sonobe et al., 2015)
		Leaf disease diagnoses	Support Vector Machine, Deep Convolutional Neural Networks	(Du et al., 2016; Ramirez-Gil et al., 2018; Zhang et al., 2018)
		Automatic pest detection	Convolutional Neural Networks, Artificial Neural Network,	(Cheng et al., 2017; Dimililer & Zarrouk, 2017; Ding & Taylor, 2016; Espinoza et al., 2016)
		Disease detection via agricultural datasets	Ensemble Learning – Ensemble-Vote, Support Vector Machine, Deep Learning, Linear Regression	(Chaudhary et al., 2016; Ferentinos, 2018; Hassanien et al., 2017; Ilic et al., 2018)
		Automated/Real time disease detection	Support Vector Machine, Bayesian Networks, Convolutional Neural Networks	(Ancin-Murguzur et al., 2018; Garcia-Santillan & Pajares, 2018; Lu et al., 2017; Stanley Tan et al., 2018)
	Prescriptive	Classification of crops and weeds for automated weed control	Support Vector Machine, Convolutional Neural Networks	(Ahmed et al., 2012; Suh et al., 2018)
		Robotic weed control	K-Nearest Neighbor, Machine Vision	(Pallottino et al., 2018; Sabanci & Aydin, 2017; Sennaar, 2017)
		Vision-based fruit detection system in aid of autonomous harvesting	Convolutional, Neural Networks, Support Vector Machines, Machine Vision	(Sennaar, 2017; Shamshiri et al., 2018)
		Classification of pesticide regulations	Logistic Regression	(Espejo-Garcia et al., 2018)

continues on following page

810

Table 3. Continued

Production Category	Type	Main Study Objectives/Impact	Technique	References
Yield, Weather, Energy & Other Farm Management Activities	Diagnostic	Determination of appropriate environmental conditions for obtaining high crop yields	Artificial Neural Networks	(Jimenez et al., 2011)
		Extraction of cropping patterns from time series data	Hidden Markov Models	(Xiao et al., 2014)
	Predictive	Yield mapping	Decision Trees, Region Merging Algorithm, Evolutionary Product Unit Neural Networks	(da Silva Junior et al., 2017; Gutierrez et al., 2008)
		Yield prediction	Artificial Neural Networks: Adaptive Neuro-Fuzzy Inference Systems, Fuzzy Logic, Time Series, Autoregressive Integrated Moving Average, Bayesian Networks, Model-Based Recursive Partitioning, Support Vector Machines, Boosted Regression Trees, Gaussian Process Regression, Random Forests, Multiple Linear Regression, Extreme Learning Machine, M5 Prime, Decision Trees, K-Nearest Neighbor	(Aghighi et al., 2018; Chapman et al., 2018; Diaz et al., 2017; Everingham et al., 2016; Farjam et al., 2014; Fernandes et al., 2011; Fortin et al., 2011; Fukuda et al., 2013; Gonzalez-Sanchez et al., 2014; Hamedani et al., 2015; Jokic et al., 2010; Khashei-Siuki et al., 2011; Khazaei et al., 2008; Kouadio et al., 2018; Rathod et al., 2018; Romero et al., 2013; Safa et al., 2015; Stastny et al., 2011)
		Temperature prediction	Artificial Neural Network	(Castaneda-Miranda & Castano, 2017; Smith et al., 2009)
		Solar generation prediction	Support Vector Machines	(Sharma et al., 2011)
		Wind power forecasting	Artificial Neural Networks: Adaptive Neuro-Fuzzy Inference System, Support Vector Machines	(Mahmoud et al., 2018; Sideratos & Hatziargyriou, 2012)
		Prediction of environmental indices affecting crop production	Artificial Neural Networks and Adaptive Neuro-Fuzzy Inference Systems	(Khoshnevisan et al., 2013)
		Prediction of output energy in crop production	Artificial Neural Networks	(Khoshnevisan et al., 2014)
		Prediction of soil properties	Linear Regression, Random Forest, Artificial Neural Networks, Support Vector Machines, Gradient Boosting Model, Cubist	(Khanal et al., 2018)
	Prescriptive	Weather prediction	Machine Vision and Various Machine Learning Techniques	(Sennaar, 2017)

Table 4. Breakdown of papers on Post-Production phase

Post-Production Category	Type	Main Study Objectives/Impact	Technique	References
Harvest & Handling	Predictive	Crop yield forecast in aid of pre-harvest sales	Lasso Approximation	(Everingham et al., 2009)
		Portable leaves recognition system	Artificial Neural Networks	(Husin et al., 2012)
		Prediction of fruit physical properties – firmness, stalk characteristics, size etc.	Data Mining: Find Laws, Artificial Neural Network, Multiple Linear Regressions	(Demir et al., 2018; Oo & Aung, 2018; Torkashvand et al., 2017)
		Determining harvest time	Artificial Neural Networks	(de Barros et al., 2018)
	Prescriptive	Post-harvest product sorting	Decision Trees, Impulse Acoustic Data Mining, Fuzzy Data Mining	(Ebrahimi & Mollazade, 2010)
		Vision-based fruit detection system in aid of autonomous harvesting	Convolutional, Neural Networks, Support Vector Machines, Machine Vision	(Fernandez et al., 2018; Sa et al., 2016; Sennaar, 2017; Shamshiri et al., 2018; Yongting & Jun, 2017)
		Harvest time estimation	Artificial Neural Networks	(Costa et al., 2018)
Storage & Processing	Predictive	Year-round temperature prediction	Artificial Neural Network	(Smith et al., 2009)
		Biomass Estimation	Random Forests, Support Vector Machines, Artificial Neural Networks	(Castro et al., 2017; Wang et al., 2016)
		Real time post-harvest classification	Support Vector Machines, K-Nearest Neighbors, Discriminant Analysis, Decision Trees, Naive Bayes	(Pour et al., 2018)
	Prescriptive	Autonomous real-time flue-curing barns	Artificial Neural Networks	(Wu et al., 2014)
		Classification of potato tubers based on solanine toxicant	Artificial Neural Networks	(Babazadeh et al., 2016)
		Evaluating of phenolic compounds and antioxidant activity of blueberries	Artificial Neural Networks	(Guine et al., 2018)
Market & Consumer	Predictive	Crop yield forecast in aid of pre-harvest sales	Lasso Approximation	(Everingham et al., 2009)
		Price forecasting	Artificial Neural Networks	(Ayankoya et al., 2016; Orge Pinheiro & de Senna, 2017; Ribeiro & Oliveira, 2011)
		Food web construction	Logic-Based Machine Learning and Text Mining	(Tamaddoni-Nezhad et al., 2013)
		Fruit vitamin phenotyping	Artificial Neural Networks	(Aquino et al., 2016)
		Predictive models in horticulture	Generalized Linear Model, Bayesian Additive Regression Tree, Boosted Classification and Regression Tree	(Logan et al., 2016)
		Estimation of color properties in aid of quality checks	Artificial Neural Networks	(Demir, 2018; Kus et al., 2017)
		Detection of internal mechanical damage of fruits	Deep Convolutional Neural Network	(Wang et al., 2018)
	Prescriptive	Trade policy making and business decision making through Big Data	TRADE-Decision Support Model	(Cameron et al., 2017)

Chapter 41
Agbiotech, Sustainability, and Food Security Connection to Public Health

Ike Valentine Iyioke
Michigan State University, USA

ABSTRACT

Supporters of agricultural biotechnology have maintained a high enthusiasm for its role in improving agricultural yields and enhancing sustainability, for instance, in Africa. However, critics are deeply skeptical. This chapter sketches some of the main arguments on both sides to provide a summary analysis. The discussion includes multiple climatic, socioeconomic, and public policy drivers that have collided with the ability of the average person to achieve food security. If food security is to be understood as a matter of human health, then its definitions and designs must recognize food's many roles in creating positive public health outcomes. Hence, the discussion expands to include an integrative model of food security linking sociocultural, public policy, and ecological aspects to public health. The chapter concludes that extensive work must be done to steer policy initiatives toward common sense sustainability paths to achieve food security and/or sovereignty.

INTRODUCTION

Food—how it is produced, stored, processed, distributed, and consumed—has posed challenges throughout human history. After air, water and food are next in importance for human existence. In a world split between resource-rich and resource-poor nations, it is difficult to ensure a sufficient, safe, and nutritious food supply. The polarity of impact only gets more pronounced when the focus shifts to considerations for income and wealth inequality and with social exclusion and disadvantages (Burns, 2004). While many rich nations experience their version of food (in)security (rather than food's availability), poor nations are inundated with a host of unmet targets from production to consumption. Either way, public health is compromised when food is not served right.

DOI: 10.4018/978-1-7998-5354-1.ch041

This chapter provides a brief description of the food security concept. This chapter discusses factors related to the switch from traditional to mechanized industrial methods, including agricultural biotechnology (or agbiotech). This analysis includes a review of the consequences attending these methods. An attempt is made to illustrate the main arguments between supporters and doubters of agbiotech. This is followed with an analysis of how both sides differ in their understanding and grounding of sustainability (i.e., risks and capabilities of biotechnology).

Because eating is an ethical act, this chapter also examines the ethical implication of food production and consumption. This includes multiple climatic and socioeconomic or public policy drivers that have collided with the ability of the average person to achieve food security. Definitions and designs for food security must recognize food's many roles in creating positive public health outcomes. The chapter concludes that a significant amount of work is needed to steer policy initiatives toward common sense sustainability paths in its aim for plentiful, accessible, and nutritious food across the globe.

BACKGROUND ON AGBIOTECH

Agricultural biotechnology is the ability to translate and apply genomic knowledge using technological and scientific techniques to accelerate breeding of complex plant, animal, and microorganism traits leading to finished products. Central to this process is the scientist's understanding of DNA, the main constituent of chromosomes of organisms, which are manipulated to increase agricultural productivity. "By identifying genes that may confer advantages on certain crops, biotechnology enhances breeders' ability to make improvements in crops and livestock (BRIEF #1, 2004)."

It is a marked departure from about 10,000 years ago since traditional farmers have improved wild plants and animals through the selection and breeding of desirable characteristics using basic methods. This practice led to the domestication of plants and animals commonly used in crop and livestock agriculture. But advancements in the twentieth century and beyond, brought forth sophisticated methods which enable breeders to select traits resulting in increased yield, disease and pest resistance, drought resistance and enhanced flavor ("What is Agricultural Biotechnology?," 2004).

Methods commonly used in agbiotech are:

- **Genetic Engineering:** Which transfers useful characteristics (such as resistance to a disease) into a plant, animal or microorganism by inserting genes (DNA) from another organism
- **Molecular Marking:** Which examines the DNA of an organism to precisely select plants or animals that possess a desirable gene, even in the absence of a visible trait.
- **Molecular Diagnostics:** Which detects genes or gene products that are very precise and specific to more accurately diagnose crop and livestock diseases.
- **Vaccination:** For protection against some infectious illnesses in for example, chickens and cattle.
- **Tissue Culturing:** The regeneration of plants in the laboratory from disease-free planting materials for crops such as citrus, pineapples, avocados, mangoes, bananas, coffee and papaya ("What is Agricultural Biotechnology?," 2004).

HOW DO YOU DECONSTRUCT THE 'FOOD SECURITY' CONCEPT?

The fusion of food and security as a concept presupposes the factorial vagaries (from production to consumption) associated with the nourishing substance that humans eat or drink to sustain life, provide energy, promote growth, and ensure good health. The term "security" evokes its antonym, "danger." Hence, food is conceptualized in terms of its susceptibility to being in "harm's way" because attempts must be made to ensure its safety and to handle it with care.[1] This attribute of fragility (delicacy/delicateness) seems to defy a simple definition for food security.

Maxwell and Smith (1992), Smith, Pointing, and Maxwell (1993), and Hoddinott's (1999) inventorying of more than 200 definitions and formulations (e.g., DEFRA, 2006) typify the difficulty with its delineation. Food security has proven to be a cornucopia of ideas that periodically melts into other forms as it is examined. The many attempts at finding an accurate conceptual meaning of food security has been due to its long evolutionary process. It is a metamorphosis that may be far from over as:

No single existing survey instrument will ever be able to collect all needed indicators at the desired periodicity, and no single institution has either the mandate or the ability to measure and monitor food security in its many dimensions on a global scale (Carletto & Banerjee, 2013, p. 31).

On both personal and collective levels, how can one tell when he/she is slipping into food insecurity? Is food security best considered by means of production (supply side), in terms of access (demand side), or both? Does enough food entail its availability? Does availability translate to access? Does access to food mean access to any type of food, including preferred or culturally acceptable foods and foods with nutritional value? Questions like these have bothered analysts. Similar to measuring health vital signs, these questions point to indicators by which food security is ascertained, quantified, and qualified as means of determining an operational definition.

Renzaho and Mellor (2010) traced this tortuous path to the 1948 Declaration of Human Rights by the United Nations General Assembly. Article 25 discusses the inalienable rights of every human, including the right to an adequate standard of living such as rights to food (United Nations, 1948). The provision was bolstered later by Article 11 of the International Covenant on Economic, Social, and Cultural Rights adopted by the General Assembly (United Nations, 1966).

However, the food security concept took on a more definitive form at the World Food Conference in 1974, resulting in the Universal Declaration on the Eradication of Hunger and Malnutrition. Hence, food security was made to mean the "availability at all times, of adequate world food supplies of basic foodstuffs to sustain a steady expansion of food consumption and to offset fluctuations in production and prices" (United Nations, 1974).

In the 1983 Food and Agriculture Organization Director General's Report, emphasis went beyond food availability to include physical and economic access to food to meet dietary needs (FAO, 1983). Citing Anderson (1990), Renzaho and Mellor (2010) highlighted the definition of food security by the United States Department of Agriculture as:

Access by all people at all times to enough food for an active, healthy life and includes at a minimum: (a) the ready availability of nutritionally adequate and safe foods, and (b) the assured ability to acquire acceptable foods in socially acceptable ways (e.g., without resorting to emergency food supplies, scavenging, stealing, and other coping strategies) (p. 1575).

Despite its frequent use, Renzaho and Mellor (2010) conclude that this definition misjudges the political and economic situations across the globe. While the nature of food insecurity tends to look alike in developing and developed countries, the environmental setting in which it occurs differs significantly. One of such similarities is the existence of droughts, but others like armed conflicts, inadequate agricultural policies, and poor governance combine to negatively impact household livelihood. "For many countries experiencing natural and man-made disasters, and whose population's livelihood relies on migration wages, kinship support, wild animal, and food hunting are part of their normal livelihood mechanism" (Renzaho & Mellor, 2010, p. 3).

In emerging economies of the Pacific region, however, the causes of food insecurity cover a wide gamut such as high population density, diminishing and high incidences of labor migration within islands and overseas, weakening soil fertility, right to own land, and natural disasters. (Renzaho & Mellor, 2010, p. 3)

Three broad shifts are reflective of the successive definitions as noted by Maxwell (1996). They ae shifts that continue to preoccupy policy makers, international organizations, and many governments: (1) global and national to household and individual; (2) food-first perspective to livelihood perspective; and (3) objective indicators to subjective perceptions.

Hovering over the categories is the aspiration to meet a satisfactory level of food security. Thus, the relevant question has been: When is food supply sufficient, acceptable, or suitable? A similar question was raised by Pinstrup-Andersen (2009, p. 5), "Is it enough to meet economic demand and if so, at what price; or is it enough to meet energy and nutrient requirements?" Answers have been varied, including, understanding food security as a "minimal level of food consumption" (Reutlinger & Knaap, 1980); as a "target level" (Siamwalla & Valdes, 1980); as "enough food for life" (Krackt, 1981); as "the basic food needed" (FAO, 1983); as "enough for active, healthy life" (World Bank, 1986); as "adequate to meet nutritional needs" (Barraclough & Utting, 1987); and, as supply "for all family members to live healthy" (Sahn, 1989). On a country-by country basis,

National food sovereignty was and still is used to measure the extent to which a country has the means to make available to its people the food needed or demanded, irrespective of whether the food is domestically produced or imported. A country that does not produce the food it needs, or its population is prepared to buy and does not have the hard currency to import what is missing, would not be food sovereign (Pinstrup-Anderson, 2009, p. 5)

A pre-eminent definition of 'food security' is the proposal at the World Food Summit that food security is attained when "all people, at all times, have physical and economic access to sufficient, safe, and nutritious food to meet the dietary needs and food preferences for an active and healthy life" (FAO, 1996).

Beyond this, suggestions have been proposed that anthropometric measures may target pertinent policies and programs. "If nutritional security is the goal of interest, estimates of access to food should be combined with estimates of access to clean water and good sanitation" (Pinstrup-Anderson, 2009, p. 5). Anthropometric measures account for factors and considerations shaping food production, access, and consumption. These include the subtle fact that the ability to acquire enough food is not necessarily the same as actual food acquisition. Also, other household needs including goods and services, often compete with food acquisition. "The extent to which individual food security results in good nutrition depends on a set of non-food factors such as … access to primary health care" (Pinstrup-Anderson, 2009, p. 6).

Nutritional adequacy, while necessary, is not enough condition for food security. Hence, an objective set of measurements would include qualitative aspects and quantitative measures along with individual preferences, consistency with local food habits, cultural acceptability, and human dignity. Whether at the level of individual, household, or country, these requirements are a function of age, state of health, size, workload, environment, and behavior (Maxwell, 1996). Certainty and stability attributes have been added to food assessment and action to deconstruct it into more complete dimensions (Coates, 2013).

Of all the assessment indices, food availability and/or accessibility presents a major challenge given the neo-Malthusian projection of the world's teeming population, estimated to reach 9 billion by 2050 (United Nations, 2015). Hence, the global demand for food is predicted to increase for decades to come. Expert forecasts project that competition for natural resources such as land, water, energy, and the wild life "will affect our ability to produce food, as will the urgent requirement to reduce the impact of the food system on the environment" (Godfray et al., 2010, p. 812).

In addition to efforts to provide food security for a quantum projection of the world's population, a demand for environmentally and socially sustainable food is desirable. This effort would have to be more thoughtful than those of the 18th and 19th century Industrial and Agricultural Revolutions, and the 20th-century Green Revolution; given that it is constrained as never before by ecological degradation and dwindling natural resources.

CAN AGBIOTECH ELIMINATE HUNGER?

Studies of the benefits of biotechnology for agriculture have rapidly proliferated. For example, biotechnology promises far greater benefits to agricultural sustainability for Africa – a continent routinely and derisively labeled as synonymous with hunger and disease. To rid Africa of such pejorative image, some authors, including Thomson (2008) and Machuka (2001) – whose views will receive focused review shortly – suggest that biotechnology holds the wand to eliminate Africa's hunger and create agricultural sustainability. Such views have been sustained even in more recent literature (for instance, Henessy, Gupta & Kowalski, 2014; Arthur & Yobo, 2014).

Thomson (2008) noted that Africa should take advantage of agbiotech breakthroughs. These include initiatives related to insect-resistant maize and cotton, virus-resistant crops, drought-tolerant crops, and improved varieties of local crops like bananas, cassava, sorghum, and sweet potatoes. Thomson (2008), in her argument that Africa has a unique set of agriculture traits, discussed the continent's "lack of a dominant farming system, predominance of rain-fed agriculture as opposed to irrigation, and prevalence of soils of poor fertility" (p. 905). In her view, this points to the cyclically deficiency of low agricultural productivity and the limited amount of organic material available to be returned to the soil after harvesting. Therefore, Africa urgently needs to "improve the nutrient status of agricultural lands, many of which are acidic, low in phosphorous and high in toxic aluminum" (Thomson, 2008, p. 905).

Thomson (2008) acknowledged that the world is awash with enough food to go around (barring endemic distribution challenges, wars, corruption, and lack of infrastructure). Nonetheless, Thomson (2008) still thinks that genetically modified (GM) crops, which provide increased yields, could hold the ace; while also recognizingd constraints to attaining this goal, including consumer concerns related to GM foods.

Though more strident, Machuka's (2001) posture is nearly identical to Thomson's as it ascribes setbacks to crop production in sub-Saharan Africa (SSA),[2] including, pests, diseases, weeds, environmental degradation, and soil nutrient depletion. He identifies also, inadequate use of synthetic and other forms of modern farming methodologies and food processing mechanisms, poor roads networks.

Due to the prime place farming occupies in generating income and sustenance for most of Africa's population, Machuka (2001) is unflinching that the ultimate answer is "biotechnology for Africa, now" (p. 17). His claim for agbiotech goes beyond substantial contributions toward increasing food production to "preserving declining resources such as forests, soil, water, and arable land" (Machuka, 2001, p. 17).

Interestingly, Machuka's approach urges that agbiotech should empower the local people by building on indigenous traditions, techniques, experience, and knowledge accumulated over the millennia. This will avert "cut and paste" approaches borne out of possible ulterior motives. Granted that they may provide short-term, quick-fix solutions to unique problems, they are not of any use to "small-scale farmers in Africa who have developed their own unique crops, cropping, and farming systems that cannot be changed without their full and careful involvement" (Machuka, 2001, p. 18)

Despite making a few valid points, many would view Thomson and Machuka's propositions as a run-of-the-mill selling pitch favoring agbiotech. Concerns revolve around their inability to factor in fundamental challenges that beset agricultural production in Africa. These include:

- The role of strangulating lending conditions by international monetary agencies (such as International Monetary Fund [IMF] and the World Bank)
- Absence of large-scale agricultural investments by many African governments
- Inconsistent and lackluster agricultural programs and policies
- Factional strife and political unrest often initiated by neocolonial and/or other foreign influences
- Effects of trade and agricultural protectionism by Western countries, particularly the U.S.
- Damaging effects of the agbiotech industry

Also, it is largely true that much of Africa relies predominantly on rain-fed agricultural practices as opposed to irrigation. Yet it is hardly convincing that the nutrient status of agricultural lands (in the 11.7 million square-mile land area and the adjacent islands) are fraught with acidity, low in phosphorous and high in toxic aluminum, and hence unproductive. On this score alone, Thomson (2008) claimed, Africa cannot afford synthetic nutrients. Curiously, both Thompson (2008) and Machuka (2001) acknowledged a surplus of food in the world if only distribution, political, and economic policy constraints got out of the way. Nevertheless, they are undeterred in their conviction that much of Africa's agricultural and sustainability challenges will evaporate with the full embrace of agbiotech.

It warrants noting that the country of South Africa was the first in the world to adopt GM technology. Before genetically modified organism (GMO) legislation was in place, the South African government issued a permit for the commercial release in 1997 of MON810 maize, which contains Monsanto's patented *Bt gene Cry1Ab* and embodies much of the controversy surrounding GMOs (AfricaFocus Bulletin, 2013). This led to Monsanto colonizing the production of staple food by large-scale commercial farmers through aggressive acquisitions in the South African seed industry and patent laws protecting Monsanto's GM technology. Also, the technology came with the promise to ease pest management, save on pesticides, and reduce loss of yield through pest damage. The promise decisively failed. Monsanto's MON89034 subsequent replacement for insect resistance, MON810, also failed. Similar disastrous outcomes have been documented across the Global South (AfricaFocus Bulletin, 2013).

There has been a long suspicion about the biotech industry's aggressive marketing of their product as a key contributor in the global fight against hunger. The 2002 famine in Southern Africa was widely viewed as an opportunity to force-feed agbiotech on the people of that region by "expanding the market access and control of transnational corporations and undermining local smallholder production" (Zerbe, 2004, p. 593).

The truth remains that this expensive technology is being deployed in lucrative commodity crops for the sake of profit. For instance, the four dominant GM crops on the market (soya, maize, cotton, and canola) are not primarily valued for their contribution to African and global food security (AfricaFocus Bulletin, 2013). It is no longer a secret that the development of new seed technology through genetic modification and other methods is presented as a key component for raising productivity of African agriculture. If truth must be told, it actually serves to lure African farmers into international value chains in which the profits from what should be common resources are concentrated in the hands of private multinational companies. (AfricaFocus Bulletin, 2012, p. 14)

It was probably with good intention that in 2007 the Bill and Melinda Gates and Rockefeller Foundations established the Alliance for a Green Revolution for Africa (AGRA). Curiously, that initiative has not only become formal U.S. foreign policy but integral to the G8 approach to the problem of food security across the African continent. AfricaFocus analysts feel dubious that AGRA's initiative has transformed into official American policy and engages large global corporations in food production on African soil with African resources. Food security refers to linking Africa's biodiverse, local foods to the global market. Yet global agricultural markets are controlled by very few corporations. It is not hard to see how such an agenda prioritizes feeding Wall Street while threatening African smallholder food producers and Africa's food sovereignty.

The preceding argument has made clear how the promise of biotechnology has failed to raise the fortunes of the world's hunger-stricken population and the smallholder farmers who struggle to feed them. Instead, it has been profiting from the insecurities of the world's hungry without solving their hunger. Agbiotech's slogan remains that it has the where-with-all to erase deepening world hunger and resolve food insecurity, particularly in the Global South. However, with the Global North's reluctance to fully embrace transgenic foods, agbiotech has swerved toward the Global South as a ready market "in much the same way as the tobacco industry shifted its market focus southward" (McMichael, 2004, p. 140).

Surely, agbiotech's promises to solve food insecurity remain largely unproven. Its methods have faced renewed challenge by the natural time of traditional processes of selection and evolution. McMichael (2004) sums up its true purpose:

- Control of technology and markets
- Reduction of global biodiversity to transgenic monocultures
- Rejection of diversity of knowledge embedded in the cultures of the world's peasant farmers

In fact, the patenting of living organisms is widely viewed by Africans as biopiracy because it gives sole ownership to the corporation that inserted one gene. It does not recognize the innovations of thousands who developed the cultivar. Benefit sharing does not occur.

PROMISE TO IMPROVE FOOD PRODUCTION OR GENE SNATCHING?

The emergence of AGRA, as well as its recent posture, has analysts scratching their heads. One manifestation of this worry is the unexpressed goal of the AGRA and U.S. agroindustry: to access African genetic wealth for gene technologies and animal or plant breeding for corporate profit. Apparently, AGRA advocates policies that access the genetic wealth of indigenous populations without recognition—neither for their knowledge nor for the genetic parent materials. Likewise, they neither have plans to share benefits with those who cultivated and bred the plants and animals over centuries (Oguamanam, 2012; AfricaFocus Bulletin, 2012).

AfricaFocus further notes AGRA's technological approach to food production which radically differs from the 1960s Green Revolution whereby hybrid seeds developed for increased yields during that era remained in the public domain, to be freely exchanged among all farmers. Acting like a cartel, AGRA-sponsored seeds are most often privatized by the corporate seed breeder (AfricaFocus Bulletin, 2012). Every year the farmer must return to buy expensive seeds and can neither replant the next generation nor save or exchange the seeds among themselves for further experimentation. Patenting of living organisms (in this case, seeds) is recognized by U.S. law and advanced through its bilateral trade agreements, even as the American government refuses to sign on to the International Treaty for Plant Genetic Resources for Food and Agriculture (IT-2004) that ensures farmers' rights to save, exchange, and breed any seeds. The treaty also disallows patents for 64 crops and fodders, an aggregate representing most crops providing human nutrition (AfricaFocus Bulletin, 2012).

There is more to be said about the world's most valuable plant genetic resources, the majority of which are found in the Global South, home of "land races." According to Thompson and Hannah (2008), land races are crop varieties that have been grown over several centuries by indigenous farmers by selecting valuable traits through an ingenious process. Scientific advances that involve extracting valuable traits from the seeds of land races have been successfully carried out by industrial plant breeders from the Global North. Hence, "biotechnology has brought this set of concerns to the forefront of public attention in conjunction with legal debates over the patentability of genes and genetic sequences and over the status of patents" (Thompson & Hannah, 2008, p. 243).

The fear that agricultural genetic diversity of crops is being lost at an alarming rate is not new. For instance, Esquinas-Alcázar (2005, p. 946) warned that "given the enormous interdependence of countries and generations on this genetic diversity, this loss raises critical socio-economic, ethical, and political questions." Citing numerous instances and fingering the U.S. and Europe as major culprits, Kelbessa (2012) exasperated over the common practice where foreign corporations, colluding with some local African intellectuals, freely obtain knowledge and resources from peasant farmers. They erect legal protection for this knowledge without acknowledging the indigenous farmers, local authorities, and community within which the knowledge originally developed. Not only do innovators of this knowledge not receive any economic compensation for their research, they are unaware that pilfering of their indigenous knowledge is widespread (Kelbessa, 2012)

It is only fair that indigenous people should be compensated for the fact that their lands hold some of the world's stock of natural biological resources even as scientists from western countries have helped to extract them via bioprospecting. According to Millum (2010, p. 25), "We must build a robust defense for this intuition if we are to put it into practice and enforce it." Anything short of that is "biopiracy." This point has been a lightning rod of sorts.

Some critics accept the basic utilitarian rationale for patents, but question whether patents in biotechnology are really beneficial. Others see the utilitarian view of patents simply as a subterfuge to allow the growth of capitalist social relations and corporate power. Still others stress the view that indigenous people who discover uses for plants and who develop germplasm through generations of trial and error have a prior claim that vitiates this utilitarian rationale. These arguments are linked with concerns about intellectual property rights in the domain of human medicine, where patenting of genes and gene processes are sometimes said to violate human dignity (Thompson & Hannah, 2008, p. 244).

Discoveries in transgenic science come in leaps and bounds. The landmark event that made the most waves may be the successful cloning[3] of Dolly the Sheep from an adult cell at a Scottish research institute in July 1996. Not surprisingly, those waves (despite the sheep's demise six years later) still reverberate. Claims include GM cows that are primed to produce milk comparable to human milk, GM chickens that will not transmit bird flu, and GM grains, fruits, grass, and vegetables that have long been around and many more that are destined to land on our dinner tables.

The frequent dose of these claims signpost scientific milestones that jolt the minds and naturally prompt curiosity. There is the promise of biotechnology that will enable humans to be smarter, improve memories, increase strength and agility, live longer, be more resistant to disease, and enjoy richer emotional lives. Despite (re)assurances on the benefits of biotechnology (and in some cases because of it), the fact is that transgenic science is a process by which scientists alter an organism's genome by transferring one or more genes from another species or breed. This is done to determine the function of the inserted gene. It is not surprising that some people have paused to ponder the unforeseen/unforeseeable consequences. In addition, individuals are considering unexplored options and possibilities. It is understandable if the feeling of wonder and questioning metamorphosizes into doubt and unwillingness to put wholesale trust on this type of science. After all, not all scientific discoveries are or have been beneficial.

AGBOITECH OR TRADITIONAL AGRICULTURAL METHODS?

A major opposition to agbiotech is the ethical dialogue approach with roots in Oromo ecotheology and represents the voiceless indigenous marginalized natives such as found in Africa. Its methods teach positive relationship between God, humanity, the natural environment and nonhuman creation. The argument of retaining the natural environment and promoting an ecological balance through well-established indigenous agrarian methods is in opposition to the characteristics of agbiotech. According to Kelbessa (2005), it is absurd that indigenous people must relinquish their identity in the quest for western development, democracy, and human rights. It is even more so because western or western-trained academics have failed to carefully study indigenous environmental knowledge. The result has been that most Africans now active in conservation do so with the Western methods of wildlife management. Thus, by promoting the European management systems, the growth of an African conservation ethic suffers (Kelbessa, 2005).

When these imports confront the African environment, they tend to relentlessly exert control over traditional African land ethics with unaccustomed practices by using natural resources as objects for exploitation and profit making.

A related threat to indigenous and local ways of life is the commercialization and privatization of knowledge. In this regard, large transnational corporations are gaining control over the production and distribution of knowledge and life as a whole.

Agricultural production through large-scale intensive farming has been the model response in the fight against hunger. However, its methods are suspect. Industrial agriculture is wasteful, highly polluting, monopolistic (concentrated in the hands of few corporations), and, in fact, a major threat to food security. Other crises it has spurned (i.e., genetic erosion, disease susceptibility, and environmental stresses) need urgent re-examination. To the contrary, "small farming continues to offer more productive, stable, biodiverse, and place-based culinary alternatives" (McMichael, 2004, p. 151).

Traditional farming methods akin to agroecology offer several advantages over the conventional agroindustrial approach. These methods provide ecological principles for the design and management of sustainable and resource-conserving agricultural systems. Altieri, Rosset, & Thrupp (1998), have summarized the advantages thus:

- Agroecology relies on indigenous farming knowledge and selected modern technologies to manage diversity, incorporate biological principles and resources into farming systems and intensify agricultural production.
- It offers the only practical way to restore agricultural lands that have been degraded by conventional agronomic practices.
- It provides for an environmentally sound and affordable way for smallholders to intensify production in marginal areas.
- It has the potential to reverse the anti-peasant bias of strategies that emphasize purchased inputs as opposed to the assets that small farmers already possess, such as their low opportunity costs of labor.

WHAT ETHICAL LINES TO DRAW?

The fact that concerns have been raised about the enduring need for mankind to have food for normal body functioning is a clear indication of its ethical obligation. Indeed, the relief of hunger is a major claim on mankind's ethical responsibilities. It should not sit well with mankind's conscience that there is more than enough food to go around but are yet unwilling to device a reliable architecture to make that possible. Policy makers within governments ought to develop strategies to promote the interests of the citizenry to whom it is accountable. According to Rush (2013, p. 37), "Ensuring national food security is clearly one such strategy. Failure to protect citizen's interests in such a fundamental way would profoundly undermine the moral legitimacy of government."

Not everyone is getting the food they need, when they need it, and how they need it. This immediately raises the ethical question: Why is food not being produced and provided appropriately? It is a presupposition that certain actions that would ensure equity and access to food have been poorly applied or ignored. It is an ethical concern that there is not a lack of food but an unwillingness to establish equitable distribution apparati due to inordinate drive for profits at the expense of the disadvantaged.

As noted, concerns over agbiotech are rife, such as the use of rDNA in manipulating plant and animal genomes and others that are general to other forms of technology. The many issues surrounding agricultural biotechnology and their embedded ethical implications come under five themes: (1) impact on human health (i.e., food safety); (2) impact on the environment; (3) impact on non-human animals; (4) impact on farming communities in the developed and developing world; and (5) shifting power relations (e.g., the rising importance of commercial interests and multinationals; Thompson & Hannah, 2008).

At first glance, the agbiotech system seems wonderful. However, its underbelly is loathful. Industrial farming no longer commands the revolutionary status it once did; its exploitative methods are unsustainable to producing safe and healthy food. As noted by the Union of Concerned Scientists (UCS), industrial agriculture regards the farm as a production line where "inputs" (i.e., seedlings, pesticides, feed, and fertilizer) result in "outputs" (i.e., corn, chickens, and cattle). Hence, the primary drive, irrespective of everything else, is to increase yield per acre or pound of meat and minimize production costs, usually by exploiting economic scale (UCS, 2001).

In hindsight, pioneers of the Industrial Age must be disappointed that no one foresaw the trail of havoc—a great source of concern to environmental ethicists—from industrial agriculture that is witnessed today. According to Horrigan, Lawrence, and Walker (2002), the ills of agbiotech make a long list. It contributes to:

Numerous forms of environmental degradation, including air and water pollution, soil depletion, diminishing biodiversity, and fish die-offs. Meat production contributes disproportionately to these problems, in part because feeding grain to livestock to produce meat—instead of feeding it directly to humans—involves a large energy loss, making animal agriculture more resource intensive than other forms of food production. The proliferation of factory-style animal agriculture creates environmental and public health concerns, including pollution from the high concentration of animal wastes and the extensive use of antibiotics, which may compromise their effectiveness in medical use. At the consumption end, animal fat is implicated in many of the chronic degenerative diseases that afflict industrial and newly industrializing societies, particularly cardiovascular disease and some cancers. The pesticides used heavily in industrial agriculture are associated with elevated cancer risks for workers and consumers and are coming under greater scrutiny for their links to endocrine disruption and reproductive dysfunction (p. 445).

It is argued that GMOs have demonstrable benefits and the potential to increase the cost-efficiency of crop production. In addition, GMOS can build wealth for farmers and seed companies. Therefore, it should not be ethically justifiable to deny the public these obvious benefits unless it could be proven that GMOs pose a hazard to human health. However, the fact that there is some chance of a hazardous outcome to the public (slight or severe), criticisms from proponents of individual rights are justified. For instance, there is the risk of allergic reaction associated with GMOs, something that is common with proteins (Thompson & Hannah, 2008). Moreover, the assertions that GMOs have demonstrable benefits of some sort, are spurious. They do not fully account for unforeseen (but probably foreseeable) future safety issues posed to humans and the environment. Similarly, it is hard to understand why some are comfortable with granting "potential benefits" of GMOs but reluctant when considering "potential harm" to the public. It is equally misleading to claim that GMOs are more valuable and cost-effective than traditional crop production. The opposite has been proven to be the case. The issue with agbiotech may be largely economic. It is also significantly ethical given that hapless small holder farmers would lose their livelihood in the ruthless fight for patent rights.

There is also the claim that the slim probability of serious health effects on 'a minute segment' of the public should not outweigh the overwhelming economic and technological benefits. In other words, the interest of a trifle percentage does not match the opportunity of achieving the classic consequentialist utilitarian goal that maximizes benefits for the majority. Such claims are a conscious effort to inaccurately label the public (represented by the smallholder farmer) as "the minority" while a handful of agbiotech businesses become "the many." Huge profits and immense political clout do not make the biotech companies representative of the interest of the public. It does not matter that corporations have become powerful institutions that inordinately drive much of the public policies. One is not persuaded that the agbiotech industry should be accorded fiduciary status. It is hubris to use the biotech industry to shape the destiny of the vulnerable class. To do so for economic gains is ethically repugnant, especially when it is done under the pretext of solving world hunger.

Also, even as it might seem harsh to prohibit GMOs without a beyond-any-shred-of-doubt evidence that they pose a hazard to human health, the reverse logic ought to be noted. Inability to provide evidence is not a lack of proof of evidence. Thus, the present argument hints at the precautionary principle. It is a disposition that considers the course of action to be taken when an activity raises threats of harm to human health or the environment, even if some cause and effect relationships are not fully established. Lessons ought to be drawn from the 1992 Rio Declaration prescription:

In order to protect the environment, the precautionary approach shall be widely applied by States according to their capabilities. Where there are threats of serious or irreversible damage, lack of full scientific certainty shall not be used as a reason for postponing cost-effective measures to prevent environmental degradation. (United Nations, 1992)

Philosophers have analyzed environmental ethics using several approaches. They are duties to posterity (our obligations to consider and lessen the negative impacts of our actions on future generations) and eco-centric ethical values (our obligations to care for nature for its own sake). A general consequence of this analysis is that they manifest themselves as impacts on human beings (Thompson & Hannah, 2008).

WHAT DOES FOOD SECURITY GOT TO DO WITH PUBLIC HEALTH?

In 1920, Charles Winslow, an influential figure in public health, described the goal of public health as preventing disease, prolonging life, and promoting health and efficient functioning. These are all key words that relate to the popular Food and Agricultural Organization's (FAO) (1996) definition of food security. Further, public health's target to reduce the impact of disease and improve health and quality of life hinge on three key concepts in the pursuit of food security: (1) prevention; (2) population; and (3) justice. Public health seeks to protect against exposure to harmful or unhealthy substances or experiences, provide basic healthy amenities (i.e., portable water and a nutritious food supply), and attend to the needs, desires, and attributes of the population as a unit (Bouldin, 2010). Likewise, the all-encompassing food security concept connotes that, "In order to have robust nutrition outcomes, food both in terms of quantity and nutritional value, is important. But, so are access to healthcare, optimal hygiene, and adequate childcare services (Fanzo, 2015, p. 17).

The causal framework for nutrition demonstrates the importance of such sectors as agriculture and food, health, education, environment, water, and sanitation (WHO-UNICEF, 2015). In sum, public health and food security are so entwined that it is impossible to discuss one in isolation of the other.

Obviously, food supply is indispensable to human life and human development is crucial to achieving food security. These two dependent variables continue to experience intractable tensions. The result is a seething food crisis that pervades even during plenty. The evidential consequence and the intergenerational links between food access and nutritional status at different stages of the life course are telling. As one in every three persons worldwide is saddled with some form of malnutrition, it has thus been called a scourge in the world (DFID, 2011). Sobering statistics by Fanzo (2015) described the daunting challenges that stand in the way to provide "plentiful, healthy and nutritious food for all in an environmentally sustainable and safe manner, while addressing the multiple burdens of undernutrition, overweight and obesity and micronutrient deficiencies" (p. 15). Rather than do the needful, the agbiotech industry exerts the power of technology for other purposes.

Nutrients are the essential ingredients the body absorbs and utilizes for nourishment, growth, health, and social well-being (Fanzo, 2014). Inadequate supply of nutrients can lead to a chain of events through the life cycle. For instance, poor nutrition *in utero* can extend into adolescent and adult life. It can also span generations. This can mean early deaths for mothers, infants, and young children. Even when they survive, potential exists for impaired or irreversible physical and social development in the young. Subsequently, the result is poor health in adulthood affecting both individual well-being and social and economic development of nations (Black et al., 2013; Hoddinot, Rosegrant, & Torero, 2012).

Figure 1. Poor nutrition and impacts throughout the life cycle

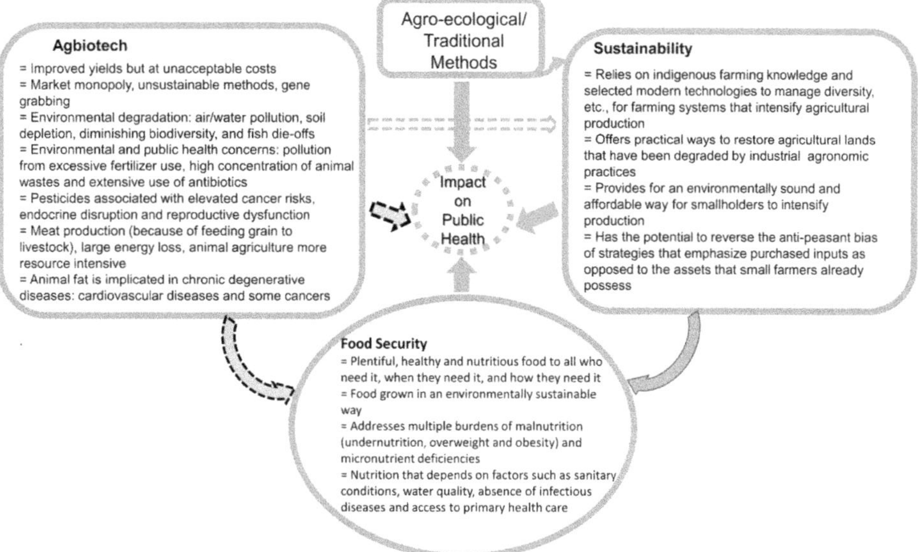

Research has unquestionably linked a swelter of impacts of erratic global climatic changes to food production. The climatic changes include more intense heatwaves, rising sea levels, blizzards with more snow storms, frequent forest fires, bizarre record rainfalls, and longer and/or shorter seasons. The conclusions of Porter et al. (2014, p. 502) is that "little is known about combined effects of climate change factors on food quality." This offers little comfort to anyone eager to see direct deleterious impacts from climate change on human health. However, that claim is probably misleading. Citing Ceccarelli et al., (2010, p. 627), the same report says that:

Climate change will have some adverse impacts on food quality through biotic and abiotic stresses. These changes may affect crop quality by altering carbon and nutrient uptake and biochemical processes that produce secondary compounds during grain development and maturation. This in turn could impact human and livestock health by altering nutritional intake and/or affect economic value by altering traits to processers or the consumers.

Climate change is primarily a problem of excessive carbon dioxide (CO_2) in the atmosphere. This carbon overload is caused mainly because humans burn massive amounts of fossil fuels like coal, oil, and gas or cut down and burn large swarths of forests which otherwise serve as a carbon sink (Union of Concerned Scientists, n.d.). In terms of agricultural production, it is hard to ignore the impacts of increased levels of CO_2. Porter et al. (2014) chronicled the effect of CO_2 on agricultural yields and human health. For example, cereals grown in elevated CO_2 show a decrease in protein (Ainsworth & McGrath, 2010; DaMatta, Grandis, Arenque, & Buckeridge, 2010; Erbs et al., 2010; Fernando et al., 2012; Högy et al., 2009; Pikki, Vorne, Ojanpera, & Pleijel, 2007). Meta-analysis of 228 experimental observations finds decreases between 10% and 14% in edible portions of wheat, rice, barley, and potato; there was a decrease of only 1.5% in soybeans, a nitrogen-fixing legume, when grown in elevated CO_2 (Taub, Miller, & Allen, 2008). Elevated CO_2 can lower the nutritional quality of flour produced from grain cereals and cassava (Erbs et al., 2010; Gleadow, Evans, McCaffery, & Cavagnaro, 2009; Högy et al., 2009). When coupled with increased crop and pathogen biomass, elevated CO_2 can result in increased severity of the *Fusarium pseudogramearum* pathogen, which leads to shriveled grains with low market value (Melloy et al., 2010). The only counter argument to this mountain of evidence is the claim by Duval et al. (2011) that elevated CO_2 can increase crop yield and overall yield of mineral.

CONCLUSION

This chapter was premised on the concentric link between public health, attainment of food security through sustainable means, and the promise of agbiotech. What has become apparent is the paradoxical reality accompanying each of the variables. Presently, agrobiotechnology research raises ethical, safety, and intellectual property rights issues. There is the question of whether we can provide plentiful, healthy, and nutritious food to all who need it, when they need it. Also, there is the lingering concern whether this can be done in an environmentally sustainable way while addressing the multiple burdens of malnutrition (i.e., undernutrition, overweight, and obesity) and micronutrient deficiencies. The drastic increase in grain yields in the past decades belies the growth in productivity and calories available per capita and pervasive malnutrition. "Though nutrition is critical to human health, it has yet to be systematically integrated into assessments of agricultural and food systems" (Remans, Wood, Saha, Anderman, & DeFries, 2014, p. 174). Likewise, the 2017 Global Hunger Index (GHI) shows that 52 out of 119 countries have levels of hunger that are serious, alarming, or extremely alarming. Despite a 27% decline since 2000, one in nine people (or 815 million worldwide) go to bed hungry each night (www.globalhungerindex.org/).

The approach of agbiotech must be revisited if its promise to wipe out hunger has failed and if its real passions are market monopoly, unsustainable methods, and gene grabbing. The combined effect of neo-colonial market influence by the Global North and the total control of crop-development agro-multinationals may be a threat to the diverse system of traditional farmers who would be forced into 'bioserfdom.'

The colossal failure of many of the newly developed or hybridized crop and plant species in the Global South is dispiriting. The report of the International Assessment of Agricultural Knowledge, Science and Technology for Development (IAASTD) approved by 57 governments in Johannesburg presents a disturbing account of the failure of industrial farming. It calls for a fundamental change in farming to better address soaring food prices, hunger, social inequities, and environmental disasters (AfricaFocus Bulletin, 2009). The report notes that small-scale farmers and agro-ecological methods provide a way to avert the current food crisis while meeting the needs of both local and international communities. More equitable trade arrangements and increased sharing of knowledge to support agroecologically-based approaches in both small farm and large-scale sectors are urgently required.

Food security cannot focus on meeting life's barest minimum. Instead, it should aim to pursue a good life. Hinderances to this goal still exist due to unsustainable agricultural practices, gauging market prices, climate change, land degradation, etc., vis-a-vis global demand (due to population increases and diet changes). Access to desired food is likely to increase substantially in the future, including a host of negative impacts on public health.

Figure 2. Agbiotech, sustainability, and food security impacts on public health

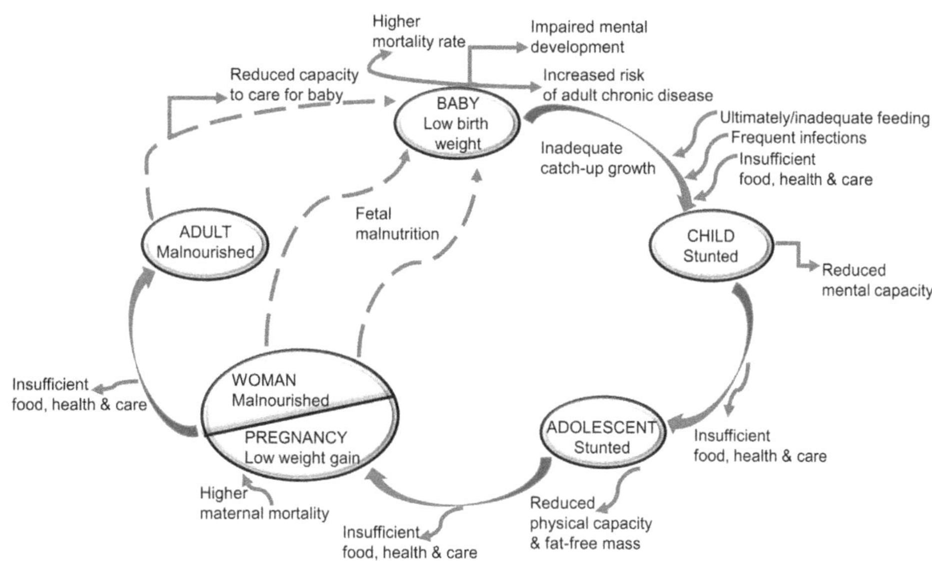

REFERENCES

AfricaFocus Bulletin. (2009, January 22). Africa: Agricultural knowledge.

AfricaFocus Bulletin. (2012). Africa: The hidden issue of "gene grabbing."

AfricaFocus Bulletin. (2013). Africa: Monopolizing maize.

Ainsworth, E., & McGrath, J. (2010). Direct effects of rising atmospheric carbon dioxide and ozone on crop yields. In D. Lobell & M. Burke (Eds.), *Climate change and food security: Adapting agriculture to a warmer world* (pp. 109–130). New York, NY: Springer.

Altieri, M. A., Rosset, P., & Thrupp, L. A. (1998). *The potential of agroecology to combat hunger in the developing world. A 2020 Vision for Food, Agriculture, and the Environment, 2020 Brief 55.* Washington, DC: International Food Policy Research Institute.

Arthur, G., & Yobo, K. (2014). Genetically Modified Crops in Africa. In M. Ahuja & K. Ramawat (Eds.), *Biotechnology and Biodiversity* (pp. 17–37). New York, NY: Springer.

Ayala, A., & Meier, B. (2017). A human rights approach to the health implications of food and nutrition insecurity. *Public Health Reviews*, *38*(10), 1–22. doi:10.118640985-017-0056-5 PMID:29450082

Barraclough, S., & Utting, P. (1987). *Food security trends and prospects in Latin America, Working paper no. 99*. Helen Kellogg Institute for International Studies, University of Notre Dame, USA.

Black, R., Victora, C., Walker, S., Bhutta, Z., Christian, P., de Onis, M., ... Uauay, R. (2013). Maternal and child undernutrition and overweight in low-income and middle-income countries. *Lancet*, *382*(9890), 427–451. doi:10.1016/S0140-6736(13)60937-X PMID:23746772

Bouldin, E. (2010). History and development of public health. In E. Andresen & E. Bouldin (Eds.), *Public health foundations: Concepts and practices* (pp. 3–24). San Francisco, CA: John Wiley & Sons, Inc.

Burns, C. (2004). *A review of the literature describing the link between poverty, food insecurity and obesity with specific reference to Australia. Centre for Physical Activity and Nutrition Research School of Exercise and Nutrition Sciences, Deakin University Melbourne*. Australia: VicHealth.

Carletto, C., & Banerjee, A. (2013). Towards better measurement of household food security: Harmonizing indicators and the role of household surveys. *Global Food Security*, *2*(1), 30–40. doi:10.1016/j.gfs.2012.11.006

Ceccarelli, S., Grando, S., Maatougui, M., Michael, M., Slash, M., Haghparast, R., ... Nachit, M. (2010). Plant breeding and climate changes. *The Journal of Agricultural Science*, *148*(06), 627–637. doi:10.1017/S0021859610000651

Coates, J. (2013). Build it back better: Deconstructing food security for improved measurement and action. *Global Food Security*, *2*(3), 188–194. doi:10.1016/j.gfs.2013.05.002

DaMatta, F., Grandis, A., Arenque, B., & Buckeridge, M. (2010). Impacts of climate changes on crop physiology and food quality. *Food Research International*, *43*(7), 1814–1823. doi:10.1016/j.foodres.2009.11.001

DEFRA. (2006). Food security and the UK: An evidence and analysis paper. Department for Environment, Food and Rural Affairs, Food Chain Analysis Group, London, UK.

Department for International Development (DFID). (2011, September). *Scaling up nutrition: The UK's position paper on undernutrition*. London, UK: DFID. Retrieved from https://assets.publishing.service.gov.uk/government/uploads/system/uploads/attachment_data/file/67466/scal-up-nutr-uk-pos-undernutr.pdf

Duval, B. D., Dijkstra, P., Natali, S. M., Megonigal, J. P., Ketterer, M. E., Drake, B. G., ... Hungate, B. A. (2011). Plant-soil distribution of potentially toxic elements in response to elevated atmospheric CO_2. *Environmental Science & Technology*, *45*(7), 2570–2574. doi:10.1021/es102250u PMID:21405117

Erbs, M., Manderscheid, R., Jansen, G., Seddig, S., Pacholski, A., & Weigela, H. (2010). Effects of free-air CO_2 enrichment and nitrogen supply on grain quality parameters and elemental composition of wheat and barley grown in a crop rotation. *Agriculture, Ecosystems & Environment*, *136*(1-2), 59–68. doi:10.1016/j.agee.2009.11.009

Esquinas-Alcázar, J. (2005). Protecting crop genetic diversity for food security: Political, ethical and technical challenges. *Nature Reviews. Genetics, 6*(12), 946–953. doi:10.1038/nrg1729 PMID:16341075

Fanzo, J. (2014). Strengthening the engagement of food and health systems to improve nutrition security: Synthesis and overview of approaches to address nutrition. *Global Food Security, 3*(3-4), 183–192. doi:10.1016/j.gfs.2014.09.001

Fanzo, J. (2015). Ethical issues for human nutrition in the context of global food security and sustainable development. *Global Food Security, 7*, 15–23. doi:10.1016/j.gfs.2015.11.001

Fernando, Panozzo, J., Tausz, M., Norton, R., Fitzgerald, G., & Seneweera, S. (2012). Rising atmospheric CO_2 concentration affects mineral content and protein concentration of wheat grain. *Food Chemistry, 133*(4), 1307–1311. doi:10.1016/j.foodchem.2012.01.105

Food and Agricultural Organization (FAO). (1983). *World food security: A reappraisal of the concepts and approaches* [Director General's Report]. Rome, Italy: FAO.

Food and Agricultural Organization (FAO). (1996). *Rome declaration on world food security*. Rome, Italy: World Food Summit.

Gleadow, R., Evans, J. R., McCaffery, S., & Cavagnaro, T. R. (2009). Growth and nutritive value of cassava are reduced when grown in elevated CO_2. *Plant Biology, 11*(1), 76–82.

Godfray, H. C. J., Crute, I. R., Lawrence, D., Pretty, J. N., Thomas, S. M., Beddington, J. R., ... Toulmin, C. (2010). Food security: The challenge of feeding 9 billion people. *Science, 327*(5967), 812–818. doi:10.1126cience.1185383 PMID:20110467

Henessy, W., Gupta, A., & Kowalski, S. (2014). Practice driving policy: Agbiotech transfer as capacity building. In S. Smith, P. Philips, & D. Castle (Eds.), *Handbook on agriculture, biotechnology and development* (pp. 314–342). Cheltenham, UK: Edward Elgar Publishing Limited. doi:10.4337/9780857938350.00028

Hoddinot, J., Rosegrant, M., & Torero, M. (2012). *Investments to reduce hunger and undernutrition. Copenhagen Consensus 2012 Challenge Paper, Hunger and Malnutrition*. Washington, DC: International Food Policy Research Institute.

Hoddinott, J. (1999). *Operationalizing household food security in developing projects: An introduction Technical Guide no. 1*. Washington, DC: International Food Policy Research Institute.

Högy, P., Wieser, H., Köhler, P., Schwadorf, K., Breuer, J., Franzaring, J., ... Fangmeier, A. (2009). Effects of elevated CO_2 on grain yield and quality of wheat: Results from a 3-year free-air CO_2 enrichment experiment. *Plant Biology*, (Suppl. 1), 1160–1169. PMID:19778369

Horn, F., & Breeze, R. (n.d.). Agriculture and food security. Agricultural Research Service, United States Department of Agriculture, Washington, DC.

Horrigan, L., Lawrence, R. S., & Walker, P. (2002). How sustainable agriculture can address the environmental and human health harms of industrial agriculture. *Environmental Health Perspectives, 110*(5), 445–456. doi:10.1289/ehp.02110445 PMID:12003747

Kelbessa, W. (2005). *The utility of ethical dialogue for marginalized voices in Africa.* Retrieved from http://pubs.iied.org/pdfs/13508IIED.pdf?

Kelbessa, W. (2012). Environmental injustice in Africa. In H. McDonald (Ed.), *Pragmatism and Environmentalism 9* (Vol. 1, pp. 99–132). New York, NY: Rodopi.

Krackt, U. (1981). Food security for people in the 1980s. *Paper prepared for discussion at the North-South Food Roundtable Meeting,* Washington DC.

Machuka, J. (2001). Agricultural biotechnology for Africa. African scientists and farmers must feed their own people. *Plant Physiology, 126*(1), 16–19. doi:10.1104/pp.126.1.16 PMID:11351064

Maxwell, S. (1996). Food security: A post-modern perspective. *Food Policy, 21*(2), 155–170. doi:10.1016/0306-9192(95)00074-7

Maxwell, S., & Smith, M. (1992). Part 1: Household food security: A conceptual review. In S. Maxwell & T.R. Frankenberger (Eds.), Household food security: Concepts, indicators, measurements: A technical review (pp. 4-72). United Nations Children's Fund, New York, NY.

McMichael, P. (2004). Biotechnology and food security: Profiting on insecurity. In L. Beneria & S. Bisnath (Eds.), *Global tensions: Challenges and opportunities in the world economy* (pp. 137–154). New York, NY: Routledge.

Melloy, P., Hollaway, G., Norton, J. L., Norton, R., Aitken, E., & Chakraborty, S. (2010). Production and fitness of *Fusarium pseudogramearum inoculum* at elevated carbon dioxide in FACE. *Global Change Biology, 16*(12), 3363–3373. doi:10.1111/j.1365-2486.2010.02178.x

Millum, J. (2010). How should the benefits of bioprospecting be shared? *The Hastings Center Report, 40*(1), 24–33. doi:10.1353/hcr.0.0227 PMID:20169653

Oguamanam, C. (2013). Intellectual Property, Ag-biotech and the Right to Adequate Food: A Critical African Perspective.

Pikki, K., Vorne, V., Ojanpera, K., & Pleijel, H. (2017). Impact of elevated O_3 and CO_2 exposure on potato tuber micronutrients. *Agriculture, Ecosystems & Environment, 118*(1-4), 55–64. doi:10.1016/j.agee.2006.04.012

Pinstrup-Anderson, P. (2009). Food security: Definition and measurement. *Food Security, 1*(1), 5–7. doi:10.100712571-008-0002-y

Porter, J. R., Liyong, X., Challinor, A. J., Cochrane, K., Howden, S. M., Iqbal, M. M., … Ziska, L. (2014). Food security and food production systems. In C. Field et al. (Eds.), Climate change 2014: Impacts, adaptation, and vulnerability, Part A: Global and Sectoral Aspects (pp. 485-533). New York, NY: Cambridge University Press.

Remans, R., Wood, S., Saha, N., Anderman, T., & DeFries, R. (2014). Measuring nutritional diversity of national food supplies. *Global Food Security, 3*(3-4), 174–182. doi:10.1016/j.gfs.2014.07.001

Renzaho, A., & Mellor, D. (2010). Food security measurement in cultural pluralism: Missing the point or conceptual misunderstanding? *Nutrition (Burbank, Los Angeles County, Calif.)*, *26*(1), 1–9. doi:10.1016/j. nut.2009.05.001 PMID:19804955

Reutlinger, S., & Knapp, K. (1980). *Food security in deficit countries.* World Bank.

Ruel, M., Garrett, J., Yosef, S., & Olivier, M. (2017). Urbanization, food security and nutrition. In Se. de Pee et al. (Eds.), *Nutrition and Health*. New York, NY: Springer. doi:10.1007/978-3-319-43739-2

Rush, E. (2013). Ethics of food security. In Q. Farmar-Bowers, V. Higgins, & J. Millar (Eds.), *Food security in Australia* (pp. 35–48). Boston, MA: Springer. doi:10.1007/978-1-4614-4484-8_3

Sahn, D. (1989). A conceptual framework for examining the seasonal aspects of household food security. In D. Sahn (Ed.), *Seasonal variability in third world agriculture: The consequences for food security* (pp. 67–77). Baltimore, MD: John Hopkins University Press.

Siamwalla, A., & Valdes, A. (1980). Food security in developing countries. *Food Policy*, *5*(4), 258–272. doi:10.1016/0306-9192(80)90055-X

Smith, M., Pointing, J., & Maxwell, S. (1993). *Household food security, concepts and definitions: An annotated bibliography. Development Bibliography No. 8.* Brighton, UK: Institute of Development Studies, University of Sussex.

Taub, D., Miller, B., & Allen, H. (2008). Effect of elevated CO_2 on the protein concentration of food crops: A meta-analysis. *Global Change Biology*, *14*(3), 565–575. doi:10.1111/j.1365-2486.2007.01511.x

The World Bank. (1986). Poverty and hunger: Issues and options for food security in developing countries. World Bank Policy Study.

Thompson, P., & Hannah, W. (2008). Food and agricultural biotechnology: A summary and analysis of ethical concerns. In U. Stahl, U. Donalies, & E. Nevoigt (Eds.), *Advances in biochemical engineering/ biotechnology* (pp. 229–264). Berlin, Germany: Springer.

Thomson, J. (2008). The role of biotechnology for agricultural sustainability in Africa. *Philosophical Transactions of the Royal Society*, *363*(1492), 905–913. doi:10.1098/rstb.2007.2191 PMID:17761472

Union of Concerned Scientists (UCS). *Why does CO_2 get most of the attention when there are so many other heat-trapping gases?* UCS.

United Nations. (1966). *The international covenant on economic, social and cultural rights.* Adopted by the General Assembly of the United Nations on December 16, 1966.

United Nations. (1974). *Report of the World Food Conference.* New York, NY: United Nations.

United Nations. (1975). *Report of the World Food Conference.* Rome: UN.

United Nations. (1992). *Sales No. E.73.II.A.14 and corrigendum.* Rio de Janeiro, Brazil: United Nations.

United Nations. (2015). *World population projected to reach 9.7 billion by 2050.* Department of Economic and Social Affairs, UN.

United Nations. (1948). *Universal declaration of human rights.* Adopted by the General Assembly of the United Nations on December 10, 1948. Retrieved from http://www.un.org/en/universal-declaration-human-rights/index.html

What is Agricultural Biotechnology? (2004). U.S. Agency for International Development, Agricultural Biotechnology Support Project II, and the Program for Biosafety Systems.

WHO-UNICEF-USAID. (2015). *Improving nutrition outcomes with better water, sanitation and hygiene: practical solutions for policies and programs.* Retrieved from https://www.unicef.org/media/files/IntegratingWASHandNut_WHO_UNICEF_USAID_Nov2015.pdf

Zerbe, N. (2004). Feeding the famine? American food aid and the GMO debate in Southern Africa. *Food Policy, 29*(6), 593–608. doi:10.1016/j.foodpol.2004.09.002

ADDITIONAL READING

Cohen, M., & Garrett, J. (2010). The food price crisis and urban food (in)security. *Environment and Urbanization, 22*(2), 467–482. doi:10.1177/0956247810380375

Fenning, T. M., & Gershenzon, J. (2003). European agbiotech crisis? *Nature Biotechnology, 21*(4), 1–2. doi:10.1038/nbt0403-360 PMID:12665816

Institute for Responsible Technology. (n.d.). Retrieved from https://responsibletechnology.org/gmo-education/

Loring, P., & Gerlach, S. (2009). Food, culture, and human health in Alaska: An integrative health approach to food security. *Environmental Science & Policy, 12*(4), 466–478. doi:10.1016/j.envsci.2008.10.006

Meyer, H. (2011). Systemic risks of genetically modified crops: The need for new approaches to risk assessment. *Environmental Sciences Europe, 7*(23), 1–11.

Morgan, K. (2009). Feeding the city: The challenge of urban food planning. *International Planning Studies, 14*(4), 341–348. doi:10.1080/13563471003642852

Ricroch, A. e., Bergé, J. & Kuntz, M. (2010). *Is the Suspension of MON810 Maize Cultivation by Some European Countries Scientifically Justified?* ISB News Report.

KEY TERMS AND DEFINITIONS

Agbiotech: A collection of scientific techniques to improve plants, animals, and microorganisms.

Agroecology: Agroecology is the study of the methods of ecological processes applied to agricultural production systems. These methods provide ecological principles applied for the design and management of sustainable and resource-conserving agricultural systems.

Food Security: When all people have physical and economic access to sufficient, safe, and nutritious food to meet the dietary needs and food preferences for an active and healthy life.

Food Sovereignty: Is a term coined by members of Via Campesina in 1996 and refers to the right of everyone to healthy and culturally appropriate food produced through ecologically sound and sustainable methods, and their right to define their own food and agriculture systems.

GMO: A GMO (genetically modified organism) is the result of a laboratory process where genes from the DNA of one species are extracted and artificially forced into the genes of an unrelated plant or animal to achieve an improved product. This process also may be called either genetic engineering (GE) or genetic modification (GM). GMOs are also known as "transgenic" organisms.

Public Health: The science of preventing disease, prolonging life, and promoting health and efficient functioning.

Sustainability: The pursuit of global environmental viability via avoidance of the depletion of natural resources to maintain an ecological balance.

ENDNOTES

[1]   Other approaches have been considered in discussing agriculture and food security. Horn and Breeze (n.d.) called attention to the growing threat on the American agriculture and food supply system, as well as its vulnerability to bioterrorism and biological warfare. They cover three major areas: (1) agriculture, the science and art of farming; (2) biological warfare, the use of disease-spreading microorganisms, toxins, and pests against enemy armed forces or civilians; and (3) terrorism, the use of terror or violence to intimidate, subjugate, and demoralize, especially as a political weapon or policy. On their part, Ayala and Meier (2017) used international human rights law as a critical role in guiding governments that are struggling to protect the health of their populations, particularly among the most susceptible groups, in responding to food and nutrition insecurity. Still, others have examined trends, unique characteristics, challenges, and distinctive factors and conditions that shape urban poverty, food insecurity, and malnutrition with a view to designing programs and policies to improve the lives of urban dwellers (Ruel, Garrett, Yosef, & Olivier, 2017).

[2]   Many authors are either unaware or nonchalant (or both) about the debasing connotation of dividing Africa between north and south of the Sahara. With the intent to project what they see as the backward "Black Africa" they expose their ignorance of the historical antecedents of the continent. The SSA reference is a fictional neo-colonial ploy promoting superficial divisions and comparisons. It gives the impression that, due to their proximity to Europe, all countries north of the Sahara are self-sufficient and have nothing in common with the rest of Africa. That is far from the truth.

[3]   This is not to confuse the meaning of cloning with that of gene modification in biotechnology. Although they are not the same, the two fall under transgenic science.

Chapter 42
Agricultural Cooperatives for Sustainable Development of Rural Territories and Food Security:
Morocco's Experience

Maria Fedorova

https://orcid.org/0000-0002-0899-6303
Omsk State Technical University, Russia

Ismail Taaricht
Cadi Ayyad University, Morocco

ABSTRACT

This chapter deals with the elaboration of a conceptual framework for agricultural cooperatives in Morocco: sustainable development of rural territories. The farming cooperative associations form an effective means for the advancement of the agricultural sector, being one of the elements of agricultural policy, which play an important role in the development of agricultural production, both plant and animal, as well as in the development process in Morocco, especially for rural development, and through it, rural income of the farmers and their social statuses. In this chapter, the authors have taken the Moroccan agriculture cooperatives as a case of cooperative longevity and survival in order to observe the evolution and processes of adaptation to the distinct economic, social, and environmental demands of a broad range of member-owners. The demands of the farming community, members, and society have resulted in social and environmental factors being as much a priority as economic aspects.

DOI: 10.4018/978-1-7998-5354-1.ch042

INTRODUCTION

Cooperative movement dates back to the end of the XIX century – the beginning of the XX century and covers over 700 million cooperatives worldwide. The homeland of cooperation is considered to be the UK. As early as 1761, sixteen weavers from East Ayrshire, Fenwick village created the Fenwick Weavers' Society, the first cooperative organization of the industrial age. In 1795, in the English village of Hull, local residents rebelled against high prices set by local millers and also cooperated to establish a fair price for the products which resulted in forming a consumer cooperative in Ayrshire in 1796.

In the mid-1990s, almost half of the world's population was provided with products and services of cooperative enterprises. According to the International Labor Organization (2007), in 47 countries, there were 330,000 agricultural cooperatives with a total number of individual members of 180 million people. Currently, almost 800 million people are the members of cooperatives, which is four times more than fifty years ago. Cooperatives provide about 100 million jobs worldwide, as well as various services to half of the world's population. International Co-operative Alliance established in 1895 to promote the cooperative model brings together 315 organizations from 110 countries (International Co-operative Alliance [ICA], n.d.).

In the EU, over 50% of agricultural products are grown, processed, and sold through cooperative marketing systems. European Community of Consumer Cooperatives (Euro Coop) brings together 2.5 million consumer cooperatives with a membership of more than 21 million people and 359 thousand employees. In the EU, agricultural cooperatives perform a large part of farming from almost full coverage (the Netherlands, Denmark, and Ireland) to 80% of agricultural organizations (France and Germany). In other EU countries, these figures are lower. In the countries with a high level of cooperation development, the total number of members in cooperative organizations significantly exceeds the number of farms since each farmer is usually a member of several cooperative societies.

Nowadays, the turnover of cooperative enterprises is $2.2 trillion. In Japan, over 90% of all farmers are the members of cooperatives. In Canada, 40% of the population are the members of at least one cooperative. In New Zealand, cooperatives are responsible for 95% of the dairy market. Romanian cooperatives keep the country's best resort facilities. Agricultural cooperatives in France have the second-largest system in the world of banking and credit institutions – Credit Agricole.

Based on the described background, this chapter considers conceptual framework for agricultural cooperatives in Morocco aimed at sustainable development of rural territories and gives some examples of such organizations.

BACKGROUND

Basic Definitions

Let us now consider some terms and definitions important for the sphere of agricultural cooperatives operation. According to the International Cooperative Alliance, a cooperative is an autonomous association of women and men, who unite voluntarily to meet their common economic, social and cultural needs and aspirations through a jointly-owned and democratically-controlled enterprise (ICA, n.d.).

A member of a cooperative is a person or a company who meets all the requirements of the current law and the organization's charter itself. Usually, cooperative member is an owner or a co-owner of a cooperative who economically contributes his capital through the purchase of a share. If everything is done according to the accepted procedure, the new member of the organization gets the right to vote.

Subsidiary liability of cooperative members is also an important term. In this case, the authors mean additional obligations that are not related to the standard list of requirements for a participant when making a contribution. Such additional responsibility may be relevant, for example, in a situation where creditors presented legal requirements to the cooperative, but the organization is not able to fulfill them in a timely manner. It is worth paying attention once again to the fact that both the size and the degree of subsidiary responsibility are determined by the charter of the structure and the legislation of this or that country.

An employee in such organizations should be understood as a person who is not a member of the organization and is employed in a certain type of activity through an employment contract.

It is also important to understand who an agricultural producer is. He is person who is engaged in the production of any product. The percentage of agricultural products from this category should be more than 50% of the total volume of products manufactured by a particular company.

A share contribution is a contribution made by a member of a cooperative to a mutual fund of an organization. This can be finance, land or any property, as well as property rights that have monetary value. There are both basic and additional shares.

Cooperative payments are payments to the participants of the organization according to the contribution and labor activity of each of them.

Johnson (2013) lists some other terms used in agricultural cooperatives studies, among which the following ones seems the most useful: agricultural co-operative – a co-operative involved in agro-allied activities; credit facilities – loanable funds provided by a financial intermediary used to enhance production activities; group farming – a system of collective agricultural practice by association of people with similar interest.

Types and Functions of Cooperatives and Supporting Organizations

Operation of agricultural cooperatives mainly provides food security in rural areas. Besides, they develop economic and social skills of people. A lot attention is now paid to the development of the territories, ecological production, and incorporating women into economic activities. The analysis of the publications and the activities of agricultural cooperatives in some countries let the authors outline the following main functions of cooperatives:

- Meeting needs and interests of the stakeholders
- Providing stakeholders with economic opportunities
- Supporting stakeholders with methods and technologies
- Providing credits for the development

cooperatives exist in some economic sectors and have corresponding variety of forms.

Agricultural production cooperatives have three main forms:

- **Agricultural Artel:** A cooperative aimed at production, selling or processing with personal participation in cooperative activities. The land of the cooperative members is also employed in its operation. Each member makes a share contribution, that is, donates money, land, or other property for public use to the cooperative.
- **Fishing Artel:** Association of fish farms operating in the same conditions as the agricultural artel.
- **Cooperative Farm:** An association established for tillage or production of livestock products. The difference from the artel is that land is not given to the mutual fund.

In all the cases, a cooperative must have at least 3-10 members (depending on the sector of the economy and the main operations and aims). Besides, generally, the number of employees of a cooperative shall not exceed the number of its members. Thus, the mandatory personal labor participation of the members is guaranteed.

Agricultural consumer cooperatives have other forms:

- **Processing Cooperatives:** Any production, including meat and dairy products.
- **Sales (Trade) Companies:** Not only the sales of products but also its packaging and storage.
- **Service Cooperatives:** Any activity related to the repair, tillage, plant protection, and even legal activity.
- **Supply Cooperatives:** Created for the joint procurement of feed, fertilizer and other goods to save money.
- Horticultural, vegetable gardening, and livestock cooperatives are created to provide services to various industries from sales to processing.

However, it should be mentioned, that the terminology differs throughout countries. For example, it is still difficult to distinguish Russian (Soviet) "kolkhoz", a production agricultural cooperative and a cooperative farm.

Agricultural cooperatives are not necessarily small organizations located in a village with an office in the basement, but also international producers and processors. Cooperatives, for example, are Valio from Finland, Fonterra from New Zealand, DMK from Germany, Dairy Farmers of America from the USA, and Friesland Campina from the Netherlands. All of them are in the TOP-20 of the largest dairy companies in the world, and the cooperative form of organization does not interfere with their development. Some of them have become powerful transnational associations with thousands of employees and billions of dollars of income. For example, the turnover of the world's largest South Korean cooperative NH Nonghyup reaches $63 billion.

In the case of the dairy industry, cooperatives can be successful producers because they are not aimed at making a profit for the organization itself. The main goal of Valio, for example, is the profit of the cooperative members, so the company is trying to keep the prices of raw milk attractive. The New Zealand Fonterra is forced to fight for raw materials which is gradually deprived of its monopoly. The high price of milk does not prevent them from competing and often contributes to modernization and innovation. In addition, the cooperative members themselves know that without successful processing there will be no demand for raw milk.

There are some organizations throughout the world which support agricultural cooperatives, such as the Food and Agriculture Organization of the United Nations (FAO), the International Fund for Agricultural Development (IFAD), and the World Food Programme (WFP), are working closely with agricultural cooperatives. Their main roles in supporting farmers organized in cooperatives are (Food and Agriculture Organization of the United Nations [FAO], International Fund for Agricultural Development [IFAD], & World Food Programme [WFP], 2012):

- Raising awareness of the role of agricultural cooperatives in reducing poverty and improving food security
- Assisting the development of agricultural cooperatives' capacities
- Supporting the development of enabling environments and better governance frameworks for agricultural cooperatives

MAIN FOCUS OF THE CHAPTER

Challenges Facing the Agricultural Cooperative Society

Among the challenges facing agricultural cooperatives are poor capitalization, corruption, illiteracy, poor inspection, and government interference (Johnson, 2013). Daman (2003) recognized internal and external factors that should be looked into in order to enhance the performance of the agricultural co-operatives.

Internal Factors

Internal factors examine the activities within the organization of the co-operative society. The areas of internal factors are focused on the inclusion of the following:

- Trained professional and motivated staff
- Dedication and selfless leadership
- Means of encouraging member's involvement and participation
- Comprehensive programs for member's education and information
- Provision for reasonable coverage of risk for loss of deposits
- Value-added activities through the use of advanced technologies

Onyima and Okoro (2009) underline the role of the cooperative member, claiming that they are the foundation of the co-operative, their support through patronage and capital investment keeps it economically healthy and their changing requirements shape the co-operatives' future. They also stated that the most important obligation of co-operative members is participation in its managing which in practice means to be kept informed about the co-operative activities, attend co-operative meetings and take their turns at the committee.

External Factors

External factors refer to the actions and decision of the agents, organizations, groups, and institution other than the co-operative society which have influence on the performance of the co-operative society (Johnson, 2013). Among the external actors, the following ones should be mentioned:

- Government support
- Market reforms
- Agriculture growth rate
- Availability of basic infrastructure
- Regulatory and development agencies and institutions

Agricultural Cooperatives in Various Countries

With the purpose to understand the overall situation with agricultural cooperatives, the authors have analyzed a number of papers devoted to rural cooperatives in various countries.

Russia

In Russia, the cooperative movement has been developing slowly. Consumer agricultural cooperatives can only be non-commercial. In this form, however, consumer cooperatives greatly helped agriculture in the late 1980s. In 1990, in the Russian Soviet Republic, consumer cooperation served 40% of the population (a quarter of retail turnover, as well as 50% of potato production and around 30% of vegetables and bread baking) and 30 million rural residents were the members of cooperatives. Then, during the 1990s, the value of cooperation in agriculture decreased rapidly.

Italy

In Italy, cooperatives have been developed both quantitatively and qualitatively. Due to the lack of common actions and objectives, their heterogeneity, and different level of economic development of northern and southern parts of the country, two opposing trends have emerged, namely, socialist, or "red" cooperatives, and Catholic, or "white" cooperatives. The predominant type was still large consumer cooperatives in urban centers, although they also operated in rural areas. In 1913, Istituto Nazionale di Credito della Cooperazione was established with the aim of funding cooperatives. Cooperatives were provided with an access to initial credit to carry out their investment activities. At the beginning of the First World War, Italian cooperatives had already acquired the features of a mass movement, even with insufficient organization. Despite the fact that many cooperatives disappeared during the war, this form of association was stronger than before, as it proved to be effective in adverse conditions. Cooperatives have become a key element in the economic restructuring of the country. In less than two years, the number of production cooperatives doubled, consumption rates remained unchanged. The loans were used to stimulate export of agricultural products and construction of agro-industrial processing plants.

Denmark

In Denmark, cooperation developed in the last two decades of the XIX century and was closely related to processing in the field of livestock. The first dairy cooperative center in Denmark was founded by the initiative of local farmers in 1882. Such cooperatives spread throughout the country. By 1888, 244 cooperatives had been established, and after a while one-third of Danish livestock farms delivered their milk to the cooperative center. Soon after, dairy cooperatives were able to compete in the butter market by moving to processing (Just, 1990; Serdyukova & Nikolaeva, 2017).

Nigeria

In the effort to improve the agricultural sector in Nigeria, the government embarked on various programs some of which were listed by Iwuchukwu and Igbokwe (2012): National Economic Empowerment and Development Strategy (NEEDS) – 1999, National Special Program of Food Security (NSPFS) – 2002, and the Root and Tuber Expansion Program (RTEP) – 2003. However, the growth rate of Nigeria's population of about 144 million at 3.2% per year, which is predicted to be doubled in less than 25 years, is a challenge in a country where more than 90% of the agricultural output is accounted for by small-scale farmers.

Japan

Japan is often considered as a country where cooperation has actually become a cult and is supported at all levels, mostly, by the state. Farmers cooperatives sell about 90% of all agricultural products (almost 100% of grain, 95% of potatoes, vegetables, fruit, and milk, 85-90% of pork, eggs, and poultry). The country has created a centralized system that protects producers from monopolistic capital. At the same time, the volume of farms that are not members of cooperatives is not more than one hectare.

One of the most striking examples of Japanese cooperation is ZEN-NOH or the National Federation of Agricultural Cooperatives of Japan. Founded in 1972 in Tokyo, the Federation is one of the most influential structures in the country. The organization has about 1,200 cooperative unions, serving about 4.78 million members and 4.8 million associate members. These cooperatives cover almost all segments of agriculture – from rice production to the construction of powerful logistics centers and international trading. The cooperative consists of nine logistics centers, markets and retail outlets, and the bank. The number of employees of the Corporation is more than 8000 people around the world (Serdyukova & Nikolaeva, 2017).

USA

The USA has become a major driver for the development of cooperation in times of crisis. Farmers' associations became the most popular during the great depression. It was this time when a powerful business giant cooperative CHS started developing. Currently, there are three thousand farm cooperatives in the USA. There are four types of agricultural associations: sales, transactions, provision of farms, and provision of credit cooperatives. The CHS cooperative is often referred as a state within a state. Established in 1929, it still remains one of the most interesting business structures in the USA. All its members, more than 1,100 cooperatives and 75,000 farmers, as well as 20,000 preferred shareholders, are free to use mineral fertilizers and fuel and have access to technology and insurance of their own risks.

Spain

In Spain, cooperatives cover only 15% of the population employed in agriculture. Most of them are based on regional legislation. At the same time, the associations are small – only one-third of local cooperatives have more than 1,000 members. There are also local cooperatives that serve their members only and large cooperatives that process products and sell them to retailers. Cooperation is characterized by the consolidation and absorption. One of the largest business groups in Spain is Mondragon which combines different types of cooperatives with powerful production subsidiaries. The Mondragon Corporation incorporates 261 organizations, including 104 cooperatives, 125 communities and branches, 8 funds, a foundation of mutual insurance, and 13 risk hedging companies. The company employs 74,000 workers. Corporate offices are located in 41 countries, the sales are carried out in 150 countries (ICA, n.d.).

Agriculture in Morocco

In Morocco, 44.6% of the population in working age is employed in agriculture covering 17.1% of the GDP (in 2010). The share of agricultural products in exports is 25%. In the agricultural production of the country, the weather factor remains a main one, therefore, irrigation is used (1.44 million hectares). Cereals, legumes, and sugar beets occupy 80% of the cultivated land. In terms of the output, the main products are wheat (3.0 million tons), tomatoes (1.2 million tons), and potatoes (1.4 million tons).

Since the 1960, a program for the construction of reservoirs and the development of water resources has allowed to provide drinking water to the population as well as agriculture and other sectors of the economy while maintaining the water resources of the country.

Meanwhile, Morocco is still an agrarian country. Despite the establishment and development of the irrigation system, weather conditions remain a decisive factor in Morocco's agricultural production. There is little use of agricultural machinery on small farms, and the output is consumed mainly by the producers themselves. The average land plot does not exceed five hectares. Many of local farmers do not have their own land and are forced to hire agricultural workers or become sharecroppers. At the other pole is the modern agricultural sector with its large and modern farms producing commercial products. The area of only 1% of agricultural enterprises is equal to or exceeds 50 hectares of land, but they provide 80% of export and 25% of all agricultural output of the country.

In 1969-1982, as the needs of the urban population in bakery products and dairy products increased, the volume of food imports increased by eight times. During the same period, exports of crops, especially citrus, tomatoes, and early vegetables, doubled. Despite the fact that in 1981-1992, the total volume of agricultural production doubled, its share in the GDP has steadily decreased. In 1991-1993, unfavorable weather conditions adversely affected the yield of grain crops. The worst indicators were observed in 1980-1988 when drought raged in Morocco. Four-fifths of the acreage is wheat, barley, legumes, and sugar beets. It was only in the 1980s that the agro-industrial sector turned to large-scale production of chicken meat and eggs. Cattle breeding has become intensive.

Fishing

Morocco's coastal waters are rich in fish resources. The country occupies a leading place in Africa for catching sardines, octopuses, and tuna. The largest fishing ports are Agadir, Tantan, and Safi. Three-quarters of the catch is sardines which are canned and exported. Since the mid-1980s, when the government began to provide significant subsidies for the development of the industry, national fisheries have reached new frontiers. In 1992, the catch in coastal waters amounted to 421 thousand tons, while in the open sea – 125 thousand tons.

Forestry

During the XX century, Morocco lost 70% of its forests. In 1914, the country had 14 million hectares of forest land, by now, its area has reduced to only 4 million hectares. Forests cover about 9% of the territory of the country. Morocco annually destroys 30 thousand hectares of forests and, although new plantations are carried out on the area of 45 thousand hectares, only 40-50% of seedlings are established.

In 1990, the production of wood amounted to 2.1 million m^3. Oak and Atlantic cedar which wood is used for decorative purposes and various crafts grow in the timber forests of the Middle Atlas region and the Rif Mountains. Cork oak forests in Garba area are the sources of commercial cork. The rest of the wood is used for the production of charcoal which is widely used in the Middle Atlas and the Reef Mountains in cooking. In the southern provinces of the country, this activity is closely related to adverse climatic conditions. Due to the nomadic life of the local population, the main agricultural activity is breeding of cattle, especially one-humped camels.

Traditional Agriculture

Morocco's traditional agriculture employs about a half of the country's population in working age which handles 70% of the country's arable land. The main production crops are citrus, olives, cereals, sugar cane, grapes, vegetables, and fruit. In addition, due to the ever-changing amount of precipitation, the area of cultivated land changes from year to year. Naturally, under such conditions, the main consumers of the products are mainly the producers. Besides, there are different farm pests in Morocco which are also infection carriers. Particularly, the raids of the locust called "cotton flea hopper" cause significant damage to agriculture.

Morocco is one of the countries that has paid attention to the agricultural cooperative associations from issuing the agrarian reform law. The laws emphasized the need for collaborative work in agriculture and the establishment of farming cooperative societies which practiced various agricultural economic activities in terms of agricultural production, agricultural equipment, credit and cooperative marketing, farm mechanization services, and others.

From a local point of view, these organizations have managed to consolidate the supply thanks to the economic and social benefits growers derive from belonging to these associations. Cooperatives show greater concern for keeping and satisfying the growers, via market prices, allowing their economic sustainability and maintaining an equity income.

As far as eco-social aspects are concerned, cooperatives have made substantial efforts as a driver adaptation to demand could not have been implemented so swiftly without the presence of these of innovation in the production and commercial sector and the improvements to production and organizations. At the same time, they play a role in the transmission of social responsibility and awareness for efficient use of natural resources to the various generations.

The longevity and survival of the cooperatives are linked to their constant and rapid adaptation to crises in which the sector finds itself or to the challenges it faces.

The Green Morocco Plan

One of the conditions for improving the efficiency of small businesses development is favorable investment climate which is measured by not only preferential tax policy but also the creation of economic conditions through a combination of many factors that ensure profitability of a company.

The Green Morocco Plan agricultural strategy launched in 2008 was designed to make agriculture the main growth engine of the national economy over the next ten to fifteen years with significant benefits in terms of GDP growth, job creation, exports, and poverty mitigation (FAO, IFAD, & WFP, 2012; Saidi & Diouri, 2017).

The Green Morocco Plan aims at developing a pluralistic agriculture that is open to foreign markets, locally diversified and especially sustainable. The strategy concerns a sector which contributes 19% of the GNP, with 15% from agriculture and 4% from agro-industry. This sector employs more than 4 million rural inhabitants and has created approximately 100,000 jobs in agriculture. This sector plays a substantial role in the macroeconomic balance of the country. It also plays an important social role as 80% of the 14 million rural inhabitants depend on revenues from agricultural production. Besides, it is important to remember that the sector is directly responsible for ensurance of food security of 30 million consumers. This reaffirms the critical role that agriculture plays in the economic and social stability of Morocco.

The Moroccan strategy has planned, for the accomplishment of its objectives, the conservation of natural resources in view of ensuring sustainable agriculture through the following steps:

- Integration of "Climatic Changes" dimension in the conception of the Green Morocco Plan;
- Conversion of nearly a million hectares from cereal crops to fruit tree plantations, which will help protect agricultural spaces;
- Experimental use of semi-desert zones to increase the usable agricultural surface area;
- Support for the water conservation irrigation systems (from the current 154,000 ha to 692,000 ha);
- Support for the use of renewable energies in agriculture (solar and wind energy, biofuels) (Sayouti & El Mekki, 2015; Oulhaj, 2013).

The implementation of the Green Morocco Plan necessitates the restructuring of the Ministry of Agriculture and Maritime Fisheries with the objective of reorganizing the resources to align itself with a new wave of changes created by the arrival of private actors; refocusing of regulatory functions; increased transfer of functional operations towards private sector; and establishment of two new entities, the Agency for Agricultural Development (ADA) and the National Office for Food Safety (ONSSA), capable of attracting growth potential and of playing the role of renewal and leadership.

The Green Morocco plan makes Morocco increasingly dependent on the world market either to export its agricultural products (tomatoes and citrus in particular) or to import its needs for cereals. Under this policy, cereal imports increased, without being covered by an adequate food export increase. In order to cope with this deterioration, we believe that grain crops must be encouraged to ensure food security, given their high share in the diet of a growing population. In order to rationalize water consumption and combat degradation of natural resources, ecological and biological practices should be adopted. As for fruit growing, GMP should encourage it on lands that are not suitable for cereals, such as mountains, hills and rugged terrains. In general, Morocco should encourage practices that locally and sustainably ensure the availability of basic foodstuffs for its population. Its food policy should also aim at increasing fish consumption, from 12 kg per capita per year to a global average exceeding 20 kg.

SOLUTIONS AND RECOMMENDATIONS

Taaricht Family Farm, Afourer

The farm with 15-year history of producing Extra Virgin Olive Oil and organic oranges. The aim of the farm is not quantity but quality. The farmers, preserving the family traditions, produce the finest Biological Extra Virgin Olive Oil from both black and green organic olives. The production of olive oil has basically not changed for the last years. The olives get picked before their ripeness. This olive juice is extracted in a traditional way of a cold spin process without use of solvents or refining methods. This preserves all the valuable ingredients of the ripe olives. After washing, the olives are mashed into a paste with a simple mortar and pestle. Extra virgin olive oil is the highest grade of virgin oil derived by cold mechanical extraction without use of solvents or refining methods. This preserves all the valuable ingredients of the ripe olives, which are crucial for the taste, smell, color and also the vitamin content of the oil. Depending on the variety, you need about 5-10 kilograms of olives for one liter of olive oil. On average, 50-70 kg of olives are harvested from an olive tree. A single tree, therefore, produces about 5-10 liters of oil per year.

In addition to producing Extra Virgin Olive Oil, they also produce organic oranges. The oranges are also grown without the usage of any herbicides or pesticides. The oranges of the farm are cultivated on the family's own plantation. Moreover, the magic about these oranges is that in this moment they are still hanging on their trees in the gardens and are only picked.

This family farm is an ecological and sustainable farm at the beginning of its way.

The Taymate Agricultural Cooperative

The cooperative was created in March 2008, comprising 16 members, unemployed young people, and women with technical and vocational skills. Its members have created a legal framework (cooperative) which enables them to exploit their skills in order to develop economic activities and thus improve their living conditions and that of their families, and thus to form a cooperative more competitive insertion in the markets. The aims of the cooperative are the following: participation in the socio-economic development of the region; involvement of marginalized groups (women and young people in situations of poverty and precariousness) in the development process; valorization of local natural resources (olive trees, olive production); creation of income-generating activities for beneficiaries and their Families; workplaces creation.

The Taymate cooperative considers that the realization of a socio-economic development program is imperative, as long as the members of the Taymate cooperative are a reliable tool to be involved as partners and not as mere beneficiaries in sustainable development while considering the social and economic gap existing between the different categories of society. The program in question will be initiated by the financing of projects whose objective is the valorization of local agricultural products.

Agricultural activities, including livestock, constitute the bulk of the economic activity of the rural community of Timoulilt; olives are among the main crops, and as a first experience, members of the Taymate cooperative worked on the transformation and marketing of green and black olives during the 2008-2009 seasons (exploitation of local potentialities).

For green olives, the test was carried out on 400 kg in 2008 and 1,000 kg in 2009 of olives which were processed in a traditional way (crushed with a flat stone) and immersed in clear water for two months to give them a very sweet taste, subsequently coated with rock salt and sold in bulk on the market of Beni-Mellal (town at 18 km from Timoulilt), this action took place in kitchen space of the local Timoulilt association for the development which has been loaned free of charge to the cooperative Taymate.

For black olives, the work was done on 1,200 kg in 2008 and 3,000 kg in 2009, purchased from the cooperative members' families, the black olives were first sorted and treated with rock salt in the house of one of the members, where once a week a group of three to four people comes back to the pile for three months, once the margins are extracted totally their taste becomes soft, then the olives are washed and mixed with a small amount of table oil. Some of the production was sold in bulk to a wholesaler in Beni-Mellal, the remainder is sold for sale in the association's premises (ATD) in 1 kg or 1/2 kg.

Women Agricultural Cooperative Toudarte, Agadir, Souss-Massa-Draa

The Toudarte (which means "life" in Berber) was founded in 2004. It specializes in the production of high-quality argan oil for cosmetic and culinary use. It is located in the center of the argan forest in the region Imsouane at 85 km of Agadir and 85 km from Essaouira. Its objectives include improvement of the socio-economic situation of rural women in Imsouane commune and promotion of their involvement in the sustainable development of their country. Currently, the cooperative is one of the biggest and most successful suppliers of argan oil in the region. The activities include production, packaging, and marketing of argan oil and its derivatives; analyzing international markets for the marketing of the products of the cooperative; production of almond oil, amlou, honey, and hammam products (shampoo, douche gel, and soap).

Employment in the co-operatives provides women with the income, which many have used to fund education for themselves or their children. It has also provided them with a degree of autonomy in a traditionally male-dominated society and has helped many become more aware of their rights. Much of the argan oil produced today is made by a number of women's co-operatives. Co-sponsored by the Social Development Agency with the support of the EU, the Union of Women Cooperatives of the Arganeraie is the largest union of argan oil co-operatives in Morocco. It comprises 22 cooperatives that are found in other parts of the region.

In Toudarte cooperative, women are given opportunities to succeed and to introduce their traditions to the rest of the world through their argan oil. It seemed almost too good to be true that in a developing country, women were forging ahead and providing for their families comfortably and with pride. The main purpose is to improve the socio-economic situation of rural women in Imsouane commune and promote their involvement in the sustainable development of their country. Cooperative Toudarte produces authentic, biological argan oil of the highest quality. More than 100 Berber women participate in the corporation, providing them a steady income, literacy classes, medical care, and an important role in local society. The production of high-quality argan oil provides them an income that is 20% above minimum wages. In addition, the cooperative takes care of literacy classes, medical care, childcare, and interest-free microcredits. Through partnerships in corporations like Cooperative Toudarte, women have paid jobs and they reach a higher social status. Women are encouraged to study and get education. More importantly, women are aware of the power of education. They can encourage their school-age daughters and help them with their homework. Illiteracy is still rife among rural women in Morocco. In a bid to improve both the economic and educational status of Berber women, a percentage of the profits made by these co-operatives is invested in the rural community. Women working in Argan co-operatives are offered free afternoon classes in literacy skills and hygienic practices.

Cooperative Toudarte is not a project just to earn money but also a place where the adherents meet to discuss different daily life matters and benefit from illiteracy classes. Moreover, it is also a place where children have support lessons. It also organizes professional trainings in cooperative management and offers different aids to the adherents in need.

Cooperative Toudarte is very important for the village Akhsmou. The production of argan oil brings new economic activities in the area where there almost no any jobs opportunities. The cooperative has become the central meeting point for approximately thousand people in 10-15 villages in the Imsouane region. The compound of the cooperative has a children playground, a crèche, a small shop, and a mosque for women.

The success of the argan co-operatives has also encouraged other producers of agricultural products to adopt the cooperative model. The establishment of the cooperatives has been aided by support from within Morocco, notably the Foundation Mohamed VI.

Multidisciplinary Social and Cultural Center in Aghenbo Village

The center is located in Atlas Mountains, about 120 km from Azilal city. It is a new one and thanks to Taghlast association gets the funds from Joud foundation. The aim of the project is to stop the migration of people from the area to big cities. Lots of people from Aghenbo village migrate to big cities because people in this area are unemployed young people and women. Although the poverty-stricken areas are spacious and bucolic, some of the land is simply not suited for crop growing.

The Association Taghlast for development, cooperation, and environmental protection decided to build a multidisciplinary social and cultural center in Aghenbo village, in high Atlas Mountains in the center of Morocco.

A lot of services and events will be provided in this center:

- A workshop for women cooperative who make traditional carpets and are engaged in knitting and weaving;
- Library for children;
- Information and internet hall;
- Meeting hall;
- educational and recreation areas for pupils.

This center is expected to give opportunities to people who live in Aghenbo village, especially women. There is a hope that people will stay in their area and will not think to immigrate to big cities.

FUTURE RESEARCH DIRECTIONS

While the authors attempted considering conceptual framework for agricultural cooperatives in various countries with a special focus on Morocco, further research is required to study country-specific experiences of cooperation in agriculture, specifically, with an aim to reveal the effects of cooperative movement on ensuring sustainable development of rural territories, improvement of farming practices, increase of agricultural production, and, ultimately, establishing food security.

CONCLUSION

This chapter examines the contributions of cooperatives towards agricultural development in Morocco. It has been shown that cooperatives boost opportunities for Moroccans by the improvement of their social and economic conditions and by creating jobs and generating income, making people more aware of their rights, the reforestation of argan forests with the support of the women's cooperatives, and the promotion of regional tourism.

Some of the above-described cases were presented at INNOSIB forums – 2017 and 2018 in Omsk, Russia and were considered very useful and of great interest for other countries. The forums are for businesses and social entrepreneurs and are aimed at sharing best practices in social-entrepreneurial sphere.

REFERENCES

Daman, P. (2003). *Rural Women, Food Security and Agricultural Cooperatives.* New Delhi: Rural Development and Management Centre.

Food and Agriculture Organization of the United Nations. International Fund for Agricultural Development, & World Food Programme. (2012). *Agricultural Cooperatives: Paving the Way for Food Security and Rural Development.* Retrieved from http://www.fao.org/3/ap088e/ap088e00.pdf

International Co-operative Alliance. (n.d.). *Statistical Information on the Cooperative Movement.* Retrieved from https://www.ica.coop/en/about-us/international-cooperative-alliance

International Labor Association. (2007). *COOP Fact Sheet #1. Cooperatives and Rural Employment.* Geneva: International Labor Association.

Iwuchukwu, J. C., & Igbokwe, E. M. (2012). Lessons from Agricultural Policies and Programmes in Nigeria. *Journal of Law. Policy and Globalisation, 5*, 11–21.

Johnson, D. S. (2013). *Contributions of Co-operative to Agricultural Development: A Study of Agricultural Co-operatives in Awka North Local Government Area.* Nnamdi Azikiwe University.

Just, F. (1990). Butter, Bacon and Organisational Power in Danish Agriculture. In F. Just (Ed.), *Co-operatives and Farmers' Unions in Western Europe – Collaboration and Tension* (pp. 137–156). Esbjerg: South Jutland University Press.

Onyima, J.K.C., & Okoro, C.N. (2009). *Co-operatives: Elements, Principles and Practices.* Awka: Maxiprint.

Oulhaj, L. (2013). *Evaluation of the Agricultural Strategy of Morocco (Green Morocco Plan) with a Dynamic General Equilibrium Model.* Marseille: Femise Research Programme.

Saidi, A., & Diouri, M. (2017). Food Self-Sufficiency Under the Green-Morocco Plan. *Journal of Experimental Biology and Agricultural Sciences, 5*(Spl-1- SAFSAW), 33–40. doi:10.18006/2017.5(Spl-1-SAFSAW).S33.S40

Sayouti, N. S., & El Mekki, A. A. (2015). Le Plan Maroc Vert et l'autosuffisance alimentaire en produits de base à l'horizon 2020. *Alternatives Rurales*, *3*(1), 78–90.

Serdyukova, M., & Nikolaeva, E. (2017). Development of Agricultural Cooperation and Small Forms of Economic Activities in Foreign Countries. *Bulletin of Chelyabinsk State University. Economic Sciences*, *406*(10), 147–155.

ADDITIONAL READING

Bailey, K. G. (1988). *The Principles of Co-operation and an Outline of Agricultural Cooperative Development*. London: Food from Britain.

Belo Moreira, M. (1984). *L'economie et la production laitiere au Portugal*. Grenoble: University of Grenoble.

Bjorn, C. (1988). *Co-operation in Denmark*. Copenhagen: Danske Andelsselskaber.

Dedieu, M.-S., & Courleux, F. (2011). *Agricultural Cooperatives: The Reference in Term of Farmer Economic Organization*. Centre for Studies and Strategic Foresight.

Ferreira da Costa, F. (1980). Etude bibliographique de la cooperation au Portugal. *Revue des Estudes Cooperatives*, 1-29.

Henriques, M. A., & Reis, J. (1993). *Heterogeneidad estructural de la agricultura portuguesa y deficit neo-corporativista. Las organizaciones profesionales agrarias en la CEE*. Madrid: MAPA.

International Labor Association. (2002). *ILO Recommendation on the Promotion of Cooperatives*. Geneva: International Labor Association.

Knapp, J. G. (1965). *An Analysis of Agricultural Co-operation in England*. London: Agricultural and Central Co-operative Association.

Moyano, E. (1988). *Sindicalismo y politica agraria en Europa*. Madrid: MAPA.

Moyano, E. (1993). *Accion colectiva y cooperativismo en la agricultura europea*. Madrid: MAPA.

Ogunnaike, O. O., & Ogbari, M. (2007). Analysis of the Effectiveness of Co-operative Society as a Tool for Satisfying Human Needs. *Nigerian Journal of Co-operative Economics and Management*, *1*(1), 11–15.

Okechukwu, E. (2006). *Manual for Co-operative Professional. Nkpor*. Optimal Press Ltd.

Tortia, E., Valentinov, V., & Iliopoulos, C. (2013). Agricultural Cooperatives. *Journal of Entrepreneurial and Organizational Diversity*, *2*(1), 23–36.

Volobueva, T. (2013). *Development of Small Economic Entities in Agriculture. Orel*. Orel State Agrarian University.

KEY TERMS AND DEFINITIONS

Agricultural Cooperative: A co-operative involved in agro-allied activities.

Cooperative: An autonomous association of women and men, who unite voluntarily to meet their common economic, social and cultural needs and aspirations through a jointly-owned and democratically-controlled enterprise.

Cooperative Payments: The payments to the participants of the organization according to the contribution and labor activity of each of them.

Credit Facilities: Loanable funds provided by a financial intermediary used to enhance production activities.

Group Farming: A system of collective agricultural practice by association of people with similar interest.

Member of a Cooperative: A person or a company who meets all the requirements of the law and the organization's charter itself; an owner or a co-owner of a cooperative who economically contributes his capital through the purchase of a share.

Share Contribution: A contribution made by a member of a cooperative to a mutual fund of an organization (finance, land, property, or property rights that have monetary value).

This research was previously published in the Handbook of Research on Globalized Agricultural Trade and New Challenges for Food Security edited by Vasilii Erokhin and Tianming Gao; pages 465-480, copyright year 2020 by Engineering Science Reference (an imprint of IGI Global).

Chapter 43
Towards the Development of Salt–Tolerant Potato

John Okoth Omondi
Ben Gurion University of the Negev, Israel

ABSTRACT

Soil salinity is a major constrain to crop production and climate change accelerates it. It reduces plant water potential, causes ion imbalance, reduce plant growth and productivity, and eventually leads to death of the plant. This is the case in potato. However, potato has coping strategies such as accumulation of proline, an osmoregulator and osmoprotector. In addition, leaching of salts below the root zone is preferred, exogenous application of ascorbic acid and growth hormones are practiced to combat salinity. Breeding and genetic engineering also play key roles in salinity management of potato. Varieties such as: Amisk, BelRus, Bintje, Onaway, Sierra, and Tobique were tolerant in North America, variety Cara in Egypt, Sumi in Korea and varieties Vivaldi and Almera in Mediterranean region. Transgenic lines of Kennebec variety, lines S2 and M48 also proved tolerance due to transcription factor MYB4 encoded by rice Osmyb4 gene.

CLIMATE CHANGE AND SALINITY

Climate change is observed and predicted as the single-most event that is changing and will continue to change the cause of the world's future. It is a major challenge to agriculture. As the climate 'forcing mechanisms' shape climate through processes such as: variation in solar radiation, continental drifts and changes in greenhouse gas concentration, they encourage increase in global temperatures, melting of ice-caps, rising ocean levels, unpredictable and variable amount of rainfall, more cyclones and heat waves, and increased desertification (Abumhadi et al., 2012). There are projections of increase in precipitation in winters and overall decrease in the tropics and sub-tropics (IPCC, 2007). A decrease in precipitation means a decrease in water availability and increase in evaporative demand due to rising temperatures (Vicente-Serrano et al., 2014; Wang et al., 2012). Increase in temperatures enhance evapotranspiration especially in arid and semi-arid regions. In the event that evapotranspiration exceeds precipitation, salts

DOI: 10.4018/978-1-7998-5354-1.ch043

accumulate on the soil surface (Sivakumar, 2007). This has an implication on irrigation requirement (Doll & Siebert, 2002). The decrease in precipitation causes demand for more irrigation (McDonald & Girvetz, 2013; Riediger et al., 2014) even though, in arid and semi-arid regions water available for irrigation is saline (Levy et al., 2013). This consequently exacerbates soil salinity. Additionally, a rise in sea-level due to global warming threatens low-lying coastal agricultural lands – this rise leads to flooding by oceans' saline water and salinization of groundwater (Gornall et al., 2010). Grenfell et al., (2016) predicts that 125 to 175 years from 2010 more wetlands will experience frequent flooding with saltwater. Flooding of the coastal area with saline water has a far-reaching impact. Indeed, this salt incursion reduces dissolved organic carbon in the coastal wetlands from 40 mg l^{-1} to 18 mg l^{-1} (Ardón et al., 2016). Furthermore, increased salinity in the coastal wetlands will cause accumulation of less stable carbon (Williams & Rosenheim, 2015), reduction in marsh biodiversity, and lead to development of more salt tolerant plant communities (Grenfell et al., 2016).

SOIL SALINITY

Salinity is a phenomenon that is causing major havoc in agricultural production (Figure 1) (D'Odorico et al., 2013). The earliest salinity effect in agriculture was recorded around 2400 to 1700 BC in the ancient Mesopotamia, currently Southern Iraq (Jacobsen & Adams, 1958). 6% of arable land around the world is affected by salinity or sodicity, this is 800 million hectares (FAO, 2009). Salt-affected soils have high levels of dissolved salts and or high concentrations of adsorbed sodium ions (Yadav et al., 2011). These soils are categorized into three classes: First are the saline soils having an electrical conductivity (EC) of over 4 dS m^{-1} and sodium adsorption ratio (SAR) of less than 13 or exchangeable sodium percentage (ESP) that is below 15. The second category are sodic soils which are characterized by an EC of less than 4 dS m^{-1}, SAR or ESP above 13 and 15 respectively. Finally, the saline-sodic soils, whose EC, SAR, or ESP are above 4 dS m^{-1}, 13 and 15 accordingly (United States Salinity Laboratory, 1954).

Figure 1. Global distribution of saline soils using data from the Harmonized World Soil Database. Salinity on the map is represented by electrical conductivity (dS m^{-1}) and the coloring schemes illustrate different ranges in soil salinity corresponding to the relative degree to which soil salinity constrains plant productivity
Source: D'Odorico et al., (2013)

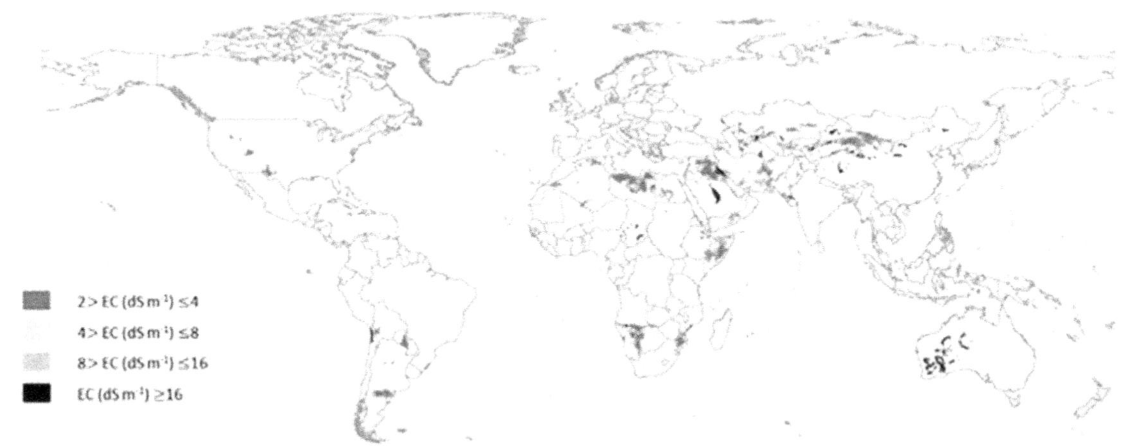

Soil salinity formation is classified into three categories (Rengasamy, 2006). The first is: groundwater associated salinity (GAS), this is prone in areas with shallow groundwater. In fact, groundwater salinity decreases with increasing groundwater depth, and as such in North-western China as an example, 2.5 m is critical (Abliz et al., 2016), although, it varies from region to region. Salts dissolved in groundwater are brought to the rhizosphere through evaporation. This is worsened by rising global temperature as it increase evaporative demand, consequently encouraging exit of salts from groundwater and their accumulation on the root-zone (Li et al., 2015). Besides, some plants have the ability to exclude salts during nutrient absorption, thus enhancing their accumulation on the root-zone (Moya et al., 2003). In other regions such as the Nile Delta, accumulation of salts on the soil surface is a factor of groundwater and rise of 3 cm year^{-1} in sea-level (Geriesh et al., 2015). This movement of salts to the soil surface is richly influenced by soil hydraulic properties (Bejat et al., 2000) and climatic conditions (Rengasamy, 2006). The second is: non-groundwater-associated salinity (NAS). Some regions have deep water table and poor drainage causing accumulation of salts on the soil solum. In addition, salts are introduced by rain, weathering, and aeolian deposits. Salt accumulation through these processes are enhanced by poor hydraulic properties of the soil. The third category is: Irrigation associated salinity (IAS). Rengasamy (2006) describes this as the salts introduced by irrigation water stored within the root zone due to insufficient leaching. The author further explains that poor quality irrigation water, low hydraulic conductivity of the soil, and high evaporative demand accelerate these conditions.

Climate change causes intense, low amount and variable pattern of precipitation (Arnell, 1999; Trenberth, 2011) creating a demand for irrigation. However, as the world population soars, there is increased demand and pressure on fresh water reducing its availability (Fischer & Heilig, 1997; Hanjra & Qureshi, 2010; WWAP, 2015). Consequently, this leads to irrigation with poor quality water, highly saline, and reduction in leaching fraction, and thus accelerating the soil salinity problem (Kitamura et al., 2006).

Salinity's negative impact is grave and cannot be underestimated. It first reduces water potential (Aziz and Khan, 2001; Romero-Aranda et al., 2001), causes ion imbalance, reduction in plant growth and productivity, and eventually death of the whole-plant (Bernstein, 1975; Parida and Das, 2005). The effect on plant growth and physiological processes is exhibited by: reduction in leaf expansion, decrease in soluble protein contents (Muthukumarasamy et al., 2000; Wang and NII, 2000), photosynthesis (Allakhverdiev et al., 2002; Khavari-Nejad & Chaparzadeh, 1998), and lipid metabolism (Hassanein, 1999), and stunted growth (Takemura et al., 2000) as the stress intensifies.

SALINITY EFFECT ON POTATO

In potato, salinity delays shoot emergence and development (Levy, 1992; Levy et al., 1993). It further decreases growth with an early indication of leaf necrosis, lowers water and osmotic potential of leaves and tubers (Gao et al., 2015; Heuer and Nadler, 1998; Levy et al., 1988) and increases sodium concentration in the roots (Prasad & Potluri, 1996) and total soluble solids (Levy et al., 1988). Finally, it decreases tuber yield (Bustan et al., 2004; Levy, 1992). Levy, (1992) observed 21 – 59% decrease in tuber yield on irrigation with saline water and different varietal response to salinity (Table 1). Decreases in tuber yield of 33.7% and 79.3% on treating plants with 1.6 dS m^{-1} and 4.8 dS m^{-1} were also reported in Korea among four varieties (Kim et al., 2013). Salinity also delays tuberization, this was proven by in vitro studies. Microtuberization was delayed by 5 to 10 days in 20 and 40 mmol NaCl and inhibited completely in 80 mmol NaCl (Zhang et al., 2005). Earlier in 2001, Silva et al. (2001) observed similar results under 100 mmol l^{-1} NaCl.

Table 1. The effect of salinity on plant height, haulm, and tuber growth of four potato cultivars

Water Source	Soil Depth (cm)	EC (dS m⁻¹) at 136 DAP	Cultivar	Plant Height (cm±S.E.)	Haulm Weight (g m⁻¹±S.E.)	Tuber Weight (g m⁻¹±S.E.)
NC	0-20	1.7±0.2	Atica	42±1.2	3962±324	1975±188
	20-60	1.8±0.4	Desiree	50±1.4	4638±140	1475±0
			Cara	45±0.5	4412±429	782±32
			Alpha	42±1.0	4475±243	1175±150
NCS	0-20	4.2±0.7	Atica	37±0.9	2500±173	1863±238
	20-60	3.8±0.8	Desiree	33±1.9	4038±305	1000±75
			Cara	37±1.1	3175±304	438±138
			Alpha	33±1.8	3350±233	638±63
S	0-20	7.3±1.0	Atica	31±1.7	1825±138	925±125
	20-60	5.1±0.6	Desiree	25±0.8	2538±184	-
			Cara	32±1.4	2225±229	213±88
			Alpha	29±1.6	2500±248	294±144

NC is common irrigation water, NCS is a mixture of common irrigation water (NC) and saline water from a local well, S is saline water from the local well, DAP is days after planting. Electrical conductivity (EC) is of the extract of saturated soil samples from root zone of potato irrigated with NC, NCS, and S.

Source: Levy, (1992)

Increasing salt concentrations alters potato physiology through decrease in number of chloroplasts and cell intercellular spaces, thickening of cell walls, rapture and complete damage to mesophyll cells and chloroplasts (Gao et al., 2015). Teixeira and Fidalgo, (2009) reported increased ammonium assimilation in potato roots and decrease in the leaves due to increased accumulation of glutamate synthetize in a salinity event (Figure 2). Although, previously, Teixeira and Pereira, (2007) observed decrease of glutamate synthetize activity in leaves and roots. In addition to the aforementioned damages, salinity predisposes potato to diseases such as: verticillium wilt, early blight (Kaufman et al., 1990; Nachmias et al., 1993), and browning of the tubers (Dzengeleski et al., 2003; Kirk et al., 2006).

Figure 2. Total GS transferase activities in potato leaves (L) and roots (R) grown under 0, 100 mM and 200 mM NaCl, expressed as nkat γ-glutamyl hydroxamate.mg⁻¹ soluble protein. Columns represent mean +S.D. of triplicates (n ≥ 3). Differences from control values are all significantly different at P < 0.05
Source:Teixeira and Fidalgo, 2009

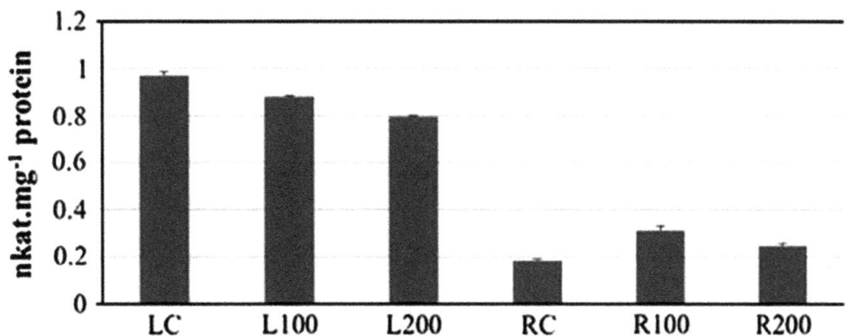

COPING STRATEGIES OF POTATO TO SALINITY

Despite all the losses caused by salinity, potato has coping strategies in salt-affected soils. Proline accumulation is one of the strategies. Proline is an osmoregulator and osmoprotector which accumulates during salt stress in potato (Figure 3) (Martinez et al., 1996; Prasad and Potluri, 1996; Rahnama and Ebrahimzadeh, 2004). The second coping mechanism is: up-regulation of proteins. Aghaei et al. (2008) observed up-regulation of osmotine-like proteins, heat-shock proteins, TSI-1 protein and calreticulin proteins and down-regulation of photosynthesis related proteins in two cultivars of potato. Evers et al. (2012) would later observe up-regulation of cell rescue and transcription factor related genes and down-regulation of photosynthesis-related genes. Moreover, potato increases activity of antioxidant enzymes such as: ascorbate peroxidase, catalase, and glutathione reductase against reactive oxygen species (ROS) in salinity situations (Aghaei et al., 2009; Hamdi et al., 2009; Rahnama and Ebrahimzadeh, 2004, 2005).

Figure 3. NaCl effects on growth and proline contents in shoot (A, C) and calli (B, D). A.B: Growth: C, D: proline content; AG: Agria; DIA: Diamant; K: Kennebec; AJ: Ajax. Agria and Kennebec: Relatively salt tolerant; Daimant and Ajax: Relatively salt sensitive. Vertical bars represent standard errors
Source: Rahnama and Ebrahimzadeh, (2004)

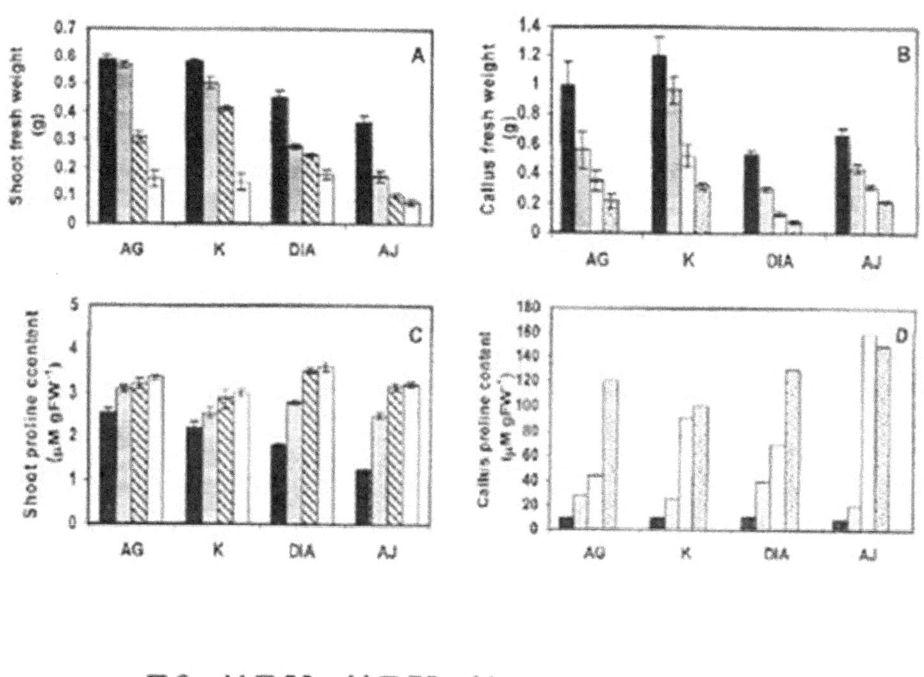

AMELIORATION OF SALINITY STRESS IN POTATO

Inasmuch as potato can defend itself to an extent towards salinity, tuber yield is yet to raise under saline conditions, and hence other methodologies are used to combat salinity. Jesus et al., (2015) details several opportunities for salt phytoremediation (Figure 4). One of which is leaching the salts below the root zone (Corwin et al., 2007; Qadir & Oster, 2004). That means irrigating with excessive water (Hanson et al., 2006) although, the water resource is dwindling globally. Therefore, other strategies of dealing with salinity in potato are supposed to be used in conjunction to irrigation. A study conducted by Back-hausen et al. (2005) found that high air humidity reduces salinity effect – high air humidity reduces Na[+] accumulation and increases non-photochemical quenching (NPQ) and thus reducing the overall rate of photosynthetic electron flow. Application of 60 Mt ha[-1] of poultry manure was observed to reduce salinity stress in potato and increase tuber yield (Oustani et al., 2014). In addition, Richardson et al. (2001) noted that supplemental Ca[++] could alleviate salinity stress effects by inhibiting degradation of nuclear of the root cell. Application of low to medium concentrations of Ca[++] are encouraged, however, higher concentrations of 2 gm Ca[++] per plant in saline conditions reduce potato yields (Abdel-Naby et al., 2001). Similarly, potassium deficiency was shown to encourage salt damage in micropropagated potato plantlets (Alhagdow et al., 1999) and therefore its supply reduces salinity effect (Elkhatib et al., 2004).

Figure 4. Techniques for enhanced salt phytoremediation grouped by type. AMF - arbuscular mycorrhizal fungi; PGPB - plant growth-promoting bacteria
Source: Jesus et al., (2015)

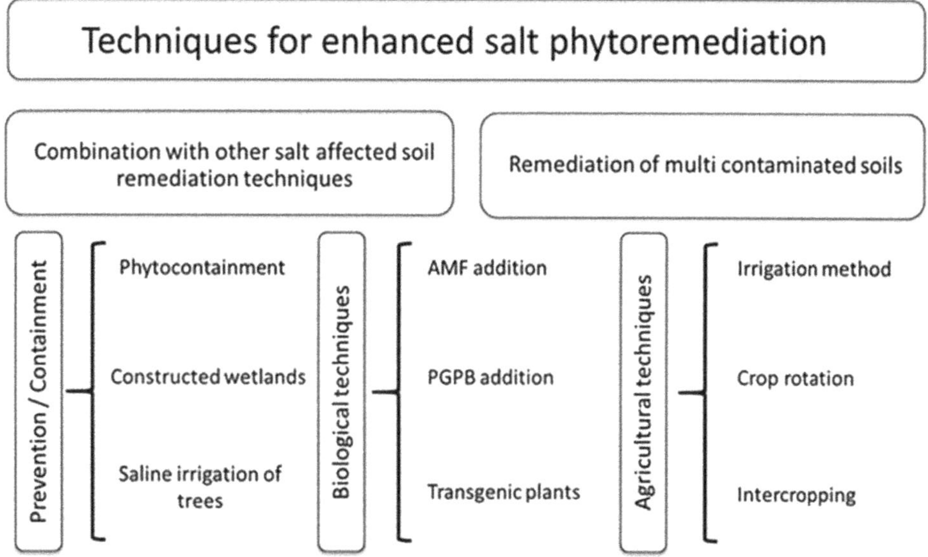

Exogenous application of ascorbic acid was noted to increase tolerance of potato towards salinity and protected chloroplasts from salt damage (Sajid & Aftab, 2009). Salicylic acid application succeeded in reducing salinity effect in potato (Sajid & Aftab, 2012) as it lowered oxidative damage caused by salinity. Furthermore, exogenous application of abscisic acid and or its method of application modified the response of potato to salinity (Etehadnia et al., 2008).

Besides exogenous application of growth hormones, breeding and genetic engineering is being used to alleviate salinity effects in potato. In tetrasomic tetraploid potatoes, DREBIA gene expression was observed to significantly reduce salinity (Celebi-Toprak et al., 2005). Another gene from rice, Osmyb4 encoding transcription factor MYB4 found in two transgenic lines of potato S2 and M48 (Variety Kennebec) caused reduction of salinity effects (Aydin et al., 2014). Further gene studies indicate that bacterial mannitol 1-phosphate dehydrogenase (mtlD) gene expression in potato increases mannitol which lead to enhanced salt tolerance (Rahnama et al., 2011). Glutamate synthetase (GS) plays a major role in regulating proline accumulation in salt stress potato, and in turn GS1 gene has been shown to be responsible for GS activity in salt affected potato (Teixeira et al., 2006). Overexpression of GalUR gene which is associated with ascorbate pathway was observed to enhance ascorbic acid content in transgenic potato variety, Taedong Valley, by minimizing oxidative stress caused by salt (Upadhyaya et al., 2011). In 2012, potato variety 'Marfona' was created via gamma irradiation (Yaycili & Alikamanoglu, 2012). This variety which was 27.5% genetically different from the control plants was proven to tolerate salinity.

Selection of potato cultivars tolerant to salinity is an age-old practice. Khrais et al. (1998) assessed 130 European and North America potato varieties for salinity. They eventually asserted that varieties: Amisk, BelRus, Bintje, Onaway, Sierra, and Tobique were the most tolerant to salinity. Other similar studies were conducted across the globe. In Egypt, variety Cara was tolerant among the four tested varieties by Elkhatib et al. (2004); in Korea, variety Sumi was tolerant among five tested varieties (Kim et al., 2013) and in the Mediterranean region, ten varieties were tested and only Vivaldi and Almera were found to be tolerant to salinity (Levy & Tai, 2013). Cultivars Desiree and Russett Burbank were also found to express tolerance towards salinity in the Netherlands (Jaarsma et al., 2013).

FUTURE RESEARCH DIRECTIONS

Potato is the third most important food crop in the world after rice and wheat. It is relatively sensitive to abiotic stress of excessive salt content in the soil. However, comparatively little work has been done with respect to abiotic stress of soil salinity on potato (Londhe, 2016). Further, it is expected to increase in salt affected soils across the globe due to climate change which influence on salinity is immense. As these changes occur, potato cultivation may be severely influenced and need coping strategies to be enhanced. Potato is means of food security and livelihood of many poor and marginal farmers. Increase in further agriculture area is not possible and cultivation of potato on abiotic stress affected soils due to salts is essential. The further research in this direction should be concentrated on development of salt tolerant potato varieties and better management practices for its cultivation on salt affected soils.

Precision nutrient application packages need to be developed and tested for various agro-ecological regions of salt affected soils. Further it is necessary to synchronizing potato growth stages with their nutrient requirement for optimal growth and yield and thereafter point application of nutrients either through drip irrigation or foliar could reduce accumulation salts in the soils. Research is needed on studying the pathway through which excess salts affects potato quality is crucial; the salt absorbed by potato could be channeled and not accumulate in the tubers such that during cooking it enhances taste and flavor.

CONCLUSION

Climate change exacerbate salinity leading to decrease in potato tuber yield. As this happens, the world population is also increasing thereby worsening the already impaired food security situation. This situation is of high concern owing to the fact that potato is a major food crop around the globe and a staple food in many countries. Therefore, addressing the climate change factors that intensify salinity is the first step towards reducing or alleviating salinity, followed by control or remediation measures in areas already experiencing the problem, and finally using the potato itself – its tolerance to salinity, breeding, selecting, and engineering it towards that.

REFERENCES

Abdel-Naby, A., El-Beltagy, M. S., Abou-Hadid, A., Helmy, Y. I., & El-Abd, S. O. (2001). Effect of Salinity Stress Modified by Calcium Application on Potato Plants. *Egyptian Journal of Horticulture*, *28*(4), 519–530.

Abliz, A., Tiyip, T., Ghulam, A., Halik, U., Ding, J. L., Sawut, M., … Abliz, A. (2016). Effects. of shallow groundwater table and salinity on soil salt dynamics in the Keriya Oasis, Northwestern China E*nviron. mental. Earth Science*, *75*(3), 1–15. doi:10.100712665-015-4794-8

Abumhadi, N., Todorovska, E., Assenov, B., Tsonev, S., Vulcheva, D., & Vulchev, D. (2012). Agricultural Research in 21 st century : Challenges facing the food security under the impacts of climate change. *Bulgarian Journal of Agricultural Science*, *18*(6), 801–818.

Aghaei, K., Ehsanpour, A. A., & Komatsu, S. (2008). Proteome Analysis of Potato under Salt Stress. *Journal of Proteome Research*, *7*(11), 4858–4868. doi:10.1021/pr800460y PMID:18855355

Aghaei, K., Ehsanpour, A. A., & Komatsu, S. (2009). Potato responds to salt stress by increased activity of antioxidant enzymes. *Journal of Integrative Plant Biology*, *51*(12), 1095–1103. doi:10.1111/j.1744-7909.2009.00886.x PMID:20021557

Alhagdow, M. M., Barthakur, N. N., & Donnelly, D. J. (1999). Salinity stress and sodium-potassium micropropagated potatoes interactions. *Potato Research*, *42*, 73–78. doi:10.1007/BF02358392

Allakhverdiev, S. I., Nishiyama, Y., Miyairi, S., Yamamoto, H., Inagaki, N., Kanesaki, Y., & Murata, N. (2002). Salt stress inhibits the repair of photodamaged photosystem II by suppressing the transcription and translation of psbA genes in synechocystis. *Plant Physiology*, *130*(3), 1443–1453. doi:10.1104/pp.011114 PMID:12428009

Ardón, M., Helton, A. M., & Bernhardt, E. S. (2016). Drought and saltwater incursion synergistically reduce dissolved organic carbon export from coastal freshwater wetlands. *Biogeochemistry*, *127*(2-3), 411–426. doi:10.100710533-016-0189-5

Arnell, N. W. (1999). Climate change and global water resources. *Global Environmental Change*, *9*(1), 31–49. doi:10.1016/S0959-3780(99)00017-5

Aydin, G., Yucel, M., Chan, M. T., & Oktem, H. A. (2014). Evaluation of abiotic stress tolerance and physiological characteristics of potato (Solanum tuberosum L. cv. Kennebec) that heterologously expresses the rice Osmyb4 gene. *Plant Biotechnology Reports*, *8*(3), 295–304. doi:10.100711816-014-0322-7

Aziz, I., & Khan, M. A. (2001). Experimental assessment of salinity tolerance of Ceriops tagal seedlings and saplings from the Indus delta, Pakistan. *Aquatic Botany*, *70*(3), 259–268. doi:10.1016/S0304-3770(01)00160-7

Backhausen, J. E., Klein, M., Klocke, M., Jung, S., & Scheibe, R. (2005). Salt tolerance of potato (Solanum tuberosum L. var. Desiree) plants depends on light intensity and air humidity. *Plant Science, 169*(1), 229–237. doi:10.1016/j.plantsci.2005.03.021

Bejat, L., Perfect, E., Quisenberry, V. L., Coyne, M. S., & Haszler, G. R. (2000). Solute Transport as Related to Soil Structure in Unsaturated Intact Soil Blocks. *Soil Science Society of America Journal, 64*(3), 818. doi:10.2136ssaj2000.643818x

Bernstein, L. (1975). Effects of Salinity and Sodicity on Plant Growth. *Annual Review of Phytopathology, 13*(1), 295–312. doi:10.1146/annurev.py.13.090175.001455

Bustan, A., Sagi, M., De Malach, Y., & Pasternak, D. (2004). Effects of saline irrigation water and heat waves on potato production in an arid environment. *Field Crops Research, 90*(2-3), 275–285. doi:10.1016/j.fcr.2004.03.007

Celebi-Toprak, F., Behnam, B., Serrano, G., Kasuga, M., Yamaguchi-Shinozaki, K., Naka, H., ... Watanabe, K. N. (2005). Tolerance to salt stress of the transgenic tetrasomic tetraploid potato, Solanum tuberosum cv. Desiree appears to be induced by the DREB1A gene and rd29A promoter of Arabidopsis thaliana. *Breeding Science, 55*(3), 311–319. doi:10.1270/jsbbs.55.311

Corwin, D. L., Rhoades, J. D., & Simunek, J. (2007). Leaching requirement for soil salinity control: Steady-state versus transient models. *Agricultural Water Management, 90*(3), 165–180. doi:10.1016/j.agwat.2007.02.007

D'Odorico, P., Bhattachan, A., Davis, K. F., Ravi, S., & Runyan, C. W. (2013). Global desertification: Drivers and feedbacks. *Advances in Water Resources, Elsevier Ltd, 51*, 326–344. doi:10.1016/j.advwatres.2012.01.013

Doll, P., & Siebert, S. (2002). Global modeling of irrigation water requirements. *Water Resources Research, 38*(4), 1–10. doi:10.1029/2001WR000355

Dzengeleski, S., Da Rocha, A. B., Kirk, W. W., & Hammerschmidt, R. (2003). Effect of soil salinity and Fusarium sambucinum infection on development of potatoes cultivar "Atlantic". *Acta Horticulturae, 19*(619), 251–261. doi:10.17660/ActaHortic.2003.619.28

Elkhatib, H. A., Elkhatib, E. A., Khalaf Allah, A. M., & El-Sharkawy, A. M. (2004). Yield Response of Salt-Stressed Potato to Potassium Fertilization: A Preliminary Mathematical Model. *Journal of Plant Nutrition, 27*(1), 111–122. doi:10.1081/PLN-120027550

Etehadnia, M., Waterer, D. R., & Tanino, K. K. (2008). The method of ABA application affects salt stress responses in resistant and sensitive potato lines. *Journal of Plant Growth Regulation, 27*(4), 331–341. doi:10.100700344-008-9060-9

Evers, D., Legay, S., Lamoureux, D., Hausman, J. F., Hoffmann, L., & Renaut, J. (2012). Towards a synthetic view of potato cold and salt stress response by transcriptomic and proteomic analyses. *Plant Molecular Biology, 78*(4-5), 4–5, 503–514. doi:10.100711103-012-9879-0 PMID:22258187

FAO. (2009). Advances in the Assessment and Monitoring of Salinization and Status of Biosaline Agriculture. *World Soil Resources Reports, 104*.

Fischer, G., & Heilig, G. K. (1997). Population momentum and the demand on land and water resources. *Philosophical Transactions of the Royal Society of London. Series B, Biological Sciences, 352*(1356), 869–889. doi:10.1098/rstb.1997.0067

Gao, H. J., Yang, H. Y., Bai, J. P., Liang, X. Y., Lou, Y., Zhang, J. L., ... Chen, Y. L. (2015). 'Ultrastructural and physiological responses of potato (Solanum tuberosum L) plantl.ets to gradient saline stress. *Frontiers in Plant Science, 5*, 1–14. doi:10.3389/fpls.2014.00787

Geriesh, M. H., Balke, K. D., El-Rayes, A. E., & Mansour, B. M. (2015). Implications of climate change on the groundwater flow regime and geochemistry of the Nile Delta, Egypt. *Journal of Coastal Conservation, 19*(4), 589–608. doi:10.100711852-015-0409-5

Gornall, J., Betts, R., Burke, E., Clark, R., Camp, J., Willett, K., & Wiltshire, A. (2010). Implications of climate change for agricultural productivity in the early twenty-first century. *Philosophical Transactions of the Royal Society of London. Series B, Biological Sciences, 365*(1554), 2973–2989. doi:10.1098/rstb.2010.0158 PMID:20713397

Grenfell, S. E., Callaway, R. M., Grenfell, M. C., Bertelli, C. M., Mendzil, A. F., & Tew, I. (2016). Will a rising sea sink some estuarine wetland ecosystems? *Science of the Total Environment. Elsevier B.V., 554-555*, 276–292.

Hamdi, M. M., Bettaieb, T., Harbaoui, Y., Mougou, A. A., & Jardin, P. (2009). Insight into the role of catalases in salt stress in potato (Solanum tuberosum L.). *Wild, 13*(3), 373–379.

Hanjra, M. A., & Qureshi, M. E. (2010). Global water crisis and future food security in an era of climate change. *Food Policy, Elsevier Ltd, 35*(5), 365–377. doi:10.1016/j.foodpol.2010.05.006

Hanson, B. R., Grattan, S. R. & Fulton, A. (2006). Agricultural Salinity and Drainage, Division of Agriculture and Natural Resources, *Publication, 3375.*

Hassanein, A. M. (1999). Alterations in protein and esterase patterns of peanut in response to salinity stress. *Biologia Plantarum, 42*(2), 241–248. doi:10.1023/A:1002112702771

Heuer, B., & Nadler, A. (1998). Physiological response of potato plants to soil salinity and water deficit. *Plant Science, 137*(1), 43–51. doi:10.1016/S0168-9452(98)00133-2

IPCC. (2007). Climate Change 2007, Mitigation of Climate Change. In B. Metz, O. R. Davidson, P. R. Bosch, R. Dave, & L. A. Meyer (Eds.), *Contribution of Working Group III to the Fourth Assessment Report of the Intergovernmental Panel on Climate Change, 2007.* Cambridge University Press. Retrieved July 31, 2016, from https://www.ipcc.ch/pdf/assessment-report/ar4/wg3/ar4_wg3_full_report.pdf

Jaarsma, R., de Vries, R. S. M., & de Boer, A. H. (2013). Effect of Salt Stress on Growth, Na+ Accumulation and Proline Metabolism in Potato (Solanum tuberosum) Cultivars. *PLoS ONE, 8*(3), e60183. doi:10.1371/journal.pone.0060183 PMID:23533673

Jacobsen, T., & Adams, R. M. (1958). Salt and silt in ancient Mesopotamian Agriculture. *Science, 128*(3334), 1251–1258. doi:10.1126cience.128.3334.1251 PMID:17793690

Jesus, J. M., Danko, A. S., Fiúza, A., & Borges, M. T. (2015). Phytoremediation of salt-affected soils: A review of processes, applicability, and the impact of climate change. *Environmental Science and Pollution Research International, 22*(9), 6511–6525. doi:10.100711356-015-4205-4 PMID:25854203

Kaufman, Z., Nachmias, A., Livescu, L., Meiri, A., & Tibor, M. (1990). Verticillium wilt of potatoes under irrigation with saline water. *Hassadeh, 70*(6), 898–901.

Khavari-Nejad, R. A., & Chaparzadeh, N. (1998). The effects of NaCl and CaCl$_2$ on photosynthesis and growth of alfalfa plants. *Photosynthetica, 35*(3), 461–466. doi:10.1023/A:1006928721986

Khrais, T., Leclerc, Y., & Donnelly, J. D. (1998). Relative Salinity Tolerance of Potato Cultivars Assessed By I n Vitro Screening Multiplication of In Vitro Material. *American Journal of Potato Research, 75*, 207–210. doi:10.1007/BF02854214

Kim, S., Yang, C., Jeong, J., Choi, W., Lee, K., & Kim, S. (2013). Physiological Response of Potato Variety to Soil Salinity. *Korean Journal of Crop Science, 58*(2), 85–90. doi:10.7740/kjcs.2013.58.2.085

Kirk, W., da Rocha, A., Hollosy, S., Hammerschmidt, R., & Wharton, P. (2006). Effect of Soil Salinity on Internal Browning of potato Tuber Tissue in Two Soil Types. *American Journal of Potato Research, 83*(3), 223-232. Retrieved 30, 2016, from http://link.springer.com/article/10.1007/BF02872158

Kitamura, Y., Yano, T., Honna, T., Yamamoto, S., & Inosako, K. (2006). Causes of farmland salinization and remedial measures in the Aral Sea basin-Research on water management to prevent secondary salinization in rice-based cropping system in arid land. *Agricultural Water Management, 85*(1-2), 1–14. doi:10.1016/j.agwat.2006.03.007

Levy, D. (1992). The response of potatoes (Solanum tuberosum L.) to salinity: Plant growth and tuber yields in the arid desert of Israel. *Annals of Applied Biology, 120*(1), 547–555. doi:10.1111/j.1744-7348.1992.tb04914.x

Levy, D., Coleman, W. K., & Veilleux, R. E. (2013). Adaptation of Potato to Water Shortage: Irrigation Management and Enhancement of Tolerance to Drought and Salinity. *American Journal of Potato Research, 90*(2), 186–206. doi:10.100712230-012-9291-y

Levy, D., Fogelman, E. & Itzhak, Y. (1988). The effect of water salinity on potatoes (Solanum tuberosum L.): Physiological indices and yielding capacity. *Potato Research, 31*(4), 601–610.

Levy, D., Fogelman, E., & Ytzhak, Y. (1993). Influence of water and soil salinity on emergence and early development of potato (Solanum tubersum L.) cultivars and effect of physiological age of seed tubers. *Potato Research, 36*(4), 335–340. doi:10.1007/BF02361800

Levy, D., & Tai, G. C. C. (2013). Differential response of potatoes (Solanum tuberosum L.) to salinity in an arid environment and field performance of the seed tubers grown with fresh water in the following season. *Agricultural Water Management. Elsevier B.V., 116*, 122–127.

Li, H., Yi, J., Zhang, J., Zhao, Y., Si, B., Hill, R., … Liu, X. (2015). Modeling of Soil Water and Salt Dynamics and Its Effects on Root Water Uptake in Heihe Arid Wetland Gansu, China. *Water, 7*(5), 2382–2401. Retrieved July 30, 2016, from http://www.mdpi.com/2073-4441/7/5/2382

Londhe, S. (2016). Cultivation of potato on abiotic stress-affected soils of India. *Current Science, 111*(1), 21-22. Retrieved July 30, 2016, from http://www.currentscience.ac.in/Volumes/111/01/0021.pdf

Martinez, C. A., Maestri, M., & Lani, E. G. (1996). In vitro salt tolerance and proline accumulation in Andean potato (Solanum spp.) differing in frost resistance. *Plant Science, 116*(2), 177–184. doi:10.1016/0168-9452(96)04374-9

McDonald, R. I., & Girvetz, E. H. (2013). Two Challenges for U.S. Irrigation Due to Climate Change: Increasing Irrigated Area in Wet States and Increasing Irrigation Rates in Dry States. *PLoS ONE, 8*(6), 1–10. doi:10.1371/journal.pone.0065589 PMID:23755255

Moya, J. L., Gómez-Cadenas, A., Primo-Millo, E., & Talon, M. (2003). Chloride absorption in salt-sensitive Carrizo citrange and salt-tolerant Cleopatra mandarin citrus rootstocks is linked to water use. *Journal of Experimental Botany, 54*(383), 825–833. doi:10.1093/jxb/erg064 PMID:12554725

Muthukumarasamy, M., Gupta, D. S., & Panneerselvam, R. (2000). Enhancement of peroxidase, polyphenol oxidase and superoxide dismutase activities by triadimefon in NaCl stressed Raphanus sativus L. *Biologia Plantarum, 43*(2), 317–320. doi:10.1023/A:1002741302485

Nachmias, A., Kaufman, Z., Livescu, L., Tsror, L., Meiri, A., & Caligari, P. D. S. (1993). Effect of salinity and its interactions with disease incidence on potatoes grown in hot climates. *Phytoparasitica, 21*(3), 245–255. doi:10.1007/BF02980946

Oustani, M., Halilat, M. M. T., & Chenchouni, H. (2014). Effect of poultry manure on the yield and nutriments uptake of potato under saline conditions of arid regions. *Emirates Journal of Food and Agriculture, 27*(1), 106–120. doi:10.9755/ejfa.v27i1.17971

Parida, A. K., & Das, A. B. (2005). Salt tolerance and salinity effects on plants: A review. *Ecotoxicology and Environmental Safety, 60*(3), 324–349. doi:10.1016/j.ecoenv.2004.06.010 PMID:15590011

Prasad, P. V., & Potluri, S. D. P. (1996). Influence of proline and hydroxyproline on salt-stressed axillary bud cultures of two varieties of potato (Solanum tuberosum). *In Vitro Cellular & Developmental Biology. Plant, 32*(1), 47–50. doi:10.1007/BF02823013

Qadir, M., & Oster, J. D. (2004). Crop and irrigation management strategies for saline-sodic soils and waters aimed at environmentally sustainable agriculture. *The Science of the Total Environment, 323*(1-3), 1–19. doi:10.1016/j.scitotenv.2003.10.012 PMID:15081713

Rahnama, H., & Ebrahimzadeh, H. (2004). The effect of NaCl on proline accumulation in potato seedlings and calli. *Acta Physiologiae Plantarum, 26*(3), 263–270. doi:10.100711738-004-0016-9

Rahnama, H., & Ebrahimzadeh, H. (2005). The effect of NaCl on antioxidant enzyme activities in potato seedlings. *Biologia Plantarum, 49*(1), 93–97. doi:10.100710535-005-3097-4

Rahnama, H., Vakilian, H., Fahimi, H., & Ghareyazie, B. (2011). Enhanced salt stress tolerance in transgenic potato plants (Solanum tuberosum L.) expressing a bacterial mtlD gene. *Acta Physiologiae Plantarum, 33*(4), 1521–1532. doi:10.100711738-010-0690-8

Rengasamy, P. (2006). World salinization with emphasis on Australia. *Journal of Experimental Botany, 57*(5), 1017–1023. doi:10.1093/jxb/erj108 PMID:16510516

Richardson, K. V. A., Wetten, A. C., & Caligari, P. D. S. (2001). Cell and nuclear degradation in root meristems following exposure of potatoes (Solanum tuberosum L.) to salinity. *Potato Research, 44*(4), 389–399. doi:10.1007/BF02358598

Riediger, J., Breckling, B., Nuske, R. S., & Schröder, W. (2014). Will climate change increase irrigation requirements in agriculture of Central Europe? A simulation study for Northern Germany. *Environmental Sciences Europe, 26*(18), 1–13.

Romero-Aranda, R., Soria, T., & Cuartero, J. (2001). Tomato plant-water uptake and plant-water relationships under saline growth conditions. *Plant Science, 160*(2), 265–272. doi:10.1016/S0168-9452(00)00388-5 PMID:11164598

Sajid, Z., & Aftab, F. (2012). Role of Salicylic Acid in Amelioration of Salt Tolerance in Potato (Solanum Tuberosum L.) Under in Vitro Conditions. *Pakistan Journal of Botany, 44*, 37–42.

Sajid, Z. A., & Aftab, F. (2009). Amelioration of salinity tolerance in Solanum tuberosum L. by exogenous application of ascorbic acid. *In Vitro Cellular & Developmental Biology. Plant, 45*(5), 540–549. doi:10.100711627-009-9252-4

Silva, J. A. B., Otoni, W. C., Martinez, C. A., Dias, L. M., & Silva, M. A. P. (2001). Microtuberization of Andean potato species (Solanum spp.) as affected by salinity. *Scientia Horticulturae, 89*(2), 91–101. doi:10.1016/S0304-4238(00)00226-0

Sivakumar, M. V. K. (2007). Interactions between climate and desertification. *Agricultural and Forest Meteorology, 142*(2-4), 143–155. doi:10.1016/j.agrformet.2006.03.025

Takemura, T., Hanagata, N., Sugihara, K., Baba, S., Karube, I., & Dubinsky, Z. (2000). Physiological and biochemical responses to salt stress in the mangrove, Bruguiera gymnorrhiza. *Aquatic Botany, 68*(1), 15–28. doi:10.1016/S0304-3770(00)00106-6

Teixeira, J., & Fidalgo, F. (2009). Salt stress affects glutamine synthetase activity and mRNA accumulation on potato plants in an organ-dependent manner. *Plant Physiology and Biochemistry. Elsevier Masson SAS, 47*(9), 807–813.

Teixeira, J., & Pereira, S. (2007). High salinity and drought act on an organ-dependent manner on potato glutamine synthetase expression and accumulation. *Environmental and Experimental Botany, 60*(1), 121–126. doi:10.1016/j.envexpbot.2006.09.003

Teixeira, J., Pereira, S., Queirós, F., & Fidalgo, F. (2006). Specific roles of potato glutamine synthetase isoenzymes in callus tissue grown under salinity: Molecular and biochemical responses. *Plant Cell, Tissue and Organ Culture, 87*(1), 1–7. doi:10.100711240-006-9103-5

Trenberth, K. E. (2011). Changes in precipitation with climate change. *Climate Research, 47*(1-2), 123–138. doi:10.3354/cr00953

United States Salinity Laboratory. (1954). Diagnosis and Improvement of Saline and Alkali Soils. *Agricultural Handbook, 60.*

Upadhyaya, C. P., Venkatesh, J., Gururani, M. A., Asnin, L., Sharma, K., Ajappala, H., & Park, S. W. (2011). Transgenic potato overproducing l-ascorbic acid resisted an increase in methylglyoxal under salinity stress via maintaining higher reduced glutathione level and glyoxalase enzyme activity. *Biotechnology Letters*, *33*(11), 2297–2307. doi:10.100710529-011-0684-7 PMID:21750996

Vicente-Serrano, S. M., Lopez-Moreno, J. I., Beguería, S., Lorenzo-Lacruz, J., Sanchez-Lorenzo, A., García-Ruiz, J. M., . . . Espejo, F. (2014). Evidence of increasing drought severity caused by temperature rise in southern Europe. *Environmental Research Letters*, *9*(4), 1-9. Retrieved July 30, 2016 from http://digital.csic.es/bitstream/10261/95049/1/BegueriaS_EnvResLett_2014.pdf

Wang, K., Dickinson, R. E., & Liang, S. (2012). Global atmospheric evaporative demand over land from 1973 to 2008. *Journal of Climate*, *25*(23), 8353–8361. doi:10.1175/JCLI-D-11-00492.1

Wang, Y., & Nii, N. (2000). Changes in chlorophyll, ribulose bisphosphate carboxylase-oxygenase, glycine betaine content, photosynthesis and transpiration in Amaranthus tricolor leaves during salt stress. *The Journal of Horticultural Science & Biotechnology*, *75*(6), 623–627. doi:10.1080/14620316.2000.11511297

Williams, E. K., & Rosenheim, B. E. (2015). What happens to soil organic carbon as coastal marsh ecosystems change in response to increasing salinity? An exploration using ramped pyrolysis. *Geochemistry Geophysics Geosystems*, *16*(7), 2322–2335. doi:10.1002/2015GC005839

WWAP. (2015). *The United Nations World Water Development Report 2015: Water for a Sustainable World*. Paris: UNESCO.

Yadav, S., Irfan, M., Ahmad, A., & Hayat, S. (2011). Causes of salinity and plant manifestations to salt stress: A review. *Journal of Environmental Biology*, *32*(5), 667–685. PMID:22319886

Yaycili, O., & Alikamanoglu, S. (2012). Induction of salt-tolerant potato (Solanum tuberosum L.) mutants with gamma irradiation and characterization of genetic variations via RAPD-PCR analysis. *Turkish Journal of Biology*, *36*(4), 405–412.

Zhang, Z., Mao, B., Li, H., Zhou, W., Takeuchi, Y., & Yoneyama, K. (2005). Effect of salinity on physiological characteristics, yield and quality of microtubers in vitro in potato. *Acta Physiologiae Plantarum*, *27*(4), 481–489. doi:10.100711738-005-0053-z

KEY TERMS AND DEFINITIONS

Amelioration: To reduce the effects of bad condition/move bad conditions to better.

Desertification: Degradation of land especially arid and semi-arid lands due to climate changes and human influence mostly deforestation and agricultural activities.

Exacerbates: Increasing the severity of a bad situation for example climate change exacerbates salinity.

Remediation: To control or rectify problems caused, in this case salinity.

Salinity: Soils whose electrical conductivity are over 4 dS m⁻¹ and sodium absorption ratio are less than 13.

Salt-Tolerance: The ability of a plant to endure high electrical conductivity and still be able to give reasonable yields.

Sodicity: Soils whose electrical conductivity are less than 4 dS m⁻¹ and sodium absorption ratio are above 13.

This research was previously published in Sustainable Potato Production and the Impact of Climate Change edited by Sunil Londhe; pages 133-151, copyright year 2017 by Information Science Reference (an imprint of IGI Global).

Chapter 44
Local Production–Based Dietary Supplement Distribution in Emerging Countries:
Bienestarina Distribution in Colombia

Jesus Gonzalez-Feliu
Mines Saint-Etienne, France

Carlos Osorio-Ramírez
National University of Colombia, Colombia

Laura Palacios-Arguello
Mines Saint-Etienne, France

Carlos Alberto Talamantes
Autonomous University of Ciudad Juarez, Mexico

ABSTRACT

The production and distribution of Bienestarina to the vulnerable population of Colombia is one of the strategies of the Colombian Institute of Familiar Wellness (ICBF) to fight malnutrition, especially among children. This case is a good example of establishing food security and social improvement logistics that merits particular attention. The chapter presents an analysis of the Bienestarina supply chain based on the four elements: steering, organization, development, and financial issues. First, an overview of social improvement logistics and the Bienestarina context is provided. Second, theoretical frameworks related to the case are presented. Third, the case is described on the basis of the proposed analysis framework. Finally, generalization issues and conclusions allow the authors proposing the first characterization of social improvement logistics.

DOI: 10.4018/978-1-7998-5354-1.ch044

INTRODUCTION

Food safety is one of the commitments which the Colombian government wants to ensure as a right of people (Dirección Nacional de Planeación, 2007). Indeed, the government must help the part of the Colombian population who is under malnutrition (i.e. due to nutrient deficiencies in their food), where children are considered as the most affected. Malnutrition of children generates several problems such as lack of concentration, and energy, decreased learning ability, and general delay in physical and mental development, among others (Cuevas García, 2005). To fight malnutrition, different strategies can be implemented by national and regional entities (Food and Agriculture Organization of the United Nations [FAO], 2010). Since several initiatives focus on bringing unused food to the most sensible families (Maldonado & Moya, 2013) or on increasing families revenues, others (mainly in Latin America) deploy dietary complements or enriched food production-distribution systems addressed to those families.

In this context, the main products used to fight malnutrition are based on flours mixtures obtained from cereals that can be locally produced. Indeed, the rates of local (at least national or regional) production for those products are high (Rozo, 2000). However, several reports state that the distribution systems related to those products present deficiencies. It is important to consider those systems in a supply chain management perspective, in order to identify the main processes but also observe the evolutions of the integrated supply-production-distribution chain.

Over 30 years, Colombia has been implementing the strategy to improve food consumption of high nutritional value through the production and distribution of food complement based on mixtures of plant origin with high nutritional content, which is called Bienestarina. The purpose of this complement is to arrive in time to children, young, elderly, poor families, ethnic groups, and other population who require sufficient nutrients which their basic food do not provide sufficiently. Production and distribution of Bienestarina to the vulnerable population of Colombia is one of the strategies of the Colombian Institute of Familiar Wellness (ICBF) to combat malnutrition, especially among children.

The aim of this chapter is to investigate the current state of the Bienestarina logistics process from a supply chain viewpoint and focus on social aspects of logistics which are not related to commercialization of a product but to make it available to sensible populations. The authors start from the theoretical framework of the four pillars of the viability of a logistics project (Gonzalez-Feliu, Malhéné, Morganti, & Morana, 2014) and examine them in the case of the Bienestarina distribution network in Colombia.

This chapter is organized as follows. First, the background and context of the research are presented. Then, the methodological issues are provided. After that, the main results of the research are summarized and discussed. In the conclusion section, practical implications of those results and further developments are proposed.

BACKGROUND

Food security is a major issue since decades and takes a special interest in developing countries, where malnutrition and hunger are one of the first causes of mortality (Valdes, 1981; Reutlinger, 1986). However, food security is in general in competition to the industrialization and performance-making of productive systems and agro-industrial developments of such countries, mainly related either to feed developed countries or to produce non-food agricultural and agro-industrial products, such as biofuels (Ewing & Msangi, 2009) and textile fibers (Fortucci, 2002), among others. In opposition to the development of such industries, the needs of local inhabitants to nourish and develop themselves, in seeking higher welfare status, feeds the public debate on the place of social improvement in the economic and sustainable development of a country (Braun & Kennedy, 1994).

The issue of social improvement is a major strategic point in emerging countries. Indeed, with the high levels of poverty and malnutrition that characterize those countries, one of the main objectives of governments, along with economic development, is an improvement of the quality of life of people. Moreover, those countries receive particular attentions of non-governmental organizations (NGOs) and other humanitarian organizations. Although humanitarian logistics is a popular subject of research (Kovács & Spens, 2007, 2009; Holguin-Veras, Jaller, Van Wassenhove, Pérez, & Wachtendorf, 2012; Holguin-Veras, Wachtendorf, Jaller, & Jefferson, 2013), it focuses on emergency response logistics and post-disasters organization, with a low scientific interest for social improvement logistics. Indeed, the first statement on the importance of logistics in supporting social improvement is found in Orbell and Dawes (1993). After that, only a few works deal with logistics contributing to the social improvement. To the best of the authors' knowledge, Stock (1990) was the first who emphasized the poor contribution of logistics research in relation to social welfare. Adivar, Atan, Sevil Oflaç, and Örten (2010) focus on the notion of the value chain for social improvement and welfare. Finally, Maldonado and Moya (2013) show the importance of combining social improvement policies with reverse logistics in developing and improving food banks actions and logistics schemes. Those authors identify different ways to reduce hunger and malnutrition, as, for example, development of food banks, different ways of increasing incomes or reducing food acquisition costs, or free distribution of dietary complements of different nature and actions.

According to the FAO (2010, 2011), deployment of the actions on improvement dietary composition of daily meals in families belonging to sensible population is crucial to their development since they decrease hunger and malnutrition. To this fact, an initiative called Latin America and the Caribbean without Hunger was launched by the FAO (2011). In this initiative, several types of stakeholders and actions were deployed. From this initiative, it was concluded that several measures could be implemented to combat malnutrition (Maldonado & Moya, 2013). The initiatives may be aggregated into five major categories:

1. Primary economic improvement: in this category, the authors included initiatives that allow the families' income increase to purchase basic food and nutritional elements. The main initiatives in this category are subsidies and income transfer actions. Those initiatives are related to financial transfers, without direct relation to logistics.
2. Cost reduction to increase accessibility to food: initiatives in this category aim to reducing the cost of basic foods for sensible groups of populations by giving income not to families but to vendors in order to make basic foods less expensive for beneficiaries. The most known examples in this category are subsidies to retailers, tax exemptions, or programs of free (or cheaper) basic baskets. Anyway, those initiatives do not have (or little) impact on logistics and freight transportation. They can indirectly increase logistic flows of retailers but do not need to deploy specific distribution channels and supply chains.
3. Food access initiatives: they aim to increase access of sensible groups of population to basic food by providing them a set of basic products. In this category, the initiatives are more heterogeneous, and the main examples are the programs on delivering healthy food to hospitals, nurseries, and schools, deployment of social retailers (which have a specific logistics based on reverse flow collection), food banks, or distribution of dietary complements to families. In all those cases, specific

supply chains are needed (or improvements of existing channels to take into account reverse flows or new products). They have a direct impact on supply, production, and distribution flows.

4. Education and monitoring initiatives: this category includes all initiatives that support and promote good habits, but also those that aim to steer and follow the risk of families and sensible groups of the population regarding malnutrition. They are, like categories 1 and 2, not directly related to logistics.

5. Promotion and development of self-production: the last, but not the least, the category is related to those actions that help families in sensible groups of population to satisfy some part or entire of their nutritional needs by themselves by providing them the agricultural resources (or access to them) to develop self-production. Although both creation and distribution of those resources need a logistical organization (sometimes being specific to those initiatives), the focus of this category is not on the distribution of products but on promotion their production for self-consumption.

As seen above, from those five categories of initiatives, two of them are related to logistic issues, but only one directly deploys specific logistic channels with an aim to distribute products in order to help sensible groups of populations, not to make profits. This chapter focuses on one of the initiatives in this category, i.e. distribution of dietary complements. The authors focus on this strategy for two reasons. The first is that it is one of the main practical solutions for emerging countries to reduce malnutrition. The second is that it has received small attention in the scientific literature.

Moreover, the case of Bienestarina in Colombia (a public-supported dietary complement addressed to children, mothers, and other inhabitants of sensible groups of the population) has received a particular attention recently (Palacios, Morana, Gonzalez-Feliu, & Devia, 2016; Peñaloza, Palacios, & Gonzalez-Feliu, 2016). The present chapter synthesizes those works and proposes a systemic vision of the distribution system of Bienestarina in relation to local production and development of local economies.

In Colombia, the government, via the Colombian Institute of Family Welfare (Instituto Colombiano del Bienestar Familiar, or ICBF), developed a series of programs to combat malnutrition by providing the families with the highest risk in terms of their dietary complement, mainly addressed to childhood. Indeed, since 1976, the ICBF produces the Bienestarina product as a dietary complement of high nutritional value as a strategy to strengthen the fundamental right to food security in the country (Dirección Nacional de Planeación, 2006). In early 2013, the ICBF launched the Bienestarina Más program, which proposed an improved product reformulation (Presidencia de la República, 2013), aimed at vulnerable Colombian population, especially among children. This product benefits children, teenagers, pregnant women, mothers, different ethnic groups, families, and seniors belonging to levels 1 and 2 of the System for the Selection of Beneficiaries for Social Programs (SISBEN), the Colombian national system for identification of beneficiaries of social subsidies (Peñaloza et al., 2016). It classifies people according to their socio-economic level into six levels, where level 1 is for homeless people and extreme poverty, while level 6 is the highest level of affluence.

The importance of this research is based on the fact that in recent years there have been irregularities in the management of Bienestarina involving distribution processes, product traceability, lead time distribution to the beneficiary (end consumer), among others. One example is the case of product expiration, according to El Nuevo Siglo (2013). 190 expired product packages were reported in the period of January-June 2012. Moreover, opposing European and North complementary food, which is based on extraction and biochemical products, Bienestarina and other Latin-American dietary complements are based on flours. The particularity of Colombian Bienestarina is that almost all flour is of domestic origin, which promotes national production and ensures a basic level of food safety (for example, Colombian corn cannot be of transgenic nature by law).

The program is entirely steered by the ICBF, a public body which directly depends on the Colombian Ministry of Social Protection. Moreover, it has the particularity that the product is entirely produced in Colombia and then distributed by a combined network of national and regional facilities, showing an important contribution to local food production and distribution. For those reasons, the authors propose to describe the case of Bienestarina following a deductive case study methodology and focusing on the description of the distribution logistic network.

MAIN FOCUS OF THE CHAPTER

Theoretical and Methodological Framework

There are many frameworks to identify and characterize supply chains. Among the most known are the SCOR model (Supply Chain Council, 2008) and the Supply Chain characterization framework by Lambert, Cooper, and Pagh (1998). The first model represents various echelons of supply chain and main categories of the processes, the processes themselves, related needs, and main tasks derived from those needs and resources of companies. The second is a global conceptual representation which includes a structure of supply chain, its main stakeholders, and its technical and managerial components (Lambert, 2001).

Those models are mainly related to business and intra-organization logistics but remain the valid tools to examine supply chain management in organizations of any type. However, they focus on logistic processes and other associated activities only, completed at private and contractual levels only. An alternative to those frameworks can be found in industrial and system engineering, where a framework to examine the viability of industrial system can be related to four main elements: steering, organization, development, and financing (Gonzalez-Feliu, Taniguchi, & d'Arcier, 2014). The authors identified those four elements on a structure-based and economic viability goal for urban logistics initiatives, proposing the first analysis framework of urban freight distribution that addressed those four elements. The authors aim to extend this framework to food distribution, by re-defining the four elements as follows:

1. Steering structure defines various stakeholders involved in steering and monitoring the deployment of food distribution systems, as well as their relations and communication processes. Different actions aimed at consultation and main tools for steering are also included in this category.
2. Organization of the process is the set of elements that allow the distribution system to be conceived and designed, as well as to ensure its daily operations. In other words, this category defines the organization and management of the whole distribution chain and its related processes.
3. Development of the distribution system is the way in which the system has spread and/or evolved during the period from its starting point to the situation when it is operational. Therefore, it is important to focus on the actions performed and constraints to which the distribution system is a subject to better understand its evolution.
4. Financial strategies need to be addressed as well. Although in private systems those strategies are well set in advance and once the system is operated, it is clear how the investments will be refunded, but not so clear in public-based systems. Moreover, it is important to know who finances and pays

for the system (mainly in social improvement logistics systems) to better understand the other three components.

From those four elements, the authors orient the analysis of the Bienestarina distribution to define its organizational model, as summarized in Figure 1.

Figure 1. Proposed framework for defining social improvement logistics systems
Source: Adapted from Gonzalez-Feliu, Malhéné, Morganti & Morana (2014)

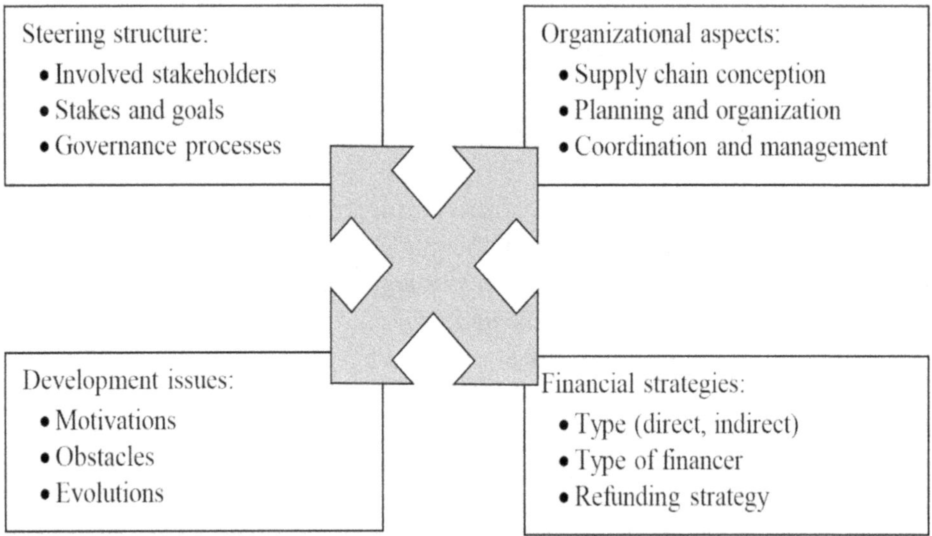

The case study has been developed via the collection of secondary and primary data to first characterize the distribution system (more details on the data collection and analysis for the characterization of the system is found in Peñaloza et al. (2016)), completed by the second data collection operation, mainly on the basis of interviews to the ICBF. Those data have been aggregated and synthesized following the theoretical framework above to build the deductive case study presented below.

The Proposed Case Study

In order to relate the theoretical framework proposed above to practice, the authors aim to develop the case study of Bienestarina distribution. Over 30 years, Colombia has been implementing the strategy to improve food consumption of high nutritional value through the production and distribution of food complements based on mixtures of plant origin with high nutritional content. This product, called Bienestarina, is addressed to populations under danger of malnutrition. In other words, the purpose of the production and distribution of this complement is to arrive in time to children, young, elderly, poor families, ethnic groups, and other population who require sufficient nutrients which their basic food do not provide sufficiently. Production and distribution of Bienestarina to the vulnerable population of Colombia is one of the strategies of the ICBF to combat malnutrition, especially among children.

This food complement, which is constituted of a mixture of flours of vegetable origin, such as corn starch, wheat, rice, soy, and milk powder, is a highly enriched source of calories, carbohydrates, proteins, natural fats, calcium, vitamins A and C, and other nutrients. It is a reinforcement to attack the problems of child malnutrition as a dietary complement and should not replace the basic food or breast milk. Bienestarina is also used as an input in the preparation of different foods such as cakes, cookies or bread, among others, which are also aimed at the target population in the different programs of the ICBF. The nutritional information about the current form of Bienestarina is presented in Table 1.

Table 1. Nutritional information for Bienestarina (per 100 g portion)

Component	Content
Energy (kcal)	360
Carbohydrates (g)	64.79
Protein (g)	20.145
Fat (g)	3.082
Total dietary fiber (g)	1.806
Calcium (mg)	700
Phosphorus (mg)	550
Iron (mg)	14.1
Vitamin A (UI)	2,000
Vitamin C (mg)	45
Niacin (mg)	7.3
Thiamine (mg)	0.5
Riboflavin (mg)	0,6
Vitamin B6 (mg)	0.9
Folic acid (mg)	160
Vitamin B12 (mg)	1.4
Zinc (mg)	8.3

Source: Colombian Institute of Familiar Wellness, 2009

The Bienestarina program was launched in 1976 by the Colombian Ministry of Social Protection (Dirección Nacional de Planeación, 2006). After that, a research on different vegetal mixed formulations, the first Bienestarina formulation, was produced and distributed in 1976. In 1989, the process of flour pre-cooking was deployed and operated. Other changes, including the ones in the formulation and the raw materials used, were introduced in 2000, 2002, 2004, and 2013. All those evolutions implied important changes in the production chain but not in the distribution one. Indeed, the distribution system is strongly dependent on the nature and activity of the subcontractor.

The entity in charge of programming, selling (to collective bodies), and managing the production and distribution of Bienestarina is the ICBF, and this for all programs. However, there are different programs and functions, and the ICBF is not able to manage every process by its own. It is why the logistic operations (for the entire supply chain of Bienestarina) are subcontracted to a private company.

This subcontract is made by a public concession. Since December 2007, the ICBF granted the concession to the Industrias Del Maiz S.A. Corn Product Andina (IDM) Company, which deployed a branch, named Ingredion, which manages production and distribution of Bienestarina and other foods of high nutritional value.

The most recent program launched in 2013 is Bienestarina Más, which proposed an improved product, mainly enriched with vitamins and other essential elements. The ICBF defines the number and locations of beneficiaries, together with public bodies. Indeed, the ICBF defines a yearly production which is derived from a number of "credits". Those credits have to be acquired by public entities (mainly municipalities, but also nurseries, hospitals, or other public institutions) who define a number of beneficiaries according to the number of credits acquired. Then, the ICBF plans a demand (making the Bienestarina supply chain being on pulled flows steering mode) and its characteristics (a type of products, quantities, and frequencies).

Knowing the demand, Ingredion is in charge of the production, which implies supply of raw materials and entire distribution process. Final destinations of the distribution process steered by Ingredion are delivery points where executing units (in general, operators in charge of bringing Bienestarina to beneficiaries) pick up the required demand.

Currently, the subcontractor (Ingredion S.A.) has two production plants, one located in Sabanagrande (Atlantico region, in the north of Colombia, near Barranquilla on the Atlantic side of the country) and Cartago (Valle region, in the west of the country, near Pereira and between Bogotá and the Pacific Ocean). The main raw products needed to produce Bienestarina are corn starch, wheat, rice, soy, and milk converted into milk powder before being mixed with other ingredients. All raw products are derived from national producers, which implies local processing and manufacturing for flours and milk powder, as well as for additives. Although it would be possible to use raw products issued from non-Colombian producers to make flours and additives, the specifications for the subcontracting impose criteria of quality, proximity, and reactivity which promote local production. However, taken into account the geography of Colombian agriculture, "local" production needs to be considered at a macro-regional level. This is also the case of milk powder, where production needs to be local to ensure the freshness of milk taken into account the need of not adding conservatives. From each production macro-region, local manufacturers produce flours and milk powder and supply them to the Bienestarina mixing plants to produce the final product.

Due to the location of the two plants, and the current number of beneficiaries (about 9 million inhabitants (Peñaloza, Palacios & Gonzalez-Feliu, 2016) spread on the entire territory of the country), the ICBF uses a division in eight macro-regions, according to the issues of regional distribution programs and operating costs of logistic, as shown in Figure 2.

To each macro-region, a number of first-tier warehouses (called primary distribution points by the ICBF) is associated. Those warehouses have the function of reception and managing the inventories to distribute the assigned beneficiaries for the entire macro-region. The demand management is made by the ICBF in function of the number of credits bought by public entities at each final destination, and then the monthly production and distribution plans. However, the inventorying operations take place at first-tier warehouses to ensure a higher inventorying capacity and a better reactivity, taken into account the geography of Colombia.

After preparing the commands in regional warehouses, the products are transported to second-tier facilities, which are called delivery points and are the interface between the distribution system and the executing units that deliver the product to the beneficiaries. There is approximatively a set of 5,000 delivery points, spread throughout the country. The Bienestarina supply chain uses different mechanisms

Figure 2. Division of logistic distribution macro-regions (MR)
Source: Peñaloza, Palacios & Gonzalez-Feliu, 2016

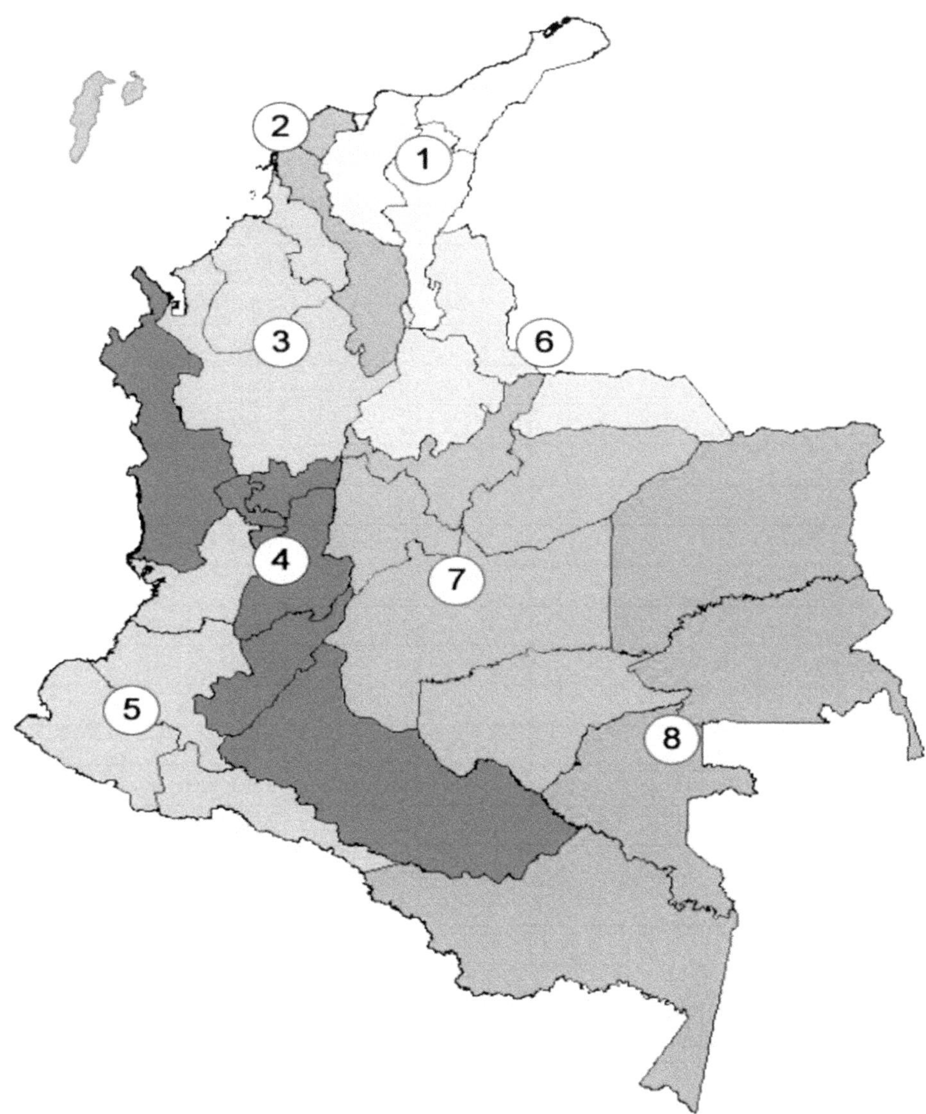

and means of transportation (land, air, and sea) to bring a product to the remote parts of the country and achieve full coverage of the territory, as shown in Table 2.

From the delivery points, products are either delivered to the executing units or those units go to the delivery points to pick up the commands. Those units are in charge of distribution of the products to the beneficiaries. Each unit has a set of beneficiaries that are assigned to it and a weekly distribution plan. Depending on a type of the beneficiaries (hospitals, nurseries, households, etc.), demand is either shipped or collected by a beneficiary. This final echelon of the chain is difficult to be steered since no trace-ability exists after the executing units pick up the goods. A recent study of the Universidad Nacional de Colombia shows that the production and distribution chain until the executing units result on negligible product loses. However, the interviews of a selected number of representatives of the executing units

Table 2. Logistic information about the Bienestarina distribution process in Colombia

Macro-region	Regional warehouse	Number of delivery points	Main transport modes
1	La Guajira	24	Land
	Cesar	238	Land, River
	Magdalena	279	Land, River
2	San Andrés	12	Land, Sea
	Atlántico	295	Land
	Bolívar	350	Land, River
3	Sucre	13	Land, River
	Córdoba	47	Land
	Antioquia	359	Land
4	Caquetá	31	Land, River
	Risaralda	44	Land, River
	Quindío	44	Land
	Chocó	115	Land, River, Sea
	Caldas	119	Land
	Tolima	177	Land
	Huila	188	Land
5	Putumayo	9	Land, River
	Nariño	72	Land, Sea
	Cauca	97	Land, River, Sea
	Valle	341	Land, Sea
6	Arauca	17	Land, River
	Santander	150	Land
	Norte de Santander	397	Land
7	Casanare	44	Land
	Guaviare	47	Land, River, Air
	Meta	124	Land, River, Air
	Boyacá	156	Land
	Cundinamarca	185	Land
	Bogotá	626	Land
8	Guainía	2	Land, River, Air
	Vaupés	7	River, Air
	Amazonas	9	Land, River, Air
	Vichada	14	Land. River, Air

Source: Authors' elaboration from Colombian Institute of Familiar Wellness (2009)

made the authors to identify some dysfunctions in this last echelon. The first is that several beneficiaries do not collect the products systematically, and a reassignment is not expected by the plans. The second is a non-negligible rate of self-consumption of the products, mainly those not claimed by the beneficiaries. The third is a difficulty to have an in-deep centralized knowledge of the entire final distribution system (an information system had not been implemented when the case study was constructed), which do not allow to have a complete product traceability. Moreover, local press reports some unfair practices, like using the product to feed farming animals instead of the population under malnutrition, but those practices have not been observed and confirmed (since they are made by a set of executing units and, being illegal, are hidden to any surveying action). However, in order to improve the efficiency of this last echelon and the entire supply chain, the ICBF has recently deployed an information system (which comes in full operation in 2017) and contributes to several research projects with Colombian leading universities.

Although the Bienestarina powder is the main product under distribution, there are other products provided to the beneficiaries. There is liquid Bienestarina (with three flavors) based on milk also produced and distributed. Moreover, some artisanal products are also produced locally. Indeed, some primary distribution points and executing units are engaged in the manufacture of food products using Bienestarina as an ingredient (cakes, biscuits, juices, etc.). Those products which need Bienestarina powder are produced locally and mainly use local agricultural products (fruits but also some flours and sugar cane products) resulting in the development of local industries. Beneficiaries of the product have a possibility to go to the executing units or corresponding primary distribution points to receive the product, just as the executing units has to go to the primary distribution point to receive the product, as shown by the purple arrows in Figure 2 with opposite way to the regular supply chain.

To summarize, the Bienestarina supply chain can be characterized as follows. The authors define the longitudinal structure of Bienestarina supply chain as shown in Figure 3. The Bienestarina supply chain counts six echelons when considering various steps from raw material (RM) suppliers to final consumers (beneficiaries):

- Only one echelon is related to the suppliers since the factories do the complete production process, so the suppliers provide the factories with raw materials only, without any industrial transformation before arriving at the factories. The only exception to this statement is that of vitamins and oligo-elements, which can be acquired from specific industrial producers.
- One echelon is related to production, although it could be decoupled in other three echelons: one for flour production, one for Bienestarina powder production (resulting in the mix of different flours, with the addition of vitamins and oligo-elements), and the third, when applicable, related to the production of elaborated products with the addition of Bienestarina. Currently, two main types of elaborated products are proposed: enriched liquid milk and cookies.
- Three echelons are related to the distribution system, which shows the importance and main place of the distribution system in the overall Bienestarina supply chain.
- The last echelon is related to the beneficiaries.

In order to illustrate the proposed characterization framework, the authors synthesized the four planning elements (steering, organization, development, and financing) (Table 3).

This exploratory overview of the Bienestarina system shows that the Bienestarina logistics follows a supply chain management structure, but there are substantial differences with respect to commercial logistics chains. The steering of the supply chain is ensured by the customer (the ICBF and the end-

Figure 3. Scheme of Bienestarina distribution chain
Source: Authors' own elaboration based on Colombian Institute of Familiar Wellness (2009)

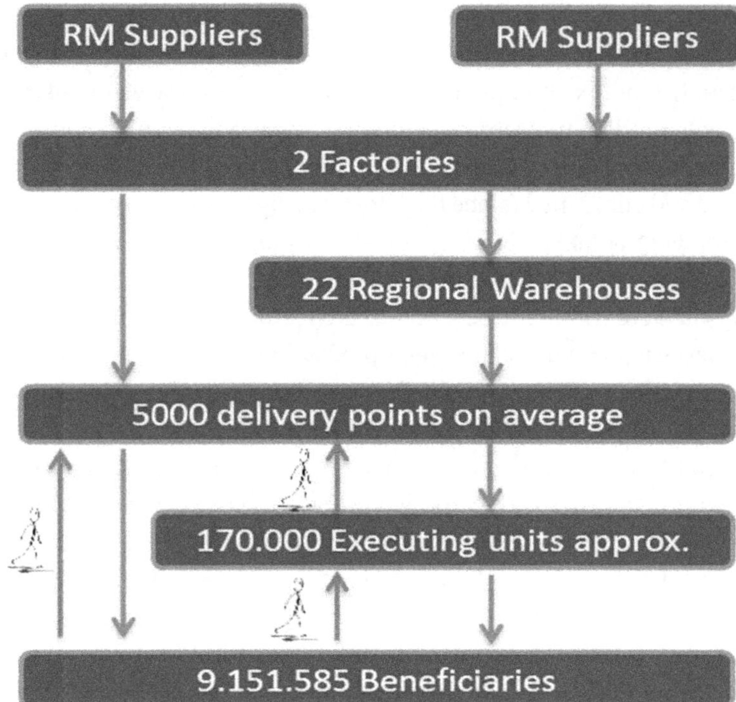

consumer (beneficiaries) are not customers). The rates of beneficiaries are established by the ICBF with local authorities (customer of the customer), adding a complex commercial/use chain with little impact on supply chain organization and steering. However, the logistics operations need to be ensured, and although there is not an evident relation between the service quality and the satisfaction of the consumer, the steering organization (ICBF) evaluates the global satisfaction of the system.

But is this system a specificity of Bienestarina or Colombian context? To give a preliminary set of elements to the discussion, the authors propose to explore other three systems: two in Mexico and one in Peru.

SOLUTIONS AND RECOMMENDATIONS

This product, exclusive of Colombia and developed and distributed under welfare programs of the Colombian Ministry of Familiar Protection, cannot be found in any other country. However, the logistics system presents similarities to other products and programs in the world. For example, in Mexico, two similar programs exist. The first is LICONSA which is aimed at production and distribution of a nutritionally-improved milk. It is not free, but its price is much lower than those of classical milk. The product is mainly distributed to sensible population locations. The second program is DICONSA which is a public company that produces and distributes flour (mainly of corn, but other variants are also produced) to public restaurants (mainly nurseries, schools, and hospitals).

Table 3. Synthesis of planning elements in the Bienestarina supply chain

Methods and structures	Steering structure	Organizational aspects	Development issues	Financial elements
Planning and control methods	The system is entirely steered and planned by the ICBF. Ingredion adjusts and executes those plans.	The entire supply chain is planned and controlled by Ingredion following global planning methods.		
Workflow and activity structure		SCM is made by Ingredion. Operations are managed by Ingredion, and only follow-up reports for yearly updating of the contract are made by the ICBF. Local agriculture at the national level is promoted.	Supply chain activities were firstly managed by the ICBF, then subcontracted. From 2007, the current system is implemented.	The service is paid by public entities through the beneficiary tickets to the ICBF, which then uses the funds to finance the supply chain costs
Organization structure		ICBF is a very hierarchical structure with many departments. Ingredion is more specialized but also has a hierarchical structure.	The organizational structure has not been strongly evolved over the years	
Information and communication structure	There is no traceability system. The steering of the supply chain is decentralized. The information exchange between the ICBF and Ingredion concerns monthly and yearly indicators of quantities delivered.	Exchanges on a number of beneficiaries between the ICBF and Ingredion, linear structure following the supply chain structure for internal transactions.		
Product flow structure	-	6-echelon supply chain: raw material suppliers, production plants, regional warehouses, delivery points, executing units, and beneficiaries	Number and variety of products and diversity of flows grow. The structure is similar for all of them.	
Management methods	Management is facilitated by Ingredion. Vertical management seems to be predominant.	Executing units are mono-personal or very small structures (no need of strong management methods); plants and warehouses use classic SCM methods.	Management has evolved over the last years towards the adoption of international SCM standards.	
Power and leadership structure	ICBF is a "customer" configuration since it purchases services from Indredion.	The supply chain has a very decentralized leadership structure which embarrasses the identification of dysfunctions and improvement opportunities.		
Risks and rewards structure	Risks are forecasted by the ICBF, but operational issues are steered and managed by Ingredion.	No rewards structure has been identified. Main risks are related to transport/traffic conditions, ruptures in raw materials, production problems and losses/bad use of products in the different echelons of the supply chain.		Risks are assumed by Ingredion but can be shared with the ICBF.
Culture and attitude	The decentralized steering and the lack of traceability have an impact on losses at the final levels.		With the increase of information about the system, collective conscience and solidarity have increased.	Not all public authorities have the same sensibility to promote the system and buy services.

Source: Authors' own elaboration

The LICONSA program was established in 1944 with the objective of increasing supply of milk by ensuring of its good quality and affordable prices for the population in a vulnerable situation.

Taking into account the results of this work and comparing them with the analysis of the logistics processes of the LICONSA supply chain (Mexican nutritional enriched-milk), some differences and similarities have been found.

Differences:

- Percentage of population served is 5.97% in Mexico and 19.14% in Colombia. In Columbia, 1 out of 5 citizens is served, while in Mexico, only 1 out of 20 citizens, respectively.
- In Mexico, the LICONSA distribution process is supported by the use of the geographic location system (SISGE). This system allows an optimization of a sale point location, in order to be more efficient in terms of delivery time, distance, routes, among others.
- Similarities:
- Production and distribution processes are managed by the public entities (the ICBF in Colombia and the SEDESOL in Mexico) which are in charge of ensuring the well-being of the population.
- Beneficiaries are the people who are in the conditions of food vulnerability.
- The last mile distribution is similar. There are established final points (sale points, executing units) which are the ones that have contact with the target population.

The authors could also establish a parallel with DICONSA (a flour-based product similar to Bienesta-rina, also for Mexican families) or with the Peruvian Glass of Milk program (Programa Vaso de Leche) (Ministerio de Desarrollo e Inclusión Social, 2013), which both aim to distribution of nutritionally-enriched menus, mainly for breakfasts or pre-dinner meals, to schools. In both cases, the main difference is that the beneficiaries are not families, but public entities, making the product traceability higher and the process easier to monitor and plan. However, in all four cases, the authors observe similar patterns, related to the four elements defined above. More precisely:

- On the financing viewpoint, all those systems start from public concern and need public support. However, the percentages of public financing capacity, as well as the mechanisms of refunding or distributing funds, are not standardized. However, it is clear that an efficient organization is needed to ensure the good use of those funds.
- On the development viewpoint, their evolution depends on that of the beneficiaries. In other words, those systems have a vocation to support the nutrition development of families. More they contribute to this nutritional development, fewer products are needed. The disappearance of those supply chains as useless would be a consequence of the good use and deployment of the food distribution systems for social improvement. However, this final stage is far to arrive, but the evolution in the number and nature of beneficiaries is a good indicator of the global performance of the social improvement logistic schemes.
- On the steering viewpoint, those systems are promoted and guided by public entities, mainly in the form of yearly or multi-yearly plans. The way those plans are actuated and deployed depends on the national (or regional) context, but in general, the logistics management is made by the ex-perts who act as subcontractors of the public entity. The role of public authorities is to monitor the subcontractors, finance the distribution system, and verify correct actuation of the yearly plans.

- Finally, the organization of the supply chain seems to be a consequence of the other three elements. Different choices can be made, but Bienestarina is following an integrated supply chain with the consequent management choices, steered by a subcontractor. This seems to be the case of LICONSA, DICONSA, and Programa Vaso de Leche, so the first statement that can be induced is the need of deploying efficient and integrated supply chains even if there is no product to sell and no economic value. However, the social value of social improvement of supply chains is clearly identifiable, and in a context of limited resources and high needs in terms of malnutrition reduction, this efficiency seems crucial.

FUTURE RESEARCH DIRECTIONS

All four initiatives seem to incite the use of local producers and are based on the extraction and transformation of raw products which are cultivated or produced in a country. However, the details on the contribution of such systems to local production economics need to be studied further.

The work completed by the authors remains preliminary. A wider comparison with other initiatives existing in Latin America and a qualitative interview-based analysis on key stakeholders of the Bienestarina supply chain would give more evidence on the characteristics of social improvement supply chains and define the main analysis framework of those systems. Moreover, further researches should be focused on traceability and operations management in order to identify the major critical points of the Bienestarina supply chain and propose management guidelines to improve their efficiency and sustainability.

CONCLUSION

The ICBF program of Bienestarina is considered one of the main actions to combat the problems of malnutrition in Colombia, which demonstrates reductions in the rates of chronic malnutrition and underweight (Colombian Institute of Familiar Wellness, Instituto Nacional de Salud, Profamilia, Ministerio de Protección Social, & DANE, 2010). This is why it is important to characterize the supply chain deployed to bring Bienestarina just in time and making compliance with the fundamental rights of the vulnerable population. For the crucial contribution of logistics to reach the main objectives of the Bienestarina plans, this case is a good example of social improvement logistics.

Via adaptation of the analysis framework of Gonzalez-Feliu et al. (2014) to Bienestarina, and a synthetic comparison of this system to similar social improvement logistics initiatives in Latin America, the authors have defined the main patterns of agroindustrial-based social improvement logistics and highlighted the importance of logistics efficiency in non-economically deployed logistics networks.

The authors observe that the logistics chain of Bienestarina presents particularities with respect to commercial logistics (by the fact that the end consumer is not the customer who pays for the product), resulting in the central role of the public entity managing and contracting the logistics system. The operator is making a service (close to that of commercial logistics, with lower costs), but the indicators for evaluating the performance of this supply chain seem different (since the customer's satisfaction is not measured, and instead the capacity of reaching families is preferred as the main measure of satisfaction). On the other hand, and with respect to humanitarian logistics in disasters, the urgent nature of distribution and suffering is perceived differently. The aim of social improvement logistics is to improve the quality of life in a medium-long term, whereas that of humanitarian logistics in disasters is to reduce suffering as quickly as possible.

Without entering to compare in-depth those three types of logistics, the authors observe that social improvement logistics seems to have particularities that make it different from other humanitarian logistics and commercial logistics. This chapter gives a first analysis by applying a combined analysis framework but remains exploratory. More in-depth analyses will be required to characterize social improvement logistics. Moreover, the question of evaluation, then of deploying suitable dashboards, on the line of current works for urban logistics (Gonzalez-Feliu & Morana, 2014; Morana & Gonzalez-Feliu, 2015) specific to dietary complement supply chains for social improvement would be an important future development of this research.

REFERENCES

Adivar, B., Atan, T., Sevil Oflaç, B., & Örten, T. (2010). Improving Social Welfare Chain Using Optimal Planning Model. *Supply Chain Management: An International Journal*, *15*(4), 290–305. doi:10.1108/13598541011054661

Braun, J., & Kennedy, E. T. (1994). *Agricultural Commercialization, Economic Development, and Nutrition*. Baltimore, MD: Johns Hopkins University Press.

Colombian Institute of Familiar Wellness. (2009). *Bienestarina: Distribución, cuidado y uso de un recurso sagrado*. Bogotá: ICBF.

Colombian Institute of Familiar Wellness. Instituto Nacional de Salud, Profamilia, Ministerio de Protección Social, & DANE. (2010). Encuesta Nacional de La Situación Nutricional En Colombia 2010 – ENSIN. Bogotá: Ministerio de Protección Social.

Cuevas García, R. (2005). *El diseño de los programas de alimentación escolar y la función de la industria alimentaria*. Retrieved November 26, 2016, from http://www.fao.org/docrep/008/y5906m/Y5906M05.htm

Dirección Nacional de Planeación. (2006). *Conpes 3443. Contratación del operador para la producción y distribución del componente nutricional (Bienestarina) en el Instituto Colombiano de Bienestar Familiar*. Bogotá: ICBF, Dirección Nacional de Planeación.

Dirección Nacional de Planeación. (2007). *Conpes 113. Política Nacional de Seguridad Alimentaria Y Nutricional (PSAN)*. Bogotá: Dirección Nacional de Planeación.

El Nuevo Siglo. (2013). *Lupa oficial a la Bienestarina*. Retrieved March 2, 2017, from http://www.elnuevosiglo.com.co/articulos/5-2013-lupa-oficial-bienestarina.html

Ewing, M., & Msangi, S. (2009). Biofuels Production in Developing Countries: Assessing Tradeoffs in Welfare and Food Security. *Environmental Science & Policy*, *12*(4), 520–528. doi:10.1016/j.envsci.2008.10.002

Food and Agriculture Organization of the United Nations. (2010). *La Iniciativa América Latina y Caribe sin Hambre*. Rome: Food and Agriculture Organization of the United Nations.

Food and Agriculture Organization of the United Nations. (2011). *Global Food Losses and Food Waste. Study Conducted for the International Congress SAVE FOOD!* Rome: Food and Agriculture Organization of the United Nations.

Fortucci, P. (2002). *The Contribution of Cotton to Economy and Food Security in Developing Countries.* Retrieved March 2, 2017, from https://www.icac.org/meetings/cgtn_conf/documents/11_fortucci.pdf

Gonzalez-Feliu, J., Malhéné, N., Morganti, E., & Morana, J. (2014). The Deployment of City and Area Distribution Centers in France and Italy: Comparison of Six Representative Models. *Supply Chain Forum: An International Journal, 15*(4), 84–99.

Gonzalez-Feliu, J., & Morana, J. (2014). Assessing Urban Logistics Pooling Sustainability via a Hierarchic Dashboard from a Group Decision Perspective. In C. Macharis, S. Melo, J. Woxenius, & T. Van Lier (Eds.), *Sustainable Logistics* (pp. 113–135). Bingley, UK: Emerald Group Publishing. doi:10.1108/S2044-994120140000006004

Gonzalez-Feliu, J., Taniguchi, E., & d'Arcier, B. F. (2014). Financing Urban Logistics Projects. In J. Gonzalez-Feliu, F. Semet, & J.-L. Frédéric (Eds.), *Sustainable Urban Logistics: Concepts, Methods and Information Systems* (pp. 245–265). Berlin: Springer. doi:10.1007/978-3-642-31788-0_13

Holguin-Veras, J., Jaller, M., Van Wassenhove, L. N., Pérez, N., & Wachtendorf, T. (2012). On the Unique Features of Post-Disaster Humanitarian Logistics. *Journal of Operations Management, 30*(7), 494–506. doi:10.1016/j.jom.2012.08.003

Holguin-Veras, J., Wachtendorf, T., Jaller, M., & Jefferson, T. (2013). Logistics and the Management of Critical Supplies Following Catastrophes. In R. Bissell (Ed.), *Preparedness and Response for Catastrophic Disasters* (pp. 131–150). Boca Raton, FL: CRC Press.

Kovács, G., & Spens, K. M. (2007). Humanitarian Logistics in Disaster Relief Operations. *International Journal of Physical Distribution & Logistics Management, 37*(2), 99–114. doi:10.1108/09600030710734820

Kovács, G., & Spens, K. M. (2009). Identifying Challenges in Humanitarian Logistics. *International Journal of Physical Distribution & Logistics Management, 39*(6), 506–528. doi:10.1108/09600030910985848

Lambert, D. M. (2001). The Supply Chain Management and Logistics Controversy. In A. M. Brewer, K. M. Button, & D. A. Hensher (Eds.), *Handbook of Logistics and Supply Chain Management* (pp. 99–126). Oxford, UK: Pergamon Press.

Lambert, D. M., Cooper, M. C., & Pagh, J. D. (1998). Supply Chain Management: Implementation Issues and Research Opportunities. *The International Journal of Logistics Management, 9*(2), 1–20. doi:10.1108/09574099810805807

Maldonado, M., & Moya, S. (2013). The Challenge of Implementing Reverse Logistics in Social Improvement: The Possibility of Expanding Sovereignty Food in Developing Communities. In J. Cheung & H. Song (Eds.), *Logistics: Perspectives, Approaches and Challenges* (pp. 1–34). New York, NY: Nova Science Publishers.

Ministerio de Desarrollo e Inclusión Social. (2013). *Programa Vaso de Leche.* Lima: Gobierno de la República del Perú.

Morana, J., & Gonzalez-Feliu, J. (2015). A Sustainable Urban Logistics Dashboard from the Perspective of a Group of Operational Managers. *Management Research Review*, *38*(10), 1068–1085. doi:10.1108/MRR-11-2014-0260

Orbell, J. M., & Dawes, R. M. (1993). Social Welfare, Cooperators Advantage, and the Option of not Playing the Game. *American Sociological Review*, *58*(6), 787–800. doi:10.2307/2095951

Palacios, L., Morana, J., Gonzalez-Feliu, J., & Devia, J. (2016). Traceability for a More Sustainable Supply Chain Management: The Case of Bienestarina in Colombia. In *Proceedings of the Third International Conference on Green Supply Chain Management*. London: Loughborough University.

Peñaloza, C., Palacios, L., & Gonzalez-Feliu, J. (2016). Characterization of the Collection and Distribution Processes of Bienestarina in Bogotá. In *Proceedings of the International Workshop on Franchising & Distribution Networks in Emerging Countries*. Saint-Etienne: Jean Monet University.

Presidencia de la República. (2013). *Bienestarina Más' llegará gratuitamente este año a 6,5 millones de beneficiarios, especialmente niños y niñas de la primera infancia*. Retrieved November 23, 2016, from http://wsp.presidencia.gov.co/Prensa/2013/Febrero/Paginas/20130228_07.aspx

Reutlinger, S. (1986). *Poverty and Hunger: Issues and Options for Food Security in Developing Countries. A World Bank Policy Study*. Washington, DC: World Bank.

Rozo, C. (2000). Complementary Foods in Colombia. *Food and Nutrition Bulletin*, *21*(1), 55–61. doi:10.1177/156482650002100109

Stock, J. R. (1990). Logistics Thought and Practice: A Perspective. *International Journal of Physical Distribution & Logistics Management*, *20*(1), 3–6. doi:10.1108/09600039010140845

Supply Chain Council. (2008). *Supply-Chain Operations Reference-Model. Overview of SCOR version, 5(0)*. Chicago, IL: Supply Chain Council.

Valdes, A. (1981). *Food Security for Developing Countries*. Boulder, CO: Westview Press.

ADDITIONAL READING

Colombian Institute of Familiar Wellness. (2013). *Logística de distribución en el territorio nacional*. Bogotá: ICBF.

Diaz-Bonilla, E., Thomas, M., Robinson, S., & Cattaneo, A. (2000). *Food Security and Trade Negotiations in the World Trade Organization*. Washington, DC: International Food Policy Research Institute.

Eisenhardt, K. M. (1989). Building Theories from Case Study Research. *Academy of Management Review*, *14*(4), 532–550.

Food and Agriculture Organization of the United Nations. (2016a). *Global Food Composition Database for Pulses. Version 1.0 -uPulses1.0 User guide*. Rome: FAO.

Food and Agriculture Organization of the United Nations. (2016b). *International Network of Food Data Systems: International Food Composition Tables/Database Directory*. Rome: FAO.

Godfray, H. C. J., Beddington, J. R., Crute, I. R., Haddad, L., Lawrence, D., Muir, J. F., ... Toulmin, C. (2010). Food Security: The Challenge of Feeding 9 Billion People. *Science*, *327*(5967), 812–818. doi:10.1126cience.1185383 PMID:20110467

IA Alimentos. (2013). *El ICBF producirá 25 mil toneladas de bienestarina en el 2013*. Retrieved January 27, 2017, from http://www.revistaialimentos.com.co/news/1223/443/El-ICBF-producira-25-mil-toneladas-de-bienestarina-en-el-2013.htm

Lutter, C. K. (2003). Macrolevel Approaches to Improve the Availability of Complementary Foods. *Food and Nutrition Bulletin*, *24*(1), 83–103. doi:10.1177/156482650302400105 PMID:12664528

Pinstrup-Andersen, P. (2009). Food Security: Definition and Measurement. *Food Security*, *1*(1), 5–7. doi:10.100712571-008-0002-y

KEY TERMS AND DEFINITIONS

Bienestarina Program: A production-distribution program of a dietary complement, called Bienestarina, steered by the Colombian government (more precisely, the Colombian Institute of Familiar Welfare (ICBF)) to fight malnutrition on sensible populations.

Commercial Logistics: A set of techniques and methods dealing with planning, design, and support of business operations that deal with procurement, purchase, inventory, warehousing, distribution, and transportation, among others, in order to bring a product or service to its final user.

Dietary Complement: A product intended for ingestion that contains a "dietary ingredient" intended to add further nutritional value to the diet. A dietary complement is ingested alone (or diluted with water) and aims to supply to deficiencies in diets by substitution to traditional foods on only the concerning elements, like some vitamins or minerals). Dietary complements may be found in many forms such as tablets, capsules, soft gels, gelcaps, liquids, or powders.

Dietary Ingredient: One or any combination of the following substances: vitamins, minerals, herbs (or botanical products), amino acids, concentrates, metabolite, constituents, or extracts. It can be used to complement diets and meals.

Humanitarian Logistics: A set of logistics operations deployed to react to emergencies (natural or human-based), and which follow a completely different logic than commercial logistics.

Social Improvement Logistics: A set of logistics operations developed to improve the social status of populations, which are of lower urgency than those of humanitarian logistics but follow aims and issues which remain different than those of commercial logistics.

Supply Chain Management: An integrated management strategy that includes the planning and management of all activities involved in sourcing and procurement, conversion, and all logistics management activities, from the extraction of raw materials to the delivery at the retailers' or end- consumers' locations, and including all the different stages.

This research was previously published in Establishing Food Security and Alternatives to International Trade in Emerging Economies edited by Vasily Erokhin; pages 297-315, copyright year 2018 by Business Science Reference (an imprint of IGI Global).

Chapter 45
State Support of Agricultural Production in Emerging Countries as a Tool to Ensure Food Security

Marina Lescheva
Stavropol State Agrarian University, Russian Federation

Anna Ivolga
Stavropol State Agrarian University, Russia

Oleksandr Labenko
National University of Life and Environmental Sciences of Ukraine, Ukraine

ABSTRACT

The chapter examines the practices of state support of agricultural production in various emerging economies in comparison with selected OECD countries. The aim of the research is to discover how agricultural protectionism and support of domestic farmers affect the level of food security on the emerging markets in the conditions of expanding globalization and liberalization of trade in food. The authors focus on the evaluation of the best practices of state support and discovery of opportunities of their utilization on the emerging markets. Content and mechanisms of state regulation are examined based on the data and evaluation methods obtained from the Organization for Economic Cooperation and Development (OECD). The authors find out that the system of state regulation is one of the key determinants of achieving food security in the conditions of turbulent emerging markets. Both the volume and priority directions of state support of agriculture are determined by financial capacities of emerging economies and current goals of their agrarian policies.

DOI: 10.4018/978-1-7998-5354-1.ch045

INTRODUCTION

International experience of development of agriculture confirms that performance is only possible based on the effective state support. Bearing in mind special role of agricultural production in ensurance of food security and sustainable social and economic development, governments of the leading countries of the world forward substantial resources on the support of domestic agricultural producers, food market regulation, rural social programs, and environment protection. Such measures undertaken as much as possible by most every country affect domestic food markets, agricultural production, and food security.

While international trade in recent decades has been gradually liberalized, trade in agricultural products and food has remained among the ones most influenced by international regulations and national policies (Božić, Bogdanov, & Ševarlić, 2011). As of Markovic and Markovic (2014), agricultural protectionism is a part of the agricultural policy of almost every country. It is focused on the selection of measures of foreign trade and economic policies to achieve the protection of agricultural sector and domestic food market from foreign competition. In a broader dimension, protectionist policies in the form of state support of agricultural production are aimed at the development of sustainable food production, ensurance of food security of a country, and sustainable management of natural resources.

As of Erokhin, Ivolga, and Heijman (2014), developed countries implement a wide range of tools that affect the competitiveness of domestic farmers and food security both directly and indirectly. Such policies support the effective elimination of price disparity and growth of farmers' incomes. The offloading of agricultural surpluses of developed countries on the world market brings down prices and creates disincentives for local producers in many developing countries where agriculture is the main source of livelihood for a major part of the population.

The case of emerging economies is different. In such countries, institutional reforms often lay behind the paces of economic growth and integration to the global market (Erokhin, 2015). Sustainability of domestic food market requires the development of institutions, but such institutional development can be extremely costly on emerging markets. In the early 1990s, due to the difficult economic situation, many emerging countries decreased the level of state support of agriculture and undertaken reductions in the protection of their domestic food markets, at considerable pain and effort, largely with a view to enhancing the supply of food products for their populations. Trade liberalization was successfully implemented in countries where this process was sustained for a long period. In the short run, trade liberalization as a way to increase food security is often painful and may be even damaging for emerging economies, which cannot compete against free trade. Liberalization froze state support and left emerging economies with very few policy instruments to protect themselves from food imports and to subsidize their agriculture.

Despite the certain progress in economic growth during the 2000-2010s, most of the emerging economies still fail to support domestic farmers on a level comparable with the developed states. In many cases, volumes of domestic support gained by farmers in emerging countries are tenfold lower than those in the developed states (Erokhin et al., 2014). Domestic production of basic agricultural products and food in many emerging countries, including such big agricultural producers as Russia, China, Brazil, India, and Argentina fails to meet demand. Providing the population with food in sufficient quantity and variety is a challenge, which includes a range of issues of food production, import dependence and export orientation of the food market, solvency and dietary patterns of the population. Many emerging economies have to rely on agricultural imports, leaving them vulnerable to global price fluctuations and affecting their export revenues, which tremendously threat food security of those nations.

BACKGROUND

State support of agriculture and its influence on food security have been investigated by many authors. In relation to the state support policies implemented in the developed countries, Josling, Anderson, Schmitz, and Tangerman (2010) focused on linkages between state support, international trade in agricultural products, and food security. Schmitz, Moss, Schmitz, Furtan, and Schmitz (2010) investigated current agricultural policies in the USA and other developed countries and elaborated prognosis of agricultural policies for the next decades. Issues of state support of agriculture in the light of liberalization of international trade in food were researched by Devereux (1999), Boehringer and Rutherford (1999), and Estevadeordal, Freund, and Ornelas (2008).

Experiences of emerging countries in the sphcrc of state support of agriculture have been studied by Petrikov (2012, 2016), Filippov (2014), Malozemov (2014), Visser, Mamonova, Spoor, and Nikulin (2015), and others. Anderson, Jha, and Nelgen (2013) impacted into research of political issues of agricultural protectionism and disarrays on international food market in relation to developing countries and emerging economies of Asia. Wittman, Desmarais, and Wiebe (2010) studied the specifics of food sovereignty in emerging countries in the conditions of growing degree of trade liberalization. As regards to the influences of trade liberalization on food security in emerging countries, Olson (2003) investigated the alternatives to the global trade order and claimed that an expansion of the Agreement on Agriculture of the World Trade Organization (WTO) would make all countries' food security increasingly uncertain and dependent on volatile international market prices and far-flung distribution chain. Liefert and Swinnen (2002) investigated changes in agricultural markets in transition economies, and later Liefert (2004) studied food security issues in Russia in the conditions of economic growth during the early 2000s. In this study, he concluded that the main food security problem was inadequate access to food by certain socioeconomic groups, which lacked sufficient purchasing power to afford a minimally healthy diet (Liefert, 2004). It is true not only for Russia but for many other emerging economies.

The specifics of the emerging markets is that they are very turbulent. There is still no clear understanding of how state support influences food security on the emerging markets in terms of four pillars of food security, i.e. availability, access, stability, and utilization. How limited tools of state support and growing openness to import of food in the conditions of trade liberalization influences domestic agricultural production, farmers and rural dwellers in the emerging countries? In all variety of conducted research, what is needed now is a rethink of international experience. The goal of the given research is an aggregation of international practices and investigation of opportunities for development of state regulation of agriculture in emerging countries with the aim to ensure food security in the conditions of import substitution and an increase of domestic agricultural production.

In this chapter, content and mechanisms of state regulation of agriculture are investigated based on the data and evaluation parameters obtained from the Organization for Economic Cooperation and Development (OECD). According to the OECD's approach, state support of agriculture includes the following elements:

- **Producer Support Estimate (PSE):** Annual monetary value of gross transfers from consumers and taxpayers to support agricultural producers, arising from policy measures, regardless of their nature, objectives or impacts on farm production or income.

- **General Services Support Estimate (GSSE):** Annual monetary value of gross transfers to services provided collectively to agriculture and arising from policy measures which support agriculture.
- **Consumer Support Estimate (CSE):** Includes explicit and implicit transfers associated with compensation to consumers of high market prices for agricultural commodities.
- Aggregated support of agriculture includes the overall amount of transfers received by agricultural producers at the expense of taxpayers and consumers (support of market price); gross transfers from taxpayers to consumers of agricultural products, and transfers at the expense of taxpayers to services provided collectively to agriculture.

OECD unites 34 countries which aggregated share in the global GDP is about 80%. Institutional and structural shifts in the evolution of basic approaches and content of state support of agriculture in those countries reflect specific features of state regulation of agriculture in the modern era of globalization in the conditions of aggravation of global challenges. They have to be considered when correcting the measures of state support of agriculture in emerging countries in order to ensure food security. In the OECD countries, almost one-third of farmers' income on average is not actually earned in agricultural markets, but rather comes from a range of government subsidies and other support measures that restrict agricultural trade and distort markets (Secretariat of the Convention on Biological Diversity, 2005). Effects of such distortions, both positive and negative ones, have to be carefully assessed in order to balance state support, protection, and liberalization policies. The research objective is to find out the key regularities of state support of agriculture in emerging countries and to discover the opportunities of using of accumulated experience for the development of a national mechanism of state regulation of agriculture in the conditions of import substitution policy and an increase of domestic agricultural production.

For the purposes of the present research, the authors used the approach of the United Nations Department of Economic and Social Affairs (DESA) and the United Nations Conference on Trade and Development (UNCTAD), i.e. considered 17 economies (Albania, Armenia, Azerbaijan, Belarus, Bosnia and Herzegovina, Georgia, Kazakhstan, Kyrgyzstan, Macedonia, Moldova, Montenegro, Russia, Serbia, Tajikistan, Turkmenistan, Ukraine, and Uzbekistan) as emerging ones. Additionally, the authors considered seven countries (China, Brazil, India, Vietnam, Laos, Cambodia, and South Africa) recognized as emerging ones by the World Bank and the International Monetary Fund. The research is based on the system methodology. It combines various methods of scientific knowledge, such as monographic, economic and statistical analysis, grouping, trend and comparative analysis.

MAIN FOCUS OF THE CHAPTER

Trade in Food in the Emerging Economies

Despite the resource-oriented model of export, most of the emerging economies are engaged in international trade in other commodities, apart from oil, including food and agricultural products. According to Liefert and Swinnen (2002), during the 1970-1980s, most of the agricultural exports went to the Soviet Union (exports of meat by Hungary, Romania, Ukraine and Kazakhstan; grain by Hungary, Ukraine, and Kazakhstan; sugar by Ukraine; and cotton by Uzbekistan and Turkmenistan). During 1995-2015,

Figure 1. Developed and developing countries and emerging economies by foreign trade turnover in food and agricultural products in 1995-2015, $ billion
Source: Authors' development based on the United Nations Conference on Trade and Development [UNCTAD] (2016)

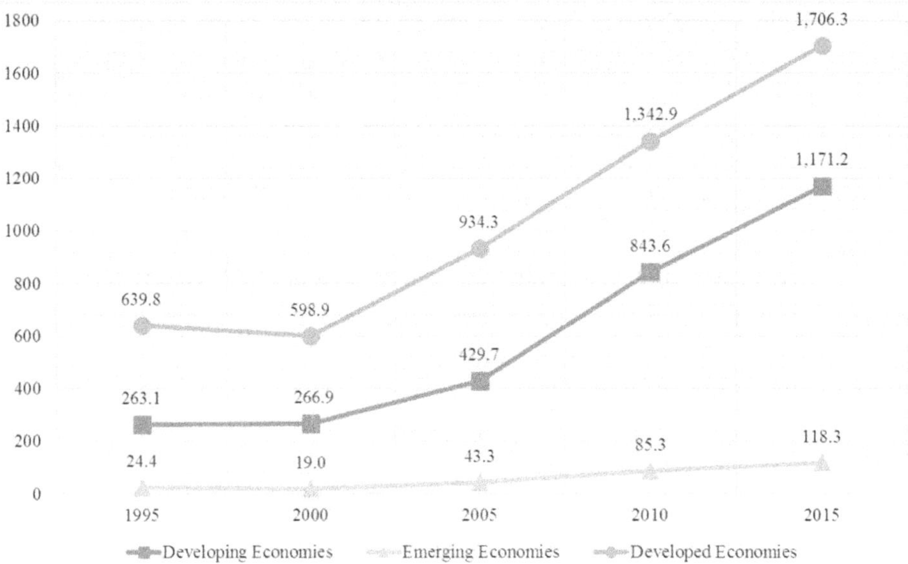

foreign trade turnover of the emerging economies continued to grow steadily and increased fivefold ($118.3 billion in 2015 in comparison with only $24.4 billion in 1995) (Figure 1).

As of Liefert and Swinnen (2002), the pre-reform trade in agriculture for the emerging economies was not market driven but rather was an integral part of countries' economic planning, i.e. resulted from politics, not economics. When most of the emerging economies liberalized trade in the early 1990s, they experienced a collapse in the export of their agricultural products to the world and dramatic rise of import flows to their domestic food markets. Export/import ratio in foreign trade turnover (FTT) in food and agricultural products in 1995 was 25/75, while developed countries had equal proportions of export and import flows in their foreign trade (Table 1). During two decades, emerging economies succeeded in balancing their foreign trade turnover to 44/56 in 2015, but import still prevails.

Table 1. Proportion of export and import flows in total trade in food and agricultural products among developed countries and emerging economies in 1995-2015, %

Group of countries	year					Change in 2015 in comparison with 1995, percentage points
	1995	2000	2005	2010	2015	
Developed economies						
share of export in FTT in food	48.5	47.3	47.2	49.6	50.6	+2.1
share of import in FTT in food	51.5	52.7	52.8	50.4	49.4	-2.1
Emerging economies						
share of export in FTT in food	25.0	26.8	31.2	34.3	44.1	+19.1
share of import in FTT in food	75.0	73.2	68.8	65.7	55.9	-19.1

Source: Authors' development based on the UNCTAD (2016)

The share of emerging economies in world trade in food and agricultural products was 3.9% in 2015. It increased by 1.3 percentage points during two decades of transition (Table 2). Share in world import was higher than the one in world export (3.5% and 4.4%, consequently).

Table 2. Shares of developed countries and emerging economies in the world trade in food and agricultural products in 1995-2015, %

Group of countries	year					Change in 2015 in comparison with 1995, percentage points
	1995	2000	2005	2010	2015	
Developed economies						
share in world trade	69.0	67.7	66.4	59.1	57.0	-8.0
share in world export	67.6	66.2	64.3	58.9	57.5	-10.1
share in world import	70.3	69.0	68.3	45.4	56.5	-13.8
Emerging economies						
share in world trade	2.6	2.1	3.1	3.8	3.9	+1.3
share in world export	1.3	1.2	2.0	2.6	3.5	+2.2
share in world import	3.9	3.0	4.1	3.8	4.4	+0.5

Source: Authors' development based on the UNCTAD (2016)

Emerging economies are oriented on the world market rather than on the internal markets. In 2015, over 68% of the total trade of the emerging economies allotted to trade with developed and developing countries, and only 31.7% – to intra-group trade. Import of food and agricultural products is even more unbalanced – over 79% of deliveries come from the developed and developing economies, not from the emerging markets (Table 3).

Such a high dependency on import deliveries from developed countries along with the drop in domestic food production during the 1990-2010s have raised concerns about food security and food sovereignty in certain emerging economies in transition, especially Russia. The level of food security and changes during transition have differed importantly between the countries. However, domestic food markets in most of the emerging economies are to a greater extent influenced by internal factors (low competitiveness of food producers, their financial instability, outdated facilities, infrastructure, lowering effective demand, etc.), than external ones. Despite certain progress of reforms, volumes of GDP and foreign trade of the emerging economies are well below than those of the developed countries, while the share of foreign trade turnover in food and agricultural products in GDP is the highest among the groups of countries under consideration (4.5% for emerging economies in comparison with 4.0% for developing and 3.7% for developed countries) (Figure 2).

Consequently, emerging economies have to concentrate on solving internal problems and increasing efficiency of domestic agricultural production. The goal is to create a profitable, market-driven agricultural economy with productivity levels and supporting infrastructure that allows it to compete effectively on the world market. In order to increase their competitiveness on the global market most of the emerging economies implement various tools of state support of agriculture.

Table 3. Proportion of intra-group and extra-group trade in food and agricultural products among developed countries and emerging economies in 1995-2015, %

Group of countries	year					Change in 2015 in comparison with 1995, percentage points
	1995	2000	2005	2010	2015	
Developed economies						
Export: intra-group trade	73.9	76.3	79.1	73.2	70.6	-3.3
Export: extra-group trade	26.1	23.7	20.9	26.8	29.4	+3.3
Import: intra-group trade	69.2	69.4	70.7	69.6	69.4	+0.2
Import: extra-group trade	30.8	30.6	29.3	30.4	30.6	-0.2
Total: intra-group trade	71.5	72.7	74.6	71.3	70.0	-1.5
Total: extra-group trade	28.5	27.3	25.4	28.7	30.0	+1.5
Emerging economies						
Export: intra-group trade	60.7	58.8	53.3	46.4	36.2	-24.5
Export: extra-group trade	39.3	41.2	46.7	53.6	63.8	+24.5
Import: intra-group trade	23.5	26.6	25.5	25.5	28.1	+4.6
Import: extra-group trade	76.5	73.4	74.5	74.5	79.1	-4.6
Total: intra-group trade	32.8	35.3	34.4	32.7	31.7	-1.1
Total: extra-group trade	67.2	64.7	65.6	67.3	68.3	+1.1

Source: Authors' development based on the UNCTAD (2016)

Figure 2. Share of foreign trade turnover in food and agricultural products in GDP in developed, developing and emerging economies in 1995-2015, %
Source: Authors' development based on the UNCTAD (2016)

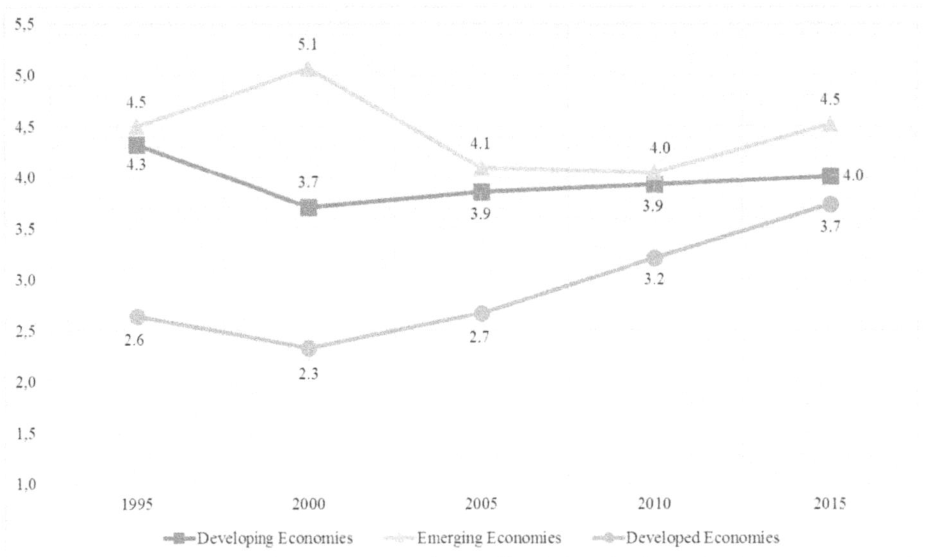

State Support of Agriculture and Effects for Food Security

Conducted analysis reveals that a system of state regulation is a key determinant of the development of agriculture. The strategic importance of support is proved by a complete synchronization of its amount with dynamics of gross agricultural production (GAP) and aggregated support of agriculture (ASA) (Figure 3).

Figure 3. GAP and ASA growth indices in selected countries (1995-1997 to 2012-2015)
Source: Authors' development based on the UNCTAD (2016)

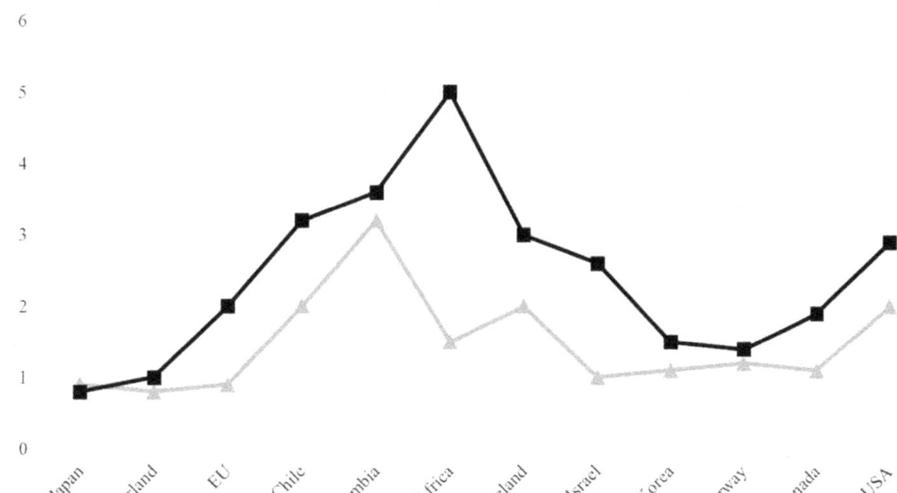

The increase of state support provides outrunning growth of gross agricultural production. When state support decreases and the index is below 1, gross agricultural production index changes correspondingly. It can be observed on the examples of Japan and Switzerland, where a decrease in state support (I = 0.7) was accompanied by a decrease in gross production (I = 0.8).

Analysis of state support in relation to the GDP allowed the authors to discover the tendency of its contraction in the majority of the countries over the previous 20 years (Figure 4).

Thus, in the EU, share of state support of agriculture in the GDP decreased from 1.5% down to 0.8%; in the USA, from 0.6% down to 0.5%; in Canada, from 0.8% down to 0.4%; in Russia, from 2.6% down to 0.7%. Exceptions to this tendency are China and Indonesia, where the relative level of support increased from 1.4% up to 3.2% and from 0.8% up to 3.6%, respectively. In Brazil, in the mid-1990s, part of incomes of agricultural producers was withdrawn in the favor of the state, but currently, agriculture benefits from the support amounted to 0.4% of the GDP. In general, among OECD countries, state support of agriculture decreased twofold (from 1.5% of the GDP in 1995 down to less than 0.8% in 2015). The most critical decrease happened in those countries, where the level of support was higher, i.e. Turkey, South Korea, Iceland, and Switzerland. However, it remains high, above 1% of the GDP.

Figure 4. State support of agriculture in selected countries in 1995 and 2015, percentage of GDP
Source: Authors' development based on the UNCTAD (2016)

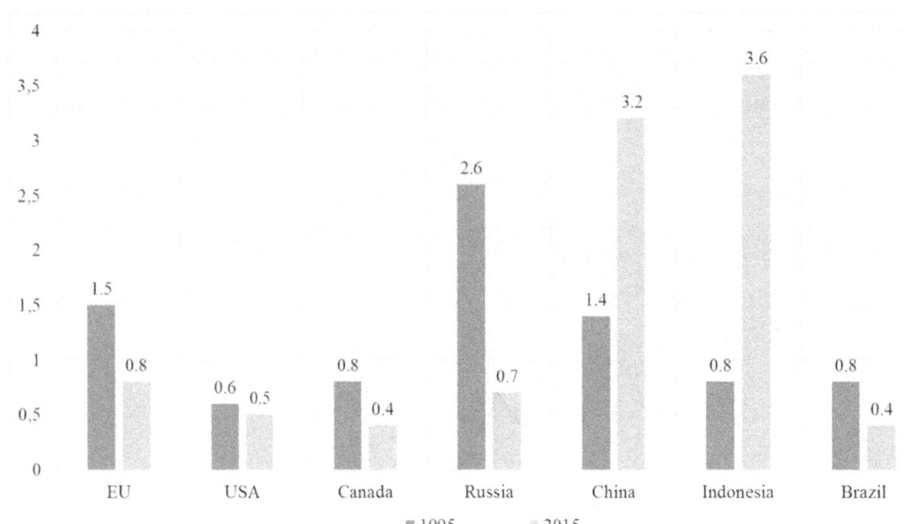

The decrease of the relative level of support does not mean the agriculture now receives less. Support in absolute terms is growing. Thus, during 1995-2015, aggregated amount of state support of agriculture among the OECD countries increased by \$23 billion (7.2%), including in the USA, by 195%; in Canada and Turkey, by 170%; in Norway, by 140%. Even more significant growth of the absolute amount of support occurred in the emerging economies, which are not the OECD members. In Brazil, withdrawal of incomes of agricultural producers in the amount of \$4.2 billion in 1995 changed to state support in the amount of \$9.4 billion in 2015. In China, the amount of support during the same period increased from only \$13 billion up to \$287 billion.

The variance of the importance of state support for farmers can be estimated by means of matching its volume with the gross product in agriculture (Figure 5). The analysis reveals that percentage ratio between the volume of state support and the gross product in agriculture in the OECD countries decreases, but fluctuates over a wide range, from negative values in Ukraine to almost 100% in Switzerland and Norway. Revealed differences between the countries are determined by the availability of natural resources, the role of agricultural sector in the national economy, the level of development, and goals of agrarian policy.

State regulation of agriculture is a complicated mechanism, which includes the tools of pressure on the structure of agricultural production, agricultural market, social sphere of rural territories, inter-industry, and inter-farm relations. In relation to this, the structure of state support and discovery of trends are the subjects of much attention. The structure of aggregate support of agriculture in the selected OECD countries and emerging economies in accordance with the methical approach described above is presented in Table 4.

In 1995, support of producers dominated in the aggregated support of agriculture. Among the OECD countries, its relative share was 78%, including in the EU – 87%, in Canada and Japan – 75%, in the USA – over 50%. As for the emerging economies, this type of support also played a critical role. Over the past 20 years, the importance of the support of producers essentially decreased. Being the members

Figure 5. Aggregated support of agriculture in selected countries in 1995 and 2015, percentage of the gross product in agriculture
Source: Authors' development based on the UNCTAD (2016)

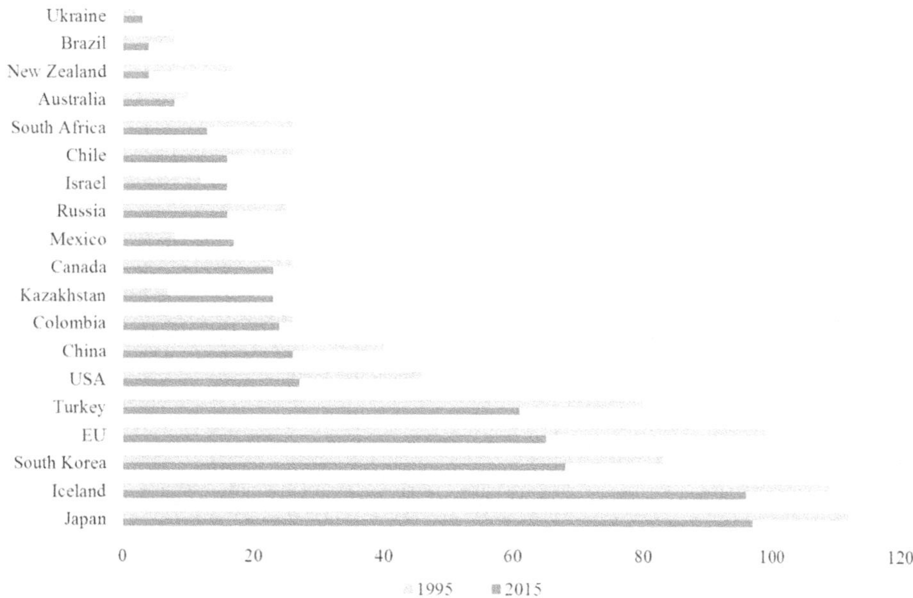

of the WTO, OECD countries are obliged to limit support of producers, which distorts market patterns. That is why they have to redirect budget transfers to support of services or support of consumers. Such a tactic gives them an opportunity to save or even increase the level of support without breaking the WTO rules. Some countries almost redirected state support on the development of infrastructure, research, and development, education in the sphere of agriculture, marketing, promotion of products, and other services. Thus, in 2015, in Australia the share of such expenses in the aggregated support of agriculture is over 50%, in Chile – 48%, in New Zealand – 73%, in Canada – 28%, in Kazakhstan – 23%, and in Israel – 20%.

It is evident that usage of such capacities of support of services not restricted by the WTO is relevant for emerging countries since many of them lose a substantial portion of actual agricultural production because of poor road networks, lack of storage and other infrastructure facilities, which is resulted in the cost of production.

As for the support of consumers, this tool is implemented massively in the USA only, where the agrifood policy is focused on the expansion of domestic and external markets of agricultural raw materials and food. Over a half of the agrarian budget of the USA is spent on food aid to low-income sections of the population in purpose to promote domestic demand. The aid is implemented in the framework of the programs of distribution of food coupons (Supplemental Nutrition Assistance Program – SNAP), free lunches in schools (The National School Lunch Program – NSLP), food for women, infants, and children (The Special Supplemental Nutrition Program for Women, Infants, and Children – WIC). The state budget also finances public awareness campaign on nutrition and research in the sphere of healthy nutrition. Each dollar of food aid generates two dollars in economic activity. Each billion of dollars in the program allows creating or supporting 18,000 of workplaces, including 3,000 workplaces in agriculture.

Table 4. Structure of aggregate state support of agriculture in the selected countries in 1995 and 2015, %

Countries	Support of producers		Support of services		Support of consumers	
	1995	2015	1995	2015	1995	2015
Australia	77	50	23	50	0	0
Brazil	176	83	-75	17	0	0
Canada	75	72	25	28	0	0
Chile	83	52	17	48	0	0
China	47	89	50	11	3	0
Columbia	91	85	9	15	0	0
EU	87	85	9	14	4	1
Iceland	87	94	9	5	4	1
Indonesia	73	89	26	6	1	5
Israel	87	80	13	20	0	0
Japan	75	85	25	15	0	0
Kazakhstan	95	76	5	23	0	0
Mexico	64	82	14	11	22	7
New Zealand	31	27	69	73	0	0
Norway	92	93	5	5	3	2
Russia	79	80	21	16	0	4
South Africa	65	57	35	43	0	0
South Korea	86	87	13	13	1	0
Switzerland	82	89	6	11	12	0
Turkey	72	85	28	15	0	0
Ukraine	142	157	-42	-57	0	0
USA	53	38	9	9	38	53

Source: Authors' development based on the UNCTAD (2016)

This experience is worthwhile implementing for the development of organizational and economic mechanisms of state regulation of agriculture in emerging countries, since the tools currently implemented in the majority of them are reciprocal and directly or indirectly focused on the increase of output, i.e. on supply, without any regulations of demand. However, as the authors referred to Liefert (2004) in the beginning of the chapter, the main food security problem for emerging countries is not the low volume of output but inadequate access to food by certain socioeconomic groups. The result is that the increase of output in agriculture is not fulfilled even at the extensive support of agriculture. One of the reasons is sensibility to domestic demand. Low effective demand does not drive production increase.

Identifying the overall tendency of decrease of support in relation to the gross agricultural production (in average, in the countries under consideration it decreased from 21% in 1995 down to 17% in 2015), it is necessary to bear in mind that such average indicators submerge differences existing between the OECD countries and emerging economies. While in the former ones the level of protectionism decreased gradually, the latter ones moved up from taxation of agriculture (it still exists in Ukraine) to ensurance of an essential level of support, which just started to catch up with the OECD countries in 2014-2015.

Change in the overall level of support of producers is followed by a change of priorities in the implementation of direct and indirect subsidies. In the late 1990s, support for domestic prices was the major measure of indirect support of agricultural producers in the OECD countries. Its share was over 45% of the overall support in the EU, the USA, Canada, Israel, Turkey, and Australia, 35% in Russia, and over 90% in Japan, Korea, Kazakhstan, and South Africa.

Support of market prices ensures higher incomes for farmers because of keeping high prices for food and making consumers support farmers by paying these high prices. In the case of agricultural surpluses because of high prices, it is possible to promote export using export subsidies, which are paid from the budget, not at the consumers' expense.

The degree of support of farmers by means of such tool is characterized by the Producer Nominal Protection Coefficient (NPC), calculated as a ratio between the average price received by producers on the domestic market and the average world market price. It shows that domestic prices for agricultural products in the USA, Canada, Mexico, and Israel are close to international ones, and did not change essentially during 1995-2015 (Figure 6).

Figure 6. Producer Nominal Protection Coefficient in selected countries in 1995 and 2015
Source: Authors' development based on the UNCTAD (2016)

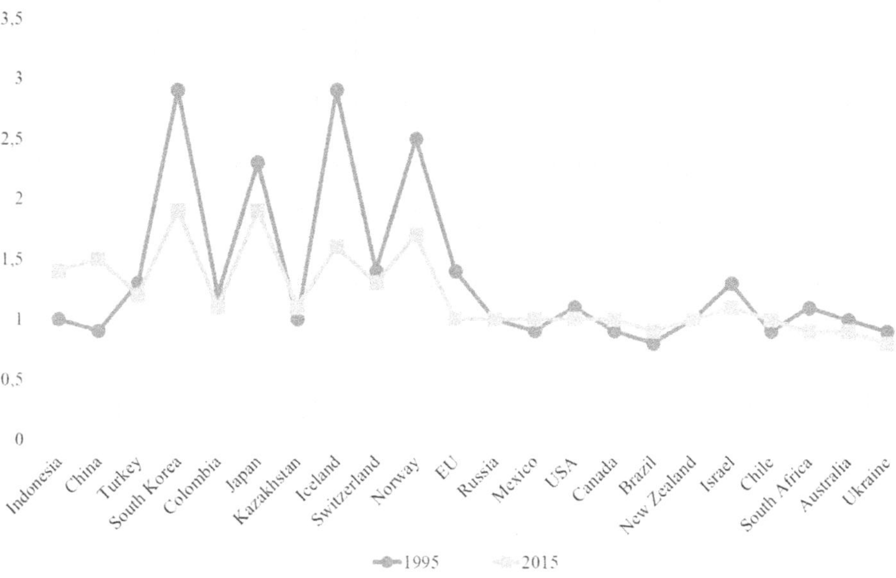

The coefficient decreased substantially in the developed countries, where it was traditionally high. Nevertheless, domestic prices in the EU, Norway, Japan, Turkey, and South Korea surpassed international price in a range from 20% to 200% in 2015. In the emerging economies, on the contrary, the coefficient rises, which is reflected in surpassing of domestic prices over the international price in a range from 2% to 20%

Those emerging countries with financial capacities replace indirect measures of support with direct ones, which do not affect consumer prices. They are implemented by the means of direct state equalization fees; compensation of disaster damages; compensation of redeployment damage (compensation of land diversion, forced cattle slaughtering, etc.); subsidies per unit area or livestock population; payments in the form of financing of procurements (for example, subsidies for purchasing of fertilizers, agricultural chemicals, and fodder); financing of target programs. Across the OECD, direct payments to farmers increased from 19% up to 37% during 1995-2015. Payments per hectare of crop area and livestock unit reached almost a half of state support of agriculture in the USA and 2/3 of the respected payments in the EU. They are increasingly used in order to stimulate implementation of certain technologies of production, including the ones with environmental restrictions. The traditional measure of support is compensation of initial costs. Its relative share in the structure of support of producers across the OECD increased from 9.5% up to 12.0%, including in the EU from 7.0% up to 14.0%.

Agricultural insurance is also one of the major tools of support of farmers' income. International experience shows that subsidizing of insurance premium and reinsurance of risks are the common and effective ways of state support of economic stability in agriculture.

In general, the share of measures, which distort trade patterns the most, decreased by 20 percentage points in the OECD countries during 1995-2015, while in the USA and the EU – more than twofold.

Along with the support of operating activities of farmers, more and more resources of agrarian budgets of the OECD countries are spent on the realization of long-term goals, such as environmental sustainability, development of infrastructure, and implementation of innovations (Table 5). Expenses on infrastructure are essentially financed from the state budgets in Turkey, Japan, Brazil, Chile, and South Korea. Kazakhstan and Canada spend the biggest amount of support on inspection and control services. Improvement of agricultural education, development and implementation into the agricultural production of innovations are priority directions for Australia, Norway, Israel, Switzerland, the EU, and the USA. In those countries, expenses for research and education comprise from 30% up to 64% of total resources spent on support services.

Facilitating organization, financing and implementation of research and development for agriculture at the expense of state budgets, governments of the most of the countries encourage innovation activities in the private sector using direct and indirect financial incentives, providing information on the results of state-funded research, developing state-private partnerships, and organizing work on information and extension support of farmers.

Over the recent years, development of information and extension services is facilitated in a way of decentralization of state services and the introduction of private entities and intermediaries in this field. Innovation brokers appeared in the EU and other countries. They formulate needs of farmers in the sphere of research, help them to get an access to technologies, or develop links in value chains. Some of them are financed from the state funds and governed by a state, through regional organizations. There are pure private systems (for example, in the Netherlands and New Zealand), where farmers pay for the services and select service providers on a commercial basis. There are mixed systems, where services provided by the state entities and private consultants are paid by the farmers either in part or in whole. Finally, there are systems managed by the farmers' organizations (for example, in France and Finland) and financed by the government, farmers' organizations, and private farmers (Kadomtseva, 2010).

SOLUTIONS AND RECOMMENDATIONS

Differences in structural content of state support of agriculture are developed under the influence of historical, political, natural, and economic conditions of various countries. They are determined by their

Table 5. Structure of state support of services in agriculture in selected countries in 1995 and 2015, %

Countries	Research and education		Inspection and control services		Infrastructure		Other	
	1995	2015	1995	2015	1995	2015	1995	2015
Australia	75	64	5	9	14	25	5	1
Brazil	23	15	4	7	58	51	15	27
Canada	41	39	22	40	12	10	24	11
Chile	28	24	1	20	64	51	7	5
China	8	29	5	6	23	37	64	28
Columbia	25	23	3	7	71	69	0	1
EU	31	37	3	6	24	30	43	27
Iceland	35	12	10	41	20	2	35	45
Indonesia	22	11	5	3	73	72	0	5
Israel	40	44	14	16	3	30	43	10
Japan	5	14	0	1	91	82	4	3
Kazakhstan	0	12	89	62	11	22	0	4
Korea	11	25	2	6	74	49	12	20
Mexico	54	48	6	11	17	38	24	3
New Zealand	65	49	24	32	11	20	14	0
Norway	56	54	18	24	11	16	14	5
Russia	12	42	8	26	15	13	64	18
South Africa	85	41	7	16	8	36	0	7
Switzerland	28	47	3	16	14	36	56	7
Turkey	1	1	3	2	75	82	21	15
Ukraine	25	45	8	30	63	11	4	14
USA	35	29	13	16	1	26	51	30

Source: Authors' development based on the UNCTAD (2016)

financial capabilities and current tasks of agrarian policies, some of which are: fulfillment of economic potential of agriculture as a sector, which ensures economic growth, and employment of population; increase of environmental sustainability of production in the conditions of natural scarcity; ensurance of food security of a country; expansion of export opportunities. Nevertheless, the analysis let the authors revealing some common tendencies in a change of role and directions of state support of agriculture in the emerging countries in the light of ensurance of food security, in particular:

- While the share of support of agriculture in the GDP decreases, its absolute value increases.
- Growth rates of state support of agriculture are synchronized with the growth rates of the gross product in agriculture. During critical periods of market slump increase of direct support of agriculture helps to stabilize production and domestic food market in order to ensure food security.
- Under an influence of globalization, the structural content of state support changes: tied price support is replaced by the untied support of producers' income.

- Importance of support of services grows, primarily of innovation activities and infrastructure.

Emerging countries have limited capabilities to provide the level support of their domestic farmers which would ensure achievement of target parameters of food security. Involvement into the international trade forces emerging countries opening their domestic food markets for imports. Effective protection of domestic farmers in emerging countries is impeded by the low import tariffs, which facilitate an easier market access for foreign agricultural products and food, lead to a reduction of domestic production, and in such a way threaten food security. Acting in the framework of the common directions of development of state support of agriculture, emerging countries should provide constant diversified aid to the direct producers of agricultural products. Measures of such support are increasingly frequently emerging into the tools of "precise pointing". They are aimed at smoothing negative consequences of unfavorable market environment because of objective and subjective circumstances. Account of those tendencies in the development of tools for state support in the emerging countries will let make the support more focused and effective and will help to adopt the measures of regulation of agriculture to the goals of ensurance of food security.

FUTURE RESEARCH DIRECTIONS

The vital issue for emerging countries in terms of achieving food security is how to secure the sustainable development of national agriculture and agribusiness in the conditions of a growing market openness and liberalization of international trade in food, taking into consideration the incomparably lower financial capabilities. Future research in this field has to be focused on exploring the ways in which emerging countries would be able to ensure the sustainable development of agricultural production and trade. The effects of the following measures on food security have to be investigated: state support of import substitution agricultural production; provision of environmental safety of domestic food and agricultural commodities; agricultural and food export increase once the domestic is saturated; logistical costs saving; optimization of all factors that affect competitiveness of domestic agricultural and food commodities in compliance with rational geographic distribution and specialization of agricultural production.

CONCLUSION

Many economies considered as emerging ones originated from the common socialist-type model of the economy (post-Soviet countries, Eastern European states, some of the Asian countries), where the dominant state and collective ownership of the means of production minimized the role of natural competitive factors (Kolodko, 1998). Foreign trade was controlled by the state, which resulted in various distortions, low level of diversification, specialization of export destinations and import channels due to political preferences. During early stages of transition, most of the economies of that type experienced a decline in output and export, significant increase in inflation, and decrease in living standards of the domestic population. Economic and trade liberalization rapidly embedded emerging economies into the international market, however, being considerably non-competitive, they had to specialize on low value-added exports and high value-added technological imports. For at least two decades after the beginning of market reforms in the 1980-1990s, most of the economies currently recognized as emerging ones have not been able to break the existing trade patterns.

Things are changing. Unimaginable growth of China, certain economic successes of Russia and Kazakhstan, the rapid increase in agricultural production and exports in Brazil and Argentina, and improvements in the region of the Eastern Europe demonstrated the potentials of the emerging economies on the global market. By the 2010s, particular countries and their strengthening alliances had been rather effective in increasing their shares in the global agricultural output and trade in agricultural products and food. New economic powers have arisen: China, Russia, Brazil, and other Eastern European and South-East Asian nations. The countries accelerated integration processes between themselves in order to ensure their food security, aggregate existing competitive advantages, and mitigate market risks. However, despite the evident achievements, there are still old problems and new challenges in terms of achieving food security. Unlike the past two-three decades of transition, coming years will manifest new factors: increasing competition between emerging countries and their alliances for better conditions of production and distribution of agricultural products and food; intensifying role of trade regulations (unification in the WTO framework and protectionism of particular domestic markets) and state support in achieving certain levels of food security; growing tensions between major global powers as to shape a new multi-polar world order.

The long-term outlook for agricultural development, trade in food and agricultural products, and food security in the emerging economies will depend on effective structural reforms, diversification and technical modernization of domestic production and exports, utilization of existing comparative advantages, and benefiting from effective state support of agriculture. As Von Braun, Serova, Seeth, and Melyukhina (1996) stated in relation to Russia, much would depend on how well incentives to increase agricultural production provided by a state are transmitted to the agriculture and food-processing sector and on the opening up of international trade opportunities.

REFERENCES

Anderson, K., Jha, S., Nelgen, S., & Strutt, A. (2013). Re-examining Policies for Food Security in Asia. *Food Security, 5*(2), 195–215. doi:10.100712571-012-0237-5

Boehringer, C., & Rutherford, T. (1999). *Decomposing General Equilibrium Effects of Policy Intervention in Multi-Regional Trade Models: Method and Sample Application*. Mannheim: Center for European Economic Research.

Božić, D., Bogdanov, N., & Ševarlić, M. (2011). *Ekonomika Poljoprivrede*. Belgrade: University of Belgrade.

Devereux, M. B. (1999). Growth and the Dynamics of Trade Liberalization. *Journal of Economic Dynamics & Control, 23*(5-6), 773–795. doi:10.1016/S0165-1889(98)00043-8

Erokhin, V. (2015). Structural Changes in International Trade in Food: Competitive Growth Models for Economies in Transition. In *Proceedings of the 3rd International Conference "Economic Scientific Research – Theoretical, Empirical and Practical Approaches"*. Bucharest: Academia Romana.

Erokhin, V., Ivolga, A., & Heijman, W. (2014). Trade Liberalization and State Support of Agriculture: Effects for Developing Countries. *Agricultural Economics*, *60*(11), 524–537.

Estevadeordal, A., Freund, C., & Ornelas, E. (2008). Does Regionalism Affect Trade Liberalization Toward Nonmembers? *The Quarterly Journal of Economics*, *123*(4), 1531–1575. doi:10.1162/qjec.2008.123.4.1531

Filippov, R.V. (2014). International Experience of Subsidizing of Agriculture as Basis of Food Security of Russia. *Naukovedenie, 20*(1).

Josling, T., Anderson, K., Schmitz, A., & Tangerman, S. (2010). Understanding International Trade in Agricultural Products: One Hundred Years of Contributions by Agricultural Economists. *American Journal of Agricultural Economics*, *92*(2), 424–446. doi:10.1093/ajae/aaq011

Kolodko, G. W. (1998). *Equity Issues in Policymaking in Transition Economies*. Washington, DC: International Monetary Fund.

Liefert, W. (2004). *Food Security in Russia: Economic Growth and Rising Incomes are Reducing Insecurity*. Washington, DC: Economic Research Service, USDA.

Liefert, W., & Swinnen, J. (2002). *Changes in Agricultural Markets in Transition Economies*. Washington, DC: Economic Research Service, USDA.

Malozemov, S. I. (2014). Experience of State Support of Agriculture in Foreign Countries. *Science and Modernity*, *32*(1), 136–141.

Markovic, I., & Markovic, M. (2014). Agricultural Protectionism of the European Union in the Conditions of International Trade Liberalization. *Economics of Agriculture*, *61*(2), 423–440.

Olson, D. R. (2003). *Towards Food Sovereignty: Constructing an Alternative to the World Trade Organization's Agreement on Agriculture*. Minneapolis, MN: Institute for Agriculture and Trade Policy.

Petrikov, A. V. (2012). It Is Necessary to Increase Adaptation of Russian Agrarian Sector to WTO Conditions. *Economy of Agricultural and Processing Enterprises*, *6*, 6–8.

Petrikov, A. V. (2016). Major Directions of Implementation of Modern Agrifood and Rural Policy. *International Agricultural Journal*, *1*, 3–9.

Schmitz, A., Moss, C., Schmitz, T., Furtan, W., & Schmitz, H. (2010). *Agricultural Policy, Agribusiness, and Rent-Seeking Behaviour*. Toronto: University of Toronto Press.

Secretariat of the Convention on Biological Diversity. (2005). *The Impact of Trade Liberalization on Agricultural Biological Diversity, Domestic Support Measures and their Effects on Agricultural Biological Diversity*. Montreal: SCBD.

United Nations Conference on Trade and Development. (2016). Statistics Database [Data file]. Retrieved from http://unctad.org/en/Pages/Statistics.aspx

Visser, O., Mamonova, N., Spoor, M., & Nikulin, A. (2015). Quiet Food Sovereignty as Food Sovereignty without a Movement? Insights from Post-socialist Russia. *Globalizations*, *12*(4), 1–16. doi:10.1080/14747731.2015.1005968

Von Braun, J., Serova, E., Seeth, H., & Melyukhina, O. (1996). *Russia's Food Economy in Transition: What Do Reforms Mean for the Long-term Outlook?* Washington, DC: International Food Policy Research Institute.

Wittman, H., Desmarais, A., & Wiebe, N. (2010). *Food Sovereignty: Reconnecting Food, Nature and Community.* Halifax, Canada: Fernwood Publishing and Food First Books.

ADDITIONAL READING

Anderson, K., Dimaran, B., Francois, J., Hertel, T., Hoekman, B., & Will, M. (2001). The Cost of Rich (and Poor) Country Protection to Developing Countries. *Journal of African Economies, 10*(3), 227–257. doi:10.1093/jae/10.3.227

Ayres, J. M., & Bosia, M. (2011). Beyond Global Summitry: Food Sovereignty as Localized Resistance to Globalization. *Globalizations, 8*(1), 47–63. doi:10.1080/14747731.2011.544203

Boyer, J. (2010). Food Security, Food Sovereignty, and Local Challenges for Transnational Agrarian Movements: The Honduras Case. *The Journal of Peasant Studies, 37*(2), 319–351. doi:10.1080/03066151003594997

Claeys, P. (2012). The Creation of New Rights by the Food Sovereignty Movement: The Challenge of Institutionalizing Subversion. *Sociology, 46*(5), 844–860. doi:10.1177/0038038512451534

Dollar, D. (2001). Globalization, Inequality, and Poverty since 1980. Washington, DC: Development Research Group, the World Bank.

Dornbusch, R. (1992). The Case for Trade Liberalization in Developing Countries. *The Journal of Economic Perspectives, 6*(1), 69–85. doi:10.1257/jep.6.1.69

Edelman, M. (2014). Food Sovereignty: Forgotten Genealogies and Future Regulatory Challenges. *The Journal of Peasant Studies, 41*(6), 959–978. doi:10.1080/03066150.2013.876998

Hospes, O. (2009). Food Sovereignty: The Debate, the Deadlock, and a Suggested Detour. *Agriculture and Human Values, 31*(1). doi:10.100710460-013-9449-3

Khanna, T., & Palepu, K. G. (2010). *Winning in Emerging Markets: A Road Map for Strategy and Execution.* Boston, MA: Harvard Business Press.

Mamonova, N. (2017). *Rethinking Rural Politics in Postsocialist Settings. Rural Communities, Land Grabbing and Agrarian Change in Russia and Ukraine.* Enschede: Ipskamp Drukkers.

Patel, R. (2009). Food Sovereignty. *The Journal of Peasant Studies, 36*(3), 663–706. doi:10.1080/03066150903143079

Spanu, V. (2003). *Liberalization of the International Trade and Economic Growth: Implications for both Developed and Developing Countries.* Cambridge, MA: Harvard University.

Ushachev, I. (2012). Measures to Secure Competitiveness of Russia's Agricultural Production in the Conditions of its Accession to WTO. *Economics of Agricultural and Processing Enterprises*, 6, 1–5.

Wehrheim, P., & Wobst, P. (2005). The Economic Role of Russias Subsistence Agriculture in the Transition Process. *Agricultural Economics*, *33*(1), 91–105. doi:10.1111/j.1574-0862.2005.00136.x

KEY TERMS AND DEFINITIONS

Agriculture: A pool of establishments engaged in growing crops, raising animals, and harvesting fish and other animals.

Developed Country: A country which has a highly developed economy in terms of bigger gross domestic product, gross national product, and per capita income, and advanced technological infrastructure relative to other countries.

Developing Country: A country which has a less developed economy in terms of smaller gross domestic product, gross national product, and per capita income relative to other countries.

Emerging Economy: An economy that is not as advanced as developed countries but progressing toward becoming advanced.

Food Market: A medium that allows buyers and sellers of agricultural raw materials, agricultural products, and food to interact in order to facilitate an exchange.

Food Security: An availability and adequate access at all times to sufficient, safe, nutritious food to maintain a healthy and active life.

State Support: A set of protective measures provided by a state to a certain industry or sector.

Trade Liberalization: A removal or reduction of restrictions or barriers on the free exchange of goods between nations.

This research was previously published in Establishing Food Security and Alternatives to International Trade in Emerging Economies edited by Vasily Erokhin; pages 55-73, copyright year 2018 by Business Science Reference (an imprint of IGI Global).

Chapter 46
New Approaches to Agricultural Production Management in the Arctic:
Organic Farming and Food Security

Mykhailo Guz

National University of Life and Environmental Sciences of Ukraine, Ukraine

ABSTRACT

Organic agriculture is a promising form of management in which the preservation of the natural foundations of life and natural processes is the determining factor in ensuring food security and sustainable development. Until recently, organic farming has been considered as something related to the traditional regions of agricultural production. However, raising food security issues make people look for new opportunities even in the severe conditions of the polar regions. In the High North, food security issues are complemented by specific challenges: climate, fragile environment, remoteness, and way of life of indigenous people. In the chapter, the author discusses the potential of organic farming as a solution to the food insecurity problem in the northern areas. The approaches to organic production management and establishment and running of an organic farm are studied. The author concludes that a green turn to more organic farming is a promising step towards food security and sustainable development of rural areas in the Arctic.

INTRODUCTION

The technology of organic farming is rapidly spreading throughout the world. The arguments that may affect the increase of organic production include profitability of organic farming and effective demand for organic products. The first argument is purely economic, which may encourage businesses to implement organic farming. The latter one is considered as a socio-economic factor that depends on the general economic development of a country (Guz & Ivolga, 2015). Until recently, organic farming has been considered as something related to the traditional regions of agricultural production. However, raising

DOI: 10.4018/978-1-7998-5354-1.ch046

food security issues make people look for new opportunities (Erokhin, 2017b) even in the severe conditions of northern part of the planet.

In the harsh environment of the Arctic, hunting and fishing have always been an important part of human existence (Sonne et al., 2017). However, in the recent decades, intensive exploration of natural resources of the Arctic and development of other kinds of economic activities have resulted in a substantial increase of Arctic population. Along with food availability issues, the inclusion of Nordic territories to the global production chains has brought along increased anthropogenic stressors on the ecosystems, environmental pollution (Muir & de Wit, 2010), and safety and quality of food.

In the High North, food security issues are complemented by specific challenges: climate, fragile environment, remoteness, and way of life of indigenous people. Food security brings together concerns over a range of interacting environmental, social, economic, political and cultural changes. These include food and water-borne diseases; increasing incidence of lifestyle diseases; high costs of healthy foods; contamination; changing ecosystems that impede access to food; high fuel costs; and loss of traditional knowledge (Nilsson, Nilsson, Quinlan, & Evengard, 2013). Exposure to long-range transported industrial chemicals (Zetterstrom, 2003), climate change, and diseases is posing a risk to the overall health and populations of Arctic wildlife (Sonne et al., 2017) and human health in the Arctic region. Arctic ecosystems, however, are being stressed by not only contaminants. Two major additional aspects to consider in the study of Arctic health are climate change and infectious diseases. Climate change acts through alteration of food web pathways for contaminants (McKinney et al., 2013), while pollution increases the risk of disease transfer from animals to humans as a large volume of marine and terrestrial wildlife is consumed by humans in the Arctic, often raw and inadequately frozen (Jenssen et al., 2015).

Arctic food security involves access by local residents to store-bought and traditional foods (Duhaime & Bernard, 2008). Access to food requires a steady income in order to ensure a consistent, year-round supply of high-quality goods in the stores and a ready supply of healthy wildlife to be harvested (Erokhin, 2017b). In terms of availability of food products, rural towns in the North can be difficult to reach, especially in winter, that is why even those communities which traditionally rely on subsistence have become increasingly dependent on costly imports of unhealthy frozen food with extended shelf life. The poor nutritional quality of many retail foods that are available in the North increases the risk of nutritional deficiencies (Kuhnlein, Receveur, Soueida, & Egeland, 2004; Gao, Erokhin, & Ivolga, 2018); furthermore, the high cost of these foods, mainly due to their transport (Beaumier & Ford, 2010; Fergurson, 2011), can impact households' food security status, particularly when local foods are not readily available (Huet et al., 2017; Gao, Ivolga, & Erokhin, 2018).

There are various drivers which may be used to ensure food security in the High North. Economic ones include changes in food prices and in people's ability to pay (Erokhin, 2017c). Social ones include changes in dietary preference and shifts in the social context in which food is produced and shared (Erokhin, Ivolga, & Lisova, 2016; Erokhin, 2018). Technological drivers include changes to infrastructure and technologies connected with both traditional and new ways of food production (Nilsson et al., 2013). Commercialization of country foods could increase accessibility of available foods in the Arctic. One of the potential solutions to the food security problem in the circumpolar territories is the development of agricultural production locally (Erokhin & Gao, 2018).

Organic agriculture is a system composed of various factors. The aim of economic science is to discover its multifold problems, analyze the current situation, elaborate scenarios of development, and search for the bifurcation points for decision making, which are efficient by Pareto optimality (distribution of resources which cannot be improved at least for one person, without having worsened thus welfare of another). Organic agriculture is appropriate for the solution of environmental problems as its spreading leads to the improvement of the majority of the ecological indexes.

The level of profitability of organic agriculture is the main factor in its spreading. However, producing organically, the one acts long-term and cares about the protection of land, water, air, plants, animals, and humans, not quick profits and high commercial yields. The adoption of any administrative decision has to be substantiated. A thorough analysis of the actual situation is always a prerequisite for a proper decision making. In organic farming, the substantial analysis is one of the principal steps in making a managerial decision. Decision making is an integral activity preceded by a number of actions, particularly, gathering the necessary information, data processing, situation analysis, selection among the available alternative decisions, and their assessment taking into account scarce resources available to organic farmers. In the conditions of the Arctic, organic farming may bring into consideration not only the lack of economic resources or the optimal combination in the production process and sustainable consumption, but also provide solutions in achieving a sustainable development of circumpolar territories (Jean-Vasile, Raluca Andreea, & Rahoveanu Adrian, 2015; Erokhin & Ivolga, 2014). In this context, the development of organic farming in the Arctic is a valuable research field.

BACKGROUND

Neither disruptions of food supply nor food insecurity problem are new phenomena in the Arctic. Northern societies have developed a number of mechanisms to respond, particularly, development of alternative sources of food and water and ways of sharing available food (Nilsson et al., 2013; Erokhin, 2017a). However, organic farming as a potential solution to combat food insecurity in the Arctic has not been extensively studied until now.

The majority of food security studies in the Arctic have focused on small, remote communities or have examined the prevalence of food insecurity at a regional scale (Boult, 2004; Ford, 2009; Huet, Rosol, & Egeland, 2012). Kondrashev, Nikitenko, Trofimova, Trofimova, and Gotsko (2016a) studied legal regulations of food security in the Arctic regions of Russia and focused on the active involvement of local inhabitants and indigenous people of the High North in establishing food self-sufficiency based on the nature management production. Kondrashev, Nikitenko, Trofimova, Trofimova, and Gotsko (2016b) analyzed strategies established by the Arctic states for development of their northern regions and put forward the measures to actively involve the population of the circumpolar territories in the self-procurement of food by utilizing of indigenous subsistence economy products.

Food security has also been discussed in the assessments of climate change (Anisimov et al., 2007; Berner & Furgal, 2005) and in relation to pollution in the Arctic (Poppel, Kruse, Duhaime, & Abryutina, 2007). Loring and Gerlach (2015) synthesized research on food security in polar regions by studying the impacts of land claims, cumulative effects of industrial development and environmental change, and health impacts of the nutrition transition among indigenous peoples. Nilsson and Evengard (2015) discussed the concepts of food security and food sovereignty and their interrelations and relevance from an Arctic perspective. Wesche and Chan (2010) studied the impacts of climate change on food security in the Western Canadian Arctic and concluded that the vulnerability of each community to changing food security was differentially influenced by a range of factors, including current harvesting trends, levels of reliance on individual species, opportunities for access to other traditional food species, and exposure to climate change hazards.

Hollesen, Matthiesen, Moller, and Elberling (2015) studied permafrost thawing in organic Arctic soils and demonstrated that the impact of climate changes on natural organic soils could be accelerated by microbial heat production with crucial implications for the amounts of carbon being decomposed. Hastrup, Rieffestahl, and Olsen (2016) analyzed how an increasing fear of contaminants had created a new sense of food insecurity in the Arctic and addressed the emerging issue of carcinogens identified in common food-items in the North. That problem seriously affects notions of food-safety in the Arctic and problems of risk and fear in relation to food with which both customers and food producers now have to deal.

In recent years, there have been many attempts to use the common food security survey modules to assess food access of indigenous people. However, these modules were not originally designed for use in mixed economies of circumpolar regions where both purchased and country (hunted, fished, and gathered) foods contribute to peoples' diets (Ready, 2016). Dresscher (2016) analyzed food security strategies and explicated how they managed to balance the subsistence hunt with the commercial one in the High Arctic. Koutouki, Booth, and Blum (2017) examined food system changes and planning from a community health and management perspective and discussed the relationship between food security, gender, livelihoods, and ecosystem capacity. Gao (2017), Erokhin (2016), and Ivolga (2014) addressed food security issues in the northern regions of Russia through the prism of sustainable rural development. Ready (2016) attempted to develop the tools that provided reliable and valid assessments of country food access, specifically including traditional knowledge and social support networks in the circumpolar territories.

There are limited research and policy discussions on how to adapt to the health effects of climate change, including to potential food security implications. The drivers that may contribute to food security in the Arctic include the development of new practices and technologies to enhance the availability of and access to local food in the Arctic, in spite of long-term environmental changes that are difficult to influence. However, to date, there exists no pan-Arctic assessment that focuses specifically on the role of organic farming in establishing food security. In this chapter, the author discusses the potential of organic farming as a solution to the food insecurity problem in the Arctic, studies the approaches to organic production management and establishment and running of an organic, and makes an effort to develop a methodology for efficient agricultural production management in the sphere of organic farming in the circumpolar territories.

MAIN FOCUS OF THE CHAPTER

Organic Farming Goes North

Despite unforgiving environmental conditions of the Arctic, farming has been developing in the circumpolar territories of Nordic countries (Dolce, 2016). There are many reasons for that. The climate is changing: Arctic temperatures over the past 100 years have increased at almost twice the global average. The diet of many indigenous Arctic peoples is also changing: traditionally meat-eaters, they are now consuming more grains and vegetables (Nobel, 2013). Also, there is a growing demand for locally grown foods. The significant fact is that the Arctic and sub-Arctic communities are isolated. On the one hand, agricultural products and food are shipped long distances from the southern parts of the planet. On the other hand, the existing supply chains are rather vulnerable to the region's litany of both natural and human-made disasters, including blizzards, earthquakes, volcanoes, and shipping strikes (Nobel, 2013).

Producing locally takes a lot of the insecurity out of the supply chain. Moreover, locally produced food results in an increased quality, as there is less risk of damage during transport or storage. Shorter distances from the farm to the consumer might also result in lower prices (Friedrich, 2018). Due to the progressing climate change, warmer weather in the Arctic is allowing farmers to grow vegetables, grains, herbs, and other plants that have typically been planted in more temperate fields (Hoag, 2016, October 31). The examples of newly established farms in the circumpolar territories are greenhouses in Nunavut, community gardens in Yellowknife, production of vegetables and berries in Greenland, vegetable farms in Northern Norway, and even crop production in Alaska (Nobel, 2013). However, the most notable and promising fact for the development of agricultural production in the High North is that many insects and diseases have not yet spread in the cold climate of the Arctic (Friedrich, 2018). That means that food production in the northern areas requires fewer pesticides compared to the traditional areas of agricultural production, facilitating the potential growth of organic farming.

Organic farming is based on the principles which reflect the specifics of any economic activity in the fragile environment of the Arctic and aim at the ensurance of sustainable development of the region (Guz & Ivolga, 2015):

- Production of high-quality food, raw materials, and other products in sufficient quantities;
- Coordination of works on the production system with natural cycles and living systems of soil, flora, and fauna;
- Recognition of the wider social and environmental impacts beyond and within the system of organic production and processing;
- Maintaining and improving soil fertility and soil biological activity through local cultural, biological and mechanical methods instead of using external factors of production (resources);
- Conservation of agro-biodiversity on the farms and their surroundings by using a sustainable system of production and protection of wildlife;
- Promoting responsible use and conservation of water resources with all of the living organisms;
- Use in systems of production and processing, as far as possible, renewable resources, preventing their loss and contamination;
- Promotion of local and regional production and movement of goods to consumers;
- Creating a harmonious balance between the production of plant and animal products;
- Provision of housing conditions in which domestic animals reveal natural behavior;
- The use of packaging materials to be re-utilized or which are decomposed by biological means;
- Ensuring all employed in organic farming and processing its output workers the quality of life that meets the requirements of a healthy and safe environment;
- Focus on the establishment of socially-oriented chain "production – processing – realization" in compliance with environmental requirements;
- Recognition of the importance and necessity of studying local experience and traditional forms of agricultural production and marketing.

In the conditions of the Arctic, organic farming is based on the principles of health, ecology, justice, and care.

The principle of health means that organic agriculture should sustain and improve the health of soil, plant, animal, human and planet as a single and indivisible whole (Erokhin, 2017a). This principle suggests that the health of a single individual and society cannot be separated from the health of the Arctic ecosystems. Healthy soils allow growing healthy plants that support the health of animals and humans. Health is the unity and integrity of living systems. It is not just the absence of disease; it is the preservation of the physical, mental, social, and environmental well-being. Immunity, resilience, and ability to recover are key characteristics of health. The role of organic farming in production, processing, distribution, and consumption is to support and improve the health of ecosystems and organisms. In particular, organic agriculture involves the production of high-quality nutritious foods that promote disease prevention as well as general well-being. According to this principle, it is necessary to avoid the use of fertilizers, pesticides, veterinary drugs, and animal food additives that may have adverse effects on health.

According to the principle of ecology, organic agriculture in the Arctic is based on the principles of natural ecological systems and cycles, working, co-existing with them and supporting them. Food production should be based on natural processes and environmentally friendly processing. Support and prosperity are achieved by the greening of the production environment.

The principle of justice means that organic agriculture is based on relationships that ensure justice with regard to the interests of the environment and life opportunities. Justice is characterized by objectivity, respect, correctness and economic attitudes, both among people and in relationships with other living beings. This principle emphasizes that all those involved in organic agriculture should follow the principles of humanity in a manner that ensures justice at all levels and to all parties – farmers, workers, processors, distributors, retailers, and consumers. Organic agriculture should create a high standard of living for each party involved and make a significant contribution to food security in circumpolar territories. Natural and environmental resources that are used in the production and consumption should be managed from the standpoint of social and environmental justice in the interests of future generations.

According to the principle of care, management of organic farming is to have preventive and responsible nature to protect the health and welfare of both present and future generations and the Arctic environment. Organic farming is a living and dynamic system that responds to internal and external needs and conditions. Those who use the methods of organic agriculture can improve efficiency and increase productivity, but health, happiness, and prosperity do not have to become risk factors. Therefore, the new technology has to be evaluated, and existing methods should be constantly reviewed. In the case of an incomplete understanding of ecosystems and agriculture, appropriate measures should be taken. This principle states that precaution and responsibility are the key components in selecting the management practices development and acceptable technologies of organic agriculture.

Management of organic farming should be adapted to local conditions, environment, culture, and scale. The impact should be reduced by reuse, recycling and efficient management of materials and energy in order to maintain and improve the environmental quality of products and resources that are protected. Organic agriculture should attain ecological balance through the design of land use, building and maintaining areas of genetic and agricultural diversity. In making management decisions regarding the further development of the economic activity, every agricultural enterprise faces the problem of initial economic assessment, which can be used to make a proper planning in the long run. Organic farming is a special area where a producer should care not only about costs and revenues but also about the quality of the environmental-friendly production, the specific market for organic food, proper packaging, labeling, storage, transportation, etc. In the North, those concerns are even much complicated due to the severe climate conditions, underdeveloped infrastructure, and unassured potential for expansion of organic food market within sparsely populated regions. There is a need for a model that would enable managers of agricultural enterprises to conduct an initial assessment of the business environment and market capacity prior making any managerial decision. Based on such a model, a manager who conducts an analysis is able to choose a proper combination of tools from a variety of those available. Within a planning process, it is recommended to carry out statistical calculation for the entire agricultural enterprise in the basis of marginal income. Thus, a multilateral relationship between the separate parts of an enterprise has to be taken into account, while the most important economic relations have to be represented in a plan and easily accessible for inspection within a relatively short period of time. Both aspects are of crucial importance when applied in practice for the purposes of establishing of an organic farm in the condition of the Arctic.

Methodology for Agricultural Production Management

In this study, a model for the analysis of the actual situation and future development of agricultural enterprise in the sphere of organic farming is developed based on the Wolfram Mathematica platform, a modern technical computing system spanning all areas of technical computing, including neural networks, machine learning, image processing, geometry, data science, visualizations, and others. Initially, Wolfram Mathematica software has been used in physics, mathematics, and engineering only. However, over the years, the use of Wolfram Mathematica has been spread to other areas of knowledge beyond technical sciences. Today, Wolfram Mathematica is efficiently used in technical, scientific, engineering, mathematical, and computing fields, as well as in social and agricultural sciences. The software has played a crucial role in many important discoveries and has become a basis of many technical documents. In the sphere of commerce, Wolfram Mathematica software plays an important role in the development of complex financial modeling and is currently widely used in many kinds of general planning and analysis of various spheres of activity. For many years, the common basic design of Wolfram Mathematica software has steadily allowed the system to expand its area of influence. Gradually, Wolfram Mathematica has gone from a software used primarily for mathematical and technical calculations to a tool widely used in various disciplines, including agricultural production.

A methodology elaborated within this study for the purposes of facilitating of production management in organic farming is based on the calculation of marginal gains across a range of agricultural products. In its turn, a technique of marginal calculations is based on the principle of marginal costs. It takes into account a yield (output) and use of production resources (input). Its main goal is to assist a manager in defining of the on-farm competitive index for the effective process of decision making during planning. Depending on the planning methodology applied, there may be used three methods to conduct marginal calculation, i.e. methodically valid marginal revenue, marginal calculation by the practical method, and standard marginal profit.

Optimization calculations (program planning and linear programming) require that a marginal revenue is calculated accurately in accordance with economic theory. Methodically valid marginal revenue is a difference between marginal value and marginal expenses.

In relation to the individual production process, the following questions arise:

- What additional amount of product a process brings with an expansion of production by one unit;
- What expenses arise from an expansion of production by one unit.

As a rule, a marginal cost is rather easy to measure since a volume of production increases in proportion to the expansion of production. To define a methodically valid marginal income, only commercial products (revenue from sales) should be estimated.

Production for domestic needs is taken into account in physical terms. It is assessed neither by a value of replacement nor by a value of the agricultural product, therefore it is not included to the sales revenue. This implies that the needs of other production processes should also be taken into account in physical terms. Sales revenue from particular processes is derived ultimately from the cost of the main and side agricultural products.

During the expansion of production, it is hardly possible to divide variable costs from those that remain constant. There are expenses, which are always variable (e.g. seeds, plant protection products, variable costs of machinery, concentrated feed, and repair of main livestock), however, depending on the decision-making situation, some costs change between constant and variable. It depends on the specifics of production planning (planning period, availability of permanent resources, and level of production expansion) and on the effects of external factors (depreciation, maintenance, costs of capital, and rents). Marginal costs of permanent and thus limited resources are only counted in the optimization of the production area (opportunity cost).

Marginal revenue is calculated by a deduction of variable costs from sales revenue. Thus, marginal revenue is the contribution:

- To cover the expenses of the resources considered in agriculture as permanent: land (rent for the use of agricultural land); labor (salaries of permanent / all employees); capital (depreciation, maintenance, interest, rental of buildings, equipment, and rights to supply);
- To form a profit and cover the cost of own production resources: equity (accrual of interest on equity); labor (rate of wages of unpaid (family) labor); management (payment for business activities of the head of a farm).

Marginal revenue shows which contribution certain manufacturing process brings in recoupment of permanent resources. Within the calculation of optimization, marginal revenue is a demonstrative indicator to determine relative economic advantages of production processes. The best process is the one in which the highest payback of limited resources is achieved. As an indicator of inter-farm comparisons, marginal revenue cannot be used since every farm has its own provision of production resources, while the expenses under consideration cannot be established similarly.

Marginal revenue is an internal indicator of efficiency. The farm does not need to wait for the calculation of profit in order to compare between the two production processes. The difference in margin revenue from one hectare of different cash crops is identical to the difference in income (usually calculated at the end of a year). Fixed and overhead costs for various crops are deducted from marginal revenue and distributed on the entire area proportionally (Beckman & Brecker, 2014a).

Decision-Making Modelling in Organic Farming

For the purpose of this study, initial data for the model are based on the application of the farm's own organic fertilizers. Several scenarios depending on the application rate have been used. In the maximum scenario, the rate of organic fertilizer is 130 tons/ha, in the minimum – 100 tons/ha. The share of replacement of green manure by biomass in obtaining an equal amount of organic matter in the soil is 40%.

Accordingly, if a farmer applies 100 tons of organic fertilizers per hectare (minimum scenario), 40 tons of green manure have to be applied (52 tons/ha in the maximum scenario, correspondingly). As regards the hummus, 78 tons/ha have to be applied in the maximum scenario and 60 tons/ha in the minimum one. Organic fertilizers are to be applied triennially for certain cash crops.

The proposed crop rotation by organic farm includes eight crops:

- Sunflower for seeds;
- Steam or green manure (viko plus buckwheat, triennially);
- Winter wheat;
- Corn for silage;
- Barley and perennial grasses;
- Perennial grass 1;
- Perennial grass 2;
- Perennial grass 3.

Where the sales price is not specified, it is assumed that this production is for on-farm use. The main feed is required for ruminants and is provided by the processes of forage production. Its assessment is possible in many cases, for example, by a relative purchase price. The definition of replacement cost is possible only in a very limited way since its replacement does not always have the same effect for ruminants (feed structure, etc.). In practice, most often, the main feeds are produced for the own use. Even where sale and purchase are possible, they exist in very small quantities. If during economic planning it is necessary to decide how the total demand for main feed can be covered with at the cheapest (in terms of expenses, working time, or capital availability), a crucial role is played by feed production cost. Therefore, an evaluation of products supplied is excessive. Composing of the animal feed balance sheets is based on nutrient content. This means that energy, protein, and other nutrients are balanced, not demand for hay or haulage. Often it is enough to balance limited nutrients only. Any loss received in the feed production shows a part of total feed costs additionally transferred per hectare of forage production (in addition to the general expenses for the livestock).

The first element of the model shows productivity of particular crops within the proposed crop rotation depending on the amount of fertilizers, prices for commodity products, and variable production costs of each crop: price of commodity products, number and value of seeds, the number and value (substitutional value) of fertilizers, variable costs of mechanization (which includes repair costs), and the cost of fuel (Table 1).

The model element "Annual balance" allows constructing a visual map of the fields taking into account the crop rotation for ten years (Figure 1).

The calculation itself is based on the method of accounting margin calculation for crops. Total costs are $1,056.3 thousand, cost of the gross output is $5,127.8 thousand, and revenue is $4,071.5 thousand (Table 2).

Introduction of a fertilizer variable allows switching between the two scenarios and assess the rates of productivity, yields, and, ultimately, revenues of a farm. Within the update on fertilizers, total costs are $1,098.9 thousand, cost of the gross output is $6,027.0 thousand, and revenue is $4,928.1 thousand (Table 3).

The model also allows making adjustments in the calculations by changing crop rotation. The model demonstrates a ten-year crop rotation cycle (Table 4).

Table 1. Model element "Initial data"

Indicators	Unit of measure	Crops							
		Sunflower	Fallow	Wheat	Silage	Barley	Grass 1	Grass 2	Grass 3
Crop productivity, fertilizers – 100 tons/ha	dt/ha	25.0	0.0	45.0	150.0	40.0	200.0	200.0	200.0
Crop productivity, fertilizers – 130 tons/ha	dt/ha	30.0	0.0	50.0	225.0	45.0	350.0	350.0	350.0
Price	$/ton	700.1	0.0	317.0	92.2	258.1	73.7	73.7	73.7
Seeds, normative	kg/ha	20.0	0.0	250.0	50.0	200.0	160.0	15.0	15.0
Seeds, price	$/kg	4.4	0.0	0.3	0.9	0.2	0.3	0.3	0.3
Fertilizers, normative	ton/ha	100.0	0.0	0.0	100.0	0.0	0.0	0.0	0.0
Fertilizers, price	$	3.7	0.0	0.0	3.7	0.0	0.0	0.0	0.0
Costs	$	132.7	0.0	132.7	110.6	121.7	55.3	55.3	55.3
Fuel, seeding	l/ha	0.7	0.0	0.7	0.7	0.7	0.7	0.7	0.7
Fuel, harvesting	l/ha	0.7	0.0	0.7	0.7	0.7	0.7	0.7	0.7
Fuel, price	$/l	0.6	0.0	0.6	0.6	0.6	0.6	0.6	0.6

Source: Author's development

Figure 1. Model element "Annual balance", visual map
Source: Author's development

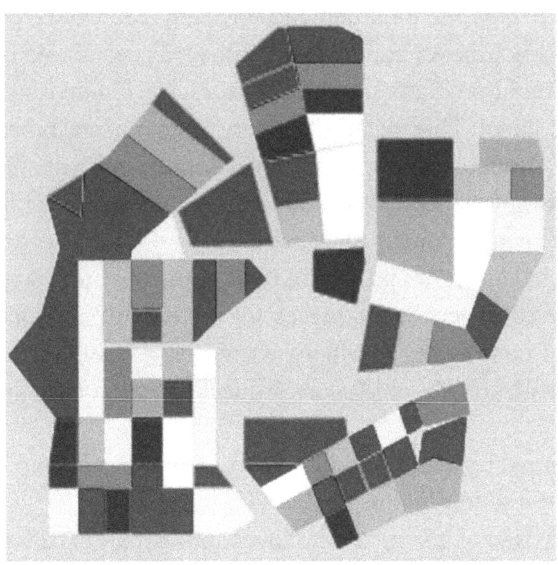

To allow a manager to make a managerial decision on the use of a particular combination of crops in the rotation and on the extension of areas under the most profitable crops, the model includes the marginal income index defined as "total balance". Using the "Area under crops" element, a manager may estimate a planned area under a particular crop for the previous ten years. Such a visibility allows a manager to optimize available agricultural land in relations to both years and crops (Table 5).

Table 2. Model element "Annual balance", data table

Crops	Area, ha	Crop yield, dt/ha	Gross output, tons	Cost, $ thous.	Seeds		Fertilizers		Other costs, $ thous.	Fuel	
					tons	$ thous.	tons	$ thous.		thous. liters	$ thous.
Sunflower	529.255	25.0	13,231.4	9,290.8	10.585	46.9	52,925.5	195.6	70.4	42.34	28.2
Fallow	320.285	0.0	0.0	0.0	0.0	0.0	0.0	0.0	0.0	0.0	0.0
Winter wheat	404.725	45.0	18,212.6	5,788.5	101.181	33.7	0.0	0.0	53.9	32.38	21.5
Silage	432.085	150.0	64,812.7	5,988.2	21.604	19.2	43,208.5	159.7	47.9	34.57	23.0
Barley	401.475	40.0	16,059.0	4,154.5	80.295	17.8	0.0	0.0	48.9	32.12	21.4
Grass 1	422.525	200.0	84,505.0	6,246.1	67.604	17.5	0.0	0.0	23.4	33.80	22.5
Grass 2	369.995	200.0	79,399.0	5,868.7	5.954	1.5	0.0	0.0	22.0	31.76	21.1
Grass 3	617.295	200.0	123,459.0	9,125.4	9.259	2.4	0.0	0.0	34.2	49.38	32.9
Winter wheat	336.740	45.0	15,153.3	4,816.2	84.185	28.0	0.0	0.0	44.8	26.94	17.9
Total	3,861.380	-	414,832.0	51,278.4	380.669	167.0	96,134.0	355.3	345.6	283.29	188.5

Source: Author's development

Table 3. Model element "Annual balance", model updated (fertilizers)

Crops	Area, ha	Crop yield, dt/ha	Gross output, tons	Cost, $ thous.	Seeds		Fertilizers		Other costs, $ thous.	Fuel	
					tons	$ thous.	tons	$ thous.		thous. liters	$ thous.
Sunflower	529.255	27.0	14,289.9	10,034.1	10.585	46.9	59,276.6	219.1	70.4	42.34	28.2
Fallow	320.285	0.0	0.0	0.0	0.0	0.0	0.0	0.0	0.0	0.0	0.0
Winter wheat	404.725	47.0	19,022.1	6,045.8	101.181	33.7	0.0	0.0	53.9	32.38	21.5
Silage	432.085	180.0	77,775.3	7,185.9	21.604	19.2	48,393.5	178.9	47.9	34.57	23.0
Barley	401.475	42.0	16,862.0	4,362.2	80.295	17.8	0.0	0.0	48.9	32.12	21.4
Grass 1	422.525	260.0	109,857.0	8,119.9	67.604	17.5	0.0	0.0	23.4	33.80	22.5
Grass 2	369.995	260.0	103,219.0	7,629.3	5.954	1.5	0.0	0.0	22.0	31.76	21.1
Grass 3	617.295	260.0	160,497.0	11,862.9	9.259	2.4	0.0	0.0	34.2	49.38	32.9
Winter wheat	336.740	47.0	15,826.8	5,030.2	84.185	28.0	0.0	0.0	44.8	26.94	17.9
Total	3,861.380	-	517,348.0	60,270.3	380.669	167.0	107,670.0	398.0	345.6	283.29	188.5

Source: Author's development

Organization of the crop rotation system in organic farming is inextricably linked to the definition of a rational structure of sown areas. Thus, it is necessary to ensure the production of agricultural products in such a quantity so to be able to fulfill contractual obligations on sales and to provide on-farm needs (seed fund, natural wages fund, forage fund, catering fund, insurance fund, marketing, repayment of loans, etc.). Among the principal measures to manage an organic farm in an efficient manner is scientifically

Table 4. Model element "Annual balance", model updated (years)

Crops	Area, ha	Crop yield, dt/ha	Gross output, tons	Cost, $ thous.	Seeds		Fertilizers		Other costs, $ thous.	Fuel	
					tons	$ thous.	tons	$ thous.		thous. liters	$ thous.
Sunflower	529.255	25.0	13,231.4	9,290.8	10.585	46.9	52,925.5	195.6	70.4	42.34	28.2
Fallow	320.285	0.0	0.0	0.0	0.0	0.0	0.0	0.0	0.0	0.0	0.0
Winter wheat	404.725	45.0	18,212.6	5,788.5	101.181	33.7	0.0	0.0	53.9	32.38	21.5
Silage	432.085	150.0	64,812.7	5,988.2	21.604	19.2	43,208.5	159.7	47.9	34.57	23.0
Barley	401.475	40.0	16,059.0	4,154.5	80.295	17.8	0.0	0.0	48.9	32.12	21.4
Grass 1	422.525	200.0	84,505.0	6,246.1	67.604	17.5	0.0	0.0	23.4	33.80	22.5
Grass 2	369.995	200.0	79,399.0	5,868.7	5.954	1.5	0.0	0.0	22.0	31.76	21.1
Grass 3	617.295	200.0	123,459.0	9,125.4	9.259	2.4	0.0	0.0	34.2	49.38	32.9
Winter wheat	336.740	45.0	15,153.3	4,816.2	84.185	28.0	0.0	0.0	44.8	26.94	17.9
Total	3,861.380	-	414,832.0	51,278.4	380.669	167.0	96,134.0	355.3	345.6	283.29	188.5

Source: Author's development

Table 5. Model element "Area under crops", hectares

Crops	Year 1	Year 2	Year 3	Year 4	Year 5	Year 6	Year 7	Year 8	Year 9	Year 10
Sunflower	529.25	336.74	617.29	396.99	422.52	401.47	432.08	404.72	320.28	529.25
Fallow	320.28	529.25	336.74	617.29	396.99	422.52	401.47	432.08	404.72	320.28
Winter wheat	741.46	937.58	926.25	759.26	1,018.77	829.08	827.25	721.76	961.34	741.46
Silage	432.08	404.72	320.28	529.25	336.74	617.29	396.99	422.52	401.47	432.08
Barley	401.47	432.08	404.72	320.28	529.25	336.74	617.29	396.99	422.52	401.47
Grasses	1,436.82	1,221.00	1,256.09	1,238.28	1,157.10	1,186.28	1,186.28	1,483.29	1,351.03	1,436.82

Source: Author's development

justified placing of crops in crop rotation. Proper implementation of crop rotation systems increase the productivity of use of farmland and fertilizers, ensures better application of plant varieties, and reduces weed infestation along with the impact of pests and diseases on crops with the minimal use of chemicals (Labenko & Perederiy, 2016).

The model element "Need for fertilizers" allows making changes in the rates of application of fertilizers according to the chosen scenario (Figure 2; Table 6).

When calculating the application rate of fertilizers, a manager relies on both the takeaway and the needs of plants in active substances, as well as considers the reserves of nutrients already available in the soil. The residual effect of the application of fertilizers under the crop-predecessor is also considered. During the calculation of the economic need for fertilizers, a manager determines the number of active ingredients required to compensate the damage caused to the balance of active substances in the soil when growing certain crops. In business and economic calculations, it is always advantageous to

Figure 2. Model element "Need for fertilizers", thousand tons, ten years
Source: Author's development

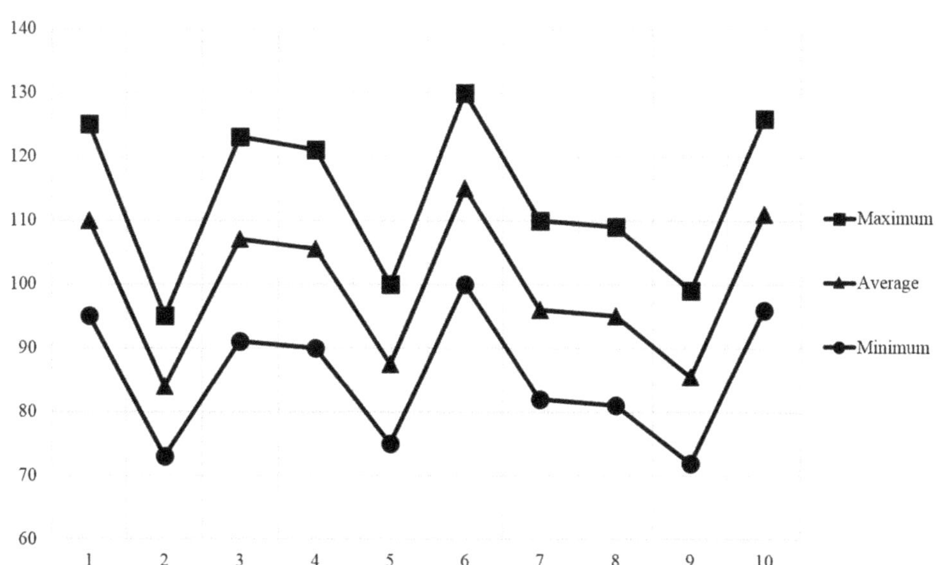

Table 6. Model element "Need for fertilizers", ten-year perspective

Crops	Year 1	Year 2	Year 3	Year 4	Year 5	Year 6	Year 7	Year 8	Year 9	Year 10
Volume of fertilizers needed, thousand tons	107.670	83.044	105.009	103.740.0	85.038	114.102	92.857	92.652	80.837	107.670

Source: Author's development

reflect the removal of active ingredients by the by-products (straw) separately, so that in the calculation practice it is possible to cover different processes (plowing or harvesting straw). Removal of the active ingredients through the parts of the plants that remain after harvesting is not considered and thus is equivalent to their return to the soil.

Properties and composition of local fertilizers of animal origin, i.e. manure, pus, and liquid manure, add to the complexity of their application through losses of nutrients. There are specific rules which a manager has to follow when applying organic fertilizers of animal origin:

- Liquid manure, pus, and bird droppings cannot be applied into the arable land from November 15 to January 15, and into the pastures from December 5 to February 5.
- Direct plowing-in of the liquid manure, pus, and poultry litter on rough fields helps to avoid losses of nitrogen. After harvesting, these fertilizers can be applied only under the field grasses, additional sowings, and winter crops and only in an amount which shall not exceed 40 kg NH4/ha or 80 kg of total nitrogen per hectare.
- In the model, the pictogram "fertilizer" allows regulating the application rate:
- Close to the soil surface application of fertilizers into the moisture. Cool and windless weather helps to avoid weathering ammonia.

- Areas with a high content of phosphate and potassium allow the application of local fertilizers of animal origin in the amount equal to the takeaway of nutrients by plants.
- Average application rate should not exceed 210 kg N/ha/year for grassland and 170 kg N/ha/year for the arable land. When stored, liquid manure loses 10% (manure – 25%) of nitrogen contained in organic matter. During application, up to 20% of the calculated total content of nitrogen is lost (Beckman & Brecker, 2014b).

Groups of agricultural animals and their maximum population per one hectare of pasture farms are presented in Table 7.

Table 7. The maximum possible location of animals in calculation per 1 hectare of pastures

Groups of animals	Type of organic fertilizer		
	Liquid manure	Manure + liquid manure	Manure of deep bedding
Dairy cows without calves (6,000 kg milk)	2.5	2.8	3.0
Dairy cows with calves (6,000 kg milk)	1.8	1.9	2.1
Cow separated from its calf	3.6	3.9	4.3
Calves up to 3 months	20.8	22.7	22.0
Heifer	6.2	6.8	7.4
Horses, 500 - 600 kg of live weight	6.0	6.5	7.1
Sheep + litter	11.3	14.5	15.9

Source: Beckman and Brecker (2014b)

Based on the assumptions and calculations presented above, a manager may recalculate maximum and minimum possible populations of various groups of agricultural animals for their retention. The model element "Yield" represents the planned total yield for each crop in years (Table 8).

Table 8. Model element "Yield", thousand tons

Crops	Year 1	Year 2	Year 3	Year 4	Year 5	Year 6	Year 7	Year 8
Sunflower	1,402.53	892.36	1,635.83	1,052.04	1,119.69	1,063.91	1,147.03	1,072.52
Winter wheat	3,447.81	4,359.75	4,307.06	3,530.58	4,737.28	3,855.22	3,846.71	3,356.18
Silage	7,453.47	6,981.51	5,524.92	9,129.65	5,808.76	10,648.30	6,848.16	7,288.56
Barley	1,666.12	1,793.15	1,679.61	1,329.18	2,196.41	1,397.47	2,561.77	1,647.53
Grasses	35,202.00	29,914.40	30,774.10	30,338.00	28,348.80	30,729.50	29,063.90	36,340.60

Source: Author's development

Using the "Fertilizer" pictogram, there is a possibility to choose any scenario for fertilization from the minimum to the maximum. In such a way, minimum possible, optimum, or maximum gross yield may be planned for a particular crop rotation.

Based on the rates of return and expenses, model element "Revenue and expenses" (enables reviewing and evaluating those rates from the point of view of the suitability of possible alternative ways of farm development. The important requirements are integrity and objectivity of facts, responsibility during consequence analysis, creativity, and persistence in the implementation of managerial decisions (Table 9).

Table 9. Model element "Revenue and expenses", $ thousand

Crops	Year 1	Year 2	Year 3	Year 4	Year 5	Year 6	Year 7	Year 8	Year 9	Year 10
Sunflower	997.2	634.5	1,163.1	748.0	796.1	756.4	814.1	762.6	603.5	997.2
Winter wheat	1,103.7	1,395.6	1,378.7	1,130.2	1,516.4	1,234.1	1,231.4	1,074.3	1,430.9	1,103.7
Silage	708.6	663.7	525.2	867.9	552.2	1,012.3	651.0	692.9	658.4	708.6
Barley	434.5	467.6	438.0	346.6	572.8	364.4	668.0	429.6	457.3	434.5
Grasses	2,708.1	2,301.4	2,367.5	2,333.9	2,180.9	2,364.0	2,235.9	2,795.7	2,546.4	2,708.1
Gross revenue	5,952.1	5,462.8	5,872.6	5,426.7	5,618.5	5,731.4	5,599.5	5,755.2	5,696.6	5,952.1
Seeds	167.0	164.7	185.0	156.0	177.1	171.6	169.3	161.2	165.0	167.0
Fertilizers	394.4	304.2	384.6	380.0	311.5	417.9	340.1	339.3	296.1	394.4
Other expenses	345.6	334.8	359.9	320.2	357.8	342.7	352.6	327.4	341.5	345.6
Fuel	188.4	177.3	187.6	172.6	184.4	183.0	184.1	182.5	183.9	188.4
Gross expenses	1,095.4	981.0	1,117.1	1,028.9	1,030.7	1,115.3	1,046.2	1,010.4	986.5	1,095.4

Source: Author's development

SOLUTIONS AND RECOMMENDATIONS

To ensure the efficient management of organic farming in the severe climate conditions and fragile environment of the Arctic, a detailed information about internal factors influencing the production and distribution processes is required. Based on those detailed input data, a manager is able to take a decision best suited to a particular situation on the market. However, as evidenced by the findings of this study, both information overload and a lack of relevant data equally complicate the processing of information flows about the existing situation and development prospects of the organic market. In the conditions of the Arctic, the issue is even more complicated due to the rapidly changing weather conditions, delays in delivery of required resources and inputs, seasonality of production and demand, and lack of knowledge and experience in the sphere of organic farming in the High North. In such conditions, a price of a mistake in a managerial decision is dramatically high. Any managerial decision has to be prepared, taken, and implemented in a proper manner and thus supported by reliable data.

A model developed and tested in this study may be used by managers of organic farms who think about starting their activities in the northern regions and even in the territories related to the circumpolar Arctic. The model is appropriate for the analysis of the actual situation and future development of agricultural enterprise, particularly, organic farming, in the unstable climate conditions and fragile environment of the Arctic. It is recommended to elaborate the model on the basis of the calculation of marginal gains across a range of agricultural products and to use Wolfram Mathematica platform. The proposed set of variables included in the model involves fertilizers, prices for commodity products, and variable production costs of each crop: price of commodity products, number and value of seeds, the number and value (substitutional value) of fertilizers, variable costs of mechanization (which includes repair costs), and the cost of fuel. To adjust the model to the changing environmental, production, economic, and market conditions of organic farming, five additional elements may be used, i.e. annual balance (corrected on the various scenarios of fertilizers applications and duration of the crop rotation cycle), area under crops, need for fertilizers, yield, and revenue and expenses.

Apart from solving a food insecurity problem, development of organic farming in the northern territories may contribute to increasing of employment of rural population and the overall efficiency of agricultural production (Erokhin & Ivolga, 2014). The implementation of the proposed model of agricultural development allows deciding on the future of rural development, including the need to address the problem of employment in private households. The agro-ecological policy should be directed to the management of land resources, environmental protection, and provision of the population with healthy products.

FUTURE RESEARCH DIRECTIONS

In the Arctic, the issue of food security brings together concerns over a range of environmental, social, economic, political, and cultural changes. This study is a preliminary attempt to investigate how those approaches to the management of organic farming which have been used in the traditional regions of agricultural production may be implemented in the conditions of the High North. The crop rotation used as a case study in the model included the crops cultivated by organic farms in the sub-polar latitudes (sunflower for seeds, steam or green manure, winter wheat, corn for silage, barley, and perennial grasses). More severe climate conditions of the circumpolar territories require additional studies of appropriate crops and crop rotations, particularly, in the greenhouses with heat-assistance. A further focus on organic farming in the light of food insecurity problem could place the issue in the larger context of social-ecological change that is affecting the resilience of the Arctic and health and well-being of its inhabitants. In such a respect, further research in the area of organic farming in the High North should involve close collaboration with current work on indicators of food and water security in the circumpolar territories, as well as other relevant initiatives. However, organic farming is only one of the possible solutions of food insecurity problem of the Arctic. Effectively addressing the food insecurity challenge in this part of the world will require continued research into food insecurity risk factors and trends in order to facilitate the identification of priority policy and action areas.

CONCLUSION

Food insecurity remains a critical issue in the Arctic. Growing scales of economic activity, when people utilize increasing volumes of natural resources, cause strengthening of human pressure on the environment and arise ecological imbalance, which, in turn, aggravates social and economic problems. Reserves of non-renewable raw materials and energy resources are limited, and environmental pollution amplifies. Finally, all those activities undermine natural and resource potential of production and negatively effect on human health. Retail foods are consumed more frequently than local foods, suggesting that food security interventions should consider the affordability of healthy retail food choices, in addition to programming increasing the availability of local foods.

One of the potential solutions to the food security problem in the circumpolar territories is the development of organic farming which provides a more positive impact on the preservation of wildlife and landscape compared to the conventional systems of agricultural production per unit of area of land used for agricultural production. In the conditions of the Arctic, organic agriculture is a perspective form of nature management, which main idea is how to secure natural basis and life processes. Organic farming is increasing its potential in the polar regions. A green turn to more organic farming is a promising step towards a food security and sustainable development of rural areas in the Arctic. In this context, an attention should be paid to the development of economic mechanisms of production and distribution of organic products in the sparsely populated northern parts of the planet.

REFERENCES

Anisimov, O. A., Vaughan, D., Callaghan, T. V., Furgal, C., Marchant, H., Prowse, T. D., ... Walsh, J.E. (2007). Polar Region (Arctic and Antarctic). In M. Parry, O.F. Canziani, J.P. Palutikof, P.J. van der Linden, & C.E. Hanson (Eds.), Climate Change 2007: Impacts, Adaptation and Vulnerability. Contribution of Working Group II to the Fourth Assessment Report of the Intergovernmental Panel on Climate Change (pp. 653-685). Cambridge, UK: Cambridge University Press.

Beaumier, M. C., & Ford, J. D. (2010). Food Insecurity among Inuit Women Exacerbated by Socioeconomic Stresses and Climate Change. *Canadian Journal of Public Health*, *101*(3), 196–201. PMID:20737808

Beckman, K., & Brecker, Y. (2014a). *Farmer: A Basic Level*. Sumy: Sumy National Agrarian University.

Beckman, K., & Brecker, Y. (2014b). *Farmer: A Professional Level*. Sumy: Sumy National Agrarian University.

Berner, J., & Furgal, C. (2005). Human Health. In J. Berner, C. Symon, L. Arris, & O. W. Heal (Eds.), *Arctic Climate Impact Assessment – Scientific Report* (pp. 863–906). Cambridge: Cambridge University Press.

Boult, D. A. (2004). Hunger in the Arctic: Food. In *Security in Inuit Communities*. Ottawa: Ajunnginiq Centre.

Dolce, J. (2016). *Farming Made Possible in Arctic*. Retrieved February 10, 2018, from https://gpnmag.com/2016/11/farming-made-possible-in-arctic/

Dresscher, S.-J. (2016). Food Security in the High Arctic while Balancing the Demands of Commercial and Subsistence Hunting. *Journal für Entwicklungspolitik*, *32*(4), 41–66. doi:10.20446/JEP-2414-3197-32-4-41

Duhaime, G., & Bernard, N. (Eds.). (2008). *Arctic Food Security*. Edmonton: Canadian Circumpolar Institute Press.

Erokhin, V. (2016). Development of Rural Territories in the Far East, Russia and Heilongjiang Province, P.R.China. *Agricultural Bulletin of Stavropol Region, 23*(3), 256–260.

Erokhin, V. (Ed.). (2017a). *Establishing Food Security and Alternatives to International Trade in Emerging Economies*. Hershey, PA: IGI Global.

Erokhin, V. (2017b). Factors Influencing Food Markets in Developing Countries: An Approach to Assess Sustainability of the Food Supply in Russia. *Sustainability, 9*(8), 1313. doi:10.3390u9081313

Erokhin, V. (2017c). Self-Sufficiency versus Security: How Trade Protectionism Challenges the Sustainability of the Food Supply in Russia. *Sustainability, 9*(11), 1939. doi:10.3390u9111939

Erokhin, V. (2018). Study of Migration Processes in Rural Areas of Northern China. *Herald of the Moscow University of Finances and Law MFUA, 1*, 182–196.

Erokhin, V., & Gao, T. (2018). Competitive Advantages of China's Agricultural Exports in the Outward-Looking Belt and Road Initiative. In W. Zhang, I. Alon, & C. Lattemann (Eds.), *China's Belt and Road Initiative: Changing the Rules of Globalization* (pp. 265–285). London: Palgrave Macmillan. doi:10.1007/978-3-319-75435-2_14

Erokhin, V., & Ivolga, A. (Eds.). (2014). Contemporary Issues of Sustainable Rural Development: International Approaches and Experiences of Eastern Europe and Russia. Stavropol: AGRUS of Stavropol State Agrarian University.

Erokhin, V., Ivolga, A., & Lisova, O. (2016). Challenges to Sustainable Rural Development in Russia: Social Issues and Regional Divergences. *Applied Studies in Agribusiness and Commerce – APSTRACT, 10*(1), 45-52.

Fergurson, H. (2011). Inuit Food (In)Security in Canada: Assessing the Implications and Effectiveness of Policy. *Queen's. Policy Review, 2*(2), 54–79.

Ford, J. D. (2009). Vulnerability of Inuit Food Systems to Food Insecurity as a Consequence of Climate Change: A Case Study from Igloolik, Nunavut. *Regional Environmental Change, 9*(2), 83–100. doi:10.100710113-008-0060-x

Friedrich, D. (2018). *Vegetable Farms 'Mushrooming' Across the Arctic*. Retrieved February 10, 2018, from http://www.highnorthnews.com/vegetable-farms-mushrooming-across-the-arctic/

Gao, T. (2017). Food Security and Rural Development on Emerging Markets of Northeast Asia: Cases of Chinese North and Russian Far East. In V. Erokhin (Ed.), *Establishing Food Security and Alternatives to International Trade in Emerging Economies* (pp. 155–176). Hershey, PA: IGI Global.

Gao, T., Erokhin, V., & Ivolga, A. (2018). Chinese Food Security Policy: Contemporary Challenges. *Agricultural Bulletin of Stavropol Region, 29*(1), 111–116.

Gao, T., Ivolga, A., & Erokhin, V. (2018). Sustainable Rural Development in Northern China: Caught in a Vice between Poverty, Urban Attractions, and Migration. *Sustainability, 10*(5), 1467. doi:10.3390u10051467

Guz, M., & Ivolga, I. (2015). Organic Agriculture as a Tool to Make Economy Green. In A. Jean-Vasile, I. Raluca Andreea, & T. Rahoveanu Adrian (Eds.), *Green Economic Structures in Modern Business and Society* (pp. 196–218). Hershey, PA: IGI Global. doi:10.4018/978-1-4666-8219-1.ch011

Hastrup, K., Rieffestahl, A. M., & Olsen, A. (2016). Food Security: Health and Environmental Concerns in the North. In M. Singer (Ed.), *A Companion to the Anthropology of Environmental Health* (pp. 257–280). Hoboken, NJ: John Wiley & Sons. doi:10.1002/9781118786949.ch13

Hoag, H. (2016, October 31). Arctic Agriculture: Farming Opportunities on the Horizon. *Arctic Deeply*. Retrieved from https://www.newsdeeply.com/arctic/articles/2016/10/31/arctic-agriculture-farming-opportunities-on-the-horizon

Hollesen, J., Matthiesen, H., Moller, A. B., & Elberling, B. (2015). Permafrost Thawing in Organic Arctic Soils Accelerated by Ground Heat Production. *Nature Climate Change*, *5*(6), 574–578. doi:10.1038/nclimate2590

Huet, C., Ford, J. D., Edge, V. L., Shirley, J., King, N., & Harper, S. L. (2017). Food Insecurity and Food Consumption by Season in Households with Children in an Arctic City: A Cross-Sectional Study. *BioMed Central Public Health*, *17*(1), 578. doi:10.118612889-017-4393-6 PMID:28619039

Huet, C., Rosol, R., & Egeland, G. M. (2012). The Prevalence of Food Insecurity is High and the Diet Quality Poor in Inuit Communities. *The Journal of Nutrition*, *142*(3), 541–547. doi:10.3945/jn.111.149278 PMID:22323760

Ivolga, A. (2014). Overview of Contemporary Issues of Sustainable Rural Development in Russia in Terms of Existing Differences between Regions. *Economics of Agriculture*, *2*, 331–345.

Jean-Vasile, A., Raluca Andreea, I., & Rahoveanu Adrian, T. (Eds.). (2015). *Green Economic Structures in Modern Business and Society*. Hershey, PA: IGI Global. doi:10.4018/978-1-4666-8219-1

Jenssen, B. M., Villanger, G. D., Gabrielsen, K. M., Bytingsvik, J., Bechshoft, T., Ciesielski, T. M., ... Dietz, R. (2015). Anthropogenic Flank Attack on Polar Bears: Interacting Consequences of Climate Warming and Pollutant Exposure. *Frontiers in Ecology and Evolution*, *3*, 1–7. doi:10.3389/fevo.2015.00016

Kondrashev, A., Nikitenko, M., Trofimova, I., Trofimova, S., & Gotsko, L. (2016a). Food Security of Arctic Territories Legal Regulation. *Journal of Siberian Federal University*, *9*(9), 2184–2193. doi:10.17516/1997-1370-2016-9-9-2184-2193

Kondrashev, A., Nikitenko, M., Trofimova, I., Trofimova, S., & Gotsko, L. (2016b). The Arctic States' Strategies and the Northern Regions' Food Security. *The Economic Annals-XXI Journal*, *162*(11-12), 32–37.

Koutouki, K., Booth, S., & Blum, S. (2017). Inuit Food Security in Canada: Arctic Marine Ethnoecology. *Food Security*, *9*(3), 1–20.

Kuhnlein, H. V., Receveur, O., Soueida, R., & Egeland, G. M. (2004). Arctic Indigenous Peoples Experience the Nutrition Transition with Changing Dietary Patterns and Obesity. *The Journal of Nutrition*, *134*(6), 1447–1453. doi:10.1093/jn/134.6.1447 PMID:15173410

Labenko, O., & Perederiy, N. (2016). Environmental Impact of Agriculture in Ukraine. *International Agricultural Management, 1*(1). Retrieved February 9, 2018, from http://ima.hswt.de/en/editions

Loring, P. A., & Gerlach, C. (2015). Searching for Progress on Food Security in the North American North: A Research Synthesis and Meta-Analysis of the Peer-Reviewed Literature. *Arctic, 68*(3), 380–392. doi:10.14430/arctic4509

McKinney, M. A., Iverson, S. J., Fisk, A. T., Sonne, C., Riget, F. F., Letcher, R. J., ... Dietz, R. (2013). Global Change Effects on the Long-Term Feeding Ecology and Contaminant Exposures of East Greenland Polar Bears. *Global Change Biology, 19*(8), 2360–2372. doi:10.1111/gcb.12241 PMID:23640921

Muir, D. C. G., & de Wit, C. A. (2010). Trends of Legacy and New Persistent Organic Pollutants in the Circumpolar Arctic: Overview, Conclusions, and Recommendations. *The Science of the Total Environment, 408*(15), 3044–3051. doi:10.1016/j.scitotenv.2009.11.032 PMID:20006375

Nilsson, A. E., Nilsson, L. M., Quinlan, A., & Evengard, B. (2013). Food Security in the Arctic: Preliminary Reflections from a Resilience Perspective. In Arctic Resilience Interim Report 2013 (pp. 113-116). Stockholm: Stockholm Environment Institute; Stockholm Resilience Centre.

Nilsson, L. M., & Evengard, B. (2015). Food Security or Food Sovereignty: What is the Main Issue in the Arctic? In B. Evengard, J. Nymand Larsen, & O. Paasche (Eds.), *The New Arctic* (pp. 213–223). Cham: Springer. doi:10.1007/978-3-319-17602-4_16

Nobel, J. (2013). *Farming in the Arctic: It Can Be Done.* Retrieved February 10, 2018, from https://modernfarmer.com/2013/10/arctic-farming/

Poppel, B., Kruse, J., Duhaime, G., & Abryutina, L. (2007). *SliCa Results.* Anchorage, AL: University of Alaska Anchorage.

Ready, E. (2016). Challenges in the Assessment of Inuit Food Security. *Arctic, 69*(3), 266–280. doi:10.14430/arctic4579

Sonne, C., Letcher, R. J., Jenssen, B. M., Desforges, J.-P., Eulaers, I., Andersen-Ranberg, E., ... Dietz, R. (2017). A Veterinary Perspective on One Health in the Arctic. *Acta Veterinaria Scandinavica, 59*(1), 84. doi:10.118613028-017-0353-5 PMID:29246165

Wesche, S. D., & Chan, H. M. (2010). Adapting to the Impacts of Climate Change on Food Security among Inuit in the Western Canadian Arctic. *EcoHealth, 7*(3), 361–373. doi:10.100710393-010-0344-8 PMID:20680394

Zetterstrom, R. (2003). Industrial and Agricultural Pollution: A Threat to the Health of Children Living in the Arctic Region. *Acta Paediatrica (Oslo, Norway), 92*(11), 1238–1240. doi:10.1111/j.1651-2227.2003.tb00489.x PMID:14696839

ADDITIONAL READING

Alston, J. M., Beddow, J. M., & Pardey, P. G. (2009). Agricultural Research, Productivity, and Food Prices in the Long Run. *Science, 325*(5945), 1209–1210. doi:10.1126cience.1170451 PMID:19729642

Anderson, D. G. (1998). Contested Arctic: Indigenous Peoples, Industrial States, and the Circumpolar Environment. *American Anthropologist, 100*(4), 1070–1071. doi:10.1525/aa.1998.100.4.1070

Cairns, R. D. (2014). The Green Paradox of the Economics of Exhaustible Resources. *Energy Policy, 65*, 78–85. doi:10.1016/j.enpol.2013.10.047

Carson, M., & Peterson, G. (2016). Arctic Resilience Report. Stockholm: Stockholm Environment Institute; Stockholm Resilience Centre.

Deichmann, U., & Fan, Z. (2013). *Growing Green: The Economic Benefits of Climate Action*. Washington, DC: World Bank. doi:10.1596/978-0-8213-9791-6

Duhaime, G. (Ed.). (2002). *Sustainable Food Security in the Arctic*. Edmonton: Canadian Circumpolar Institute.

Fuglie, K. (2010). Accelerated Productivity Growth Offsets Decline in Resource Expansion in Global Agriculture. *Amber Waves, 8*, 46–51.

Ginsberg, J. M., & Bloom, P. N. (2004). Choosing the Right Green Marketing Strategy. *MIT Sloan Management Review, 46*(1), 79–84.

Gupta, S., & Ogden, D. T. (2009). To Buy or not to Buy? A Social Dilemma Perspective on Green Buying. *Journal of Consumer Marketing, 26*(6), 376–391. doi:10.1108/07363760910988201

Hole, D., Perkins, A., Wilson, J., Alexander, I., Grice, P., & Evans, A. (2005). Does Organic Farming Benefit Biodiversity? *Biological Conservation, 122*(1), 113–130. doi:10.1016/j.biocon.2004.07.018

Illarionova, K. (2014). Green State Procurements in International Practice. *Product Quality Control, 3*, 17–25.

Kalafatis, S. P., Pollard, M., East, R., & Tsogas, M. H. (1999). Green Marketing and Ajzen's Theory of Planned Behavior: A Cross-Market Examination. *Journal of Consumer Marketing, 16*(5), 441–460. doi:10.1108/07363769910289550

Keil, K., & Knecht, S. (Eds.). (2017). *Governing Arctic Change*. Cham: Springer. doi:10.1057/978-1-137-50884-3

Kozlova, O. (2011). Marketing Analysis of Development of International Organic Market. *Bulletin of Altay State Agrarian University, 79*(5), 117–121.

Kreidler, N. B., & Joseph, M. S. (2009). How Green should You Go? Understanding the Role of Green Atmospherics in Service Environment Evaluations. *International Journal of Culture, Tourism and Hospitality Research, 3*(3), 228–245. doi:10.1108/17506180910995414

Levinson, J. C., & Horowitz, S. (2010). *Guerrilla Marketing Goes Green: Winning Strategies to Improve Your Profits and Your Planet*. New York, NY: John Wiley & Sons.

Mainieri, T., Barnett, E. G., Valdero, T. R., Unipan, J. B., & Oskamp, S. (1997). Green Buying: The Influence of Environmental Concern on Consumer Behavior. *The Journal of Social Psychology*, *137*(2), 189–204. doi:10.1080/00224549709595430

Pars, T., Osler, M., & Bjerregaard, P. (2001). Contemporary Usage of Traditional and Imported Food among Greenlandic Inuit. *Arctic*, *54*(1), 22–31. doi:10.14430/arctic760

Peattie, K., & Crane, A. (2005). Green Marketing: Legend, Myth, Farce or Prophesy. *Qualitative Market Research*, *8*(4), 357–370. doi:10.1108/13522750510619733

Petrov, A. BurnSilver, S., Stuart Chapin, F., Fondahl, G., Graybill, J.K., Keil, K., … Schweitzer, P. (2017). Arctic Sustainability Research. London: Routledge.

Pop, O., Dina, G. C., & Martin, C. (2011). Promoting the Social Corporate Responsibility for a Green Economy and Innovative Jobs. *Procedia: Social and Behavioral Sciences*, *15*, 1020–1023. doi:10.1016/j.sbspro.2011.03.232

Poto, M. (2017). Participatory Engagement and the Empowerment of the Arctic Indigenous Peoples. *Environmental Law Review*, *19*(1), 30–47. doi:10.1177/1461452917691778

Schuster, R. C., Wein, E. E., Dickson, C., & Chan, H. M. (2011). Importance of Traditional Foods for the Food Security of Two First Nations Communities in the Yukon, Canada. *International Journal of Circumpolar Health*, *70*(3), 286–300. doi:10.3402/ijch.v70i3.17833 PMID:21631967

Seyfang, G., & Longhurst, N. (2013). Growing Green Money? Mapping Community Currencies for Sustainable Development. *Ecological Economics*, *86*, 65–77. doi:10.1016/j.ecolecon.2012.11.003

Starks, Z. S. (2007). Arctic Foodways and Contemporary Cuisine. *Gastronomica*, *7*(1), 41–49. doi:10.1525/gfc.2007.7.1.41

Wiik, E., Brown, N., Bacon, S., Cantalou, J., Costigan, G., & Edwards, M. (2017). *The Rapidly Changing Arctic Environment – Implications for Policy and Decision Makers from the NERC Arctic Research Programme 2011-16. Cambridge: NERC Arctic Office*. Southampton: University of Southampton.

KEY TERMS AND DEFINITIONS

Agro-Industrial Complex: A complex of integrated industries (animal husbandry, crop production, food processing, agricultural machinery, organic farming) and supportive facilities (storage, insurance, transportation, distribution of food and agricultural products).

Food Security: A physical, social, and economic access by all people at all times to sufficient, safe, and nutritious food which meets their dietary needs and food preferences for an active and healthy life.

High North: Territories of Nordic countries (Canada, Denmark, Finland, Iceland, Norway, Russia, Sweden, and the United States) located throughout the Arctic beyond the Polar Circle.

Management: The coordination of all resources through the process of planning, organizing, directing, and controlling in order to attain stated objectives.

Managerial Decision Making: A process, which includes establishing the objective of the business enterprise, defining the problem, identifying possible alternative solutions, evaluating alternative courses of actions, and implementing the decision.

Rural Territory: An area outside larger and medium-sized cities and surrounding population concentrations, generally characterized by small towns and unpopulated regions. Rural circumpolar territories are inhabited predominantly by indigenous people.

Sustainable Development: A concept of conserving resources for future generations which major goal is the long-term stability of the economy and environment; this is only achievable through the integration and acknowledgment of economic, environmental, and social concerns throughout the decision-making process.

This research was previously published in the Handbook of Research on International Collaboration, Economic Development, and Sustainability in the Arctic edited by Vasilii Erokhin, Tianming Gao, and Xiuhua Zhang; pages 593-615, copyright year 2019 by Business Science Reference (an imprint of IGI Global).

Chapter 47
Produce Internationally, Consume Locally:
Changing Paradigm of China's Food Security Policy

Vasilii Erokhin
https://orcid.org/0000-0002-3745-5469
Harbin Engineering University, China

ABSTRACT

China is one of the world's biggest importers of agricultural products. Until quite recently, China's agricultural policy focused on food self-sufficiency. Globalizing trade in agricultural commodities, however, has brought new challenges to establishing secure supply and achieving security rather than self-sufficiency. In the face of emerging trade tensions with the USA, one of China's responses to the emerging volatility of the global market is to expand production facilities abroad and thus diversify deliveries. This chapter discusses how China's Belt and Road Initiative may serve improving food security of the country by establishing of a predictable system of agricultural production and trade across Eurasia, particularly, with the involvement of land-abundant Russia and the countries of Central Asia. The author explores possible responses to emerging threats to China's domestic food market by elaborating an approach to theoretical definitions and practical issues of ensurance of food security and adaptation of China's policy to contemporary global challenges.

INTRODUCTION

Food security is commonly defined as a condition when people have access to sufficient amounts of safe and nutritious food and are therefore consuming the food required for normal growth and development, and for an active and healthy life (Food and Agriculture Organization of the United Nations [FAO], 1992). Food security is the physical, social and economic access by all people at all times to sufficient, safe, and nutritious food that meets their dietary needs and food preferences for an active and healthy

DOI: 10.4018/978-1-7998-5354-1.ch047

life (FAO, 1992). FAO's approach is based on physical availability of food and agricultural products on the domestic market (domestic production plus import) and economic access to adequate supply by all people (purchasing power, food inflation, distribution, etc.) (Erokhin, 2017c). Jash (2015) explains FAO's dimensions of food security along the four pillars: food availability (sufficient quantities of food available on a consistent basis); food access (sufficient resources to obtain appropriate food for a nutritious diet); utilization (appropriate use based on knowledge of basic nutrition and health care as well as adequate water and sanitation); and stability (ensuring that a population, household or individual have access to adequate food at all times, without any risk of losing access to food as a consequence of sudden shocks. In this vein, food security is argued to be a complex sustainable development issue, linked to health through malnutrition, but also to sustainable economic development and environment.

Food security is usually categorized as a non-trade concern within trade policy as it incorporates factors other than those directly relevant to the operation of an international market system (Erokhin, 2017b). The concept of food security emerged after World War II, when reconstruction efforts created a global food regime that was increasingly sought through economic policies including trade liberalization and the opening of economic markets (Schanbacher, 2010). In the current global dynamics, food security is increasingly assessed in the light of concerns over global trade in agricultural commodities, distribution of agricultural production facilities and food products, and insufficient production to meet the future needs in food. An increasing number of developing countries have transitioned from being net food exporters to net food importers (Valdes & Foster, 2012). Liberalization of international trade has become a significant source of tension in contemporary agricultural change with the incorporation of agriculture into the world trading system (Lee, 2007). In the conditions of globalization, where liberalization of food trade and the reduction of administrative protection of food producers are mandated by the rules of the WTO, many countries have lost a part of their sovereignty over food policies (Lawrence & McMichael, 2012). Some of them (primarily, developing ones) have become food dependent, others managed to benefit from easier access to foreign markets and unified framework of global trade in food. In general, globalization has refocused attention from trade-based food self-sufficiency to availability-based food security.

Many countries are now concerned about the sustainability of their food supply. As a counter to liberalization, they are now re-examining their strategies for achieving food self-sufficiency rather than food security, and are seeking measures to improve the sustainability of food supplies, while also protecting their domestic food markets from increasing imports (Valdes & Foster, 2012). In an attempt to decrease the reliance on imports, some countries reduce the availability and access to food for the population. Abundant food stocks in some countries coexist with shortages in some others, while unexpected price surges and influences of other factors push millions of people into poverty, aggravating income inequalities and threatening food security. Price instability is detrimental not only to poor countries, where deteriorating living conditions of people may raise food conflicts, but even to some developing countries. International trade plays a vital role in stabilizing food supplies and food prices, but importing and exporting countries also worry about the unreliability of world markets. Even high-income countries feel threatened by volatile food markets, and want to guarantee food availability and accessibility in the long run (Saravia-Matus, Gomez, Paloma, & Mary, 2012).

Being the most populous country in the world with the biggest internal market for food and agricultural products, China is one of the most demonstrative examples of a country extremely concerned about food security and sustainability of food supply. In China, understanding of food security differs from the internationally accepted one of the FAO, particularly, in the context of food self-sufficiency

(Zhang & Cheng, 2016; Gao, 2017). Luan, Cui, and Ferrat (2013), Ghose (2014), and Zhang (2011) treat food security as self-sufficiency by stressing the ensurance of physical and economic access to food products of high quality and sustainability of such access in the long-term. Food security is thus accepted as increasing of domestic food production up to the certain threshold set by the government. In 1996, China announced the 95% self-sufficiency rate as the bottom line of its food security (State Council of the People's Republic of China [State Council], 1996). In 2008, the government pledged to achieve absolute self-sufficiency in major cereals, including wheat, rice, and corn (State Council, 2008).

Such a focus on self-sufficiency looks rationale. China is a country where agricultural sector is intended to feed over 1.3 billion people, where the incomes of over 737 million rural people depend on agricultural production, and where 42.6% of labor is employed in agriculture (Mukhopadhyay, Thomassin, & Zhang, 2018). Tian (n.d.) defines the following special concerns of China on national food security: (1) rural people still earn over a half of their income from farming; (2) share of food in total spending is high; (3) food price is one of the critical elements of consumer price index. The core to understand China's food security policy is controllability perceived by policymakers in three aspects. First is to avoid over-dependence on foreign trade by means of the development of domestic production and stockholding and regulations on domestic utilization of staple foods. Second is to avoid external-induced shocks to domestic food market by practicing domestic food price and border interventions and food stock measures. Third is to ensure social stability by means of preventing of combating income disparity, preventing volatility of food prices, and targeting support policies to rural and urban poor.

Reformulated food security strategy announced in 2013 prioritized domestic production and supply and aimed at moderating food imports. Many experts, however, claim that food self-sufficiency policy has not really improved food security of China. Zhang and Cheng (2016) reveal that, in an attempt to increase domestic production, Chinese farmers excessively use chemical fertilizers and thus threaten the long-term sustainability of agricultural sector. Despite numerous support measures, the government still failed to sufficiently compensate farmers because of the rapidly rising production cost. Eventually, agricultural producers were discouraged to switch to cash crops and continued growing wheat and corn.

Arable land scarcity and political emphasis on self-sufficiency in staple foods has resulted in a lack of agricultural capacity (ChinaPower, 2017). In pursuing food self-sufficiency and avoiding over-dependence on imports, one of the possible solutions for China is the diversification of the sources where the country obtains food and agricultural products. This chapter investigates Belt and Road Initiative (BRI) as a potential tool to diversify food imports to China by means of expansion of joint ventures abroad and overseas agricultural investments. The goal is to review China's agricultural production, food supply and demand, assess their implications for food security of the country in the long run, and discuss possible responses to emerging threats to food security in the conditions of trade tensions with the USA and expansion of the BRI format to Russia and the countries of Central Asia.

BACKGROUND

Until the 1990s, China's agricultural policies were focused on taxing farmers and thus reallocating resources from agricultural sector to support rising industrial production. When China became a member of the World Trade Organization (WTO) in 2001, increased competition under a liberalized trade scheme initiated a transformation of trade policies of the country along with agricultural support policies. A special attention was paid to establishing food self-sufficiency and placing agricultural development at the top of the agenda.

Since the start of economic reforms in China in the late 1970s, domestic agricultural sector has achieved remarkable growth in terms of production of major crops, vegetables, fruits, meat, and aquatic products. By now China has achieved self-sufficiency on major kinds of food and agricultural products on the level of about 91-97% of domestic consumption. Nevertheless, food self-sufficiency policy has brought several critical concerns. Zhang and Cheng (2016) identify four key pressures, namely, widening gap between demand and supply on the domestic food market, emerging threat to sustainability of China's agricultural sector due to degradation of limited arable land and heavy use of fertilizers, prevalence of cash crops production and consequent distortion of domestic agricultural market and income growth for farmers, and expansion of overseas operations of large state-owned agricultural as domestic competition intensified. Economic development along with progressing urbanization and transformation of food consumption patterns are likely to bring increased demand for major crops, including corn, rice, soybeans, and wheat (Gro Intelligence, 2018). Particularly, by the 2030s, the demand for corn is projected to rise up to 300 million tons per year (currently, it is about 250 million tons), for soybeans – up to 180-190 million tons (about 100 million, respectively).

In 2013, China transformed its agricultural policy by merging self-sufficiency and security approaches. The central focus of the food security strategy has been shifted from ensuring grain (rice, wheat, corn, soybean, root tubers, and coarse grains) self-sufficiency to self-sufficiency in cereals (wheat, rice, and corn) and absolute security of the staples (rice and wheat) (Zhang & Cheng, 2016). Second critical change is that since that time, food security has been ensured by not only domestic supply, but also moderate imports. The updated concept envisaged more active utilization of global food market and international agricultural resources in order to effectively coordinate and supplement domestic supply.

China's current agricultural imports are limited to a few agricultural products and national suppliers, particularly, the USA. The country heavily depends on food imports being the world's top importer of soybeans, cotton, palm oil, and sugar. About 80% of consumed soybean and other agricultural products, such as milk and sugar, are imported to China. Soybean imports significantly increased from 0.3 million tons in 1995 to 95 million tons in 2017, presently accounting for two-thirds of the world's soybean market (Cui & Shoemaker, 2018). China is one the world's biggest importer of palm oil, sugar, meat, fish, fruits, and feeding stuff for animals. Supply and demand are roughly in balance for grains such as rice, corn, and wheat. But thwarting its goal of food security, China must import 100 million tons of soybeans, mainly as feedstock for farm animals, making China the world's biggest importer of the oilseeds (Gro Intelligence, 2018). The World Bank (2018) forecasts that due to positive population growth coupled with growing incomes and changing diets in China, the demand for oilseeds, meats, milk, and sugar will continue to increase. The goal of new food security policy is to diversify agricultural imports via multiple channels, regions, and approaches. Its purpose is to reduce risks caused by overdependence on a few suppliers by several means: nurturing potential markets, exporting agricultural products, and supporting agricultural development in the countries with huge potential for production increase (Zhang & Cheng, 2016).

Collaboration with such countries land-abundant countries as Russia, Ukraine, Belarus, and the countries of Central Asia within the BRI is considered as a tool to diversify import flows to China, particularly, in relation to food and agricultural commodities. Recent studies of China's contemporary trade policy in relation to the BRI by Bondaz, Cohen, Godement, Kratz, and Pantucci (2015), Zhang (2016), Shah (2016), and Wong, Chi, Tsui, and Wen (2017) acknowledged that the BRI could be an active driver of China's new food security strategy. He, Huang, and Zhang (2016) made an empirical research on agricultural trade between China and the BRI countries and concluded that both sides should strengthen and diversify the trade cooperation on agricultural products on the basis of existing bilateral and multilateral mechanisms to achieve common development. The BRI focuses on the improvement of connectivity and collaboration among the countries of Eurasia through the increase of China's role in global affairs. Having interregional character, it potentially involves over 50 countries of Asia, Europe, and the Middle East (Bondaz et al., 2015) and seeks to rebuild the historical Silk Road through the development and upgrading of regional infrastructure projects (Erokhin, 2017a). China aims at promotion of cross-continental partnership along the overland and maritime routes in five areas: policy communication, road connectivity, unimpeded trade, money circulation, and cultural understanding. Expansion of joint ventures in the sphere of agricultural production in the neighbor countries may improve food security of China amid the uncertain geopolitical environment and rising protectionist wars between China and the USA.

MAIN FOCUS OF THE CHAPTER

Agricultural Production in China

In the early 1990s, many experts predicted that China would not be able to ensure the growing demand of its population in food, while the growth of China's agricultural import would fuel the food prices surge globally. When China accessed the WTO in 2001, there were concerns if domestic agricultural sector would withstand international competition, as well as if agricultural imports would take over domestic food market (Huang & Yang, 2017). By now, however, China has succeeded to achieve self-sufficiency on major agricultural commodities up to 91-97% of domestic consumption (Mahendra Dev & Zhong, 2015; Kravchenko & Sergeeva, 2014). Today, China feeds 20% of the world's population on only 7% of the world's agricultural land (Cui & Shoemaker, 2018).

Self-sufficiency has been achieved by means of the rapid development of agricultural sector. Compared to the pre-reform period of 1970-1978, when annual average growth rate of agricultural production was 2.7%, in the years of reforms (1979-1984) the growth rate almost doubled (Table 1).

Development of agricultural sector has been affected by many factors, the most important of which have been institutional innovations in rural areas, technological breakthrough, market reforms, and agricultural investments. Institutional reforms started in 1978 with the introduction of responsibility system, according to which land plots were attached to particular rural households depending on the number of workers. At the start of the reform, such solution allowed substantial increasing of labor productivity by 40-50% (Fan, 1997). In the late 1980s, introduction of land contracts and ensurance of land tenure rights both encouraged agricultural investments.

Due to the scarcity of fertile land, agricultural production has been intensifying. There has been developed a system of agricultural science, technologies, and innovations. China has established the world's largest network of information consulting offices in rural areas (Huang & Yang, 2017). Government invested in the development of irrigation and flood prevention, construction of transport infrastructure in rural areas, and development of distribution infrastructure. All those efforts allowed involving small farms into network relationship with food processing enterprises, distributors, and consumers. Along with the

Table 1. Annual average growth rates of agricultural production, population, and GDP per capita in China in 1970-2017, percentage

	1970-1978	1979-1984	1985-1995	1996-2000	2001-2005	2006-2010	2011-2017	Average in 1970-2017
GDP in agriculture	+2.7	+7.1	+4.0	+3.4	+4.3	+4.5	+4.1	+4.6
Wheat	+2.8	+4.7	+1.7	-0.7	+1.1	+2.5	+2.0	+1.9
Cotton	-0.4	+19.3	-0.3	-1.9	+5.3	-0.9	-2.1	+3.2
Oils and fats	+2.1	+8.9	+17.2	+8.0	+2.0	-2.7	+9.8	+8.8
Friuts	+6.6	+8.0	+12.5	+8.2	+29.2	+6.0	+12.8	+12.6
Meat	+4.4	+8.5	+10.0	+7.3	+5.1	-3.1	+7.7	+6.6
Fish	+5.0	+7.4	+12.6	+6.8	+3.9	+3.6	+11.0	+8.3
Population	+1.8	+1.4	+1.4	+0.9	+0.6	+0.5	+0.5	+1.0
GDP per capita	+3.1	+7.4	+8.3	+7.2	+9.0	+10.6	+7.5	+8.3

Source: Author's development based on National Bureau of Statistics of China (2019)

Figure 1. Dynamics and projections of yields of major crops in China, tons per hectare
Source: Author's development based on Gro Intelligence (2018)

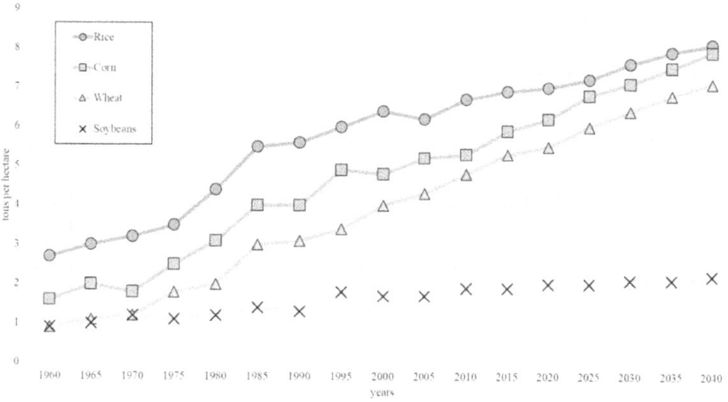

expansion of irrigation, investments in the improvement of soil fertility allowed increasing productivity. Yields have increased steadily for all major crops, including rice, corn, wheat, and soybeans (Figure 1).

One of the critical concerns, however, is that the growth in productivity has damaged environment and decreased the quality of land (Zhang, Chen, & Vitousek, 2013). The yield of soybean is lower than that of other major crops, about 1/3 of wheat and 1/4 of rice and corn. With China's shift to importing rather than growing soybean, a total of 50 million hectares of fertile cropland (40% of China's total arable land) freed up for growing other higher yielding crops (Cui & Shoemaker, 2018). A common way to boost domestic agricultural production is to expand farm acreage. China's total farm area has increased since the 1960s, particularly, for corn (Figure 2), but currently, only 12.8% of the total national land area is available for agricultural production (Chen, 2007).

Despite the overall growth, China's land and water issues remain the primary constraints to the expansion of agricultural production. Pressures from increased urbanization has prevented expansion

Figure 2. Dynamics and projections of farm area by crop, million hectares
Source: Author's development based on Gro Intelligence (2018)

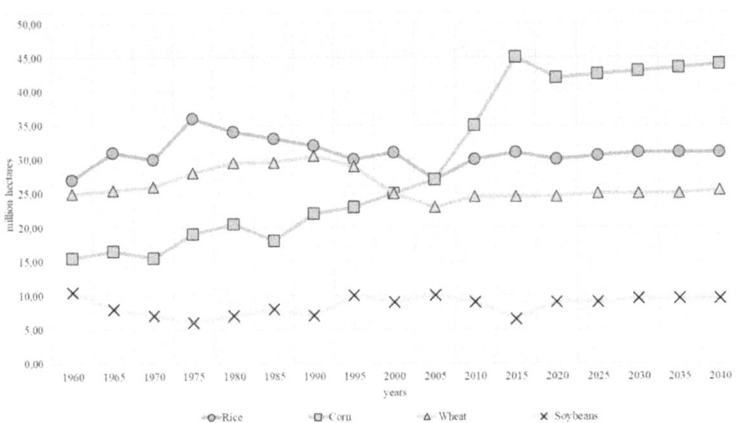

in the arable area, and competition for land is high. China's agricultural sector is dominated by small households (Ma, 2011), which provide the bulk of domestic product in agriculture. Land area per capita is only 0.08 ha, which is far below the world average of 0.22 ha per capita (Nath et al., 2015). As of 2016, the number of households is above 200 million, and the average size of a household is 0.66 ha (264 ha in the USA and 37 ha in the EU, respectively) (Gao, Ivolga, & Erokhin, 2018).

The growth in farmland alone without improvements in farming techniques is insufficient to keep pace with growing Chinese demand (Gro Intelligence, 2018). Significant portions of China's yield gains have been obtained by means of overuse of pesticides and fertilizers, which, in turn, caused problems with water and air pollution. The volume of contaminated soil in China is increasing while the environmental remediation industry is still in its infancy (Kennedy, Zhong, & Corfee-Morlot, 2016).

Realizing the emerging threats to sustainable development of agricultural production, the government has implemented several measures, including direct payments to farmers, subsidies to improved seeds and animal breeds, subsidies to purchase of farm machineries, raising rural incomes via reducing taxes and fees, promoting agricultural research and development (Liu, Xu, Su, & Tao, 2012; Yi, Sun, & Zhou, 2015). The investment in modernization of agricultural production reached $450 billion, which aimed mechanization of farms and land consolidation (Gro Intelligence, 2018).

Overseas Farming

One of the components of the contemporary food policy of China is the expansion of overseas agricultural investment which totaled $26 billion in over 100 countries worldwide as of 2016 (Gro Intelligence, 2018). The main task for China's overseas agricultural investment lies in establishing a global system for production, marketing, transportation, storage, processing, and manufacturing (Zhang & Cheng, 2016). China has been diversifying where it obtains crops that Chinese farmer are not able grow in sufficient quantities domestically.

Zhang and Cheng (2016) recognize private sectors and enterprises as the main forces of investment in foreign agricultural resources. In terms of investment destinations, neighboring countries can supply agricultural products that are in shortage in China. According to Gro Intelligence (2018), China's

Figure 3. Locations of major Chinese land purchase agreements
Source: Gro Intelligence (2018)

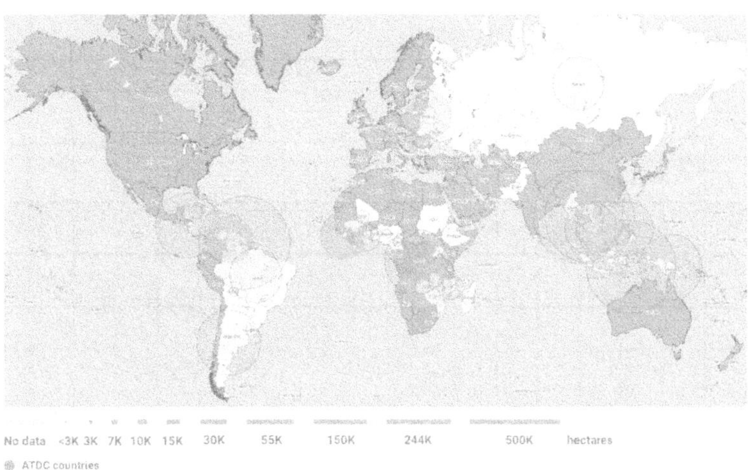

agricultural expansion has resulted in 6.6 million hectares of land being acquired around the world over the past 15 years, primarily, in Southeast Asia, Africa, and Latin America (Figure 3).

China's overseas agricultural investment is led by large agricultural enterprises with government support (Zhang & Cheng, 2016). China supports its agricultural companies to grow into internationally competitive corporations that can address growing concerns about food security of the nation (Zuo, 2014). At the same time, China is also actively establishing overseas agri-business and investment associations to enhance coordination and cooperation among Chinese companies to improve risk management and conflict resolution (Zhang & Cheng, 2016). Particularly, in Africa, China runs Agriculture Technology Demonstration Centers (ATDC) which serve as aid platforms for local farmers, transferring technology and Chinese know-how, and thereby helping to increase local food supplies (Gro Intelligence, 2018). In South America, China is increasing soybean plantations to meet its demand for soybeans. Chinese companies participate in the development of logistics and transport infrastructure to link plantations with seaports, which would allow easier shipments to China via the Panama Canal and Pacific Ocean.

The BRI and Diversification of Agricultural Imports

Among promising sources of agricultural imports to China are the countries located along the overland Silk Road Economic Belt (SREB), a network of the BRI economic corridors, which goes from China through the countries of Central Asia to Russia and then through Ukraine and Belarus to Eastern, Central, and Western Europe (Figure 4).

Within the BRI, collaboration with such countries land-abundant countries as Russia, Ukraine, Kazakhstan, Belarus, and countries of Central Asia is considered as a tool to diversify import flows to China, particularly, in relation to food and agricultural commodities. Russia, Belarus, Kazakhstan, Kyrgyzstan, and Armenia are the members of the Eurasian Economic Union (EAEU) established with an aim to ensure free movement of goods, services, labor and capital between the states, as well as to provide for common policies in macroeconomic sphere, transport, industry and agriculture, energy, foreign trade and investment, customs, technical regulation, competition and antitrust regulation. China has already

Figure 4. China's collaborations in agricultural imports along the SREB
Source: Author's development

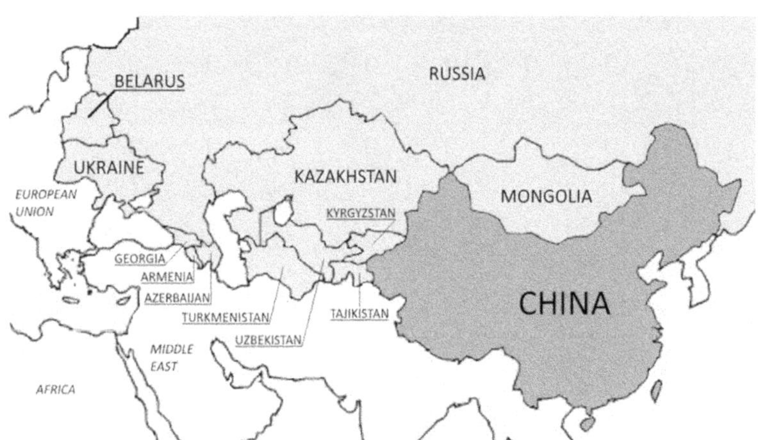

become the most important trade and investment partner for the EAEU countries, including Russia, as well as for all five economies of Central Asia (Kazakhstan, Kyrgyzstan, Tajikistan, Turkmenistan, and Uzbekistan) (Golam & Monowar, 2018).

Russia, the leading member of the EAEU, is leaning towards China for trade and investment in many areas, including in agriculture. Chinese companies has increasingly been signing leases and other temporary agreements to use fertile land, primarily, in the Far East and Siberia, Russia's main soybean growing regions. Russia has already made 1 million hectares of arable land available to foreign investors, which could become a boon for China as it struggles to diversify its suppliers amid the trade tensions with the USA (Zheng, 2018). China has already reduced its soybean purchases from the USA and as result bought a record 850,000 tons ($188.4 million) of them from Russia in 2017 (Table 2).

In 2016, Russia became the world's biggest exporter of wheat, but surprisingly, China's wheat imports from Russia started only in 2017 and in very small amount. Among the countries under study, China's major supplier of crops is Ukraine with $369.6 million of maize and $148.7 million of barley in 2017 (Table 3).

Agricultural sector of Belarus is oriented on cattle farming and vegetable production, therefore, China's import of milk, cream, and dairy products from Belarus increased from $0.5 million in 2015 up to almost $7.3 million in 2017 (Table 4).

Since early 2010s, Kazakhstan has been emerging as a supplier of wheat and oilseeds to China (Table 5). In 2017, Kazakhstan dominated in sunflower seed import of China (90% of total import of sunflower seed) and also emerged as the fourth-largest supplier of wheat after the USA, Australia, and Canada (6% of total import of wheat) (The World Bank, 2018).

Kazakhstan has a strong potential in increasing wheat and sunflower seed production by increasing their yields. More importantly, there is a potential to increase soybean production, but this potential is limited by the area of agricultural land under irrigation, most of which is now used for production of vegetables. For production on rain-fed lands, Kazakhstan is disadvantaged on precipitation and sun radiation, which both are critical in soybean production, therefore, increase in soybean import from Kazakhstan to China is possible only by account of reallocation of land resources and reduction in pro-

Table 2. China's agricultural import from Russia in 1995-2017, $ million

Product	1995	2000	2005	2010	2015	2016	2017	Average in 1995-2017
Live animals	0.05	0.01	0.31	3.80	21.30	37.21	19.41	11.73
Meat and edible meat offal	0.03	2.66	5.95	20.46	n.d.	n.d.	n.d.	13.76
Milk, cream, and milk products	0.92	1.34	0.03	0.02	0.73	2.42	2.74	1.17
Fresh, chilled, or frozen fish	111.55	335.17	1,062.34	1,227.58	1,100.59	1,264.16	1,282.76	912.02
Dried, salted, or smoked fish	0.10	0.05	0.66	0.70	0.71	0.27	0.24	0.39
Crustaceans, mollusks, and aquatic invertebrates	3.95	8.00	23.91	12.91	69.44	94.86	40.01	36.15
Fish, prepared and preserved aquatic invertebrates	n.d.	0.04	0.15	0.18	0.83	2.42	122.82	21.07
Wheat and meslin	0.05	n.d.	n.d.	n.d.	n.d.	n.d.	4.52	2.29
Rice	n.d.	n.d.	n.d.	n.d.	0.82	1.22	0.96	1.00
Maize	n.d.	n.d.	n.d.	n.d.	14.40	10.23	0.28	8.30
Cereals, excluding wheat, rice, barley, and maize	4.13	0.01	n.d.	0.18	1.92	0.14	0.15	1.09
Meal and flour of wheat and flour of meslin	n.d.	0.00	0.01	0.45	5.98	4.29	12.63	4.67
Cereal preparations, flour of fruits or vegetables	n.d.	n.d.	0.00	0.01	4.21	5.50	4.20	3.48
Vegetables	n.d.	0.03	0.74	1.02	0.78	1.69	2.40	1.11
Prepared and preserved vegetables, roots, tubers	n.d.	0.11	0.21	n.d.	0.13	1.05	0.22	0.34
Fruits and nuts	n.d.	1.68	15.74	9.23	82.68	34.38	25.47	28.20
Preserved fruits and fruit preparations	n.d.	n.d.	1.96	1.78	6.63	4.58	5.43	4.08
Sugar, molasses, and honey	0.06	n.d.	0.00	n.d.	1.59	1.66	1.55	1.22
Confectionery sugar	n.d.	n.d.	n.d.	0.04	0.60	0.60	1.55	0.70
Chocolate and food preparations with cocoa	n.d.	n.d.	0.28	0.06	7.40	4.44	21.89	6.81
Feeding stuff for animals	7.69	73.30	28.13	94.21	117.40	106.84	97.44	441.49
Oil seeds and oleaginous fruits	8.05	8.12	0.04	0.20	152.51	147.31	188.38	72.09

Source: United Nations Conference on Trade and Development [UNCTAD], 2019

duction of other crops. Animal husbandry sector also competes for a part of soybean output and thus limits the expansion of exports.

In Kyrgyzstan, the products with the highest export potential to China include fruits and nuts (cherries, apricots, plums, and walnuts), live animals, and sugar (Table 6).

Kyrgyzstan has certain potential to increase supplies of agricultural commodities to China in terms of both volume and variety. There are, however, several key constraints. Fruit production is high-seasonal, low-scale, and lacks farming technologies. Most of the facilities, including cold storage, cleaning, drying, processing, and packaging are outdated. Kyrgyzstan's farmers have low capacity to comply with China's strict sanitary and phytosanitary regulations, as well as requirements on packaging and labeling.

Table 3. China's agricultural import from Ukraine in 1995-2017, $ million

Product	1995	2000	2005	2010	2015	2016	2017	Average in 1995-2017
Milk, cream, and milk products	0.01	n.d.	0.85	3.08	0.52	2.30	12.77	8.89
Barley	n.d.	n.d.	n.d.	n.d.	184.36	61.95	148.68	131.66
Maize	n.d.	n.d.	n.d.	n.d.	876.81	508.31	369.58	584.90
Meal and flour of wheat and flour of meslin	n.d.	n.d.	n.d.	n.d.	2.75	0.17	22.53	8.48
Cereal preparations, flour of fruits or vegetables	n.d.	n.d.	n.d.	0.20	0.69	1.31	1.08	0.82
Preserved fruits and fruit preparations	n.d.	n.d.	0.79	4.86	0.39	0.27	2.07	1.68
Confectionery sugar	n.d.	n.d.	n.d.	n.d.	2.31	2.16	3.39	2.62
Chocolate and food preparations with cocoa	n.d.	n.d.	n.d.	0.07	3.21	2.08	2.11	1.87
Feeding stuff for animals	n.d.	n.d.	n.d.	2.44	5.23	2.44	3.93	3.51
Oil seeds and oleaginous fruits	n.d.	n.d.	n.d.	0.35	0.48	1.45	9.24	2.88

Source: UNCTAD, 2019

Logistics, transport, and export networks are underdeveloped and do not allow increase transportation without substantial losses in volumes and quality of the cargo.

Such problems are similar to Uzbekistan, many of which agricultural products (primarily, cherries, grapes, apricots, and plums) are not allowed to be imported to China due to low quality control and quarantine restrictions. In 2017, China's import of fruit and nuts from Uzbekistan decreased to $16.5 million from $25.4 million in 2016 (Table 7).

The countries of Central Asia have made substantial efforts to increase agricultural production and diversify their exports to China. The production volumes, however, are very small to meet China's demand in food. In 2015, China initiated extensive purchases of nuts and oilseeds in Mongolia to tackle the existing gap, and Mongolia has thus overtaken many of Central Asian economies as a supplier of fruits and nuts, oilseeds, and meat to China (Table 8).

Table 4. China's agricultural import from Belarus in 1995-2017, $ million

Product	1995	2000	2005	2010	2015	2016	2017	Average in 1995-2017
Milk, cream, and milk products	n.d.	0.32	n.d.	1.24	0.48	0.84	7.27	2.03
Cereal preparations, flour of fruits or vegetables	n.d.	n.d.	n.d.	n.d.	0.01	0.52	0.28	0.27
Preserved fruits and fruit preparations	n.d.	n.d.	n.d.	0.01	0.04	0.02	0.07	0.04
Fruit and vegetable juices	n.d.	n.d.	n.d.	n.d.	0.02	0.01	0.01	0.01
Confectionery sugar	n.d.	n.d.	n.d.	n.d.	0.00	0.03	0.03	0.03
Chocolate and food preparations with cocoa	n.d.	n.d.	n.d.	n.d.	0.01	0.47	0.37	0.28
Feeding stuff for animals	n.d.	n.d.	0.35	0.25	1.16	0.10	0.03	0.38
Edible products and preparations	n.d.	n.d.	n.d.	n.d.	n.d.	0.01	0.07	0.04

Source: UNCTAD, 2019

Table 5. China's agricultural import from Kazakhstan in 1995-2017, $ million

Product	1995	2000	2005	2010	2015	2016	2017	Average in 1995-2017
Live animals	n.d.	0.02	n.d.	0.04	0.57	n.d.	n.d.	0.21
Fresh, chilled, or frozen fish	0.03	0.07	0.06	0.56	1.59	2.03	4.29	1.23
Wheat and meslin	n.d.	n.d.	n.d.	8.76	27.65	53.76	56.60	36.69
Meal and flour of wheat and flour of meslin	n.d.	n.d.	n.d.	0.17	0.25	2.82	2.58	1.46
Cereal preparations, flour of fruits or vegetables	n.d.	n.d.	n.d.	0.01	0.04	0.25	0.26	0.14
Fruits and nuts	n.d.	0.01	0.35	n.d.	20.74	n.d.	0.11	5.30
Preserved fruits and fruit preparations	n.d.	n.d.	n.d.	n.d.	0.02	0.02	8.74	2.93
Confectionery sugar	n.d.	n.d.	n.d.	0.05	0.16	0.37	0.33	0.23
Chocolate and food preparations with cocoa	n.d.	n.d.	n.d.	0.58	0.19	0.94	0.63	0.59
Feeding stuff for animals	n.d.	n.d.	0.49	0.76	0.60	0.24	1.77	0.77
Margarine and shortening	n.d.	n.d.	n.d.	n.d.	0.06	0.08	0.06	0.07
Edible products and preparations	n.d.	n.d.	n.d.	n.d.	0.04	0.02	0.01	0.02
Oil seeds and oleaginous fruits	n.d.	n.d.	0.02	1.29	27.52	31.39	45.44	21.13

Source: UNCTAD, 2019

Table 6. China's agricultural import from Kyrgyzstan in 1995-2017, $ million

Product	1995	2000	2005	2010	2015	2016	2017	Average in 1995-2017
Live animals	0.06	n.d.	n.d.	n.d.	n.d.	0.26	1.48	0.60
Cereal preparations, flour of fruits or vegetables	n.d.	n.d.	n.d.	n.d.	0.02	0.12	0.14	0.09
Vegetables	n.d.	n.d.	n.d.	0.20	0.01	0.02	0.06	0.07
Fruits and nuts	0.04	0.50	0.06	0.85	3.46	1.79	1.76	1.21
Preserved fruits and fruit preparations	n.d.	n.d.	n.d.	n.d.	0.01	n.d.	0.20	0.10
Sugar, molasses, and honey	n.d.	n.d.	n.d.	n.d.	0.51	0.54	0.72	0.59
Chocolate and food preparations with cocoa	n.d.	n.d.	n.d.	n.d.	0.10	0.00	0.01	0.05
Feeding stuff for animals	n.d.	n.d.	n.d.	n.d.	0.08	0.11	0.16	0.12

Source: UNCTAD, 2019

The World Bank (2018) outlines three groups of constraints the countries of Central Asia face in terms of exporting their agricultural commodities to China: production and processing, technical barriers, and institutional constraints. Production and processing constraints include low yields resulting in low production volumes, low quality and insufficient quantity of planting materials and inputs, underdeveloped system of irrigation, logistical constraints, and outdated processing and packaging practices. Technical barriers include the lack of adequate sanitary and phytosanitary capacities, mismatch between national

Table 7. China's agricultural import from Uzbekistan in 1995-2017, $ million

Product	1995	2000	2005	2010	2015	2016	2017	Average in 1995-2017
Live animals	n.d.	n.d.	n.d.	n.d.	n.d.	n.d.	0.35	0.35
Cereal preparations, flour of fruits or vegetables	n.d.	n.d.	n.d.	n.d.	0.15	0.02	0.10	0.09
Vegetables	n.d.	n.d.	0.04	0.05	0.01	0.01	0.02	0.03
Fruits and nuts	n.d.	0.01	n.d.	0.54	19.43	25.42	16.46	12.37
Preserved fruits and fruit preparations	n.d.	n.d.	n.d.	n.d.	n.d.	n.d.	3.53	3.53
Fruit and vegetable juices	n.d.	n.d.	n.d.	n.d.	0.03	0.06	0.18	0.09
Feeding stuff for animals	n.d.	n.d.	n.d.	n.d.	2.29	2.05	2.06	2.13

Source: UNCTAD, 2019

Table 8. China's agricultural import from Mongolia in 1995-2017, $ million

Product	1995	2000	2005	2010	2015	2016	2017	Average in 1995-2017
Live animals	n.d.	0.00	n.d.	1.12	1.93	1.74	0.26	1.01
Meat and edible meat offal	0.03	0.07	n.d.	3.87	3.61	12.54	48.95	11.51
Fresh, chilled, or frozen fish	0.02	0.04	0.27	0.13	0.21	0.07	n.d.	0.12
Fruits and nuts	n.d.	0.11	0.50	0.75	37.67	75.84	89.20	34.01
Fruit and vegetable juices	n.d.	n.d.	n.d.	0.01	0.00	0.05	0.01	0.02
Feeding stuff for animals	2.30	0.27	0.24	0.49	2.55	6.85	8.30	3.00
Edible products and preparations	n.d.	n.d.	n.d.	n.d.	n.d.	0.42	1.07	0.75
Oil seeds and oleaginous fruits	0.00	0.02	0.13	0.20	25.38	14.77	38.39	13.15

Source: UNCTAD, 2019

and China's quality standards, and lack of compliance with specific China's regulations, including labeling and packaging requirements. Finally, institutional constraints are related to weak inland transport infrastructure, lack of export infrastructure, cumbersome customs procedures, and low spending on agricultural research and extension.

SOLUTIONS AND RECOMMENDATIONS

Maintaining food security has become the top priority of China. According to Jash (2015), to gain stability, China needs to implement better farming practices, reduced wastage of resources, greater environmental management, and increased mechanization. Offshore sourcing of food both in terms of agricultural investment as well as global food market, will help to ensure China greater food security. China's main policy should be to adhere to the principle that agriculture is the foundation of the national economy. Food production needs to be made more efficient and greater investment to be laid on education, research, innovation science, and technology.

Taking into account the existing production constraints and infrastructure barriers, China should consider collaboration with Russia and Central Asia in the following three directions:

- Increase purchases of the agricultural commodities abundant in Russia, the EAEU, and Central Asia to avoid overdependence on the USA, diversify deliveries, and establish reserves.
- Development of agricultural production in available lands in Russia (Far East and Siberia) and Kazakhstan (high-productive farming in northern and southern parts of the country) with the following export of agricultural commodities and processed food products to China.
- Joint investment projects in agricultural sector.

First solution is the easiest one which may increase food supply and diversify the sources in the short run. However, in relation to cereals and meat, China implies rather strict sanitary, phytosanitary, and veterinary regulations. For many farmers in Russia, the EAEU, or Central Asia, it is difficult to meet the standards adequately due to the technological backwardness of agricultural production. Particularly, Russian farmers complain about the restriction of the territories and particular suppliers allowed to export grain to China made by the General Administration of Quality Supervision, Inspection, and Quarantine of China (AQSIQ). There are also constraints to import pork from Russia, which should be revised. In the Far East of Russia, there have been established several pork production complexes, from which pork may be exported to the northern provinces of China. Another constraint related to the increase in agricultural imports is underdeveloped transport and logistics infrastructure, which is a weak point in all countries under study. Actually, one of the BRI's goal is to improve connectivity between China and the countries of Eurasia, including transport networks. China prefers operating through large logistics companies (Cofco, for instance), which aggregate big shipments, instead of establishing deals with dozens of small scattered suppliers. In Russia and Central Asia, however, Cofco and other Chinese companies will have to establish the logistics networks from scratch. Russia has recently announced subsidies for container shipments of agricultural commodities to China (up to 50% of transportation costs). As a response, China should provide Russian suppliers with subsidized tariffs on in-China transportation, privileged access to storage facilities and establishment of consolidated warehouses, free legal support, electronic platforms for promotion of agricultural products and foods, and simplified customs regime for agricultural imports from Russia and Central Asia.

Second way is a long-term oriented solution to diversify supply chains of high value-added agricultural products. Currently, China heavily depends on the USA on a number of cash crops, soybeans, and other high value-added agricultural products. Development of overseas agricultural production is an alternative to, first, reduce imports spending on value-added foods, and second, establish supply chains controlled by Chinese agricultural producers and operators. Russia's initiatives on attraction of Chinese farmers to the Far East and Siberia are very attractive. Russia has the world's highest level of land per capita (0.85 hectare), while in China, land per capita ratio is only 0.08 hectare. Russia's Far East and Kazakhstan's Northeast have vast farmland area and border China, which, along with low local taxes reduces planting costs (Niu, 2018). Although the lands have not been used in a regular manner and therefore require substantial investment in start of agricultural production, they are fertile and ecologically clean which means they can be used in the production of high-quality and value-added agricultural products. There is an agreement between Russia and China, according to which Chinese farmers are allowed to rent agricultural lands in the Far East to cultivate vegetables, legumes, and cereals, breed cattle, and process agricultural raw (Pitsuk & Chen, 2017). The problem is that in the Far East, there has been political resistance, including from residents, to Chinese companies renting land for agricultural production. The concerns regard the large influx of Chinese workers and a dissatisfaction with Chinese farming methods like using too many pesticides and fertilizers (Zheng, 2018).

One of the possible ways to reduce resistance is to implement joint investment projects in agricultural sector instead of direct land leases. The most promising areas are production of soybeans, cash crops, and meat, including pork and poultry. China should develop investment collaboration with the countries of Central Asia and the EAEU in the improvement of technical crops, feed production, soil fertility, production of organic fertilizers, and environmental protection. There should be established joint agricultural parks and zones for the development of collaboration in the spheres of crop production (grain, soybeans, oilseed, vegetables, and fruits) and animal husbandry (production of meat and milk with a focus on organic farming).

FUTURE RESEARCH DIRECTIONS

The region of Russia, Ukraine, and the countries of Central Asia is expected to gain an increased share in China's agricultural import in the future. Enabling those countries to convert their natural advantages into competitive advantage and to become significant sources of agricultural imports for China requires complementary investments in farming, processing, logistics, trade, and transport infrastructure. The long-term forecast of China-Russia and China-Central Asia collaboration in agricultural sector is needed to build a helpful scenario of such relations and plan investments for China-oriented development of their agricultural sector.

To expand overseas agricultural investments, China strategically places ATDCs in the countries where agricultural productivity is low and has room to improve, as well as in places where China already owns land or has a high probability of acquiring it. Further investigation is required to reveal the effects of such platforms not only on local food supplies but also on deliveries of agricultural commodities and food products to China. It is necessary to identify the determinants of competitiveness for the selected agri-food value chains in Russia, EAEU and Central Asia countries and suggest policy reforms and investments that could facilitate expansion of agricultural imports from those countries to China.

CONCLUSION

Over the past few decades, China has experienced a transition from a food shortage to an achievement of security status on the provision with food staples. However, despite the remarkable achievements, China still faces both domestic problems in the sphere of sustainability of its achieved food security (instability of agricultural production growth rates, low income in agriculture, rural poverty, etc.) and new external challenges (trade policy of major food exporters, particularly, the USA, and volatility of global markets). China needs to learn from its decades of experience in international agricultural cooperation and initiate the new model to keep up with global changes. It aims to further liberalize China's agricultural sector to enhance the country's food security. Based on the principle of mutual beneficial cooperation, China will give economic and technological support to develop the agricultural sector in neighboring countries. China needs to enhance connectivity with neighboring countries, establish more cross-border trade centers and free trade zones, and improve environmental conditions for cross-border investment. China should fund agricultural development in developing countries and also sign bilateral agricultural cooperation agreements.

In this chapter, the author reviewed the promising directions of diversification of agricultural import for China by means of the collaboration with Russia and the countries of EAEU and Central Asia. Russia and the countries of Central Asia are well-positioned to supply China's demand for food due to their geographical proximity, untapped yield potential in many crops, and good growing conditions for highly demanded food products. The sustainability of China's food security may be ensured by the increase in purchases of those agricultural products in which China experiences deficit, the launch of agricultural production on the underutilized lands in the countries of Eurasia, as well as the implementation of joint investment projects in agriculture in the framework of the BRI.

ACKNOWLEDGMENT

This chapter is supported by the Fundamental Research Funds for the Central Universities (grant no. HEUCFJ170901, 3072019CFP0902).

REFERENCES

Bondaz, A., Cohen, D., Godement, F., Kratz, A., & Pantucci, R. (2015). *One belt, one road: China's great leap outward*. London, UK: European Council on Foreign Relations.

Chen, J. (2007). Rapid urbanization in China: A real challenge to soil protection and food security. *Catena*, 69(1), 1–15. doi:10.1016/j.catena.2006.04.019

ChinaPower. (2017). *How is China feeding its population of 1.4 billion?* Retrieved from https://chinapower.csis.org/china-food-security/

Cui, K., & Shoemaker, S. (2018). A look at food security in China. *NPJ Science of Food, 2*. doi:. doi:10.103841538-018-0012-x

Erokhin, V. (2017a). How to shape the market: China's one belt one road initiative. In M. Malovic, & K. Roy (Eds.), *The state and the market in economic development: In pursuit of millennium development goals* (pp. 144–156). Brisbane, Australia: The IIDS Australia Inc.

Erokhin, V. (2017b). Self-sufficiency versus security: How trade protectionism challenges the sustainability of the food supply in Russia. *Sustainability*, 9(11), 1939. doi:10.3390u9111939

Erokhin, V. (2017c). Trade in agricultural products and food security concerns on emerging markets: how to balance protection and liberalization. In V. Erokhin (Ed.), *Establishing food security and alternatives to international trade in emerging economies* (pp. 28–54). Hershey, PA: IGI Global.

Fan, S. (1997). Production and productivity growth in Chinese agriculture: New measurement and evidence. *Food Policy*, 22(3), 213–228. doi:10.1016/S0306-9192(97)00010-9

Food and Agriculture Organization of the United Nations. (1992). *Food, nutrition, and agriculture*. Rome, Italy: Food and Agriculture Organization of the United Nations.

Gao, T. (2017). Food security and rural development on emerging markets of Northeast Asia: Cases of Chinese North and Russian Far East. In V. Erokhin (Ed.), *Establishing food security and alternatives to international trade in emerging economies* (pp. 155–176). Hershey, PA: IGI Global.

Gao, T., Ivolga, A., & Erokhin, V. (2018). Sustainable rural development in Northern China: Caught in a vice between poverty, urban attractions, and migration. *Sustainability, 10*(5), 1467. doi:10.3390u10051467

Ghose, B. (2014). Food security and food self-sufficiency in China: From past to 2050. *Food and Energy Security, 3*(2), 86–95. doi:10.1002/fes3.48

Golam, M., & Monowar, M. (2018). Eurasian Economic Union: Evolution, challenges, and possible future directions. *Journal of Eurasian Studies, 9*(2), 163–172. doi:10.1016/j.euras.2018.05.001

Gro Intelligence. (2018). *China's road map to food security.* Retrieved from https://gro-intelligence.com/insights/chinas-roadmap-to-food-security

He, M., Huang, Z., & Zhang, N. (2016). An empirical research on agricultural trade between China and "The Belt and Road" countries: Competitiveness and complementarity. *Modern Economy, 7*(14), 1671–1686. doi:10.4236/me.2016.714147

Huang, J., & Yang, G. (2017). Understanding recent challenges and new food policy in China. *Global Food Security, 12*, 119–126. doi:10.1016/j.gfs.2016.10.002

Jash, A. (2015). *China's quest for food security: Challenges & policies.* Retrieved from https://papers.ssrn.com/sol3/papers.cfm?abstract_id=2773903

Kennedy, C., Zhong, M., & Corfee-Morlot, J. (2016). Infrastructure for China's ecologically balanced civilization. *Engineering, 2*(4), 414–425. doi:10.1016/J.ENG.2016.04.014

Kravchenko, A., & Sergeeva, O. (2014). China policy in the area of food security: Modernization of agriculture. *Pacific Rim: Economics, Politics, Law, 32*(4), 57–65.

Lawrence, G., & McMichael, P. (2012). The question of food security. *International Journal of Sociology of Agriculture and Food, 19*(2), 135–142.

Lee, R. (2007). *Food security and food sovereignty.* Newcastle upon Tyne, UK: Centre for Rural Economy, University of Newcastle upon Tyne.

Liu, M., Xu, Z., Su, F., & Tao, R. (2012). Rural tax reform and the extractive capacity of local state in China. *China Economic Review, 23*(1), 190–203. doi:10.1016/j.chieco.2011.10.002

Luan, Y., Cui, X., & Ferrat, M. (2013). Historical trends of food self-sufficiency in Africa. *Food Security, 5*(3), 393–405. doi:10.100712571-013-0260-1

Ma, L. (2011). Sustainable development of rural household energy in Northern China. *Journal of Sustainable Development, 5*(4), 115–124.

Mahendra Dev, S., & Zhong, F. (2015). Trade and stock management to achieve national food security in India and China? *China Agricultural Economic Review, 7*(4), 641–654. doi:10.1108/CAER-01-2015-0009

Mukhopadhyay, K., Thomassin, P. J., & Zhang, J. (2018). Food security in China at 2050: A global CGE exercise. *Journal of Economic Structures*, *7*(1), 1. doi:10.118640008-017-0097-4

Nath, R., Luan, Y., Yang, W., Yang, C., Chen, W., Li, Q., & Cui, X. (2015). Changes in Arable land demand for food in India and China: A potential threat to food security. *Sustainability*, *7*(5), 5371–5397. doi:10.3390u7055371

National Bureau of Statistics of China. (2019). *Statistical database*. Retrieved from http://www.stats.gov.cn/english/Statisticaldata/AnnualData/

Niu, S. (2018). *China reaches into Russia's Far East in hunt for crop supplies*. Retrieved from https://www.bloomberg.com/news/articles/2018-09-05/china-reaches-into-russia-s-far-east-in-hunt-for-crop-supplies

Pitsuk, I., & Chen, J. (2017). To the question of development of cooperation Chinese people's Republic of and Khabarovsk Territory (Aspect of security food security). *Electronic Scientific Journal. Scientists Notes of Pacific National University*, *8*(2), 345–350.

Saravia-Matus, S., Gomez y Paloma, S., & Mary, S. (2012). Economics of food security: Selected issues. *Bio-Based and Applied Economics*, *1*(1), 65–80.

Schanbacher, W. D. (2010). *The politics of food: The global conflict between food security and food sovereignty*. Santa Barbara, CA: Praeger Security International.

Shah, A. (2016). *Building a sustainable "Belt and Road"*. Retrieved from http://www.cirsd.org/en/horizons/horizons-spring-2016--issue-no-7/building-a-sustainable-%E2%80%98belt-and-road-

State Council of the People's Republic of China. (1996). *The Grain Issue in China, White Paper*. Beijing: Information Office of the State Council.

State Council of the People's Republic of China. (2008). *Mid- and long-term grain security plan (2008-2020) Policy guideline*. Beijing, China: Information Office of the State Council.

The World Bank. (2018). *Central Asia. China (and Russia) 2030 – Implications for agriculture in Central Asia*. Washington, DC: The World Bank.

Tian, W. (n.d.). *China's experiences in domestic agricultural support*. Retrieved from https://www.adelaide.edu.au/global-food/documents/food-security-in-china.pdf

United Nations Conference on Trade and Development. (2019). *Statistics database* [Data file]. Retrieved from http://unctad.org/en/Pages/Statistics.aspx

Valdés, A., & Foster, W. (2012). *Net food-importing developing countries: Who they are, and policy options for global price volatility*. Geneva, Switzerland: International Centre for Trade and Sustainable Development. doi:10.7215/AG_IP_20120823

Wong, E., Chi, L. K., Tsui, S., & Wen, T. (2017). One belt, one road: China's strategy for a new global financial order. *Monthly Review. An Independent Socialist Magazine, 68*(8). Retrieved from https://monthlyreview.org/2017/01/01/one-belt-one-road/#en1

Yi, F., Sun, D., & Zhou, Y. (2015). Grain subsidy, liquidity constraints and food security: Impact of the grain subsidy program on the grain-sown areas in China. *Food Policy*, *50*, 114–124. doi:10.1016/j.foodpol.2014.10.009

Zhang, F., Chen, X., & Vitousek, P. (2013). Chinese agriculture: An experiment for the world. *Nature*, *497*(7447), 33–35. doi:10.1038/497033a PMID:23636381

Zhang, H., & Cheng, G. (2016). China's food security strategy reform: An emerging global agricultural policy. In F. Wu, & H. Zhang (Eds.), *China's global quest for resources. Energy, food, and water* (pp. 23–41). London, UK: Routledge.

Zhang, J. (2011). China's success in increasing per capita food production. *Journal of Experimental Botany*, *11*(1), 3707–3711. doi:10.1093/jxb/err132 PMID:21551079

Zhang, J. (2016). *What's driving China's one belt, one road initiative?* Retrieved from http://www.eastasiaforum.org/2016/09/02/whats-driving-chinas-one-belt-one-road-initiative/

Zheng, S. (2018). *Russia offers 2.5 million acres of land to Chinese farmers, but will it ease Beijing's soybean shortage?* Retrieved from https://www.scmp.com/news/china/diplomacy-defence/article/2159713/russia-offers-25-million-acres-land-chinese-farmers

Zuo, M. (2014). *China turning state-owned farms into agricorporations to take on world players.* Retrieved from https://www.scmp.com/news/china/article/1573077/china-turning-state-owned-farms-agricorporations-take-world-players

ADDITIONAL READING

Afonso, O. (2001). *The Impact of International Trade on Economic Growth*. Porto: University of Porto.

Anderson, K., Jha, S., Nelgen, S., & Strutt, A. (2013). Re-examining Policies for Food Security in Asia. *Food Security*, *5*(2), 195–215. doi:10.100712571-012-0237-5

Anderson, K., Martin, W., & van der Mensbrugghe, D. (2010). China, the WTO and the Doha Agenda. In D. Greenaway, C. Milner, & S. Yao (Eds.), *China and the World Economy* (pp. 1–20). London: Palgrave Macmillan. doi:10.1057/9781137059864_1

Asian Development Bank. (n.d.). *Agriculture and Food Security Issues in Asia and the Pacific*. Retrieved January 25, 2019, from https://www.adb.org/sectors/agriculture/issues

Beloglazov, G. (2007). Food Security of the People's Republic of China and its Russian Vector. *Russia and Pacific RIM*, *3*, 75–83.

Cass, D. Z., Williams, B. G., & Barker, G. R. (2003). *China and the World Trading System: Entering the Millennium*. New York, NY: Cambridge University Press. doi:10.1017/CBO9780511494482

Chaisse, J., & Gorski, J. (Eds.). (2018). *The Belt and Road Initiative: Law, Economics, and Politics*. Leiden: Brill Nijhoff. doi:10.1163/9789004373792

Chang, X., DeFries, R. S., Liu, L., & Davis, K. (2018). Understanding Dietary and Staple Food Transitions in China from Multiple Scales. *PLoS One, 13*(4), e0195775. doi:10.1371/journal.pone.0195775 PMID:29689066

Cheng, G. (2007). China's Agriculture within the World Trading System. In I. Sheldon (Ed.), *China's Agricultural Trade: Issues and Prospects* (pp. 81–104). Beijing: International Agricultural Trade Research Consortium.

Dohmen, H. (1976). China's Foreign Trade Policy. *Inter Economics, 11*(7), 197–201. doi:10.1007/BF02929005

Dorosh, P. A. (2004). Trade, Food Aid and Food Security: Evolving Rice and Wheat Markets. *Economic and Political Weekly, 36*(39), 4033–4042.

Erokhin, V. (Ed.). (2016). *Global Perspectives on Trade Integration and Economies in Transition*. Hershey, PA: IGI Global. doi:10.4018/978-1-5225-0451-1

Erokhin, V. (Ed.). (2017). *Establishing Food Security and Alternatives to International Trade in Emerging Economies*. Hershey, PA: IGI Global.

Erokhin, V. (2017). Factors Influencing Food Markets in Developing Countries: An Approach to Assess Sustainability of the Food Supply in Russia. *Sustainability, 9*(8), 1313. doi:10.3390u9081313

Erokhin, V. (2018). Contemporary Foreign Trade Policy of China in the Region of Central and Northeast Asia. In A. C. Ozer (Ed.), *Globalization and Trade Integration in Developing Countries* (pp. 27–54). Hershey, PA: IGI Global. doi:10.4018/978-1-5225-4032-8.ch002

Erokhin, V., & Gao, T. (2018). Competitive Advantages of China's Agricultural Exports in the Outward-Looking Belt and Road Initiative. In W. Zhang, I. Alon, & C. Lattemann (Eds.), *China's Belt and Road Initiative: Changing the Rules of Globalization* (pp. 265–285). London: Palgrave Macmillan. doi:10.1007/978-3-319-75435-2_14

Erokhin, V., & Ivolga, A. (2012). How to Ensure Sustainable Development of Agribusiness in the Conditions of Trade Integration: Russian Approach. [IJSEM]. *International Journal of Sustainable Economies Management, 2*(1), 12–23. doi:10.4018/ijsem.2012040102

Erokhin, V., Ivolga, A., & Heijman, W. (2014). Trade Liberalization and State Support of Agriculture: Effects for Developing Countries. *Agricultural Economics – Czech, 60*(11), 524-537.

Estevadeordal, A., Freund, C., & Ornelas, E. (2008). Does Regionalism Affect Trade Liberalization Toward Nonmembers? *The Quarterly Journal of Economics, 124*(4), 1531–1575. doi:10.1162/qjec.2008.123.4.1531

Gale, F., Hansen, J., & Jewison, M. (2015). *China's Growing Demand for Agricultural Imports*. Washington, DC: U.S. Department of Agriculture, Economic Research Service.

Henneberry, S. R., & Diaz, C. C. (2015). Food Security Issues: Concepts and the Role of Emerging Markets. In A. Schmitz, P. L. Kennedy, & T. G. Schmitz (Eds.), *Food Security in an Uncertain World* (pp. 63–79). Bingley: Emerald Group Publishing Limited. doi:10.1108/S1574-871520150000015005

Huang, J., & Rozelle, S. (2006). The Emergence of Agricultural Commodity Markets in China. *China Economic Review*, *17*(3), 266–280. doi:10.1016/j.chieco.2006.04.008

Huang, J., Wei, W., Cui, Q., & Xie, W. (2017). The Prospects for China's Food Security and Imports: Will China Starve the World via Imports? *Journal of Integrative Agriculture*, *16*(12), 2933–2944. doi:10.1016/S2095-3119(17)61756-8

Kneller, R., Morgan, C. W., & Kanchanahatakij, S. (2008). Trade Liberalization and Economic Growth. *World Economy*, *31*(6), 701–719. doi:10.1111/j.1467-9701.2008.01101.x

Ozer, A. C. (Ed.). (2018). *Globalization and Trade Integration in Developing Countries*. Hershey, PA: IGI Global. doi:10.4018/978-1-5225-4032-8

Raynolds, L., Murray, D., & Wilkinson, J. (2007). *Fair Trade: The Challenges of Transforming Globalization*. London: Routledge. doi:10.4324/9780203933534

Schmitz, A., & Meyers, W. H. (Eds.). (2015). *Transition to Agricultural Market Economies. The Future of Kazakhstan, Russia and Ukraine*. Boston, Oxfordshire: CABI. doi:10.1079/9781780645353.0000

Spoor, M., & Robbins, M. J. (Eds.). (2012). *Agriculture, Food Security, and Inclusive Growth*. The Hague: Institute of Social Sciences.

Windfuhr, M., & Jonsen, J. (2005). *Food Sovereignty: Towards Democracy in Localized Food Systems*. Heidelberg: FIAN ITDG Publishing. doi:10.3362/9781780441160

Wittman, H., Desmarais, A., & Wiebe, N. (2010). *Food Sovereignty: Reconnecting Food, Nature and Community*. Oakland, CA: Food First Books.

Yanikkaya, H. (2003). Trade Openness and Economic Growth: A Cross-Country Empirical Investigation. *Journal of Development Economics*, *72*(1), 57–89. doi:10.1016/S0304-3878(03)00068-3

Yu, W., Elleby, C., & Zobbe, H. (2015). Food Security Policies in India and China: Implications for National and Global Food Security. *Food Security*, *7*(2), 405–414. doi:10.100712571-015-0432-2

Yu, Y., Feng, K., Hubacek, K., & Sun, L. (2016). Global Implications of China's Future Food Consumption. *Journal of Industrial Ecology*, *20*(3), 593–602. doi:10.1111/jiec.12392

Zhang, H. (2016). Food in Sino-U.S. Relations. From Blessing to Curse? In F. Wu & H. Zhang (Eds.), *China's Global Quest for Resources. Energy, Food and Water* (pp. 100–118). London: Routledge.

Zhang, W., Alon, I., & Lattemann, C. (Eds.). (2018). *China's Belt and Road Initiative: Changing the Rules of Globalization*. London: Palgrave Macmillan. doi:10.1007/978-3-319-75435-2

Zhou, Z. (2010). Achieving Food Security in China: Past Three Decades and Beyond. *China Agricultural Economic Review*, *2*(3), 251–275. doi:10.1108/17561371011078417

Zhou, Z., Liu, H., Cao, L., Tian, W., & Wang, J. (2014). *Food Consumption in China: The Revolution Continues*. Cheltenham: Edward Elgar Publishing. doi:10.4337/9781782549208

KEY TERMS AND DEFINITIONS

Belt and Road Initiative: A development strategy proposed by the Chinese government in 2013 and focused on the improvement of connectivity and collaboration among the countries of Eurasia through the increase of China's role in global affairs.

Central Asia: The region in Asia which extends from China in the east to the Caspian Sea in the west and consists of Kazakhstan, Kyrgyzstan, Tajikistan, Turkmenistan, and Uzbekistan.

Eurasian Economic Union: The international economic union of five countries located in northern Eurasia (Armenia, Belarus, Kazakhstan, Kyrgyzstan, and Russia) established in 2015 with an aim to ensure free movement of goods, services, labor and capital between the states, as well as to provide for common policies in macroeconomic sphere, transport, industry and agriculture, energy, foreign trade and investment, customs, technical regulation, competition and antitrust regulation.

Food Market: The supply and demand of agricultural commodities and food products within a single country (domestic) or between countries (international).

Food Security: A condition when people have access to sufficient amounts of safe and nutritious food and are therefore consuming the food required for normal growth and development, and for an active and healthy life.

Food Self-Sufficiency: An extent to which a country can satisfy its food needs from its own domestic production.

Foreign Trade: The system of international commodity-money relations composed of foreign trade activities of all countries worldwide.

This research was previously published in the Handbook of Research on Agricultural Policy, Rural Development, and Entrepreneurship in Contemporary Economies edited by Andrei Jean Vasile, Jonel Subic, Aleksander Grubor, and Donatella Privitera; pages 273-295, copyright year 2020 by Business Science Reference (an imprint of IGI Global).

Chapter 48
Determinants of Agricultural Production in Romania:
A Panel Data Approach

Alina Zaharia
The Bucharest University of Economic Studies, Romania

Simona Roxana Pătărlăgeanu
The Bucharest University of Economic Studies, Romania

ABSTRACT

Agriculture plays an important part in the worldwide challenges, such as sustainable development, climate change, high level of greenhouse gas emissions, food security and safety, overpopulation, social welfare, and natural resource depletion. This chapter examines a panel data approach to determine the contribution of several factors on the agricultural output in terms of value and of yield. Different regression models were established for the analysis at territorial level in Romania. Some findings suggest a negative influence of the excessive drought years on the cereals yield while a statistical relevance could not be found for the influence of the excessively rainy years. Still, further studies should be conducted on analyzing the influence of the environmental and social factors on the agricultural economic output.

INTRODUCTION

The factors influencing agriculture are highly relevant for decision making in terms of their wide implications for food security and safety, sustainable management of natural resources, and climate change. While the global population is continually increasing, policy makers try to identify ways of ensuring food security and safety by investigating the relationship between agricultural inputs and outputs (Burja, 2012; Teryomenko, 2008). The liberalization of trade has increased competition on local markets and has required more attention given to production costs, resource management, farm size, agricultural policies. Despite increased competition, the trade liberalization could contribute to diminishing the degradation of natural capital by internalizing its effects on production (Lopez, 1994).

DOI: 10.4018/978-1-7998-5354-1.ch048

Moreover, climate change impacts the agriculture and the land use and, consequently, policies regulate new sustainable agricultural practices. Several studies have indicated the positive effects of climate change on agriculture, such as extension of the arable area to the North, introduction of new crop species; negative effects have also been documented such as increase in temperature and extreme weather events (Vijayasarathy & Ashok, 2015; Olesen, 2006). Hence, analyses of agricultural determinants are explored by a vast literature which will be thoroughly discussed in the literature review section of this paper.

It becomes increasingly necessary to continually analyze the factors influencing agricultural production in order to better understand their impact on agricultural outputs. The impact of agricultural activities on environment and social dimensions should be considered. As a result, new sustainable strategies and practices might emerge.

The objective of the paper is to explore the relationships between the agricultural determinants and outputs in general, as well as, the cereals' ones in particular. The authors argue that economic and social indicators, technical and material capital, financial support, human capital, natural resources, climate variability represent the main determinants of agricultural output.

The main questions that underpin this research are: Which are the main drivers of the Romanian agricultural output? Which are the main influences of the agricultural output's drivers at territorial level in Romania?

To the best of authors knowledge, few studies focus on discussing the influencing factors of the Romanian agricultural output from an econometric point of view. Unlike previous studies, which focused on more specific relationships with fewer variables, this paper undertakes an overview of the Romanian agriculture sector over 1997-2014 periods. Hence, improved understanding of this subject will hopefully lead to identifying the directions for increasing the agricultural output.

BACKGROUND

The gross value added of agriculture, forestry and fishing represented 1.7% of the EU total gross value added while in Romania this indicator reached the EU peak of 6.4% of total gross value added in 2013 (Eurostat, 2016). The employment level is 2.75 million Romanian persons occupied in this sector in 2013 and 2.5 million persons self-employed – the highest in the EU – reaching to a share of 24.16% in 2013 (Eurostat, 2016).

In addition, food security and safety is a more and more discussed issue all over the world. In simplistic definitions, food security refers at assuring the necessary quantity of food for the population while food safety refers at assuring the so needed quality of food. It is interesting to emphasize the existence, in general, of enough food available for the population, still the lack of its quality and the access to it raise many problems. By access, the specialists refer mainly to the affordability (Hazell & Wood, 2008), to *the access to sufficient, affordable and nutritious food* (European Commission, 2016a). Still, by solving the problem of assuring food security by providing for the population enough money to afford the healthy and the necessary food, it might arise:

Income increases => land conversion for cultivation => overconsumption => overpopulation => environmental issues (natural resource depletion, loss of biodiversity, agricultural and food waste, pollution) => climate change (social, economic and environmental problems).

The climate change has intensified since the industrial revolution when fossil fuels started to be intensively used in all sectors of economy and pollution started to increase drastically. It is a worldwide known problem for which policy makers, experts, farmers, etc. identified the main causes and impacts and now they try to find solutions and apply policies for mitigating and adapting to climate change (Zaharia & Antonescu, 2014). Climate change affects the agricultural activities considerably, as the status of environmental inputs represents a vital condition for increasing the agricultural yields and agricultural output values, as well as for assuring social, environmental and economic stability.

Climate change produces changes in temperature, precipitation, availability of resources and cropping systems, as well as increased climatic variability (Olesen & Bindi, 2004). These global changes have positive and negative effects. Olesen (2006) states that, among the positive ones, we could find the emergence of new crop species and varieties, expansion of agricultural area, increased crop production, cultivation of some crops in winter. Among the negative ones, the following could be identified: water shortages, diminution of soil organic matter, emergence of extreme weather events, and variability in crop yields. In light of these positive and negative effects, the Southern areas will still emerge as the most affected regions (Olesen, 2006).

Equally, agricultural activities contribute to climate change through the emissions they generate (Olesen, 2006). The greenhouse gas emissions have drastically increased since the end of the 19th century, mainly due to massive industrialization and use of fossil fuels (Zaharia & Antonescu, 2014). According to the European Commission (2016b), currently, the EU share in the total global emissions is approximately 11%. Zaharia and Antonescu (2014) suggest that the EU policies on the reduction of pollution are contributing to the diminishing emissions on a downward trend, including the ones from agriculture. Thus, the EU GHG emissions registered decreases of 18.33% overall and of 23.12% in agriculture over 1990-2011 (Zaharia & Antonescu, 2014). In 2013, the European Union's agriculture contributed 9.55% to the overall EU GHG emissions while Romania's agriculture contributed 0.38% to the overall EU GHG emissions. In addition, Romania's agriculture contributed 4.004% to the GHG emissions produced by the EU agriculture and 6.31% to the overall Romanian GHG emissions (European Commission, 2016c).

As a result, the agricultural sector is very important for the three dimensions of sustainable development: social, economic and environmental ones. In these circumstances, European Union adopted and is implementing a series of sustainable policies, regulation and measures for increasing the overall performance of agriculture, the farmers' income and the agricultural yields and values, as well as for mitigating and adapting to climate change and assuring food security and safety.

One of these EU directions is the "Europe 2020 Strategy" (European Commission, 2010), by which the European Union establishes the targets on the reduction of GHG emissions by each Member State for contributing to climate change mitigation. In addition, this strategy establishes the guidelines for increasing the resource efficiency, for protecting the biodiversity and the natural capital and for increasing the practices of organic farming. European Commission presents indicators for all these issues. This important EU growth strategy is also applied in Romanian agriculture through the Rural Development Strategy 2014-2020 and financial supported by the National Rural Development Programme 2014–2020. The Romanian sustainable development measures introduced through these strategic documents are based on a series of 26 agricultural needs, such as: education and counseling of farmers and of agricultural occupied population; linking the agricultural research, production and market; modernization of farms, processing units, infrastructure; protection and improvement of natural resources; diminishing the pollution and adapting to climate change (The Romanian Ministry of Agriculture and Rural Development, 2016). Based on these needs this Programme gives financial supports for rural projects.

Another important policy for EU agriculture is the Common Agricultural Policy. In 1962 the European Union created the CAP which, over time, has been reformed repeatedly in order to face the challenges in the agricultural sectors of the member states (European Commission, 2014a). Currently, this policy focuses on improving and conserving the natural capital while developing a sustainable market-oriented agriculture. CAP seeks to ensure food security and safety, as well as farmers' income among its objectives (European Commission, 2016d; Popescu, 2014). Romania shall beneficiate of 20 billion euro for improving the agri-food sector and the rural areas during 2014-2020. CAP finances the agricultural activities through direct payments, market measures and rural investments (European Commission, 2014b).

In this context, many studies pay close attention to the influence of climatic factors, the development level of technical and material inputs, the educational level of the persons occupied in agriculture, the investments and financing of the agricultural sector, and the overall factors which could induce high values of agricultural outputs.

Agriculture has several agricultural drivers that could be divided according to the global, national and local scale. Hazell and Wood (2008) present as global drivers: trade liberalization, climate change, international agreements on these issues in all economic sectors, *rapid globalization of science and knowledge access*, as national drivers: legislative framework, population income, infrastructure and market access, and, as local drivers, the climate variability and the agricultural production system. In addition, the above-mentioned authors state that the international trade and the globalization of markets increase competition and increase the difficulties of small farms to enter and remain on the market. So, due to this matter, the costs of the small agricultural producers increase.

Zaharia and Antonescu (2014) consider the relationship of interdependency between agriculture and climate change because the agriculture produces GHG emissions and other negative effects which contribute to climate change and the latter influences negatively and positively the agricultural activities by weather changes, agricultural system changes, natural resources changes. Their study also concluded that even though "there is no dependency between the Romanian arable land and the Romanian GHG emissions, there are other factors which could influence the pollution level, such as: synthetic fertilizers, bad management of manure, type of cultivated crops, burning crop residues" (Zaharia & Antonescu, 2014). Figure 1 presents this relationship illustrated by the above mentioned authors.

Figure 1. The interdependency between agriculture and climate change
Source: Zaharia and Antonescu, 2014.

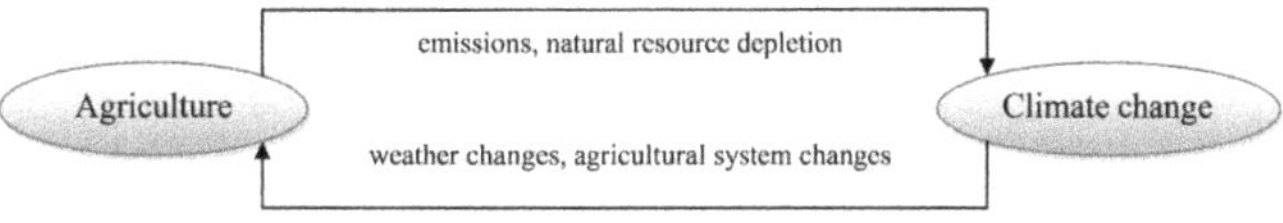

Two main types of GHG emitted by agricultural activities have the highest values of all GHG emissions from agriculture: nitrogen protoxide and methane. These are very dangerous and powerful in creating the greenhouse effect which contributes to climate change. Moreover, the nitrogen protoxide is 300 times more harmful than the CO_2 (Romanian National Institute of Statistics, 2016a). Howbeit, the agricultural GHG emissions are released by practicing a varied group of activities, such as applying pesticides and fertilizers, manure management, burning crop residues, cereals cultivation (mostly the rice) (Zaharia & Antonescu, 2014).

So far, the main looked upon determinants of agriculture were mainly the global ones, therefore, in the following, the authors discuss the main focus of this chapter: the national and local determinants of agriculture, which will be thoroughly investigated in this paper.

MAIN FOCUS OF THE CHAPTER

Analyzed Issues

Many studies show the importance of infrastructure for agriculture development as the productivity growth of crops is explained by increases in investments for public infrastructure (Mamatzakis, 2003). Expanding to the digital world, the development of geospatial applications is becoming more helpful for the farmers in planning the location of land operations (Wiebensohn & Jackenkroll, 2013). More-over, water and sewage infrastructure contribute to the increases in the welfare of the rural inhabitants (Piasecki & Jurasz, 2015).

Nevertheless, the natural capital represents the main influencing factor of crop productivity and value. Nowadays, European Union follows the evolution of indicators on the state of natural resources in all member states. Soil and water quality, climate variability and land changes are continually monitored in the context in which the use of these resources should be planned for a better sustainability of agricultural inputs and for increasing their efficiency. The resource efficiency is an EU objective because it might,

reduce the risk of vulnerability to future resource volatility or scarcity, reduce the costs through pro-ductivity savings and mitigate the environmental and social problems linked with unsustainable use of resources, such as pollution. (European Commission, 2011)

The Romanian legislation regulates the investigation, evaluation, monitoring restoration, and conservation of natural resources. The soil has many vital functions, such as: food production, water storage, source of raw materials, biodiversity, geological and archaeological heritage, represents the physical environment for human activities (Romanian National Agency for Environmental Protection, 2016). In this context, EU tries to create databases with the evolution of soil quality indicators: texture, organic matter content, pH, electric conductivity, soil water retention, groundwater level. Nevertheless, the soil state encounters many problems, such as: erosion, organic matter degradation, soil biodiversity loss, compaction, salinization, contamination, landslides and floods, sealing (Romanian National Agency for Environmental Protection, 2016). So, soil productive potential should be emphasized and improved. Crop rotation helps maintaining soil fertility and control of pests and diseases, and it has a role in terms of crop diversification by increasing their efficiency and the conservation of plant genetic resources (Voicu & Dobre, 2003).

The water is also a vital natural resource because without it the agriculture faces real challenges in conditions of actual pollution and increasing desertification. The water depends on the environment conditions as one of the major aspects in providing the necessary water for healthy increasing proportions of agriculture products (Giovannucci Scherr, Nierenberg, Hebebrand, Shapiro, Milder, & Wheeler, 2012).

Climate parameters represent also an influencing factor of agricultural output in time and space. The states of these parameters determine the suitability of one culture or another, of the applied production system and the supplementary investments and expenses which have to be made for improving productivity. All of these would eventually impact the final agricultural outcome (Voicu & Dobre, 2003).

The agricultural producer can only act within the limits imposed by the natural conditions and, where possible, further improvements could be made by using the technical capital. This may conduct to increased costs, but so needed for the achievement of desired level of production. Studies indicate negative effects of technical capital on food safety and environment. The decrease of emissions from agricultural soils is due to diminishing the use of mineral and organic fertilizers and pesticides. The soil emissions are mainly related to fertilizers, waste decomposition, sewage sludge application, cultivated crop (Anderl, 2009).

All these presented factors should be combined according to the type of crop culture used and to the type of production system applied. The allocation decisions and the combination of inputs are made exclusively by the farmer, considering the past prices on the market (Voicu & Dobre, 2003).

The national and local drivers influence also the outcome of agriculture in what concerns the productivity and its value. Popescu and Zaharia (2015) analyzed the relationship between energy consumption, technical progress and value added in the European Union's agriculture and found that the value added of agriculture, forestry and fishing is correlated with the energy consumption, with tractors, and with fertilizers and pesticides consumption, all reported to 1000 ha agricultural area. The authors concluded that there is no statistical correlation to day between the Romanian area equipped for irrigation and the value added in agriculture, forestry and fishing.

Another study (Carvalho, 2006) emphasizes the importance of soil and water management, intensive irrigation, fertilizers, pesticides and agricultural land increases in assuring the future food security in a context in which the negative effects of the previous presented factors and the status of the environmental factors, such as the soil and water quality, would greatly impact the agricultural output. The application of pesticides and chemical fertilizers negatively influence the cost of production, the human and biodiversity health, as well as the natural capital in its entire. As the weeds, insects and other types of pests increase their resistance to control chemicals; the latter is increasing to be applied while raising the costs and damaging the agricultural product nutrient structure. Also, the pesticides and the fertilizers damage the quality of soils, water and atmosphere. Nevertheless, a better control and use of these substances could diminish their negative impact on human health and environment.

Several researchers have analyzed the determinants of agricultural production at national level. Abugamea (2008) investigated the agricultural production outcome in relation with the input cost, the labor force and the cultivated land by using time series econometrics procedures. The authors find a significant effect on agricultural production both from capital (negative) and labor (positive).

Moreover, Teryomenko (2008) explored several parametric and non-parametric methods for establishing and analyzing the determinants of agricultural productivity, namely the farm size, the farm specialization, the expenses on inputs such as electricity, repairs, labor. The results of Teryomenko's study indicate that farm size influence the agricultural productivity up to a point where more rented land could generate decreases of productivity and that the policies pursued by authorsities which might influence positively or negatively the analyzed variables could generate changes on the productivity level.

Another study (Ekbom, 1998) focuses its analysis on the material, human and capital inputs to explore the influence on agricultural productivity by using a Cobb-Douglas production function and the research concludes that in Kenya is statistically significant correlation between agricultural productivity and the following factors: farm size, distance, labor availability, costs of fertilizers, on-farm non-agricultural incomes, access to credits, and soil conservation quality. Likewise, it was found that the productivity of energy, substitution of labor by capital and crop output per hectare influence the mixed farming in EU. As previously seen, the evaluation of production efficiency is as a result of climatic conditions and variability of farms (Špička, 2014).

Burja (2012) concludes that the agricultural holdings from the West region are the least productive while the ones from the South Muntenia region are similar in efficiency as those from the EU. *Above average performance is recorded by the South-West Oltenia and South-East regions.* Other study (Nowak, Kijek, & Domańska, 2015) suggests that Romania has a low agricultural technical efficiency and that its determining factors are the age of the head of the household, the soil quality and the surcharges for investments while the farm size seems to be irrelevant. One negative influencing factor of the Romanian agriculture is the labor force which is characterized by many families who work for their subsistence farms, by the aging population with a low level of education (Tocco, Davidova, & Bailey, 2014).

Methodological Background

This study focuses on analyzing the determinants of agricultural production at national and territorial level in Romania by applying panel data and secondary data analyses in EViews 7 software for explaining the influencing factors of agricultural crop values on eight Romanian development regions during 1997-2014. The data was provided by the Romanian National Institute of Statistics, the European Commission (Eurostat and Farm accounting data network) and the ESPON database portal.

The indicators considered in this paper are: agricultural values, agricultural crop values, cereal yield – as endogenous variables -, irrigated area, the number of villages, final energy consumption in agriculture, physical agricultural tractors per agricultural ha, the labor cost per employee, civil economically active population, chemical and natural fertilizers, pesticides, greenhouse gas emissions from agriculture, gross domestic product per capita, population density, the actual heating degree-days per year, and the type of season to illustrate the climate variability (rainy, dry – dummy variables) – as explanatory variables.

The cereals crop was chosen as it represents one of the most important agricultural cultures worldwide, because of their importance in assuring food security. Thus, cereals are easy to cultivate, transport, store, and give more than 60% of the nutritional value required by the human body (Cereal Science and Technology, 2016). Cereals have economic, social and environmental significance. Also, corn and wheat are the two cereal cultures prevailing in Romania that are belonging to the cereals group.

The corn is the predominant culture in Romania due to the fact that it can be used both as food and as fodder. It is an expensive culture to set up; still, it needs no high degree of mechanization which makes it accessible to the numerous Romanian individual households. Unlike corn, the wheat requires a higher degree of mechanization, which leads to higher volume of payments made to service providers. (Gavrilescu & Giurcă, 2000: p. 111-113)

THE ROMANIAN LAND USE AND THE LAND IMPROVEMENTS

Since 1997 the land fund use has changed due to various factors. The shift from the socialist economy (centrally planned economy) to a market economy has influenced this change as the restructuring of the Romanian economy has negatively impacted the agricultural activities. The cropland abandonment has been affected due to several determinants, such as topography, migration, market access, tractors density, public policies (Müller, Leitão, & Sikor, 2013). According to the Romanian National Institute of Statistics (2016b), the total land of Romania is 23839071 hectares, of which 14630072 hectares agricultural land and 9208999 hectares non-agricultural land. The agricultural land has diminished by 1.11% while the non-agricultural land has increased by 1.81% in 2014 compared to 1997. The decreases of the Romanian agricultural land could be explained by the shift in the type of usage. So, although the arable land and the meadows land have registered small increases by 0.58% and by 4.39% during 1997-2014, the land with orchards, the vineyards and the pastures has significantly decreased by 25.87%, 26.86% and 4.04% during 1997-2014. Figure 2 illustrates the evolution of the Romanian agricultural land structure evolution.

Figure 2. The evolution of the Romanian agricultural land use during 1997-2014
Data source: Romanian National Institute of Statistics, 2016.

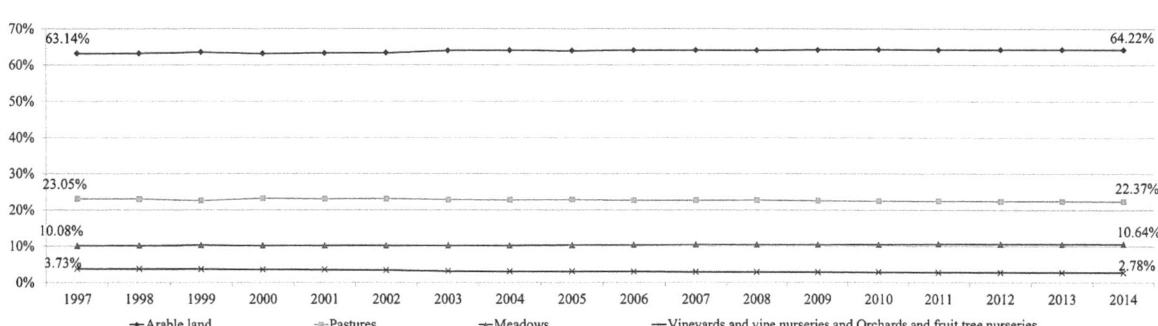

The lowest shares of arable land of each regional agricultural land are found in Center region (40%) and in the North-West region (50%) in the analyzed time frame. The arable land of the Center region is the 2nd smallest region as arable surface of all the eight regions while the North-West region is placed on 6th. Even though the Bucharest-Ilfov region has the smallest area of arable land, this region has the highest share of arable land in the Bucharest-Ilfov agricultural land.

Equally, the highest regional shares of agricultural area are found in the South Muntenia region (16%) and in the South-East (15%) while, as expected, in the Bucharest-Ilfov region has the lowest share of 1%. The situation is similar when analyzing the arable land structure.

In addition, the land improvements and quality represent important factors which contribute to the cereal yield and, further, to the agricultural value. As all the EU member states, Romania registered loses in the agricultural land because of various factors. The Romanian land improvements have increased since 1997. The erosion and soil improvements have slightly increased as area, by 1.86%. Yet, on regional level the changes are a bit bigger as in the case of the irrigated area and the drainage works in hectares. The Romanian actual irrigated area has improved by 15.11% while the area with drainage works has increased by 8.17% during 1997-2014. The land use and the status of the natural resources' quality contribute to the agricultural crop outcome. Therefore, their analysis, in accordance with other determinants, is important for developing the performance of the Romanian agriculture.

THE CAUSAL RELATIONSHIP BETWEEN THE AGRICULTURAL DETERMINANTS

The support for Romanian rural development has slightly increased in terms of financial support in 2013 since 2010, but this has slightly decreased in terms of supported farms. The number of Romanian farms, presented in Table 1, has decreased between 2005 and 2013, maybe due to the changes in the legislative framework as well as the economic crises. It is interesting to highlight the slight increase of the number of farms with more than 50% of production self-consumed by the holder until 2010, although the European Union supports agriculture directed to market. Nevertheless, the number of farms with more than 50% of production self-consumed by the holder has decreased less than the total number of farms since 2005.

Table 1. Total number of Romanian farms by region

GEO/TIME	2005	2007	2010	2013	2005	2007	2010	2013
	Total No. of Farms				More Than 50% of Production Self-Consumed by the Holder (no.)			
Romania	4256150	3931350	3859040	3629660	3444760	3172280	3589530	3178490
North-West	591510	533770	528460	499860	465490	404800	489710	421780
Centre	440710	398540	394650	358470	348760	321640	348480	292020
North-East	854870	807460	790790	754530	701530	662920	749070	684120
South-East	532150	501420	460330	433040	414010	374010	420470	363620
South - Muntenia	847560	762890	800830	753590	697700	621860	738580	671780
Bucharest – Ilfov	63860	62410	33490	25320	48670	53880	29270	18480
South-West Oltenia	608160	580610	576600	557850	527040	518410	561030	525410
West	317330	284260	273890	247000	241560	214760	252930	201280

Source: (European Commission, Eurostat database, 2016).

Romania has more than half of its farms producing for at least 50% to self-consumption. In 2013, the lowest share of farms with more than 50% of production self-consumed by the holder in total number of holdings was registered in Bucharest-Ilfov region (72.99%) while the highest share was listed in the South-West Oltenia region; The Romanian average share was 87.57%. This indicator could show the development degree of holdings because when the self-consumption increases it could mean the economic downfall of the holder of the farm. In addition, it is well-known the Romanian farm structure: that there are the subsistence farms above EU average.

The total agricultural value (the agricultural output) and, in particular, the crop output (the agricultural crop value) followed a varying and increasing trend since 1997 that it could be explained by the modification of moneys' value as well as by the agricultural market in a specific year. Both indicators have augmented by 9 times in 2014 compared to 1997.

The agricultural greenhouse gas emissions have decreased by 15% while the final energy consumption by 53.29% during 1997-2014, as illustrated in Figure 3.

Figure 3. Some key Romanian indicators relevant for agriculture
Source: Romanian National Institute of Statistics, 2016.
Note: AV/1000ha – agricultural value per 1000 ha, ACV/1000ha – agricultural crop value per 1000 ha, GHGa – agricultural greenhouse gas emissions, YC – cereal yield, LCE – labor cost per employee, FECa – final energy consumption in agriculture

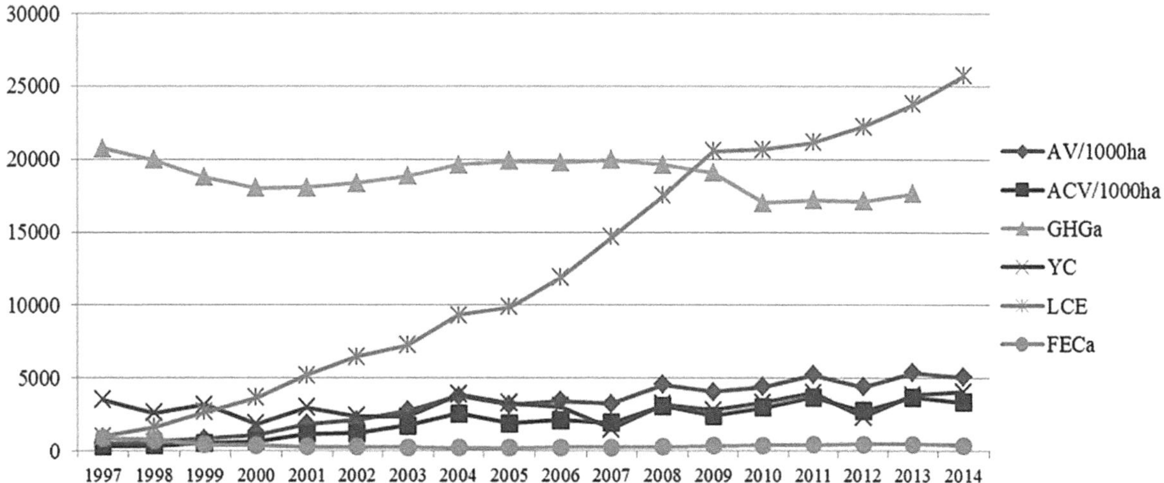

The population density recorded a slight decrease since 1997 while the GDP per capita has almost doubled during 1997-2013. The material and economic capital, which might influence the agricultural productivity, has also varied overtime. The tractors density has increased since 1997 as well as the technological development of the field. The fertilizers and pesticides have started to be carefully monitored for a better protection of the environment and the human health. Both the chemical and the natural fertilizers have decreased 29.26% and 15.49% during 1997-2014. Likewise, the insecticides, the herbicides and the fungicides have significantly reduced by 76.84%, 45.74% and 67.02% since 1997. The labor cost per employee has gotten up during the analyzed period while the number of employees working in agriculture has significantly decreased, by 69.4%, during 1997-2014.

Again, the climate variability influence considerably the agricultural crop value and the cereal yield; this is why, in the analyses, the authors took into consideration also the type of the season (excessively dry, excessively rainy) and, as much as possible, the actual heating degree-days.

Further, in order to determine the correlation matrix between the variables influencing the crop output, it must be tested the stationarity of each variable for model validity. The authors chose the augmented Dickey-Fuller test for unit roots in order to eliminate the autocorrelation and to test the stationarity of data (Asteriou & Hall, 2007).

Testing for Units Roots by Using the Augmented Dickey-Fuller Test

Table 2 presents the results of the unit root tests briefly.

If the null test hypothesis (that the analyzed variable has a unit root, meaning that the data is non-stationary) is rejected, than the data is stationary and the further steps of the analysis could be followed. Otherwise, the data is non-stationary and, before continuing the analysis, the data must be processed by applying the required difference.

Table 2. The results of the unit root test for the analysis of agricultural output determinants

EViews Code	Variable Name	Null Test Hypothesis in Level	Conclusion
av	Agricultural output	accepted	non-stationary data
acv	Agricultural crop value (crop output)	Rejected (trend and intercept)	stationary data***
yc	Cereal yield	Rejected (trend and intercept)	stationary data***
agrl	Agricultural land	Rejected (trend and intercept)	stationary data***
sirr	Irrigated area	accepted	non-stationary data
feca	Final energy consumption agriculture	accepted	non-stationary data
ghga	GHG agriculture	accepted	non-stationary data
gdp	GDP pps pcr inhabitant	accepted	non-stationary data
lfc	Labour force total costs	accepted	non-stationary data
ceapop	Civil economically active population	accepted	non-stationary data
ir_fp	Inflation rate food products	Rejected (trend and intercept)	stationary data***
ur	Unemployment rate	accepted	non-stationary data
pd	Population density	accepted	non-stationary data
pdagrl	Population density on agricultural land	Rejected (trend and intercept)	stationary data***
pat	Physical agricultural tractors per agr.ha	accepted	non-stationary data
cf	Chemical fertilizers	accepted	non-stationary data
nf	Natural fertilizers	accepted	non-stationary data
p	Pesticides	Rejected (trend and intercept)	stationary data**
subv	Subsidies	accepted	non-stationary data
hdd	Actual heating degree-days per year	accepted	non-stationary data

*10% significance; ** 5% significance; ***1% significance
Note: See Appendix, Table 9 for the legend

The analysis was initially performed in level with the option of trend and intercept at maximum lags 3. The pesticides data is stationary without trend and intercept at 5% significance level.

The Correlation Matrix for the Agricultural Output in Romania

The correlation for the agricultural output (expressed in thousands lei) takes into consideration the previous possible analyzed determinants, when it was conducted the unit root test for stationing the data.

The correlation matrix shows the influence of one variable to another. As it can be observed, the crop value is correlated with the yield of cereals, the agricultural area, the inflation rate of food products, the population density per agricultural land, the difference of the tractors' number and the pesticides. The cereal yield is correlated with the agricultural area, the irrigated area, the number of tractors and the 2nd difference of the population density.

Further, the Granger causality test is conducted to identify in which way these variables influence each other. The null hypothesis of this test is that the independent variable does not affect the dependent variable. Patra and Poshakwale (2006) recommend using 6 lags in order to determine the optimal results. However, in this case, as the dimension of the sample is quite small, the analysis will be made with 2 lags.

Table 3. The transformation of the non-stationary data into the stationary ones

EViews Code	Applied Difference	Significance	Trend	Intercept	None
dav	1st	1%	x	x	
dsirr	1st	1%			x
ddfeca	2nd	1%			x
ddghga	2nd	1%	x	x	
ddgdp	2nd	1%			x
dlfc	1st	1%	x	x	
dceapop	1st	1%			x
dur	1st	5%	x	x	
ddpd	2nd	5%			x
dpat	1st	5%	x	x	
dcf	1st	5%	x	x	
dnf	1st	1%			x
dsubv	1st	5%			x
dhdd	1st	5%	x	x	

Note: See Appendix, Table 9 for the legend

The difference of the agricultural value (dav) is influenced by the yield of the cereals (yc) and the difference of subsidies (dsubv) with 99% significance, as well as by the difference in the irrigated area (dsirr) by more than 95%. Also, the crop output (acv) is influenced by the yc, the dsubv and by the pesticides (p) with more than 90% significance. The yield of cereals (yc) is influenced by the difference of subsidies (dsubv) with more than 90% significance.

The 2nd level difference of the greenhouse gas emissions from agriculture (ddghga) are influenced by the difference of the unemployment rate (dur), by the 2nd level difference of the GDP per capita (ddgdp), by the difference of the labor force costs in agriculture (dlfc), by the difference of the chemical fertilizers (dcf) and by the difference of the agricultural value (dav) with a significance of more than 90%.

The 2nd level difference of the energy consumed in agriculture (ddfeca) is influenced by the agricultural crop value (acv), by the agricultural land and by the inflation rate at food products (ir_fp) with a significance of more than 89%.

These relationships could represent a focus for the decision makers at the level of political, legislative and agricultural activities.

THE RELATIONSHIP BETWEEN SOCIAL, ECONOMIC, AND ENVIRONMENTAL DIMENSIONS ON TERRITORIAL LEVEL

A series of Romanian indicators are explored at territorial level by using the panel data approach. This section presents the analysis conducted in EViews. Economic, social and environmental indicators are explored with the hope of shedding new light on the Romanian agriculture's performance at territorial level and its impact on environment.

For the purpose of this small scale research, it is important to understand what the development regions are. These are not administrative units of Romanian territory, but regions created for helping the planning and the distribution of the EU funds in Romania. This country has 8 development regions (Ministerul Dezvoltării Regionale şi Administraţiei Publice, 2016):

- **North - East Region – Counties:** Bacău, Botoşani, Iaşi, Neamţ, Suceava,Vaslui;
- **South - East – Counties:** Brăila, Buzău, Constanţa, Galaţi, Vrancea, Tulcea;
- **South - Muntenia – Counties:** Argeş, Călăraşi, Dâmboviţa, Giurgiu, Ialomiţa, Prahova, Teleorman;
- **South - West Oltenia – Counties:** Dolj, Gorj, Mehedinţi, Olt, Vâlcea;
- **West – Counties:** Arad, Caraş–Scverin, Hunedoara, Timiş;
- **North - West – Counties:** Bihor, Bistriţa-Năsăud, Cluj, Sălaj, Satu–Mare, Maramureş;
- **Center – Counties:** Alba, Braşov, Covasna, Harghita, Mureş, Sibiu;
- **Bucureşti – Ilfov:** Bucharest municipality and the Ilfov county.

Except the Bucureşti-Ilfov region, which has around 0.8% of Romanian territory, the rest of the regions have around 12-15% of Romanian territory.

The Panel Unit Root Test and the Correlation Matrix

The panel unit root test provides the necessary results for establishing the existence of non-stationary data. These types of variables should be transformed to stationary data in order to have valid further analysis. It is used the summary method to apply this test at automatic leg length. Table 4 presents the results of the panel unit root test and it explains the data transformation in what concerns the stationarity.

Table 4. The panel unit root test for the data stationarity

EViews Code	Type of Data	Conclusion - Action
av, cf,	stationary data*	Null hypothesis rejected (trend and intercept) – summary
acv, yc, qc, sirr	stationary data***	Null hypothesis rejected (trend and intercept) – summary
yc	stationary data***	Null hypothesis rejected (trend and intercept) – summary
sc	stationary data**	Null hypothesis rejected (intercept) – summary
nov	stationary data*	Null hypothesis rejected (none) – summary or 1st difference, trend and intercept*** => *dnov*
p	stationary data**	Null hypothesis rejected (intercept) – summary
ceapop, pd, pdagrl	stationary data***	Null hypothesis rejected (none) – summary
pat	non-stationary data	1st difference, trend and intercept*** => *dpat*
nf	non-stationary data	1st difference, intercept*** => *dnf*
lce	non-stationary data	1st difference, intercept*** or trend and intercept* => *dlce*
lfc	non-stationary data	1st difference, trend and intercept*** => *dlfc*
rgdp	non-stationary data	1st difference, trend and intercept*** => *drgdp*
hdd	stationary data***	Null hypothesis rejected (intercept) – summary

*10% significance; ** 5% significance; ***1% significance
Legend: See Appendix, Table 9

The data is non-stationary if the analyzed variable has a unit root (the null test hypothesis is accepted) by using the summary method. If the null hypothesis is rejected, then the data is stationary. Those variables which present non-stationary data have been transformed by difference at 1st, 2nd or 3rd level for model validity. The analysis was initially performed in level with the option of trend and intercept by using the summary test type in EViews.

In Appendix, Table 10, the descriptive statistics of the panel data are presented and it could be noticed that the mean cereal yield is 3039.1 kg/ha during 1997-2014. The maximum of 4381 kg cereals/ha was registered in the Bucharest-Ilfov region in 2004 and the minimum of 834 kg cereals/ha was registered in the South-West region in 2007. The 2007 excessive draught year negatively influenced the cereal yield. Although, the majority of development regions registered favorable cereal yields in 2004, the Bucharest-Ilfov region registered a low agricultural crop value in 2004. This year did not have excessive draughts or excessive rains and the inputs used were relatively high in values.

In addition, big differences between the maximum values and minimum ones could be observed for several determinants, such as the difference in the labor costs.

After transforming the data to be able to use it, the correlation matrix is listed in Appendix, Table 11. The correlation's coefficients are stained according to the maximum level of 40% and the probabilities are marked with *, ** or *** according to the 10%, 5% or 1% significance.

Moreover, the Granger causality test was performed to identify the possible causal relationships between the considered variables and their direction of action. The results show that the agricultural value (*av*) is influenced by the cereal yield (*yc*), the cereals production (*qc*), the civil economically active population (*ceapop*), the difference between the labor force costs (*dlfc*), the agricultural crop value (*acv*), the irrigated area of land (*sirr*), the population density on the agricultural land (*pdagrl*), the number of villages (*nov*) and the population density (*pd*) at a significance level of more than 99%, as well as by the difference of the labor cost per employee (*dlce)* at a significance level of more than 95% and by the pesticides (*p*) at a significance level of more than 90%. Agricultural value influences the *dlfc, acv*, the difference of the regional GDP (*drgdp*), *qc*, cultivated area with cereals (*sc*) and *yc*.

Equally, agricultural crop value (*acv*) is causally influenced by *yc, av, qc, dlfc, dlce, sirr* and *sc* at a significance level of more than 99%, as well as by *ceapop, nov, pdagrl* and *pd* at a significance level of more than 95%. Vice versa, the agricultural crop value influences the *dlfc, drgdp, av, qc, sc* and *yc*.

The cereal yield (*yc*) is influenced by the *dlce* and *p*, at a significance level of more than 99%, as well as by *av* and *acv* at a significance level of more than 95% and by *dlfc, ceapop* and *hdd* at a significance level of more than 90%. The cereal yield (*yc*) influences *av, acv, qc, drgdp, sc, pd, ceapop* and *dlce*.

The regional GDP (*rgdp*) is influenced by the agricultural value, including also the crop value, by the civil economically active population, by the population density (*pd and pdagrl*), by the number of villages, by the cereal yield.

The Panel Data Analysis

The panel data analysis includes 6 models considering the correlation matrix and the Granger causality test. Table 5 and table 6 present the determinants of cereal yield and of agricultural output value considered for the regression models and the related results.

The models analyzed in table 5 (M1, M2, M3 and M4) have been established without the dummy variables regarding the type of the season. After testing all the possible panel models, the suitable one was the fixed cross-sectional model with no period for the M2, M3 and M4 models. The fixed cross-

Table 5. Determinants of the cereal yield and of the crop output for the Romanian development regions – Linear regression model without dummy variables

Variable	M1 1998-2014	M2 1998-2014	M3 1998-2014	M4 1998-2009
Agricultural output	endogenous			
Crop output		endogenous		
Cereal yield	1645.439***	782.6529***	endogenous	endogenous
Irrigated area			-0.0063***	-0.0061***
The modification of the physical agricultural tractors per agricultural ha			434904.2***	416804.4000***
Chemical fertilizers			1018.661**	1069.3680**
The modification of the natural fertilizers			14.90256**	26.6795*
Pesticides			-100.6186***	-56.7003
The modification of the labor cost per employee	671.0702**	-124.0245		
Civil economically active population	-9434.669***	-30689.53***		
The number of villages	5181.596***	24222.01***		
Actual heating degree-days per year				0.2972
Intercept	-5038207.***	-27016382	3306.585***	2174.7330*
R-squared	0.521576	0.876810	0.406106	0.378747
Hausman test	-	Valid, but not statistically relevant	Valid, but not statistically relevant	Valid, but not statistically relevant
Redundant fixed effects (F)	-	80.2338***	2.8849***	2.0117*
Durbin-Watson	0.326846	1.2147	2.3231	2.6353
Chosen model	Cross-sectional: none; Period: none	Cross-sectional: fixed; Period: none	Cross-sectional: fixed; Period: none.	Cross-sectional: fixed; Period: none.

***1% significance **5% significance *10% significance

Note 1: See Appendix, Table 9 for the legend.

sectional model indicates the consistency of the regression model, meaning that, as the sample size increases, the model is more accurate.

The R-squared tendency towards 1 shows the validity of each model and the tendency of Durbin-Watson test towards 2 indicates the existence of relatively small correlation among the model variables. So, the chosen panel model for M2, M3 and M4 are consistent and it could be relevant in practice.

As can be seen in M2, the crop output is positively correlated by the cereal yield and by the number of villages. The difference in the labor cost per employee and the number of civil economically active population influence negatively the agricultural crop value. These findings are sustained by the reality practices because, sometimes, as the employees and their related costs are increasing, the agricultural crop value might be negatively influenced due to price rises.

The positive influence of the labor cost per employee on total agricultural output from model 1 could be explained by the increase in its productivity. Maybe, the increase of this cost is generated by the improvements in education and/or experience which, further, it leads to productivity rises, and, therefore, fewer number of employees. The other 3 variables are similar to the ones from M1.

As the number of persons working in agriculture or the ones depending on a lower surface of agricultural land increases, the value of agricultural production is smaller. The population density per agricultural area was considered in the analysis as an indicator of food security. Still, due to its high correlation with many considered variables, there were no concluding results.

The 3rd and 4th regression models display the positive determinants of cereal yield (the difference of the physical agricultural tractors used in agriculture per ha, the chemical fertilizers, the difference of the natural fertilizers and the actual heating degree-days) and the negative ones (the irrigated area and the pesticides). Yet, the 4th model was analyzed on short timeline. Table 6 illustrates the negative effects which appeared in the North-West and South-West Oltenia regions in what concerns the cereal yield.

Table 6. Cross-section fixed effects of model 3

Romanian Development Region	M3 Effect
North - West	-153.0868
Center	52.73498
North - East	32.58526
South - East	741.7025
South - Muntenia	332.7986
Bucharest - Ilfov	174.8243
South - West Oltenia	-1528.382
West	321.1813

As the cereal yield depends on the climate variability, 2 models of regressions are analyzed in Table 7 by considering 2 scenarios: model 5 (M5) indicates the regression results by taking into account the years with excessive draughts; model 6 (M6) indicates the regression results by taking into account the excessively rainy years.

The negative and positive determinants of cereal yield explained by the M5 and M6 regressions are as the ones from M3 and M4. The dummy variable of M5 (the excessive draughts years) indicates a negative influence on the cereal yield. This result could be correlated with the reality. With an opposite effect, the dummy variable of M6 (the excessively rainy years) did not registered a statistical relevance as the p-value is 43.7%, which is a lot more than the 5% accepted significance level.

As previous, all possible regression models were tested in order to choose the right one, that of the fixed cross-sectional model without random period for the 2 explored models. The R-squared tendency towards 1 shows the validity of each model and the Durbin-Watson test indicates the existence of relatively small correlation among the model variables. So, the chosen panel model for M5 and M6 is consistent and it could be relevant in practice. The redundant fixed effects test (F) indicates the effects on each region. These are presented in the Table 8 which summarize the results regarding the cross-section fixed effects (at regional level).

Table 7. Determinants of cereal yield considering the type of the yearly season - Linear regression model

Variable	M5 1998-2014	M6 1998-2014
Yield cereal	endogenous	endogenous
Irrigated area	-0.005743***	-0.005996***
The modification of the physical agricultural tractors per agricultural ha	397786.1***	424095***
Chemical fertilizers	874.9874**	1029.805**
The modification of the natural fertilizers	15.17281***	15.35443**
Pesticides	-85.48199**	-94.75368**
Ddry	-428.392***	
Drainy		122.3217 (p-0.437)
Intercept	3609.936***	3238.207***
R-squared	0.443735	0.409550
Adjusted R-squared	0.374202	0.335744
Durbin-Watson test	2.5136	2.3070
Hausman test	Not statistically valid	Not statistically valid
Redundant fixed effects(F)	2.4814**	2.7174**
Chosen model	Cross-sectional: fixed; Period: none	Cross-sectional: fixed; Period: none

***1% significance **5% significance *10% significance

Note 1: The analyzed determinants are estimated according the type of season, which is represented by dummy variables for the years with excessive draughts and excessive rain (Ddry and Drainy).

Table 8. Cross-section fixed effects for M5 and M6

No.	Romanian Development Region	M5 Effect	M6 Effect
1	North - West	-155.5458	-109.5532
2	Center	43.11479	64.89199
3	North - East	15.08060	37.98230
4	South - East	647.9279	701.3351
5	South - Muntenia	297.3141	322.6093
6	Bucharest - Ilfov	138.9700	180.3643
7	South - West Oltenia	-1356.052	-1531.176
8	West	331.4499	339.4943

The fixed cross-sectional model indicates the consistency of the regression model, meaning that, as the sample size increases, the model is more accurate. In addition, the error term from the equation is not constant. The models register different effects on regional level.

CONCLUSION AND FUTURE RESEARCH DIRECTIONS

The agriculture is the new old key for continuous economic development in Europe as it can be a vital tool for reducing unemployment while achieving food security and safety. Agriculture is a strong option to stimulate growth, overcome poverty, and enhance food security which helps in accelerating growth within an economy. Moreover, agriculture plays an important part in worldwide challenges, such as climate change, high level of greenhouse gas emissions, food security and safety, overpopulation and natural resource depletion.

This chapter presented an overview of the Romanian agriculture sector over 1997-2014 periods and explores the influences of the agricultural output determinants at the Romanian territorial level. The results indicate a mean cereal yield of 3039.1 kg/ha during 1997-2014 while the maximum yield registered 4381 kg cereals/ha in the Bucharest-Ilfov region in 2004 and the minimum yield registered 834 kg cereals/ha in the South-West region in 2007. The majority of development regions registered favorably yields of cereals in 2004 as many agricultural inputs were used and no excessive draughts and rains were recorded. However, as expected, 2007 was a year with excessive draught, which negatively influenced the yield from cereals.

The Granger causality test suggests that the value of the agricultural output influences the difference of the regional GDP, the difference between the labor force costs, the cereals quantity and surface, as well as the cereal yields while it is causally influenced by the cereal yield, the civil economically active population, the difference between the labor force costs, the irrigated area of land, the population density and the number of villages at a significance level of 99%. The cereal yields influence the agricultural values, the difference of the regional GDP and the difference of the labor cost per employee while the difference in the labor cost per employee and the pesticides determine the yields of cereals by considering the significance error of 1%.

Moreover, the panel data approach consisted in analyzing 6 models based on the least correlated variables explained by the correlation matrix. 5 out of 6 problems were finally analyzed with the fixed cross-sectional model which indicates consistency of the regression models. Also, the findings suggest a negatively influence of the excessive draughts years on the cereal yield while it could not be found a statistical relevance for the influence of the excessively rainy years.

However, the limit of this research is the lack of available data on many agricultural indicators during time and/or at territorial level. The regression models indicated a high level of correlation which raises a question mark regarding the validity of the models in practice. Anyhow, the determinants could represent a starting point in analyzing and forecasting the farm activities. Future research might explore further the determinants of the agricultural production on every category of crop and of livestock. Likewise, it should be considered into the analysis more socio-environmental indicators for sustainable management of agricultural resources.

REFERENCES

Abugamea, G. H. (2008). A Dynamic Analysis for Agricultural Production Determinants in Paletsine: 1980-2003. In *Proceedings of International Conference on Applied Economics, ICOAE* (pp. 3-10). Academic Press.

Anderl, M. (2009). Emisiile în aer produse de agricultură în Austria şi România. *Pro Environment, 2*, 84–92.

Asteriou, D., & Hall, S. G. (2007). *Applied econometrics: A modern approach using eviews and microfit* (revised edition). Palgrave Macmillan.

Burja, C. (2012). Determinants of the agricultural productivity growth among Romanian regions. *Annales Universitatis Apulensis Series Oeconomica, 1*(14).

Carvalho, F. P. (2006). Agriculture, pesticides, food security and food safety. *Environmental Science & Policy, 9*(7), 685–692. doi:10.1016/j.envsci.2006.08.002

Cereal Science and Technology. (2016). *The economic importance of cereal grains.* Retrieved from http://cereal-scientech.blogspot.ro/2011/12/economic-importance-of-cereal-grains.html

Ekbom, A. (1998). Some determinants to agricultural productivity: An application to the Kenyan highlands. In *World Conference of Environmental Economics* (pp. 25-27). Academic Press.

ESPON Database Portal. (2016). Retrieved from http://database.espon.eu/db2/home;jsessionid=b7c0e44c4a7260687a2df61e4e09

European Commission. (2010). Europe 2020 - A European strategy for smart, sustainable and inclusive growth. Brussels: EC.

European Commission. (2011). *Analysis associated with the Roadmap to a Resource Efficient Europe.* Part I, Commission staff working paper, Brussels, 20.9.2011, SEC(2011) 1067 final, Accompanying the document Communication from the Commission to the European Parliament, the Council, the European Economic and Social Committee and the Committee of Regions, Roadmap to a Resource Efficient Europe, COM(2011) 571 final, SEC(2011) 1068 final.

European Commission (2014a). *Agriculture and Rural Development, The CAP, Overview, The EU explained: Agriculture.* Retrieved from http://ec.europa.eu/agriculture/index_en.htm

European Commission (2014b). *Agriculture and Rural Development, Romania, Common Agricultural Policy.* Retrieved from http://ec.europa.eu/agriculture/cap-in-your-country/index_ro.htm

European Commission (2016a). *International Cooperation and Development, Food and agriculture, Food and nutrition security.* Retrieved from https://ec.europa.eu/europeaid/sectors/food-and-agriculture/food-and-nutrition-security_en

European Commission. (2016b). *Climate Action-Policies-Greenhouse gas emission.* Retrieved from http://ec.europa.eu/clima/policies/g-gas/index_en.htm

European Commission (2016c). *Sustainable Development indicators, Climate change, Greenhouse gas emissions by sector.* Retrieved from http://ec.europa.eu/eurostat/data/database

European Commission. (2016d). Overview of CAP Reform 2014-2020. Agricultural Policy Perspectives Briefs, no.5, December 2013, pp 1-10. Retrieved from http://ec.europa.eu/agriculture/policy-perspectives/policy-briefs/index_en.htm

Eurostat. (2016). Retrieved from http://appsso.eurostat.ec.europa.eu/nui/submitViewTableAction.do

Gavrilescu, D., & Giurcă, D. (Eds.). (2000). Economie agroalimentară. editura Expert şi Bioterra, 111-113.

Giovannucci, D., Scherr, S. J., Nierenberg, D., Hebebrand, C., Shapiro, J., Milder, J.,Wheeler, K. (2012). *Food and agriculture: The future of sustainability. The sustainable development in the 21st century (SD21).* Report for Rio, 20.

Hazell, P., & Wood, S. (2008). Drivers of change in global agriculture. *Philosophical Transactions of the Royal Society of London. Series B, Biological Sciences, 363*(1491), 495–515. doi:10.1098/rstb.2007.2166 PMID:17656343

Lopez, R. (1994). The environment as a factor of production: The effects of economic growth and trade liberalization. *Journal of Environmental Economics and Management, 27*(2), 163–184. doi:10.1006/jeem.1994.1032

Mamatzakis, E. C. (2003). Public infrastructure and productivity growth in Greek agriculture. *Agricultural Economics, 29*(2), 169–180. doi:10.1111/j.1574-0862.2003.tb00155.x

Ministerul Dezvoltării Regionale şi Administraţiei Publice. (2016). *Dezvoltare regionala, Programe europene 2007-2013, Programul Operational Regional 2007-2013, Regiuni de dezvoltare.* Retrieved from http://www.mdrap.ro/dezvoltare-regionala/-2257/programul-operational-regional-2007-2013/-2975

Müller, D., Leitão, P. J., & Sikor, T. (2013). Comparing the determinants of cropland abandonment in Albania and Romania using boosted regression trees. *Agricultural Systems, 117*, 66–77. doi:10.1016/j.agsy.2012.12.010

Nowak, A., Kijek, T., & Domańska, K. (2015). Technical efficiency and its determinants in the European Union agriculture. [Zemědělská Ekonomika]. *Agricultural Economics, 61*(6), 275–283.

Olesen, J. E. (2006). *Climate change as a driver for European agriculture. SCAR-Foresight in the field of agricultural research in Europe.* Expert paper.

Olesen, J. E., & Bindi, M. (2004). Agricultural impacts and adaptations to climate change in Europe. *Farm Policy Journal, 1*(3), 36–46.

Patra, T., & Poshakwale, S. (2006). Economic variables and stock market returns: Evidence from the Athens stock exchange. *Applied Financial Economics, 16*(13), 993–1005. doi:10.1080/09603100500426523

Piasecki, A., & Jurasz, J. (2015). Development of water and sewage infrastructure on rural areas in Poland. *Development, 15*(3).

Popescu, G. (2014). The common agricultural policy-in the traps of land property. *Calitatea, 15*(8), 8-15.

Popescu, G., & Zaharia, A. (2015). Analysis of technical progress, energy consumption and value added in European Union's agriculture. *2nd International Multidisciplinary Scientific Conference on Social Sciences and Arts, 3*, 49 - 56.

Romanian National Agency for Environmental Protection (2016). *Areas-Soil.* Retrieved from http://www.anpm.ro/sol-subsol

Romanian National Institute of Statistics. (2016a). Retrieved from http://statistici.insse.ro/shop/?page=tempo3&lang=ro&ind=PMI114B

Romanian National Institute of Statistics. (2016b). Retrieved from http://statistici.insse.ro/shop/

Špička, J. (2014). The regional efficiency of mixed crop and livestock type of farming and its determinants. *AGRIS On-Line Papers in Economics and Informatics*, *6*(1), 99–109.

Teryomenko, H. (2008). *Farm Size and Determinants of Agricultural Productivity in Ukraine* (Doctoral dissertation). National University.

The Romanian Ministry of Agriculture and Rural Development. (2016). *National Rural Development Programme 2014 – 2020, The Romanian village has future!* Retrieved from http://www.madr.ro/pndr-2014-2020/implementare-pndr-2014-2020/documente-aprobate.html

Tocco, B., Davidova, S., & Bailey, A. (2014). labor adjustments in agriculture: Evidence from Romania. *Studies in Agricultural Economics (Budapest)*, *116*(2), 67–73. doi:10.7896/j.1406

Vijayasarathy, K., & Ashok, K. R. (2015). Climate Adaptation in Agriculture through Technological Option: Determinants and Impact on Efficiency of Production. *Agricultural Economics Research Review*, *28*(1), 103. doi:10.5958/0974-0279.2015.00008.7

Voicu, R., & Dobre, I. (2003). *Organizarea şi strategia dezvoltării unităţilor agricole*. Bucureşti: Editura ASE.

Wiebensohn, J., & Jackenkroll, M. (2013). Evaluation and modelling of a standard based spatial data infrastructure for precision farming. In *Proceedings of the EFITA-WCCA-CIGR Conference* (*Vol. 2427*, p. C0107). Academic Press.

Zaharia, A., Antonescu, A. (2014). Agriculture, greenhouse gas emissions and climate change. *14th International Multidisciplinary Scientific GeoConference SGEM*, 3.

KEY TERMS AND DEFINITIONS

Agricultural Crop Value: The value generated by all the crop products in a year.

Agricultural Inputs: All type of entry resources for a process, activity, and business.

Agricultural Outputs: All type of results generated by a process, activity, and business.

Cereal Yield: The ratio between the cereal production and surface.

Cross-Section Fixed Effects: The effects determined by the differences between different spaces.

Panel Data: It represents an econometric technique used to estimate cross-sectional and time effects of several factors on a variable.

Romanian Development Regions: Regions created for helping the planning and the distribution of the EU funds in Romania.

This research was previously published in Agrifood Economics and Sustainable Development in Contemporary Society edited by Gabriel Popescu; pages 1-27, copyright year 2019 by Engineering Science Reference (an imprint of IGI Global).

APPENDIX

Table 9. Data Legend

EViews Code	Variable Name	Data Source	Website
av	Agricultural output	The Romanian National Institute of Statistics	www.insse.ro
acv	Agricultural crop value (crop output)	The Romanian National Institute of Statistics	www.insse.ro
yc	Cereal yield	The Romanian National Institute of Statistics	www.insse.ro
agrl	Agricultural land	The Romanian National Institute of Statistics	www.insse.ro
sirr	Irrigated area	The Romanian National Institute of Statistics	www.insse.ro
feca	Final energy consumption agriculture	The Romanian National Institute of Statistics	www.insse.ro
ghga	GHG agriculture	The Romanian National Institute of Statistics	www.insse.ro
gdp	GDP pps per inhabitant	European Commission	eurostat
lfc	Labour force total costs	The Romanian National Institute of Statistics	www.insse.ro
lce	The labor cost per employee	European Commission	eurostat
ceapop	Civil economically active population	The Romanian National Institute of Statistics	www.insse.ro
ir_fp	Inflation rate food products	The Romanian National Institute of Statistics	www.insse.ro
ur	Unemployment rate	The Romanian National Institute of Statistics	www.insse.ro
pd	Population density	The Romanian National Institute of Statistics	www.insse.ro
pdagricl	Population density on agricultural land	The Romanian National Institute of Statistics	www.insse.ro
pat	Physical agricultural tractors per agricultural ha	The Romanian National Institute of Statistics	www.insse.ro
cf	Chemical fertilizers	The Romanian National Institute of Statistics	www.insse.ro
nf	Natural fertilizers	The Romanian National Institute of Statistics	www.insse.ro
p	Pesticides	The Romanian National Institute of Statistics	www.insse.ro
subv	Subsidies	European Commission	eurostat
hdd	Actual heating degree-days per year	European Commission	eurostat
qc	Production of cereals (tonnes)	The Romanian National Institute of Statistics	www.insse.ro
sc	Cultivated area with cereals	The Romanian National Institute of Statistics	www.insse.ro
rgdp	Regional GDP	The Romanian National Institute of Statistics	www.insse.ro
nov	The number of villages	The Romanian National Institute of Statistics	www.insse.ro
ddry	Years with excessive draughts	Dummy variable – introduced by authors	
drainy	Years with excessive rain	Dummy variable – introduced by authors	

The matrix correlation was performed for 1997-2014 time frames; 144 observations included after adjustments, unbalanced sample, pairwise samples (pairwise missing deletion) (see Table 11).

Table 10. Descriptive Statistics Of Panel Variables

Indicators	AV	ACV	YC	SC	SIRR	QC	DPAT	CF	DNF	P	DLCE	DLFC	CEAPOP	PD	PDAGRL	DRGDP	HDD	NOV
Mean	5779436.0	3738187.0	3039.1	698465.0	31623.1	2108581	0.0	0.2	1.5	4.3	1452.7	17749.8	349.9	2.4	3.9	783.0	2936.8	1625.7
Median	6049575.0	3816415.0	3127.5	700953.0	3582.5	2051773	0.0	0.1	0.0	3.9	1248.0	16659.4	355.7	0.8	1.4	650.0	2858.2	1800.0
Maximum	15613379.0	11539817.0	4381.0	1412613.0	305404.0	5588606	0.0	2.0	64.9	11.2	3048.0	107920.3	721.8	13.7	23.9	6600.0	3754.8	2445.0
Minimum	138343.4	75522.2	834.0	29782.0	12.0	47194	0.0	0.0	-18.7	1.2	96.0	-76707.6	35.6	0.6	1.1	-3500.0	2410.9	91.0
Std. Dev.	3896944.0	2682861.0	792.5	375581.2	56884.8	1302584	0.0	0.4	10.2	2.0	857.7	25417.5	164.3	4.2	6.8	1115.7	361.0	665.7
Skewness	0.25	0.51	-0.54	-0.12	2.47	0.52	-2.81	2.60	3.94	1.06	0.42	-0.42	-0.21	2.26	2.28	1.53	0.53	-1.26
Kurtosis	2.14	2.66	2.94	2.18	9.44	2.98	19.65	8.59	23.77	4.44	2.11	7.16	2.71	6.14	6.27	12.97	2.22	3.85
Jarque-Bera	5.98	6.91	6.89	4.44	346.56	6.55	1750.7	349.93	2795.2	39.5	8.51	101.95	1.61	182.18	189.3	398.51	7.58	42.27
Probability	0.05	0.03	0.03	0.11	0.00	0.04	0.00	0.00	0.00	0.00	0.01	0.00	0.45	0.00	0.00	0.00	0.02	0.00
Observations	144	144	144	144	126	144	136	144	136	144	136	136	144	144	144	88	104	144

Source: own computation with Eviews, 2016

Table 11. Matrix Correlation

Correlation Probability	AV	ACV	YC	SC	SIRR	QC	DPAT	CF	DNF	P	DLCE	DLFC	CEAPOP	PD	PDAGRL	DRGDP	HDD	NOV	DNOV
av	1																		
	-----																		
acv	0.9905	1																	
	***	-----																	
yc	0.3061	0.3552	1																
	***	***	-----																
sc	0.4139	0.4270	-0.0493	1															
	***	***	0.5574	-----															
sirr	0.1464	0.1536	-0.2346	0.5390	1														
	0.1018	*	***	***	-----														
qc	0.5166	0.5601	0.3945	0.8640	0.2986	1													
	***	***	***	***	***	-----													
dpat	0.2198	0.2069	0.3623	0.1260	-0.0408	0.1719	1												
	**	**	***	0.1438	0.6608	**	-----												

continues on following page

Table 11. Continued

Correlation Probability	AV	ACV	YC	SC	SIRR	QC	DPAT	CF	DNF	P	DLCE	DLFC	CEAPOP	PD	PDAGRL	DRGDP	HDD	NOV	DNOV
cf	-0.0164	0.0044	-0.0496	0.2506	-0.0075	0.2007	0.0723	1											
	0.8449	0.9583	0.5550	***	0.9332	**	0.4027	-----											
dnf	0.2087	0.2375	0.2040	0.1310	0.0673	0.2635	0.0027	0.1794	1										
	**	***	**	0.1284	0.4692	***	0.9754	**	-----										
p	-0.3914	-0.3942	-0.2090	0.2387	0.0374	0.1245	-0.1151	-0.1405	-0.0881	1									
	***	***	**	***	0.6778	0.1370	0.1822	*	0.3080	-----									
dlce	0.1795	0.1492	-0.0434	-0.0194	0.0857	-0.0342	-0.0679	-0.0673	0.0193	-0.2767	1								
	**	*	0.6158	0.8225	0.3559	0.6927	0.4324	0.4366	0.8232	***	-----								
dlfc	0.1645	0.1242	-0.0165	0.2300	0.1901	0.1796	-0.0101	-0.0816	0.0742	0.0237	0.4430	1							
	*	0.1496	0.8487	***	**	**	0.9067	0.3451	0.3908	0.7839	***	-----							
ceapop	0.2369	0.2069	-0.1738	0.7028	0.1767	0.5365	0.1679	0.1421	-0.0195	0.5410	-0.1189	0.1604	1						
	***	**	**	***	**	***	*	*	0.8221	***	0.1678	*	-----						
pd	-0.5012	-0.4748	-0.0014	-0.6446	-0.1836	-0.5628	-0.2920	-0.1975	-0.0394	-0.1487	-0.0001	-0.1642	-0.6872	1					
	***	***	0.9868	***	**	0.0000	***	**	0.6488	*	0.9994	*	***	-----					
pdagrl	-0.5009	-0.4749	0.0064	-0.6531	-0.1918	-0.5700	-0.2748	-0.1980	-0.0418	-0.1622	0.0007	-0.1691	-0.6889	0.9984	1				
	***	***	0.9391	***	**	***	***	**	0.6293	*	0.9938	**	***	***	-----				
drgdp	-0.3693	-0.3336	-0.0076	-0.3031	-0.0883	-0.2773	-0.0862	-0.1072	-0.1398	-0.0505	0.0883	-0.2294	-0.3729	0.4166	0.4123	1			
	***	***	0.9440	***	0.4545	***	0.4248	0.3204	0.1941	0.6403	0.4135	**	***	***	***	-----			
hdd	0.0365	0.0079	0.1359	-0.1845	-0.3202	-0.0938	0.1905	-0.1828	0.1327	0.3084	-0.3110	-0.0586	0.3072	-0.2869	-0.2804	-0.1935	1		
	0.7129	0.9363	0.1689	*	***	0.3438	*	*	0.1975	***	***	0.5705	***	***	***	0.1530	-----		
nov	0.5018	0.4580	-0.0668	0.6037	0.0045	0.4979	0.2650	0.3037	0.0387	0.2408	-0.0039	0.1538	0.8558	-0.8599	-0.8573	-0.4087	0.4097	1	
	***	***	0.4263	***	0.9604	***	***	***	0.6551	***	0.9639	*	***	***	***	***	***	-----	

Source: Own computation with Eviews, 2016.

***1% significance **5% significance *10% significance

Note: Accepted correlation for the regression models at more than 0.4 coefficient; Rejected correlation for the regression models

Chapter 49
Farm Security for Food Security:
Dealing with Farm theft in the Caribbean Region

Wendy-Ann Isaac
The University of the West Indies – St. Augustine, Trinidad and Tobago

Wayne Ganpat
The University of the West Indies – St. Augustine, Trinidad and Tobago

Michael Joseph
The University of Trinidad and Tobago, Trinidad and Tobago

ABSTRACT

Agricultural production in the Caribbean is being threatened by many factors such as decreasing availability of arable land, climate change effects such as increased incidences of flooding and drought, labour shortages, and competition from importers. However, one of the most important threats to agricultural production is the often under-recognised and under-reported area of farm theft (referred to as praedial larceny in the Caribbean). It involves the theft of agricultural produce (crops, livestock and fisheries) and farm equipment. One of the main reasons why this threat is so important is that theft of this type is very hard to prove. If indeed perpetrators are caught, and prosecuted successfully, the penalty is practically negligible. This paper examines the current status of farm theft in the Caribbean region, explores some of the main factors influencing farm theft, reviews some of the strategies attempted in the Caribbean and other places around the world and makes several suggestions to create a more secure food region. While the discussion calls on food producers to take several best practice actions to mitigate losses to praedial larceny, it emphasises that the primary responsibility is with government-led actions in the areas of modernised policies, updated laws and enhanced enforcement efforts.

DOI: 10.4018/978-1-7998-5354-1.ch049

INTRODUCTION

Nobody wannu plant the corn
Everybody want to raid the barn
Who yuh a guh blame it on
When is a next man yuh a depend pon
Well yuh wrong
Nobody wannu plant the corn
Everybody want to raid the barn
Haffi sing yuh owna song
Can't compete with careless John.....

These lyrics, written by Anthony B, aptly reflect the unremitting challenge facing the typical farmer in the Caribbean region. Referred to as praedial larceny throughout the Caribbean, farm theft is one of the most extensive among all crimes committed in the region in terms of the number of persons and families affected. Praedial larceny refers to the theft of agricultural produce such as crops, livestock, and fisheries. This term also covers the theft of agricultural equipment such as spray cans, brush cutters, water pumps and other irrigation equipment. It can also be extended to the theft of agriculture inputs and secondary products such as feed and fodder. Praedial larceny has been cited as one of the major challenges impacting the growth of the agricultural sector throughout the Caribbean and has been described as the "Achilles heel" of the agricultural sector across the world. Estimates indicate that the Caribbean region is losing over USD $321 million annually to praedial larceny and it has now become one of the most pervasive and entrenched crimes in business and livelihoods (Caricom, 2011).

A Caricom 2010 study reported that among regional stakeholders there is general consensus (more than 90%) that praedial larceny was the single most discouraging and serious disincentive threatening food security in the region. Farmers throughout the region have been clamouring their Governments to introduce legislation to combat this increasing threat. However, there are concerns by the farming community throughout the region that praedial larceny is not being treated as a very serious crime. Praedial larceny is the only crime at a regional level that consistently trends upwards (Little, 2011). Praedial larceny has moved from the theft of small amounts to large amounts of produce involving in some instances truckloads of bananas in or an entire field of pineapples or other vegetable and root crops or even the entire harvest of a freshwater fish pond. Thieves may also pose serious dangers to farm families and farm workers as many cases of threats on lives of farmers or even homicide have been reported. Some farmers have abandoned their entire enterprise due to heavy losses and the high cost paid for security.

According to Smith (2010), this type of criminal activity typically occurs in a changing social landscape, affected by demographic changes, trends and by the introduction of new policing practices. No longer can the notion of the stereotypical praedial larcenist be viewed as a rural criminal or as a "piper" as many refer to them. The activity has now moved to the status of organized crime, extending away from rural areas into more urban settlements where agriculture is practised. This organized activity now requires a different set of skills and practices for policing the urban landscape (Smith, 2010)

This chapter provides an overview of the problem of praedial larceny facing the Caribbean region, tracing the historical roots of the problem. The chapter examines the drivers and nature of this, now organised criminal activity, focusing on the opportunistic and professional nature of praedial larceny.

It finally explores the various strategies being used throughout the Caribbean to address this growing scourge to move toward farm security for food security.

OVERVIEW OF FARM THEFT (PRAEDIAL LARCENY) IN THE CARIBBEAN

A study titled "An Analysis of the State of Praedial Larceny in Member States of CARICOM" conducted in collaboration with the Caribbean Disaster Emergency Management Agency (CDEMA) under the umbrella of the Agricultural Sector Disaster Risk Management Committee (ASSC/TMAC) found that in terms of the number of persons and families affected by praedial larceny, it is the most extensive among all crimes committed in the Caribbean (Food and Agriculture Organization, 2013) Farm theft was for decades, not taken seriously and perceived as petty by many, but has however, transformed itself into a very serious and complicated crime, with now organized overtones, impacting food security and vulnerable populations in the region (Beckford & Campbell, 2012). Considered a "rural crime", its neglect has been attributed to social disorganisation. This theory begins with the fundamental assumption that places with high levels of expressions of cohesion and solidarity have lower rates of crime, however, places which display less order and more disorganisation tend to have higher rates of crime (Donnermeyer & Scott, 2013).

It has been recognised as a problem not only in the Caribbean, and there is a growing body of academic studies conducted in America, Australia, Britain and Scotland which relate specifically to this rural crime (Sugden, 1999; Barclay, 2001; Donnermeyer & Barclay, 2005; Yarwood & Gardener, 2005; Jones, 2008; Spore, 2009; Smith, 2010; Little, 2011). These studies all show that farm theft is regarded as one of the major deterrents to agricultural production. In many cases, this crime has been one of the major contributing factors to the exodus of farmers from the sector. Little (2011) indicated that it has been recognized by the highest level of leadership in the Caribbean as one of the major constraints to sustainable agricultural development in the region. These losses from praedial larceny can be classified under the categories of financial, physical or prevention/solution (Little, 2011). According to a 2010 survey carried out among regional stakeholders, more than 90% agreed that praedial larceny was the single most discouraging aspect of agriculture and has become a disincentive to investment in the sector and a threat to livelihoods in farming and fishing communities (Little, 2011). The report further indicated that on average, 82% of farmers and fishers affected are commercial or semi-commercial producers. The report also revealed that 18% of the value of farm output regionally is taken by thieves, resulting in the loss of over USD $321 million annually (Caricom, 2011), while worldwide losses are estimated as high as USD $5 billion on an annual basis (Swanson et al., 2000). In some countries in Europe, the loss is between 6 and 18% of agricultural output.

The CARICOM (2011) study revealed the following estimated country losses.

- **Trinidad and Tobago:** Losses of USD $22.6 million annually.
- **Jamaica:** Losses in excess of USD $55 million annually.
- **Belize:** Losses in excess of USD $300,000 annually.
- **St. Vincent and the Grenadines:** Losses of USD $2.3 million annually.
- **Bahamas:** Losses to its marine fish industry of US $16 million annually.

Losses due to praedial larceny can be so devastating that many farmers quit farming altogether. As thieves become better organized and armed, farmers not only suffer loss of their agricultural products and income, but also risk their lives trying to scare off thieves or defend their crops and livestock. Many of the countries spend millions in praedial larceny prevention programmes, some of which will be described later in this chapter. Indeed, St. Lucia is spending in excess of USD $400,000 annually on piloting activities to prevent praedial larceny.

CHANGING ECOLOGY OF FARM THEFT IN THE CARIBBEAN

As a complicated crime, it is extremely difficult to prove and therefore difficult to arrest and convict the perpetrators (FAO, 2013). With rising crime in many Caribbean territories, Governments focus on what Dingwall and Moody (1999) refer to as "mean streets myopia", where they focus their "criminological gaze" on urban criminality, such as drug and gang related crimes (Smith, 2010). Dingwall and Moody (1999) argue that criminologists have long viewed crimes against agricultural operations as unreal and as such it is not of interest to the police or to criminology scholars and thus has been neglected (Swanson, Chamelin & Territo, 2000; Smith, 2010). Many farmers refuse to report this crime due to frustration with inaction by police, who oft times dismiss farm related crime in rural areas as trivial or motiveless. According to Little (2010), only 45% of incidences are reported to the police regionally and very often farmers take matters into their own hands and often end up on the other side of the law. Many farmers are afraid to report for fear of reprisals. Data have also shown that just over 35% of produce stolen at the regional level is used for household food and other needs in the home while around 27% is disposed of in the trafficker (higgler/huckster) trade which is dominated by rural women, most of whom are single, vulnerable household heads and with no other source of income (FAO, 2013).

An FAO brief on praedial larceny in the Caribbean explains that offenders operate in a complex, social and economic environment encompassing varied groups of individuals who have become organized and entrepreneurial by developing livelihoods and businesses from the stealing of agriculture produce, equipment, and materials (Food and Agriculture Organization of the United Nations, 2013). There is a growing body of literature on examining the changing ecology of agricultural crime, criminality and policing (Donnermeyer & Scott, 2013; Smith et al., 2013; Smith & McElwee, 2013). The basic ideology, described by Smith, Laing and McElwee (2013) and Smith and McElwee (2013), around which the policing of rurality is governed posits that urban areas are the natural habitat for the serious and organised criminal. There is less crime in rural areas - known as the rural idyll thesis, with the socially constructed perception of the rural criminal as a loveable, rural rogue and small time thief. Furthermore, the policing of rurality suggests that the majority of rural crime is committed by urban criminals - known as urban marauder thesis; rural crime is somehow less serious than urban crime and therefore requires less of a policing presence. These ideologies are however changing, and as Smith (2010) explains, rural crime is now organized, semi-organized or committed by outsiders or sometimes committed by "rogue farmers" or "exploitative farmers" themselves (Wilkinson, Craig & Gaus 2010). The Caribbean region has in the last 20 years or so noted increasingly, this changing ecology of praedial larceny in terms of frequency of incidences, the large volumes of crop, livestock and fish stolen, and the highly organized and often violent behaviours of the thieves. The significance of the loss resulting has become a disincentive to investment in agriculture and fishing and a danger to farmers, fisher folks, aquaculturists, their employees and families (Little, 2010).

Each criminal group has developed its own dynamics in a distribution chain where the crime enters undetected into the normal processes of legitimate industry, especially of domestic fresh food distribution (FAO, 2013). Smith (2010) and McElwee (2009) refers to this as "illegal rural enterprise"; the most pervasive and hidden type of entrepreneurial criminality. In some cases it involves insider knowledge, thus adding to its complexity of the complicity of rural communities (Smith, 2010). Similar rural criminal activity has been described by Sergi and Lavorgna (2012) and Smith et al. (2013) in Europe. Here there has been in the last decade, an escalation in rural crimes such as the theft of farm machinery and tools, and into unregulated butchery practices. These are all evidence of the danger that serious and organised crime groups can pose to rural areas when they seek to expand their criminal activities in the current economic recession.

Table 1. describes the typology of most farm related crimes throughout the Caribbean (adapted from Smith, 2010). Smith (2010) categorises farm crimes as situation-specific and context-bound, wildlife crime as predatory (carried out by organised gangs of urban criminals), illegal rural enterprise (symbiotic/entrepreneurial) and village crime (opportunistic or context-bound).

Table 1. A typology of rural related farm crimes in the Caribbean adapted from Smith (2010)

Farm Crime (Predatory/Organised/ Context Bound)	Wildlife Crime (Predatory)	Illegal Rural Enterprise (Symbiotic/ Entrepreneurial)	Village Crime (Opportunistic/ Context Bound)
Theft – farm equipment (irrigation lines, tractors, diesel, water pumps, weed whackers, fertilizer and pesticides etc.) Vandalism – to farm and buildings and fences, damage to crops Fire-raising – buildings and farms Cruelty to livestock	Hunting out of season for wildlife – agouti, manicou, lappe, deer Illegal fishing for tilapia etc. Trapping Theft of turtle eggs etc.	Theft of livestock/sheep, goat, cattle, poultry and small stock Theft of seedlings, fruits and vegetables Squatting on private lands Drug cultivation – cannabis farming	Petty theft (pipers) – generally opportunistic Illegal trespassers and shooters Breaking and entering Dumping of rubbish on farmland

Further to this, there is a hidden cost to agriculture production, productivity, and food security when farmers decide to leave the sector or when high quality genetic breeds of livestock and crop varieties are stolen from breeding stations and agriculture research facilities and sold as food (FAO, 2013). Further, there are the likely consequences for public health and subsequent industry fallout should tainted, un-certified produce gain entry into the domestic food chain, which has been the case where crops which have been sprayed with chemicals are stolen by thieves (George Ramtahal, Personal Communication, November 2015). Although not officially reported, because of the difficulty of detection by farm owners, many farms may be the location for clandestine drug operations, especially marijuana as in the case in St. Vincent and the Grenadines, where, after the loss of preferential market access for their banana in the 1990s, it is alleged that several farmers got into the illegal production of marijuana in the more remote mountainous parts of the country. Several authors have described the growing trend of this type of illegal activity globally (Muhammad, 2002; Weisheit & Fuller, 2004; Barclay & Donnermeyer, 2011; Garriott, 2011).

On average 82% of farmers and fishers affected are commercial or semi-commercial producers between the ages of 45 and 50 years. Poor and vulnerable farming populations are also targeted victims. Ninety-eight percent of all producers surveyed have experienced loss of produce from theft - more than 332,000 fisher folk families, and well over 1,000,000 crop and livestock farm families. In addition, farmers have been killed and others have been known to have received threats and physical attacks by persons who have returned to the communities after serving time in prison for praedial larceny. Farmers' crops have also been damaged by these same persons.

The crime, therefore, has potentially high, though undetermined, social costs to welfare in farming communities, livelihoods, and household food security. Concomitant with this, more than 90% of producers regionally agree that it is the single greatest disincentive to investment in the sector.

Policing programmes to combat praedial larceny have now become an integral consideration in determining how agriculture producers, processors, and distributors function in the region in an effort to secure their on-farm investments. For example in Trinidad and Tobago, the praedial larceny squad was established to manage theft in many farming areas. However, in this country, the burden of proof appears to lie with the Police Service. It is required that they produce evidence (the allegedly stolen goods). The problem is: these goods are usually highly perishable. Proper storage is required but often not available. Compounding matters is the fact that the judiciary is burdened by huge backlogs of cases resulting in untimely delays. By the time the cases reach the courts, there is no evidence; crops rot or animals die.

Many governments in the region have also been strengthening policies in order to build strategies which will secure the economic gains from public investment in the sector.

HISTORICAL PERSPECTIVES ON FARM THEFT IN THE CARIBBEAN

Farm theft, better known as praedial larceny, can be traced historically from the Plantation economies of many of the Caribbean islands (Engledow, 1945; Shepherd, 1945; Eisner, 1961; Grossman, 1997 and Bryan, 2000). Eisner (1961) suggested that the problem of praedial larceny, like that of illegitimacy, has its origin in slavery and both have been held responsible for poverty. Bryan (2000) noted that the crime was considered a 'typically black perversion' reflective of the structural problems in the countryside, however, he mentioned that one observer referred to it as the 'rotten and unscientific state of relations between labour and capital', and this is what lay at the root of the problem. Grossman (1997) cited the seriousness of this long-standing problem in Engledow (1945) supplement to the Moyne Commission Report:

No circumstance affecting home-grown food production is more widely or more forcibly brought to notice than what in these colonies is known as praedial larceny. It affects agriculture in many ways.....Praedial larceny is, indeed, a profound handicap to agricultural development.

A report on agriculture in St. Vincent in 1953 similarly mentions *the wave of praedial larceny which prevails and so discourages peasants from growing more food.*

In St. Vincent, Shepherd (1945) reported that *bitter complaints volunteered by many settlers indicate that the losses are serious and that the prevalence of theft is a deterrent to the more extensive planting of food crops.* He also revealed that the problem of theft was more severe with food crops than with export crops. This probably accounts for the reason why farmers up to today still focus on the production of banana over extensive food crops, in what can be described as a culture of dependency (Isaac et al. 2012). According to Shepherd (1945):

Food crops are usually confined to land least suited to the staple cash crop and as these areas are fre-quently the most remote from the cultivator's home, they are seldom under continuous observation. Food crops can be consumed by the thief, and even if sold are unlikely to arouse suspicion. But cash crops, such as sugar-cane, seed cotton and arrowroot rhizomes, require processing: the number of buyers is limited, and in most cases they are registered, and required to keep an account of their transactions: thus the thief runs a greater risk of detection.

Eisner (1961) noted that this crime was ranked equally important with technical inefficiency as the "drawback to the system of peasant proprietorship". Reported as a criminal offence since the 1850s, statistics show that in many Caribbean islands it was compounded by land tenure status. This was be-cause many rural farmers did not always own or cultivate the parcel of land. Landlords were also away from their estates for long periods of time. These situations facilitated praedial larceny as detection rates were very low and as Eisner (1961) suggested, "detections bear no proportion to commission". Eisner (1961) reported that in Jamaica in 1905, "the average value assigned to the stolen property in 2,349 cases brought into court amounted to only 1.03 shillings". Given the high cost associated with going to court for farm theft related cases, it was not worth the time for small farmers to pursue cases and hence the actual reports and costs associated with this crime were underreported. According to Eisner (1961), in Jamaica in 1883, it was claimed that only one-twentieth of all cases were brought into the court, and in spite of the various measures adopted, the number of convictions for this crime continued to fall. Eisner (1961) also reported that a Baptist minister offering evidence to the 1897 Royal Commission, explained that the problem was not as serious as the complainers suggested, citing the large acreages of canes, banana and coconuts left unprotected in all parts of the island, and yet rarely touched by the poor.

Bryan (2000) citing the reasons for praedial larceny, reported that it was sometimes attributed to ignorance or to hunger. Supporting the hunger thesis, he points to the decline of praedial larceny when crops were good, and the rise of praedial larceny during periods of severe drought. Bryan (2000) also stated that there was evidence pointing to the marketability of stolen produce as a major incentive to praedial larceny, including larceny of citrus, logwood and pimento, all export commodities in Jamaica. He cited an example of a planter, who reported that his grapefruits were never touched until a market for them appeared in the United States.

Bryan (2000) cited Justice Gibbons on the relationship between logwood stealing and local merchants. According to Gibbons:

Since I require the production of the wharf books in a case of logwood stealing at May Pen, when I was informed by an overseer of Denbeigh, that the Lord Penrhyn had been robbed of 60 tons (£300) during the then season, I have observed that no prosecutions have been instituted. There is no disguising the fact that Mr. W. C. the Custos, is a large shipper of logwood.........I have observed a suspicious connec-tion between larceny of produce, particularly logwood and pimento from a small cultivator tried before me, there was no doubt of the thief having sold the stolen pimento to a local buyer who was himself the employer of the buyer and the party who ultimately profited by the theft of pimento....So, too, in several cases of logwood stealing it has appeared that the stolen logwood was readily purchased at the local wharf belonging in almost every case to a magistrate. These facts which have only casually come to my notice are doubtless well known to the bulk of the people (Bryan, 2000, pp. 25).

In Jamaica, praedial larceny was consistently regarded as an offence typically committed by members of the working classes. Thus, Act 32 of 1889 disallowed casual roadside buying and selling of produce, although this 'tended to restrict legitimate trade'. Law 37 of 1896 (the Produce Protection Law) tried to limit the offence from the receiving end (Bryan, 2000).

The punishment for this crime was corporal punishment or flogging (with the cat-o'-nine-tails in Jamaica and Trinidad and Tobago), an important method which was used to intimidate and terrorise the black population into obedience up to the end of the nineteenth century according to Bryan (2000). After the abolishment of this method of punishment in 1886 however, it was observed that there was no increase in the offence. A report in 1896 describes a wealthy banana producer and shopkeeper, advocating, "Flog the Negro; that is the only thing they are afraid of………." The same report mentions a boy receiving twelve lashes for stealing one orange.

Bryan (2000) mentioned Robert Love's anger over the legislation which proposed the continuation of flogging for praedial larceny in 1896. Love's anger was triggered from his belief that flogging was another example of class legislation since it was well known that only blacks were likely to be victims of the lash. In an editorial Love declared:

Whilst a thief who lifts a shop, or robs a bank, may be punished by a few months imprisonment, the poor wretch who steals a 2lb yam, or a stick of logwood, must, besides imprisonment, be lacerated by a cat-o'-nine tails….We hate this law because we are convinced that it was intended to operate on a class only. How many white men will be whipped for praedial larceny? Not one. Why? Because the circumstances are such that they are not exposed to the commission of the offence. We hate this law because, while its penalty will brutalise the offender, it will leave him no less an offender…… By a strange species of reasoning, they propose to drive out of us by the lash, the evil which they had driven into us, by the lash, for nearly 300 years.

In Trinidad, Brereton (2010) informed that in ordinance 6 of 1868—just thirty years after the end of slavery—corporal punishment was allowed as the punishment for praedial larceny and the practice of Obeah. An earlier Brereton (1979) document reported that in 1882,

One person was sentenced to four floggings of 36 lashes each by a Couva magistrate, and it was the governor who remitted three of them. A petition organised by a Methodist minister in 1883 to abolish flogging (—the great and disgusting vice of slavery in the brutal practice of flogging to blood the labouring population for petty larceny and other crimes) failed completely; indeed, an 1893 Ordinance actually extended the practice by making flogging mandatory for a second conviction for praedial larceny.

The situation in St. Vincent and other Eastern Caribbean countries showed changes, in that advanced plantation production technologies served as a deterrent to the praedial larcenist. The British and EU governments, the main importing countries of banana, imposed pressures for improved fruit quality, thus mandating technological innovations in harvesting and packing (Grossman, 1997). These technological innovative practices provided banana production another advantage over local food crop production that is related to the perennial problem of crop theft according to Grossman (1997). This movement from plantation crops, however, led to an emphasis on crop theft in other food crops and now this acted as a deterrent for many farmers getting into production (Shepherd 1945; Rubenstein 1975, 1987). According to Grossman (1997),

A thief could easily go into someone else's food garden under cover of night, dig up provisions, put them in a sack, and carry them to Kingstown the next day to sell to hucksters without being discovered. In contrast, technological innovations in harvesting and packing banana have made them less susceptible to theft than food crops. St. Vincent and the other Windward Islands have been forced to adopt a succession of complicated, intricate, labour-intensive processing methods-field packing, paco pack, and, most recently, cluster packing. Given the increasingly intricate, detailed steps required in these systems, stealing banana at night, processing and packing them according to specifications, and then selling them to the St. Vincent Banana Growers Association (SVBGA) the next day are extremely difficult - yet one more advantage of banana production over local food crop production.

In a historical review from colonial Zanzibar, Grassman (2011) describes a situation where crop theft was considered a 'hobby' (Makinde) or a means of economic sustenance since squatters who lived on large plantations harvested whatever they wanted from the landlord's plantation anytime he was absent. In the 1920s, crop theft was the most common form of property crime. These squatters were often in possession, with the landlord's consent, of large surpluses of coconut or clove, which they sold in the market as they wished (Grassman, 2011).

INFLUENCING FACTORS FOR FARM THEFT

There has been little attention paid to the study of patterns and causes of agricultural crimes in the Caribbean. However, there are several factors that contribute to, and encourage the growing spread of this crime. Several studies have however been conducted within recent years on farm crime in Australia, the United Kingdom, and the United States. These studies have consistently found that most farm crime is property-related, including the theft of livestock, spare parts, tractors and other machinery, fuel, tools, agrichemicals, and farm produce and the destruction of property (vandalism) (Barclay, 2001; Anderson & McCall, 2005; Donnermeyer & Barclay, 2005; Mears et al., 2007a; Jones, 2008; Barclay & Donnermeyer, 2011; Bunei et al., 2013).

A review of literature on agricultural crime found that crime against farms is widespread and costly to farmers (Barclay, 2001; Grassman, 2011; Little, 2011; FAO, 2013). Studies have shown that: (1) larger farms tend to experience more victimization than smaller ones in more developed countries (McCall, 2003; Mears et al., 2007b). However, this is not the case in the Caribbean where, regardless of size, farms are not immune to victimization (Little, 2011; FAO, 2013); (2) farmers use few security measures and are reluctant to report crimes (Jones, 2008; Little, 2011; Dickson, 2013); and (3) although farms are isolated, farm property can be easily accessed from public roads and have many portable commodities and items which are easy to steal (Barclay, et al., 2001). Studies have also indicated that employee theft can be a problem (Swanson et al., 2000; Donnermeyer & Barclay, 2005), especially for farm operations that hire part-time or immigrant or low-paid workers (Anderson & McCall, 2005; Little, 2011; FAO, 2013).

Most of the literature from these studies shows that farm crime is linked to the specific nature of physical, social, geographic, and cultural environments of farming communities and areas (Barclay, 2001; Barclay et al,. 2001; Barclay & Donnermeyer, 2002; Barclay et al., 2004; Anderson & McCall, 2005; Mears et al., 2007a; Jones, 2008; Barclay & Donnermeyer, 2011; Grassman, 2011). According to Barclay et al. (2001), unemployment and drug abuse are the most common social problems linked to farm crime. A study conducted in Australia by Anderson and McCall (2005) showed that isolated farmlands, larger farms with higher incomes, and proximity to urban centres, were the greatest predictors of being a victim of various types of farm crime. Although isolated farmlands and proximity to urban centres seem to be contradictory correlates of agricultural crime, they are not. The isolation refers to the distance from one farm to another, which affects guardianship. Hence, there is a large flow of non-local people (especially by road) in farm areas near towns. Additionally, a farm family's house may be too far from storage buildings, supplies, livestock and other valuable property to be seen, and farm neighbours can still be far enough away from each other so as not to notice intruders and thieves.

Similar studies conducted by Mears et al. (2007a) in the United States found that farm properties which are highly attractive, portable and have value, such as fruits and nuts, were more likely to experience theft. Further, proximity in terms of target and offender has been shown by several studies to be linked to high rates of farm crime victimization. Mears et al. (2007a) and Barclay (2001) found that farm theft was related to the number of employees on the farm, with some farm workers being responsible for crime directly, or by passing information to criminals for a fee. Further, Swanson et al. (2000) argued that farmers themselves constitute a source of support for farm theft and may readily purchase stolen commodities at a bargain price. The fact is that property crime on farms is highly situational, with certain factors being strongly associated with certain types of farm crimes (Barclay et al., 2001).

Even though most empirical studies on agricultural crime have been conducted in Australia, the United Kingdom, and the United States (Anderson & McCall, 2005; Barclay, 2001; Barclay et al. 2001; Jones, 2008; Mears et al., 2007b), factors that explain the various types of crime in developing countries such as the Caribbean region, have not been thoroughly investigated. Indeed, farm crime presents major problems to farm economies in these countries. Thus, such crimes must be given the due attention they deserve if agricultural theft is to be effectively reduced and managed in a growing and increasingly globalised economy.

Cohen and Felson (1979) described the routine activity theory, one of the main theories of environmental criminology, which is derived from an earlier Hawley (1950) theory of human ecology. The routine activity theory explores the temporal aspects of human behaviour in community environments. It includes perspectives such as situational crime prevention and the crime prevention through environmental design model (CPTED) and Newman's (1972) notion of defensible space. This theory suggests that criminal offences are directly related to patterns of daily social interaction of both victims and offenders in time and space, which define in part the situation or context under which crime occurs (Cohen & Felson, 1979). Tittle (2000); Felson (2002); Brantingham and Brantingham (1995) and Barclay et al. (2001), all describe the concept of place to the study of crime. They argue that in order for a crime to occur, three elements must converge. These three elements are (1) a motivated offender, (2) the absence of a capable guardian, and (3) the presence of a suitable target. As the authors explain, they involve proactive environmental techniques such as target hardening, controlled access and effective surveillance in an attempt to dissuade offenders and reduce the opportunistic potential for the crime. In this theory, a motivated offender is anyone who has the tendency or inclination to commit the crime, whereas the target refers to the object, person, place or property against which the crime occurs. Capable guardianship according to Cohen and Felson (1979) includes anyone or any object (that is, forms of physical security) which can limit the chances of an offender committing a crime. The routine activity theory indicates that offenders are motivated to make their decisions based on the characteristics of the target. The choice of the target is based on its value, accessibility, visibility, concealability, removability and disposability (Bunei et al., 2013). Bursick and Grasmik (1993) discussed the work of Cohen and Felson (1979) by referring to guardianship as both a human (human presence or physical guardianship) and a non-human (for example, locks, alarms) phenomenon. Guardianship is the availability of others who may prevent crimes by their mere presence or by offering assistance to ward off an attack. Capable guardianship can include neighbours, friends, relatives, passers-by, plus physical measures for example locks, alarms, and remote cameras; all of which can act as substantial obstacles to offenders (Clarke & Felson, 1993; Clarke, 1995). Barclay and Donnermeyer (2011) in a later study challenged these mainstream criminological theories and concepts of social disorganisation and collective efficiency. They rationalise on the importance of developing perspectives for place-based or ecological theories of crime. The aim is to develop a critical criminology of agriculture and food, exploring studies of rural 'others'. In addition, giving greater analytic attention to divisions and marginalities of peoples living in smaller and more isolated places based on gender, race, and lifestyles, among other factors (Barclay & Donnermeyer, 2011).

According to Bunei et al. (2013), the nature of rural communities together with transformations in their socio-economic and cultural makeup may tend to increase the number of offenders and reduce guardianship, thus exposing the farm property to greater risks. Mears et al. (2007b) describe the vulnerability of farms to criminal activity relative to their remoteness and isolation, increasing chances of theft from perpetrators including neighbours and employees. These authors argue that there is a traditional reluctance by farmers to seek help from law enforcement, which may serve to increase the opportunities for farm crime victimization from reprisals. This, Muhammad (2002) lamented, is due to the tendency for many rural communities to keep community problems within the community.

The routine activity theory stresses the importance of the exposure due to the isolation of property as a key ingredient in assessing vulnerability. Guardianship on a large farm where a great deal of the property is far from the location where the owner lives, tends to be minimal and is not effective in reducing the vulnerability of property (Mears et al., 2007b). Agricultural crimes occur at specific places on agricultural operations and these places reflect the visibility of property from a road by other people (opportunistic) as well as from the place where the farmer lives (guardianship).

In a later publication, Barclay and Donnermeyer (2011) noted that improvements in roads, the increasing cost of farm machinery and farm inputs, increasing reliance on transient or seasonal workers, and encroachment of urbanization into formerly rural and remote areas, have increased visibility, attractiveness and accessibility of farm properties. A study conducted in Kenya, found farm theft to be associated with high market integration and market availability (Omiti et al., 2007). This phenomenon somehow resembles the situation in many Caribbean countries. From the perspective of routine activity theory, this represents an increase in the attractiveness of the target. There is oft times little or no interest in the legitimacy of the source of the produce based on market availability and as a result, there is an imbalance in their daily demand and supply of fresh food and the buyer is often clueless. According to the FAO (2013), one of the major drivers for farm theft in the Caribbean lies in maintaining the supplier/producer relationship, in which, reliability of supplies, freshness, smaller amounts not requiring storage and an acceptable price necessitates what can be referred to as an organized trade. Praedial larcenys' most readily identified business feature is, therefore, the ability of the supplier to combine large volumes, timely delivery and a level of determination to ensure his delivery, that does not rule out the use of violence (FAO, 2013). Hence, sometimes overnight, a farmer's entire crop can be harvested to maintain this supplier/buyer relationship. Residing near major transportation routes would also increase a farmer's vulnerability to farm theft because potential offenders can easily navigate between urban and rural areas.

Barclay et al. (2001) examined ecological factors in conjunction with crimes occurring on farms over a two year period to identify those factors that influenced a farm's vulnerability to victimization. The ecological factors they identified included; the terrain of the property, the cover, the layout of the property, the visibility between the house and shed on the property and the distance of the property from a public road or a highway and the nearest town or service centre. These were all drivers to increase the risk of farm crime.

In a rather interesting study on "illegal pluriactivity" in the farming community by Smith and McElwee (2013), the authors describe a case study in which the minority of farmers are presented as "rogue-farmers" or criminal-entrepreneurs operating across legal and illegal domains and an anti-authority attitude is embedded in their *modus operandi*. Here, the farmer is part of a wider entrepreneurial network which exploits an alternative shadow work economy. A similar situation is now growing throughout the Caribbean. These criminal acts are all unified by the concept of illegal pluriactivity because they provide alternative income generation strategies which supplement their legitimate incomes.

HHB & Associates Limited, Media and Market Research Consultants (2007) examined the nature and extent of praedial larceny in Trinidad and Tobago by interviewing a random sample of 750 farmers – 700 from Trinidad and 50 from Tobago. They determined that the hardest hit areas were Wallerfield and Sangre Grande; 21% - 30% of victims were located in these areas. They also found out that within a six month period, the incidence of theft can be as frequent as one to four times for equipment, two to four times for livestock and two to six times for crops. The incidence of praedial larceny was highest among vegetable farmers (17%) and lowest among those with large animals (for example, Cattle - 2%). The time of attacks was significant during both day and night, although attacks at night were notably higher. They also found that praedial larceny is under-reported to the police with reports ranging from 19% for root crops and 90% for fertilizers. The study discovered that farms with road frontage, as well as those with easy access, were more likely to fall victim to praedial larceny. Another factor which contributed to the increased incidence of praedial larceny was whether or not non-family members were employed. The research showed that farms which employed non-family members were more likely to fall victim to praedial larceny than those which employed family members only. The most frequently cited reason for praedial larceny, however, was the ready market for stolen goods and the farmers' recommendations for combating praedial larceny were to have stiffer penalties for praedial larceny and more police patrols.

Risk management of praedial larceny according to FAO (2013), therefore requires significant inputs from the criminal justice system, traceability systems for proof of ownership under the law, information sharing for deterrence and for capacity building, networking and intelligence gathering on the nature and reduction of the risk.

The major weaknesses and deficiencies in the legislation and the criminal justice system related to praedial larceny (FAO, 2013) include:

1. Deficiencies in the social and economic consequences among the critical players, including the police and judiciary, resulting in the failure to treat praedial larceny as a serious offence. Fines and penalties awarded under the law have not proven to be a deterrent to the thieves. The low priority given to the hearing of praedial larceny cases by the Courts and the ease with which bail is granted to repeat offenders undermines efforts to reduce praedial larceny.
2. Unfamiliarity and underutilization by the police of relevant legislative acts that can be used for prosecution, including the Trespass Act and the Unlawful Possession Act, which may be applied when the source of the produce is not identified in a timely manner.
3. Lack of reporting due to frustration with inaction by authorities means only 45% of incidences are reported to the police regionally. Thieves are therefore fairly confident they will face limited or no consequences.

4. Insufficient proof of ownership. Data management for traceability of produce is inefficient at the farm level. Ineffective registration processes do not permit produce to be followed from the source to the consumer and the monitoring of movement of produce within countries is not enforced

5. Information sharing on praedial larceny is absent at the community level, so the data and information are inadequate to provide guidance to the Police in critical areas such as hotspots, preferred subsectors and commodities or to build intelligence on the habits of suspicious or known perpetrators.

6. Farmer organizations and farmers are not sufficiently vigilant in information sharing and networking and do not adequately support the receipt book system including proper record keeping and the reporting of incidences or suspicious activities.

STRATEGIES FOR MITIGATING FARM THEFT

It is accepted that farm theft is a worldwide phenomenon. Many countries have established different methods to combat this problem. Since 1983, The United Nations Food and Agriculture Organization Praedial Larceny Prevention Act of 1983 granted agricultural wardens the power to detect offenses and arrest suspects in the Caribbean. The routine activities theory suggests that reducing criminal opportunities serves a key role in reducing the prevalence of crime (Brantingham & Brantingham, 1993; Felson, 2002; Barclay et al., 2001).

Early methods of dealing with praedial larceny in many Caribbean islands included a traditional folk belief that if the maljo bean (*Canavalia ensiformis*) is planted around crops it prevents petty theft (Winer, 2009). This bean is also reportedly planted in West African gardens in order to protect (them) from praedial larceny.

Globally, law enforcement agencies refer to the 3D's when attempting to mitigate the impacts of crime. Craig (2011) explained that these include: deterrence, detection, and delay. Deterrence involves the use of lighting, gates, fencing, no trespass signs, security systems and dogs. Detection includes systems to alert you when someone enters your property, which may include the use of motion lights, cameras, sensors and detectors, visual surveillance by your employees or neighbours. Delay is part of the strategy to slow access to your property or equipment and may include the use of cables across field lanes, fencing, locking doors on equipment storage facilities, parking equipment away from public viewing when left in fields overnight (Craig, 2011).

Strategies have also been recommended for farmers to review their operation from a thief's viewpoint and ask, what would be the easiest method to enter and steal items. Farmers should be cognizant of potential targets and conceal them as thieves have many strategies when identifying potential targets. One such strategy they use is calling addresses to see if anyone is home. It is recommended not putting your name on your mailbox which can provide easy access to phone numbers. They may even scout areas, observing farms to establish patterns of use. Altering daily routines can act as a deterrent, making movements unpredictable to thieves.

Asking for the credentials of any unknown or unexpected visitors is also important.

Record keeping is important, especially for keeping tabs on employees who manage your locks and keys on the farm. Records should be kept of all locks, the location of each lock and the number of keys that exist for each lock. Keep a list of any employee that has each key and inventory all keys periodically. It is important not to issue keys for convenience to employees and only provide a key when necessary and then follow through on proper return (Craig, 2011). It's also important that farmers take an inventory of all their equipment, taking pictures where necessary of distinguishing marks and recording serial numbers that can assist in recovery in the case of theft.

Locks should be of the highest security quality, with keys that are not easily reproduced and pick resistant, marking all keys with "Do Not Duplicate". It is important also to use locks with an added security measure of hasps that fold over, which will prevent access to mounting screws.

Precaution must be taken when leaving large equipment such as tractors in the fields by removing keys, locking doors if possible and never leaving equipment within easy access to roads. Use of a lockable fuel cap is also recommended as reports have been made of fuel theft from parked farm vehicles.

In 2007 at The Public Consultation on Food Prices held in *Trinidad*, the Association of Professional Agricultural Scientists of Trinidad and Tobago (APASTT) presented a novel proposal designed primarily to secure food production and also mitigate praedial larceny. The proposal included the following features:

- The establishment of Designated Agricultural Zones. These zones would be provided with the necessary physical infrastructure: roads, electricity, and water. There would be controlled access to the zones.
- From the outset, the zones must be established with inputs from the Police service regarding security concerns;
- There must be close collaboration between the entities in the zone and the Police Service;
- Farmers would be provided with performance leases for the lands within the zones;
- Farmers would be encouraged to form co-operatives as economic units within the zones;
- Each economic enterprise must be registered, and have its own labels and bar-code;
- All vehicles transporting produce out of the zones must have the appropriate signage;
- All produce leaving the zones must be labeled;
- Each zone must be mapped along with all relevant data to produce Geographical Information Systems (GIS). This system should be made available to the Police Service;
- The officers of the Praedial Larceny Squad would be provided with hand-held devices linked to the GIS. This would facilitate verification of information during stop and search exercises.

The *Jamaican* Government addressed the problem of praedial larceny by establishing a receipt book system which was used by farmers and agricultural traders to demonstrate legal proof of sale or purchase of agricultural products. They also initiated a Praedial Larceny Public Education Program which aimed at increasing awareness about unacceptable levels of praedial larceny. In addition, all persons involved in agricultural transactions had to register with the Rural Agricultural Development Authority (RADA) and Island Special Constabulary Force (ISCF) officers would be assigned to various parishes to preside over the implementation of the Praedial Larceny Program.

In *St. Lucia*, the Agriculture Ministry attempted to address the praedial larceny problem by implementing a "four-pronged strategy". The first arm of this strategy involved the enactment of stronger legislation to deal with praedial larceny and to regulate the sale of agricultural produce. The second arm aimed at a national identification program and licensing of bona fide farmers and traders. Thirdly, the government set upon working with Local Government and sought funding through the European Union Social Recovery Program to re-introduce the Rural Constabulary. Finally, the government embarked on an intensive public sensitization program to educate the public on the seriousness of praedial larceny.

A similar situation exists in *Antigua/Barbuda* where "the agriculture sector continues to lose millions of dollars through the effects of praedial larceny" (Hilson Baptiste, Minister of Agriculture, Lands,

Housing and the Environment, Antigua/Barbuda, 2009). This Government also introduced an agricultural receipt book system and farmers were encouraged to register their business or form cooperatives. A public education program was also established to increase awareness of praedial larceny and to educate farmers to use prompt action in detecting and reporting praedial larceny.

When dealing with praedial larceny there are several considerations that must be addressed through a multisectoral and multifaceted approach to ensure appropriate integration of policy issues. These may include (FAO, 2013):

- Issues of land tenure and proof of ownership of land and produce under the law. Programs for alternative livelihoods to manage the perceived relationship between vulnerable and poor households and praedial larceny in rural populations and along rural/ urban livelihood chains.
- Public education and communication strategies that empower and build resilience in farmers and fisher folks and their organizations at all levels - regional, national and community - in praedial larceny prevention and reduction.
- Information systems that provide clarity in the relationships in the legitimate businesses in the trafficker (higgler/huckster) trade between islands.

Some specific actions should revolve around:

- Policy and legislative frameworks to support the work of the police and the judiciary through the criminal justice system and the Agriculture Ministry.
- Mainstreaming of praedial larceny into the work of Agriculture Ministries and technical partners for implementation of a Plan of Action for praedial larceny prevention.
- Integration of praedial larceny prevention into the planning and monitoring systems of the National Agriculture Strategy and the national strategies for crime prevention.
- Information generation and knowledge management at the Ministries of Agriculture and partners including baseline data and mechanisms for knowledge-based planning and evaluation such as mapping praedial larceny hotspots.
- Capacity building for praedial larceny prevention among all stakeholders, Ministries of Agriculture in collaboration with regional and national farmers and fisher-folks and their organizations.
- Strategic partnerships for development and implementation of the Plan of Action for praedial larceny prevention.
- Use of the Comprehensive Disaster Management Strategy framework to provide additional co-ordination for praedial larceny at the regional level. The processes of CDM already provide a mechanism for management and sharing.
- Research to identify solutions to praedial larceny – The University of the West Indies to lead.

CONCLUSION

Praedial larceny can be labelled as a scourge for food producers; it is a very complex and serious problem affecting the agricultural sector worldwide. It involves a wide range of agricultural produce and equipment and its complexity lies in the fact that it is very difficult to prove that a crime has been committed. In the past, the problem of praedial larceny was not given the attention it deserved, but as the global problem of food availability and food security comes to the forefront, more attention is being paid to this problem. In addition, farmers are now being shown more respect and their voices are being heard- they are saying that they are fed up with this problem. Steps are currently being made to mitigate this serious crime as can be seen by the various programs being set up by governments of different countries throughout the region to combat or reduce the prevalence of praedial larceny.

In developing countries, food producers generally struggle to keep financially afloat, producing food under disadvantageous conditions which include: unfavourable weather conditions, frequent pests and disease outbreaks, limited or no support from the government, trade barriers and unfair regulations. Most farmers barely make ends meet, far less generate profits which can be reinvested to move them further along the continuum to full commercial operation. It is in these circumstances that any theft of farm produce or equipment becomes a serious blow to farmers, and if it is a regular occurrence it has the effect of causing the farmer to become impoverished; unable to feed one's family or frustrates movement away from subsistence to commercial farming or make profits to have a better standard of living.

Praedial larcenists do an injustice to farmers. While farmers can do somethings at the farm level to restrict the level of praedial larceny, actions at the higher level can be more effective. This chapter reviewed several actions that have been tried which may be useful for countries struggling with this scourge to consider. Moreover, several suggestions are put forward; actions at government level which brings agriculture, legal and enforcement agencies to the table can be most productive.

One bag of hot pepper taken by a thief may not be much in the eyes of the general public, but to a poor farmer it may determine whether his children will get all their school books in the new school term!

REFERENCES

Anderson, K. M., & McCall, M. (2005). *Farm Crime in Australia*. Canberra, Australia: Australian Institute of Criminology. Retrieved on October 5th, 2015 from www.aic.gov.au/publications/current%20 series/cfi-120/cfi119.aspx

Anderson, S. (1997). Crime and social change in Scotland. In G. Dingwall & S. Moody (Eds.), *Crime and conflict in the countryside* (pp. 24–41). Cardiff, UK: University of Wales Press.

Barclay, E. M., & Donnermeyer, J. F. (2002). Property Crime and Crime Prevention on Farms in Australia. *Crime Prevention and Community Safety: An International Journal.*, *4*(4), 47–61. doi:10.1057/ palgrave.cpcs.8140169

Barclay, E. M., & Donnermeyer, J. F. (2011). Crime and Security on Agricultural Operations. *Security Journal*, *24*(1), 1–18. doi:10.1057j.2008.23

Barclay, E. M., Donnermeyer, J. F., Doyle, B. P., & Talary, D. (2001). *Property Crime Victimization and Crime Prevention on Farms. Report to the New South Wales Attorney General's Crime Prevention Division*. Armidale, Australia: The Institute for Rural Futures, Incorporating the Former Rural Development Centre. University of New England.

Barclay, E. M., Donnermeyer, J. F., & Jobes, P. C. (2004). The dark side of gemeinschaft: Criminality within rural communities. *Crime Prevention and Community Safety: An International Journal*, *6*(3), 7–22. doi:10.1057/palgrave.cpcs.8140191

Barclay, L. (2001). *A review of the literature on agricultural crime: report to the criminology research council*. Institute for Rural Futures, University of New England. Retrieved on December 19th, 2015 from: www.criminologyresearchcouncil.gov.au/reports/barclay.pdf

Beckford, C. L., & Campbell, D. R. (2012). *Domestic Food Production and Food Security in the Caribbean: Building Capacity and Strengthening Local Food Production Systems*. Palgrave Macmillan.

Bekele, I., Singh, R., Mustapha, N., & Ramsaroop, M. (1998). Incidence of Praedial Larceny in Food Crop Production in Trinidad: Major Highlights. *Proceedings of UWI, Ag. 50*.

Bouffard, A. L., & Muftíc, R. L. (2006). The "Rural Mystique": Social disorganization and Violence beyond Urban Communities. *Western Criminology Review, 7*, 56–66.

Brantingham, P., & Brantingham, P. (1981). *Environmental Criminology*. Prospect Heights: Waveland Press.

Brantingham, P. & Brantingham, P. (1995). Criminality of Place: Crime Generators and Crime Attractors. *European Journal on Criminal Policy and Research, 3*(3).

Brereton, B. (1979). *Race Relations in Colonial Trinidad 1870-1900*. Cambridge, UK: Cambridge University Press.

Brereton, B. (2010). The Historical Background to the Culture of Violence in Trinidad and Tobago. *Caribbean Review of Gender Studies, A Journal of Caribbean Perspectives on Gender and Feminism, 4*, 1-16.

Bryan, P. (2000). *The Jamaican People 1880-1902, Race, Class and Social Control*. The University Press.

Bunei, E. K., Rono, J. K., & Chessa, S. R. (2013). Factors Influencing Farm Crime in Kenya: Opinions and Experiences of Farmers. *International Journal of Rural Criminology, 2*(1), 75–100.

Bursik, R. J., & Grasmik, H. G. (1993). *Neighborhoods and Crime: Dimensions of Effective Community Control*. New York: Lexington Books.

Caricom. (2011). Food Security in Caricom. *Caricom View*. Retrieved from http://www.caricom.org/jsp/communications/caricom_online_pubs/caricom_view_jul_2011.pdf

Clarke, R.V. (1995). Situational Crime Prevention. *Crime and Justice, 19*, 91-150.

Clarke, R. V., & Felson, M. (Eds.). (1993). *Routine activity and rational choice*. New Brunswick, NJ: Transaction Publishers, Inc.

Cohen, L. E., & Felson, M. (1979). Social change and crime rates trends: A routine activities approach. *American Sociological Review, 44*(4), 588–608. doi:10.2307/2094589

Craig, P. H. (2011). *Protecting you Farm from Theft. PennState Extension, Cumberland County*. Retrieved on July 7th, 2011 from: http://extension.psu.edu/cumberland/news/2011/protecting-your-farm-from-theft

Dickson, D. (2013). Praedial Larceny - A Serious Crime. Trinidad and Tobago Chamber of Industry and Commerce. *Feature, 13*(1), 26–27.

Donnermeyer, J., & Scott, J. (2013). How Rural Criminology Informs Critical Thinking. *International Journal for Crime, Justice and Social Democracy.* Retrieved from http://eprints.qut.edu.au/68038/2/C1_Donnermeyer_Rural_Criminology_Pub_Paper.pdf

Donnermeyer, J. F., & Barclay, E. M. (2005). The policing of farm crime. *Police Practice and Justice Research, 6*(1), 3–17. doi:10.1080/15614260500046913

Eisner, G. (1961). *Jamaica 1830 - 1930, A Study in Economic Growth.* Manchester, UK: Manchester University Press.

Engledow, F. L. (1945). *West India Royal Commission: Report on Agriculture, Fisheries, Forestry and Veterinary Matters. Cmd. 6608.* London: His Majesty's Stationery Office.

Felson, M. (2002). *Crime and everyday life* (3rd ed.). London: Sage.

Food & Agriculture Organization (2013). *Praedial Larceny in the Caribbean.* Issue Brief #3.

Garriott, W. (2011). *Policing methamphetamine: Narcopolitics in rural America.* New York University Press.

Grassman, J. (2011). *War of Words, War of Stories: Rural Thought and Violence in Colonial Zanzibar.* Indiana University Press.

Grossman, L. S. (1997). *The Political Ecology of Bananas: Contract Farming, Peasants and Agrarian Change in the Eastern Caribbean.* Chapel Hill, NC: The University of North Carolina Press.

Hawley, A. (1950). *Human Ecology: A Theory of Community Structure.* New York: Ronald Press.

Isaac, W., Joseph, M., Ganpat, W., Wilson, M., & Brathwaite, R. (2012). The Caribbean's Windward Islands banana industry: A heritage of dependency. *The Journal of Rural and Community Development, 7*(2), 98–117.

Jones, J. (2008). *Farm crime on Anglesey: Local partner's and organisations.* Views on the Issue, second report, January 2008. Retrieved on December 12th, 2015 from http://www.aber.ac.uk/en/media/jane-jones---second-report.pdf

Little, D. (2011). *Praedial Larceny: Its Consequences For Caribbean Agriculture.* Caricom View. Retrieved on June 3rd, 2015 from http://www.caricom.org/jsp/communications/caricom_online_pubs/caricom_view_jul_2011.pdf

Marshall, B., & Shane, J. (2005). *Crime in rural areas: A review of the literature for the Rural and Evidence Research Centre.* London: University College London.

Mawby, R. I. (2004). Myth and reality in rural policing: Perceptions of the police in a rural country of England. *Policing: An International Journal of Police Strategies & Management, 27*(3), 431–446. doi:10.1108/13639510410553158

McCall, M. (2003). *Results from the 2001-02 National Farm Crime Survey.* Australian Institute of Criminology, Trends and Issues in Crime and Criminal Justice, No.266.

McElwee, G. (2006). Farmer's as entrepreneurs: Developing competitive skills. *Journal of Developmental Entrepreneurship, 11*(3), 187–206. doi:10.1142/S1084946706000398

McElwee, G., & Vik, J. (2011). Diversification and entrepreneurial motivations of farmers in Norway. *Journal of Small Business, 49*(3), 390–410. doi:10.1111/j.1540-627X.2011.00327.x

Mears, D. P., Scott, M. L., & Bhati, A. S. (2007a). Opportunity theory and agricultural crime victimization. *Rural Sociology, 72*(2), 151–184. doi:10.1526/003601107781170044

Mears, D. P., Scott, M. L., & Bhati, A. S. (2007b). *Policy, theory and research from an evaluation of an agricultural crime prevention program.* Washington, DC: The Urban Institute.

Muhammad, B.L. (2002). *Rural Crime and Rural Policing Practices (Multicultural Law Enforcement).* An applied research project submitted to the Department of Interdisciplinary Technology as part of the School of Police Staff and Command Programme.

Newman, O. (1972). *Defensible Space.* New York: Macmillan.

Omiti, J. (2007). *Participatory prioritization of issues in smallholder agricultural commercialization in Kenya.* Nairobi: KIPPRA.

Rubenstein, H. (1975). The Utilization of Arable Land in an Eastern Caribbean Valley. *Canadian Journal of Sociology, 1*(2), 157–167. doi:10.2307/3339805

Rubenstein, H. (1987). Remittances and Rural Underdevelopment in the English Speaking Caribbean. *Human Organization, 42*(4), 295–306. doi:10.17730/humo.42.4.07091084145384 71

Saugeres, L. (2002). Of Tractors and Men: Masculinity, Technology and Power in a French Farming Community. *Sociologia Ruralis, 42*(2), 143–159. doi:10.1111/1467-9523.00207

Sergi, A., & Lavorgna, A. (2012, September). Trade Secrets: Italian Mafia expands its illicit business. *Janes Intelligence Review,* 44-47.

Shephard, C. Y. (1945). *Peasant Agriculture in the Leeward and Windward Islands.* Trinidad: Imperial College of Tropical Agriculture.

Sherman, L. W., Gartin, P. R., & Buerger, M. E. (1989). Hot spots of predatory crime: Routine activities and the criminology of place. *Criminology, 27*(1), 27–56. doi:10.1111/j.1745-9125.1989.tb00862.x

Smith, R. (2010). Policing the Changing Landscape of Rural Crime: A Case Study from Scotland. *International Journal of Police Science & Management, 12*(3), 18–30. doi:10.1350/ijps.2010.12.3.171

Smith, R., Laing, A., & Mcelwee, G. (2013). The Rise of Illicit Rural Enterprise within the Farming Industry. *International Journal of Agricultural Management, 2*(4), 185–188. doi:10.5836/ijam/2013-04-01

Smith, R., & McElwee, G. (2013). Confronting Social Constructions of Rural Criminality: A Case Story on "Illegal Pluriactivity" in the Farming Community. *Sociologia Ruralis, 53*(1), 112–134. doi:10.1111/j.1467-9523.2012.00580.x

Spore Magazine. (2009). *Theft: Tactics for battling crime*. Technical Centre for Agricultural Land Rural Cooperation (CTA). Retrieved on March 21st, 2016 from: http://spore.cta.int/images/stories/pdf/SE139-web.pdf

Sugden, G. (1999). Farm crime: out of sight, out of mind: a study of crime on farms in the county of Rutland, England. *Crime Prevention and Community Safety: An International Journal, 1*(3), 29–36. doi:10.1057/palgrave.cpcs.8140023

Swanson, C. R., Chamelin, N. C., & Territo, L. (2000). *Criminal investigation*. Boston: McGraw Hill.

Swanson, C. R., & Territo, L. (1980). Agricultural Crime: It's Extent, Prevention and Control. *FBI Law Enforcement Bulletin, 49*(5), 8–12.

Weisheit, R. A., Falcone, D. N., & Wells, L. E. (2006). Crime and policing in rural and small-town America (3rd ed.). Waveland Press.

Wilcox, P., Land, K. C., & Hunt, S. (2003). *Criminal Circumstance: A Dynamic Multicontextual Criminal Opportunity Theory*. New York: Walter de Gruyter.

Wilkinson, M., Craig, G., & Gaus, A. (2010). Forced Labour in the UK and Gangmaster Licensing Authority. Report for the Contemporary Research Centre, University of Hull.

Winer, L. (2009). *Dictionary of the English / Creole of Trinidad and Tobago*. McGill-Queen's University Press.

Yarwood, R., & Gardener, G. (2005). Fear of Crime, Cultural Threat and the Countryside. *Area, 32*(4), 403–411. doi:10.1111/j.1475-4762.2000.tb00156.x

This research was previously published in Agricultural Development and Food Security in Developing Nations edited by Wayne G. Ganpat , Ronald Dyer, and Wendy-Ann P. Isaac; pages 300-319, copyright year 2017 by Information Science Reference (an imprint of IGI Global).

Section 5

Sustainable Consumption and Alternative Diets

Chapter 50
A Review on Impact of Changing Climate on Sustainable Food Consumption

Tosin Kolajo Gbadegesin
University of Ibadan, Nigeria

ABSTRACT

Food security is of great importance in the politics of sustainable consumption and production (SCP) because of its implication on environment and people. The changing climate is adding to world resource problems such as food security, water scarcity, pollution, soil degradation, etc. Greenhouse gas (GHG) emissions and land use demand by agriculture has continued to influence what people quantity and quality of available food. This review used resources from all relevant literatures to examine impact of changing climate on sustainable food consumption by identifying effect of changing climate on nutrition, food production, and food consumption, and provides recommendations on sustainable food consumption measures. The review is of the opinion that food consumption patterns are changing in the face of population growth, economic development, and environmental challenges. Such shifts place increased pressure on already depleted natural resources due to the resource-intensive production and transportation requirements of these products.

INTRODUCTION

Feeding a global population of nine to ten billion people by 2050 presents an enormous challenge and at the same time humanity is facing a variety of serious sustainability challenges. On the environmental side, it is global warming and resource scarcity, on the social side, it is increasing inequity. At the same time, focus on growth, innovations and technological solutions builds a locked-in situation in a system, hindering an effective targeting of these challenges if not contributing to them. Outside the effects on humans, further stress is placed on the ecosphere and biodiversity (FAO, 2012; IPCC, 2012).

DOI: 10.4018/978-1-7998-5354-1.ch050

Food security is a major issue in the politics of sustainable food consumption and production (SCP) because of its impact on the environment, health of the people and the economy. Several key issues high on policy development agendas worldwide show how far-reaching the problem is. Serious environmental challenges associated with food production and consumption include water scarcity, soil abjection, eutrophication of water bodies, climate change, water pollution, and loss of habitats and biodiversity. Food consumption is responsible for most of the global water use as well as for generation of about one fifth of greenhouse-gas emissions (GHGs) (Bazilian et al., 2011).

Latest efforts by international and national policy makers have sought to urge individuals to engage in several ranges of environmental friendly practices to address both discrete environmental problems and global challenges of great importance such as climate change (Hanss & Böhm, 2012). The concept sustainable consumption was first coined in Oslo in 1994 in line with the Brundtland commission definition of "sustainable development" and includes both consumption and production. It was seen as the use of goods and services to meet basic needs and improve quality of life, while reducing the use of natural resources, toxic materials and emissions of waste and pollutants over the life cycle, in order to meet the needs of the present and future generations (Brundtland Commission, 1987). Similarly, sustainable consumption has attracted attention under the headline of Sustainable Consumption and Production (SCP). It received support with respect to implementation at the World Summit of Sustainable Development held in Johannesburg in 2002 where each participating countries pledged themselves to promoting SCP, with developed countries taking the lead (Gerbens-Leenes et al., 2010; Fuchs & Lorek 2005).

Over the years, the importance of sustainable food consumption policies has been increasingly expressed at international policy level. In 1992, Rio Declaration on Environment and Development calls upon States to reduce and eliminate unsustainable patterns of production and consumption in order to achieve sustainable development and a higher quality of life. There is also Agenda 21 with its chapter 4 on sustainable consumption and production. Similarly, in 1999, UN Guidelines for Consumer Protection gives governments a comprehensive framework for policy setting for more sustainable consumption and production. And in 2002, at the World Summit on Sustainable Development in Johannesburg, the summit called for development of a 10-year plan to speed-up the move towards sustainable consumption and production patterns (Fuchs & Lorek 2002; Lorek, Spangenberg & Oman 2008).

Gerbans-Leenes & Nonhebel, (2002); Schafer, Herde & Kropp (2007) have examined the environmental impact of different food consumption patterns in terms of energy and land use. Results demonstrated higher use of energy for food of animal origin, processed food and greenhouse cultivations, compared with plant food, fresh products and open-air cultivations. Accordingly, diets rich in meat consumption were found to consume energy and devour lands (Gerbans-Leenes & Nonhebel, 2002). Schafer, Herde & Kropp (2007) stated that present food consumption patterns are unsustainable, as they endanger not only the carrying capacity of the earth, but human health as well. Food production and consumption is increasing the rate at which natural resources such as water and energy are depleted. Chemical materials such as pesticides and fertilizers are also overused in the process (WHO, 2004).

Climate change is one of the most challenging threats facing the world (UNFCCC, 2007). Most notable consequences include shortfall in rainfall, droughts, high temperature, flooding and unpredicted weather. Developing countries are usually the most vulnerable because their economies as it is more dependent on climate sensitive natural resources making them less able to deal with the impacts of climate change (UNFCCC, 2007). This creates a vicious circle, as malnourished population is less resistant to the effects of climate change, such as the spread of diseases. Climate change is equally expected to negatively affect both crop and livestock production systems in most regions, although some countries may actually benefit from the changing conditions (Church & Lorek, 2007).

Climate changes together with other environmental constraints are affecting food production and consumption and they will likely undermine the possibility of meeting world food demands. By 2050, a year in which global population is projected to reach 9 billion people, the dynamics between population, diet, and climate change will amplify challenges facing global food systems (IPCC, 2014; UNFCCC, 2007). The effects of changing climate are already visible in some places. For example, drought in Eastern and Southern Africa left more than 1 million children undernourished in 2013. Food prices in those areas have skyrocketed and many farmers have struggled to produce crops (IPCC, 2014). Also, by 2050, it is predicted that heat waves, floods and other climate change effects will not be the only worry as there is an evidence of global warming affecting diet and nutrition (Godfray, Beddington, Crute, Haddad, Lawrence, Muir & Toulmin 2010).

It is noted that geographic limits and yields of different crops may be altered by changes in precipitation, temperature, cloud cover and soil moisture as well as increases in CO_2 concentrations. High temperatures and reduction in rainfall affect soil moisture, reducing the quantity of water available for irrigation and impair crop growth in non-irrigated regions (IPCC, 2014). Climate change influence food production due to resulting geographical shifts and yield changes in crops, reduction in the quantity of water available for irrigation, and loss of land through sea level rise and associated salinization (Prasad, Staggenborg & Ristic, 2008).

It is noted that higher levels of CO_2 in the atmosphere also mean that wheat; rice, maize, potatoes and other staples will grow with lower levels of protein and by 2050 extra 150 million people in 47 countries will be at greater risk of malnutrition (Collier, Conway & Venables 2008). For example, climate influences the seasonality of food production and consumption, epidemics of diarrheal disease, and water use for mothers whose ready access to clean drinking-water in coastal regions declines as sea-levels rises (IPCC, 2012).

The UN stated that four out of five people on the planet depend mostly on grain staples and legumes for dietary protein, and estimated that poor nutrition already accounts for around three million deaths among young children every year (UNFCCC, 2007) while Fuchs & Lorek (2002) experiments shows that higher CO_2 levels in the atmosphere are associated with protein losses of around 5%. Prasad et al., (2008) showed how droughts, floods and other weather events linked to climate change hurt global crop yields and lead to a less healthy diet composition in addition to making food less available overall. Lorek et al., (2008) found that on average the consumption of vegetables and fruits will decline 4% by 2050 due to climate change compared to a projection of consumption without global warming. The decline is expected to hit low and medium-income countries more compared to high-income countries across the globe (IPCC, 2014).

IPCC(2012); Beddow et al., (2012) stated that rising temperatures and particularly greater intensity and frequencies of heat waves, droughts and floods will threaten global food security by reducing vegetable and fruit yields, hit grain crop harvests such as wheat in one of the most populous and poorest nations on the planet. Approximately, about 1.3 billion ton or one third of food gets lost or wasted globally per year. These occur throughout the food value chain, through waste of edible foods in medium and high-income countries while in lower income countries, it is lost at earlier stages such as during storage and transport.

Summarily, greenhouse gas emissions and land use demand by agriculture has a significant impact on what people eat and global food systems. To achieve food security at a time of climate change, policies promoting sustainable food consumption need to be developed. Consumption activities that help reduce the ecological and social problems associated with conventional production and consumption need to be encouraged (Bazilian, Rogner, Howells, Hermann, Arent, Gielen, Steduto, Mueller, Komor, Tol & Yumkella, 2011).

RESEARCH METHODOLOGY

The aim of this review is to contribute to knowledge on impact of changing climate on sustainable food consumption. Using resources from all relevant literatures, this review theoretically examines sustainable food consumption by identifying impact of changing climate on nutrition, food production and food consumption and provides recommendations on meeting the growing food demand in this era of climate change.

EFFECT OF CHANGING CLIMATE ON FOOD PRODUCTION

Effect of Changing Temperature

Agriculture is perhaps the most sensitive of all food security activities affected by climate change as increase in temperature affect the moisture availability through evaporation. Evaporation increases by about 5% for each 1℃ increase in main annual temperature and this is significant in tropical regions where most crops are generally constrained by water availability (WHO, 2004). Meteorological records show that heat waves have been more frequent since the end of the last century, and it is expected that this trend will continue over coming decades. Together with limited rainfall, this directly impacts the performance of some crops. The adaptation of crops to these occasional temperature increases varies depending on the geographical region. The impact is more in temperate zones than in hotter zones where agriculture is already at the limit of its ability to adapt, and where it might be faced by conditions that have never been experienced before (Thornton, Ericksen, Herrero & Challinor, 2014). Increasing temperatures have different effects on farming in different parts of the world and productivity may increase in medium and high latitudes due to longer growing seasons (FAO, 2010).

In Europe, crops traditional to the south, such as maize, sunflower and soy, could flourish at higher latitudes, leading to harvests increase of around 30% by 2050, depending on the crop (El-Fadel, Ghanimeh, Maroun & Alameddine, 2012). A 2℃ increase in temperature in medium latitudes could lead to a 10% increase in wheat production, but would result in a corresponding loss in lower latitude (Battisti & Naylor 2009). However, in semi-arid and tropical regions, where farming conditions are extreme, an increase in temperature could lead to reduction in harvests, increasing the stress of high temperatures, with increased water loss through evaporation, further increasing water stress for plants (Tirado et al., 2010). Soil fertility can also be impaired by increased air temperatures. Furthermore, losses from evaporation and longer growing seasons could result in increased water demand in the Middle East, North Africa and South-East Asia. Maize is usually one of the crops mostly affected by increased temperatures and changing rainfall (FAO, 2006).

Crahay (2010) found that agricultural output might decrease by 10% by 2055, mainly in Africa and Latin America, affecting over 170 million small-scale farmers in these regions. The effect of changing climate on pests may add to the effect of other factors such as the overuse of pesticides and the loss of biodiversity which already contribute to plant pest and disease outbreaks. Higher temperatures resulting from climate change may spread insects and pathogens to a wider range of latitudes (Beddow et al., 2012).

Effect of Changes in Rainfall Patterns

Water is crucial for plant life. Any change in rainfall patterns would impact directly on agriculture, 80% of which is dependent on rainwater. While it may be difficult to predict the effects of global warming on rainfall in a particular region, most of the forecasts produced conclude that there will be an increase in rainfall at high latitudes in winter, with lower rainfall in tropical and subtropical regions (Elliott, Deryng, Müller, Frieler, Konzmann, Gerten & Glotter 2014).

In a nation like India, rainfall is expected to be lower in the dry season, with higher rainfall throughout the rest of the year (Beddow et al., 2012). Drought is a regional phenomenon, with different characteristics depending on the climatic region, frequency and duration. Lack of rainfall causes water stress in plants and, as with heat waves, the areas most affected will be those already suffering extreme water shortages (Elliott et al., 2014). Dryness of the soil stops root growth and decomposition of organic material which further decrease soil fertility. However, droughts have further effects, as they increase soil erosion due to reduced plant cover; this is of particular concern on mountain sides (El-Fadel et al., 2012). Important effects of climate change will be an increase in the severity of droughts, both in terms of their duration and frequency, such as the one that affected the Horn of Africa in the late 2011, with famine affecting 13 million people (Battisti & Naylor 2009). Forecasts suggest that by 2050, the proportion of the earth subject to constant drought will increase from 2% to 10%, with the area suffering from extreme droughts increasing from 1% to 30% by the end of the 21st century (WHO, 2013). Samuel et al., (2017) estimated that rainfall shortages in certain African countries dependent on cultivation of non-irrigated and semi-humid crops could reduce production by 50% by 2020, exposing 70% of the population dependent on such crops on the continent to serious food insecurity.

Irrigated crops account for 20% of cultivated land globally and 40% of the food produced. Usually, the water used is drawn from rivers; as a result availability depends on weather in remote areas. One example of this is agriculture along the length of the Nile, which depends on rainfall in its highest stretch in Ethiopia (Elliott et al., 2014). In other regions, river flows depend on ice melting (FAO, 2008). In medium and high latitudes, mild winters result in lower precipitation in the form of snow, resulting in reduced water flow in spring (Samuel et al., 2017). Almost a sixth of the world's population lives around the Ganges and Indus river basins, using their waters for domestic and agricultural purposes. Both rivers depend on melting of glaciers in the mountains, and this in turn is being influenced by global warming. This phenomenon may result in seasonal flows in rivers, decreasing in the dry season and increasing in the rainy season with greater risks of flooding (Mason & Calow, 2014). Combined with increasing populations in the area, this could result in water shortages in future. In other situations, water shortages are not due to low rainfall, but to surface run off, evaporation and deep percolation (FAO, 2010).

Similarly, Mougou, Mansour, Iglesias, Chebbi & Battaglini, (2011) stated that there will be an increase in the amount of water falling as torrential rain over coming years. Mougou et al., (2011) further stated that excess water can damage crops, ruining harvests and flooding can devastate large expanses of cultivated land. Nelson, Rosegrant, Koo, Robertson, Sulser, Zhu & Ringler, (2009) stated that tropical cyclones may become more intense over the coming decades, with stronger winds and higher rainfall. These cyclones can have serious social and economic impact, particularly on developing countries. For example, in the Indian Ocean region like Myanmar, Bangladesh and India where majority of the people are domiciled in river deltas. Increasing populations in these areas make them extremely vulnerable to the risk of flooding, which will be aggravated by loss of harvests. However, inland regions may benefit from these weather systems as they decay to heavy rain. For example, for Cyclone Eline which devastated agriculture in Madagascar in 2000, but whose subsequent rains helped to offset drought in the south of Africa (Crahay, 2010).

Effect of Rising Sea Level

Over the past one hundred and fifty years, sea level changes have been observed at tide gauge stations, and for the past twenty years, with satellite altimeters. Rising sea levels are inevitable consequences of climate change. There are two main factors responsible for this increase: thermal expansion of the oceans and an increase in the volume of water due to ice melting from warming (Florida Oceans and Coastal Council, 2010). Although these effects should be taken into account at present, they are not expected to occur in the short term, given the rate of ice melting in the major ice shelves at present (Stéphane, Colin, Robert, Nicholls & Jan, 2013). The fourth IPCC report estimated that sea levels could rise by between 0.1m and 0.5m. The most vulnerable regions to such changes are those in river deltas and island states in South-East Asia, which could suffer flooding of crops and salination of underground water sources (Samuel et al., 2017). IPCC also predicted a global sea level rise (SLR) by 52-98 cm by 2100, which would threaten the survival of coastal cities & entire island nations (Florida Oceans and Coastal Council, 2010).

For the past, proxy data are shown in light purple & tide gauge data in blue. For the future, the IPCC projections for very high emissions (red) and very low emissions (blue) are shown.

Effects of Changes in Atmospheric Composition

The levels of carbondioxide in the atmosphere and effect on climate change are interlinked during most of the Earth's history. The present global carbon dioxide levels are at 38% higher than the levels that hovered around 280 ppm during the last 2.1 million years (Ahn and Brook 2009; Goodwin et al., 2009). Human activities of this age such as fossil fuel burning, deforestation, draining of wetlands, adoption of modern technology in farming and livestock rearing etc., are the main factors responsible for the present degraded state of the global environment. A higher concentration of carbondioxide (CO_2) in the atmosphere may have a direct effect on physical processes in plants, such as photosynthesis and transpiration. Increased CO_2 in the atmosphere increases photosynthesis by between 10% and 50%; this is beneficial (Horisch et al., 2009). However, comparing the overall effect of CO_2 on fertility with the results of climate change, it is believed that the former is much more critical for determining whether harvests increase or decrease. Damage from consumption of the toxic emissions from CO_2 by the surrounding vegetation can affect the quality and aesthetic value of plants and reduce their economic value (Westenbarger & Frisvold, 1994). If CO_2 fertilization remains high, climate change will benefit agriculture in Europe and the USA. However, in Africa and India, despite the increased fertilization levels resulting from higher CO_2, climate change will result in harvests falling by 5% by 2050 (Goodwin et al., 2009). Ozone hampers photosynthesis and accelerates leaf ageing, impacting on harvests. These effects are particularly visible in agricultural products, reducing their market value (Caesens et al., 2009). When CO_2 settles in the atmosphere, the resulting water can become harmful to vegetation and aquatic life (Johnson and Fegley, 2002).

Figure 1. IPCC 2100 Sea Level Rise Projection. Source: Church, Clark, Cazenave, Gregory, Jevrejeva, Levermann, Merrifield, Milne, Nerem, Nunn, Payne, Pfeffer, Stammer & Unnikrishnan, 2013

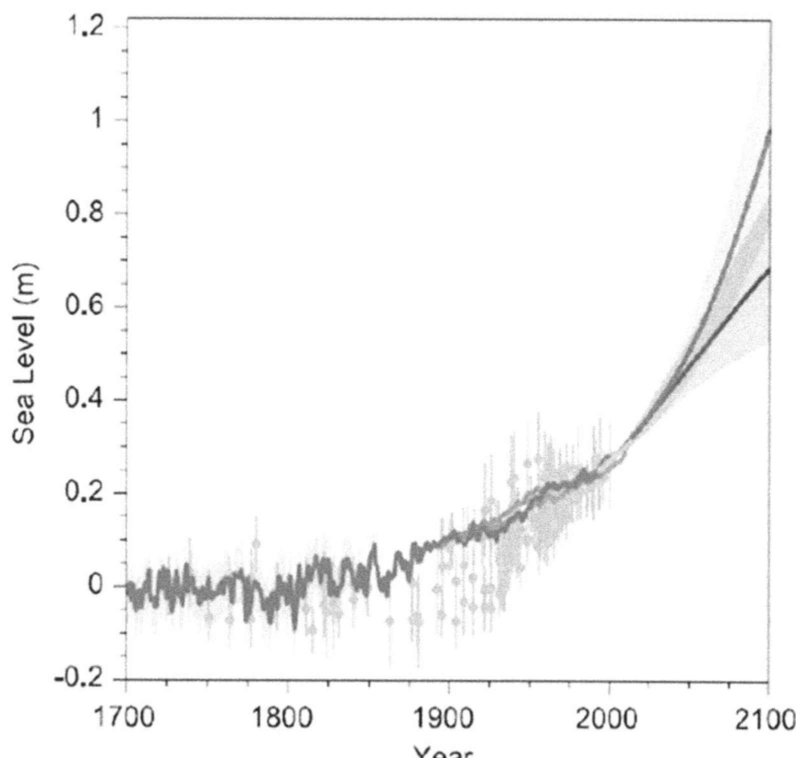

Effect of Ground-Level Ozone

Ground-level ozone is obtained primarily from chemical reactions between human-induced emissions. Ozone formation increases with increase in temperature, particularly above 32^0C (90^0F) (Ainsworth, Yendrek, Sitch, Collins & Emberson, 2012). Apart from being a human cardiorespiratory toxin, ground-level ozone is also a plant toxin, preventing crop photosynthesis and growth, and reducing the weight and yields of grain (Bell, Goldberg, Hogrefe, Kinney, & Knowlton, 2007). Open-air experiments showed that the ozone concentrations of 54-75ppb found in polluted regions decrease yields by 8-25% in rice, soybean, and wheat (Ashmore, 2005). Globally, the current levels of ozone pollution are expected to have reduced maize, wheat, and soybean yields by 6-9%. Efforts from government in the area of regulation are believed to contribute to reduction in ozone levels over the coming decades in developed countries (R. Soc. 2008). Many developing countries, especially in Africa and Asia, can anticipate increased ozone levels due to greater emissions and warming (Tirado et al., 2010).

EFFECT OF CHANGING CLIMATE ON NUTRITION

The link between climate change and nutrition is multifaceted. The common expectation is that climate change will have an effect on nutrition outcomes through its impact on the underlying drivers of nutritional status (Mueller, Gerber, Johnston, Ray, Ramankutty & Foley, 2012). The seasonality of climate, climate and weather shocks, year-to-year variability and longer-term shifts all influence directly and indirectly, the four environments which underpin nutrition: food, social, health and living environments (Mueller et al., 2012). Climate influences the seasonality of food production and consumption, epidemics of diarrheal disease, and the time utilization of mothers whose ready access to clean drinking-water in coastal regions declines as sea-levels rise (Tilman and Clark 2014). Droughts affect human nutrition not only by seriously reducing crop harvests but also by reducing grazing and fodder for livestock, thus lessening the availability of milk and meat. Drought inhibits plant growth and development by disturbing the uptake and absorption of essential minerals. This is reflected in the final crop yield, and may also affect the nutritional content of roots/tubers, foliage and seeds (WHO, 2013).

Beyond its effect on yields, increase in CO_2 levels is changing the nutritional composition of crops. Experiments in which food crops are grown at elevated CO_2 levels, both in chambers and in open-field conditions using free air CO_2 enrichment methods, showed reductions in protein content in the edible portion of these crops. Grains and tubers including rice, wheat, barley, and potatoes experience 7-15% reductions in protein content, whereas legumes and crops show either very small or insignificant reductions (Long, Ainsworth, Leakey, Nosberger & Ort, 2006). When these nutrient changes are modelled across current diets, more than 200 million people are expected to fall below thresholds of recommended protein intake, and protein deficiency levels among those already below this threshold will worsen (Myers et al., 2014).

Crops grown at elevated CO_2 also exhibit lower concentrations of important minerals. CO_2 concentrations of 550ppm can lead to 3-11% decreases of zinc and iron concentrations in cereal grains and legumes and 5-10% reductions in the concentration of Phosphorus, Potassium, Calcium, Sulphur, Magnesium, Iron, Zinc, Copper, and Manganese across a wide range of crops under more extreme conditions of 690ppm CO_2 (Medek, Schwartz & Myers, 2017). These reductions in zinc content are expected to place about 150-200 million people at risk for zinc deficiency and will aggravate existing deficiencies in more than 1 billion people (Long et al., 2006). In addition, roughly 1.4 billion children ages 1-5 and women of child bearing age, which represent 59% of the world total in these groups, live in countries where current anaemia rates exceed 20% of the population and where dietary iron intake is expected to decrease by 3.8% or more as a result of these CO_2-mediated nutrient changes (Myers et al., 2014). Overall, hundreds of millions of people are expected to be placed at risk of zinc, iron, and/or protein deficiencies as a result of rising CO_2 concentrations in the atmosphere, and about two billion people already experiencing zinc or iron deficiency are likely see those deficiencies exacerbated by this effect (Samuel et al., 2017).

Similarly, Selenium affects the level of nutrients absorbed by plants when they are growing. It's an essential element for humans, boosting immune systems and preventing cognitive decline (Myers, Wessells, Kloog, Zanobetti & Schwartz, 2015). A lack of selenium has also been known to inhibit the proper growth of children's bones in some selenium deficient areas of China (Long et al., 2006). A recent study has projected that, as a direct result of climate change, 66% of croplands will lose 8.7% of their Selenium (Myers et al., 2014).

Nutrient content of seafood is also affected by changing climate. This occurs by changing the nutritional composition of phytoplankton communities with consequent effects on the food chain (Myers, 2015). Warming leads to reduced long-chain polyunsaturated fatty acid content in phytoplankton and in cold-water pelagic fish, such as sprat and anchovy. Another study suggested that uptake of minerals such as iron becomes more limited in warmer and more acidic waters, though further examination of impacts on micronutrient composition is needed (Crahay, 2010). The direct effects of CO_2 emissions combined with attendant changes in climate lead to substantial uncertainties regarding the implications for the availability of food and nutrition. For fisheries, the compounding complexity of how the entire marine food chain will be affected leads to perhaps even greater uncertainty (WHO, 2013).

IMPACT OF CLIMATE CHANGE ON FOOD CONSUMPTION

Climate change could have a pronounced effect on incomes and urban consumers' access to food. Long-term climate changes and trends may act as a drag on economic growth and job creation through mechanisms including higher mortality, lower performance, and social unrest, limiting households' ability to earn incomes and improve their purchasing power. Reduced economic growth could make it more difficult for governments to manage food prices and fend off higher and more volatile food prices. This would result in food becoming more expensive for poor households. At the same time, climate change impacts on the economy and natural resource-based activities may threaten some livelihood activities underpinning food security especially in areas with high concentrations of people and economic activities (Dell et al., 2009).

Heat extremes could impact incomes and food access through reducing labour productivity and affecting sensitive sectors. Increase in temperature will take an especially heavy toll on manual workers especially in Middle East North Africa (MENA) countries as heat extreme affect tourism sector (DARA, 2012). For example, the proportion of the workforce expected to be particularly affected between 2010 and 2030 by reduced productivity ranges between 10-20% in most MENA countries. Tourism being one of the climate sensitive sector is likely to shift in seasonality, as visitors would avoid hot months, and is projected to decline around 8% for MENA region by 2050 (Bigano et al., 2008).

According to Parsons (2009), by the 2030s, it is believed that urban areas will face disruptive extreme events that threaten incomes, health and food security. The study further stated that heat waves are expected to become more common and more intense. Heat extremes threaten health in several ways. Most relevant to food security are the impacts of heat stress on human physiology (Parsons, 2009). Exposure to heat stress increases the risk of dehydration, strokes and heart disease as the human body has to work harder to maintain an average body temperature and dehydration can affect food metabolism (Parsons, 2009). Preventing heat stress requires avoiding strenuous activity and drinking enough water, but this is a challenge for people in certain occupations and living conditions (Schellnhuber et al., 2014).

Extreme climate events may present shocks to food safety, affecting utilization. Under scenarios of prolonged heat extremes, non-refrigerated foods will spoil more quickly if electricity supply is strained, breaks in the cold chain may raise spoilage in chilled foods too (Kolahi, Rastegarpour, Abadi & Gachkar, 2010). Periods of high temperature also result in higher incidences of common forms of food poisoning, such as salmonellosis (Confalonieri et al., 2007). A study in Beirut projected climate change driven increases of 16-28% in food and water-borne related morbidity by 2050 (El Fadel et al., 2012). And diarrhoeal disease could increase between 6-15% by 2040 if health infrastructure does not improve from its current status (Kolstad & Johansson, 2010).

Climate variability and extremes could affect harvests and global food prices which would make food security of urban populations less stable. With food accounting for 60% of household spending in the poorest countries (e.g. Yemen) and 35-45% of spending in middle-income countries (e.g. Algeria, Iraq) food price volatility has a large impact on the welfare of population (Kolahi et al., 2010). Global agricultural production is expected to continue rising, yet all regions can expect increasing risk of harvest failure due to climate shocks (Abou-Hadid, 2014). Expected increases in population and incomes combined with climate change mean prices for most food commodities are expected to rise by 2050 (Nelson et al., 2010). This contrasts with the second half of the 20th Century, when food prices fell. While an increase in food prices is enough to threaten the food security for those struggling with current costs, many more will feel the impact if food markets become more volatile and countries are unable to increase trade to offset unpredictable price spikes brought on by climate shocks (DARA, 2012).

Imports vital to stability of local food markets may be further affected by climate change. For instance, while it is not possible to forecast developments on international grain supply chains, rising sea levels and increasing extreme events including storms and wave surges could potentially disrupt deliveries of supplies, for example if port infrastructure is damaged. Such events would likely push up prices, and possibly make food temporarily more scarce (Tacoli et al., 2013). Food losses during transport and storage will remain high and vulnerable to climatic events unless infrastructure is well designed and maintained. Poorly constructed warehouses mean supplies are at risk from flooding and disease. For food that requires cooling, electricity systems are at risk from load-shedding as well as storms, and water-cooled systems are vulnerable to drought. With food storage and transportation systems already saddled with problems in many countries, climate change is expected to present more challenges. Temperature rises and more extreme weather events may lead to more post-harvest losses, for example if higher humidity of stored foods rises above safe levels, it will increase fungal or pest infection (Kitinoja, 2011).

Losses of perishable foods including fruit and vegetables are already high, and more extreme temperatures could obstruct efforts to bring these down. This could limit potential export revenues and also impede strategies to raise domestic consumption of fruit and vegetables needed to improve diets. Countries that rely heavily on open storage to store grain such as Egypt could experience higher losses of cereals (USDA, 2014).

SOLUTIONS AND RECOMMENDATIONS

There is need for nutrition transition from meat-based consumption that is occurring in low and middle-income countries and that has world-wide consequences for supply, thus putting enormous stress on ecosystems. This transition can occur from switch in a diet rich in animal proteins to a diet that is closer to health guidelines and that at the same time puts less pressure on the environment. Investment should be made on renewable energy technology especially in development of solar dryer as it has the tendency to reduce quantities of wasted foods.

According to European Commission (2007), understanding factors influencing food choice such as biological determinants, economic determinants, physical determinants, social determinants, psychological determinants, attitudes, beliefs and knowledge about food plays crucial part in people's consumption approach. Consumers also need to be empowered to choose instead of being told what to or not to eat, and food should be safe. As food consumption is a daily routine, consumer choices are also daily routines.

It should be noted that calories are not good enough without micronutrients. Cognitive and physical development depends on eating the right things. This review call on policymakers to take steps to reduce greenhouse gas emissions along the lines of the Paris Agreement, which commits countries to working to keep global atmospheric temperatures from going beyond 2°C (3.6°F) by 2100. Meeting this agreement would help prevent some of the most dramatic effects of climate change on sustainable food consumption. Governments should equally adjust public health and food programs to meet the expectations of malnourished population.

Also, strategies to maintain adequate diets need to focus on as countries with less capacity to cope with food security challenges must be given attention. Efforts aimed at reducing vulnerability to nutrient deficiencies by supporting diverse and nutritious diets in children, enriching the nutritional content of staple crops and breeding crops less sensitive to these emissions effects need to be supported.

It is noted that the world's climate change and nutrition communities have overlapping agendas, this situation should improve. More collaboration between the two communities could generate a better understanding of climate-related risks to nutrition while also engaging the nutrition community in concerns about the impact of food systems and dietary choices on greenhouse gas emission. It would be ideal to identify dietary choices that are both good for health and good for the planet. The climate and nutrition communities should engage in dialogue that can stimulate collaboration between them and improve the coherence of their respective policy agendas.

This review also suggests that the three areas in sustainable food consumption: the food we consume, the means of transport we choose, and the type of housing we live in should be given balanced attention. These areas together are vulnerable to impact of climate change and efforts should be made to address all the areas. Also, since feeding nine to ten billion people by 2050 presents an enormous challenge, a number of options such as closing the yield gap, increasing the production potential of crops, reducing waste, changing diets and expanding aquaculture etc. are particularly important, all of which need to be coordinated in a multifaceted and linked global strategy to ensure sustainable and equitable food security.

Embedding risks associated with changing climate to the food supply system could help reduce long term costs and increase efficiency, for example by minimizing the impact of heat extremes on post-harvest losses in food storage and distribution. Climate risk management could also help mitigate the potential for cascading impacts, where risks to key bottlenecks in the food supply system result in widespread consequences.

People in remote rural areas and rapidly growing and informal urban areas have the greatest challenges in accessing safety nets and basic services. Rural and urban poor people who are unable to find, afford, or safely consume food predictably are already living in risk, and are vulnerable to climate impacts on food systems. Addressing the needs of these communities is likely to require both more resources and reforms in policies and systems but is likely to provide benefits towards increased social stability. Food subsidy programmes should be put in place in continents such as Africa and Asia.

FUTURE RESEARCH DIRECTIONS

It is evident research on the interaction of climate change, food, and agriculture is growing every day, there are many pressing areas that require additional study in order to enable researchers, policymakers, and others to fully adopt a sustainable food consumption approach. Areas such as application of climate-smart technologies for food production, development of seedlings better able to cope with changing climate, frameworks for sustainable food consumption implementation and creation of habitat suitable for continuous food production need to be accorded attention. Also, climate change should not divert attention from fundamental food security and development aims and objectives, and achievement of the Sustainable Development Goals. Instead, risk associated with climate change should be mainstreamed into food systems to help address underlying vulnerabilities, weaknesses, and risks from other sources.

CONCLUSION

As climate change policies have become more of a priority over the years, it is expedient to look at ways it connects with sustainable food consumption. Also, fostering sustainable food consumption should be an integral part of the sustainable development strategy. Therefore, this review looked at different climatic factors affecting food production and made recommendations on approaches toward sustainable food consumption. It offers insights for researchers, politicians, and activists who intend to contribute to this objective.

Climate change poses risks and challenges to the whole food value chain, from production through to distribution and to consumption (DARA, 2012). Seizing the imperative to adapt to the challenges of climate change can be an opportunity to reform and strengthen food systems and food security, and also the human security, stability, and longer term sustainable development of nations from most-vulnerable to least-vulnerable. Similarly, climate risks to food security especially for poor rural producers can be reduced by helping them to cope with droughts through improved programmes that anticipate and reduce the impact of shocks and help affected people recover quickly. Also, by improving access to appropriate techniques and technology, utilizing climate-smart technologies and by adopting climate-smart food policies, farm productivity would increase and people will be more equipped to deal with climate challenges affecting sustainable food consumption.

REFERENCES

Abou-Hadid, A. F. (2014). *Arab Environment: food security*. Beirut, Lebanon: Arab Forum for Environment and Development.

Ahn, J., & Brook, E. J. (2009). Atmospheric CO2 and climate on millennial time scales during the last glacial period. *Science*, *322*(5898), 83–85. doi:10.1126cience.1160832 PMID:18787135

Ainsworth, E. A., Yendrek, C. R., Sitch, S., Collins, W. J., & Emberson, L. D. (2012). The effects of tropospheric ozone on net primary productivity and implications for climate change. *Annual Review of Plant Biology*, *63*(1), 637–661. doi:10.1146/annurev-arplant-042110-103829 PMID:22404461

Ashmore, M. R. (2005). Assessment of response of future vegetation to ozone. *Plant, Cell & Environment*, *28*, 949–964. doi:10.1111/j.1365-3040.2005.01341.x

Battisti, D. S., & Naylor, R. L. (2009). Historical warnings of future food insecurity with unprecedented seasonal heat. *Science*, *323*(5911), 240–244. doi:10.1126cience.1164363 PMID:19131626

Bazilian, M., Rogner, H., Howells, M., Hermann, S., Arent, D., Gielen, D., ... Yumkella, K. (2011). Considering the energy, water and food nexus: Towards an integrated modelling approach. *Energy Policy*, *39*(12), 7896–7906. doi:10.1016/j.enpol.2011.09.039

Beddow, J., Pardey, P., & Seeley, M. (2012). *Changing Agricultural Climate: Implications for Innovation Policies*. Food Policy Research Center. University of Minnesota. Available at: https://www.foodpolicy. umn.edu/policy-summaries-and-analyses/changing-agricultural-climate-implications-innovation-policies

Bell, M. L., Goldberg, R., Hogrefe, C., Kinney, P., Knowlton, K., Lynn, B., ... Patz, J. A. (2007). Climate change, ambient ozone, and health in 50 U.S. cities. *Climatic Change, 82*(1-2), 61–76. doi:10.100710584-006-9166-7

Bigano, A., Bosello, F., Roson, R., & Tol, R. S. (2008). Economy-wide impacts of climate change: A joint analysis for sea level rise and tourism. *Mitigation and Adaptation Strategies for Global Change, 13*(8), 765–791. doi:10.100711027-007-9139-9

Brundtland Commission. (1987). Report on World Commission on Environment and Development: Our Common Future. UN Document: Gathering a body of Global Agreements.

Caesens, E., Rodriguez, M. R., Figueroa-Irizarry, I., Gillard, T., Pershing-Foley, Z., & Rosenblum, P. (2009). Climate Change and the Right to Food: A Comprehensive Study. Columbia Law School Human Rights Institute, Heinrich-Böll-Stiftung.

Carlsson-Kanyama, A., & Gonzalez, A. (2009). Potential contributions of food consumption patterns to climate change. *The American Journal of Clinical Nutrition, 89*(5), 1704S–1709S. doi:10.3945/ajcn.2009.26736AA PMID:19339402

Church, C., & Lorek, S. (2007). Linking policy and practice in sustainable production and consumption: An assessment of the role of NGOs. *International Journal of Innovation and Sustainable Development, 2*(2), 230–240. doi:10.1504/IJISD.2007.016936

Church, J. A., Clark, P. U., Cazenave, A., Gregory, J. M., Jevrejeva, S., Levermann, A., ... Unnikrishnan, A. S. (2013). Sea Level Change Supple¬mentary Material. In *Climate Change 2013: The Physical Science Basis. Contribution of Working Group I to the Fifth Assessment Report of the Intergovernmental Panel on Climate Change*. Available from www.climatechange2013.org

Collier, P., Conway, G., & Venables, T. (2008). Climate change and Africa. *Oxford Review of Economic Policy, 24*(2), 337–353. doi:10.1093/oxrep/grn019

Confalonieri, U., Menne, B., Akhtar, R., Ebi, K. L., Hauengue, M., Kovats, R. S., ... Woodward, A. J. (2007). Human health. In Climate Change 2007: Impacts, Adaptation and Vulnerability. Contribution of Working Group II to the Fourth Assessment Report of the Intergovernmental Panel on Climate Change. Cambridge, UK: Academic Press.

Crahay, P. (2010). The Threats of Climate Change on Under-nutrition. A neglected issue that requires further analysis and urgent actions. In: United Nations Standing Committee on Nutrition (SCN). *SCN News, 38*, 2010.

DARA. (2012). *"Labour Productivity Indicator." Climate Vulnerability Monitor: A Guide to the Cold Calculus of a Hot Planet* (2nd ed.). Madrid, Spain: DARA.

Dell, M., Jones, B., & Olken, B. (2009). Temperature and Income: Reconciling New Cross-Sectional and Panel Estimates. *The American Economic Review, 99*(2), 198–204. doi:10.1257/aer.99.2.198

El-Fadel, M., Ghanimeh, S., Maroun, R., & Alameddine, I. (2012). Climate change and temperature rise: Implications on food-and waterborne diseases. *The Science of the Total Environment, 437*, 15–21. doi:10.1016/j.scitotenv.2012.07.041 PMID:22903000

Elliott, J., Deryng, D., Müller, C., Frieler, K., Konzmann, M., Gerten, D., ... Wisser, D. (2014). Constraints and potentials of future irrigation water availability on agricultural production under climate change. *Proceedings of the National Academy of Sciences of the United States of America*, *111*(9), 3239–3244. doi:10.1073/pnas.1222474110 PMID:24344283

European Commission. (2007). Food consumer science. Lessons learnt from FP projects in the field of food and consumer science. Brussels: Author.

FAO. (2006). *Food Security; Policy Brief.* Rome: Food and Agriculture Organization of the United Nations.

FAO. (2008). *Climate change and food security: a framework document.* Rome, Italy: Food and Agricultural Organization of the United Nations.

FAO. (2010). Final Document: *International Scientific Symposium Biodiversity and Sustainable Diets: United Against Hunger.* Rome: Food and Agriculture Organisation.

FAO. (2012). *IFAD, the state of food insecurity in the world 2012.* FAO.

Florida Oceans and Coastal Council. (2010). *Climate Change and Sea-Level Rise in Florida: An Update of The Effects of Climate Change on Florida's Ocean and Coastal Resources, Dec. 2010.* Retrieved from http://www.floridaoceanscouncil.org/reports/ClimateChange andSeaLevelRise.pdf

Fuchs, D., & Lorek, S. (2002). Sustainable Consumption Governance in a Globalizing World. *Global Environmental Politics*, *2*(1), 19–45. doi:10.1162/152638002317261454

Fuchs, D., & Lorek, S. (2005). Sustainable Consumption Governance - A History of Promises and Failures. *Journal of Consumer Policy*, *28*(3), 261–288. doi:10.100710603-005-8490-z

Gerbens-Leenes, P. W., Nonhebel, S., & Krol, M. S. (2010). Food consumption patterns and economic growth. Increasing affluence and the use of natural resources. *Appetite*, *55*(3), 597–608. doi:10.1016/j.appet.2010.09.013 PMID:20854862

Godfray, H. C. J., Beddington, J. R., Crute, I. R., Haddad, L., Lawrence, D., Muir, J. F., ... Toulmin, C. (2010). Food security: The challenge of feeding 9 billion people. *Science*, *327*(5967), 812–818. doi:10.1126cience.1185383 PMID:20110467

Goodwin, P., Williams, R. G., Ridgwell, A., & Follows, M. J. (2009). Climate sensitivity to the carbon cycle modulated by past and future changes in ocean chemistry. *Nature Geoscience*, *2*(2), 145–150. doi:10.1038/ngeo416

Hallegatte, S., Green, C., Nicholls, R. J., & Corfee-Morlot, J. (2013). Future Flood Losses in Major Coastal Cities. *Nature Climate Change*, *2*(9), 802–806. doi:10.1038/nclimate1979

Hanss, D., & Böhm, G. (2012). Sustainability seen from the perspective of consumers. *International Journal of Consumer Studies*, *36*(6), 678–687. doi:10.1111/j.1470-6431.2011.01045.x

Horisch, B., Hemming, N. G., Archer, D., Siddall, M., & McManus, J. F. (2009). Atmospheric carbon dioxide concentration across the mid-pleistocene transition. *Science*, *324*(5934), 1551–1554. doi:10.1126cience.1171477 PMID:19541994

IPCC. (2012). *IPCC, 2012: Change Adaptation. A Special Report of Working Groups I and II of the Intergovernmental Panel on Climate Change. Cambridge UK and New York, USA.* Cambridge, UK: Cambridge University Press.

IPCC. (2014). Summary for policymakers. In *Climate change 2014: Impacts, adaptation, and vulnerability. Part A: Global and sectoral aspects. Contribution of Working Group II to the Fifth Assessment Report of the Intergovermental Panel on Climate Change* (pp. 1–32). Cambridge, UK: Cambridge University Press.

Johnson, N. M., & Fegley, B. Jr. (2002). *Tremolite decomposition and venus. Planetary chemistry laboratory.* St. Louis, MO: Earth and Planetary Science Dept., Washington University.

Kitinoja, L. (2011). Developing and promoting sustainable postharvest technologies for India and Africa. Centre for Alleviation of Poverty through Sustainable Agriculture Palawija Newsletter, 28(3).

Kolahi, A. A., Rastegarpour, A., Abadi, A., & Gachkar, L. (2010). An unexpectedly high incidence of acute childhood diarrhea in Koot-Abdollah, Ahwaz, Iran. *International Journal of Infectious Diseases, 14*(7), e618–e621. doi:10.1016/j.ijid.2009.10.001 PMID:20116314

Kolstad, E. W., & Johansson, K. A. (2011). Uncertainties associated with quantifying climate change impacts on human health: A case study for diarrhoea. *Environmental Health Perspectives, 119*(3), 299–305. doi:10.1289/ehp.1002060 PMID:20929684

Long, S. P., Ainsworth, E. A., & Leakey, A. D. (1918–21). Food for thought: Lower-than-expected crop yield stimulation with rising CO2 concentrations. *Science, 312.*

Lorek, S., & Fuchs, D. (2011). Strong Sustainable Consumption Governance - Precondition For A De-growth Path? *Journal of Cleaner Production.*

Lorek, S., Spangenberg, J., & Oman, I. (2008). *Sustainable Consumption Policies Effectiveness Evaluation (SCOPE2) - Conclusion.* Vienna: Sustainable Europe Research Institute SERI.

Mason, N., & Calow, R. (2014). *The real water crisis: inequality in a fast changing world.* Working Paper. Overseas Development Institute.

Medek, D. E., Schwartz, J., & Myers, S. S. (2017). Rising CO2 poses a threat to global protein intake. *Environmental Health Perspectives.*

Mougou, R., Mansour, M., Iglesias, A., Chebbi, R. Z., & Battaglini, A. (2011). Climate change and agricultural vulnerability: A case study of rain-fed wheat in Kairouan, Central Tunisia. *Regional Environmental Change, 11*(S1), 137–142. doi:10.100710113-010-0179-4

Mueller, N. D., Gerber, J. S., Johnston, M., Ray, D. K., Ramankutty, N., & Foley, J. A. (2012). Closing yield gaps through nutrient and water management. *Nature, 490,* 254–257.

Myers, S. S., Smith, M. R., Guth, S., Golden, C. D., Vaitla, B., Mueller, N. D., ... Huybers, P. (2017). Climate Change and Global Food Systems: Potential Impacts on Food Security and Undernutrition. *Annual Review of Public Health, 2017.* doi:10.1146/annurev-publhealth-031816-044356 PMID:28125383

Myers, S. S., Wessells, K. R., Kloog, I., Zanobetti, A., & Schwartz, J. (2015). Effect of increased concentrations of atmospheric carbon dioxide on the global threat of zinc deficiency: A modelling study. *The Lancet. Global Health, 3*(10), e639–e645. doi:10.1016/S2214-109X(15)00093-5 PMID:26189102

Myers, S. S., Zanobetti, A., Kloog, I., Huybers, P., Leakey, A. D., Bloom, A. J., ... Usui, Y. (2014). Increasing CO2 threatens human nutrition. *Nature, 510*(7503), 139–142. doi:10.1038/nature13179 PMID:24805231

Nelson, G. C., Rosegrant, M. W., Koo, J., Robertson, R., Sulser, T., Zhu, T., & Ringler, C. (2009). *Climate change: Impact on agriculture and costs of adaptation* (Vol. 21). International Food Policy Research Institute.

Nelson, G. C., Rosegrant, M. W., Palazzo, A., Gray, I., Ingersoll, C., Robertson, R., & Tokgoz, S. (2010). *Food security, farming, and climate change to 2050: Scenarios, results, policy options.* Washington, DC: International Food Policy Research Institute.

Parsons, K. (2009). Maintaining health, comfort and productivity in heat waves. *Global Health Action, 2*(1), 2057. doi:10.3402/gha.v2i0.2057 PMID:20052377

Prasad, P. V. V., Staggenborg, S. A., & Ristic, Z. (2008). Impacts of drought and/or heat stress on physiological, developmental, growth, and yield processes of crop plants. In L. H. Ahuja & S. A. Saseendran (Eds.), *Advances in Agricultural Systems Modeling* (pp. 301–355). Madison, WI: Academic Press.

Schafer, M., Herde, A., & Kropp, C. 2007. Life events as turning points for sustainable nutrition. *Proceedings: SCP cases in the field of food, mobility and housing*, 115-130. http://www.scorenetwork.org/files//9594_Proceedings_worshop.07.pdf

Schellnhuber, H. J., Reyer, C., Hare, B., Waha, K., Otto, I., & Serdeczny, O. (2014). *Turn Down the Heat.* Washington, DC: World Bank.

Smith, P., Martino, D., Cai, Z., Gwary, D., Janzen, H., Kumar, P., ... Smith, J. (2008). Greenhouse gas mitigation in agriculture. *Philosophical Transactions of the Royal Society of London. Series B, Biological Sciences, 363*(1492), 789–813. doi:10.1098/rstb.2007.2184 PMID:17827109

Soc, R. (2008). *Ground-Level Ozone in the 21st Century: Future Trends, Impacts and Policy Implication. Sci.Policy Rep. 15/08.* London: R. Soc.

Tacoli, C., Bukhari, B., & Fisher, S. (2013). *Urban poverty, food security and climate change.* Human Settlements Working Paper No. 37. I. H. S. Group. International Institute of Environment and Development.

Thornton, P., Ericksen, P. J., Herrero, M., & Challinor, A. J. (2014). Climate Variability and Vulnerability to Climate Change: A Review. *Global Change Biology, 20*(11), 3313–3328. doi:10.1111/gcb.12581 PMID:24668802

Tilman, D., & Clark, M. (2014). Global diets link environmental sustainability and human health. *Nature, 515*, 518–522.

Tirado, M. C., Clarke, R., Jaykus, L. A., McQuatters-Gollop, A., & Frank, J. M. (2010). Climate change and food safety: A review. *Food Research International, 43*(7), 1745–1765. doi:10.1016/j.foodres.2010.07.003

UNFCCC. (2007). *Climate Change: Impacts, Vulnerabilities And Adaptation In Developing Countries.* United Nations Framework Convention on Climate Change. Retrieved from https://unfccc.int/resource/docs/publications/impacts.pdf

USDA. (2014). *Egypt grain and feed annual 2014. G. A.I. Network.* Washington, DC: United States Department of Agriculture Foreign Agriculture Service.

Westenbarger, D. A., & Frisvold, G. B. (1994). Agricultural exposure to ozone and acid precipitation. *Atmospheric Environment, 28*(18), 2895–2907. doi:10.1016/1352-2310(94)90338-7

WFP. (2009). *Emergency Food Security As-sessment Handbook* (2nd ed.). Rome: World Food Programme.

WHO. (2004). *Global Strategy on Diet, Physical Activity and Health.* Rome: World Health Organisation. Available at http://www.who.int/dietphysicalactivity/strategy/eb11344/en/index.html

WHO. (2013). *Diet, Nutrition and the Prevention of Chronic Diseases.* Report of a joint WHO/FAO expert consultation. Technical report series 916. Geneva: World Health Organization.

ADDITIONAL READING

Di Falco, S., Yesuf, M., Kohlin, G., & Ringler, C. (2011). Estimating the Impact of Climate Change on Agriculture in Low-Income Countries: Household Level Evidence from the Nile Basin, Ethiopia. *Environmental and Resource Economics, 52*(4), 457–478. doi:10.100710640-011-9538-y

Giesen, R. H., & Oerlemans, J. (2013). Climate-model induced differences in the 21st century global and regional glacier contributions to sea-level rise. *Climate Dynamics, 41*(11-12), 3283–3300. doi:10.100700382-013-1743-7

Goodwin, P., Williams, R. G., Ridgwell, A., & Follows, M. J. (2009). Climate sensitivity to the carbon cycle modulated by past and future changes in ocean chemistry. *Nature Geoscience, 2*(2), 145–150. doi:10.1038/ngeo416

IFPRI. (2015). *Global Nutrition Report 2014: Actions and Accountability to Accelerate the World's Progress on Nutrition.* Washington, D.C.: IFPRI.

IPCC. (2007). *Climate change impacts, adaptation and vulnerability summary for policy makers (Contribution of working Group II to the forth assessment Report of the IPCC).* Cambridge, MA: Cambridge University Press.

Muamba, F., & Kraybill, D. (2010). Weather Vulnerability, Climate Change, and Food Security in Mt. Kilimanjaro. Poster prepared for presentation at the Agricultural & Applied Economics Association 2010 AAEA, CAES, & WAEA Joint Annual Meeting. Denver, Colorado, 25-27 July, 2010.

Stehfest, E., Bouwman, L., van Vuuren, D. P., den Elzen, M. G. J., Eickhout, B., & Kabat, P. (2009). Climate benefits of changing diet. *Climatic Change, 95*(1-2), 83–102. doi:10.100710584-008-9534-6

Steinfeld, H., & Gerber, P. (2010). Livestock production and the global environment: Consume less or produce better? *Proceedings of the National Academy of Sciences of the United States of America, 107*(43), 18237–18238. doi:10.1073/pnas.1012541107 PMID:20935253

KEY TERMS AND DEFINITIONS

Carbon Dioxide (CO$_2$): A colorless gas with density higher than 60% of dry air.

Climate Change: Change in weather patterns and related changes in oceans, land surfaces and ice sheets, occurring over time scale.

Diet: The kind of food a person, animal or community habitually eats.

Environmental Challenges: Refers to the existence of crises in the environment in such a way that it can cause damage to man or his environment.

Food Consumption: The quantity of food eaten by a person so as to allow growth and provide energy to the body.

Food Production: Process of preparing food by converting raw materials into ready-made food products.

Greenhouse Gas (GHG): Is a gaseous compound in the atmosphere that absorbs and emits radiant energy within the thermal infrared ray.

Nutrition: The process of providing or obtaining food necessary for health and growth.

This research was previously published in Global Food Politics and Approaches to Sustainable Consumption edited by Luke Amadi and Fidelis Allen; pages 54-76, copyright year 2020 by Engineering Science Reference (an imprint of IGI Global).

Chapter 51

Comparing the Effects of Unsustainable Production and Consumption of Food on Health and Policy Across Developed and Less Developed Countries

Josue Mbonigaba
University of KwaZulu-Natal, South Africa

ABSTRACT

The unsustainable food consumption across high-income countries (HICs) and low-income countries (LICs) is expected to differ in nature and extent, although no formal evidence in this respect has been documented. Documenting this evidence is the aim of this chapter. Specifically, the chapter seeks to answer the following questions: 1) Do the contexts in less developed countries (LDCs) and developed countries (DCs) make the nature and extent of unsustainability in food consumption different? 2) Do the mechanisms of the linkage between unsustainability of food consumption and health outcomes independent of countries' contexts? 3) Are current policies against unsustainable food consumption equally effective in DCs and LDCs? These questions are answered by means of a systematic review of the literature for the period 2000-2017. The findings are that the nature and extent of unsustainability is quite different across contexts of LICs and HICs.

INTRODUCTION

Unsustainable activity refers to actions that result in outcomes now that are due to worsen over the next period (Hobson, 2002). Consequently, in terms of production processes, unsustainable development has been referred to as processes resulting in the satisfaction of the current generation's needs without a guarantee of the same benefits for the next generation (Johnson et al., 2014:422). Unsustainable food consumption is defined in a similar fashion. It refers to food consumption/production levels and patterns

DOI: 10.4018/978-1-7998-5354-1.ch051

that are likely to result in a continual decrease in welfare across generations. This welfare is expected to be lost in three domains as reported in the literature, these being environmental degradation, economic inefficiency, and negative social outcomes (Lefin, 2010). In the environmental domain, for example, food consumption/production becomes unsustainable when biodiversity that is crucial to the welfare of the next generation is reduced through food consumption/production processes. In the economic domain, the technical and allocative inefficiencies that arise from current consumption/production processes deprive the next generation of resources through wastage (Clapp, 2017;91). The unsustainability of food consumption in the social domain emerges from consumption/production processes that are degrading the environment whilst at the same time resulting in sicknesses, social conflicts and lower human capital formation, among many others social ills (Hobson, 2002, Hertwich and Katzmayr, 2003).

To date, the literature has referred anecdotally to the possibility that the nature and extent of unsustainability in food consumption might differ in both nature and extent depending on the livelihood and lifestyles of communities (Barnidge et al., 2011, Connell, 2010, Vermeir and Verbeke, 2006, Lehota, 2004, Schloster et al., 2012, Capone et al., 2014), on the economic processes (Vermeir and Verbeke, 2006), and on socio-cultural-political set ups (Vermeir and Verbeke, 2006, Thøgersen, 2010, National insitute of consumer research, 2010, Nemecek et al., 2016, Lorek and Fuchs, 2013). In this chapter the "nature of unsustainability" refers to specific features of unsustainability. As an example, a type of production process might result in deforestation in one setting, while it might lead to greenhouse gas emission in another setting. Furthermore, unsustainability might arise predominantly from inefficiency in production processes (weak unsustainability) or it might stem from consumption behaviours (strong unsustainability). With reference to the "extent of unsustainability", this chapter refers to quantities of damages arising from unsustainability. The differences in extent across different settings might arise from mitigating or aggravating factors affecting unsustainability that prevail in these different settings. The effects of consumption/production processes and institutions on unsustainable food consumption mean that differences in these processes imply differences in the vulnerability of the various populations and their coping strategies (Gautam and Andersen, 2016, Alemu, 2010, Charles et al., 2010), which in turn have a bearing on the environmental, economic and social domains of unsustainability.

DCs and LDCs more generally differ in many respects regarding food consumption/production processes and in institutional set-ups (Herrero and Thorntonb, 2010:20880, Thøgersen, 2010). DCs use mechanized and industrial agriculture in their food production processes (Mózner, 2013) and have more established regulations concerning environmental degradation (Charles et al., 2010). Economic and social behaviours are likely to be different to those in LDCs due to established social security systems in DCs that mitigate the impacts of unsustainable food consumption. In these countries over nutrition and consumption of saturated fats from meat products prevail (Herrero and Thorntonb, 2010). Diseases in these countries are predominately non-communicable such as heart diseases, diabetes and obesity-related disorders, which are related to the consumption of high-energy foods and fats (McKenzie and Williams, 2015b). In LDCs, agriculture is less mechanized and largely traditional (Pretty et al., 2013) and the population is increasing rapidly. Hunger and deficiency in micronutrients in diets are characteristic of the majority of the population (Randolph et al., 2007, Seligman et al., 2009, Alinov, 2010, Oni, 2010, Pretty et al., 2003). Furthermore, these countries suffer from very limited or an absence of social security systems and safety nets. Diseases for the majority of people in these countries are largely infectious.

These differences imply different consequences of unsustainability either directly or through the indirect effects of these set-ups, which also mean that standard policies across DCs and LDCs might not be equally effective (Connell, 2010, Randolph et al., 2007, Hobson, 2002). Because set-ups and lifestyles in these countries are expected to impact on the nature and extent of unsustainability in food consumption/production (Mont and plepys, 2005, Kjærga et al., 2013), it follows that the patterns and extent of unsustainability are likely to be related to specific settings (Hobson, 2002, Mackay and Wolbring, 2013a, Hawkes, 2006, Mackay and Wolbring, 2013b). In spite of this possibility and its relevance for policy making, whether or not the nature and extent of unsustainability follows these contexts has not been investigated across DCs and LDCs. Therefore, through a systematic review of the literature, this chapter analyses the evidence to answer the question as to whether patterns of unsustainability and mechanisms causing ill health follow consumption/production processes and institutional set-ups in DCs and LDCs. Also investigated in this chapter is whether policies have been equitable in the context of differences in institutions, consumption behaviours and production processes across DCs and LDCs. The chapter ends with suggestions for new ways in which policies can be managed to impact effectively on unsustainability at a global level, by addressing factors in specific countries.

The rest of the chapter is structured such that the next section deals with the methodology, section 3 presents the findings and the chapter ends with a discussion of the findings and the conclusions.

MATERIALS AND METHODS

A systematic review of the literature was conducted in line with the standard practice of literature review (Littell et al., 2008, Khalid et al., 2003). Different databases were searched using search strategies to yield the maximum number of materials to be screened. The following terms or their combinations were used: "unsustainable food consumption" and "health" OR "policy", OR "high-income countries" OR "low-income countries", OR "developing countries", OR "developed countries" or "low-resource counties", OR agriculture OR farming, OR sustainable, OR context OR livelihood OR production OR institutional. Databases searched included EBSCOhost, Econlit, Cochrane Library, Medline, Social Sciences Citation Index, and Web of Science databases. For the search to yield sufficient material to screen, the period covered by the review was 2000-2017. References in the retrieved literature were searched to identify and search for additional studies. Finally, a search of gray literature was conducted to identify documents that are non-academic in nature to provide information especially on policies.

Overall, this search process resulted in identifying 1565 documents. These included journal articles, books, book chapters, working papers and conference proceedings. The number of the final papers reviewed was arrived at after a screening of titles and the abstracts for relevance to the focus of this chapter. The screening was done independently by research assistants and then by the main investigator. The main investigator, based on the screenings of his own and assistants', decided on the documents to include in the review. The screened document was included in the review if a source analysed (un)sustainability of food consumption/production or its relation to health, if it reported evidence for DCs or LDCs or both; or if it was peer reviewed or published by a reliable source such as policy making bodies; and if it reported on evidence relevant to the chapter's research question(s). With regard to DCs and LDCs, a country was classified as DC or a LDC if at the time of a source's publication, a country covered was classified as such by the World Bank. The screening process resulted in 75 documents being included in the final review.

The study classified the screened documents under three themes, each related to a research question under investigation. These themes were 1) "unsustainability of food consumption", 2) "unsustainability of food consumption and health"; and 3) "unsustainability of food consumption and policies". Because some papers covered more than one research question under investigation, these appeared under more than one theme. In the end, 44 documents focused or had sections focusing on the first theme, 40 focused or had sections focusing on the second theme, while 34 focused or had sections focusing on the third theme. The critical review of the evidence of studies classified under each theme resulted in answers to the three research questions. The extent of unsustainability under theme 1 was reviewed in terms of mitigating or aggravating factors within DCs or LDCs. The evidence arising from this methodology is reported next.

RESULTS AND DISCUSSION

(Un)sustainability of Food Consumption: DCs vs. LDCs

There have been many studies focusing on the unsustainability of food consumption/production in DCs and LDCs (Table 1). These studies used a variety of methods to characterize and explain the unsustainability of food consumption/production. The most common methods used by the studies were qualitative, consisting of analysing information through discussion with people or document reviews (see for example Reisch et al., 2013, Thøgersen, 2010). Some studies reported on evidence from specific countries whilst most of the studies reported results on DCs and LDCs as groups. A few studies used quantitative methods, notably descriptive statistics, inferential methods or their combination (Amendah et al., 2014, Grunert et al., 2014 for instance). Data sources included food balance surveys (FBS) constructed by the Food and Agriculture Organisation of the United Nations (FAO) based on national accounts, households or individual budgetary and dietary surveys. Other sources of data included the United Nations Environment programme (UNEP), Biodiversity International, Water Footprint Network, IFAD, and the World Food Programme (WFP). Studies included micro- (individuals or households) and macro-level (cross-country) analyses and covered different geographical regions of the world.

The evidence about unsustainability in food consumption from these studies can be analysed according to three pillars of unsustainable consumption, these being environmental, economic and social unsustainability (Table 1). Indicators of environmental unsustainability included loss of biodiversity, greenhouse gas emissions, water shortage, non-responsiveness of soil to chemicals, soil erosion, extreme weather conditions, ecosystem loss, ocean acidification and sea level rise. Social unsustainability was dominated by illnesses that arise from unsustainable consumption such as heart diseases and stunting. In very few studies in LDCs, social unsustainability included also social conflicts over land, unsustainable strategies to cope with food shortages such as contracting debts, selling assets, and dropping children from school (Alemu, 2010, Alinov, 2010). Economic inefficiencies consisted of wastes in food production, food markets distortions, unequal distribution of food, price distortions and externalities (Horrigan et al., 2002 for example).

In DCs, unsustainability in the form of environmental degradation stemmed mainly from industrial agriculture. This type of agriculture resulted in losses of biodiversity in the food consumption/production process, non-response of soil microorganisms due to overuse of chemicals, and greenhouse gas emissions of which DCs contributed 14% of global output due to meat production (Thøgersen, 2010, vonMeyer-Höfer et al., 2015, Hart et al., 2013 for instance). In the form of social unsustainability, the evidence revealed heart related diseases, diabetes, respiratory diseases, and hypertension as the most salient feature of social unsustainability related to food consumption/production in DCs (Kearney, 2010, Reisch et al., 2013). Economic inefficiency consisted of waste of cereals, which were processed industrially to get output used to feed livestock rather than feeding these cereals directly to the livestock.

Table 1. Nature and extent of unsustainability across DCs and LDCs: summary of studies

	Studies	Environmental Degradation		Economic Inefficiency		Social Unsustainability		Data Sources Methodology	Contextual, Institutional Factors ant Extent
		LDCs	DCs	LDCs	DCs	LDCs	DCs		
1	(Alinov, 2010)	Environment degradation through traditional survival methods	NA	Insufficiency of of food, limited micronutrient	NA	Selling productive assets, dropping kids out of school	NA	Secondary survey data analysed with statistical methods	Social ill more prevalent in LDCs than in DCs, aggravated by absence of infrastructure in LDCs
2	(Amendah et al., 2014)	Environment degradation through traditional survival methods	NA	Insufficiency of food, limited micronutrient	NA	Selling productive assets, dropping kids out of school	NA	Household survey, use desctiptive statistics and logistic regression analysis	Absence of food more acute in LDCs than in DCs, aggravated by lack social safety nets
3	(Brown and Jacobson, 2005)	Destruction of rainforest to plant palm tree	NA	Costly to treat illness from saturated oil from palm tree	NA	Ill health from consumption of palm oil	NA	Source of data is documentary analysed and argue in relation to research question	Deforestation in LDCs, oil processing in DCs, extent: trade aggravate situation for LDCs
4	(Thøgersen, 2010)	NA	Green gas house emission, loss of biodiversity	NA	Pricing distortions	NA	NA	Data on published research analysed using qualitative methods	LDCs benefit less of subsidies as buffer to price shocks than Dcs
5	(Reisch et al., 2013)	NA	Mechanized agriculture, use of pesticides	NA	Process of globalization resulting in inequalities	NA	Heart related diseases	Source of data is documentary analysed and argue in relation to research question	Mechanized agriculture more in DCs than in LDCs, LDCs, food in high energy increasing in LDCs
6	(Kearney, 2010)	Degradation of through limited usage input	Excessive water and land use in dunstrial sector	NA	NA	NA	Saturated consumption fat leading to heart related diseases	Source of data is documentary analysed and argue in relation to research question	Governments in LDCs and policies in these countries are less responsive to these issues than in DCs
7	(Han and Hansen, 2012)	NA	NA	NA	NA	Health effect of food consumption and behaviour	High energy meat consumption leading to cardio vascular diseases	Literature Meta-analyses	Increasing consumption of unhealthy food in urban area of LDCs is due to aggravate health outcomes
8	(vonMeyer-Höfer et al., 2015)	Depletion of resources, unequal access, loss of biodiversity in LDCs	NA	Depletion of resources, unequal access, loss of biodiversity in LDCs	NA	Unequal access to resources In LDCs	NA	Online consumers survey analysed within the context theory of planned behaviours and structural equation modelling in China and India	LDCs suffer more unequal access to resources than in DCs
9	(Vermeir and Verbeke, 2006)	NA	NA	NA	Consumption processes that result in higher prices	NA	Consumption behaviour in high energy food	Survey data Documents reviews	Policy intervention on more prevalent in DCs than in LDCs
	(Hart et al., 2013)	NA	Degraded environment as a result of degradation	NA	Not halting the loss of biodiversity in the production process	NA	Exposure to pollution resulting in respiratory diseases	Source of data is documentary analysed and argue in relation to research question	DCs institutions own promoting fresh food non existing in LDCs

continues on following page

Table 1. Continued

Studies	Environmental Degradation		Economic Inefficiency		Social Unsustainability		Data Sources Methodology	Contextual, Institutional Factors ant Extent
	LDCs	DCs	LDCs	DCs	LDCs	DCs		
10 (Vogit, 2014)	NA	Process where prod and consumer relate in DCs	NA	More power from producers when they are not connected to food	NA	Increase in consuming unhealthy food with no influence of consumer	Source of data is documentary analysed and argue in relation to research question	DCs institutions own promoting fresh food non existing in LDCs
11 (Grunert et al., 2014)	NA	Consumption of environment unfriendly food and unhealthy	NA	NA	NA	Consumption related social unsustainability in terms caaaaardio vascular diseases	Online survey data Data analysed were hierarchal regression	Prevalent in DCs and in LDCs but LDCs have less mitigating set ups
12 (McKenzie and Williams, 2015b)	System that lead to water and sold degradation, loss of biodiverse	System that lead to water and sold degradation, loss of biodiverse	Productivity growth due to decreased owing soil degradation	Productivity growth due to decreased owing soil degradation	Absence of balanced nutrients	Over consumption of meat products	Source of data is documentary analysed and argue in relation to research question	Absence of governance and management of unsustainability more prevalent in LDCs
13 (Bryceson, 2004)	Livelihood that do not cater for environmental shock	NA	Inefficient in food production system	NA	Livelihood results in insufficiency of food	NA	Source of data is documentary analysed and argue in relation to research question	Policy based on contextual vulnerability less prevalent in LDCs than in DCs
14 (Hobson, 2002)	NA	Environmental impacts of consumption pattersn	NA	Inefficient use of land in terms of production	NA	Ignorance Toxic materials and waste emission	Documentary, conceptual, argumentative	Politically dominant approach to prevent unsustainable actions more in DCs than in LDCs
15 (Horrigan et al., 2002)	NA	Consumption process that degrade environment in DCs	NA	Externality of unsustainable production not included in pricing	NA	Production process that results in health outcome	Source of data is documentary analysed and argue in relation to research question	More institutions to deal with these issues in DCs than in LDCs
16 (Johnson et al., 2014)	Production that results in Poverty and nutrition	Loss of biodiversity Large scale acquisition of land	Allocative inefficiency as some community do not get basic food	NA	Production systems that result in hunger in LDCs	Increased consumption rich in energy and meat in LDCs and DCs	Nutrition survey Uses a causal model	Institutional in DCs are more socially inclusive that those in LDCs
17 (Mózner, 2013)	Production that do not allow calories intake	Production and consumption that damage environment	Production inefficient	Demand for land based resources in other countries	Hunder and food poverty	High beef meat consumption	Biophysical methodology	Institutions that treat environmental issues and health simultaneously, less prevalent in LDCs than in DCs
18 (Nemecek et al., 2016)	NA	Production system that degrades environment	NA	Poor production methods. unfair market through international trade	Health and other social dimension		Source of data is documentary analysed and argue in relation to research question	LDCs suffer more effects of international trade in food than DCs
19 (Clapp, 2017)	Crop that are associated with deforestation	Crop that are associated with a lot of water usage	High food price		Hunger, famine, aggravated	NA	Documentary, reviewed with argumentative approach	Food output and modern agriculture more limited in LDCs than in DCs
20 (Randolph et al., 2007)	Process that produce livestock are beneficial	NA	Not maximizing productivity per animal	NA	Insufficient production of animal stock	NA	Documentary, analytical	Livestock production, limited in LDCS than DCs

continues on following page

Table 1. Continued

Studies	Environmental Degradation		Economic Inefficiency		Social Unsustainability		Data Sources Methodology	Contextual, Institutional Factors ant Extent
	LDCs	DCs	LDCs	DCs	LDCs	DCs		
21 (Garnett, 2014)	NA	Environment degradation from the supply chain	Unequal distributing of the product in LDCs and DCs	Pricing and subsidies distortions	System that produce food that not culturally acceptable	NA	Documentary, argumentative	Institutions to minimize environment degradation less prevalent in LDCs compared to DCs
22 (Cullet, 2004)	NA	NA	Production process that do not assure fairness in food distribution		Technological development not aimed at providing food security	NA	Documentary, qualitative analysis	Legal regime needed to take account of the food needs is less established in LDCs
23 (International Institute of Social Studies, 2015)	NA	NA	NA	NA		Consumption of unhealthy processed product	Online surveys from consumers Descriptive statistics and hierarchical regressions	Limited institutions to respond to consequences in LDCs
24 (Pretty et al., 2003)	Technologies that sustain environment	NA	Limited agricultural productivity	NA	NA	NA	Survey data Analysis of based on the questionnaire	Insufficient means to acquire inputs, lack of institutional
25 (Freibauer et al., 2011)	NA	biofuel and industrial materials compete with food for biomass	NA	Less variety of food.		Absence of non-sustainable diets	Documentary, argumentative analysis	Instituting that balance diets
26 (Godfray et al., 2010)	Competition for land and water resources	Completion of land and water aggravated by climate change		Feeding grain to live stock rather than feeding them directly to human is inefficient	High growth of population, income inequality	Change in consumption patterns	Literature Reviews of the evidence	Adopting new technologies Is a challenge
27 (Capone et al., 2014)	Food systems that degrade environment	Food systems that degrade environment			Food systems that result in hunger		Documentary argumentative Research	Institutions that moderate good production system more prevalent in DCs
28 (Alemu, 2010)	Production process that result in poverty	NA	Farming activities generating less income	NA	Strategies that might affect some other aspects of well-being	NA	Data from general households survey analysed with descriptive stats	Institutions aimed at understanding socioeconomic fabric of the population more available in DCs
29 (Alinov, 2010)	Production process affected by climate shock	NA	Suffer price instability of the food system	NA	Production process result in food insecurity	NA	Used a survey, analysed using descriptive statistics	Institutions that cater for the most vulnerable household to price and climate shock
30 (Risku-Norja, 2011)	NA	Production process that degrade environment	NA	NA	NA	Consumption of animal food	Documentary, analysis	
31 (Stewart et al., 2013)	NA	Production system that do not provide enough food to urban population in LDCs	NA	Inefficiency in urban food market	Production system that do not provide enough food to urban population in LDCs	NA	Documentary, literature analysis	Urban population more growing in LDCs than in DCs
32 (Dobermann and Nelson, 2013)	Absence of agro-ecological intensification	Unsustainable use of waters and land soil nutrients		Absence of agro ecological intensification process	absence of economic, social and Eco local principles of farmers need	Process that don not consider social context of famers	Documentary review, argumentative	Inequity in terms of accessing inputs

continues on following page

Table 1. Continued

	Studies	Environmental Degradation		Economic Inefficiency		Social Unsustainability		Data Sources Methodology	Contextual, Institutional Factors ant Extent
		LDCs	DCs	LDCs	DCs	LDCs	DCs		
33	(Carlsson-Kanyama and Gonzalez, 2009)	NA	Agricultural practice that are damaging in DCs	NA	Losses in production due wastage in energy	NA	Agricultural practice leading to unhealthy diets in DCs	Documentary, argumentative analysis	Institutions that control the greenhouse emissions
34	(Pretty and Noble, 2006)	Production lacking technology that are not harmful in LDCs	NA	Urbanisation is causing shift in consumption and pricing		Processes that result in insufficiency of food in LDCs	NA	Interview with farmers analyse using descriptive statistics	Political involvement is the way forwards
35	Bert et al. (2017)	NA	Food consumption that lead to unsustainable production n DCs	NA	Process do not use efficiently resources	NA	Process not producing health food	Documentary, argumentative analysis	Institution on heath information and better nutrition more available in DCs
36	(Lorek and Fuchs, 2013)	Governance that does not take care of sustainability	Governance that does not take care of sustainability	NA	Policy that focus on growth only without considering environment	Governance that does not take account of social burden of consumption	NA	Argumentative analysis	Incorporate external costs into prices, technological innovation
37	(Kasa, 2008)	NA	Process resulting in overconsumption	Process that result in diversified foods	Beef consumption process might result in shortage of global		Process allowing social issue to arise from beef consumption	Documentary, argumentative methods	Information's and discouragement
38	(Seyfang and Smith, 2007)	NA	Technologies that do not safeguard environment	NA	Markets that are not transformed for sustainable choice	NA	The lack of a social and active citizenship	Documentary, argumentative community level factor	Institution that incorporate social culture into consumption
39	(Temme et al., 2015)	NA	Process that do not replace plant-based product by high energy food	NA	NA	NA	Absence of sustaible diets	Survey,, energy and nutrient intake observed and analysed	Public health institution combine sustaible message
40	(Friedl et al., 2014)	NA	Increase in consumption that degree environment	NA	Influence of these on energy use	NA	Create obesity, disability and chronic diseases	Survey, household analysis of sustainable consumption and regression analysis	Public canteen to cater for fresh food more prevalent in DCs
41	(Amendah et al., 2014)	Consumption system that degraded envir in LDCs	NA	Buying good on credit	NA	Removing children from school	NA	Secondary data analysis from another study using descriptive methods	Public insition that cushion social ills
42	(Herrera-Estrella, 2000)	Process that make water and soil dwindling	NA	Limited use of efficient methods	NA	Crop yields are significantly lower	NA	Literature Critical analysis	Limited capacity to store food that are produced
43	(Khan et al., 2014)	Production system not taking account of climate change in LDCs	NA	Productions are inefficiency	NA	Food insecurity in sub-sharan Africa	NA	Literature Document reviews	Use push pull technology to allow the dealing
44	(Herrero and Thorntonb, 2010)	Livestock Taking land	livestock	NA	Overconsumption	Some part	All of the developed world	Literature Documents review	Developed and developing

NA means that there is no evidence in the study referring to that types of unsustainability

Different patterns of unsustainability were observed in LDCs. Although there was some sort of environmental unsustainability in the form of carbon emissions from industrial agriculture, this was not the predominant one. The environment in these countries is degraded rather through traditional methods of food consumption/production, which result in deforestation, soil erosion from rain, and soil deterioration because of limited technological inputs. Regarding social unsustainability, the evidence revealed hunger and limited variety in food, deficiency in micronutrients (Amendah et al., 2014), and conflicts over land tenure as the most common features of social unsustainability. Furthermore, LDCs suffer limited food output which leads to strategies that are likely to perpetuate and complicate social unsustainability. These strategies consist of contracting debts to get food (Alinov, 2010, Gautam and Andersen, 2016) and removing children from school to help in work related to food search. Economic inefficiency is more abundant in LDCs and included inappropriate storing of food, and misuse of land by planting inappropriate crops (Pretty et al., 2003).

These patterns of unsustainability across DCs and LDCs stem from their food consumption/production processes and their institutional makeup. In DCs, most of the evidence (about 40% of reviewed studies) focus on environmental degradation in terms of loss of biodiversity, water resources, and the non-response of soil to microorganisms. This degradation stem from mechanized agriculture linked to industrial production of processed high-energy food in these countries. Mass processing of high-energy food is mainly driven by increasing consumption in these products in urban areas of LDCS due to globalization and less regulated trade of these products (see for example Brown and Jacobson, 2005). Consumption of high-energy food is in contrast stable and likely to decrease in DCs. It is also worth to note that declining population in DCs which takes place jointly with increasing incomes per capita result in more high-energy meat products per capita. The resulting outcome is the development of cardiovascular diseases. Such outcomes clearly follow the production process and other contexts (declining population and high income). Similarly, the patterns observed in LDCs stem from their contexts of production and social conditions. Even if some features of industrialized agriculture as well as rising incomes in the developed world are observed in some parts of LDCs (Connell, 2010, Bryceson, 2004, Bulte and Soest, 2001), there are notable differences. The evidence shows that soil degradation through erosion, traditional agricultural methods, limited use of technology and excessive degradation of soil productivity, characterize these countries. These outcomes stem from traditional agricultural practices involving deforestation as a way to gain agricultural land and firewood (Pretty et al., 2003). These traditional methods result further in very low crop yields amidst growing populations and inefficiencies in production processes, which result in hunger and malnutrion. The absence of or very limited safety nets, the illiteracy rate, and the lack of strong institutions complicate matters, resulting in conflicts over land in the quest for survival, which lead to injuries and deaths. Furthermore, hardship in these countries leads to the adoption of survival strategies such as dropping children from school, contracting debts and selling assists (Gautam and Andersen, 2016) which are likely to worsen the well-being of future generations.

The evidence revealed further that, even in case of the unsustainability being the same in nature across LDCs and DCs, the extent of the damages is higher in LDCs. In these countries' contexts, insufficiency of food and food insecurity prevail side- by -side with urban situations similar to those in DCs. While some urban population of DCs are being exposed to high energy food and suffer the same illness as in DCs, they suffer additional inconvenience specific to their predicaments such as limited social infrastructures. DCs' production process established in LDCs through multinationals add to the vulnerability of the environment and people in these countries, a situation that is aggravated by the interdependence and trade through globalization. The evidence also indicate that production processes in DCs influence environment degradation in LDCs when food processing in DCs require the use raw food commodities in LDCs (Brown and Jacobson, 2005 for example). The extent of damages in LDCs is further inflated by absence or limited safety and social systems, environmental management policies, and health systems to cater for these impacts. LDCs suffer most of food price shocks and unequal distribution of the food products, and benefit less from subsidies by their governments than DCs. Low literacy rates and low health literacy rates amid fast urban migration in LDCs increase unawareness of health risks associated with exposure to processed food than is the case in DCs. Evidence of land competition exists in DCs and LDCs, but might not result in serious injuries due to regulation and the definition of property rights in DCs (Barnidge et al., 2011).

Briefly, the institutions, settings and social contexts in DCs and LDCs shape the features of unsustainability as well as the extent of this unsustainability. The consumption/production processes in DCs results in greenhouse gas emissions, the overproduction/consumption of unhealthy food, long term non-communicable diseases but with a trend and movement towards decreasing these patterns. The institutional setting mitigates these impacts through social safety nets and proper regulation more than institutions in LDCs do.

Unsustainability of Food Consumption and Health: DCs vs. LDCs

The reviewed literature also revealed that consumption/production processes in DCs and LDCs determine mechanisms leading to ill health (Table 2). Starting with the review of diseases arising from unsustainable consumption/production, the diseases included communicable and non-communicable diseases. The review revealed that diseases most common to DCs were predominantly non-communicable such as cardiovascular and respiratory diseases. The review showed also that these non-communicable diseases were prevalent in urban settings of LDCs. Nevertheless, infectious, short term diseases, were the most prevalent diseases in LDCs while DCs suffered mainly from non-communicable diseases of a long term duration. LDCs also suffered diseases arising from injury, emotional stress and fatigue. Although many factors can be responsible for these diseases, income levels, lifestyles systems, and contexts, which are believed to differ across DCs and LDcs, are likely to determine the mechanisms linking food production/consumption to these illness

A close analysis of the evidence about how these diseases occur reveals that non-communicable diseases in DCs occur through a long-time exposure to risk of air pollution or some type of consumption for a long period of time. Over an extended period, the exposure to polluted environment produces the effects that lead to respiratory diseases. Other diseases occur in these countries, as noted earlier, because people eat a lot of processed industrial food. The long-term effects of consuming this type of food is the development of heart diseases, obesity and diabetes, which have serious long-term consequences for the population.

In contrast, the review of the evidence suggests that diseases in LDCs are predominantly infectious diseases. In the rural parts of these countries, exposure to air pollution is less serious. Rather, a different kind of pollution in the form of debris prevails. This type of pollution arises from soil erosion which in turn happens as a result of deforestation which is such that when it rains, debris gets dumped into rivers whose water is used for drinking and cooking in households. The use of this water culminates in infectious waterborne diseases such as cholera and diarrhea and other infectious diseases. The common crowding and the absence of sanitation in these circumstances aggravate the situation by facilitating contamination. Furthermore, deforestation in these countries results in mudslides when it rains, leading to injuries and deaths. The other mechanism leading to diseases arises from survival strategies. People face shortages of food and consequent nutritional deficiencies lead to fatigue, dizziness and poor immune function. It should be noted that on way of responding to the shortage of food in order to survive is to try and get more arable land. This often results in clashes between communities, which lead to injuries and deaths. Working an excessive number of hours a day in an effort to satisfy household needs for food is also a mechanism leading to ill health in these countries. Finally, as in DCs, increasing numbers of people are exposed to air pollution and to the consumption of processed food following a process of urbanisation, implying that this segment of the population is set to suffer from respiratory diseases as well.

A review of the mechanisms through which these diseases occur suggests some patterns in these mechanisms and inherent types of diseases. While diseases patterns can be attributed to a myriad of factors, these factors are in fact embedded in types of unsustainable production/consumption. The extensive production of processed food in fact results in air pollution. Not only air pollution, but also the inhalation of chemicals used in the production of food such as vegetables. The greater availability of processed meat products results in the overconsumption of these products, which results in diseases such as heart diseases. Prolonged exposure to air pollution gives rise to other chronic diseases such as respiratory diseases. The evidence of these linkages explains why the problem of chronic non-communicable diseases is most prevalent in DCs and among the well-off urban populations of LDCs.

In the poor parts of LDCs in contrast, processes that lead to diseases are different. In these countries, traditional agriculture is inefficient with respect to land usage, which results in very limited crop yields. The associated deforestation not only results in loss of biodiversity but also in degradation of land through erosion. The aggravating factors in these countries are weak institutions, the high growth rate of the population and the fact that firewood is the main source of energy. As reported in the literature these factors are related to health outcomes in many ways. First, low crop yields means that people have not enough food, and limited food leads to deaths and disease associated with malnutrition. Second, sections of the population are exposed to contaminated water resulting in waterborne infectious diseases aggravated by prevailing poor sanitation, third, coping strategies include fighting to get better land for crops, and in social and psychological behaviours that result in drug addiction and prostitution. This evidence now makes it clear why we have more hunger-related deaths, diseases of malnutrition and more infectious diseases in these countries.

Briefly, the evidence discussed above suggests that consumption and production processes result in different mechanisms leading to ill health. These processes in addition to existing institutions and ways of life result in patterns of diseases that are different across DCs and LDCs. It was shown in particular that DCs and urbanized areas of LDCs experience similar mechanisms leading to chronic diseases with some exceptions of food insecurity (Ekpenyong, 2015), while the rural parts of the developing world are likely to suffer mainly short-term and infectious diseases. The evidence in particular showed that production processes result in diseases of overconsumption, while mechanisms of production lead to diseases of poverty. Since processes, circumstances and institutions determine the nature and extent of unsustainability and mechanisms leading to ill health, policy making should take into account differences in these processes across DCs and LDCs.

Table 2. Mechanisms of linkage to health in DCs and LDCs: summary of the studies.

Study no	Study	Production	Consumption	Mechanism	Type of Ill Health	LDCs	DCs	Contextual and Institutional Factors	Methodology
1	(Kasa, 2008)	Production of beef degrades health and environment	Process focusing on animal product	Long exposure to air pollution	Respiratory diseases	NA	✓	DCs have more food processing in DCs but LDCs also exposed	Source of data is documentary analysed and argue in relation to research question
2	(Amendah et al., 2014)	Food shortage	Insufficient food	Working excessive hours in informal, conflicts over land tenure	Fatigue, emotional stress, injury	✓	NA	Mechanism more unique to LDCs	Source of data is documentary analysed and argue in relation to research question
3	(Barnidge et al., 2011)	Shortage of land, poor distribution of structural factor	Absence of sustainable consumption	Involvements in conflicts to get	Different types of injury	✓		Conflicts over land is a mechanism more unique to LDCs	Qualitative participatory methods to get perception from community
4	(Gauker. 2010). (Reisch et al., 2013)	Chemicals effects consumed in the food	Chemicals effects consumed in the food	Chemical infected food leading to resistance to antibiotics	Heart diseases and respiratory diseases		✓	Some regulations exist to stop mechanism	Source of data is documentary analysed and argue in relation to research question
5	(Godfray et al., 2010)	Production process that tend to safeguard livestock as a capital in LDS	Lifestyles that reduce the consumption of meat	Insufficient calorie intake Drinking contaminated water	Chronic diseases, diseases of poverty	✓	✓	Insufffient food intake, contaminated water mechanism unique to LDCs	Documentary, argumentative method
6	(vonMeyer-Höfer et al., 2015)	NA	unwariness of health motives in choosing consumption in china and india	Consumption of high saturated fat	Herat diseases	✓	NA	DCs have more saturated fat but LDCs also exposed	Online consumer survey analysed with econometric analysis
7	(Reisch et al., 2013)	Social: Food shortage	Deforestation	Injury due to mud sliding as a result of deforest	Various types of diseases	✓	✓	Injury due to mud sliding unique to LDCs	Documentary analysis
8	(Kearney, 2010)	Production of food rich in animal products	High saturated food	Increase in consumptions of saturated fat	Cardio diseases and diabetes	NA	✓	DCs have more food processing in DCs but LDCs also exposed	Systematic reviews
9	(Pretty et al., 2003)	Food shortage	Health saturated fats	Shift towards diversified diets	Heart diseases	NA	✓	DCs have more food processing in DCs but LDCs also exposed	Analysis of survey data and qualitative information
10	(Han and Hansen, 2012)	Degradation of environ related food	Food choices that are unsustainable	Compelled to consume these foods. Pyscho-social	Heart diseases	NA	✓	DCs have more food processing in DCs but LDCs also exposed d	Databases of empirical studies, evidence of which is synthetized
11	(Vermeir and Verbeke, 2006)		Consumption processes that do not take into account social responsibilities	Attitude behaviour and perception	Obesity and	✓	✓	DCs have more food processing in DCs but LDCs also exposed	These more placed in DCs
12	(Freibauer et al., 2011)	Production of waste	Overconsumptions	Waste, overconsumption	Heart diseases	✓	✓	DCs have more food processing in DCs but LDCs also exposed	Documentary evidence
13	(Vogit, 2014)	Production process not allowing consumer	Consumption patterns showing limited consumer	Getting food from supermarkets	Chronic illness	NA	✓	DCs have more of the mechanism but LDCs also exposed	Documentary, argumentative analysis
14	(Temme et al., 2015)	Not based of dietary patterns resulting in sustainable	Not linking public health to consumption	Getting high energy food	Chronic diseases	✓	✓	DCs have more of the mechanism but LDCs also exposed	Survey, energy and calorie s intake observed
15	(Friedl et al., 2014)	Process of consumption that affect prod process	Consumption process that affect heath	Overproduction of food	Chronic diseases	✓	✓	DCs have more of the mechanism but LDCs also exposed	Source of data is documentary analysed and argue in relation to research question

continues on following page

Table 2. Continued

Study no	Study	Production	Consumption	Mechanism	Type of Ill Health	LDCs	DCs	Contextual and Institutional Factors	Methodology
16	(Thøgersen, 2010)	Absence of organic food	Consumption of food that is not organics	Heath problem and consumption of animal fat	Chronic diseases	✓	✓	DCs have more of the mechanism but LDCs also exposed	Documentary, analysis
17	(Risku-Norja, 2011)	Production in animal rich energy food	Production of unhealthy food	Increasing overnatution in animal meat	Chronic	✓	✓	DCs have more of the mechanism but LDCs also exposed	Documentary, analysis
18	(Oni, 2010)	Poverty and food insufficiency	Absence of sufficient food	Food insecurity and hunger	Chronic and infectious	✓	NA	Limited food and related illness unique to LDCs	Source of data is documentary analysed and argue in relation to research question
19	(McMichael et al., 2007)	Livestock production consume more energy	Consumption results in fat	Increase in meat consumption		✓	✓	Policy that prevent both health risk and environment degradation	Documentary
20	(Mont and plepys, 2005)	Consummers influence productive process	Consumes consume unsustainably	Health problems	Short and chronic diseases	✓	✓	Instruction that motivate behaviour	Documentary analysis
21	(Mózner, 2013)	Production options not orientated towards health	Consumption options not orientated toward health	Overocumption of unhealthy animal products	Cardio	NA	✓	Intuitions linking consumption to health	Biophical methods
22	(World Health Organisation, 2003a)	Contribution to greenhouse gas emissions	Consumption of energy dense diet	Over consumption	Chronic diseases	✓	✓	Food policy to deal with health issues	Documentary evidence, descriptive analyses
23	(World Health organisation, 2003b)	Production process that result in ovary affect health	Insufficient consumption	Insufficient calories	All sorts of diseases	✓	NA	Institutions in DCs	Documentary analysis
24	(Godfray and Garnett, 2014)	Deforestation, water use overfishing, pollution and biodiversity loss	Growing populations and increasing demand for food	Insufficient food or over consumption of unhealthy food	All sort of diseases	✓	✓	Adopt intensification that is coherent through governance	Argumentative methods
25	(McKenzie and Williams, 2015a)	Process that results in food insecurity in LDCs, and more unhealthy food in DCs	Process that lead to over consumption and under nutrient	Overconsumption and under consumption	Underweight And overweight in LDCs overweigh in DC	✓	✓	DCs have more saturated fat but LDCs also exposed	Documentary, argumentative research
26	(Horrigan et al., 2002)	Factory style animal agriculture affect health	Process involving consumption of animal fact in LDCs and DCs	Degenerative disease in LDCs and DCs	Chronic heart related diseases	✓	✓	DCs have more saturated fat but LDCs also exposed	Documentary, argumentative
27	(Pretty et al., 2003)	Use of nonrenewable unhealthy inputs	Very limited consumption and food insecurity	Through inhalation, through hunger	Infectious disease	✓	NA	DCs have more saturated fat but LDCs also exposed	Questionnaire data, analysed using descriptive statistics
28	(Herrero and Thorntonb, 2010)	NA	More avaaibility in processed food	Consumption of high-energy processed food		✓	✓	DCs have more saturated fat but LDCs also exposed	Source of data is documentary analysed and argue in relation to research question
29	(DeBon et al., 2010)	Not taking account of urban migration	NA	Persistence inefficiency in agriculture resulting in limited food	Food insecurity and unhealthy food	✓ NA		Persistence inefficiency in agriculture resulting in limited food more in LDCs	Documentary analysis
30	(Johnson et al., 2014)	Biodiversity loss and ecosystem degradation	Obesity, suffering micro-nutrition	Eating patterns, poverty, eating meat product, urbanisation	Heart disease and others		✓ Long	DCs have ways of avoiding but process being initiated in LDCs	Source of data is documentary analysed and argue in relation to research question

continues on following page

Table 2. Continued

Study no	Study	Production	Consumption	Mechanism	Type of Ill Health	LDCs	DCs	Contextual and Institutional Factors	Methodology
31	(Clapp, 2017)	Insufficient production in food of some types	Insufficient type of healthy diet	Overconsumption of unhealthy of available but unhealthy food	Heart diseases	NA	✓	DCs have more saturated fat but LDCs also exposed	Documentary, argumentative analysis
32	(Carlsson-Kanyama and Gonzalez, 2009)	Processes not taking into account healthy diets	Consumptions process not informed by campaign	Consumption of unhealthy diets	Non communicable disease		✓	DCs have more saturated fat but LDCs also exposed	Documentary sources analysed with argumentative methods
33	(Seligman et al., 2009)	Food insecurity	Food insecurity and health outcomes in DCs	Diet in high energy food ases	Heart diseases	✓	✓	DCs have more saturated fat but LDCs also exposed	Survey data analysed quantitatively
34	(Kjærga et al., 2013)	Not including health promotion strategies in production	NA	Production process not taking care of health consideration	Malnutrition	✓	✓	Production process not taking care of health consideration more in LDCs	Documentary analysis
35	(Vermeir and Verbeke, 2006)		Consuming high fat meat	Attitude and behaviour	Obesity, heart diseases			Attitude and behaviour more looked at in DCs	Documentary
36	(Europian public health association, 2017)	Process that follows unhealthy consumption	Consumption process affect environment	Consumption of unhealthy product influencing production	Chronic diseases	✓	✓	Consumption of unhealthy product influencing production more in DCs	Documentary, argumentative analysis
37	(Hawkes, 2006)	Insufficient taking into account agriculture and health	NA	Hunger and obesity happening simultaneous	Hunger related diseases	✓	✓	Hunger and obesity happening simultaneous in LDCs	Source of data is documentary analysed and argue in relation to research question
38	(Mackay and Wolbring, 2013b)	Not linking production and health	Not linking consumption and health	Hunger and obesity happening simultaneous	Hunger related diseases	✓	✓	Hunger and obesity happening simultaneous	Documentary
39	(Ekpenyong, 2015)	Production process orientated towards urban consumption	Food insecurity in urban areas	Hunger and obesity happening simultaneous	Chronic diseases and poverty diseases	✓	✓ NA	Institution that deal with food security more in DCs	Relied on secondary data based on growth analysis
40	(Connell, 2010)	Not linking livelihood and health	Not linking livelihood and health	Injury and other possible outcomes	Chronic and other diseases	✓	NA	Net to operationalize livelihood and health to go hand in hand	

NA means that there is no evidence in study referring to that types of unsustainability

Unsustainability of Food Consumption and Policies: DCs vs. LDCs

In spite of differences across LDCs and DCs, a review of the evidence on the response policies, however, revealed that these policies took into account neither the differences in institutional set-ups nor the production processes that shape mechanisms to ill health and unsustainable food consumption. Most of the policies reviewed consisted of policies to increase output while safeguarding the environment. These were policies such as watershed and irrigation management, integrated ecological demonstrations (Pretty et al., 2003), bans on pesticides, support for organic agriculture, ecological farming to implement Agenda 21, placing value on the natural capital and taxing unsustainable use. Other policies were aimed at sustainable consumption that safeguards the environment, such as restrictions on international trade in processed food while nurturing healthy lifestyles, and labelling processed food to make the consumer aware of the unsustainability of certain food (Table 3).

To be effective and equitable under prevailing circumstances in DCs and LDCs, policies need to incorporate aspects of differences in institutional settings and production processes that impact on unsustainability. To assess whether policies took into account production processes and policies across DCs and LDCs, policies were evaluated with respect to the source of the policy, the proposer of the policy, the issue of focus, and the involvement of local political institutions.

With respect to the context from where policy proposals emanate, a review of the evidence revealed that most policy proposals arise from research and from policy makers in DCs (Table 3). The evidence reviewed showed that most of the policy documents and policy research papers make up about 90% of the reviewed documents. This evidence implies that policies did not take into account, at least sufficiently, the effects of institutions and consumption/production processes in LDCs.

With respect to the issues of focus, policies focused on issues such as reducing unsustainable food consumption through trade, placing a value on natural resources and taxing unsustainable use (Griggs, 2013), self-sufficiency and limiting international trade in processed food (Kearney, 2010, Clapp, 2017), labeling of processed food, emphasizing nutritional consideration in agricultural practices, and reducing the production of saturated animal products (Pretty et al., 2003). Policies that refer to the use of biological fertilizer, soil conservation, and biotechnological meant to meet food shortages in LDCs, did not specify how these are to be practical given the current predicament in these countries. The evidence indicated that these countries are characterized by poor soil quality as a result of inefficient usage practices aggravated by climatic conditions, lack of economic resources as well as issues relating to keeping stock, but how these would be effectively overcome were not addressed.

An analysis of these issues shows that, in spite of the fact that contexts in LDCs countries lead to more impact of unsustainability, policy has been disproportionally directed towards the DCs issues. For instance, reducing unsustainable food consumption by restricting international trade in some of the processed foods traded is likely to work for DCs. For the majority of the population in DCs, this policy appears to be irrelevant since the production processes in these countries result in shortages of food. They would, therefore, be better off consuming processed food via international trade than consuming no food at all. Furthermore, valuing and taxing the usage of natural resources is less relevant in LDCs due to limited expertise to value different types of natural resources in these countries. Given that the issues focused on are more likely to reflect the institutions and realities in DCs, the evidence suggest inequities within these policies.

Table 3. Policy equity across LDCs and DCs.

	Study	Source: Policy Design Context	Degradation	Social Unsustainability Policy	Econo Inefficiencies	Data Methodology	Areas of Focus	Policy	Suitability to LIC ? Suitability to LIC ?
1	(Brown and Jacobson, 2005)	Policy makers		Negative effects of palm oil on health		Reports and document information Descriptive analysis	Developed country	Labels dangers of product. discourage processing	No. No related measure from source Yes. Policy directly targeted at consumption in DCs
2	(Garnett et al., 2016b)	Research in DCs	Completion of land water and energy	Food shortage	NA	Documentary, argumentative analysis	Developed country	Sustainable intensification	Most relevant to both DCs and LDCs
3	(Seyfang and Smith, 2007)	Research	Degraded environment	Social concerns	NA	Reports	Developed country	Combine environment and social policy	Most relevant to DCs
4	(Carlsson-Kanyama and Gonzalez, 2009)	Research	Green gas house emission	NA	NA	Documentary, review and analysis	Developed country	Reduce meat consumption, encourage energy efficient food	Most relevant to DCs
5	(Reisch et al., 2013)	Research in DCs and LDcs	Environment degradation	Reduced meat consumption	Wastages	Documentary, analysis of documentary evidence	Developed country	Avoid product by airplane	Most relevant DCs
6	(Pretty et al., 2003)	Research focusing in LDCs	Negative effects of sustainable agriculture	NA	NA	Survey questionnaire analysed, reports Qualitative analysis and descriptive statistics	Developed country	Political involvements	Most relevant to DCs
7	(Griggs, 2013)	Research general	Negative effect on environment	NA	NA	Online survey	Developed country	Taxing unsustainable use	No. inability to place a sound taxation system Yes. Taxation enforcement possible
8	(Kearney, 2010)	Research paper for DCs and LDCs	NA	Health degradation due to shifts	NA	Documentary review, argumentative	DCs and LDCs	Consider trade, agricultural and health factors	Relevant to both countries but mostly DCs
9	(Pretty et al., 2003)	Research Paper	Soil erosion	Hunger, poverty	Low productivity	Survey data Descriptive statistics	LDCs	National policy reforms	Non conducive, social and political conditions NA
10	(vonMeyer-Höfer et al., 2015)	Research in LDCs	NA	Health related are the key issues, food insecurity	NA	Structural equation modelling online survey and theory of planned behaviour	China and india	Change prices of food and improve the safety information	No, pricing information important to significantly reduce commotion No, pricing more important for poor community Bu marginally affected
11	(Vermeir and Verbeke, 2006)	Research in DCs	NA	Unsustainable consumption based on behaviours	NA	Surveys, descriptive and inferential methods	DCs	Change diets, marketing to influence behaviours	More relevant to DCs
12	(Kasa, 2008)	Research in DCs and LDCs	NA	Increase in beef consumption through trade	NA	Documentary, argumentative analysis	DCS LDCs	Regulate international trade in	Most relevant to DCs
13	(Europian public health association, 2017)	Policy documents	Consumption	diets that damage health and associated with		Documentary evidence Critical analysis	Europe	Reduce green gas house. Increase plant based consumption	Most suitable to DCs and LDCs
14	(Thøgersen, 2010)	Research in DCs	NA	Consumption practices	NA	Documentary, analysis of documentary evidence		Deal with institutional and culture practices	Most relevant to LDs

continues on following page

Table 3. Continued

	Study	Source: Policy Design Context	Degradation	Social Unsustainability Policy	Econo Inefficiencies	Data Methodology	Areas of Focus	Policy	Suitability to LIC ? Suitability to LIC ?
15	(Kesavan and Swaminathan, 2008)	Research in LDCs	Degradation	Food shortage	NA	Documentary, review and analysis	LDCs in Asia	Ecofriendly agriculture and on farm enterprise to intensify crop	Most relevant to LDCs
16	(Godfray and Garnett, 2014)	Research in DCs and LDCs	Degradation	Food shortage Over consumption	Wastages of resources e	Documentary evidence, argumentative analysis	DCs and LDCs	Moderate demand, reducing waste, good governance, sustainable intensification	Most relevant to DCs
17	(Herrero and Thorntonb, 2010)	Research in DCs and LDCs	Degradation	Food consumptions	NA	Documentary, argumentative analysis	DCs and LDCs	Combination of policy proposed	Most relevant to DCs
18	(Horrigan et al., 2002)	Research in Dcs	Water wastage, pesticides	Health issues	Externalities of unsustainable consumption	Documentary, argumentative methods	DCs	Pollution policies, consumption policies	Most relevant to DCs
19	(Britsih Dietitic Association, 1013)	Policy document in UK	NA	overconsumption	NA	NA	Developed country	Pricing, of unsustainable food	Most relevant for DCs
20	(Stewart et al., 2013)	Research	NA	NA	NA	NA	Developed country	Increase veg consumption	NA
21	(Lorek and Fuchs, 2013)	Research in DCs	Degradation	Overconsumption	NA	Documentary, review of stats	DCs	Focus on the consumption patterns	Most relevant DCs
22	(Oni, 2010)	Research	NA	NA	NA	NA	Developed country	Government should play a bigger role in address food policy	LDCs less involved in policy make king
23	(Sonigo et al., 2012)	Research	NA	NA	NA	NA	Developed country	NA	NA
24	(Clapp, 2017)	Research in DC	Trade in unsustainable food	Insufficiency of food	NA	Documentary, conceptual and argumenta tie methods	Europe	Selective self f-sufficient policies	Most relevant for DCs .
25	(Pretty and Noble, 2006)	Research in DCs and LDCs	Traditional methods	Low crop yield, hunger	NA	Commentary evidence Critical analysis	LDCs	Institutional, international and local, and institutional	Most relevant to DCs
26	(UNEP, 2012)	Research in DCs and LDCs		Unsustainable Diets	NA	Documentary evidence	LDCs and DCs	Reduce subsidies unsustainability	Most relevant
27	(Hobson, 2002)	Research paper in DCs	Consummation induced environment tal degradation	NA	NA	Interview with consumers	DCs	Reduce unsustainable consumption	More relevant for DCs
28	(Ekpenyong, 2015)	Reach paper in LDCs	NA	Urban poverty, food insecurity	NA	Secondary data, descriptive research design	Nigeria	Nutrition projects needed in cities	More relevant to LDCs

continues on following page

Table 3. Continued

	Study	Source: Policy Design Context	Degradation	Social Unsustainability Policy	Econo Inefficiencies	Data Methodology	Areas of Focus	Policy	Suitability to LIC ? Suitability to LIC ?
29	(Charles et al., 2010)	Research paper in Dcs and LDs	Water mismanagement in DCs	Food insecurity in DCs	Economic inefficiencies in DCs and LDCs	Documentary reviews	DCs and LDCs	Increase yield without expanding land	More relevant for both DCs a and LDCs
30	(Dobermann and Nelson, 2013)	Policy document in DCs and LDCs	All sorts of degradation	NA	NA	NA	DCs and LDCs	All environment policies aimed	More oriented to DCs due to health
31	(Freibauer et al., 2011)	Policy in DCs and LDCs	Resource scarcity due increasing demand	Unhealthy eating patterns	NA	Documentary, meta-review of documents	DCs and LDcs	Control food supply chain, change mindset, new technologies	Most relevant to DCs
32	(Johnson et al., 2014)	Research paper	NA	Unsustainable diets	NA	Survey, descriptive analysis and causal model	DCs	Find and respond factors of unsustable consumption	Most relevant to DCs
33	(vonBraun, 2007)	Policy document	NA	Food shortage and prices increase	NA	NA	DCs and LDCs	increase market access, impact food prices	Most relevant to DCs than to LDCs
34	(Europian commisison, 2015)	Policy documents	Environment degradation	Food shortage	Inefficiency	NA	LDCs	Variety of policies proposed	Most relevant

NA means that there is no evidence in study referring to that types of unsustainability

With respect to political involvement, most policy proposals involve political stakeholders in DCs than they do in DCs ones. Political governance has been found to be important in enforcing policies. Given that the role of political governance in countries is not taken into account by policy makers, it follows that policies that seek to deal with unsustainability would not be effective. Briefly, the above evidence and the implied equity for DCs and LDCs suggest that policies on unsustainable food production/consumption have not been guided by production processes and characteristics. Policies have been formulated more on the basis of insights on issues as they are in DCs rather than those in the developing world. New ways of dealing with unsustainable food consumption that are equitable for both DCs and LDCs need to be sought.

Discussion of the Evidence and the Way Forward

Institutional set-ups, people's lifestyles and their interactions have been found to be instrumental in determining food consumption/production processes. These processes are in turn crucial in explaining the unsustainability in food consumption/production as well as mechanisms leading to ill health. A reviewed literature indicated that these institutions and consumption/production processes in DCs and LDCs influence unsustainability of food consumption to a different extent. In spite of these differences and their implications for the nature and extent of unsustainability in food consumption/production across these countries, limited research has delved into assessing the possible role of institutions and consumption/production processes in these countries in determining the patterns of the nature, extent and mechanisms of unsustainability in food consumption/production. The questions in this study that have been asked specifically in this respect are 1) whether there is evidence for institutional set-ups and consumption/production processes influencing the nature and extent of unsustainability across DCs and LDCs; 2) whether mechanisms arising from these production processes link to ill health in different ways across these countries; and 3) whether policies dealing with unsustainable consumption/production have been equitable in taking into account different institutional and production processes across DCs and LDCs. These questions were answered by means of a systematic review of the literature.

The evidence revealed that declining populations, increasing income per capita and industrial-orientated food consumption/production processes in DCs result in the overproduction of processed food, which degrades the environment while hampering the health of people through overconsumption in high-energy diets. In contrast, DCs, which have a higher population growth rate, suffer from limited technology in food production processes, and from hunger and inadequate micro-nutrients alongside a degraded environment. The extent of unsustainability is deeper in LDCs as it is associated with the absence of safety nets, resulting in increased impoverishment and limited human capital formation for the next generation. This situation is aggravated by the movement of rural-to-urban migration (Ekpenyong, 2015:31), which exposes the urbanized part of the population in these countries to issues similar to those suffered by the population in DCs. The evidence revealed further that mechanisms leading to ill heath are different. LDCs suffer ill health that is both short- and long-term in nature due to direct exposure to degraded environments, but also due to malnutrition and hunger. Most of the contexts in LDCs give rise to burdens of diseases that are essentially infectious. The unsustainable situation in DCs culminates instead in long-term and non-communicable diseases.

In spite of these differences, policies have not been equitable. Policies have been developed from within the context of DCs and have largely ignored issues in LDCs due to limited involvement in policy making by stakeholders in LDCs. This oversight has been happening in spite of the recognition that policies tailored to issues in LDCs work (Pretty et al., 2003:217). The important role of paying attention to institutions, political and socio-cultural outcomes has also been highlighted as instrumental in policy equity (McKenzie and Williams, 2015a, Garnett et al., 2016a). Given that these differences in institutions across LDCs and DCs has not been contemplated, it follows that policies have not addressed equitably the issues of low food productivity and hunger and their ramifications in LDCs. The proposals to date, aimed at feeding the population projected to be 9 billion people in 2050 in a sustainable manner do not address many of the issues in LDCs, such as decreasing farm productivity and limited crop diversity. Most of the additional growth in population is, however, projected to come from these countries. Without localized sustainability policies, some LDCs will depend on the more generalized policy making, which is doomed to be ineffective in addressing prevailing issues equitably.

This situation calls for a change in the policy response to the challenges of sustainable food consumption brought about by different consumption and production processes across DCs and LDCs. Policies that focus on specific aspects in these countries, would involve local political bodies and country-specific polices tackling both underfeeding and overfeeding in LDCs. While geopolitical issues do not allow to take needs and possibilities for poorest countries (Freibauer et al., 2011:16, UNCTAD, 2011) change is needed for these countries to be considered in a more integrated policy frameword. As a way forward, a unified policy framework is needed that incorporates aspects such that these policies work for both DCs and LDCs. According to the status quo, these policies are inclined towards DCs and need to change to include focus on issues affecting most parts of LDCs, such as the shortage of food, inclusion of localized policy proposals and reforms, and ensuring a buy-in from political stakeholders in these countries.

REFERENCES

Alemu, Z. G. (2010). *Livelihood strategies in rural South Africa: Implications for poverty reduction. International Association of Agricultural Economists (IAAE).* Foz do Iguacu, Brazil: Triennial Conference.

Alinov, L. (2010). Livelihoods strategies and household resilience to food insecurity: An empirical analysis to Kenya. In Promoting Resilience through Social Protection in Sub-Saharan Africa. Dakar, Senegal: Academic Press.

Amendah, D. D., Buigut, S., & Mohamed, S. (2014). Coping strategies among urban poor: Evidence from Nairobi, Kenya. *PLoS One*, *9*(1), 1–8. doi:10.1371/journal.pone.0083428 PMID:24427272

Barnidge, E., Baker, E. A., Motton, F., Fitzgerald, T., & Rose, F. (2011). Exploring community health through the Sustainable Livelihoods Framework. *Health Education & Behavior*, *38*(1), 80–90. doi:10.1177/1090198110376349 PMID:21169478

Birt, C., Buzeti, T., Grosso, G., & Justesen, L. (2017). Healthy and Sustainable Diets for European Countries. European Public Health Association – EUPHA. https://biblio.ugent.be/publication/8521128/file/8521129.pdf

British Dietetic Association. (2013). *Policy on sustainable food*. Author.

Brown, E., & Jacobson, M. F. (2005). *Cruel Oil: How palm oil Harms health, rainforest & wildlife*. Center of Science in the Public Interest.

Bryceson, D. F. (2004). Agrarian vista or vortex: African rural livelihood policies. *Review of African Political Economy, 31*(102), 617–629. doi:10.1080/0305624042000327831

Bulte, E. H., & Soest, D. P. V. (2001). Environmental degradation in developing ountries: Households and the reverse environmental Kuznets Curve. *Journal of Development Economics, 65*(1), 225–235. doi:10.1016/S0304-3878(01)00135-3

Capone, R., Bilali, H. E., Debs, P., Cardone, G. & Driouech, N. (2014). Food system sustainability and food Security: Connecting the Dots. *Journal of Food Security, 2*, 13-22.

Carlsson-Kanyama, A., & Gonzalez, A. D. (2009). Potential contributions of food consumption patterns to climate change. *The American Journal of Clinical Nutrition, 89*(5), 1704S–1709S. doi:10.3945/ajcn.2009.26736AA PMID:19339402

Charles, H., Godfray, J., Crute, I. R., Haddad, L., Lawrence, D., Mui, J. F., ... Whiteley, R. (2010). The future of the global food system. *Philosphical Transactions of the Royal Socieity B, 365*(1554), 2769–2777. doi:10.1098/rstb.2010.0180 PMID:20713383

Clapp, J. (2017). Food self-sufficiency: Making sense of it, and when it makes sense. *Food Policy, 66*, 88–96. doi:10.1016/j.foodpol.2016.12.001

Connell, D. J. (2010). Sustainable livelihoods and ecosystem health: Exploring methodological relations as a source of synergy. *EcoHealth, 7*(3), 351–360. doi:10.100710393-010-0353-7 PMID:21104294

Cullet, P. (2004). Intellectual property rights and food security in the South. *The Journal of World Intellectual Property, 7*(3), 261–286. doi:10.1111/j.1747-1796.2004.tb00209.x

Debon, H., Parrot, L., & Moustier, P. (2010). Sustainable urban agriculture in developing countries. A review. *Agronomy for Sustainable Development, 30*(1), 21–32. doi:10.1051/agro:2008062

Dobermann, A. & Nelson, R. (2013). *Opportunities and solutions for sustainable food production.* Academic Press.

Ekpenyong, A. S. (2015). Urbanization: Its implication for sustainable food Security, health and nutritional nexus in developing economies - A case study of Nigeria. *Journal of Studies in Social Sciences, 11*, 29–49.

European Commission. (2015). *Sustainable food consumption and production in a resource-constrained world.* https://ec.europa.eu/research/scar/pdf/scar_3rd-foresight_2011.pdf.

Freibauer, Mathijs, Brunori, Damianova, Faroult, Gomis, O'Brien, & Treyer. (2011). Sustainable food consumption and production in a resource-constrained world. Belgium: European Commission-Standing Committee on Agricultural Research (SCAR).

Friedl, B., Omann, I., & Pack, A. (2014). *Socio-economic drivers of (non-) sustainable food consumption. An analysis for Austria.* Academic Press.

Garnett, M. C., Appleby, A., Balmford, I. J., Bateman, T. G., Benton, P., Bloomer, B., ... Vermeulen, H. C. J. (2016a). Sustainable intensification in agriculture: Premises and policies. *Scinece, 30*, 1–2.

Garnett, T. (2014). *What is a sustaiable healthy diet Discussion paper.* Food Climate Research Network.

Garnett, T., Appleby, M., Balmford, A., & Bateman, I. (2016b). Sustainable Intensification in Agriculture: Premises and Policies. *Science, 30*, 1–2. PMID:23828927

Gauker, C. (2010). *The impacts of sustainable and industrial agriculture on human health*. Academic Press.

Gautam, Y., & Andersen, P. (2016). Rural livelihood diversification and household well-being: Insights from Humla, Nepal. *Journal of Rural Studies, 44*, 239–249. doi:10.1016/j.jrurstud.2016.02.001

Godfray, H. C. J., Crute, I. R., Haddad, L., Lawrence, D., Muir, J. F., Nisbett, N., ... Whiteley, R. (2010). The future of the global food system. *Philosophical Transaction of the Royal Society B, 365*, 2769-2777.

Godfray, H. C. J. & Garnett, T. (2014). Food security and sustainable intensification. *Philosophical Transaction of the Royal Society B, 369*, 1-12.

Griggs, D. (2013). *Sustainable development goals for people and planet*. Academic Press.

Grunert, K. G., Hieke, S., & Wills, J. (2014). Sustainability labels on food products: Consumer motivation, understanding and use. *Food Policy, 44*, 177–189. doi:10.1016/j.foodpol.2013.12.001

Han, Y., & Hansen, H. (2012). Determinants of Sustainable Food Consumption:A Meta-Analysis Using a Traditional and a Structura Equation Modelling Approach. *International Journal of Psychological Studies, 4*(1), 22–44. doi:10.5539/ijps.v4n1p22

Hart, K., Allen, B., & Karsten, J. (2013). *EU policy options to encourage more sustainable food choices*. Academic Press.

Hawkes, C. (2006). The links between agriculture and health: An intersectoral opportunity to improve the health and livelihoods of the poor. *Bulletin of the World Health Organization, 84*(12), 984–990. doi:10.2471/BLT.05.025650 PMID:17242835

Herrera-Estrella, L. R., & Alvarez-Morales, A. (2000). Genetically Modified Crops and Developing Countries. *EMBO Reports, 2*(4), 256–258. doi:10.1093/embo-reports/kve075 PMID:11306538

Herrero, M., & Thorntonb, P. K. 2010. Livestock and global change: Emerging issues for sustainable food systems. *Proceedings of the National Academy of Sciences of the United States of America, 110*.

Hertwich, E., & Katzmayr, M. (2003). *Examples of sustainable consumption*. Academic Press.

Hobson, K. (2002). Competing discourses of sustainable consumption: Does the rationalisation of lifestyles' make sense? *Environmental Politics, 11*(2), 95–120. doi:10.1080/714000601

Horrigan, L., Lawrence, R. S., & Walker, P. (2002). How sustainable agriculture can address the environmental and human health harms of industrial agriculture. *Environmental Health Perspectives, 110*(5), 445–456. doi:10.1289/ehp.02110445 PMID:12003747

International Institute Of Social Studies. (2015). *Global governance/politics, climate justice & agrarian/ social justice: linkages and challenges*. Author.

Johnson, J. L., Fanzo, J., & Cogill, B. (2014). Understanding sustainable Diets: A descriptive analysis of the determinants and processes that influence diets and their impact on health, food security, and environmental sustainability. *Advances in Nutrition, 5*(4), 418–429. doi:10.3945/an.113.005553 PMID:25022991

Kasa, S. (2008). Globalizing unsustainable food consumption:Trade policies, producer lobbies, consumer preferences, and beef consumption in Northeast Asia. *Globalizations, 5*(2), 151–163. doi:10.1080/14747730802057480

Kearney, J. (2010). Food consumption trends and drivers. *Philosophical Transaction of the Royal Society B, 365*(1554), 2793–2807. doi:10.1098/rstb.2010.0149 PMID:20713385

Kesavan, P. C. & Swaminathan, M. S. (2008). Strategies and models for agricultural sustainability in developing Asian countries. *Philosophical Transaction of the Royal Society B, 363*, 877-891.

Khalid, S., Khan, M. B., Regina, K., Jos, K., & Gerd, A. (2003). Five steps to conducting a systematic review. *Journal of the Royal Society of Medicine*, 96. PMID:12612111

Khan, Z. R., Midega, C. A. O., Pittchar, J. O., Murage, A. W., Birkett, M. A., Bruce, T. J. A., & Pickett, J. A. (2014). Achieving food security for one million sub-Saharan African poor through push-pull innovation by 2020. *Philosophical Transactions of the Royal Society of London. Series B, Biological Sciences*, 369. PMID:24535391

Kjærga, B., Land, B., & Pedersen, K. B. (2013). Health and sustainability. *Health Promotion International, 29*, 10–15. PMID:23300191

Lefin, A. L. (2010). *Food consumption and sustainable development: An introduction.* Institut pour un Développement Durable.

Lehota, A. L. (2004). National and international trend of food consumption and behaviour. *Marketing, 1*, 7–14.

Littell, J. H., Corcoran, J., & Pillai, V. (2008). *Systematic reviews and meta-analysis.* New York, NY: Oxford University Press. doi:10.1093/acprof:oso/9780195326543.001.0001

Lorek, S., & Fuchs, D. (2013). Strong sustainable consumption governance – precondition for a degrowth path? *Journal of Cleaner Production, 38*, 36–43. doi:10.1016/j.jclepro.2011.08.008

Mackay, R., & Wolbring, G. (2013a). *Sustainable Consumption of Healthcare: Linking Sustainable Consumption with Sustainable Healthcare and Health Consumer Discourses.* The 3rd World Sustainability Forum.

Mackay, R., & Wolbring, G. (2013b). *Sustainable Consumption of Healthcare: Linking Sustainable Consumption with Sustainable Healthcare and Health Consumer Discourses.* Academic Press.

Mckenzie, F. C., & Williams, J. (2015). Sustainable food production: Constraints, challenges and choices by 2050. *Food Security, 7*(2), 221–233. doi:10.100712571-015-0441-1

Mcmichael, A. J., Powles, J. W., Butler, C. D., & Uauy, R. (2007). Food, livestock production, energy, climate change, and health. *Lancet, 370*(9594), 1253–1263. doi:10.1016/S0140-6736(07)61256-2 PMID:17868818

Mont, O., & Plepys, A. (2005). Motivating sustainable consumption. *Sustainable Development Research Network, 29*, 30.

Mózner, Z. V. (2013). *Towards Sustainable food consumption? An Ecological footprint in Hungary* (PhD thesis). Corvinus University of Budapest.

National Institute Of Consumer Research. (2010). *Sustainable Consumption and some contemporary European issues*. Author.

Nemecek, T., Jungbluth, N., Canals, L. M., & Schenck, R. (2016). Environmental impacts of food consumption and nutrition: where are we and what is next? *Int J Life Cycle Assess, 21*, 607-620.

Oni, O. A. (2010). *Food Poverty and Livelihoods Issues in Rural Nigeria*. Academic Press.

Pretty, J., Noble, A., Bossio, D., Dixon, J., Hine, R. E., & Morison, I. L. (2013). Resource-conserving agriculture increases yields in Developing Countries. *Environmental Science & Technology, 40*(4), 1114–1119. doi:10.1021/es051670d PMID:16572763

Pretty, J. N., Morison, J. I., & Hine, R. E. (2003). Reducing food poverty by increasing agricultural sustainability in developing countries. *Agriculture, Ecosystems & Environment, 95*(1), 217–234. doi:10.1016/S0167-8809(02)00087-7

Pretty, J. N., & Noble, D. (2006). Resource-Conserving Agriculture Increases Yields in Developing Countries. *Environment Science and Technology*.

Randolph, T., Schelling, E., Grace, D., Nicholson, C. F., Leroy, J., Cole, D., ... Ruel, M. (2007). Role of livestock in human nutrition and health for poverty reduction in developing countries. *Journal of Animal Science, 85*(11), 2788–2800. doi:10.2527/jas.2007-0467 PMID:17911229

Reisch, L., Eberle, U., & Lorek, S. (2013). Sustainable food consumption: an overview of contemporary issues and policies. *Sustainability: Science, Practice, & Policy, 9*, 7–24.

Risku-Norja, H. (2011). *From environmental concerns towards sustainable food provisioning. Material flow and suitable food consumption scenario studies on sustainability of agri-food systems* (Doctoral dissertation). Faculty of agriculture and Forestry, Faculty of Agriculture and Forestry, University of Helsinki.

Schloster, H., Deboer, J., & Boersema, J. J. (2012). Can we cut on the meat of the dish? Constructing consumer-oriented pathway towards meat substitution. *Appetite, 158*, 39–49.

Seligman, H. K., Laraia, B. A., & Kushel, M. B. (2009). Food Insecurity Is Associated with Chronic Disease among Low-Income NHANES Participants. *Journal of Nutrition and Diseases, 5*, 304-310.

Seyfang, G., & Smith, A. (2007). Grassroots innovations for sustainable development: Towards a new research and policy agenda. *Environmental Politics, 16*(4), 584–603. doi:10.1080/09644010701419121

Sonigo, D. P., Bain, M. J., Kong, M. M. A., Fedrigo, M. D., Withana, M. S., Watkin, M. E., ... Dresner, D. S. (2012). *Policies to encourage sustainable consumption Full*. France Europian Commsion.

Stewart, R., Korth, M., Langer, L., Rafferty, S., & Silva, N. R. D. (2013). What are the impacts of urban agriculture programs on food security in low and middle-income countries? *Environmental Evidence, 2*(1), 7. doi:10.1186/2047-2382-2-7

Temme, E. H., Bakker, H. M., Seves, M., Verkaik-Kloosterman, J., Dekkers, A. L., Raaij, J. M. V., & Ocké, M. C. (2015). How may a shift towards a more sustainable food consumption pattern affect nutrient intakes of Dutch children? *Public Health Nutrition, 18*(13), 2468–2478. doi:10.1017/S1368980015002426 PMID:26344035

Thøgersen, J. (2010). Country differences in sustainable consumption: The case of organic food. *Journal of Macromarketing, 30*(2), 171–185. doi:10.1177/0276146710361926

UNCTAD. (2011). Sustainable agriculture and food security in LDCs. *Least Developed Countries Series, 20*, 1-2.

UNEP. (2012). *The Critical Role Of Global Food Consumption Patterns In Achieving Sustainable Food Systems And Food For All.* A UNEP Discussion Paper.

Vermeir, I., & Verbeke, W. (2006). Sustainable food consumption: Exploring the consumer "attitude–behavioral intention" gap. *Journal of Agricultural & Environmental Ethics, 19*(2), 169–194. doi:10.100710806-005-5485-3

Vogit, M. (2014). *Meanings attached to food and sustainable food consumption* (Master's thesis). Uppsala University, Department of Earth Sciences.

Vonbraun, J. (2007). The world food situation: New riving forces and required actions. *IFPRI's Bi-Annual Overview of the World Food Situation presented to the CGIAR Annual General Meeting.*

Vonmeyer-Höfer, M., Juarez Tijerino, A. & Spiller, A. (2015). *Sustainable food consumption in China and India.* Global Food Discussion Papers, No. 60.

World Health Organisation. (2003a). Diet, nutrition and the prevention of chronic diseases. *World Health Organization Technical Report Series*, 916. PMID:12768890

World Health Organisation. (2003b). *Poverty and Health.* Paris: OECD.

This research was previously published in Food Systems Sustainability and Environmental Policies in Modern Economies edited by Abiodun Elijah Obayelu; pages 124-158, copyright year 2018 by Engineering Science Reference (an imprint of IGI Global).

Chapter 52
Sustainable Food Consumption in the Neoliberal Order:
Challenges and Policy Implications

Henry E. Alapiki
University of Port Harcourt, Nigeria

Luke A. Amadi
University of Port Harcourt, Nigeria

ABSTRACT

In recent decades, we have seen the rise of the sustainable food consumption field and its push for disciplinary space in development studies. This chapter turns to the original impetus of sustainable food consumption and the question of how neoliberal order can be reconciled with the need to save the ecology. Beyond the fundamental objectives, there is a need to assess the links between the global food system, as influenced by neoliberal order, and the signs that it leads to adversity for low-income countries. A review of relevant literature in the sustainable consumption field is explored using content analysis to examine links between neoliberal food consumption dynamics, the logic of global food politics, and the emerging terminological shifts from food consumption to food system. The world systems theory and the Marxian political ecology framework are used to show that sustainability is notable for emphasizing resource efficiency and equitability, which can be useful when sustainability challenges are matched with ecological policies. This chapter makes some policy recommendations.

INTRODUCTION

Since the end of the Cold War sustainable food consumption has been a major concern in development studies. In the Earth Summit of 1992 in Rio de Janeiro, world leaders came to a conclusion that "the major cause of the continued deterioration of the global environment is the unsustainable pattern of consumption and production" (UN, 1992). The phases of food production encompass agriculture, food

DOI: 10.4018/978-1-7998-5354-1.ch052

processing, warehouse/retail, consumption (including storage and preparation) and waste management (Åström, et al., 2013).

This process provides some lucid explication of the patterns of sustainable or unsustainable food consumption. In particular, the inverse relationship between increasing food consumption in the affluent North and ecological breakdown in the poor South has resulted in the destruction of the environment. This partly includes the emergence of genetically modified(GM) seeds or genetically engineered(GE) foods which suggests that "genetic engineering is one type of genetic modification that involves the intention to introduce a targeted change in a plant, animal or microbial gene sequence to effect a specific result" (NRC, 2004). The notion is that "genetic engineering has increased the number and type of substances that can be intentionally introduced into the food supply"(NRC,2004).

A critical perspective suggests that the reliance on technology by the affluent societies including globalization, free trade and the methods of production impact directly on climate change variables like green house /carbon emission, deforestation, land grab and degradation arising from capitalist farming, plantation agriculture and the use of organic fertilizers (Wise, 2015).

For neo liberal proponents, consumption represents the liberal ideals of freedom of choice in a market society. The consumer is the King of modern freedoms according to which he/she freely chooses from a broad offering of goods and services (Lock & Ikeda, 2005). The U.S. food system provides a remarkably varied food supply to the U.S. consumer at lower cost than nearly anywhere else in the world' (National Research Council, 2015). However, freedom of choice results in lower costs but leads to choices that might not be sustainable. With billions of people on earth, freedom of choice might not comply necessarily with ecological requirements.

By 2050, the world's population is projected to grow by one-third, reaching between 9 billion and 10 billion people (FAO, 2010). Meting the food needs of this population draws policy attention to sustainable food consumption. This has pressured scholarly engagement with the question of sustainable food consumption as food is inevitably at the center of both human survival and sustainable development.

The objective of this chapter is to stimulate synergies to mitigate unsustainable consumption and related efforts to strengthen proactive policy initiatives. In particular, the chapter suggests ways to provide food for an increasing population on sustainable basis. The central argument is that unsustainable consumption and lifestyles of the affluent societies framed in the context of the neo liberal policies, may lead to increasing and unsustainable food demands which consequently have deleterious effects on both food system and the environment.

Sustainable Food Consumption

Recent trends suggest that debates on sustainable food consumption have moved to the center of development discourse (Lock & Ikeda, 2005). A number of factors account for this emphasis. First is that food is essential for human life and secondly its consumption is interwoven with the natural environment which has implications for sustainability. In their views, Jongen and Meerdink (1998) and Vitterso et al., (1999) recount that "close to half of all human impact on the environment, such as loss of biodiversity, is directly and/or indirectly related to food production and consumption".

Since the end of the Cold War, neo liberal ideology has dominated much of the thinking in most of the powerful industrialized societies and in supranational institutions such as the World Bank and International Monetary Fund, which in turn have imposed this ideology on countries in the global South.

Such trajectories claim that the exercise of "freedom of choice" and "consumer sovereignty" creates a dynamic and democratic society (Lock & Ikeda, 2005).

Neo liberalism is first and foremost a belief in the ability of unrestricted market forces to achieve the best possible economic outcomes for all people. Other neo liberal doctrine includes the primacy of economic growth, reduction of regulatory capacity and size of governments, the importance of free trade to economic growth and individual choice (Steger, 2002). In this worldview, the whole notion of democracy is reduced to the freedom to choose between various goods and services in the market place. Conway and Heynen (2006:20) argue that neoliberalism emerged as a shift from the Keynesian economic model. They pointed out that a critical element of the neoliberal order is the fact that it represents a similar bout of suffering and impoverishment for the poor in the global South just like colonialism and post colonialism, modernization which results in dependency and "development of underdevelopment". Agnew (2005) recounts that neoliberalism is propagated by America as its global project including institutionalization of globalization. This has been increasingly linked to the rise in global food system and the politics of sustainable food consumption.

Within consumption and neoliberalism, there are a number of insightful debates which underscore the increasing effects of unsustainable consumption. Debates on finite resources suggest that global resources are in a decline. Hinrichsen, Salem & Blackburn, (2002) argue for instance that global fresh water is in decline and this exerts pressure on water resource use following the rise of global water politics in the West. This is accompanied by global environmental insecurity threats including climate change, ecological breakdown and the need for ecological security (Roggers,1995). With the rise in environmental insecurity, meeting future food security challenges requires a shift in thinking from "food production and consumption" to sustainable food consumption (Schor, 2005). Milner (2012) had identified the consequences of consumption suggesting the basis of sustainable consumption. The recently emergent field of sustainable consumption attempts to remedy deficiencies in the overall food consumption patterns particularly in the context of equitable and resourceful consumption. Lucia Reisch, Ulrike Eberle, and Sylvia Lorek (2013) argue that the unsustainable consumption dynamics of current arrangements arises from the industrialization and globalization of agriculture and food processing. This suggests that the shift of consumption patterns to dietary animal protein, the resurgence of processed products, results in increasing gap on a global scale between rich and poor, and the paradoxical lack of food security amid an abundance of food.

Against this background, the chapter puts the domain of sustainability frontal in the food consumption agenda as the foundational basis for alternative policy options.

THEORETICAL FRAMEWORK

Food consumption has been explored from divergent theoretical perspectives. To live sustainably in a highly capitalist society driven largely by profit motives remains a development challenge. Since the end of the Cold War, the global food system has become a powerful paradigm for understanding the link between human activities and sustainable consumption.

The rise in capitalist food corporations which exploit the poor societies as sources of raw materials, point out the need to investigate inequality in capitalist resource extraction. Luke Amadi (2012) recounts that pioneering work in this field was undertaken by Harry Braverman in his work *Labour and Monopoly Capital*. Baraverman notes that capitalism is founded on the ability of capitalists to extract surplus labor from production activities and that in the process of development of capitalism, any vestiges of worker control over production that might give them the ability to regulate how much surplus value is produced have been removed (Amadi, 2012). As Braverman argued that the capitalist mode of production systematically destroys all-around skills where they exist, and brings into being skills and occupations that correspond to its needs (Amadi, 2012). This forms part of the wider theoretical basis of "development of underdevelopment" a strand of dependency debate advanced in the World Systems theory popularized by Wallerstein (1976). The systems theory argues that any country's development conditions and prospects are primarily shaped by economic processes, commodity chains, division of labour and geo-political relationships operating at the global scale (Klak, 2013:121).

Another key relevance of this theory is its exploration of the dynamics of entrenched economic interests of the global food corporations and patterns of food chains linked to capitalism.

In a distinct manner, capitalism has been an integral part of the food consumption and underdevelopment logic. Nesheim, et al; (2015) argue that the food system is woven together as a supply chain that operates within broader economic, biophysical, and sociopolitical contexts. This suggests a complex interplay of cross sectorial entities such as health, environmental, social, and economic effects linked to food distribution chain in a globalizing world. The food system is both advantageous and disadvantageous, the system supplies food across all other sectors but in an increasingly unequal manner with divergent implications. The major detrimental effect as Nesheim, et al;(2015:6) suggest is unhealthy dietary patterns considered as a risk factor resulting in mortality and morbidity. They identified additional effects of the food system to include "climate, land, and water resources depletion". They identify the depletion of resources (e.g., water) and flow of outputs (e.g., nitrogen from fertilization, pesticides, and greenhouse gases) to the environment as a result of food system activities" (Nesheim, et al., 2015:6). This remains a persistent challenge to sustainable consumption.

The less developed societies such as the sub- Saharan Africa(SSA), Latin America and South Asia have been vulnerable to undernourishment including challenges posed by food insecurity (Shopouri, et al; 2010). This partly arises from alienating land owners from their lands particularly in agrarian societies, while degradation results in the washing away of top soil nutrients (leaching), use of organic chemicals and depletion of soil nutrients, due to intensive or unsustainable agricultural production methods (Moomaw, et al., 2012). This is a strand of the imperialism debate. This capitalist trend also forms the basis of the emerging ecology and world systems debate (O'Connor, 1998). This is a central basis of mitigating capitalism's war on nature (Harvey, 2005).

In particular, the ecological effects which are expressed in varying degrees between the high income societies and the poor societies have been less lucid. This has equally made the Marxian political ecology theory a useful framework to examine the consequences of unsustainable food consumption.

Since the 1970s following the rise in environmental movements, unsustainable consumption has been under serious attack by the ecological Marxist scholars. These scholars argue that the traditional role of the State, in protecting its citizenry from environmental degradation is seriously put into question (Peet & Watts, 1996; Bryant & Bailey, 1997; O'Connor, 1998; Robbins, 2004; Amadi, Igwe & Wordu, 2014). This is premised on the notion that capitalism is implicitly profit motivated. Critical of ecological factors is to capture relations between food consumption and natural environment, Akenji & Begsson (2014) argue that beyond being an "overarching objectives of, and essential requirements for sustainable development", consumption is central to the actualization of environmental protection and poverty reduction. Political ecology as a strand of Marxism argues that capitalist resource extraction taints nature (Peet & Watts, 1996; Amadi & Igwe, 2015). They point out the role of capitalists in the global food system and the attendant decimation of the natural resources as 'every-thing' in nature becomes a commodity, resulting in nature marketization and commodification. This is equally linked to the dialectical materialistic contradictions of food systems between the affluent and poor societies in which the material conditions of resource expropriation are largely exploitative (Ake, 1981). This creates a complex environmental system one which is at variance with ecological justice and socially responsible consumption.

Whereas the World systems perspective in which core/periphery asymmetry exists—suggests a regulatory dynamic in which the periphery provides the raw materials which are exploited by the advanced / core societies in an unequal scale, resulting in "development of underdevelopment" (Wallerstein, 1976; Amadi, 2012). The ecological Marxists clearly explore the patterns of deleterious effects including inequality in natural resource exploitation. Thus, the world systems theory and Marxian political ecology perspectives provide useful theoretical tools for this study.

METHODOLOGY

The methodology to achieve integrated analysis of sustainable food consumption requires a deepened exploration of the conceptual and theoretical issues raised in the literature. And how the issues relate to both consumption patterns of the affluent societies of the North and associated deleterious effects.

This at the same time aims at providing on the ground evidence which suggests patterns of such effects of unsustainable consumption. This includes anthropogenic problems linked to consumption notably economic resource exploitation, green-house emission, health implications of consumption and related ecological breakdown.

On these bases, this study is framed within the content analysis methodology. Content analysis according to Holsti (1969:14) is, 'any technique for making inferences by objectively and systematically identifying specified characteristics of messages'. Content analysis transcends "identifying characteristics of messages" rather reviews and analyses key issues in the literature. This becomes suitable for a broader elucidation of the literature as the aim is to deepen the investigation and in a distinct manner advance new knowledge.

Amadi and Imoh-Ita (2017) argue that content analysis examines and analyses contents or set of data for relevant research objectives. This methodology is important as it critically identifies sets of data in relation to the subjects under investigation and in particular, provides evidence of how the neoliberal food system results in unequal resource access and extraction between the North and South.

The ensemble of divergent perspectives into a unified whole provide a coherent account of the challenges associated with unsustainable consumption patterns. This helps to strengthen the arguments advanced in the study in line with various perspectives on the subject of sustainable food consumption.

Specific methods of selecting relevant data for the study was adopted which includes both online and direct library resource materials. The online search of secondary data such as seminal conceptual, empirical and theoretical data that provide on the ground evidence of the research problems was identified and selected. This is premised on identifying and explaining how such patterns of consumption have posed challenges to sustainable food consumption. The extensive search was specifically based on scholarly journals published on the proquest and Ebsco data bases since the post -Cold War era. This timeline of relevant publications from different schools of thought on neo liberal food consumption dynamics, sets of data on conceptual issues related to the study including global corporation, food politics, sustainable consumption patterns etc was relevant to access a robust set of data for possible generalization. This helps to deepen knowledge of the neo liberal consumption patterns, understand the logic of capitalist consumption and need for policy response to redress the problems identified.

The search yielded 300 results on themes related to the study. However, specific themes directly linked to the research was chosen and a total of 120 works were found useful. A number of similar relevant data were sourced from institutional publications which included the United Nations Food and Agriculture Organization (FAO) reports which for instance suggests that in order to ensure food security needs, additional 70% food must be available by 2050, from an already severely depleted natural resource base (Moomaw, et al., 2012). Others institutional literature included the FAOSTATS,World Bank,UN etc.

This aims at exploring causal connections between food and sustainable consumption and to explore prevailing perspectives in the on-going debate. And to explain how these identified problems could be explored within the political ecology framework to advance a new scholarship and policy agenda.

The rest of the chapter is structured as follows; conceptual clarifications, global corporation, food politics and sustainable consumption, conclusion, recommendations and future research directions.

Figure 1. Per capita consumption of major food items in developing countries, 1961-2005

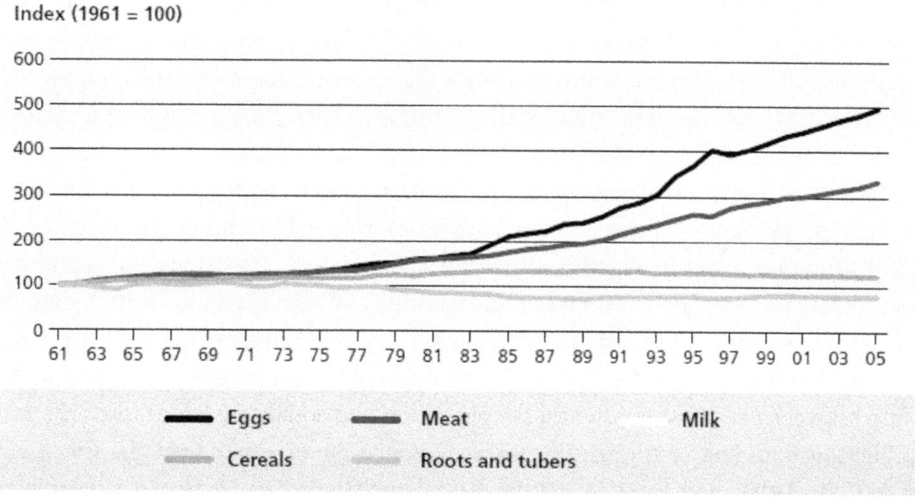

Source: FAO, 2009b.

Conceptual Clarifications

The conceptual literature builds on relevant studies in the broad field of consumption. It corroborates dominant debates on sustainable consumption (Koten,1995; Harvey, 2005; Schor, 2005; Davidson & Hatt, 2005; Stiglitz,2010; Milner, 2012; Amadi, Igwe & Wordu, 2014) and advances a novel argument which suggests the need for sustainable food consumption.

There is a widespread assumption that the term food is a common place to everybody. However the conceptual exploration of the term sustainable food consumption is important to understand the interwoven contextual use of the concept and beyond this, to offer a way of understanding the linkages between food system and unsustainable consumption. Thus, concepts like "food system" and "sustainable consumption" form part of broader elucidation of consumption dynamics deployed to explore the processes, practices and social relations which shape capitalist food production and consumption.

The contemporary food system is a dynamic, fast-changing, multidimensional enterprise, particularly influenced by technological advancement (IOS & NRC,2015). In the global food system dynamics and in scholarly debates, there have been absence of consensus on common theoretical approach to the study of sustainable food consumption. Thus, theoretical exploration of what contexts and ways consumption could be classified as sustainable and how it could be classified as unsustainable is less clear. This has increasingly stimulated global concern on collective efforts at institutionalizing effective mechanisms and common grounds to understand the key drivers of unsustainable food consumption, which this study is one.

On its part, sustainable food consumption offers a means of conceptualizing the global capitalist power and equality in food consumption. Although as an offshoot of the definition provided by the Brundtland Commission Report, sustainable food consumption could be seen as a consumption that meets the needs of the present consumers without tainting food resources for the future generation.

The UK Sustainable Development Commission in its 2005 report, posits that "sustainable food and drink" include safe, healthy, and nutritious consumption which meets the needs of the poor at a global scale. A related account suggests that sustainable food styles must fit into people's everyday lifestyles and should allow for socio-cultural diversity (Eberle, et al., 2006).

Inequality has also been linked to unsustainable food consumption. UNEP (2012: 12) suggests that, "food demand is only met in the aggregate, as there are profound disparities in access to food across geographic regions and across the spectrum of incomes at both the household and country levels". There are variations in access to food including cultural and religious barriers, government policies and control mechanisms, demographic factors linked to food consumption dynamics.

The neo Malthusian perspective argues that population growth partly accounts for low food availability and consumption function among the poor societies. Beyond this perspective are the implications of capitalist consumption patterns which is les explored. This gives rise to various analytical, theoretical and conceptual difficulties. For example, while capitalist system is riddled with inequality (Harvey, 2005; Muller, 2013), the same capitalist system and its protagonists propagate sustainable and equitable resource consumption (Lock & Ikeda, 2005). Where these propositions are concerned with addressing the relationship between capitalist production, exploitation and equality, natural resource extraction and ecological breakdown are less critiqued. For instance, since the emergence of the green consumerism paradigm in the late 1980s and early 1990s, in the United States, its impressive response during the decade, has deepened. However, it appears the state of green consumption and business transactions have been less revolutionary.

The critical implications of unsustainable consumption is ever scant in development studies as several people in the poor societies are marginalized in the event of asymmetrical appropriation of food resources including the deleterious food consumption patterns of the affluent societies. This includes disproportionate food consumption of the industrialized societies like the United States (Schor, 2005). There is introduction of genetically modified (GM)foods or genetically Engineered (GE) foods (Paalberg, 2013), groceries, burger etc, which could have carcinogenic effects including the rise in obesity.

This reaffirms the importance of inclusive dynamics in food consumption and a critique of the new paradigm of global capitalist food system. According to Marx (1978), capitalism breeds both love and crisis. This points out the inevitable contradictions surrounding food consumption including recent conceptual and terminological shifts associated with food consumption such as ecological conscious consumer behavior (ECCB)' (Straughan & Roberts, 1999), green purchase behavior and the green consumer (Jansson, Marell, & Nordlund, 2010; Akehurst & Akenso, 2012),, food security (Shopouri,etal;2011), 'pro-environmental consumer behaviour'(Riley, Kohlbacher & Hofmeister, 2012), 'green consumer values(Haws, Winterich & Naylor, 2014),environmental sustainability measurement (Amadi & Imohita, 2017) etc, have attracted novel scholarly interest as issues of sustainable food consumption have increasingly become a globalized phenomenon. For instance, in 2015 a committee was appointed by the Food and Nutrition Board of the Institute of Medicine (IOM) in collaboration with the Board on Agriculture and Natural Resources of the National Research Council (NRC) to develop a report and an analytical framework to assess the health, environmental, social, and economic aspects of the U.S. food system. The committee took into account the complexity of the system and recognized that "the U.S. food system is embedded in a global system that is broadly interconnected" (IOM and NRC,2015).

In particular, the report "provided insights into how aspects of the food system influences modern life" (IOM and NRC,2015). This includes changes and adaptation to Western consumption patterns of packaged foods, lifestyles, beverages, blended drinks including alcohol at the expense of traditional or indigenous patterns of production and consumption and the rise in GM foods often liked to food modernization.

Proponents of modernization of agriculture argue that there is need to encourage GM foods in the South particularly in Africa.Robert Paalberg (2008) and similar advocates argue that African farmers need to grow more crops through GM seeds and subsequently increase the potential productivity of African farmers. Paalberg (2008)contends that Africa is 'starved of science'as they are 'kept out of biotechnology' and that the central basis for advancing food production in Africa should be revamping agriculture in line with modernization models, that this has been a key to Africa's economic growth.

Right or wrong, much of Paalberg's debate perhaps falls within Gidden's (1990) thesis on "societal consequences of modernization".Critiques argue that GM foods and similar modernization thesis may not bring the poor out of poverty nor check unsustainable consumption. Masters, et al;(2004:8) have explored the unintended effects of genetically engineered foods on human health and found that "all evidence evaluated to date indicates that unexpected and unintended compositional changes arise with all forms of genetic modification, including genetic engineering".

Thus, food consumption has become a central trend in economic advancement, identity, lifestyle, interaction between one another and the increasing consumption dichotomy among the societies of the global North and South (Davidson & Hatt, 2005; Milner, 2012).

Among the developed societies, Milner (2012) had identified the relevance of consumption in contemporary development dynamics and argued that Norway has been an example of a society with a modest consumption pattern unlike the United States. This has increasingly resulted in complexities in the study of contemporary food system. Such complexities include the issues of world hunger, sustainable production, inequality and poverty.

FAO (2015) reports that 'world hunger is on the rise: the estimated number of undernourished people increased from 777 million in 2015 to 815 million in 2016". Global food politics which needs to be reconciled with freedom of choice and the imbalance between food consumption in the high and low income countries. FAO estimates for 2016 indicate that the global prevalence of undernourishment in 2016 may have actually risen to 11 percent (FAO, 2017). According to the food first and World Watch institute, global hunger hits an increasing percentage since the 1990s to the 2000s particularly in food insecure areas.

Beyond food consumption, food production has also been a core challenge in understanding the underlying triggers of unsustainable consumption. Sustainable production entails the mode of manufacturing food from 'process to production' including packaging such as canned foods or similar modes of food processing mechanisms etc. A central issue has been the dynamics of equitable and responsible use of resources in the cause of food production. This has been more critical in the neo liberal order where ecological factors which should have been given priority attention appears less prioritized (Korten, 1995). This disproportionate mode of food consumption results in inequality (Schor, 2005).

Figure 2. Number of People and shares of population living in poverty in low-and-middle-income countries

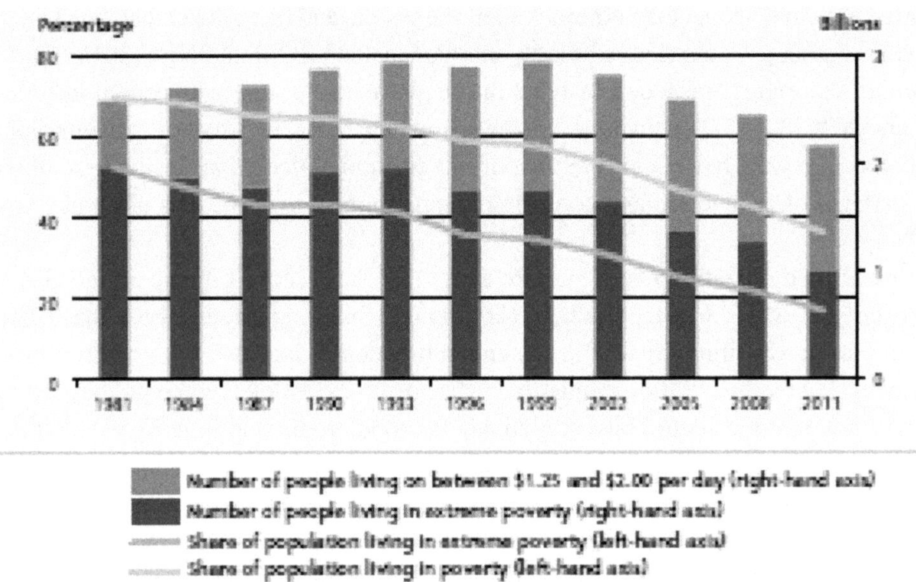

Note: The figure refers to the international poverty lines of $1.25 a day (extreme poverty) and $2.00 a day (poverty) as measured in constant 2005 PPP dollars.
Source: Authors' compilation using World Bank (2015a). See Annex table A1.

The rise of the consumer culture is typified in the capitalist system (Schor, 2005). Equally from the perspectives on environmentally significant consumption, Stern (1997:20) argues that 'consumption consists of human and human-induced transformations of materials and energy'. He recounts that this transformation is critical to the environment and humans to the extent that it makes materials or energy less available for future use.

Growing poverty remains a central concern in global food politics as most people of the South are poorer today than 100 and 50years ago(Weinsten,2008). In both urban and rural contexts poverty remains pervasive. The urban poor live in slums and squatter settlements, without food and adequate access to clean water, sanitation, and health care (Hinrichsen, et al., 2002). Thus,the poor who are predominantly in the less developed societies have been at the margins of popular discourse on global food politics. Martin Ravallion (2001) estimates that, worldwide, 30% of poor people live in urban areas. By 2020 the proportion is projected to reach 40%, and by 2035 half of the world's poor people are projected to live in urban areas.

In 1988, the World Bank estimated that some 330 million urban poor in the developing world were living on less than US$1 a day (World Bank 1991). In 2000 the estimate had increased to 495 million (Hinrichsen et al., 2002). Sub-Saharan Africa has some of the world's highest levels of urban poverty, reaching over 50% of the urban populations in Chad, Niger, and Sierra Leone. Chen and Ravallion (2001) measured absolute poverty in terms of household consumption expenditure percapita in the Middle East, North Africa, South Asia and Sub Saharan Africa. Their findings suggest the prevalence of inequality in income and consumption distribution. The study pointed out that the region with highest poverty incidence relative to $1perday line is sub Saharan Africa(SSA) followed by South Asia, that this group accounted for 70% of those living below 1$ per day in 1998.East Asia came Third in terms of incidence of poverty with Latin America.

Green consumerism which results in green economy has often been advocated as it legitimizes sustainable consumption. However, it has also been criticized in capitalist contexts as it results in "ecological calamity", or "disaster capitalism" (Klein, 2008). It becomes "an opportunity for corporations to turn the very crisis that they generate through their accumulation of capital via the exploitation of nature" (Klein, 2008). This according to Estavo and Prakash (1998) has resulted in the waste of nature and production of rot and decay. Eastwood (2006:118-119), has created nexus between capitalist production and consumption in the contexts that "capital accumulation relies not only on the production of goods, but also on the production of the willing consumer". This corroborates the perspective that consumption in a distinct manner promotes production and vice vasa.

The concept of food security has been part of the wider terminological shifts food consumption had witnessed. Food security includes a situation in which all people always 'have physical, social and economic access to sufficient, safe and nutritious food that meets their dietary needs and food preferences for an active and healthy life" (FAO, 2010). There are linkages between food security and climate change including biofules and land grab by the affluent countries (Lawrence, et al;2011)

Hinrichsen, et al; (2002) argue that about 50% of the world's poor are living in food insecure areas with low subsistent level. There are issues of resource depletion. For instance fresh water shortages soars and accounts for resurgence of several water related diseases where access to clean water is scarce, sanitation is poor. This is reinforced in related accounts on ecological breakdown while related environmental consumption challenges arising from fossil fuel and industrial pollution are critical. The pollution rate recorded in the high income countries between 1900 to 2015, suggest the imminent dangers of unsustainable food consumpton.

Global Food Politics and Sustainable Consumption

Food in global contexts has divergent interpretations. At the aftermath of the second world war food became a major instrument of foreign policy. However following the end of the Cold War a period of competitive world food prices and a return to a more "free market" food policy remerged. The scenario has persisted resulting to a rise in Western food hegemony. The contention remains the need to understand how sustainable a food system is and in particular, the failure of the neo liberal food system to deliver sustainable and equitable consumption.

Christopher Rosin,Paul Stock and Hugh Campbell (2011) analyze the contemporary global food system in the context of its failure to actualize food security. This includes complexities and contradictions surrounding dominant dynamics of production linked with industrial capitalism. Thus, world food systems cannot be discussed in isolation of globalization, free trade and the logic of capitalist mode of production as well as persistent inequality.

Global food politics linked to the neoliberal policy prescriptions of the World Trade Organization (WTO), the World Bank, and the International Monetary Fund (IMF)have resulted in persistent and unmitigated unequal natural resource consumption which has been at variance with sustainable and equitable development. Capitalist consumption is perhaps contradictory as it includes the politics of market and competition informed by the logic of liberalism which preaches freedom and capitalism which is riddled with inequality and exploitation.

In the United States, Natural Resources Defense Council (2010) contends that a typical American meal contains ingredients from five foreign countries, and even domestically grown produce travels an average of 1,500 miles before it is sold. In Germany,260 million tons of CO^2 equivalents are emitted per year, i.e. 3.2 tons per inhabitant to feed the country's 80 million persons (Fuchs & Lorek, 2001).

Capitalist exploitation is linked to the patterns of economic relationship between the North and South. By the latter part of the nineteenth century, places as diverse as Malaysia (rubber producer), India (cotton producer), Egypt (cotton producer),Argentina (beef and wheat producer), Ghana (cocoa producer), and Cuba (sugar producer) had become specialized in the production of one or more export crops for European (and later U.S.) markets(Wolf, 1997).This results in unequal exchange and poverty on a grand scale.This is reinforced in the unequal labour relationships which shape the economic relationship of the 'North' and ' South' and have become issues of scholarly concern in contemporary sustainable consumption debate(Amin, 1972).

Paalberg (2008) argues that because Western consumers derive no benefits from biotechnological advances in agriculture they inflict a frivolous "imperialism of rich tastes" on African farmers.

This points out that the prevailing food system ignored the divergent effects of unsustainable consumption. This compels the need for provision of food for an increasing population on sustainable basis. In the 'North', increasing food consumption must take adequate audit of the environment which is perhaps less examined. Paul Stern (1997) argued that consumption is central to development of every society especially within ecological contexts. This includes chemical residues in crops and livestock, aflatoxin/ mycotoxin contaminants which reduce the quality and acceptability of food, evidence of contaminants which in turn, adversely affects the poor societies as they rely on 'finished' food products from the high income societies.

Equally, the rise in Western food corporations and capitalist resource consumption have increasingly become an opportunity for the corporations to accumulate and exploit nature in a bid for profit and investment revenue. In this particular case, as the global food system makes food available, the affluent societies benefit to the exclusion of the poor, through access and hegemonic control mechanisms. A sustainable food system entails meeting present food consumption and nutrition security needs which should not undermine food and nutrition security for future generations. The sustainability of food system is influenced by anthropogenic and non- anthropogenic factors. These complexities are situated within the interwoven contexts of dynamics of 'food production, distribution, consumption, nutritional health, socio-economic and environmental factors related to the quantity, quality and affordability of food, as well as health and wellbeing'(UN, 2015).

Globalization of food consumption gained relevance at the instance of the US hegemony. Globalization fosters unequal wealth distribution, favors a small economic elite, leaving out the majority who are economically vulnerable (Rees, 1998).This is perhaps evident in the rise of global food corporations-food supply chains, stores and outlets that consume disproportionate resources notably, Nestlé (Switzerland), PepsiCo (USA), Kraft (USA), ABinBev (Brazil), ADM (USA), Coca-Cola (USA), Mars Inc. (USA), Unilever (Netherlands), Tyson Foods (USA), Cargill (USA)(Berne Declaration,2013), have resulted in dependency linked to globalization as they extract natural resources from the developing economies at a relatively cheap rate and export finished products at a higher economic rate (Bello, 2004;Amadi, 2012; Wise, 2015).

Figure 3. Shares of the population in low- and middle-income countries living in extreme poverty, by region

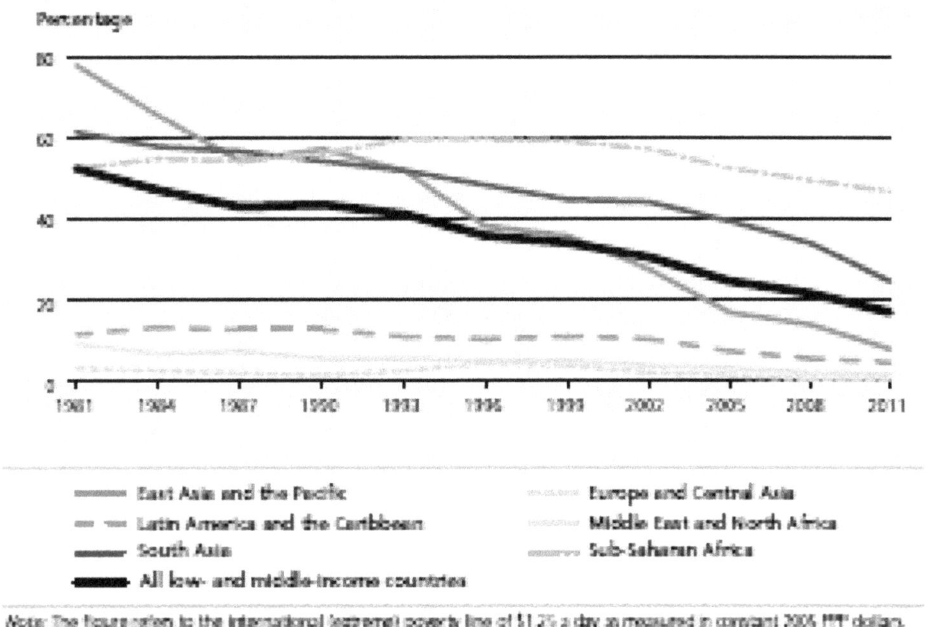

A recent beach clean -up and audit at Freedom Island in Manila Bay, Philippines by the Greenpeace showed that Nestlé, Unilever and Indonesian company PT Torabika Mayora are the top three contributors of plastic waste discovered in the area, contributing to the 1.88 million metric tonnes of mismanaged plastic waste in the Philippines per year(Tiu, 2017).Thus, food corporations seem not to have fully recognized the challenges of environmental degradation and complexities of ecological breakdown and social distortions .Despite the alleged claim on green corporate social responsibility(Amadi & Imohita, 2017).

This provides useful insights on contemporary global food dynamics. On this basis, corporate interest dominates much of the mainstream burgeoning thinking on neo liberal food consumption with less emphasis on the imminent long term dangers of the ecological consequences(Korten, 1995).

Another critical dimension contemporary global food politics had taken is necessitated by the rise in global integration of national economies as globalization takes consumption to a new level. Paehlke (2003) argues that the result is a fully integrated global system dominated by corporate actors. Essentially global food politics dominates much of the advanced industrialized societies. Wapner, (1996) argues that the emergence of international and global economic institutions diminishes state sovereignty and reduces the state's capacity to intervene in economic activities.

In this regard, global food politics remains a complex matrix of interactions advancing from colonial and post -colonial era to the neo colonial era including imperialism and globalization. In most post-colonial societies of the Third World a circle of economic exploitation through trade is linked to a systemic exploitation through the colonial marketing boards (Ekekwe, 1986). Accordingly, in Latin America, Janvry (1981) recounts the unequal patterns of resource extraction through, agro-export production by the Spanish and Portuguese colonizers which extended to the post- independence era. Pointing out that the newly independent states of Latin America re-entered the global economy as suppliers of agricultural commodities to Europe and the United States and as purchasers of manufactured goods.

Figure 4. Meat consumption and share of net imports in consumption, least-developed countries, 1961-2005

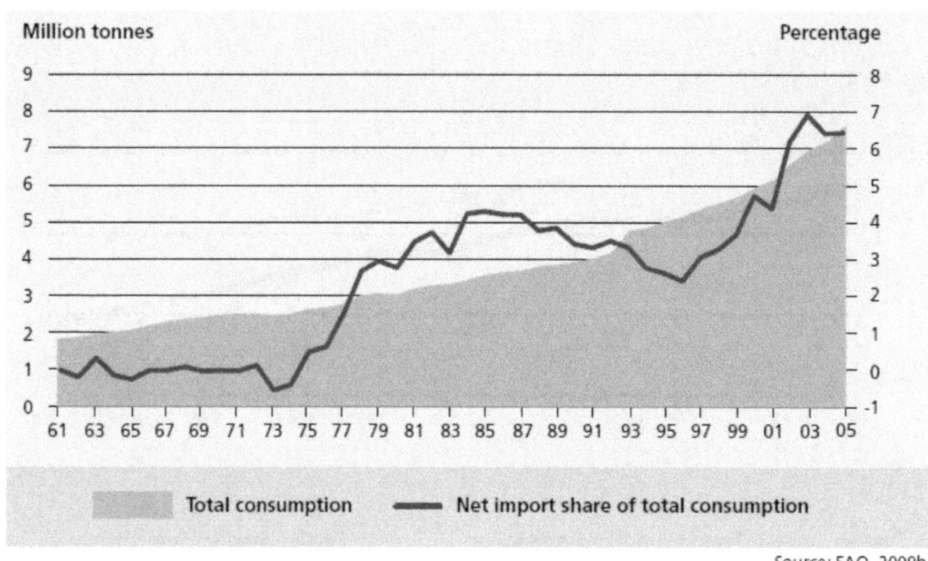

Source: FAO, 2009b.

The implications of the free market debate has equally favored the economies of the developed capitalist societies as most developed countries, including the United Kingdom, the United States, France, Germany, and Japan, used tariffs, subsidies, and other interventionist measures in order to promote industrialization (Chang, 2003:426).

Paalberg (2013) argues that farm subsidies shape contemporary international agricultural trade. However, highly indebted developing countries are precluded from using these measures as they are subject to the neoliberal policy prescriptions of the IMF and the World Bank leading to structural adjustment programs designed to ensure loan repayment (Chang, 2003). In Africa, for example, exports diversification and development of manufacturing sector have been negatively impacted by the neoliberal reforms imposed by the IMF and the World Bank which emphasizes comparative advantage in raw material and primary product exports (Stein, 2003).

There are issues of consequences of overconsumption in the industrialized countries(Schor,2005) This is in line with the disproportionate consumption debate by the industrialized societies which have been examined in seminal writings (Shove,2003;Hobson, 2003, Schor, 2005; Milner, 2012). In the United States the NRDC (2010)estimates that 'in California, which imports food distributed throughout the nation, the smog-forming emissions from importing fruits and vegetables are equivalent to the annual emissions from 1.5 million cars". This is linked to the need for ecological footprints of the North (Rees, 1998). The several limitations posed by capitalist international trade particular in relation to the rual peoples of the tropics have been examined (Carlsson-Kanyama, 1997)

Another key component of unsustainable consumption is food wastage. This includes water and similar consumables. The USDA estimates 'that 27% of all food produced for people in the United States is either thrown away or is used for a lower-value purpose, like animal feed. This suggests the need for policy response and strategies to mitigate the waste of food. Again, the patterns of waste management and processes of discarding the waste has ever more demanding sustainability implications. For instance,

Table 1. Per capita consumption of livestock products by region, country group and country, 1980 and 2005

REGION/COUNTRY GROUP/ COUNTRY	MEAT		MILK		EGGS	
	1980	2005	1980	2005	1980	2005
	(kg/capita/year)		*(kg/capita/year)*		*(kg/capita/year)*	
DEVELOPED COUNTRIES	76.3	82.1	197.6	207.7	14.3	13.0
Former centrally planned economies	63.1	51.5	181.2	176.0	13.2	11.4
Other developed countries	82.4	95.8	205.3	221.8	14.8	13.8
DEVELOPING COUNTRIES	14.1	30.9	33.9	50.5	2.5	8.0
East and Southeast Asia	12.8	48.2	4.5	21.0	2.7	15.4
China	13.7	59.5	2.3	23.2	2.5	20.2
Rest of East and Southeast Asia	10.7	24.1	9.9	16.4	3.3	5.1
Latin America and the Caribbean	41.1	61.9	101.1	109.7	6.2	8.6
Brazil	41.0	80.8	85.9	120.8	5.6	6.8
Rest of Latin America and the Caribbean	41.1	52.4	109.0	104.1	6.5	9.4
South Asia	4.2	5.8	41.5	69.5	0.8	1.7
India	3.7	5.1	38.5	65.2	0.7	1.8
Rest of South Asia	5.7	8.0	52.0	83.1	0.9	1.5
Near East and North Africa	17.9	27.3	86.1	81.6	3.7	6.3
Sub-Saharan Africa	14.4	13.3	33.6	30.1	1.6	1.6
WORLD	30.0	41.2	75.7	82.1	5.5	9.0

Source: FAO, 2009b.

most of the wastes 'end up in landfills where it releases even more heat-trapping gas in the form of methane as it decomposes'(Martin,2008;NRDC,2010).

Capitalist mode of production and unsustainable patterns of consumption have been declared the primary causes of environmental deterioration (Akenji & Bengtsson,2014). This was clearly recognized at the United Nations Conference on Environment and Development (UNCED) in 1992, and has been reconfirmed in all high-level sustainability meetings since then (Akenji & Bengtsson,2014). In sustainability discourse, ecological justice provides a platform for capitalist corporations to retrace the perverse ecological crisis they engender through their accumulation ethos in the context of exploitation of nature for profit maximization. Panitch and Leys (2007) argue, that there is need for multiple moves in 'political education: from blind consumerism to a mobilization against specific corporations to an organized understanding of the unsustainable logic of the capitalist system in toto".

Technological advancement is another issue of relevance in sustainable food consumption. In recognition of the interwoven contexts of the natural environment and food, the challenge to sustainable food consumption results in the novel turn technological advancement had taken in recent decades pointing to the ecological modernization perspectives which are "confident" of the ability of capitalism to transform itself in the face of ecological crisis(Sparaagen,1997). This partly accounts for the rise in GE foods in the industrialized societies since the early 2000s. Genetically modified foods (GMs) or genetically engineered crops(GE) and its products derive from genetically engineered organisms. They are among a number of biotechnological developments intended to improve shelf life, nutritional content, flavor, color, and texture, as well as agronomic and processing characteristics.

Scholarly literature suggests two key perspectives on the GEs namely the proposing perspective which argue for the technological, nutritional and economic relevance of GE foods (Sears, 1981, Gupta & Tsuchiya, 1991; Heyman, et al., 1998, Georges, 2001) and the opposing perspectives which hold a contrary view on the sustainability of the GE foods (Gepts, 2006; Wang, et al. 2006; Altieri, 2008; Frison, 2009;Jacobsen, et al. 2013). Altieri (2008) argued on resilience and sustainability of non GE crops suggesting that agro-ecological farms contain a high level of biodiversity and are self-supporting systems in harmony with their environment.

Similarly, Frison (2009) argued that contemporary agro-systems with low biodiversity offer low-diverse diets which in turn lead to high incidence of lifestyle illnesses such as obesity, Type II diabetes, heart diseases and cancer. There is a debate which contends that the persistence of GE has resulted in the loss of crop and livestock biodiversity including deteriorated genetic loss and vulnerability (Gepts, 2006).

In many instances, states in industrial societies are constrained by the logic of capital or the need to subsidize industry so that the corporate organizations can continue to make a profit, keep people employed, and in turn generate revenues for the state through taxation. The constraints placed on capitalist states are only exacerbated when the priorities of economic growth become codified in international trade agreements. The regulations of NAFTA, for example, make it much more difficult for states to protect natural resources, or to support locals in doing so (Schnaiberg & Gould, 1994; O'Connor,1998; Roberts & Grimes, 2002, Moore, 2000, Chew, 1995; Chase-Dunn, 1989; Davidson & Hatt, 2005, p.238).

Carmen Gonzalez (2004) recounts that inequality remains a core neo liberal threat to sustainable development. For instance, close to a billion people go hungry in the world every day, with 10 children dying of starvation every minute (Pinstrup-Andersen, 2010b). This not only suggests the urgency of sustainable food consumption rather points to food equality which underscores the primacy of equal access to food consumption across regions and in gender contexts. Data below suggests that women are most affected with food insecurity issues.

Figure 5. Women are slightly more likely to be food insecure than men in every region of the world

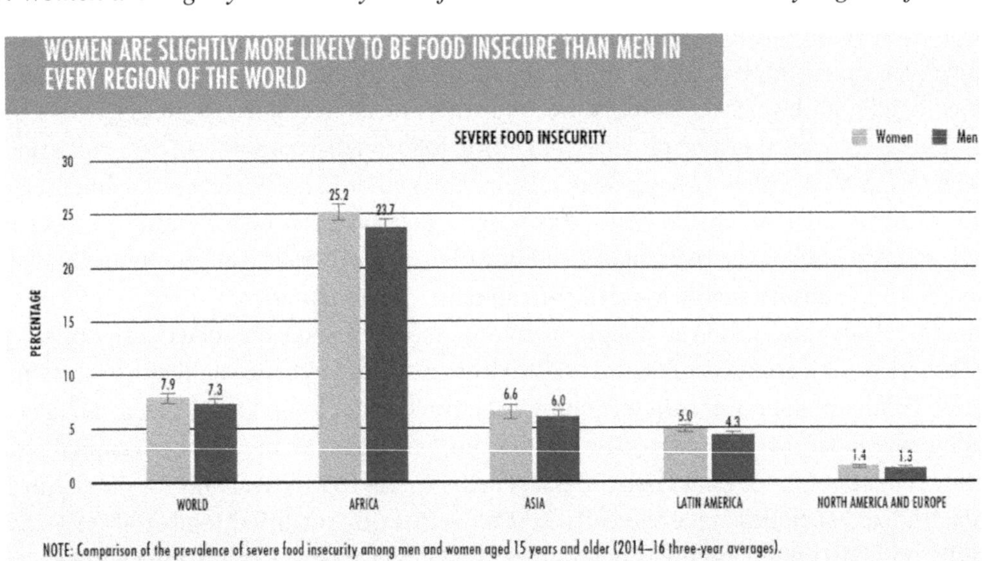

Globalization has been a central factor to consumption disparity creating a wide gap between the affluent and poor societies. This includes issues of international trade networks, globalization of capital concentration, technological advancement and innovation, Western hegemonic power, information flow and diffusion of values. This relates to the expansion of capitalism replicated in global land grab, plantation agriculture (capitalist farming) and land degradation which have been at issue in unsustainable consumption debates (Wise, 2015). The global convergence of consumption pattern has given rise to emphasis on the North-South divide with emphasis on influence of the North on consumption response and behavior of the South as the latter adapt to the behavior of the former.

Contemporary society is confronted with the challenge of attaining sustainable food consumption for its growing population. Sustainable food consumption is no longer optional, rather mandatory. Since the Rio summit of 1992 sustainable consumption has become a global issue in development discourse. Similarly Goal 2 of the Sustainable development Goal(SDGs)which is Zero Hunger, points to the saliency of sustainable and equitable consumption. To strengthen this paradigm, there have been growing literature on aspects of sustainable consumption most notably green consumerism, eco- friendly consumption, ecological justice, consumption culture etc.

To redirect the prevailing global food politics requires collective policy engagement. Thus, while sustainable food consumption discourse plays a key role in recreating the dominant notion of consumption and patterns of lifestyle, the affluent societies typically fail to distinctively, attenuate the deleterious consumption patterns. In Sweden, the Swedish Environmental Protection Agency pointed out that the 'use and misuse of nature's resources account for environmental unsustainability. For instance, food consumption alone accounts for 20% of the greenhouse emission in Sweden (Lönnroth, 2010).

Figure 6. Per capita and meat consumption by country, 2005

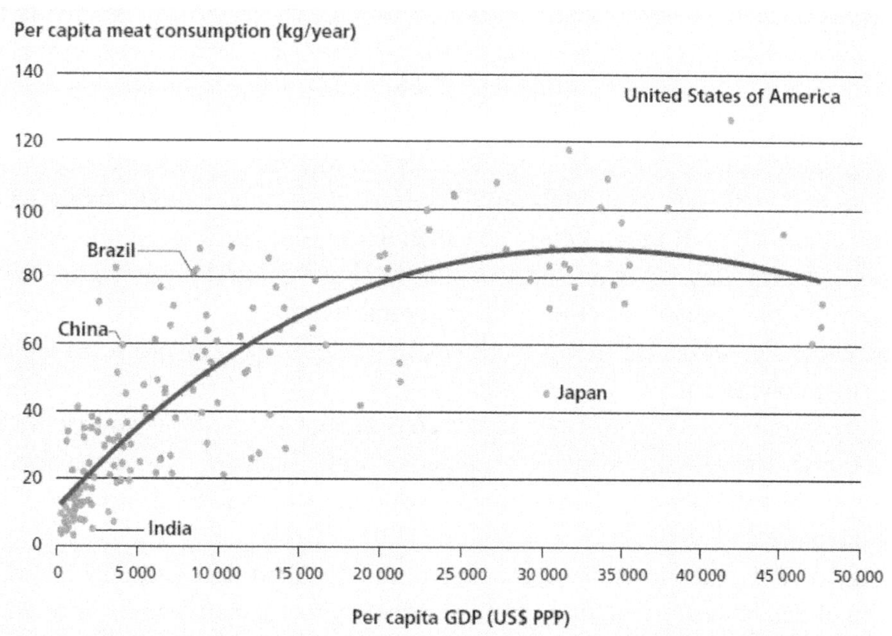

Note: GDP per capita is measured at purchasing power parity (PPP) in constant 2005 international US dollars.
Source: Based on data from FAOSTAT (FAO, 2009b) for per capita meat consumption and the World Bank for per capita GDP.

RECOMMENDATIONS

Although sustainable consumption policies and practices are still in its early stages, there is urgent need for food reform. This chapter has attempted to chronicle some of the scholarly evidence of unsustainable consumption. Since we cannot retain the natural environment amidst unsustainable consumption and marketization of nature and since capitalism is built on profitability, how can the overarching sustainability and consumption be framed to resolve the challenges of deleterious environmental implications? The logic of sustainable consumption helps to resolve the problem and allows for a better policy intervention more generally linked to equality in food consumption. The important question now becomes, how to overcome the challenges of both inequality and deleterious effects of unsustainable food consumption.

The emergence of the field of sustainable food consumption has provided useful insights pushing for disciplinary space in addressing these problems. Beyond this, a return to the original impetus of sustainable food consumption one which seeks for equality and resource efficiency within the capitalist system has not been satisfactorily resolved particularly in ecological contexts as sustainable consumption remains contestable.

In this regard, no single set of policies can meet all the challenges of global food subsystem particularly in the international capitalist system. A broader reconstructive consumption which goes beyond greening project is necessary one which links sustainable consumption with production for an equitable democratization is suggested.

Policy instruments to promote sustainable food systems which range from wide perspectives and strategies, should include the need to return to local food systems as they are eco- friendly, healthy and largely interconnected with green consumerism. The eco- friendly debate on food consumption contends that the natural environment cannot be divorced from mode of consumption and suggests instead the preservation the ecosystem. Thus, "eco-friendly consumption", is a strand of sustainability" that "is seen as an act of equitable development, which aims to meet the material needs and at the same time create a healthy environment (Vlaemincka, et al;2014). However a critical dimension has been the notion that 'food is heavily politicised and considered a global industry worth approximately USD 4.8 trillion yearly' (World Bank, 2006).

The ecological justice thesis had emerged to offer a direct and serious challenge to unsustainable capitalist consumption (Korten, 1995; Hobson, 2003; Harvey, 2005; Eastwood, 2006; Akenji & Begsson, 2014; Amadi, et al., 2014). Korten (1995) had called for an ecological revolution one which includes environmental sustainability, economic justice, biological and cultural diversity. Specifically, to serve the needs of the people and not corporations or governments.

Thus, the entire line of debate in this work emphasizes the need for pro poor, inclusive and eco-friendly consumption pattern.

Eco friendly consumption is a pro-environment consumption pattern which forms part of the alternative consumption debate. It is akin to green consumerism which includes reduction in food toxins, global warming emissions, reduction in biodiversity loss, wildlife preservation, protection of the ecosystem and natural habitats etc.

Green consumerism aims to promote consumption in "natural state" namely eco-efficient access and extraction of natural resources, eating fresh and healthy meals including fruits or vegetables. Thus natural resources if sustainably consumed can add value in many ways to the environment.

The "ecosystem first" consumption dynamics is a pro-environment research agenda which aims to protect the ecosystem needs of the present and future generations in the cause of consumption without tainting the environment. It protects species that inhabit the system. As it aims at ecological conscious consumer behaviour (ECCB) (Straughan & Roberts, 1999)., green purchase behaviour and the green consumer (Jansson, Marell, & Nordlund, 2010; Akehurst & Akenso,2012; Riley, Kohlbacher & Hofmeister, 2012).

Ecological foot print in consumption maintains a clean and healthy consumption dynamic. The aim is to check emission and related green -house effects associated with capitalist consumption.

Strict state regulation based on command-and-control policies to weak state intervention relying on market-based instruments and to private voluntary initiatives could prove helpful in mitigating unsustainable choices and 'consumer freedom' that guides capitalist consumption patterns (Reisch et al., 2013).

Sustainability measurement (Amadi & Imohita, 2017) suggests "ecological accounting" to check unequal and deleterious resource consumption. The point this chapter continues to argue is that sustainability is notable for its critical emphasis on resource efficiency and equitability. And that such hugely significant insights could only be useful where sustainability challenges are matched with ecological policies as some of the foundational questions of development, particularly the relationship of food consumption to sustainability have not been adequately resolved.

The fundamental objectives of this chapter require collaborative policy framings involving relevant stakeholders including the global food giants, policy makers and corporations. Getting the capitalist corporations to account for their mode of natural resource extraction remains at issue. Korten (1995) suggests that neo liberal consumption patterns are linked to global consolidation of corporate power. He provides useful critique of neo liberal consumerism, market deregulation, free trade and privatization. Bakan (1995) had explored this within the context of 'pathological pursuit of profits' pointing out the evidence of capitalist exploitation that drives corporations.

The chapter re-emphasizes the global dichotomy in food system among the affluent North and the poor South. In particular, there is need to rethink the consumption culture and the patterns of lifestyles of the affluent societies. Policy response in this direction should argue instead for resource renewal and ecological justice. This orientation has given rise to the need for new policy initiative with the question of food and consumption policies in the modern societies including global and regional conferences, the involvement of international food and research institutes and NGOs.

The underlying practices and understanding of what policies that are driving these trends in the is critical. Much of these require new policy intervention which this chapter emphasizes at intervals.

Perhaps one of the greatest contributions of sustainable food consumption is the need for resource accountability and equality to check the access and resource control dynamics of the powerful nations. Against the idealization of sustainable consumption, terms such as green consumerism as explicated, consistently emphasize the socially just and equitable mode of consumption. Thus, sustainable consumption is not a set of abstract term insulated from ecological and social reality. Rather, it constitutes the reality of everyday living, "food is life" and should be protected in equitable contexts.

Thus, idealist orientation which conceives food as mere "thing" within abstract contexts, devalues food from the actual development realm and rather suggests a mundane and naïve rhetoric. In particular, while sustainable food consumption is critical to resource efficient development, it points out that humanity must assimilate resource renewal, ecological justice and eco-friendly dynamics. This implicates the capitalist material accumulation which appears to be at variance with the ideal values and norms of sustainable food consumption. This points out the inevitability of new constitutive relationships between 'food' and 'consumption', in the liberal order in a manner which puts sustainability at the center of policy discourse.

So, while the dominant neo liberal consumption patterns remain largely materialistic in orientation, this arguably vitiates sustainable consumption. Harvey (2005)provides one of the most influential treatise in this direction leading to his contention on "creative destruction" .Thus, pattern of food consumption that meets generational needs of humanity and preserves the natural environment is inevitable.

FUTURE RESEARCH DIRECTIONS

Although this chapter tackled an important aspect of sustainable development that could result in further thought provoking debates, several important research themes are worth investigating for a future study. The point the chapter has been aiming at is that the dilemma surrounding international political economy of food consumption may likely worsen the existing inequalities and gaps in well-being across the North and South. Emphasis should be laid on strategies to bridge this gap. Future research should critically examine modernization of agriculture to either provide a nuanced critique or otherwise. A new research engagement with "green revolution" is suggested to help the developing societies to boost food production in a sustainable manner. Novel trends such as GM or GE seeds or crops should be re-examined in further research to understand the future policy direction of food system.

Against, the rise in capitalist farming and plantation agriculture are themes of scholarly relevance and should be given research attention including dynamics and patterns of the use of organic fertilizers. Thus, future research direction should insist on theorizing the possible strategies or alternative policy options for inclusive and green consumption.

CONCLUSION

Based on the key issues raised in this chapter in line with the methodological tools and over- all objective of the study, a number of evidence suggesting how sustainable food consumption has been compromised particular since the post 1992 Rio summit and its agenda 21 the plan of action for implementation of sustainable development was provided.

The neoliberal consumption patterns and trade regimes are not entirely free with regards to the poor societies. While it fosters protectionism in the developed countries in which they open their markets to highly subsidized foreign competition, the poor societies are increasingly restricted with highly stringent conditions. This impedes economic diversification, on the contrary, fosters dependency and inequality. Thus the developing societies are tailored in line with Western food systems in the international capitalist system. This has dominated the ideals of the Breton Woods institution.

There is need for urgent policy response. Thus, food provision alone as propagated by neo liberal proponents is not enough but creating the enabling policy framework to mitigate the adverse environmental challenges is important.

The mainstream notion of consumption reinforces the liberal ideals of freedom of choice in a market society seemingly at the expense of the ecosystem. Capitalism encourages profit maximization regardless of ecological and environmental costs. The chapter demonstrates that this increasingly taints the ecosystem, creates global disparity and inequality. Yet the dominant notion is that there is no alternative. While the chapter does not suggest alternative order, are there no alternative ways of mitigating the rise in unsustainable consumption? This forms the basis for the argument on sustainable food consumption.

REFERENCES

Agnew, J. (2005). *Hegemony The New Shape of Global Power*. Philadelphia: Temple University Press.

Ake, C. (1981). *A Political Economy of Africa*. London: Longman.

Akehurst, G., Afonso, C., & Gonçalves, H. (2012). Re-examining green purchase behavior and the green consumer profile: New evidences. *Management Decision, 50*(5), 972–988. doi:10.1108/00251741211227726

Akenji, L., & Begsson, M. (2014). *Making Sustainable Consumption and Production the Core of the Sustainable Development Goals*. Discussion Paper Institute for Environmental Global Strategies.

Altieri, M. (2008). *Small farms as a planetary ecological asset: Five key reasons why we should support the revitalization of small farms in the Global South*. Third World Network.

Amadi, L. (2012). Africa: Beyond the "new" dependency: A political economy. *African Journal of Political Science and International Relations, 6*(8), 191–203. doi:10.5897/AJPSIR12.022

Amadi, L., & Igwe, P. (2016). Maximizing the Eco Tourism Potentials of the Wetland Regions through Sustainable Environmental Consumption: A Case of the Niger Delta, Nigeria. *The Journal of Social Sciences Research, 2*(1), 13–22.

Amadi, L., Igwe, P., & Wordu, S. (2014). Sustainable Development, Greening and Eco-efficiency. A Political Ecology. *Journal of Sustainable Development Studies, 7*(2), 161–196.

Amadi, L., & Imoh-Ita, I. (2017). Intellectual capital and environmental sustainability measurement nexus: A review of the literature *Int. J. Learning and Intellectual Capital, 14*(2), 154–172. doi:10.1504/IJLIC.2017.084071

Amin, S. (1972). Underdevelopment and Dependency in Black Africa Origins and Contemporary Form. *The Journal of Modern African Studies, 10*(4), 503–524. doi:10.1017/S0022278X00022801

Åström, S., Roth, S., Wranne, J., Jelse, K., & Lindblad, M. (2013). *Food consumption choices and climate change*. Swedish Environmental Research Institute.

Bakan, J. (2004). *The Corporation: The Pathological Pursuit of Profit & Power*. Toronto: Penguin Group.

Bello, W. (2003). *De-globalization:Ideas for a New World Economy*. Fernwood.

Berne Declaration. (2013). *Agropolicy. A handful of corporations control world food production*. Available at http://www.econexus.info/sites/econexus/files/Agropoly_Econexus_BerneDeclaration.pdf

Brenkert, G. (1998). The Marketing Challenge: Towards Being Profitable and Socially Responsible. *Journal of Business Ethics, 7*(7), 497–507.

Bryant, R., & Bailey, S. (1997). *Third world political ecology: An introduction*. London: Routledge.

Carlsson-Kanyama, A. (1997). Weighted average source points and distances for consumption origin-tools for environmental impact analysis? *Ecological Economics, 23*(1), 15–23. doi:10.1016/S0921-8009(97)00566-1

Chang, H. (2003). Kicking Away the Ladder: Development Strategy in Historical Perspective. In Re-thinking Development Economics. Anthem Press.

Chase-Dunn, C. (1989). *Global Formation*. Cambridge, MA: Blackwell.

Chen, S., & Ravallion, M. (2001). How did the World's Poor Fare in the 1990s? *Review of Income and Wealth, 4*(3).

Chew, S. (1995). Environmental Transformations: accumulation,Ecological Crisis and Social Movements. In D. Smith & J. Borocz (Eds.), *A New World Order?Global Transformations in the Late Twentieth Century*. Westport, CT: Praeger Publishers.

Conway, D., & Hynen, N. (2006). *Globalization's Contradictions: Geographies of Discipline,destruction and Transformation*. New York: Routledge.

Davidson, D., & Hatt, K. (2005). *Consuming Sustainability Critical Social Analysis of Ecological Change*. Fernwood Publishing.

Eastwood, L. (2006). Contesting the Economic Order: Resisting the Media Construction of Reality. In S. Best & A. J. Nocella (Eds.), *Igniting a Revolution: Voices in Defense of Mother Earth*. Edinburgh, UK: AK Press.

Eberle, U., Hayn, D., Rehaag, R., & Simshäuser, U. (Eds.). (2006). *Ernährungswende. Eine Herausfor-derung für Politik, Unternehmen und Gesellschaft* [Nutrition Change: A Challenge for Politics, Business, and Society]. Munich: Oekom. (in German)

Ekekwe, E. (1986). *Class and State in Nigeria*. London: Longman.

Estavo, G., & Prakash, M. (1998). *Grassroots Post-Modernism: Remaking the soil of cultures*. Zed Books.

FAO. (2002). The State of Food Insecurity in the World 2001. Rome: FAO.

FAO. (2010). *Biodiversity for a World without Hunger*. Retrieved from http://www. fao.org/biodiversity/biodiversity-home/en/

FAO. (2012). *Food Outlook Global Market Analysis*. FAO.

FAO. (2015). *The State of Food and Agriculture. Social protection and agriculture: Breaking the cycle of rural poverty*. FAO.

FAO. (2017). *The State of Food Security and Nutrition in the World*. FAO.

Frison, E. (2009). Director General calls for investment in true food security. *Biodiversity News*. Retrieved from http://www.bioversityinternational.org/news_and_events/news/news/article

Fuchs, D., & Lorek, S. (2001). Sustainable Consumption Governance in a Globalizing World. *Global Environmental Politics, 2*(1), 19–45. doi:10.1162/152638002317261454

Georges, M. (2001). Recent progress in livestock genomics and potential impact on breeding programs. *Theriogenology, 55*(1), 15–21. doi:10.1016/S0093-691X(00)00442-8 PMID:11198079

Gepts, P. (2006). Plant genetic resources conservation and utilization: The accomplishments and future of a societal insurance policy. *Crop Science, 46*(5), 2278–2292. doi:10.2135/cropsci2006.03.0169gas

Giddens, A. (1990). *The consequences of Modernity*. Stanford, CA: Stanford University Press.

Gonzalez, C. (2004). Trade Liberalization, Food Security and the Environment: The Neoliberal Threat to Sustainable Rural Development. *Transnat'l L. & Contemp. Probs., 14*(4), 419.

Gupta, P., & Tsuchiya, T. (1991). *Chromosome Engineering in Plants: Genetics, Breeding Evolution*. Amsterdam: Elsevier.

Harvey, D. (2005). *Brief History of Neoliberalism*. New York: Oxford University Press.

Haws, K., Winterich, K., & Naylor, R. (2014). Seeing the world through GREEN-tinted glasses: Green consumption values and responses to environmentally friendly products. *Journal of Consumer Psychology, 24*(3), 336–354. doi:10.1016/j.jcps.2013.11.002

Heyman, Y., Vignon, X., Chesne, P., Le Bourhis, D., Marchal, J., & Renard, J. P. (1998). Cloning in cattle: From embryo splitting to somatic nuclear transfer. *Reproduction, Nutrition, Development, 38*(6), 595–603. doi:10.1051/rnd:19980602 PMID:9932293

Hinrichsen, D., Salem, R., & Blackburn, R. (2002) Meeting the Urban Challenge. Population Reports, Series M, No. 16. Baltimore, MD: The Johns Hopkins Bloomberg School of Public Health, Population Information Program.

Hobson, K. (2003). Consumption, Environmental Sustainability and Human Geography in Australia: A Missing Research Agenda? *Australian Geographical Studies, 41*(2), 148–155. doi:10.1111/1467-8470.00201

Holsti, O. (1969). *Content Analysis for the Social Sciences and Humanities*. Addison-Wesley.

IOM (Institute of Medicine). (2015). *A framework for assessing effects of the food system*. Washington, DC: The National Academies Press.

Jacobsen, S., Sorensen, M., Soren, M., & Weiner, J. (2013). Feeding the world: Genetically modified crops versus agricultural biodiversity. *Agronomy for Sustainable Development, 0138-9*. doi:10.100713593-013

Jansson, J., Marell, A., & Nordlund, A. (2010). Green consumer behavior: Determinants of curtailment and eco-innovation adoption. *Journal of Consumer Marketing, 27*(4), 358–370. doi:10.1108/07363761011052396

Janvry, L. (1981). *The Agrarian Question and Reformism in Latin America*. Johns Hopkins University Press.

Jongen, W., & Meerdink, G. (1998). *Food Product Innovation: How to Link Sustainability and the Market*. Wageningen Agricultural University.

Klak, T. (2013). World System theory core,semi-peripheral and peripheral regions. In The companion to Development Studies. Routledge.

Klein, N. (2008). *The Shock Doctrine The Rise of Disaster Capitalism*. Metropolitan Books Henry Holt and Company.

Korten, D. (1995). *When Corporations Rule the World*. West Hartford, CT: Kumarian Press Inc.

Lawrence, G., Lyons, K., & Tabatha, W. (2010). *Food Security, Nutrition and Sustainability*. New York: Earthscan.

Lock, I., & Ikeda, S. (2005). *Clothes Encounters: Consumption, Culture, Ecology and Economy. In Consuming Sustainability Critical Social Analysis of Ecological Change*. Fernwood Publishing.

Lönnroth, M. (2010). The Organization of Environmental Policy in Sweden - A Historical Perspective. *The Swedish Environmental Protection Agency Report, 6404*, 319.

Lukaszewski, A. (2004). Chromosome manipulation and crop improvement. In *Encyclopedia of Plant and Crop Science*. New York: Marcel Dekker. doi:10.1081/E-EPCS-120005593

Martin, A. (2008, May 18). One Country's Table Scraps, Another Country's Meal. *The New York Times*.

Marx, K. (1978). *The Marx-Engels Reader*. New York: Norton.

Masters, B. (2004). *Safety of Genetically Engineered Foods: Approaches to Assessing Unintended Health Effects*. Washington, DC: The National Academies of Sciences.

Milner, D. (2012). *Consumption and Its Consequences*. Cambridge Polity Press.

Moomaw, W., Griffin, T., Kurczak, K., & Lomax, J. (2012). *The Critical Role of Global Food Consumption Patterns in Achieving Sustainable Food Systems and Food for All, A UNEP Discussion Paper*. United Nations Environment Programme, Division of Technology, Industry and Economics.

Moore, J. (2000). Environmetal Crisis and the Methabolic Rift in World –historical perspective. *Organization & Environment, 13*(2), 2. doi:10.1177/1086026600132001

Muller, J. (2013). Capitalism and Inequality, What the Right and the Left Get Wrong. *Foreign Affairs, 92*(2), 30–51.

Nesheim, M., Oria, M., & Yih, P. (Eds.). (2015). *A Framework for Assessing Effects of the Food System*. Washington, DC: The National Academies Press.

NRC (National Research Council). (2004). *Safety of Genetically Engineered Foods: Approaches to Assessing Unintended Health Effects*. Washington, DC: The National Academies Press.

NRC (National Research Council) & IOM (Institute of Medicine). (2015). A framework for assessing effects of the food system. Washington, DC: The National Academies Press.

O'Connor, J. (1998). *Natural Causes: Essays in Ecological Marxism*. Guiford Press.

Paalberg, R. (2013). *Food Politics: What Everyone Needs to Know*. Oxford University Press.

Paarlberg, R. (2008). *Starved for Science: How Biotechnology is Being Kept Out of Africa*. Harvard Univ. Press. doi:10.4159/9780674041745

Paehlke, R. (2003). Egalitarian Perspectives on Sustainability. In UNESCO's Encyclopaedia of Life Support Systems (vol. 36). UNESCO.

Panitch, L., & Leys, C. (Eds.). (2007). Coming to Terms with Nature: Socialist Register 2007. Fernwood.

Peet, E., & Watts, W. (1996). Liberation Ecology: Development, Sustainability and Environment in an Age of Market Triumphalism. In R. Peet & M. Watts (Eds.), *Liberation Ecologies:Environment,Develo pment,Social movements* (pp. 1–45). London: Routledge. doi:10.4324/9780203286784

Pinstrup-Andersen, P. (2010). *The advantages of genetic engineering in agriculture include increased food production and reduced hunger - benefits for hungry and malnourished in developing countries outweigh disadvantages.* Retrieved from http://www.monsanto.com/biotech GM/asp/experts.asp?id=P

Ravallion, M. (2001). *On the urbanization of poverty.* Washington, DC: World Bank. doi:10.1596/1813-9450-2586

Rees, T. (1998). *Mainstreaming Equality in the European Union: Education, Training and Labour Market Policies.* Routledge.

Reisch, L., Eberle, U., & Lorek, S. (2013). Sustainable food consumption: an overview of contemporary issues and policies. *Sustainability: Science, Practice, & Policy, 9*(2), 7–25.

Riley, L., Kohlbacher, F., & Hofmeister, A. (2012). A cross-cultural analysis of pro-environmental consumer behavior among seniors. *Journal of Marketing Management, 28*(3-4), 290–312. doi:10.1080 /0267257X.2012.658841

Robbins, P. (2004). *What is political ecology? In Political ecology: A critical introduction* (pp. 5–16). Malden, MA: Blackwell Publishing.

Roberts, J., & Grimes, P. (2002). World system Theory and the environment: Towards a new Synthesis. In Sociological Theory and the Environment: Classical Foundations, Contemporary Insights. New York: Rowman and Littlefield.

Rogers, K. (1997). *Ecological Security and Multinational Corporations.* Kluwer Academic Publishers.

Rosin, C., Stock, P., & Campbell, H. (Eds.). (2011). Food Systems Failure The Global Food Crisis and the Future of Agriculture. London: Routledge.

Schnaiberg, D., & Gould, K. (1994). *Environment and Society The Enduring conflict.* New York: St Martin's.

Schor, J. (2005). Prices and quantities: Unsustainable consumption and the global economy. *Ecological Economics, 55*(3), 309–320. doi:10.1016/j.ecolecon.2005.07.030

Sears, E. (1981). Transfer of alien genetic material to wheat. In L. T. Evans & W. J. Peacock (Eds.), *Wheat Science, Today and Tomorrow* (pp. 75–89). Cambridge, UK: Cambridge University Press.

Shapouri, H., Gallagher, P., Nefstead, W., Schwartz, R., Noe, R., & Conway, R. (2010). *Energy balance for the corn–ethanol industry. Agricultural Economic Report 846. Office of the Chief Economist.* Washington, DC: U.S. Department of Agriculture.

Shopouri, S., Rosen, M., Peters, S., Tandon, F., Mancino, G. L., & Bai, J. (2011). *International Food Security Assessment, 2011-12. GFA- 22*. United States Department of Agriculture-Economic Research Service. Retrieved from http://www.ersusda.gov/Publications/GFA22/GFA22.pdf

Spaargaren, G. (1997). *The ecological modernisation of production and consumption: in environmental. sociology*. Wageningen, The Netherlands: Landbouw University Wageningen.

Steger, M. (2002). *Globalism: The new Market ideology*. New York: Rowman and Littlefield Publishers.

Stein, H. (2003). Rethinking African Development. In Rethinking Development Economics. Anthem Press.

Stern, P. (1997). *Environmentally Significant Consumption*. National Academy Press.

Stiglitz, J. (2010). *Free Fall: America, Free Markets and the Sinking of the World Economy*. New York: W.W. Norton.

Straughan, R., & Roberts, J. (1999). Environmental segmentation alternatives: A look at green consumer behavior in the new millennium. *Journal of Consumer Marketing, 16*(6), 558–575. doi:10.1108/07363769910297506

Swedish Environmental Protection Agency (SEPA). (2010). *The Climate Impact of Swedish Consumption*. Author.

Tiu, J. (2017). *Nestlé, Unilever, P&G Among Worst Offenders for Plastic Pollution in Philippines Beach Audit*. Available at https://www.ecowatch.com/plastic-pollution-philippines-beach-audit-2488280848.html

UN. (2015). *The Zero Hunger Challenge – Advisory notes for action*. The UN Secretary General's High level Task Force on Global Food and Nutrition Security. Retrieved from http://www.un.org/en/issues/food/taskforce/pdf/HLTF%20 %20ZHC%20Advisory%20Notes.pdf

UNEP. (2012). *The critical role of global food consumption patterns in achieving Sustainable Consumption*. Nairobi, Kenya: UNEP.

United Nations Commission for Environment and Development (UNCED). (1992). *Agenda 21*. Oxford Press.

Vlaemincka, P., Jiangb, T., & Vrankena, L. (2014). Food labeling and eco-friendly consumption: Experimental evidence from a Belgian supermarket. *Ecological Economics, 108*.

Wallerstein, I. (1976). World System Analysis:the second Phase'. *RE:view, 13*(2).

Wang, S., Just, D., & Pinstrup-Andersen, P. (2006). *Tarnishing Silver Bullets: Bt technology adoption, bounded rationality and the outbreak of secondary pest infestations in China*. Paper presented at American Agricultural Economics Association annual meeting, Long Beach, CA.

Wapner, P. (1996). *Environmental Activism and World Civic Politics*. State University of New York Press.

Weinstein, B. (2008). Developing Inequality. *The American Historical Review, 113*(1), 1–18. doi:10.1086/ahr.113.1.1

Wise, T. (2015). Two roads diverged in the food crisis: Global policy takes the one more travelled. *Canadian Food Studies, 2*(2), 9–16.

Wolf, E. (1997). *Europe and the People Without History*. Berkeley, CA: University of California Press.

World Bank. (1991). *Urban policy and economic development: An agenda for the 1990s*. Washington, DC: World Bank. Retrieved from http://wwwds.worldbank.org/servlet/WDSContentServer/WDSP/IB/1999/0/10/000178830_9810 9014 2135/Rendered/PDF/multi_page.pdf

World Bank. (2006). *The World Bank Annual Report*. Retrieved from http:// siteresources.worldbank.org/INTANNREP2K6/ Resources/2838485 1158333614345/AR06_final_LO_RES.pdf

KEY TERMS AND DEFINITIONS

Capitalist Consumption: A materialistic pattern of consumption informed primarily by profit motives and value augmentation at the expense of the natural environment or ecosystem.

Eco-Efficiency: The less wasteful use of the ecosystem's natural resources.

Green Consumer: A natural resource friendly consumption pattern that does not taint the environment.

Political Ecology: A Marxian theory which underscores the primacy of resource equality as a critique of the neo Malthusian debate.

Sustainable Food Consumption (SFC): A development term linked to socially just and ecologically friendly consumption pattern.

This research was previously published in Food Systems Sustainability and Environmental Policies in Modern Economies edited by Abiodun Elijah Obayelu; pages 90-123, copyright year 2018 by Engineering Science Reference (an imprint of IGI Global).

Chapter 53

Food and Environment:
A Review on the Sustainability of Six Different Dietary Patterns

Pedro Pinheiro Gomes

National Statistics Institute, Portugal

ABSTRACT

Recent studies related the link between food consumption and impacts on environment and health. These may present variations according to the dietary patterns of different populations. This chapter assesses the impacts of six dietary patterns while emphasizing protein overconsumption and sustainability of food systems in a world where one billion people are hungry and several more suffer from conditions related to obesity. The chapter shows the nutritional disparity existent in different dietary patterns and potential to make changes. Changes in dietary patterns are an opportunity to contribute for environmental and health benefits. The analysis was based on a set of environmental indicators such as greenhouse gas (GHG) emissions and land use demand, while providing a nutritional balance. The methodology comprehended a life cycle assessment in order to quantify the GHG emissions and the land use demand for food production. Finally, a review is made to focus on the benefits of shifting from current diet patterns to more sustainable ones, such as the Mediterranean.

FOOD AND ENVIRONMENT

With the fast growth of cities and the increase in world population food needs keep increasing in order to face the demands. This demand is responsible for the increase of pressures over the environment. The priorities for the communities' well-being become interlinked with those regarding environmental conservation (Johns and Eyzaguirre, 2001; Chan et al, 2011). Nutrition is the most fundamental aspect for the human needs; deficient nutrition can lead to health problems such as malnutrition, infectious diseases, contamination and also obesity (FAO, 2011). Environmental contamination from industrial sources such as heavy metals and organochlorines can contribute to people's nutrition and health. The main challenge of food for the 21st century is to try to understand how diets can respect the body's needs of nutrients and energy while maintaining the balance of ecosystems and respect cultural differences between communities.

DOI: 10.4018/978-1-7998-5354-1.ch053

The quality of the environment is vital to the quality of food, since in every region, each species is adapted to the local conditions, if these change, the ecosystems will be impacted, thus, plants and animals will also have to adapt in a direction that may be less productive and even lead to extinction (OECD, 2011). Not every impact is easily predictable, for instance, it is common sense that a forest fire will have severe impacts on the ecosystem, however, what are the effects of climate changes on the productivity? Although several sources point out that many cultivated plants will react positively to the predicted increase of carbon dioxide in the atmosphere, weeds will also react favourably, which can lead to a decrease in soil, thus, leading to the increase in the use of pesticides with potential negative impacts over agriculture. These risks will contribute to a decrease in food safety, especially to those who depend on agriculture for food and income (Oenema et al., 2007; Cassman et al, 2003). The quality of environment in which food is produced also translates, according to FAO (2011) into three classes of potential croplands: prime, good and marginal. About 81% of the cultivated land is classified either as prime or good, which means that 19% have its productivity determined by adding other inputs, this percentage of cultivated lands add negative impacts to the environment and the balance of ecosystems.

The conversion of lands with low productivity in terms of food production will decrease its capacity to provide other goods and services.It is precisely in such situations that land use and its proper management has impact on both food production and environmental sustainability. Regarding water, its quality is essential for populations in terms of consumption and use for agriculture and livestock production. However, it is also used for activities like production and processing of food, its preparation and also for disposal of waste. Since agriculture is highly dependent on water, its scarcity will affect either the quality of produced food, or the water availability needed for livestock. The current patterns of use of water for agriculture are unsustainable with several negative impacts requiring an efficient approach for its use (FAO, 2011). The production or value of crops per volume of water utilized will be a decisive factor into the choices in land management for agriculture. This indicator is currently low (OECD, 2008) since the losses of water are around 50% due to ineffective practices or lack of investment in new technologies such as low pressure sprinklers or drip irrigation.

In a world where it's expected to have less availability of water for agriculture due to the effects of climate changes and with the fertility of soil decreasing with the abundant use of inputs to force high productivities, it is essential to establish efficient pratices for water consumption, while maintaining the soils structure without the use of inputs and pesticides that damage not only surface water but also groundwater. Regarding climate change and its effects on water, it is expected to impact the availability in many regions, affecting the precipitation, hydrologic flows and recharges of groundwater, water quality will also be compromised due to the flooding of fertile coastal regions due to sea level rise (IPCC, 2014). An European Commission study (EC/JRC, 2009), showed that food consumption represented 27% of all environmental impacts in the EU-27, and enhanced a prominent role of meat production on environmental impacts generated along the food chain.

The environment has influence on the quality of food, but the food systems also have impacts over the environment since these use natural resources and depend on human activities. There's still a wide use of fossil fuels to produce, process and transport food which contributes to an increase of carbon dioxide emissions into the atmosphere, the use of imputs lead to the emission of nutrients to water bodies. Food production will always have impacts on the environment since activities such as agriculture and livestock production are open systems based on natural processes, meaning that there's the need of a system in order to manage, control, prevent and if possible avoid effects on the environment (Vermeulen et al., 2012). In Table 1 are synthesized main environmental damages related to each cycle of food, from its production to its waste.

Table 1. Negative Impacts of food activities on the environment

Environmental Impact	Food Production	Food Processing and Packaging	Food Distribution	Food Consumption	Waste Management
GHG Emissions	Fertilizers; Irrigation; Machinery; Livestock; Land Conversion	Machinery	Machinery	Cooking	Landfills
Air	Pastures; Livestock	Exhaust	Exhaust	Cooking	Waste
Biodiversity	Land Conversion; Habitat Fragmentation	Paper and Card		Fuel Use	Pollution
Soil	Erosion; Compaction; Salinization	Pollution	Pollution		Pollution
Water	Eutrophication; Pollution	Pollution	Coastal Degradation		Pollution

Source: Adapted from Ingram (2011)

WATER AND SOIL QUALITY

A food system affects the water resources in several manners, through the overuse of inputs which leads to pollution by nutrients, pesticides, other chemicals, bacteria and organic waste. The pollution can be local, mainly from organic sources, such as waste or effluents or assuming regional and global scale with nutrient and chemical pollution, which, not only affects the quality of water used for agriculture but also drinking water, leading to health risks.

Excessive fertilization, urbanization and livestock production are the main drivers for water pollution with increases in Nitrogen and Phosphorus in the soil which eventually will runoff to the water bodies (Seitzinger et al, 2010; Hall and Richards, 2013). The soils have drivers related to water pollution, the excessive use of inputs such as nutrients and chemicals and emissions from industries will contaminate the soils with heavy metals, copper and zinc, used often in the livestock production. These substances can reduce the productivity of soils, and the effect is persistent, since the removal of contaminants, a process known as "remediation" is very expensive and is often costlier than prevention.

GREENHOUSE GAS EMISSIONS

Emissions occur throughout all activities related to food, such as changes in land use, use of fossil fuels and even energy related diets. Total emissions account for more than 10 gigatonnes of CO2eq in 2010, resulting in around 25% of total greenhouse gas emissions in the reported year (FAO, 2014). Agriculture contributes around 80% of total emissions, due to deforestation and animal sources, such as emission of methane (FAO, 2014). The distribution of food represents an important source of emissions due to the transport, refrigerators leakages and also the preparation of food itself. Mitigation plans for emissions will have to contemplate the food systems in order to have a significant contribution to the environment.

FOOD SYSTEMS DISPARITY

Food security was redefined in the World Summit on Food Security in 2009 (FAO, 2009) depending on four main standards: 1) Food availability, where quantities should be enough to meet the demands; 2) Food Access: Whether physically and economically to support a nutritious diet; 3) Food Use: where the use is related with means and knowledge related to basic nutrition and well being and finally 4) Stability in food availability regarding its access and use. These four pillars should be the back bone of a proper food system while adding a fifth one: Food Sustainability.

Food systems are the main concern of the 2030 Agenda for Sustainable Development, the global commitment is focused to eradicate poverty and hunger while maintaining investments to develop quality of life and economical development. These systems are intended to be "resource-oriented" since they depend largely on natural resources such as land, soil, terrestrial and marine biodiversity (Lang et al, 2009). These resources need to be used efficiently in order to guarantee a sustainable management, since these are also sources of a number of environmental impacts, such as the loss of biodiversity, water degradation and depletion and the emission of greenhouse gas, therefore, the stakeholders related to food systems need to be aware that they influence directly and indirectly the health and quality of life of communities, which also makes them possible agents of change of the current systems (Garnett et al, 2016; Fraser, 2005).

Globalization increased the demand for food, meaning that a system, more than just a way to organize the processes, is a needed requirement since the majority of food that reaches families' plate is no longer produced by families themselves, but it goes (sometimes from long distances) from producers to consumers. Current systems are failing in terms of security, quality of the food itself and threatening sustainability by using more natural resources and inputs to increase productivity to meet the world demands. Food production has more than doubled; diets are energy intense in order to make them affordable, which is often not the equivalent to healthy, or sustainable (Lawrence and Burch, 2007). There is more variety of food, in terms of tastes, presentations, brands and even segments of the brands themselves in the shape of prices, such as the premium brands, well-known brands, low brands and even in terms of presentation with the growth of the "gourmet" sections regarding its marketing. Several local, national and even multinational companies related to food have emerged; some of them used the financial crisis of 2008 to promote these cheaper segments of food to expand their businesses and areas of influence. However, nearly 1 billion people daily are hungry and over 2 billion have nutrient deficiencies and over 2 billion people overweight or even obese, meaning that around 5 billion people have unhealthy patterns which will challenge the sustainability of food systems (Berdegué et al, 2005; Sutton et al, 2013). With the increase in world population, the scenario is not positive; in order to reach the international targets, changes need to be made, to provide access to healthy food to everyone. The main focus should be the markets, at local, regional and even global level to protect the most vulnerable population clusters and rely on information for societies suffering from overconsumption, in order to assist them make the right choices.

It is important to rely on statistics to understand the food systems are and how to assess the equality or inequality between them. The data from Table 2 demonstrate the high dependence of food from nutrients such as Nitrogen and Phosphorus and its impact on the environment and health, especially, natural resources and associated toxicity issues as well as health problems related to deficiencies in nutrition (USGS, 2013; Allen et al, 2011). Land use and the loss of biodiversity still are the main challenges, while the loss of nutrients due to the intensive use of soil leads to the decrease inequality of food (FAO,

2007).. Nonetheless it's also important to highlight the overuse of nutrients as inputs also cause toxicity issues. Higher crop yields have been proposed as an alternative to a more sustainable way of agriculture. However, progress has been slow, since these methods have other problems associated, namely, the pollution of waters due to the use of nutrients and chemicals. Food systems will meet several challenges at short, medium and long term with the population growth, increasing the demand for food, the economy growth in developing countries will change the dietary patterns to more unsustainable ones, with red meat consumption, fish, vegetables and processed foods and drinks (Gustavsson et al, 2011). Climate change is the long term barrier, which will impact weather conditions and the natural resources vital for food production.

Table 2. Minerals needed in food systems and their relation to the environment

Nutrients	Share of Agriculture or Food in use	Deficiency Issues Reported Related to Food	Toxicity Issues
Nitrogen (N)	80%	Protein	Reported
Phosphorus (P)	90%	Reported	Reported
Potassium (K)	85%	Reported	No
Sulphur (S)	60%	Protein	No
Magnesium (Mg)	10%	Reported	No
Calcium (Ca)	10%	Reported	No
Iron (Fe)	1%	Reported	No
Zinc (Zn)	2%	Reported	Reported
Copper (Cu)	1%	Unknown	Reported
Molybdenum (Mo)	1%	Unknown	Reported
Manganese (Mn)	1%	Unknown	No
Boron (B)	12%	Reported	Unknown
Selenium (Se)	10%	Reported	Reported
Iodine (I)	1%	Reported	Unknown
Cobalt (Co)	1%	Reported in deficiencies of B12 vitamin	Unknown

Source: Adapted from USGS (2013)

The efficient management of food systems will be an imperative, as it is stated in the Sustainable Development Goals, and it goes through the prevention of resource degradation by adapting good practices such as diminishing overexploitation, increasing the efficient use of resources while decreasing the environmental impact of food production, higher agricultural yields without increasing environmental impacts, reducing the use of pesticides, higher productivity of feed conversion, efficient use of energy and water, reduction of food losses throughout the chains and alerting to the impact of overconsumption in diets (Galal, 2002;Verburg et al, 2012).

DIETARY PATTERNS

The six dietary patterns selected for this analysis were based on a study from Auestad and Fulgoni (2015), based on several other studies comparing the method of analysis, the region, the environmental impacts, the conclusions and also the study limitations in order to allow improvement for future analysis. The selection of the studies was subjective, and is intended to cover different global realities. Diet 1 is based on the pattern consumptions of New Zealand, Diet 2 in Indian patterns, Diet 3 of rural China patterns, Diet 4 is be representative of a Northern European pattern, Diet 5 an example of a standard European pattern and Diet 6 should be representative of the American pattern.

Greenhouse gas emissions as an environmental indicator is a measure of the energy-driven procedures applied to the production of food composing the dietary pattern. The more resources are spent and the more processing is applied to the food, more energy will be spent leading to a trend to deforestation patterns for conversion to intensive agriculture. These are the main drivers to increase carbon dioxide emissions, thus, making the first choice indicator in terms of environmental analysis.

Diet 1 has higher costs to the communities; however the tradeoff between food quality, security and price results in higher environmental protection; the reduction of the use of milk increases the cost of food. Diet 2 presents several sources for greenhouse gases; however it also presents threats, since the dietary pattern is varied, and since it refers to a country in its developing stage, if it enters in an industrialized pattern of eating with consumption of meat, probably environmental impacts will increase severely. Diet 3 is in the exact opposite of the industrialized pattern, where the dietary pattern is the minimum required for survival in which meat consumption will translate into a more balanced diet. However, the tradeoff will be higher values of greenhouse gas emissions. Diet 4 is an example of what could be a sustainable diet with less consumption of meat and more consumption of fruits and vegetables. Diet 5 and especially Diet 6 are meat oriented, which will reflect in higher emissions and consequently more energy and resources are spent; these are the diets further from sustainability.

SUSTAINABLE DIETS

The main challenge regarding diets is to simultaneously provide enough food, in quantity and in a safe way, while conserving nutritional and cultural values to meet the present needs and for the future generations (Kastner et al, 2012). However, there is another dimension to satisfy, which is the environment in the figure of the protection of natural resources, making the diet fully sustainable. FAO provided estimates referring that for 2050, in order to satisfy the needs of the population, there will be the need to increase food production by 60% focusing on animal products (FAO, 2010). While increasing the efficiency of the food systems and reducing waste can cut this number, the biggest shift must be the promotion, not only of healthier diets, but essentially on sustainable diets. FAO recently begun collecting information in order to design methods to assess in different regions, what could be an harmonized concept for a sustainable diet (FAO, 2010).

Table 3. The environmental impacts associated with six dietary patterns

Diet	Study, Year, Reference	Diets	Environmental Impacts	Key Results	Conclusions	Limitations of Study
1	Wilson et al., 2013, New Zealand	Diet modeling study (16 diets) to meet New Zealand nutrient recommendations for men with inputs for energy, macronutrients, and 10 select micronutrients in foods, food prices, food wastage, and food-specific GHGe. Models designed to 1) minimize cost and meet nutritional needs; 2) minimize GHGe and meet nutritional needs; 3) be relatively healthy diets (Mediterranean and Asian style); 4) be familiar New Zealand meals.	GHGe determined for 76 food items. GHGe data were scant for New Zealand foods, so used UK GHGe data; estimates made for some foods. Sensitivity analysis conducted.	Increasing dietary variety and likely acceptability of modeled diets had increased daily cost when optimized for both low-cost and low GHGe. Several diet scenarios had small number of foods (e.g., 9, 10, or 14 foods). All modeled low-cost and low-GHGe diets had likely health advantages over the current New Zealand model. Diets that included ''more familiar meals'' for New Zealanders had higher costs.	Low-cost, low-GHGe modeled diets are complementary but with trade-offs of higher daily food costs. This is partly because of reduction in higher GHGe foods, such as eggs and milk; pushes food choices to more costly alternative foods containing nutrients such as calcium. Milk is a relatively efficient beverage for nutrient provision (i.e., nutrients per GHGe generated).	Diet-related GHGe limited to 76 food items. LCA for GHGe of foods in New Zealand limited; substituted data from the UK, with approximations for foods not covered.
2	Pathak et al., 2010, India	Five common nutritionally balanced diets in India: 1) vegetarian, 2) lacto-vegetarian (vegetarian with milk), 3) ovo-vegetarian (nonvegetarian with egg), 4) nonvegetarian with poultry meat, 5) nonvegetarian with mutton	GHGe (g CO2eq/d) were determined using LCA (production, processing, transportation, and preparation) based on published data	GHGe were 40% higher for nonvegetarian vs. vegetarian meals. Nonvegetarian meal with mutton had 1.8 times more GHGe than vegetarian, 1.5 times more than nonvegetarian with chicken and ovo-vegetarian, and 1.4 times more than lacto-vegetarian. In nonvegetarian meal with mutton, GHGe from mutton (35%) were similar to those from rice (34%). In lacto-vegetarian meal, 49% GHGe were from rice, 22% were from milk.	A change in food habits could offer a possibility for GHGe mitigation. Some potential options to reduce GHGe from food may be consumption of locally produced foods; less mutton; substitute meat and milk with vegetable protein	Diet-related GHGe limited to 16 food products. LCA for GHGe covered on farm production, transport, processing, and preparation (consumer) but not storage and handling losses during production or storage at households. LCA for GHGe from different sources.
3	Zhen et al., 2010, rural Guyuan, China	Habitual diets	Land requirements for 8 food categories (25 foods/ sub categories) determined per capita (m2) and per household (m2 per household)	Food consumption pattern in Guyuan depends on wheat; more mixed for China. Less meat consumed than plant foods; land requirement for meat was only 5.7% of arable land (national average, 8.4%). Animal protein intake was 7.5% of total protein, below recommended 30% protein intake.	In Guyuan, food consumption met only basic energy needs for survival, with protein, especially animal protein, and fat below recommendations. Meat consumption expected to increase with projected increasing incomes of local people, thus toward a more balanced diet.	Several uncertainties and assumptions in estimates of food consumption and land requirements.

continues on following page

Table 3. Continued

Diet	Study, Year, Reference	Diets	Environmental Impacts	Key Results	Conclusions	Limitations of Study
4	Saxe et al., 2012, Denmark	Habitual Danish diet, based on >300 foods/beverages	GHGe based on:	GHGe were lower in diets with less meat and dairy. Type of meat in diet can impact GHGe. Within methodologic constraints, local produce may help reduce GHGe. May be negative effects from organic vs. conventional farming. Alcoholic beverages, sweets, and hot drinks (coffee, tea, cocoa) in habitual diet accounted for 22% of diet-based GHGe (meat at 37%). Theoretical vegetarian diet did not reduce GHGe more than optimized omnivore diet.	A well-designed diet could lead to lower climate impact and improved health. A change to Nordic diets (less animal foods, more fruits and vegetables) could support climate change mitigation, but must be cautious with diet recommendations. Reducing alcoholic drinks, hot drinks, and sweets by 50% would reduce GHGe the same as reducing meat intake by 30%.	Diet-related GHGe limited to 31 food categories. LCA for GHGe only farm to retail and from different sources (Danish LCA food database and from literature).
		Recommended diet:	LCA farm to retail;			
		New Nordic diet (more local foods; 75% organic foods)	LCA ISO 14040 (GHGe/ kg food; based on consequential LCA method);			
		Theoretical scenarios, compared to 3 base diets:	Converted to CO2eq (IPCC 2007);			
		1) Conventional farming	Accounted for wasted and spoiled food;			
		2) Conventional farming with factor for transport of imported foods;	31 food categories, derived from >300 foods/ beverages			
		3) Organic farming with factor for transport of imported foods;	GHGe reported as:			
		Other scenarios:				
		4, 5) Type of meats varied				
		6, 7) Amounts and types of organic foods varied	kg CO2eq/person per year			
		8) Ovo-lacto version of scenario 7				
5	Vieux et al., 2012, France	Habitual diet based on a French national diet survey (2006–2007)	GHGe based on:	GHGe were lower with 240 fewer kcal and less meat intake (when kcal not replaced with other foods). GHGe were moderately reduced when meat and deli kcal replaced with kcal from dairy or mixed dishes. GHGe were negated or slightly higher when meat and deli kcal were replaced with kcal from fruits and vegetables.	GHGe linked to amount of food and kcal eaten. Substituting fruits and vegetables for meat (especially deli meat) may be desirable for health but is not necessarily the best approach to decreasing diet-associated GHGe.	Diet-related GHGe limited to 73 foods. LCA for GHGe only farm to retail, via conventional production and distribution.
		Theoretical diets:	LCA farm to retail;			
		Habitual diet with	LCA ISO 14040;			
		1) 240 fewer kcal	g CO2eq/100 g of edible portion food;			
		2) 20% less meat/deli with a) no replacement of kcal or b) replacement of kcal with fruits/vegetables, dairy, or mixed dishes	73 representative foods			
		3) Red meat limited to 50 g/d; no deli with a) no replacement of kcal or b) replacement of kcal with fruits/ vegetables, dairy, or mixed dishes	GHGe reported as:			
			g CO2eq/d			

continues on following page

Table 3. Continued

Diet	Study, Year, Reference	Diets	Environmental Impacts	Key Results	Conclusions	Limitations of Study
6	Eshel and Martin, 2006, USA	Food consumption based on per capita food disappearance	GHGe based on:	Energy efficiency of animal-based portion of diets: lacto-ovo-vegetarian, omnivore with poultry > average US diet > omnivore with red meat, omnivore with fish. GHGe estimates from theoretical diets (tons CO_2eq/person per year): omnivore with red meat > mean US diet > omnivore with fish > lacto-ovo-vegetarian > omnivore with poultry.	A mixed diet at average US calorie intake has 1485 kg CO_2eq higher emissions than the same number of calories from plant foods.	Diet-related GHGe limited to CO_2eq from agricultural production (on farm). GHGe from direct energy (primarily fossil fuel) and non-CO_2emissions from numerous sources. Theoretical diets described as "semirealistic."
		Theoretical diets: semirealistic mixed diets with animal-based foods at 0–50% daily kcal based on:	Farm only ($CO_2$from direct energy use + non-$CO_2$from agricultural production; NH4, CH4, N2O);			
		1) Average, habitual US diet	LCA ISO 14040 (consequential LCA method)			
		2) Lacto-ovo-vegetarian	GHGe reported as:			
		3) Omnivore with fish source	g CO_2eq/kcal;			
		4) Omnivore with red meat	Tons of CO_2/person per year;			
		5) Omnivore with poultry	Energy efficiency (% fossil fuel energy input retrieved as edible energy from protein output)			

Source: Adapted from Auestad and Fulgoni (2015)

Mediterranean Diet

The Mediterranean Diet is very well known by its characteristics as healthier diet, having been subjected to several analyses to assess its impacts not only on health, but also environment. For the latter, it is suggested that it presents a lower environmental impact with other available options. This diet involves several countries (Portugal, Spain, Italy, Greece, France, Morocco, Cyprus and Croatia, the main motive for which is considered cultural heritage. However, recent studies show that there's a decline of this diet as an option in the Mediterranean area, since this region is passing through a transition in terms of diet to a more energy-related one (Gussow, 1995; Belahsen and Rguibi, 2006).

Figure 1. The Mediterranean Diet
Source: Estruch et al, 2013

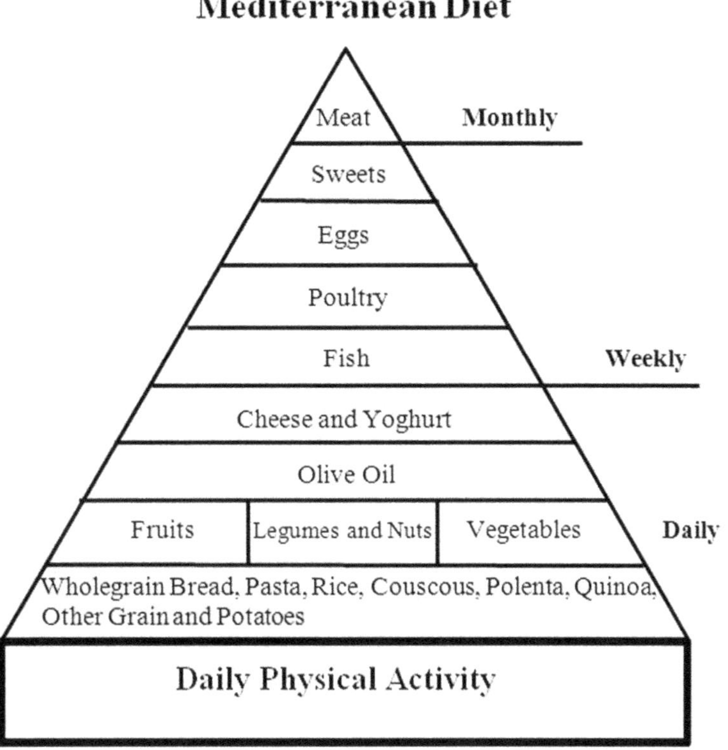

As it is possible to analyze it from Figure 1, the Mediterranean diet is more than just quantity and quality of food, it also incorporated physical exercise into the daily quantities of food. In fact, the basis of the pyramid is daily exercise from moderate to vigorous in order to maintain activity throughout the entire life. Both exercise and correct servings of food allow a proper weight and protect health from nutrient deficiency and diseases related to overconsumption and obesity, namely heart related diseases (Estruch et al, 2013). Analyzing the environmental component related to food of the Mediterranean Diet Pyramid, the monthly consumption of meat will reduce the amount of energy and water used to produce it, thus, reducing GHG emissions, while maintaining the necessary nutritional values to daily food consumption.

A diet rich in protein and calories has several negative impacts on both health and environment. Eating meat was always regarded as a symbol of economic well-being and after an economic crisis in 2008 which affected the very core of families' consumption, the steady recover verified in the financial and economical systems are re-shifting the diets into ones with patterns of industrialization. While improving the food systems in the Mediterranean area may contribute to enhance its influence in the communities, promoting information among communities and alerting stakeholders in food systems the need to promote sustainable diets should be the steps to take to minimize or even mitigate the negative externalities caused by unsustainable diets. The threat to the Mediterranean Diet was evident in the 2005 Mediterranean Strategy on Sustainable Development (UNEP/MAP, 2005): "Mediterranean agricultural and rural models, which are at the origins of Mediterranean identity, are under increasing threat from the predominance of imported consumption patterns. This trend is illustrated in particular by the decline of the Mediterranean dietary model despite its benefits on health. The prospective scenario for the expected impacts of trade liberalization, climate change and the lack of efficient rural policies offers a gloomy picture in some southern and eastern Mediterranean countries, with the prospect of aggravated regional imbalances, deeper ecological degradation and persistent or accrued social instability."

The price of food is one of the key drivers for its consumption nowadays since it is also related to security and access, two of the main pillars of food systems (Kharas, 2010). In lower income countries, expenditure on food accounts for 40-50% of the household budget (FAO, 2014), meaning that people will condition their food choices on how much energy they can get at the minimum possible. This is one of the reasons that also made fast food popular, since people can get calories at a cheap price; however, it also shifts diets to less sustainable ones.

CONCLUSION AND RECOMMENDATIONS

Feeding the world population will require strategies that comprehend multicultural and transversal communication, while considering health and environment related aspects towards more sustainable patterns to use natural resources while ensuring food security.

The activities surrounding food systems have a considerable impact on the environment, mainly due to the overuse of natural resources. The main impacts are on biodiversity, especially due to changes in land use and ecosystems for intensive agriculture and monocultures. IIts impacts will be on air, soil and water quality with the loss of nutrients and water contamination., Energy use and greenhouse gas emissions not only are a measure of the inefficiency of the food systems, but also the main driver for climate changes, which will impact the systems in all the above referred situations.

The lack of proper food systems can have serious problems, such as the increase of vulnerability of agro-systems to resist climate changes and pests and diseases resulting in loss of productivity. The loss of productivity will only result in higher needs of inputs to face the growing demand due to the population increase and the growth of the food industry as a business characterized by the existence of quantity and variety. The regeneration rates of the natural resources will also be lower since the natural systems are overloaded with the increasing use of inputs and the overconsumption of stocks.

It is important to rethink food systems in order to contemplate sustainability by cutting food losses and waste, alerting regarding the consumption of energy-intensive foods such as red meat, processed food and the way urban environments affect the way people consume further from a sustainable way. Reconnecting to the rural roots could develop in the consumers the consciousness that there's the need to promote healthier lifestyles while empowering small producers. There is a lack of information on how local, regional and national food systems interact between themselves, understanding this dynamic would improve the efficiency between producers and consumers. Reinforce investments in education, technology and environmental services are always good measures to sustainability regarding environmental protection and create the conscience that current practices are negative and leading to food inequalities.

From the Diets analysed it was possible to show that Nordic and Mediterranean diets are possible solutions towards the sustainable pattern since they focus on variety, but especially focus on less consumption of meat. A linear comparison of the different food patterns will have several limitations, the choice of the method by each author is different, thus, the quantification of environmental impacts will have different sources of error. However the added value are the different sources of greenhouse gas registered in each pattern, further studies should be based on a single method, but focusing on the application of the method to different realities in order to establish a common ground to define sustainability.

REFERENCES

Allen C.R., Fontaine J.J., Pope K.L., Garmestani A.S. (2011) Adaptive management for a turbulent future. *Journal of Environmental Management, 92*, 1339-1345.

Auestad, N., & Fulgoni, V. L. (2015). What current literature tells us about sustainable diets: Emerging research linking dietary patterns, environmental sustainability, and economics. *Advances in Nutrition, 6*(1), 19–36. doi:10.3945/an.114.005694 PMID:25593141

Belahsen, R., & Rguibi, M. (2006). Population health and Mediterranean diet in southern Mediterranean countries. *Public Health Nutrition, 9*(8A), 1130–1305. doi:10.1017/S1368980007668517 PMID:17378952

Berdegué, J.A., Balsevich, F., Flores, L., & Reardon, T. (2005). Central American supermarkets' private standards of quality and safety in procurement of fresh fruits and vegetables. *Food Policy, 30*, 254-269.

Cassman, K. G., Dobermann, A., Walters, D. T., & Yang, H. S. (2003). Meeting cereal demand while protecting natural resources and improving environmental quality. *Annual Review of Environment and Resources, 28*(1), 315–358. doi:10.1146/annurev.energy.28.040202.122858

Chan, L., Receveur, O., Sharp, D., Schwartz, H., Ing, A., & Tikhonov, C. (2011). *First Nations Food, Nutrition and Environment Study (FNFNES): Results from British Columbia (2008/2009). Prince George.* University of Northern British Columbia.

EC/JRC. (2009). *Environmental impacts of diet changes in the EU. Technical Report, European Commission (EC), Joint Research Centre (DG JRC).* Brussels: IPTS.

Estruch, R., Martínez-González, M. A., & Corella, D. (2013). Effects of a Mediterranean-style diet on cardiovascular risk factors: A randomized trial. *Annals of Internal Medicine, 2006*(145), 1–11. PMID:16818923

FAO. (2007). *Paying farmers for environmental services.* Rome: Food and Agriculture Organization of the United Nations.

FAO. (2009). *Linking people, places and products. A guide for promoting quality linked to geographical origin and sustainable geographical indications.* Rome: FAO/SINER-GI.

FAO. (2010). *Report of the Technical Workshop on Biodiversity in Sustainable Diets.* Rome: FAO.

FAO. (2011). *The state of the world's land and water resources for food and agriculture. Managing systems at risk.* Rome: Food and Agriculture Organization of the United Nations.

FAO. (2014). Agriculture, Forestry and Other Land Use emissions by sources and removals by sinks. Rome: FAO.

Fraser, E.D.G., Mabee, W., & Figge, F. (2005). A framework for assessing the vulnerability of food systems to future shocks. *Futures, 37*, 465-479.

Galal, O. M. (2002). The nutrition transition in Egypt: Obesity, Under-nutrition and the Food Consumption Context. *Public Health Nutrition, 5*(1a), 141–148. doi:10.1079/PHN2001286 PMID:12027277

Garnett, T., Appleby, M.C., Balmford, A., Bateman, I.J., Benton, T.G., Bloomer, P., … Godfray, H.C.J. (2013). Sustainable intensification in agriculture: Premises and policies. *Science, 341*, 33-34.

Gussow, J. D. (1995). Mediterranean diets: Are they environmentally responsible? *The American Journal of Clinical Nutrition, 61*(suppl), 1383S–1389S. PMID:7754992

Gustavsson, J., Cederberg, C., Van Otterdijk, R., & Meybeck, A. (2011). *Global Food Losses and Food Waste.* Rome: Food and Agriculture Organization of the United Nations.

Hall, A. J., & Richards, R. A. (2013). Prognosis for genetic improvement of yield potential and water-limited yield of major grain crops. *Field Crops Research, 143*, 18–33. doi:10.1016/j.fcr.2012.05.014

Ingram, J. (2011). A food systems approach to researching food security and its interactions with global environmental change. *Food Security, 3*, 417-431.

IPCC. (2014). *Mitigation of Climate Change.* Contribution of Working Group III to the Fifth Assessment Report of the Intergovernmental Panel on Climate Change.

Johns, T., & Eyzaguirre, P. B. (2001). Nutrition for sustainable environments. *SCN News, 21*, 24–29.

Kastner, T., Rivas, M. J. I., Koch, W., & Nonhebel, S. (2012). Global changes in diets and the consequences for land requirements for food. *Proceedings of the National Academy of Sciences of the United States of America, 109*(18), 6868–6872. doi:10.1073/pnas.1117054109 PMID:22509032

Kharas, H. (2010). *The Emerging Middle Class in Developing Countries.* Development Centre Working Paper No. 285. Organization for Economic Co-operation and Development.

Lang, T., Barling, D., & Caraher, M. (2009). *Food policy: integrating health, environment and society.* Oxford, UK: Oxford University Press. doi:10.1093/acprof:oso/9780198567882.001.0001

Lawrence, G., & Burch, D. (2007). Understanding supermarkets and agri-food supply chains. In D. Burch & G. Lawrence (Eds.), *Supermarkets and agri-food supply chains: transformations in the production and consumption of foods.* Cheltenham, UK: Edward Elgar.

OECD. (2008). *Environmental Performance of Agriculture in OECD Countries Since 1990*. Paris: OECD Publishing.

OECD. (2011). *Evaluation of Agricultural Policy Reforms in the European Union*. Paris: OECD.

Oenema, O., Oudendag, D., & Velthof, G. L. (2007). Nutrient losses from manure management in the European Union. *Livestock Science, 112*(3), 261–272. doi:10.1016/j.livsci.2007.09.007

Seitzinger, S. P., Mayorga, E., Bouwman, A. F., Kroeze, C., Beusen, A. H. W., Billen, G., ... Harrison, J. A. (2010). Global river nutrient export: A scenario analysis of past and future trends. *Global Biogeochemical Cycles, 24*(4), n/a. doi:10.1029/2009GB003587

Sutton, M.A., Bleeker, A., & Howard, C.M. (2013). *Our nutrient world: the challenge to produce more food and energy with less pollution*. Edinburgh, UK: NERC/Centre for Ecology & Hydrology.

UNEP/MAP. (2005). *Mediterranean strategy for sustainable development: a framework for environmental sustainability and shared prosperity. Tenth Meeting of the Mediterranean Commission on Sustainable Development (MCSD)*, Athens, Greece.

USGS. (2013). *Mineral Commodity Summaries: (various elements)*. Washington, DC: U.S. Geological Survey.

Verburg, P.H., Mertz, O., Erb, K.H., Haberl, H., & Wu, W. (2013). Land system change and food security: towards multi-scale land system solutions. *Current Opinion in Environmental Sustainability, 5*, 494-502. DOI: .cosust.2013.07.003 doi:10.1016/j

Vermeulen, S.J., Campbell, B.M., & Ingram, J.S.I. (2012). Climate Change and Food Systems. *Annual Review of Environment and Resources, 37*, 195-222.

This research was previously published in Food Systems Sustainability and Environmental Policies in Modern Economies edited by Abiodun Elijah Obayelu; pages 15-31, copyright year 2018 by Engineering Science Reference (an imprint of IGI Global).

Chapter 54

Re–Thinking Meat:
How Climate Change Is Disrupting the Food Industry

Jeff Anhang

The World Bank Group, USA

ABSTRACT

This chapter describes how among vegetarian, vegan and animal advocates, it has been a common practice for many decades to cede the terms "meat" to livestock producers, and to ask people to sacrifice meat. Yet during those decades, global consumption of livestock products has exploded. People have often overlooked the fact that "meat" has been defined for centuries as an essential food that includes vegan versions, and plant-based meat has always been framed as equivalent or superior to animal-based meat. In fact, replacing animal-based foods with better alternatives is said to be the only pragmatic way to stop climate change quickly as needed. However, it is unlikely to happen through efforts to reduce meat consumption. It is much more likely to happen through efforts to disrupt meat production and consumption by making and marketing meat and other foods directly from plants.

INTRODUCTION

The invitation to write this chapter started with the following introductory claims: "Our understanding about the benefits and negatives related to the consumption of meat… is influenced by dietary habits and social norms but also by their marketing. There is however ample scientific evidence that excessive meat consumption is not good for the natural environment and can be detrimental to human health".

However, this chapter explains why the abovementioned claims are themselves detrimental. First, vegan food producers sometimes market their products as "meat" (Field Roast, 2017), and dictionaries define "meat" as an essential food that includes plant-based meat (Merriam Webster Dictionary, 2017); so a critique of "excessive meat consumption" is unnecessarily ambiguous if it does not specify whether the meat in question is animal-based or plant-based. Second, the abovementioned claims imply that moderate animal-based meat consumption could be good for the natural environment, when there is plenty

DOI: 10.4018/978-1-7998-5354-1.ch054

of evidence to the contrary. Third, those claims wrongly imply that it could be good for the environment for people to switch from consuming animal-based meat to consuming dairy products and eggs. Fourth, those claims suggest that advocating against excessive meat consumption could be successful, but this is contradicted by history. Fifth, those claims omit any reference to climate change, though plenty of evidence indicates that climate change is unique among environmental risks in being large-scale, transboundary, potentially irreversible, and potentially catastrophic in the near term.

While this chapter provides evidence to contradict the abovementioned claims and their implications, it also proposes ways in which some common views of animal- and plant-based meat might be constructively reassessed.

SHORT HISTORY OF "MEAT"

In English, the word "meat" was used in the early Middle Ages as a generic term to describe foods in general. Later in the Middle Ages, the word gradually became focused on various types of flesh used for food, including the flesh of vegetables (Online Etymology Dictionary, 2017). These days, food companies market products such as "grain meat" (Wegmans, 2017) and "nut meat" (Vegie Delights, 2017), practically always as being equivalent or superior to animal-based meat.

The phenomenon by which plant-based meat is considered equivalent or superior to animal-based meat is not new. Soyfoods started to be considered superior foods in China during the Han dynasty (206 BC–220 AD), when soy sprouts began to be used alternately as both food and medicine. During this period, the introduction of the hand-turned stone mill helped in developing and expanding the production of soymilk, fermented black soybeans, fermented soybean paste, soy sauce, and fermented tofu (Shurtleff et al., 2014).

Starting in the ninth century AD, a form of soymeat called Yuba was created from the film formed when soybeans are boiled; this began first in China and soon after in Japan (Tsutsumi & Tsutsui, 2009). Around the same time, soybean oil and cake – as well as tofu – also started to be created in China (Shurtleff et al., 2014). The earliest known document to use the word "tofu" was written by Tao Ku around the year 965 (Shurtleff et al., 2014). The document was called Qing Yilu – which translates to "Anecdotes, Simple and Exotic" – and it framed soyfoods as superior to animal-based foods. Several centuries later in China, an encyclopedic document entitled Jujia Biyong Shilei Quanji – which translates to "Essential Arts for Family Living" – described methods of making plant-based sausage using wheat gluten. From then through to modern times, soybeans have been rarely used in whole form in Asian cuisine (Shurtleff et al., 2014).

In modern times, disruption of one industry occurs after another has become prevalent. However, this was not always so. In fact, the history of meat shows that its production generally developed in phases of evolution and consolidation, rather than through rapid disruption.

Originally, in Paleolithic societies, people's success in hunting wild animals was never assured; shooting an arrow and missing the target was often as likely as success. As technology for hunting improved, success still was highly variable, notably dependent on seasonality, local climatic conditions, and the local availability of desired animals (Chiles & Fitzgerald, 2017). Later, after the transition from hunting to animal agriculture, animals were first used for draft labor, eggs, milk, wool, and soil fertilization more than for meat. Feed crops were generally considered too valuable to feed to animals. Livestock products were mainly reserved for rich people, and even for them, they often provided a minor contribution to diets overall (Chiles & Fitzgerald, 2017).

The evolution of democracy brought with it a positive political connotation when animal-based meat was taken up by the non-rich. At the same time, vegetarianism became denigrated as being for poor and/or non-Western people. However, vegetarianism was still common due to widespread poverty and the lack of industrialized processes to produce, process, refrigerate, and transport animal-based foods.

Industrialization of livestock production brought refrigeration, transportation, large-scale production, and reduced prices. It also meant that consumption of animal-based foods was no longer dependent on seasonality, local climatic conditions, and the local availability of desired animals. Animal-based foods became symbols of prosperity and health (Chiles & Fitzgerald, 2017). This occurred even though modern European genes may have favored vegetarianism (Ye et al., 2017). Yet while the size and marketing prowess of the livestock sector have increased year after year for many years, plant-based diets have persisted all over the world, even among people who do not live in poverty.

SACRIFICING MEAT

As described above, the origins of the word "meat" indicate that plant-based meat has long been a rival to animal-based meat. This suggests that there is no good reason for ceding the term "meat" to livestock producers and asking people to sacrifice meat. Indeed, since "meat" is commonly defined as an essential food, livestock producers would be expected to benefit by having a monopoly on the marketing of "meat". As evidence of this, a conglomerate representing livestock producers in the European Union has lobbied for the word "meat" to be reserved for animal-based products (Mammoser, 2017). Another tactic used by some livestock producers – and by some people who cannot imagine giving up animal-based meat – is to call plant-based meat "fake".

Yet plant-based meat need not involve any more processing than does whole-wheat bread, which nobody calls fake. In fact, plant-based meat has almost always been produced by artisanal methods – whereas animal-based meat has long been produced in developed economies primarily in factory settings, using hormones and antibiotics. Producers of plant-based meat never use hormones or antibiotics, and they also often avoid genetically modified organisms – which are rarely avoided in animal-based meat production. With that in mind, and given the long history of plant-based meat, animal-based meat could be considered less authentic than plant-based meat. In other words, animal-based meat could be considered an ersatz version of meat when compared to plant-based meat.

However, among vegetarian, vegan, and animal advocates, it has been common practice for many decades to cede the terms "meat" and "milk" to livestock producers, and to ask people to sacrifice meat and milk. Yet during those decades, global consumption of livestock products has exploded six-fold (Renner, 2014), twice as fast as human population growth. Further evidence for a case not to cede the term "meat" to livestock producers exists in a major trend to market plant-based meat for sustainability (Retail News Insider, 2014 and 2017). Therefore, some part of vegetarian, vegan, and animal advocacy might merit re-thinking.

Perhaps the most popular campaign that advocates for people to sacrifice meat is the Meatless Mondays campaign. By touting "meatless" eating in its name, the campaign overlooks the fact that dictionaries define meat as an essential food that includes vegan versions. The Meatless Mondays campaign prioritizes a prescription from medical authorities who have indicated that a 15 percent reduction in saturated fat is needed for good medical health (Kamila, 2011). According to the campaign, this can be fully achieved if people give up consuming meat just one day per week. However, by its name and otherwise, the Meatless Mondays campaign fails to emphasize that dairy products often contain even more saturated fat per serving than does meat, and eggs too contain a significant amount of saturated fat; nor does the campaign indicate what change in consumption is needed for good climatic health.

For example, for consumers concerned about saturated fat, a fitness website has estimated that a 3.5-ounce fast-food hamburger contains approximately 4 grams of saturated fat (Myfitnesspal, 2017a). The same website has also estimated that 100 grams (equivalent to 3.5 ounces) of quiche Lorraine contains 8 grams of saturated fat. Yet the Meatless Mondays campaign can and does lead some people to switch from a hamburger to quiche Lorraine, which can worsen both public health and climate change.

If the Meatless Mondays campaign were to clarify that it frowns upon eggs and dairy products as well as animal-based meat, then it could potentially yield a 13 percent replacement of livestock products with better alternatives. Yet 13 percent less livestock products would be far less than the amount of replacement that is actually needed to reverse climate change – which is somewhere between 50 to 85 percent, depending on whose analysis is used (Goodland, 2014).

However, it seems unlikely that Meatless Mondays will ever yield even 13 percent less livestock products. After all, the campaign frames what is needed as a sacrifice, so the required action is likely to suffer the same fate as everything that promotes sacrifice – i.e., people who sacrifice livestock products one day are likely to crave them more the next day. Indeed, the Meatless Monday campaign anachronistically touts its basis in American rationing during World War I (Meatless Monday, 2017), after which a major expansion in meat production occurred in the U.S. (The National Provisioner, 2016). Yet no consumer product is successfully sold by pressing people to use it just one day a week. For example, consumers might be wary of choosing Pepsi Cola at all if its marketing promoted it as a one-day-a-week drink, conceding that Coca Cola remains the drink of choice the rest of the week.

In fact, while Meatless Mondays has expanded around the world since 2003, the worldwide consumption of livestock products did not fall in the subsequent decade; it rather continued to rise (Nierenberg & Reynolds, 2012). It continued to rise even during 2007-2012 which is especially striking when considering the wave of economic downturns in one region after another during this period. By comparison, in earlier times in history, the consumption of livestock products dropped markedly during economic downturns (Hawkins, 1974).

Actual trends in global meat consumption are surely more important than the trend of organizations to adopt Meatless Mondays. Perhaps the organizers of Meatless Mondays would achieve more success by framing alternatives to livestock products as better products, rather than a sacrifice. If alternatives to livestock products might seem hard to promote, then one might consider as an example the fact that bicycles may be hard to promote to car-lovers, but bike advocates normally do not frame bike-riding as a sacrifice.

The Meatless Monday campaign promotes sacrificing meat to reduce health risks, energy and water usage, and carbon emissions. Yet goals for such reductions are common in the case of many consumer products, and they usually do not motivate major action to replace any products. In contrast, emergencies normally motivate major action – and both the UN Intergovernmental Panel on Climate Change and the UN International Energy Agency have warned that greenhouse gas emissions must be reduced significantly by 2020 (Stromberg, 2012) or at the latest 2026 (Dechert, 2016), or else climate change may no longer be controllable. Therefore, climate change may be the most compelling motivation on which to dwell.

An alternative to the Meatless Mondays campaign is a campaign that has a similar but more sophisticated name, namely Meat Free Monday, founded and operated by three members of a famous family, Mary, Stella and Paul McCartney. By replacing "Meatless" with "Meat Free", they have moved from using a term that connotes taking something away to an expression that raises the idea of being free. Unlike the Meatless Mondays, the Meat Free Monday campaign was launched specifically to address climate change (Lean, 2014). The Meat Free Monday campaign has made it clear that it does not support switching from animal-based meat to eggs or dairy (e.g. Meat Free Monday, 2017b). Sometimes the Meat Free Monday campaign has clearly stated that it promotes "plant-based meats" (e.g. Meat Free Monday, 2017a).

So there are several ways in which the Meatless Monday campaign could easily improve itself to become more relevant – notably by using a more positive and climate-oriented approach to its advocacy; by clarifying that it does not support switching from animal-based meat to eggs or dairy; and by promoting plant-based meat.

In recent years, activists have promoted the idea of getting people to sacrifice animal-based meat by taxing it. Yet people who favor animal-based meat far outnumber those who do not, so it is likely to be political suicide for politicians to propose taxing animal-based meat in almost every jurisdiction in the world. Moreover, in any particular jurisdiction, taxing animal-based meat to combat climate change would contradict the fact that climate change can be managed effectively only with a global approach. Anyway, tax is generally imposed on an industry to get it to do something only when there is not a business case to do it – yet there is a business case for replacing livestock products with better alternatives (Goodland & Anhang, 2009).

A CASE TO REPLACE

A vivid example of how detrimental it can be to advocate for "less meat" was displayed during a meeting in 2015 where public comments were made on recommendations for U.S. dietary guidelines. Those comments can be seen and heard in a video of the meeting (Health.gov, 2015). A man representing McCormick Spices played to the crowd, saying: "let's spice up the guidelines!" He proposed that consumers would buy his company's products "not because they have to but because they want to". Some speakers at the meeting said they were attending on behalf of a broad coalition representing "millions of Americans" anxious for the dietary guidelines to incorporate recommendations for "less meat" to improve environmental sustainability. One couldn't help wondering who would win a contest between millions of "less meat" consumers *versus* hundreds of millions of meat consumers. Indeed, a number of speakers representing livestock interests spoke as if they represented the average consumer, and they pitched livestock products as center-of-the-plate foods in the most positive terms possible.

In contrast, none of those promoting "less meat" pitched anything easily perceived by an average consumer as center-of-the-plate foods. Instead, they pressed for meat to be replaced with things like "fruits and vegetables" and "more plants". They left it to the audience to puzzle over how vegetables and fruits might be something other than side dishes and desserts, and how a plant could be a center-of-the-plate food. Contradicting the claim by the "less meat" speakers that they spoke for a broad coalition, virtually all but one of them were clearly Caucasian. In contrast, many speakers outside that coalition were clearly African American, Asian American, and Hispanic American.

One speaker said "less meat" is needed because emissions of methane and nitrous oxide from livestock production "may double by 2070… making it impossible to meet climate change targets" and "Americans are eager for good science-based information". Yet according to the most prominent climate authorities, the world must significantly reduce greenhouse gases by 2020 (Stromberg, 2012) or at the latest 2026 (Dechert, 2016), or else climate change may no longer be controllable. So, the "less meat" speakers failed to define correctly what is needed. They also failed to explain that Americans cannot act to meet climate targets on their own. That is because greenhouse gas emissions and climate change are large-scale and do not respect borders. Climate targets can be met only if people in much more populous countries participate, especially China and India. Yet it is even less possible to sell "less meat" in China and India than it is in the U.S., as there is much less perception in those countries that there is an excess of meat consumption.

"Less meat" proponents also failed to talk about how widely-cited assessments of food and climate change by the Food and Agriculture Organization of the United Nations (FAO) and others have focused on *all* livestock production, not just meat production. Yet promotion of "less dairy products" and "less eggs" would be even less acceptable than "less meat" in China and India – particularly in India, where dairy products are especially preferred.

So, it seems that what is needed is some sort of positive, internationally acceptable marketing of center-of-the-plate and other vegan products. They could be called something like "Happy Better Vegan Foods". In part because positive marketing of center-of-the-plate products is already being undertaken by plant-based food producers who market products such as "grain meat" and "nut meat," it seems that recommendations for changing U.S. dietary guidelines were mistaken in prescribing "smaller meat portions" without qualifying them as animal-based meat portions.

If a term such as "Happy Better Vegan Foods" would be used, then what is needed could be framed as preferable, delicious center-of-the plate foods and vegan alternatives to dairy products and eggs. This could inspire consumers to choose what is needed not because of dietary guidelines, but because they want to – the holy grail prescribed by the man from McCormick Spices.

A variation on the "less meat" theme came from a speaker advocating for the "humane" raising of animals. She spoke of her concern for greenhouse gas emissions, saying: "The FAO has evidence to show that 14.5 percent of anthropogenic greenhouse gas emissions come from livestock production". Therefore, this speaker claimed, "there is an overwhelming case" to accept recommendations for "less meat". However, the FAO report that originated the cited 14.5 percent emissions estimate actually promotes more livestock production, to be facilitated by "technologies and practice currently used by the 10 percent of producers with the lowest emission intensity" (Gerber et al., 2013, p. xiii). The lowest emission intensity producers are those with the most confined operations – which means that they raise animals in the least humane way possible.

The FAO's livestock-climate analysis cited by the "less meat" speakers was used in the recommendations for "less meat" that they cited, but it elicited no criticism from them. Yet the FAO's livestock-climate analysis has been written by livestock specialists, not environmental specialists, and the organisation is just one of nineteen UN specialized agencies.

In contrast, Bill Gates (2013) argues for the replacement of most livestock products with better alternatives, referencing the work of environmental specialists employed by two other UN specialized agencies – the World Bank and International Finance Corporation (IFC) – who have explained how livestock account for much more greenhouse gas than the FAO asserts (Goodland & Anhang, 2009). One of those environmental specialists – Goodland (2012) published a critique of the FAO's partnership with the global livestock industry which appeared in The New York Times. Whether "less meat" activists use the FAO's analysis or not, if they otherwise want to address climate change properly, then they might serve themselves and others well by defining the key problem as being the need to reduce emissions significantly before climate tipping points occur, and by settling on a calculation of how much livestock reduction is needed to avoid those tipping points.

Our world is at stake, so there is an ethical need to act without worrying what policymakers or consumers might accept. In a past case, it turned out that such worrying was undue (Shaw & Stroup, 1995), and it similarly involved large-scale emissions that do not respect borders. Specifically, in the 1990s, environmentalists worried whether policymakers and consumers would accept (under the Montreal Protocol) eliminating coolants and aerosols that destroy the ozone layer. People loved their spray cans, refrigerators and air conditioners just as much as people today love consuming livestock products. Yet decisions were made to frame alternative products as positive things, and to talk about spray cans as much as refrigerators and air conditioners – and to define exactly what was needed – and it worked (Parry, 2011).

As with coolants and aerosols, it should not matter that "less meat" proponents are vastly outnumbered. So were Steve Jobs and Bill Gates long ago but they didn't tone down out of fear of what policymakers or consumers might accept. They just went ahead with marketing happier and better things – which made their competitors' products obsolete in only a few years – and the same can be done with Happy Better Vegan Foods.

The case promoted by "less meat" proponents at the meeting for public comments on the proposed U.S. dietary guidelines ended up not being reflected in new U.S. dietary guidelines. This might not be considered surprising. After all, Steve Jobs and Bill Gates didn't market fewer mainframe computers; instead they marketed Happier Better Cheaper Computers. Similarly, rather than promoting less meat, greater success might well come from promoting plant-based meat to replace animal-based meat.

PEAK LIVESTOCK

The FAO's report entitled "Livestock's Long Shadow" (Steinfeld et al., 2006) contemplates actions to manage a projected doubling in livestock production to feed the projected 9 billion people who will be alive in 2050. Specifically, "Livestock's Long Shadow" projects that "the production of meat will double between now and 2050" (Steinfeld et al., 2006, p. 388). Yet the FAO's projection is based on a presumed large-scale expansion of the livestock sector, which would lead to "further destruction of natural habitats like rainforests" and would "not solve food insecurity", according to the Soil Association (Soil Association, 2010, p. 8 and p. 3).

The FAO's projection presumes that it is possible for the livestock sector to continue expanding. In contrast, a projection that demand for animal products could decline through at least 2030 has been published by the International Food Policy Research Institute (IFPRI) in its report entitled "Feeding the Future's Changing Diets" (Msangi & Rosegrant, 2011). The IFPRI co-published with FAO a report 15 years ago that kicked off the "Livestock Revolution", projecting inevitably more livestock (Delgado et al., 1999). So, it is particularly striking to see the IFPRI now projecting such a different future.

In thinking about whether livestock production is bound to expand or contract, it is worthwhile noting that there are presently more than 173 billion animals raised for food each year (Chomping Climate Change, 2015). In fact, it has been said that replacing livestock products with better alternatives may be the only pragmatic strategy to reverse climate change before it is too late (Goodland, 2014). That is because livestock and feed production are estimated to occupy 45 percent of all land on earth (Thornton et al., 2011) – that's all land, both arable and non-arable, not excluding ice caps or mountaintops or anything else. Much of that 45 percent of all land was once forested, and could be forested again, yielding many more trees to absorb excess carbon from our atmosphere.

In 2006, the FAO published a report estimating that livestock were responsible for 18 percent of anthropogenic greenhouse gas emissions – yet that report prescribed no less livestock, but rather more factory farming: "The principle means of limiting livestock's impact on the environment must be… intensification" (Steinfeld et al., 2006, p. 236). That report's lead author and a co-author later wrote to confirm that prescription (Steinfeld & Gerber, 2010). The FAO subsequently published a 2013 report that reduced its livestock emissions estimate from 18 percent to 14.5 percent, and paired that estimate with prescriptions to facilitate 70 percent more livestock production by 2050 (Gerber et al., 2013).

However, livestock products can be replaced with better alternatives in order to reverse climate change before it's too late (Goodland, 2014). If livestock are not replaced with better alternatives voluntarily, then climate change is likely to force it. Notably, a one degree Celsius rise in temperature above optimum in a growing season causes a 10 percent decline in grain yields (Brown, 2011). This is already happening in some regions.

Spikes in the prices of grains used to feed animals have started to make animal-based meat production unprofitable. For example, at the start of 2017, it was forecast that the average U.S. pork producer would lose money for the year, after having been unprofitable in 2016, and before that in 2012-2013, and in 2008-2009 (Plain, 2017). The phenomenon of ongoing unprofitability has occurred in Chinese pork production (Day, 2015). In the U.S., the production of feedlot beef – the vast majority of beef in the U.S. – has been unprofitable for the past two years (Soderlin, 2017). Indeed, as of January 2017, few countries in the world could claim long-term profitability in cattle enterprises, even though beef prices rose to record highs in 2013-2014 (Behrendt & Weeks, 2017).

While poultry production may be profitable for now, poultry are expected to suffer the worst of any livestock under climate change, as they are particularly sensitive to temperature-associated environmental challenges, especially heat stress (Bhadauria at el., 2014). In fact, heat stress from climate change may have only just started to be felt. As conservative an organization as PriceWaterhouseCoopers (2012) has warned of a possible six degree Celsius rise in global temperature this century – that's a 10.8° Farenheit rise – which implies a 60 percent decline in agricultural outputs.

Energy specialists may aim for continued expansion of the fossil-fuel based sector until Peak Oil is reached– that is, when oil demand can no longer be satisfied as a result from a terminal decline in production (Heinberg, 2017). Livestock specialists may similarly aim for expansion of the livestock sector until "Peak Livestock" is reached. However, there are some notable differences between the oil and livestock industries. As the production of oil takes place underground and underwater, it is relatively unaffected by climate change. On the contrary, agriculture is more exposed to the impacts of climate change than any other industry as the production of livestock and crops to feed them takes place aboveground and largely outdoors. According to Chomping Climate Change (Admin, 2015): "Until recently, evidence was slim that climate change was causing dire hardship and large-scale die-offs in the raising of livestock and crops that feed them. However, there has recently been a noticeable spike in such hardships and die-offs all over the world". This has helped to create a point of inflection, whereby after many years of expansion of the livestock sector, there suddenly appears to be a trend favoring the replacement of animal-based foods with plant-based ones.

While a point of inflection seems to be taking hold (e.g., see Sciponi, 2016), projections are still commonly cited not only for a doubling in livestock production, but also for 70 percent more food; and in some places, it is even being noted that the FAO projects a potential need for 100 percent more food worldwide by 2050 (WFP, 2009). Yet such FAO projections have been called a "big fat lie" (Soil Association, 2010). After all, human population is not projected to increase by 70 percent or 100 percent by 2050.

The UN Population Division's medium-variant projection for human population in 2050 is 9.77 billion (up from around 7.55 billion in 2017), while its low-variant project for human population in 2050 is 8.8 billion (UN, 2017)[1]. This is 30 (medium-variant) or 17 (low-variant) percent more people than exist in 2017. If 17 to 30 percent more people exist in 2050 than today, then there is no obvious good reason why the world would need 70 percent more food. The UN Population Division has not expressed any opinion on whether its low- or medium-variant projection is more likely to be fulfilled. So even if nothing is done to reduce the incidence of overweight and obese people — and the most recent data indicates that a shocking 2.2 billion people are overweight or obese today (The GBD 2015 Obesity Collaborators, 2017) — it seems that between 25 and 30 percent more food would be needed in 2050, not 70 percent more food.

Yet the UN's projections do not factor in any potential for population contraction due to sea-level rise due to climate change (ENS, 2013). Sea-level rise driven by climate change is said to imperil 1700 cities in the U.S. alone, including New York, Boston, and Miami (Strauss, 2013). Much poorer cities across the world face a similar risk, which they are much less capable of managing (ENS, 2013). This suggests that fewer people may well exist in 2050 than today, which by itself should mean that the world would need less food, not more.

Whether or not fewer people exist in 2050 than today, disruptive climate events are already causing declines in agricultural output in every region of the world. These declines are projected to worsen over time in both magnitude and geographic scope. This is helping to create a new business case – connected to climate change – for making meat directly from crops, rather than from feeding many times the same amount of crops to animals.

Trends in the food industry have historically been supply-led, rather than demand-driven. For instance, food industry leaders – rather than consumers – have been responsible for such innovations as chicken nuggets, Big Macs, and bacon-wrapped pizza. In fact, supply-led trends are generally the norm in most categories of consumer products. For example, consumers did not (nor could they) originate trends favoring digital TVs, iPhones, or drones; those trends were originated by industry leaders. However, while consumers have not originated those trends, they have had the power to help drive or stop their spread. So, to drive a trend, it is essential to engage consumers.

Large-scale die-offs of livestock and feed crops due to climate change now provide extra reason for food industry leaders to be interested in replacing animal-based foods with plant-based ones. Food industry leaders have generally ignored vegetarian or vegan advocacy based on concerns over public health and animal rights – but they cannot ignore climate change. In other words, climate change is uniquely and unmistakably advancing a business case for disruption of the food industry.

CULTURE CHANGE?

While a business case connected to climate change is developing for making meat directly from plants rather than from animals, animal-rights activists rarely incorporate this in their advocacy. Instead, they generally advocate for a change in culture – otherwise known as "culture change" – whereby people in the future would reject the systemic aggression and violence used in raising and slaughtering animals to become food.

When animal-rights activists advocate for transformations in the age of climate change, it would seem ethically sound for them to recognize that culture change is normally generational, taking typically 50-100 years to achieve, under the best of circumstances, with reversals not uncommon (e.g., one can think of the "Dark Ages" or today's "Brexit"). So, activists working toward such culture change could be acting perversely, if they could better succeed with a climate strategy. An approach that seeks culture change might not only extend the misuse of animals for decades longer than under a climate change strategy, but could mean that activists would be resigning themselves to the possibility of extinction of much of life on earth.

Conversely, a strategy could better succeed by recognizing the origin and positive associations of the word "meat", and by aiming to disrupt rather than reduce its consumption. An interesting perspective on such a strategy has been enunciated by Ethan Brown, the founder and CEO of a company named "Beyond Meat". Mr. Brown said in a televised interview in 2014: "We've been having meat as humans for about 2.3 million years so there is a great familiarity with it, the way it crosses across the teeth, the way it bites, etc. and we don't want to walk away from that. You know, fried chicken tastes great. Steak tastes great. Let's just take the amino acid, the fats, from another source and recreate those so we can take an animal entirely out of the equation. I also think about what happened with the automotive sector where we had horse-drawn carriages, the internal combustion engine came along and basically obviated the need for the horse in that equation. We're trying to do the same with animal protein" (CBS This Morning, 2014). Mr. Brown also invoked climate change in that interview: "And here's an important statistic, so people have a certain hopelessness about climate change, they say: 'I don't know what to do?', but, in fact, 51 percent of greenhouse gas emissions can be attributed to livestock" (CBS This Morning, 2014).

In other words, the best strategy to address climate change – and to disrupt the meat industry – may involve engaging people to persuade them to do something that fits their existing priorities, rather than advocating something that requires them to change their priorities. Less meat or meatless diets, vegan diets and animal rights rank nowhere on most people's lists of priorities. Conversely, climate change is among the very top few priorities for many policymakers, industry leaders and other individuals across the world.

So, activists can implement a quick, global strategy of engaging people to learn how climate change imperils life on earth in the near term, but can be reversed through plant-based meat and other plant-based foods. Already, momentum has been building in efforts to replace animal-based foods with plant-based ones, often with references to climate change.

Companies that have tried sticking with animal agriculture have already started to go out of business (e.g., see Genoways, 2015), while financiers of plant-based food companies have started to become the envy of investors everywhere (Wortham & Miller, 2013). A similar phenomenon has occurred in every disrupted industry. For example, in many poor countries, about 20 years ago, only a few percent of people had telephones; a few years later, 25 percent had mobile access; a few years later, the figure was 70-80 percent (Sullivan, 2007). These days, analogue telephones and their manufacturers can scarcely be found anymore, anywhere in the world.

Surveys consistently show that consumers buy food items primarily on the basis of price and quality. Included in quality are ease and speed of preparation and delivery, cleanliness of retail outlets and good taste. Only a relatively small percentage of consumers have ever chosen foods on any other basis, and there is no sign that this will change anytime soon. While activists have a long track record of agitating for less or no meat, the results show more meat-eating year after year, not less.

Climate-friendliness is now sometimes included as part of marketing of food quality to consumers. Indeed, there is no practical alternative for consumers to reverse climate change – especially if it is true that livestock products are responsible for at least 51 percent of anthropogenic greenhouse gas emissions.

One reason why animal advocacy has not reduced global consumption of animal products is that most activists do not account for the way people normally decide to try different foods. Most people will happily experiment one meal at a time, and will then repeat if the new meal made them happy. In contrast, promoting a vegan/vegetarian diet will appear to most people as abrupt and radical as if McDonald's were to promote a "meatarian" diet. Instead, McDonald's has conquered one country after another by marketing "Happy Meals". In order to match or beat McDonald's success, animal advocates might do well to promote something even more positive, such as "Happier Meals" – marketing plant-based meat burgers as the best ones to choose any day of the week or year.

CONCLUSION

Authoritative projections indicate that climate change may no longer be reversible if emissions are not cut significantly by 2020 (Stromberg, 2012) or at the latest 2026 (Dechert, 2016). Yet according to the International Energy Agency, the amount of renewable energy infrastructure that is needed to stop climate change could only be fully developed long after 2026, and will cost at least $53 trillion (Kramer, 2013).

A faster and much more economical strategy begins with recognizing that livestock production accounts for at least half of human-caused greenhouse gas (De Schutter, 2014) and uses 45 percent of all land on earth (ILRI, 2011). Replacing livestock products with better alternatives offers a unique dual opportunity to reduce greenhouse gas emissions while freeing up land to enable more trees to capture excess atmospheric carbon.

Better alternatives to livestock products are generally made from grains and legumes, such as wheat, peas, sorghum and beans. Such foods are better than livestock products because any food that comes directly from a plant will generally be responsible for much less greenhouse gas than are livestock products. According to an article in Nature (Petherick, 2012), improvements in the way livestock are raised can achieve only 4 percent reduction in greenhouse gas emissions through 2030. That is much less reduction in emissions than every other industry is being called upon to achieve, and indeed is a trivial amount relative to what the food industry needs to accomplish (Goodland, 2013).

People can change their food choices literally overnight. That is a key reason why replacing animal-based foods with better alternatives is said to be the only pragmatic way to stop climate change quickly as needed. However, it is unlikely to happen through efforts to reduce meat consumption. It is much more likely to happen through efforts to disrupt meat production and consumption by making and marketing meat and other foods directly from plants.

REFERENCES

Behrendt, K., & Weeks, P. (2017). *How are global and Australian beef producers performing?* Meat & Livestock Australia. Retrieved from https://www.mla.com.au/globalassets/mla-corporate/prices--markets/documents/trends--analysis/agri-benchmark/revised_mla_agribenchmark-beef-results-report_jan-2017.pdf

Bhadauria, P., Kataria, J. M., Majumdar, S., Bhanja, S.K., & Divya, G.& Kolluri. (2014). Impact of hot climate on poultry production system-A review. *Journal of Poultry Science and Technology*, 2(4), 56–63.

Brown, L. R. (2011). *World on the edge: How to prevent environmental and economic collapse*. New York, NY: Norton.

CBS This Morning. (2014). Beyond Meat CEO Ethan Brown on the benefits of meat substitutes. Retrieved from https://www.cbsnews.com/videos/beyond-meat-ceo-ethan-brown-on-the-benefits-of-meat-substitutes-2/

Chiles, R. M., & Fitzgerald, A. J. (2017). Why is meat so important in Western history and culture? A genealogical critique of biophysical and political-economic explanations. *Agriculture and Human Values*. Retrieved from https://link.springer.com/article/10.1007/s10460-017-9787-7 doi:10.100710460-017-9787-7

Chomping Climate Change. (2014). Why it's a big fat lie that the world needs 70 percent more food by 2050. Retrieved from http://www.chompingclimatechange.org/updated-analysis/why-its-a-big-fat-lie-that-the-world-needs-70-percent-more-food-by-2050

Chomping Climate Change. (2015). Has climate change caused "Peak Livestock"? Retrieved from http://www.chompingclimatechange.org/updated-analysis/has-the-world-reached-peak-livestock/

Day, C. (2015). Smaller Chinese hog herd, opportunity for U.S. National Hog Farmer. Retrieved from http://www.nationalhogfarmer.com/marketing/smaller-chinese-hog-herd-opportunity-us

De Schutter, O. (2014). Ending hunger - the rich world holds the keys. *The Ecologist*, 25(March). Retrieved from http://www.theecologist.org/blogs_and_comments/commentators/2333245/ending_hunger_the_rich_world_holds_the_keys.html

Dechert, S. (2016). *1.5 degree climate chances "Not dead yet," but gone within a decade*. Planetsave. Retrieved from http://planetsave.com/2016/09/24/1-5-degree-climate-chances-not-dead-yet-but-gone-within-a-decade

Delgado, C., Rosegrant, M., Steinfield, H., Ehui, S., & Courbois, C. (1999). *Livestock to 2020: The next food revolution*. Food, Agriculture and the Environment Discussion Paper 28. Washington D.C.: International Food Policy Research Institute (IFPRI), Food Agriculture Organization (FAO) and International Livestock Research Institute (ILRI).

Environment News Service (ENS). (2013). 10 Coastal cities at greatest flood risk as sea levels rise. Retrieved from http://ens-newswire.com/2013/09/03/10-coastal-cities-at-greatest-flood-risk-as-sea-levels-rise

Field Roast. (2017) FAQ. Retrieved from http://fieldroast.com/faq

Gates, B. (2013). *Food is ripe for innovation*. Mashable. Retrieved from http://mashable.com/2013/03/21/bill-gates-future-of-food/#n7CpGZPdiGqi

Genoways, T. (2015). *Fear in a handful of dust*. New Republic. Retrieved from https://newrepublic.com/article/121558/what-climate-change-doing-texas-cattle-ranch

Gerber, P. J., Steinfeld, H., Henderson, B., Mottet, A., Opio, C., Dijkman, J., . . . Tempio, G. (2013). Tackling climate change through livestock: A global assessment of emissions and mitigation opportunities. Food and Agriculture Organization of the United Nations (FAO), Rome, Italy.

Goodland, R. (2012). FAO yields to meat industry pressure on climate change. *New York Times*, 11 July. Retrieved from bittman.blogs.nytimes.com/2012/07/11/fao-yields-to-meat-industry-pressure-on-climate-change/?_r=0

Goodland, R. (2013). Lifting livestock's long shadow. *Nature Climate Change*, 3(1), 2. doi:10.1038/nclimate1755

Goodland, R. (2014). How to reverse climate change before it's too late. *Meatanomics*. Retrieved from https://meatonomics.com/2014/09/04/how-to-reverse-climate-change-before-its-too-late

Goodland, R., & Anhang, J. (2009). Livestock and climate change: What if the key actors in climate change are... cows, pigs and chickens? *World Watch*, (November/December), 11–19. Retrieved from https://www.worldwatch.org/files/pdf/Livestock%20and%20Climate%20Change.pdf

Hawkins, A. (1974). *Tighten your belt: Food prices to soar with world demand. The Afro-American*, 10 August. Retrieved from https://news.google.com/newspapers?nid=2211&dat=19740810&id=uSomAAAAIBAJ&sjid=YP4FAAAAIBAJ&pg=1821,526870&hl=en

Health.gov. (2015). *Public meeting for oral testimony on the Scientific Report of the 2015 Dietary Guidelines Committee*. U.S. Office of Disease Prevention and Health Promotion. Retrieved from https://health.gov/DietaryGuidelines/2015/public-meeting.asp

Heinberg, R. (2017). *The Peak Oil President?* Post Carbon Institute. Retrieved from http://www.post-carbon.org/the-peak-oil-president

International Livestock Research Institute (ILRI). (2011). Livestock and climate change. Retrieved from https://www.ilri.org/node/6432

Kamila, A. Y. (2011). Natural foodie: Sebago Brewing Co. launches Meatless Monday menu. *Portland Press Herald*. Retrieved from http://www.pressherald.com/2011/06/29/sebago-brewing-co_-launches-meatless-monday-menu_2011-06-29

Kramer, S. (2013). $53 trillion of clean energy needed to meet global 2C target. Earthtechling. Retrieved from http://earthtechling.com/2015/11/53-trillion-of-clean-energy-needed-to-meet-global-2c-target

Lean, G. (2014). Sir Paul McCartney: Why I have a beef with meat-eating. *Telegraph*. Retrieved from http://www.telegraph.co.uk/news/earth/environment/globalwarming/11231472/Sir-Paul-McCartney-why-I-have-a-beef-with-meat-eating.html

Mammoser, G. (2017). Meat producers are concerned vegan bacon is deceiving consumers. *Vice*. Retrieved from https://munchies.vice.com/en_uk/article/aey4ba/the-way-you-eat-pizza-says-a-lot-about-you-according-to-body-language-experts

Meat Free Monday. (2017a). Mark Ruffalo and Lily Cole back #MFMclimatepledge in NYC. Retrieved from https://www.meatfreemondays.com/pledge-brunch-spotlights-un-climate-summit-pledge-campaign/

Meat Free Monday. (2017b). Vegan Quarter puts plant-based food centre stage. Retrieved from https://www.meatfreemondays.com/vegan-quarter-puts-plant-based-food-centre-stage/

Meatless Monday. (2017). History. Retrieved from http://www.meatlessmonday.com/about-us/history

Merriam Webster Dictionary. (2017). Meat. Retrieved from https://www.merriam-webster.com/dictionary/meat

Msangi, S., & Rosegrant, R. W. (2011). Feeding the future's changing diets: Implications for agriculture markets, nutrition and policy, 2020. *Paper presented at the Leveraging Agriculture for Improving Nutrition and Health Conference*, New Delhi, India. Retrieved from http://www.foresightfordevelopment.org/sobipro/download-file/46-953/54

Myfitnesspal. (2017a). Calories in hamburger fast food. Retrieved from http://www.myfitnesspal.com/food/calories/45914216

Myfitnesspal. (2017b). Calories in Traditionnelle Quiche Lorraine. Retrieved from http://www.myfitnesspal.com/food/calories/traditionnelle-quiche-lorraine-510312963

Nierenberg, D., & Reynolds, L. (2012). Disease and drought curb meat production and consumption. Vital Signs, Worldwatch Institute. Retrieved from http://vitalsigns.worldwatch.org/vs-trend/disease-and-drought-curb-meat-production-and-consumption

Online Etymology Dictionary. 2017. Meat (n.). Retrieved from http://www.etymonline.com/index.php?allowed_in_frame=0&search=meat

Parry, W. (2011). Climate success story: Saving the ozone layer. *Live Science*. Retrieved from https://www.livescience.com/17347-climate-success-montreal-protocol-ozone.html

Petherick, A. (2012). Light is cast on a long shadow. *Nature Climate Change*, 2(10), 705–706. doi:10.1038/nclimate1703

Plain, R. (2017). More hogs and higher prices — unusual, but desirable. *National Hog Farmer*. Retrieved from http://www.nationalhogfarmer.com/marketing/more-hogs-and-higher-prices-unusual-desirable

PriceWaterhouseCoopers (PWC). (2012). *Too late for two degrees?* Retrieved from https://www.pwc.com/gx/en/sustainability/publications/low-carbon-economy-index/assets/pwc-low-carbon-economy-index-2012.pdf

Renner, M. (2014). Peak meat production strains land and water resources. *Vital Signs, Worldwatch Institute*. Retrieved from http://vitalsigns.worldwatch.org/vs-trend/peak-meat-production-strains-land-and-water-resources

Retail News Insider. (2014). *From lab to table: The future of food*. Retrieved from http://www.retailnewsinsider.com/2014/06/01/from-lab-to-table-the-future-of-food

Retail News Insider. (2017). *Supply solutions: Sourcing Sophistication for today's new retail landscape*. Retrieved from http://www.retailnewsinsider.com/2017/07/06/supply-solutions-sourcing-sophistication-for-todays-new-retail-landscape/

Sciponi, J. (2016). *Bill Gates and NY Met David Wright see money in meatless venture.* Fox Business. Retrieved from http://www.foxbusiness.com/features/2016/10/31/bill-gates-and-ny-met-david-wright-see-money-in-meatless-venture.htm

Shaw, J. S., & Stroup, R. L. (1995). *Should we worry about ozone?* National Center for Policy Analysis. Policy Report No. 191. Retrieved from http://www.ncpa.org/pdfs/st191.pdf

Shurtleff, W., Huang, H. T., & Aoyagi, A. (2014). *History of soyfoods in China and Taiwan, and in Chinese cookbooks, restaurants, and Chinese work with soyfoods outside China. Extnsively annotated bibliography and sourcebook.* Lafayette, CA: Soyinfo Center.

Soderlin, B. (2017). *More cattle, lower prices: Ranchers and feeders hope consumers respond by buying more beef.* Omaha World. Retrieved from http://www.omaha.com/money/more-cattle-lower-prices-ranchers-and-feeders-hope-consumers-respond/article_f7dd3bbc-2b41-5c05-a5e7-4f55a24483a1.html

Soil Association. (2010). *Telling porkies: The big fat lie about doubling food production.* Bristol, UK: Soil Association. Retrieved from http://stopogm.net/sites/stopogm.net/files/webfm/plataforma/Telling-Porkies.pdf

Steinfeld, H., & Gerber, P. (2010). Livestock production and the global environment: Consume less or produce better? *Proceedings of the National Academy of Sciences of the United States, 107*(43), 18237–18238. doi:10.1073/pnas.1012541107 PMID:20935253

Steinfeld, H., Gerber, P., Wassenaar, T., Castel, V., Rosales, M., & de Haan, C. (2006). *Livestock's long shadow: environmental issues and options.* Rome, Italy: Food Agriculture Organisation.

Strauss, B. H. (2013). Rapid accumulation of committed sea-level rise from global warming. *Proceedings of the National Academy of Sciences of the United States, 110*(34), 13699–13700. doi:10.1073/pnas.1312464110 PMID:23898210

Stromberg, J. (2012). Climate change tipping point: research shows that emission reductions must occur by 2020. Smithsonian.com. Retrieved from http://www.smithsonianmag.com/science-nature/climate-change-tipping-point-research-shows-that-emission-reductions-must-occur-by-2020-162222340

Sullivan, N. P. (2007). *You can hear me now: How microloans and cell phones are connecting the world's poor to the global economy.* San Francisco, CA: Jossey-Bass.

The GBD 2015 Obesity Collaborators. (2017). Health effects of overweight and obesity in 195 countries over 25 years. *The New England Journal of Medicine, 377*, 13-27.

The National Provisioner. (2016). Meat industry timeline: 1917-1941. Retrieved from http://www.provisioneronline.com/articles/103508-meat-industry-timeline-1917-1941

Thornton, P., Herrero, M., & Ericksen, P. (2011). *Livestock and climate change. Livestock Exchange Issue Brief, 3.* Nairobi, Kenya: International Livestock Research Institute. Retrieved from https://cgspace.cgiar.org/bitstream/handle/10568/10601/IssueBrief3.pdf

Tsutsumi, A., & Tsutsui, N. (2009). Yuba ~ it's a traditional healthy food. The Kyoto Project. Retrieved from http://thekyotoproject.org/english/yubaits-a-traditional-healthy-food

United Nations. (2017). *World population prospects 2017*. Retrieved from https://esa.un.org/unpd/wpp/

Vegie Delights. (2017). Products: Nutmeat. Retrieved from www.vegiedelights.com.au/product/nutmeat

Wegmans. (2017). Field Roast: Grain Meat Sausages, Vegetarian, Smoked Apple Sage. Retrieved from https://www.wegmans.com/products/natures-marketplace/frozen-foods/sausage/grain-meat-sausages-vegetarian-smoked-apple-sage.html

World Food Programme (WFP). (2009). *World must double food production by 2050: FAO chief*. Retrieved from https://www.wfp.org/content/world-must-double-food-production-2050-fao-chief

Wortham, J., & Miller, C. (2013, April 28). Venture capitalists are making bigger bets on food start-ups. *New York Times*. Retrieved from http://www.nytimes.com/2013/04/29/business/venture-capitalists-are-making-bigger-bets-on-food-start-ups.html

Ye, K, Gao, F., Wang, D., Bar-Yosef, O., & Keinan, A. (2017). Dietary adaptation of FADS genes in Europe varied across time and geography. *Nature Ecology & Evolution*, *1*, 0167. doi:10.103841559-017-0167

KEY TERMS AND DEFINITIONS

Animal-Based Meat: Food that consists of animal flesh.

Disruption: Appearance of disturbances, problems or alternatives which interrupt the usual course of an event, activity or process.

Meat Free Monday: A campaign launched by Paul, Mary and Stella McCartney to address climate change by promoting the consumption of plant-based foods on Monday.

Meatless Monday: A non-profit initiative and global movement to cut the consumption of meat on Monday.

Peak Livestock: The moment in time when livestock production reaches its peak and is consequently reduced due to factors beyond the control of the producers, such as lower demand or climate change disruptions.

Plant-Based Meat: Food that consists of flesh from plants.

Yuba: A form of soymeat created from the film formed when soybeans are boiled.

ENDNOTE

[1]   The United Nations low-variant population projection is for 10.6 billion people in 2050 or 40 percent more people than in 2017. This does not justify a 70 percent increase in food demand either.

This research was previously published in the Handbook of Research on Social Marketing and Its Influence on Animal Origin Food Product Consumption edited by Diana Bogueva, Dora Marinova, and Talia Raphaely; pages 311-326, copyright year 2018 by Business Science Reference (an imprint of IGI Global).

Chapter 55
Normality, Naturalness, Necessity, and Nutritiousness of the New Meat Alternatives

Diana Bogueva
Curtin University, Australia

Kurt Schmidinger
Vienna University, Austria

ABSTRACT

In the West, meat is acceptable, tasty, delicious, palatable, and enjoyable. It has a well-established position in the consumers' food habits shaping the taste of the affluent eating culture and accepted as normal, natural, necessary, and nutritious. Although recent scientific evidence recognizes that meat has a high negative environmental impact, there is still lack of attention on the fact that we live on a planet with limited resources which need to be preserved. Part of this is a transition to more sustainable consumption habits and diets. This chapter examines the social readiness and acceptability of new meat alternatives as normal, natural, necessary, and nutritious amongst Gen Y and Gen Z consumers. It concludes that a reduction in meat consumption should be an essential part of creating a more sustainable diet in light of the projected increase of the world population, expected human health benefits, and improved environmental wellbeing of the planet.

INTRODUCTION

In this day and age, consumption, and especially meat consumption, has moved beyond its primary utilitarian function of serving basic human needs. The culture of the wealthiest societies is imbued with the idea of excessive meat consumption as absolutely normal part for everyone's equal opportunities to have abundant access to meat protein, often taken for granted and constantly fulfilling consumers' voracious appetites. Over the past fifty years, global meat production and consumption have increased five to ten-fold and the trends are expected to rise by 2050 (Ritchie & Roser, 2018). In a Western diet

DOI: 10.4018/978-1-7998-5354-1.ch055

type, the prevalent excessive, unsustainable meat eating is based on consumption levels from daily to at least 4–5 days a week (Bogueva, Marinova, & Raphaely, 2017). In a wealthy country like Australia, meat consumption has reached 116 kg per person a year (Ritchie & Roser, 2018). Such consumption levels are environmentally harmful and have major repercussions on several related global crises linked with water, climate, and energy (Steinfeld, Gerber, Wassenaar, Castel, Rosales & de Haan, 2006).

It is indeed indisputable that all serious environmental problems the world is facing today, including climate change, resource depletion, degradation of the planet's ecosystems, biodiversity depletion, and pollution of air, water and soil, are human-made (Cook, Oreskes, Doran, Anderegg, Verheggen, Maibach, … Green, 2016; Raphaely & Marinova, 2016; Springmann, Mason-D'Croz, Robinson, Garnett, Godfray, Gollin, … Scarborough, 2016; Myers, Gaffikin, Golden, Ostfeld, Redford, Ricketts … Osofsky, 2013; Steinfeld, Gerber, Wassenaar, Castel, Rosales & de Haan, 2006) and connected with our consumption and production patterns. The Earth's ecosystems cannot survive without urgent changes in human behaviour.

The environmental problems are further compounded with health issues caused by people's voluntarily dietary choices of high animal protein intake. This leads to early mortality risk (Sarich, 2013), higher incidence of heart disease (Quintana Pacheco, Sookthai, Wittenbecher, Graf, Stübel, Johnson … Kühn, 2018), diabetes (Mari-Sanchis, Gea, Basterra-Gortari, Martinez-Gonzalez, Beunza, & Bes-Rastrollo, 2016; Bernard, Levin, & Trapp, 2014), cancer (Lippi, Mattiuzzi, & Cervellin, 2016), including colon cancer (Singh & Fraser, 1998; Giovannucci, Rimm, Stampfer, Colditz, Ascherio, & Willett, 1994), prostate cancer (Dagnelie, Schuurman, Goldbohm, & Van den Brandt, 2004; Giovannucci, Rimm, Colditz, Stampfer, Ascherio, Chut, & Willett, 1993; Kolonel, 1996), breast cancer (Carroll & Braden, 1985), and obesity (You & Henneberg, 2016). Future dietary change directions need to be identified to reduce the burden of diseases and predisposing factors.

There is a pressing need for re-evaluation of consumer dietary choices. As the effects from meat consumption and production are detrimental, humanity's long-term survival prospects are dependent on shifting to alternative proteins, including new plant-based meat alternatives, emerging insect or algae-based foods and lab-grown meat products (Schmidinger, Bogueva, & Marinova, 2018). Meat alternatives will have to play an essential role in replacing meat products or supplementing them, so that people consume less animal-based meat. The market for new meat alternatives is still developing. Those producing and promoting these new products are trying to influence consumers by portraying the new meat alternatives as good, sustainable options, with the hope to establish them as regular food choices.

This chapter aims to fill in the gap in understanding consumer attitudes toward what is normal, natural, necessary and nutritious in relation to meat alternatives. It also aims to explore the future prospects for their acceptability.

BACKGROUND

From soy-based tofu to chopped nuts, almond and peanut meatless meat, plant-based blood and lab-grown steaks, science continues to work to take the animal out of the flesh. It is not about culinary delights, experiments, or something special, but about looking for global solutions to global problems. According to data gathered by the Food and Agriculture Organization of the United Nations, by 2050 the world's population will grow by 34 per cent reaching 9.1 billion and will require a 70 per cent increase in food production (FAO, 2009). Scientists are trying to find food alternatives that will save humankind from starvation and feed the next generation of humans because most of the world's population is estimated to suffer from food shortages (Hincks, 2018; Breene, 2016). Besides world nutrition, these food alternatives should also solve other global problems associated with industrial mass meat production, including: alarming animal welfare issues, high water and land usage, massive contribution to global greenhouse gas emissions, rainforest destruction and conversion into feed and grazing land, water contamination, loss of biodiversity and soil erosion, risks of new global pandemics, rise of antibiotic-resistant bacteria, lifestyle diseases and many more (Schmidinger, 2012, Steinfeld, Gerber, Wassenaar, Castel, Rosales & de Haan, 2006) .

Creating animal-free meat is actually not a new invention for the consumer market. Created during the Han dynasty in China (206BC–220AD), the first meat alternative – tofu, was known as "small mutton" (Du Bois, Tan, & Mintz, 2008). In Medieval Europe, during Lent people were replacing mincemeat with chopped almonds and grapes and diced bread was made into imitation cracklings and greaves (Adamson, 2004). Around 1877, the American medical physician and inventor John Kellogg developed meat replacements from nuts, grains, and soy as an alternative to feed patients with his vegetarian Sanitarium foods (Shurtleff & Aoyagi, 2004; 2014).

CAN GEN Y AND GEN Z HELP SOLVING THE MEAT PROBLEM?

Gen Y or Millennials (born between 1977 to 1995) and Gen Z or Centennials, or iGen (born between 1996 and 2009) can definitely be instrumental in resolving the humanity's insatiable appetite for meat. Currently the Millennials and Centennials are not only the two largest generations in the world considered as the present and future buying and decision-making power, but they are also the imminent leaders (Bresman & Rao, 2017) and the world's most environmentally, health and well-being conscientious generations ever born (Nielsen, 2015; Chang, 2017; Bogueva & Marinova, 2018). Anxiously they attribute global warming to human activity, want to be drivers in health and environmental discoveries and support environmentally friendly policies (Pew Research Centre, 2011). They are armed with their duty and a desire to protect the environment. In exploring the best possible innovative ways to do so, as adopting meat alternatives in their diets, these two generations are the hope to solve the carnivore's dilemma of humanity.

METHODOLOGY

Due to the massive expansion of the internet and social media into all aspects of the digital life of Gen Y and Gen Z target market population, the research study was conducted through an online-based survey. The online transfer of traditional research methods and techniques was used to adapt the whole study to the new technological environment in which the target groups are naturally habituating. Using the online research method, we were able to obtain information in a cost-effective and quick way, and were able to easily target and reach the specific respondent groups. The used qualitative online survey consisted of predominantly open-ended questions as we were interested to explore the opinions, knowledge, perceptions, and concerns of individuals in regard to meat alternatives. These open-ended questions allowed the participants to provide unstructured responses which became an important part of the research. They allowed the participants to share their own explanations, unique opinions and attitudes, feelings, provide additional comments that they considered relevant to the research in relation to its specific topic.

Indicators for the quality of the online survey are the value of the data obtained and the participants' satisfaction with the included questions. The survey had a high response rate of 75.6% – it was successfully completed by 227 respondents out of 300 invited people. We targeted adult people born between 1980 and 2000 and employed in both part or full-time work. The number of participants in this study was purposely limited for data processing purposes as the survey included a lot of open-ended questions.

The research explored in this chapter is based on four assumptions in regard to new meat alternatives. We assumed that for most participants, meat alternatives are abnormal, unnatural, unnecessary and not nutritious and we were seeking approval or disapproval of these assumptions. The central aim of the research was to discover what is considered and accepted as normal, natural, necessary and nutritious by the participants who are representatives of Millennial and Centennial consumers. The research is inspired by similar 3N or 4Ns classifications used for common rationalisation in defence of meat eating with the justification that it is natural, necessary, normal and nice (Joy, 2010, p. 97; Piazza, Ruby, Loughnan, Luong, Kulik, Watkins, & Seigerman, 2015). The three persistent reasonings individuals employ to diffuse their guilt when consuming animal products, described by Joy as part of a carnism ideology are: Normal, Natural, and Necessary (Joy, 2010). The additional N added in a study lead by Piazza is "Nice" and the defending justifications behind each of the 4Ns of meat-eating are: Natural – "humans are natural carnivores", Necessary – "meat provides essential nutrients", Normal – "I was raised eating meat" and Nice – "It's delicious" (Piazza, Ruby, Loughnan, Luong, Kulik, Watkins, & Seigerman, 2015).

The current study looks at psychological perception and barriers among consumers in regard only to meat alternatives and their food content, taste and quality as well as previous consumer experience. Together they form a concept of the ways the acceptability of new meat alternatives could be enhanced.

FINDINGS

When it comes to food, all people believe they are experts in what is normal, natural, necessary and nutritious. In total, 227 respondents – 111 females and 116 males, born between 1980 and 2000 and representatives of the two generations (Table 1), shared their expertise about meat alternatives and gave very thoughtful and informative responses in regard to the researched topic.

Table 1. Survey demographics

Generation	Number Male	Number Female	Total Number	Total Percentage
Gen Y Millennials	61	58	119	52.4%
Gen Z Centennials	55	53	108	47.6%
Total	116	111	227	100%

The majority of participants were consuming meat at a different frequency ranging from daily consumption (44.5%), few times per week (34.8%), sometimes or occasionally (12.8%) and 7.9% were abstaining from meat (Table 2).

Table 2. Meat consumption frequency

Frequency	Number	Percentage
Never, I don't eat meat	18	7.9%
Yes, sometimes on occasion	29	12.8%
Yes, few times per week	79	34.8%
Yes, daily	101	44.5%
Total:	227	100%

Meat alternatives are not a novelty, especially plant-based ones, and this was clearly stated by the majority of the survey participants who were asked to explain what they thought new meat alternatives were. A large number, namely 199 (87.7%) of the participants, demonstrated and shared a clear idea about the essence of new meat alternatives. The presented answers not only named some of the meat alternatives available worldwide and on the Australian market but also stated their ingredients, such as tofu, tempeh, quorn, lentils, mushrooms, beans, chickpeas etc. They also offered some focused and meaningful explanations as shown in Table 3.

In addition to the informed majority, there was a small number of 28 (12.3%) participants who were lacking knowledge about the nature of the new meat alternatives as shown in Table 4. Interestingly, many of them linked the new meat alternatives to other, not so common in mass consumption internal animal parts or meat from wild animals.

It was clear that the attitudes and understanding demonstrated by the survey participants about new meat alternatives was positioned at the intersection of the concepts of normality, naturalness, necessity and nutrition. These four concepts are discussed in turn below.

ARE MEAT ALTERNATIVES NORMAL?

If something is claimed to be normal, it means it is perceived as typical, expected, established, standard by which behaviours are measured and being consistent with the traditional norm within a culture and society. The survey participants are equally divided around the idea whether consumption of meat alternatives is normal or abnormal. Just below half of the sample – 112 (49.3%) of the survey participants, consider meat alternative as a normal part of their diet compared to 115 (50.7%) who believe the consumption of meat alternatives is not normal. These opinions are also relatively evenly distributed between the two generations as shown in Figure 1. However, a slightly higher proportion of Gen Z considered eating meat alternatives as not normal.

A substantial number of the participants claim that they are open-minded about new meat alternatives and they are willing to try them if they are not already eating them as part of their diet. Many partici-pants expressed united view about the idea that meat alternatives are essential for humankind because of their environmental benefits. One of the participants stated: "Meat alternatives are a good alternative, especially looking at the environmental benefits we often ignore (when choosing food) and prefer to use meat instead of creating a difference". Selected other opinions and reasons representing the normality of consuming meat alternatives are presented in Table 5.

Table 3. What do you think new meat alternatives are?

1	Meat alternatives should be healthy (which meat-free does not necessarily equate to), sustainable and environmentally friendly and also taste good
2	Food that does not contain animal products but that tastes or is similar to a meat product, e.g. vegetarian sausages and fake bacon
3	An alternative to meat that offers similar qualities to real meat, i.e. tofu
4	Products that can either be used to substitute meat or provide an alternative with similar nutritional properties
5	Vegetable-based ingredients made to taste like meat or something exotic like insects
6	Vegan options that fit meat profile, offering similar/close to nutritional level
7	Meat produced by science that does not need animals
8	Vegetarian meat, manufactured/artificial meat
9	I would see it 2 ways – as other food groups that provide the same nutritional value as meat or it could also be an actual product that vegans/vegos could use to replace meat, i.e. Quorn
10	Protein based alternatives to meat (vegan, vegetarian options) which can include anything from nuts to vegetables etc.
11	Substitutes for meat – either imitation or just an alternative that has the same nutrients
12	Something that can provide the same nutritional content as meat. Needs to be high in protein, it needs to mix well with other food groups and needs to taste good
13	Lab-grown meats
14	Plant-based products made to look, smell and taste like meat
15	Both – alternative ingredients that are made to mimic meat, e.g. soy-based protein sausages, and substitutes, e.g. mushroom instead of meat in a burger
16	Products that mimic the taste, texture and protein content of meat but are in fact plant-based
17	Food items with similar nutritional value to meat, similar flavour profiles and textures that are made from non-animal sources of protein, such as soy or gluten. These products may also look like meat
18	New meat alternatives are the food we can use and can taste as if there were meat in your dish but in fact there is not meat
19	Plant-based foods appropriate for those looking to adopt a meat-free diet
20	Chemically produced food that mimics the taste, smell and texture of meat, also aimed to reduce overconsumption of animals
21	Any meat substitutes like plant-based food, insects, anything that is not from animal origin
22	Innovative solutions to replace meat as the main source of protein and other nutrients
23	Meat alternatives replicate the feel, texture and taste of meat, like Quorn, fake bacon, fake chicken, etc.
24	Vegan products that are made to taste similar to traditional counterparts, the same taste without the impact
25	Possible alternatives to meat, such as tofu, and vegetable products used to imitate the nutrients, flavours and textures that are present in some meat products
26	Meat obtained from other sources, such as plants or even insects.

As one of the participants in the study stated: "What is normal today may be not so normal tomorrow as we are evolving in our food preferences". If positioned well, meat alternatives could be accepted as normal as they could serve various valuable purposes, including helping a person in a transition from a meat diet to a more plant-based diet, because of health reasons, animal welfare and environmental concerns. Meat alternatives can help with the reduction or elimination of meat consumption, can be comfort food, for vegetarian and vegan socialising purposes around the BBQ gatherings or to blend in at Australia Day or Thanksgiving.

Table 4. What do you think new meat alternatives are?

1	Introduction of some less common animal parts
2	No idea. Some type of meat perhaps
3	Different animals / different part of the animal
4	Maybe internal organs like liver, kidney as alternative to meat
5	New combinations
6	Other internal parts of meat that are given to the animals
7	Kangaroo
8	Feral animals and other uncommon animal parts
9	Different animals
10	Not sure what you mean by meat alternatives
11	Some rubbish food with no real meat in it like kidney and liver
12	Dairy products, flour made products
13	Perhaps some wild meat
14	No idea at all, I think wild meat
15	Internal parts of meat, dog's food
16	New way of cooking
17	No idea what meat alternatives are
18	Internal organs that are not for human consumption yet
19	Something that real human can't consume such as animal intestines or it will be artificial
20	Perhaps new options from different types of meat
21	Different animal parts not so popular among normal people
22	No idea at all, perhaps different type of meat cuts
23	I think it is some different part of the animal
24	Internal parts of meat used as type of food some nations around the world traditionally eat
25	Kangaroo, other not popular meat parts
26	Feral animals, kangaroo
27	Different animal parts not eaten by human before
28	Not sure what meat alternatives are. I hope some other meaty parts like kidneys, tripe, liver.

ARE MEAT ALTERNATIVES NATURAL?

Despite the main meaning of natural as something derived from nature and created without human intervention, in relation to food and especially meat, the word natural is more complex in nature and conveys much broader meanings. It is used as a metaphor for good and wholesome, and is also culturally defined. Although half of the survey participants are accepting meat alternatives as normal, only 78 (34.4%) of them think meat alternatives are natural to consume. The remaining participants – 149 (65.6%), consider meat alternatives as unnatural. Some of the popular arguments in both directions are presented in Table 6.

Figure 1. Is consumption of meat alternatives normal?

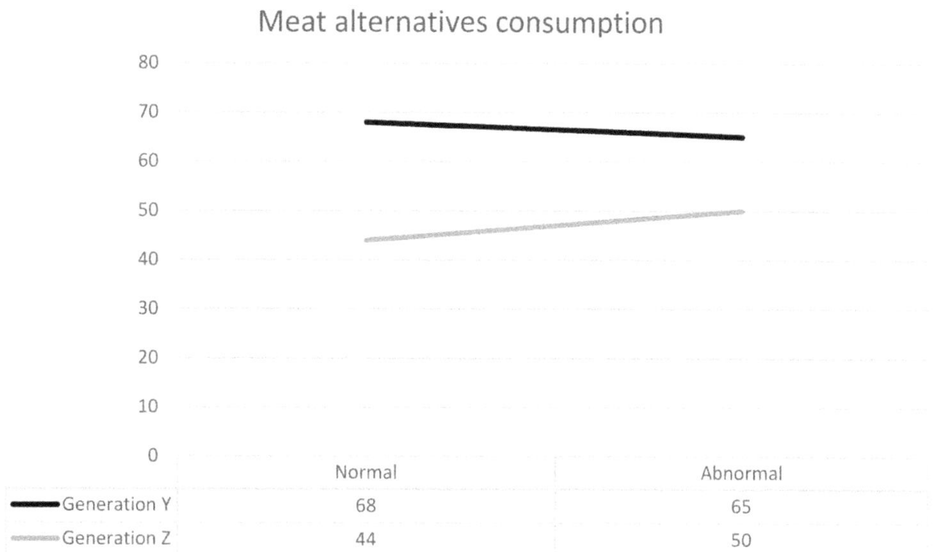

Table 5. Reasons for meat alternatives being normal to consume

1	It must be normal as we are all overeating not only meat, but vegetables as well and soon we will be left without any food
2	Normal as I make an effort to not eat too much meat, so I like alternatives. My flatmates are vegetarian, so we all get veggie burgers, tofu bacon and even quorn 'chicken' nuggets. I have tried crickets once but that's not something I can imagine eating all the time. But who knows…
3	Fairly normal, I am reducing my meat intake and branching out into vegetarian foods, so like to try new alternatives
4	It's becoming normal and quite fashionable, especially amongst young people
5	It's normal and about adjusting one's mentality to the endless possibilities that nature offers
6	Now meat alternatives are absolutely normal. I have only recently stopped eating meat and the reason for this was primarily because of the impact meat industry has on the environment – having always previously eaten meat, I like to have options to have meals I enjoy with meat alternatives
7	It is normal to eat them as we need to change the way we are eating, it is necessary if we want to save our environment, change human impact on our planet
8	For me is normal as one of my favourite restaurants has soybean meat alternatives and it mimics actual meat products so well I can't really tell the difference. I'm always interested to see how food can be manipulated into different forms
9	Eating plant-based products is normal for me, I buy some occasionally to avoid eating meat
10	Normal for me, but not normal for the greater part of humanity as people have lots of prejudice about what they are putting into their mouth
11	They are normal, high in protein and good sources of iron and zinc. I also find them tasty and recently living with a vegetarian, I have enjoyed eating these meat alternatives and adding them to my everyday salads and diet
12	More normal as we need a variety of food and we all need to be willing to try new products
13	It is absolutely normal to consume them if this is to change the way we are eating to save our environment and our planet
14	Consumption of substitutes of meat is becoming more and more normal for many. Maybe there is a need of a push or advertising of it. Even when I eat meat only few times a week I still have the taste and the respect for it.
15	It is normal to eat alternatives to meat and to change the way we are eating, and it is not normal to hurt animals for our food
16	I eat tofu and tempeh sometimes and I found them normal, although they have not much taste and need some supplements to be edible
17	Sometimes is normal to eat in some circumstances, but I don't think it is normal for everyone in our society as people love eating meat

Table 6. Natural/unnatural to consume meat alternatives

Natural	Unnatural
I think it is natural and it's a really sustainable and smart solution – I would rather eat crickets than cows	Not natural. Our ancestors survived eating natural stuff and our generations are spoilt by scientific advancement that may or may not actually be beneficial for the human race and human health. People in the old days didn't have all these allergies and health problems. We don't need another chemically produced food, but to return back to nature and eat as our ancestors.
It would be as natural as eating meat itself; if it's insects then it's a living being same as a cow, chicken etc. I don't see any of those options being unnatural to consume.	Maybe some of the meat alternatives are unnatural. I like to eat healthier if possible and I have problem with the chemically processed food.
Natural and important for the sustainability and future of our planet.	Not normal. The normality of eating meat alternatives I believe comes with the societal acceptance and at the moment this is not the norm. I prefer to be part of the society and to follow its norms.
Natural food made of plants or insects. People may not like them, but they are good healthy protein alternative.	Abnormal right now as meat alternatives are pretty new and undiscovered yet, but with time perhaps they become more natural and common to eat.
It is very natural as we are an adapting world and not everyone wants to eat the same products anymore. As long as we are getting our nutrients from somewhere that's most important	It is not natural for us, because we are used to eat meat and we are taught to eat meat as something very natural for humans. My family was always fed on meat and we never questioned it.
I feel it's a natural progression as livestock is not sustainable in the foreseeable future	Not sure what do you mean by meat substitutes to be natural. They never will be as people will associate them with engineering and modifications.
If it tasted like the most popular meats like beef, lamb, and it became the social norm then it would become more "natural" for humans to adopt it. As people are becoming more socially aware of the consequences of eating meat, it is becoming more and more popular.	Not necessarily natural, but certainly more beneficial in times of meat scarcity.
I think we are seeing a big cultural shift towards people being curious about meat alternatives and I think it is quite natural for many of us to want to gravitate towards a more plant-based diet	Nothing natural about these foods. We are living in a civilised society not in the jungle searching for some insects and larvae.
Probably a good idea as meat could become expensive in the future as well as plant-based food can help reduce cholesterol	Natural is to eat meat, I grew up with this idea, we have to eat meat and to have two veggies with it, now everybody is pro meat alternatives.
It is natural. I feel like it makes sense for us to move away from consuming meat now that we know the negative effects it has on the environment	Better for the environment maybe, but not natural for your tummy. All meat alternatives are heavily processed to mimic meat.
All young people like me, my friends lately are very much interested in meat alternatives and this is a natural process of acceptance of a plant-based diet. The rest of the alternatives, cultured meat especially and the insects to some extent as we are all eating seafood which is similar stuff to crickets, but in the sea.	Not considering them as natural as they are chemically produced to imitate meat
Meat alternatives are important for us to know and enjoy as the humanity is concentrating too much on meat	It is not natural for humans as we consume meat as a natural thing. My mum was telling me: Eat your meat darling:)
Completely natural, there is no reason to consume anything that sustains as long as it doesn't harm anyone else. If anything, eating alternatives is more natural than our current system of mass farming. Technology in food is a natural human advancement, but the cost of it is not worth it	Pretty natural for some people, but for me not natural because I can't abandon my meat for other food. I am a man and I like the taste, the smell, the blood if you want of the real juicy meat, not the imitation.
I don't see why it wouldn't be natural. Cultures all around the world eat various things, something what is 'natural' is just what we have become accustomed to. If people only ate the things suggested, these would be deemed 'natural'.	People think they are natural, I am still not sure about it. Maybe I need more time, but also, I feel I am forced to accept meat alternatives as natural, even I am uncertain about it. I feel there is a push from my peers, sometimes I think it is fashionable.
We really need more of those smart solutions to become natural for all the people especially in Australia, even embracing the crickets.	Natural ingredients, I believe, they use to make it, but the final result is not so natural to eat. Probably need some improvements in the presentation also as it is totally sick looking, shrank and ugly when not freshly made.
Fairly natural as people these days are developing new allergies and the growing research that shows diets high in meat aren't always good.	Meat alternatives can be natural for some nations and people with specific dietary requirements, but not natural for the majority of the Australians and the normal food consuming society worldwide.

The participants in the study are clearly divided into two opposite poles in terms of their understanding whether it is natural or not natural to consume meat alternatives. While the first group, the proponents of the naturalness of consuming meat alternatives opinionated that embracing such diet is good for human health, animal welfare and the sustainability of our planet, the second group was not so categorical in the unnaturalness of eating meat alternatives. Some key concerns highlighted were about the unnaturalness of meat alternatives because they are a product of scientific advancement, chemicals, engineering and modifications, which was not perceived positively by the participants.

ARE MEAT ALTERNATIVES NECESSARY?

The understanding of necessity as essential, fundamental, indispensable for maintaining a minimum standard and an important element for human survival is the meaning shared by the research partakers. The majority of the participants – 198 (87.2%), are united and believe in the idea that meat alternatives are necessary to consume for the sake of our planet's future, for sustainable animal raising, to deal with resource scarcity, for feeding the growing population and for maintaining humankind's physical health (Table 7).

Table 7. Necessity of meat alternative consumption

1	I definitely think there needs to be some sort of change within human feeding habits. The production and distribution of the meat industry are extremely detrimental to the environment, let alone the lack of rights given to the animals themselves. Thus, it is quite necessary for humanity to embrace new-meat alternatives that are more sustainable for our future.
2	I believe given the current population growth and food production issues it will become an increasing necessity for humanity to explore and consume these new types of meat alternatives.
3	Consuming new meat alternatives is definitely a vital part of the future. Humans cannot continue to consume and deliver meat as there is an exponential growth in human population. There isn't enough land to be able to cater for all meat types ethically. Alternatives are critical for us to save Earth in the future and humanity.
4	I think it's important for lots of different reasons; we evolve and, in some ways, go back to basics in finding meat substitutes. We live in a world where we are aware more than ever of our wellbeing, heath and the part our diet plays in this. Also, meat alternatives bring up lifestyle, health but also sustainability issues and simple choice
5	Eating less meat and choosing meat alternatives would be a benefit to lessen inappropriate farming methods
6	Necessary is to make cultured meat as this will be in huge need in near future when we will create food wars because of not enough meat and other food resources.
7	Humans need to look at new protein sources in order to increase biodiversity and be more environmentally sustainable
8	Essential. We know that meat as it is processed today is unsustainable for the planet. We need alternatives if we want to keep some meat in our diet without destroying everything.
9	Depends on availability, to be honest. If nothing else is available, there is no doubt you will eat it.
10	With the increasing amount of added hormones in meat, it seems somewhat natural to try other products.

The rest of the participants – 29 (12.8%), who consider the consumption of meat alternatives unnecessary, base their arguments on the abundance of meat in Australia and the country being one of the largest meat exporters in the world. Some also believed that the meat scarcity scenario is still far away.

ARE MEAT ALTERNATIVES NUTRITIOUS?

Nourishing, healthy and efficient as food is the meaning behind nutritious. The majority of the survey participants – 188 (82.8%), shared immense uncertainty about the meat alternatives' nutritional values. Their arguments gravitated around two major concerns. One of them is the vitamins and mineral content of the meat alternatives, especially the sufficiency of iron, zinc and vitamin B12. The other concern the participants gravitated around is the protein content in comparison to real meat. This was complimented by the fear for their own health based on the view that mimicked meat is too processed and chemically produced to be nutritious. Table 8 shows some of the shared opinions.

Table 8. Nutritiousness of meat alternative consumption

Yes	No	Unsure
Meat alternatives have essential nutrients we all can benefit from.	Chemically produced foods can mimic being nutritious, but actually they are not.	I have no idea, but I imagine that they are nutritious otherwise why they will produce them as alternatives to meat.
The ingredients are nutritious, so I suppose they are nutritious.	Meat alternatives can't beat the nutritional benefits of meat like iron, zinc, B12.	I have no idea about the nutritious component of the meat alternatives. Maybe they are good, but I will doubt it because of the way they are produced.
As long as they share the characteristics similar to meat protein then all meat alternatives are acceptable and nutritious.	If meat alternatives are nutritious for someone it's okay as this is their choice, but personally for me they are not nutritious, more likely a combination of who knows what type of chemicals.	I'm not knowledgeable about the nutritional value. I sometimes read the ingredients on the packages and I can't recall anything bad there, especially in the meat alternatives I tried. I can't be certain I read it 100% properly, but I assume.
The nutrition depends on the nutrition of the alternative protein made. Often they are all good.	Nutritious is maybe too much to be used to describe meat alternatives.	I have absolutely no idea if these alternatives are having similar iron, zinc and magnesium content to say if they are nutritious.
Depending on the ingredients included, it can be more nutritious than meat.	It's not nutritious. What nutrients you can find in crickets and bugs? The whole thing is too much under question.	They must have the proper nutrition and I am not sure about that and not sure how they will make me feel after I try them.
I don't think vegan meat is very nutritious, but the insects were used by the Aborigines and they are certainly nutritious.	Can be nutritious, but I have a big doubt about it.	It could be nutritious, I don't really know, as they are so much meaty looking for me. I don't like it when people think I am vegetarian and I'll enjoy them, and they cook me a veggie sausage at the BBQ. It is not the problem they are plant-based made, but the look they have imitating real meat stuff.
Meat alternatives are nutritious with similar flavour, taste, textures and look like meat.	I think real veggies are more nutritious to consume. Meat alternatives look too processed and not nutritious at all.	Nutritious aspect is difficult to describe as I am not familiar with all the meat alternatives on the market.
I believe they are nutritious enough, but people don't know about meat alternatives. They are a less popular choice and not enough advertised as a correct choice.	Can't beat the nutritional benefits of meat like iron, zinc, B12.	I have no idea about it as I am not eating them. I prefer to cook veggie food instead from raw ingredients.
Highly nutritious and tasty for us as consumers to eat.	Not nutritious I think. They definitely can't have the properties of meat with enough iron and B12 like meat.	More unsure of the nutritional value of alternative meat then to be certain about it. Maybe if I have more info… I'll have some opinion about it.

The existing knowledge gap about meat alternatives is worth filling in as most of the participants are convinced about the necessity of meat alternatives because of their environmental benefits for the planet and human health.

MANLINESS AND MEATINESS OF MEAT ALTERNATIVES

The research revealed the specific need of reconceptualization the appearance of meat alternatives. When issues related to manliness and meatiness were mentioned, the look of the meat alternatives was in the centre of the discourse. Quite a few of the male survey participants, predominantly representatives of generation Y, found meat alternatives not so masculine to consume. The meat issue as a genuine consumer concern was clearly outlined in the respondents' answers (Table 9).

Table 9. Manliness and meat alternatives

1	Not natural and not masculine at all for me as real men eat real meat.
2	I reckon these (meat alternatives) are food for pussies. They are like veggies.
3	These are not meat at all as they taste, look and smell like no meat and there is no blood in it when you want to cook them.
4	For humans is natural to eat meat not some alternatives to it. We are hunter-gatherers, not pussy.
5	I am a man and I like the taste, the smell, the blood, if you want, of the real juicy meat, not the imitation.

Although the less meaty appearance of meat alternatives bothered some male participants, the resemblance to meat in the appearance of meat alternatives emerged as an issue for some female participants (Table 10).

Table 10. Meatiness of meat alternatives

1	I have a real problem with their look mimicking meat and when they are cooked they look not so appealing.
2	If they didn't duplicate the look of normal meat I believe they would be more acceptable by people with my believes against animal killing.
3	I never will eat them, they are made to imitate meat and I don't like it as I care about the animal welfare.
4	I feel kind of uncomfortable with the similar to meat appearance of meat alternatives.
5	It's fine for meat eater, I reckon, not for vegetarians like me as I prefer not to eat something that seems like meat

THE INSECTS DILEMMA

Most of the participants objected to the eating of insects. Being an unpopular meal dictated by our affluent culture, the insect dilemma was pretty much discussed as a choice or necessity in this research. A solid number – 112 (75.2%) out of 149 (65.6%) of the survey participants sharing the opinion that meat alternatives are not natural to consume, feel some sort of disgust when hearing the word insects (Table 11). Contrary to the opinion shared by the survey participants, many scientists believe that entomophagy (known as insect-eating) will not only benefit human health, but also the planetary health as insects are an environmentally friendly source of human protein (Sogari, 2015; van Huis, Itterbeeck, Klunder, Mertens, Haloran, Muir, & Vantomme, 2013; Bennington-Castro, 2017), with low production cost, short life cycle, low space requirement (van Huis, 2013) and good nutritional quality (Rumpold & Schlüter, 2013).

Making people look at insects simply as a source of food will be an incredible challenge. While 80% of the world's population traditionally, freely and regularly eats insects as normal, natural, necessary and nutritious (Carrington, 2010; Guynup & Ruggia, 2004), in the Western world, this is perceived more as a strange delicacy, which more often provokes negative feelings (Verbeke, 2015; Hartmann & Siegrist, 2017) and disgust rather than any positive reactions (Ruby, Rozin, & Chan, 2015), and draws food neophobia (Gere, Székely, Kovács, Kokai, & Sipos, 2017). Maybe we should think of a new name for edible insects to eliminate the disgusting factor or presenting them in more familiar forms to enhance the willingness of people to try (Megido, Gierts, Blecker, Brostaux, Haubruge, Alabi, & Fransis, 2016; Tan, Verbaan, & Stieger, 2017) as a solution to the insect dilemma.

Table 11. Attitude to insect consumption

Against Insect Consumption	Pro Insect Consumption
I lived most my childhood in China. I ate a lot of weird things when I was little – water beetles, snakes, rabbits, racoons. I might not feel comfortable eating something that looks like insect anymore, but I'm willing to try things that does not look like insects.	Regarding insects, I have tried on holidays in Asia, but never considered to make them part of my diet. I'm not reluctant and don't think this is weirder than eating other animals but I wouldn't know where to buy them.
… the crickets and larvae are totally sick	I think it's natural enough to eat insects and bugs, as people have done all over the world for hundreds of thousands of years. However, I think the more chemically-based manufactured 'meats' are, perhaps less natural for humans to eat.
I am not in favour of the idea to eat insects, they are kind of gross. I think people are not grass feeders, so insects and cultured meat are something we all have to be reluctant about to consume, as we have better options with plant-based alternatives.	People just need to get over the stigma of eating insects.
If it is insects I don't feel that it's very human to eat at all.	Sounds lovely as insects are a good source of protein.
Not normal for us to eat gross insects and larvae.	Insects have a branding problem.
The insect options are under big question. We have to starve ourselves before trying it.	Crickets and larvae, algae can be highly nutritional and beneficial for us to eat.

FUTURE RESEARCH DIRECTIONS

What used to be normal, natural, necessary and nutritious, should no longer be perceived in the same way, because in our ever-changing world we must be able to assess the pressing problems, including our over-consumption, overuse of resources, the human and the planetary health, and to learn how to resolve them quickly and in a timely manner. Humankind needs to be open to new ideas and to break through its traditional beliefs in order to learn from the mistakes of the past and remove the barriers to offering new opportunities. Attention to what the generations in power want, their awareness of the necessity of new meat alternatives and the actions they are willing and ready to take should be at the centre of any future discussions and research.

CONCLUSION

New meat alternatives are regarded as normal and necessary by most of the survey participants, but are unnatural, and not nutritious for the majority of them. Especially the perception about meat alternatives being "unnatural" obviously in contrast to "natural" meat, shows a notable discrepancy between consumers' ideas of a natural meat production versus the actual unnatural reality in industrial intensive livestock facilities as described in many publications (such as Ewbank, Ray, Kim-Madslien, & Hart, 1999 or Webster, 2010). Replacement with new meat alternatives does not have the same respect in people's minds and palates. The idea of mass use as different protein is still at the beginning of a long journey before being accepted as normal, natural, necessary and nutritious.

Over the next few decades, people will have to change their eating habits, food-related gender norms and stereotypes, and give up their prejudice about food because the health of the planet and their own health are likely to remain a big issue.

REFERENCES

Adamson, M. W. (2004). *Food in medieval times*. Westport, CT: Greenwood Press.

Bennington-Castro, J. (2017). How crickets could help save the planet. *NBC News*. Retrieved from https://www.nbcnews.com/mach/environment/how-eating-crickets-could-help-save-planet-n721416

Bernard, N., Levin, S., & Trapp, C. (2014). Meat consumption as a risk factor for type 2 diabetes. *Nutrients*, *6*(2), 897–891. doi:10.3390/nu6020897 PMID:24566443

Bogueva, D., & Marinova, D. (2018). What is more important perception of masculinity or personal health and the environment? In D. Bogueva, D. Marinova, & T. Raphaely (Eds.), *Handbook of research on social marketing and its influence on animal origin food product consumption* (pp. 148–162). Hershey, PA: IGI Global. doi:10.4018/978-1-5225-4757-0.ch010

Bogueva, D., Marinova, D., & Raphaely, T. (2017). Reducing meat consumption: The case for social marketing. *Asia Pacific Journal of Marketing and Logistics*, *29*(3), 477–500. doi:10.1108/APJML-08-2016-0139

Breene, K. (2016). *Food security and why it matters*. World Economic Forum. Retrieved from https://www.weforum.org/agenda/2016/01/food-security-and-why-it-matters/

Bresman, H., & Rao, V. D. (2017). A survey of 19 countries shows how generations X, Y, and Z are — and aren't — different. *Harvard Business Review*. Retrieved from https://hbr.org/2017/08/a-survey-of-19-countries-shows-how-generations-x-y-and-z-are-and-arent-different

Carrington, D. (2010). Insects could be the key to meeting food needs of growing global population. *The Guardian*. Retrieved from https://www.theguardian.com/environment/2010/aug/01/insects-food-emissions

Carroll, K. K., & Braden, L. M. (1985). Dietary fat and mammary carcinogenesis. *Nutrition and Cancer*, *6*(4), 254–259. doi:10.1080/01635588509513831 PMID:6443636

Chang, R. (2017). Survey: Generation Z's best students seek careers in STEM and healthcare. *The Journal*. Retrieved from https://thejournal.com/articles/2017/07/12/survey-generation-zs-best-students-seek-careers-in-stem-and-healthcare.aspx

Cook, J., Oreskes, N., Doran, P. T., Anderegg, W. R. L., Verheggen, B., Maibach, E. W., ... Green, S. A. (2016). Consensus on consensus: A synthesis of consensus estimates on human-caused global warming. *Environmental Research Letters*, *11*(4), 048002. doi:10.1088/1748-9326/11/4/048002

Dagnelie, P. C., Schuurman, A. G., Goldbohm, R. A., & Van den Brandt, P. A. (2004). Diet, anthropometric measures and prostate cancer risk: A review of prospective cohort and intervention studies. *BJU International*, *93*(8), 1139–1150. doi:10.1111/j.1464-410X.2004.04795.x PMID:15142129

Du Bois, C. M., Tan, C.-B., & Mintz, S. W. (2008). *The world of soy*. National University of Singapore: National University of Singapore Press.

Ewbank, R., Ray, P., Kim-Madslien, F., & Hart, B. (Eds.). (1999). *Management and welfare of farm animals*. Wheathampstead, UK: Universities Federation for Animal Welfare.

Food and Agriculture Organization of the United Nations (FAO). (2009). *How to feed the world in 2015*. Retrieved from http://www.fao.org/fileadmin/templates/wsfs/docs/expert_paper/How_to_Feed_ the_World_in_2050.pdf

Gere, A., Székely, G., Kovács, S., Kokai, Z., & Sipos, L. (2017). Readiness to adopt insects in Hungary: A case study. *Food Quality and Preference*, *59*, 81–86. doi:10.1016/j.foodqual.2017.02.005

Giovannucci, E., Rimm, E. B., Colditz, G. A., Stampfer, M. J., Ascherio, A., Chut, C. C., & Willett, W. C. (1993). A prospective study of dietary fat and risk of prostate cancer. *Journal of the National Cancer Institute*, *85*(19), 1571–1579. doi:10.1093/jnci/85.19.1571 PMID:8105097

Giovannucci, E., Rimm, E. B., Stampfer, M. J., Colditz, G. A., Ascherio, A., & Willett, W. C. (1994). Intake of fat, meat, and fiber in relation to risk of colon cancer in men. *Cancer Research Journal*, *54*(9), 2390–2397. PMID:8162586

Guynup, S., & Ruggia, N. (2004). *For most people eating bugs is only natural*. National Geographic Channel, National Geographic. Retrieved from https://news.nationalgeographic.com/news/2004/07/0715_040715_ tvinsectfood.html

Hartmann, C., & Siegrist, M. (2017). Insects as food: Perception and acceptance. Findings from current research. *Ernährungs-Umschau*, *64*(3), 44–50. doi:10.4455/eu.2017.010

Hincks, J. (2018). The world is headed for a food security crisis. Here's how we can avert it. *Time Magazine*. Retrieved from http://time.com/5216532/global-food-security-richard-deverell/

Joy, M. (2010). *Why we love dogs, eat pigs and wear cows: An introduction to carnism*. San Francisco, CA: Red Wheel/Weiser.

Kolonel, L. N. (1996). Nutrition and prostate cancer. *Cancer Causes & Control*, *7*(1), 83–44. doi:10.1007/ BF00115640 PMID:8850437

Lippi, G., Mattiuzzi, C., & Cervellin, G. (2016). Meat consumption and cancer risk: A critical review of published meta-analysis. *Critical Reviews in Oncology/Hematology*, *97*, 1–14. doi:10.1016/j.critrevonc.2015.11.008 PMID:26633248

Mari-Sanchis, A., Gea, A., Basterra-Gortari, F. J., Martinez-Gonzalez, M. A., Beunza, J. J., & Bes-Rastrollo, M. (2016). Meat consumption and risk of developing type 2 diabetes in the SUN Project: A highly educated middle-class population. *PLoS One, 11*(7), e0157990. doi:10.1371/journal.pone.0157990 PMID:27437689

Megido, R. C., Gierts, C., Blecker, C., Brostaux, Y., Haubruge, E., Alabi, T., & Fransis, F. (2016). Consumer acceptance of insectbased alternative meat products in Western countries. *Food Quality and Preference, 52*, 237–243. doi:10.1016/j.foodqual.2016.05.004

Myers, S. S., Gaffikin, L., Golden, C. D., Ostfeld, R. S., Redford, K. H., & Ricketts, T. H. … Osofsky, S. A. (2013). Human health impact of ecosystem alteration. *Proceedings of the National Academy of Sciences of the United States of America, 110*(47), 18753–18760. 10.1073/pnas.1218656110

Nielsen. (2015). *The sustainability imperative*. Nielsen Research. Retrieved from http://www.nielsen.com/au/en/insights/reports/2015/the-sustainability-imperative.html

Pew Research Centre. (2011). *The generation gap and the 2012 election*. Retrieved from http://www.people-press.org/2011/11/03/section-8-domestic-and-foreign-policy-views/

Piazza, J., Ruby, M. B., Loughnan, S., Luong, M., Kulik, J., Watkins, H. M., & Seigerman, M. (2015). Rationalizing meat consumption. The 4Ns. *Appetite, 91*, 114–128. doi:10.1016/j.appet.2015.04.011 PMID:25865663

Quintana Pacheco, D. A., Sookthai, D., Wittenbecher, C., Graf, M. E., Stübel, R., Johnson, T., … Kühn, T. (2018). Red meat consumption and risk of cardiovascular diseases—is increased iron load a possible link? *The American Journal of Clinical Nutrition, 107*(1), 113–119. doi:10.1093/ajcn/nqx014 PMID:29381787

Raphaely, T., & Marinova, D. (Eds.). (2016). *Impact of meat consumption on health and environmental sustainability*. Hershey, PA: IGI Global. doi:10.4018/978-1-4666-9553-5

Ritchie, H., & Roser, M. (2018). *Meat and seafood production & consumption*. Retrieved from https://ourworldindata.org/meat-and-seafood-production-consumption

Ruby, M. B., Rozin, P., & Chan, C. (2015). Determinants of willingness to eat insects in the USA and India. *Journal of Insects as Food and Feed, 1*(3), 215–225. doi:10.3920/JIFF2015.0029

Rumpold, B. A., & Schlüter, O. K. (2013). Nutritional composition and safety aspects of edible insects. *Molecular Nutrition & Food Research, 57*(5), 802–823. doi:10.1002/mnfr.201200735 PMID:23471778

Sarich, C. (2013). Harvard says reducing red meat consumption can extend life by 20%. *Natural Society*. Retrieved from http://naturalsociety.com/reducing-red-meat-consumption-extend-life-20-percent/#ixzz2zdnAhdzY

Schmidinger, K. (2012). *Worldwide alternatives to animal derived foods – Overview and evaluation models – Solutions to global problems caused by livestock* (Doctoral thesis). University of Natural Resources and Life Sciences, Vienna, Austria.

Schmidinger, K., Bogueva, D., & Marinova, D. (2018). New meat without livestock. In D. Bogueva, D. Marinova, & T. Raphaely (Eds.), *Handbook of research on social marketing and its influence on animal origin food product consumption* (pp. 344–361). Hershey, PA: IGI Global. doi:10.4018/978-1-5225-4757-0.ch023

Shurtleff, W., & Aoyagi, A. (2004). *Dr. John Harvey Kellogg and Battle Creek Foods: Work with soy.* Lafayette, CA: Soyinfo Center. Retrieved from http://www.soyinfocenter.com/HSS/john_kellogg_and_battle_creek_foods.php

Shurtleff, W., & Aoyagi, A. (2014). *History of meat alternatives (965 CE to 2014): Extensively annotated bibliography and sourcebook.* Lafayette, CA: Soyinfo Center. Retrieved from http://www.soyinfocenter.com/pdf/179/MAL.pdf

Singh, P. N., & Fraser, G. E. (1998). Dietary risk factors for colon cancer in a low-risk population. *American Journal of Epidemiology, 148*(8), 761–774. doi:10.1093/oxfordjournals.aje.a009697 PMID:9786231

Sogari, G. (2015). Entomophagy and Italian consumers: An exploratory analysis. *Progress in Nutrition, 17*(4), 311–316.

Springmann, M., Mason-D'Croz, D., Robinson, S., Garnett, T., Godfray, H. C. J., Gollin, D., … Scarborough, P. (2016). Global and regional health effects of future food production under climate change: A modelling study. *Lancet, 387*(10031), 1937–1346. doi:10.1016/S0140-6736(15)01156-3 PMID:26947322

Steinfeld, H., Gerber, P., Wassenaar, T., Castel, V., Rosales, M., & de Haan, C. (2006). *Livestock's long shadow: Environmental issues and options.* Rome, Italy: Food and Agricultural Organization of the United Nations. Retrieved from www.virtualcentre.org/en/library/key_pub/longshad/A0701E00.pdf

Tan, H., Verbaan, Y., & Stieger, M. (2017). How will better products improve the sensory-liking and willingness to buy insect-based foods? *Food Research International, 92*, 95–105. doi:10.1016/j.foodres.2016.12.021 PMID:28290303

van Huis, A. (2013). Potential of insects as food and feed in assuring food security. *Annual Review of Entomology, 58*(1), 563–583. doi:10.1146/annurev-ento-120811-153704 PMID:23020616

van Huis, A., Itterbeeck, J. V., Klunder, H., Mertens, E., Haloran, A., Muir, G., & Vantomme, P. (2013). *Edible insects: Future prospects for food and feed security.* Rome, Italy: Food and Agriculture Organization of the United Nations (FAO). Retrieved from https://www.researchgate.net/publication/311424459_Edible_insects_Future_prospects_for_food_and_feed_security_Food_and_Agriculture_Organiation_of_the_United_Nations_FAO_Rome_Italy

Verbeke, W. (2015). Profiling consumers who are ready to adopt insects as a meat substitute in a Western society. *Food Quality and Preference, 39*, 147–155. doi:10.1016/j.foodqual.2014.07.008

Webster, J. (2010). *Management and welfare of farm animals.* London, UK: John Wiley and Sons.

You, W., & Henneberg, M. (2016). Meat consumption providing a surplus energy in modern diet contributes to obesity prevalence: An ecological analysis. *BMC. Nutrition (Burbank, Los Angeles County, Calif.), 2*, 22. doi:10.118640795-016-0063-9

ADDITIONAL READING

Bogueva, D., Marinova, D., & Raphaely, T. (2017). Reducing meat consumption: The case for social marketing. *Asia Pacific Journal of Marketing and Logistics*, *29*(3), 477–500. doi:10.1108/APJML-08-2016-0139

Breene, K. (2016). *Food security and why it matters*. World Economic Forum. Retrieved from https://www.weforum.org/agenda/2016/01/food-security-and-why-it-matters/

Du Bois, C. M., Tan, C.-B., & Mintz, S. W. (2008). *The world of soy*. National University of Singapore: National University of Singapore Press.

Joy, M. (2010). *Why we love dogs, eat pigs and wear cows: An introduction to carnism*. San Francisco, CA: Red Wheel/Weiser.

Piazza, J., Ruby, M. B., Loughnan, S., Luong, M., Kulik, J., Watkins, H. M., & Seigerman, M. (2015). Rationalizing meat consumption. The 4Ns. *Appetite*, *91*, 114–128. doi:10.1016/j.appet.2015.04.011 PMID:25865663

Schmidinger, K., Bogueva, D., & Marinova, D. (2018). New meat without livestock. In D. Bogueva, D. Marinova, & T. Raphaely (Eds.), *Handbook of research on social marketing and its influence on animal origin food product consumption* (pp. 344–361). Hershey, PA: IGI Global. doi:10.4018/978-1-5225-4757-0.ch023

Springmann, M., Mason-D'Croz, D., Robinson, S., Garnett, T., Godfray, H. C. J., Gollin, D., ... Scarborough, P. (2016). Global and regional health effects of future food production under climate change: A modelling study. *Lancet*, *387*(10031), 1937–1346. doi:10.1016/S0140-6736(15)01156-3 PMID:26947322

KEY TERMS AND DEFINITIONS

Generation Y (Gen Y): (referred also as the Millennials) People born between 1977 and 1995; they have grown with technologies such as the internet, computers, and video games and are considered to be technologically savvy.

Generation Z (Gen Z): (referred also as the Centennials or iGen) People born between 1996 and 2009 (although the end of this generation is not clearly defined); they have grown with social media and are considered independent and entrepreneurial.

Natural: Derived from nature, not made or caused by humankind.

Necessary: Required, compulsory, mandatory, inevitable.

New Meat Alternatives: A meat analogue, substitute, vegetarian meat, or vegan meat, a food product which replaces nutritionally animal meat and may or may not imitate meat qualities, such as taste, texture, flavor, and appearance.

Normal: Conforming to a standard; usual, typical, or expected.

Nutritious: Efficient as food to provide essential nutrient; nourishing.

This research was previously published in Environmental, Health, and Business Opportunities in the New Meat Alternatives Market edited by Diana Bogueva, Dora Marinova, Talia Raphaely, and Kurt Schmidinger; pages 20-37, copyright year 2019 by Business Science Reference (an imprint of IGI Global).

Chapter 56
New Meat Without Livestock

Kurt Schmidinger
University of Vienna, Austria

Diana Bogueva
Curtin University, Australia

Dora Marinova
iD https://orcid.org/0000-0001-5125-8878
Curtin University, Australia

ABSTRACT

This chapter summarizes the global problems associated with livestock production and meat consumption and shows solution strategies through replacing animal products with plant-based alternatives. The positive effects of plant-based alternatives on human health and the environment are reviewed together with approaches for reducing world hunger. Psychological strategies for nutritional transitions towards more sustainable consumption patterns and criteria for market success of meat alternatives are presented. This is followed by an overview of meat alternatives – from soy[1], lupine or wheat based, to bleeding burgers and artificial intelligence concepts. Marketing strategies and best practice policy suggestions complete the chapter.

INTRODUCTION

Global mass production of livestock and the consumption of animal products are the major cause of a wide range of serious problems – environmental, health-related, concerning animal welfare and world nutrition. Environmentally, livestock production is a, or the, leading factor in land use, water consumption, pollution, rainforest destruction, climate change, loss of biodiversity and soil erosion (Steinfeld et al., 2006). The main reason for most of these problems is the inefficiency of livestock, where the largest share of the feed calories is used in the animals' metabolism and converted to excrements instead of food for human consumption. Such lengthened food chains, namely plant to animal to human, are heavily inefficient in resource use compared to short food chains, namely plant to human (see Figure 1). This inefficiency also explains why mass production of livestock is associated with world hunger (see later for more detail).

DOI: 10.4018/978-1-7998-5354-1.ch056

Most of the 70 billion animals (excluding sea creatures) produced annually for food consumption live in confined conditions raising severe concerns for their welfare. Although animal welfare is beyond the scope of this chapter, it is a major consideration for the wellbeing of all living beings on this planet. Intensive livestock production is a major risk factor for new global pandemics originating from industrial types of facilities as well as for antibiotic resistances while excessive consumption of meat, eggs and dairy is associated with lifestyle diseases, such as obesity, type 2 diabetes, cancer and heart disease (Schmidinger, 2012).

Given the convincing evidence about the negative impacts of animal-based dietary choices (Raphaely & Marinova, 2016), the question arises how to make consumers consume less of such food and whether a meat-free future is possible. This chapter explores plant-based alternatives to meat and other animal products together with strategies to encourage their acceptability. It also outlines criteria for market success which can trigger positive responses from the consumers and beneficial outcomes.

Figure 1. Livestock's long food chain
Note: Lengthening the food chain by livestock production leads to a loss of a big share of calories from plants within the metabolism of the farmed animals, only a small share of the plant calories is converted to animal products, the major share is converted to excrements and lost for human nutrition.

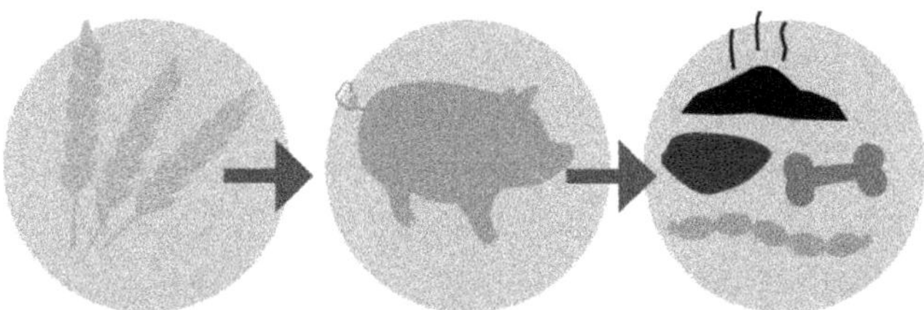

MAKING CONSUMERS EAT LESS ANIMAL PRODUCTS

Promoting plant-based food diets has a solid environmental and especially health case and is increasingly finding space in the EU countries. This is the case in the food guidelines of Sweden (Fischer et al., 2016), France (ANSES France, 2017), the UK Eatwell Guide (Public Health England, 2017) and Germany (DGE, 2017). Producing, distributing, selling and promoting meat is a seriously lucrative business, which relies heavily on the well-established forms of animal mass production at a minimum cost for the producer and especially on the ever-increasing consumption of meat and other foods of animal origin. The existing marketing and advertising efforts aim at bolstering further the intake of animal-based proteins (Bogueva and Phau, 2016). This is despite the clear evidence about the positive consequences, for both human health and the environment, of dietary changes toward healthier and more sustainable plant-based intake (Raphaely and Marinova, 2016; Bogueva et al., 2017; Springmann et al., 2016) and meat alternatives (Schmidinger, 2012). A major shift is clearly necessary.

In principle, a shift could be achieved with existing foods which do not contain animal products, but new plant-based innovations can assist such a transition and make it more realistic (Aiking and de Boer, 2006). As it stands, at the moment the consumption of new alternatives has a long way to cut across existing habits before achieving mass popularity globally. Within any given society, the majority of people tend to adhere to an average diet. In traditional societies, this diet uses more plant-based ingredients, but globalisation triggers widespread westernisation of consumer tastes and with it higher intake of animal products (Hossain, 2016). Furthermore, improvements in people's earning capacity in developing countries also result in preferences for animal-based food (Raphaely & Marinova, 2014). On the other hand, people are influenced by the food choices made by others – relatives, friends, peers, celebrities, as well as advertising, availability and accessibility of products.

Stability/Energy Minimum Hypothesis

The *Stability/Energy Minimum Hypothesis* is a model derived from the theory of Balluch (2009). Adapted to nutritional aspects it shows the need for concerted actions instead of relying only on behaviour changes by billions of individuals.

The basic assumption of this hypothesis is that most individuals in a society try to live in a way that requires least effort or minimum energy. In Figure 2 this is represented by the trough, the area around the minimum of the curve. Applied to eating habits, this means that people tend to eat what is cheap, widely available, socially accepted and tastes well. In industrialised societies, this overwhelmingly involves animal-based products. Living as a vegan, an individual might be excluded from eating in certain restaurants. It may also cause stressful situations when attending business lunches or being invited for dinner or barbecue where vegan options are not served. Furthermore, it may cost more energy and longer shopping times to find the right foods. When abroad in a country with a foreign language, it will be harder to identify all ingredients of food products or dishes. It could be harder for vegetarian parents to find all-day school places offering a varied vegetarian menu for their children. Furthermore, for the children it might cost more energy to avoid becoming an outsider by not joining their friends in going to fast-food restaurants and eating non-vegetarian burgers.

Figure 2. Stability/energy minimum hypothesis in industrialised countries
Note: This graph shows how much energy an individual needs to keep up a certain diet. The political and economic system shape the curve. The trough (in red) is the minimum energy area. Outside the minimum, the individuals have to invest perpetual energy not to "roll back" into the trough, so their position is not stable.

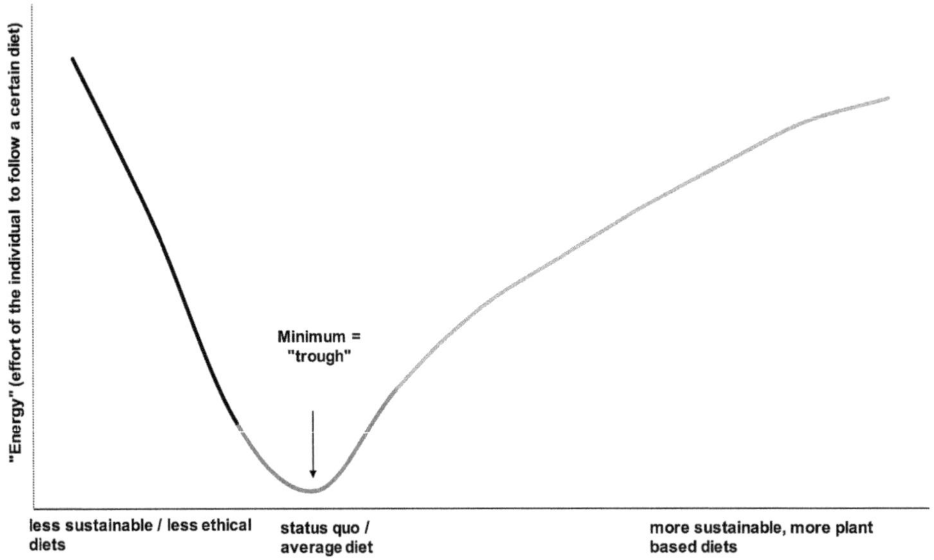

Many individuals who originally were willing to change, tend to "save energy" and revert back to behaviour that makes their lives easier and matches that of the majority of the society to which they belong. In Figure 2, the red minimum represents the behaviour which requires the minimum energy associated with heavy use of animal-based foods in industrialised societies. The right side from the curve's minimum represents a more sustainable/ethical diet, while the left side is a less sustainable diet. Both require more individual energy than adhering to the average diet of a western society. The problem of minimum energy arises from both sides of the curve. A vegan or vegetarian diet is an example from the more sustainable right hand-side of the curve. Eating dogs may be acceptable in some parts of the world (see Figure 3), but would require more energy in the West where such animals are considered pets and domestic companions. This is an example of a less ethical diet from the left hand-side of the curve.

Figure 3. Dog meat sold in the streets of Hanoi, Vietnam, March 2017

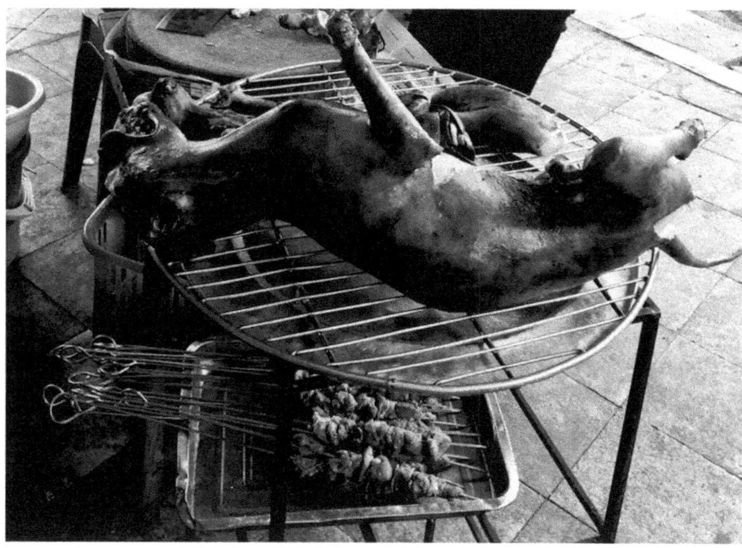

Living outside the trough around the minimum of the curve (see Figure 2) costs energy and requires more effort than following the nutritional mainstream. Such individuals need a lot of motivation and perseverance not to roll back and keep their position stable in the long term.

Shifting to a More Sustainable Diet

In Figure 4, the trough of the curve is pushed to the right, towards a more sustainable form of eating within a society. A wider range of new and attractive plant-based foods offered in markets, supermarkets, shops, restaurants and canteens can help push the trough towards a more sustainable consumption if these new choices become easily available, cheaper and their marketing is successful. The reminder of the chapter presents ideas how to make possible and pleasant to eat more sustainably, which pushes the minimum energy trough to the right and with it the majority of individuals in a society towards a more sustainable nutrition.

Figure 4. Push to a more sustainable diet
Note: Changed conditions in a society (e.g. food markets, political actions etc.) can push the energy minimum to the right, to a more sustainable diet

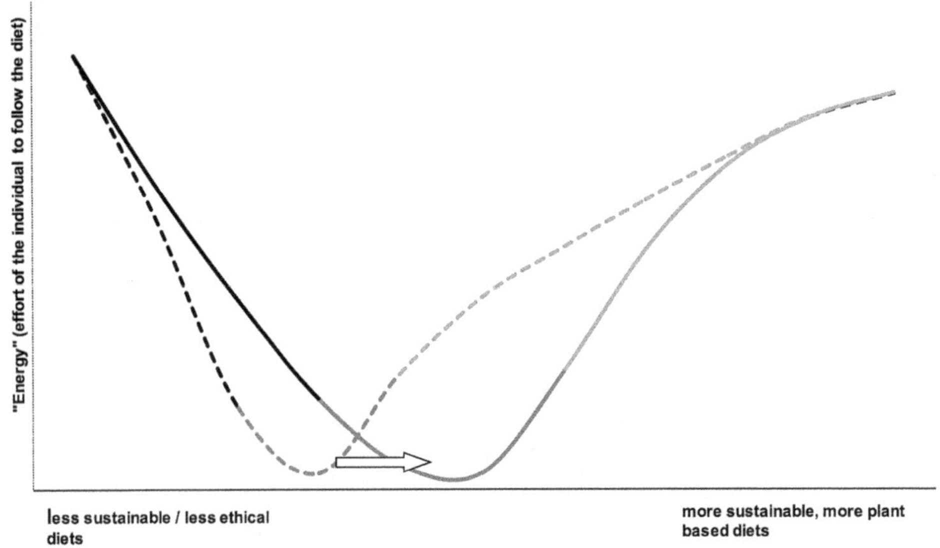

Figure 5 shows a further variation of this model taken from Schmidinger (2012). In it, communities within a society define their own, more sustainable "rules" of nutrition, and the process of adhering to these agreements leads to social acceptance and affirmation creating local troughs in the right part of the curve. Examples are the vegan movements in Europe or the US since 2012 – it has become trendy to live without animal products (e.g. Harvard Medical School, 2016). Being part of such movements and adhering to their vegan agreements form local troughs in the curve on the right of the status quo minimum.

Let's use the example of the vegan movement and illustratively draw an optimistic picture for its future. The more like-minded people form such vegan groupings, the easier it is for each individual to stick to the lifestyle of the group. Figuratively, the more individuals such a social grouping consists of, the more "weight" will be exerted on the curve and the deeper such a local minimum will become. The markets will respond with new varieties of vegan products and food offers, labelling them as vegan. Politics will change due to the influence of vegan voters; the media will react, making the vegan lifestyle even more attractive, and the vegan energy minimum (the trough on the right of the curve) will become deeper and deeper. Such local minimums could eventually also lead to a shift of the energy minimum to the right as shown in Figure 4. Ideally if the more sustainable local minimums become deeper than the current minimum, many individuals from the current trough will roll over to the new minimum to the right of the curve. This will make the old trough disappear with not many individuals there and less weight and the curve from the old minimum will go directly up. Finally, this will lead to a new trough further right than before, and thus a more sustainable diet is achieved.

If broad target groups of people or even the majority of society are to shift to the right of the respective curves as postulated by the Stability/Energy Minimum-Hypothesis, many actions would be required. Given the seriousness of the problems associated with the consumption of animal-based products, it is important that such a transition occurs smoothly with wide social acceptance. People however are generally reluctant to make drastic changes in their diets, even when their personal health is threatened (Blanchard

Figure 5. Push to a more sustainable diet
Note: Local minimums might also attract groups of individuals to practise a more sustainable diet. The more popular such a diet becomes, the deeper and relatively more stable the local minimums are. An optimum final consequence might be that such a new local minimum becomes deeper than the original minumum, making people roll over from the old to the new (more sustainable) minimum trough as shown in Figure 4.

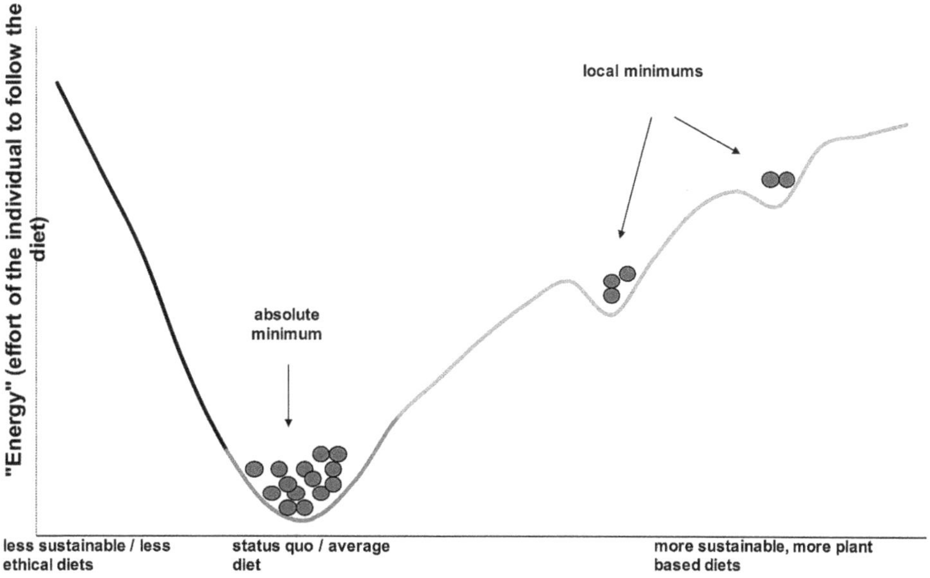

et al., 2008). What criteria should the new plant-based food options fulfil? What requirements should the new plant-based alternatives to animal products, including alternatives to beef, veal, pork, poultry, lamb, mutton, venison, eggs and dairy products, satisfy to be accepted by the majority of consumers? Would even cultured meat grown in vitro in labs become an acceptable alternative? The section below lays out criteria for the success of alternatives to animal products in order to shift the average consumer diet towards more sustainable nutrition.

SUCCESS CRITERIA FOR ALTERNATIVES TO ANIMAL PRODUCTS

The original definition of "meat" refers to the core of a food as distinctive to its husk, shell or to a drink (Merriam–Webster, 2017). More recently however the word "meat" began to be associated with the flesh of an animal used for food. Irrespective of the term's etymology, what is important in this day and age is to break the largely spread assumption that when we eat meat we need to consume animal-based products. We need to reclaim the word together with encouraging food choices healthier for consumers and the planet. Hence, we refer to the entire spectrum of sustainable food options which do not involve livestock as the *new meat*. This includes traditional fruit and vegetables, classical products using tofu as well as new plant-based products, such as vegetarian sausages and soy mince, and meats produced in laboratory conditions. They all share the common characteristic of being animal-free food products.

In order for the new meat to be socially acceptable and to become a preferred option for consumers, it needs to satisfy several criteria. Below is a list of five main criteria informed by the work of Molnár (1989), de Boer and Hoek (2006) and Schmidinger (2012) developed predominantly for western consumers and individuals who are in a position to make food choices.

1. **Sensual Properties and Flavour – Taste, Texture, Satiety Feeling and Aroma:** In the perception of the majority of people within society, the flavour of alternatives to animal products should completely satisfy their preferences. Textures can be fibre-like – such as in meat products, gel-like – such as in yoghurt, coagulated – such as in cheese, and so on (O'Kane, 2006). Hence the alternatives to animal products must fulfil various texture tasks. Meat-like sensory properties and luxury aspects are relevant for plant-based alternatives with higher protein content in a product improving satiety sensations (Hoek, 2006). For example, favoured properties for vegetarian meat products are: brown, soft, smooth, crispy, seasoned, spicy and meat-like flavour (Elzerman, 2006).

2. **Price:** Alternatives to animal products should be affordable, preferably cheaper than the livestock-based products. The lengthened food chain and the losses of plant food calories through metabolism make animal products costly in principle. Model calculations for pea-based meat alternatives show that they should be cheaper than pork (Apaiah, 2006). Applications for the byproducts of, for example, pea- or soy-based meat alternatives exist (Willemsen, 2006), but should be economically optimised. Efficient alternatives to the byproducts of livestock production, such as leather, gelatine or pet food, need to be found (Willemsen & Apaiah, 2006), although many already exist while others need to be improved and made economically viable.

3. **Marketing, Target Groups and Advertising:** Alternatives to animal products should appeal to a wide target group, not only to vegans, vegetarians or health-conscious people! In fact, the target should be the general or average consumer. Information about new foods should "evoke feelings like comfort, familiarity, happiness, ease, low price and popularity" (Goodland & Anhang, 2009, p. 17). Advertising campaigns should "pitch the theme of eating all week long a line of food products that is tasty, easy to prepare and includes a superfood, such as soy" that will enrich the consumers' lives (Goodland and Anhang, 2009, p. 17). Availability in supermarket and discount stores as well as advertising, especially at the point of sale, are essential and have massive room for improvement (Ruiz, 2007). Also, plant-based alternatives should be placed side by side on the same shelf with livestock products to achieve the same exposure to consumers (Goodland and Anhang, 2009).

4. **Health:** Fruits and vegetables have numerous health benefits and their consumption should continue to be encouraged. The new plant-based foods should also be healthier than the animal products in an overall health appraisal. This should be valid at a personal level as well as being a public health consideration. Their use could minimise the risk of formation of new pandemics, antibiotic resistance (Raphaely et al., 2016) and development of salmonella, E. coli and other infections (Review of Antimicrobial Resistance, 2015). They should also be able to outperform animal products in terms of personal health issues. With reference to cultured meat, for example, it should be possible to optimise the fatty acid or amino acid composition of the final product and leave out cholesterol, Neu5GC and other unwanted compounds, making a healthier meat than those currently existing.

5. **Shelf Life and Hygiene:** Existing plant-based meat-, egg- or dairy-alternatives typically have a longer shelf-life than their equivalent livestock products – a fact that easily can be verified in any supermarket. For example, dried products, such as textured vegetable protein (TVP) chunks, have shelf lives of a year or longer. In fact, manufacturers of meat products use plant-based solutions as

a natural way to extend shelf life, control bacteria development and improve food safety (Pelligrini, 2014). With the majority of foodborne diseases originating from animal products, plant-based foods carry lower risk and hence, their shelf life is longer representing weighty advantages for the consumer and the food industry alike.

PRODUCTS MAKING THE CHANGE POSSIBLE

There is plenty of more or less well-known plant-based alternatives to meat, milk and eggs on the market, but certain innovations – recent or still being developed, could have a bright future. Some common or promising livestock-free solutions are presented below. The focus is on meat alternatives (sometimes even difficult to distinguish visually as shown in Figure 6), but similar innovations are also available to replace egg or dairy products.

Figure 6. Plant based chicken drumsticks

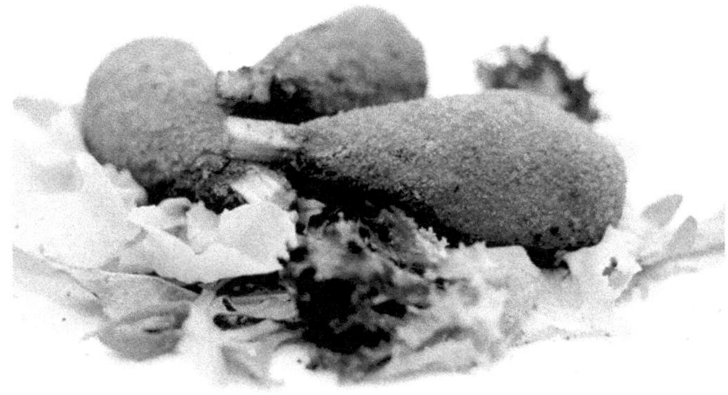

Classic Plant-Based Meat Alternatives

The most common base materials for meat alternatives are wheat gluten (also called seitan) and soy-based ingredients, such as tofu and textured soy protein (abbreviated as TSP or TVP), also called soy meat. Seitan is obtained simply by rinsing wheat dough and washing out the starch until the protein components gliadin and glutenin are isolated from the wheat. Tofu is a worldwide well-known traditional Asian foodstuff, where a coagulant (traditionally nigari salt) is added to soy milk and the resulting protein solids are pressed into a desired form. Soy meat is produced using hot extrusion of defatted soy proteins, resulting in expanded high protein chunks, nuggets, strips, grains and other shapes. The fibrous, insoluble, porous soy meat can soak up water or other liquids a multiple of its own weight.

Unlike tofu, seitan and even more soy meat show consistencies which are remarkably similar to the stringy fibres that make up animal-based meat. Often, you find products made of mixes of soy- and wheat-based protein ingredients. The disadvantage of this mix is that these products are not suitable for consumer groups suffering from soy allergies or gluten intolerance (coeliac disease). For the other consumers, such mixes represent perfect meat-like textures as well as optimised protein contents and quality. The protein quality can be explained by the fact that the profiles of the essential amino acids contained in soy and wheat complete each other well and compensate the deficiencies of their individual amino acid profiles.

Another classical plant-based meat alternative is tempeh which has a very old tradition in Indonesia. Controlled fermentation of soaked, hulled, hacked and damped soybeans with a Rhizopus mold binds them together into a compact, firm white patty form. The protein content makes tempeh a suitable ingredient for meat alternatives, whereas its texture is not meat-like. Experiments to produce tempeh based on barley and oats instead of soy have also been made (Swedish-Research-Council, 2008).

Other Meat Alternatives

These ingredients are innovative, some already available on the market, others on the way to being commercialised. The list of such alternatives is long and expanding in response to rising consumer interest, mainly from vegans and vegetarians. Below is a selection of such new meats.

Quorn, based on the so called Mycoprotein, is a commercially successful meat alternative range introduced by the English company Marlow Foods. Mycoprotein is a fermented fungus which is processed and textured to produce meat alternatives. Quorn products include steaks, burgers, chicken breasts as well as sliced meats and ready meals. It is marketed in European countries, USA, South Africa and Australia.

Sweet lupines have become another, increasingly popular base ingredient for meat or dairy alternatives, especially in Europe. Meatless was one of the first companies to use lupine-based fibres for the production of meat substitutes. The already completed Like Meat project funded by the European Union similarly used lupines as one of its experimental base materials.

Sprouted soybeans are used commercially, even though on a small scale, especially by the Hungarian company Yaso. Rice protein and pea protein have also been introduced for the production of meat alternatives together with vegetable fibres used by companies like Wiefleisch or the former company Proviand, taken over by the German veggie meat specialist Like Meat.

Using fresh mushrooms could be another option, as the company Fresh'shrooms has shown. Algae similarly holds huge potential for meat alternatives. Nuts (e.g. pecans) and garbanzo beans are the main ingredients for meat alternatives produced by Neat.

Science-Intensive Plant-Based Alternatives

This category of new meats includes innovations underpinned by scientific work which aims at reproducing the appearance of animal products to our senses A plant-based, perfect *bleeding beef burger* is the flagship of Impossible Foods in the USA, using heme (haem) from plants as a "bloody" juice. The burger exhibits a meat-like exterior fulfilling the equation: plants + science = meat. With funding from Google and Bill Gates (Woods, 2015), the company was able to create plant-based meats that give people the texture, flavour, aroma, taste and nutritional benefits of animal meat, without the negative health and environmental impacts of livestock products (Belvedere, 2016; Herships, 2016; Fellet, 2015; Gates, 2013).

The Not Company in Chile also explores path-breaking ways. Currently it focuses on dairy alternatives, but the same ideas will be applied to meat analogues. The company uses Guiseppe – the smartest food scientist on earth, who studies the perceptions about foods by humans (Sunder, 2016). However, Giuseppe is not a person, but an artificial intelligence robot that replicates the taste, texture and even smell of animal-based products by copying their molecular structure. Guiseppe uses plant-based ingredients for its food creations with the aim to achieve high nutritional values with low ecological impacts. Unlike humans, Giuseppe's knowledge is ever-increasing as the robot never forgets anything it has learned.

Real Meat of the Future out of the Lab

Besides plant-based meat alternatives, there are even more futuristic approaches. The concept is called *in vitro* meat or cultured meat, and the process is in principle as follows. Starting cells are taken painlessly from live animals; they are put into plant-based culture media, including growth factors, where they start to proliferate and grow independently from the animal. This all should happen in large bioreactors which can be monitored and controlled. To achieve a fibrous and three-dimensional texture, various concepts are applied – using edible scaffolds to which the cells could attach, 3-D-printing to print meat or electrical stimulation on the cells as a training to build muscle-like fibres.

Mark Post and his team in the Netherlands were the first to produce a burger in vitro, with financial support from the Google founder Sergey Brin. The burger was presented in 2013 in London and while still extremely expensive at an estimated cost of around US$ 300,000, it was a striking achievement (Shen, 2013). Memphis Meats recently produced several cultured meat balls. Modern Meadow are US-based projects also working on cultured meat. In Israel, Supermeat with Yaakov Nahmias and the Kitchen FoodTech Hub similarly pursue cultured meat efforts. The list of organisations and initiatives which are active in this domain includes New Harvest, the Good Food Institute, Future Food and the Modern Agriculture Foundation. They are making good progress with a lot of publicly available information.

MARKETING OF FUTURE FOOD ALTERNATIVES

Currently worldwide there exist many plant-based meat alternatives and plant-based protein products – enough to fill up a meatless butcher shop. The producers are concentrated mainly in (Shurtleff & Aoyagi, 2014; Schmidinger, 2012): USA and Canada in North America, Germany, the Netherland, UK, Italy, Czech Republic, Austria, France and Hungary in Europe, Australia and New Zealand in the Asia Pacific, Taiwan, China and Thailand in Asia, Brazil and Argentina in South America. Meat alternatives are projected to be soon stretched out of their niche market segment and as per the Allied Market Research (2016) forecast this trend is going to grow substantially offering many business opportunities (The Economist, 2017). Similarity to animal flesh-food composition, appearance and flavour is one reason for these plant-based food alternatives starting to make their way and gradually becoming popular amongst consumers. Another reason is their improved performance in relation to human health – they are cholesterol-free, have lower risks for numerous chronic diseases, such as cancer and cardiovascular disease. They also perform better in response to environmental concerns. In countries, such as USA, Germany and UK, these new meat alternatives are gaining good market shares and are no longer limited to a display at the back shelves of the supermarket. Nevertheless, the new meat alternatives still require more intense and competitive market strategies to establish themselves in the consumers' mind and to break out of their niche label into the mainstream.

Marketing strategies used by new meat producers usually follow the traditional mix around the 4P – product, promotion, place and price (Luca & Suggs, 2010; Thackeray & McCormack Brown, 2010), focused on increasing awareness about the existence of new cutting edge innovative plant-based products and promoting them among consumers. Some however are utilising novel approaches. Injecting culturally relevant concepts which resonate with people, through social media (e.g. Facebook) into brand communication was used by the advertising campaign of Alternative Meat Co (2017). The campaign ridiculed the Lambasador used by livestock advertisers to create a cultural identity of the multicultural Australian society around eating lamb on Australia Day. Alternative Meat Co used a mocking advertisement highlighting the increasing number of Australians who represent the changing food trends towards reduced meat consumption. The advertisement encourages people to try an alternative, e.g. vegetables, on Australia Day in line with the social trend away from animal-based products. This online advertisement received more than 1.1 million views, 13.5 thousand shares, 11 thousand likes and 5 thousand comments (Australian Meat Co, 2017). Tofurky can replace the turkeys traditionally consumed on Thanksgiving in USA (Shurtleff and Aoyagi, 2014).

Endorsement by celebrities is a marketing strategy employed by the California-based start-up Impossible Foods (Woods, 2015; Belvedere, 2016; Herships, 2016; Fellet, 2015). Promoting famous vegetarians who symbolise strength and masculinity is also a good way to increase the attractiveness of new meats. The list of names includes Mike Tyson – the undisputed heavyweight boxer champion, Carl Lewis – the nine-time Olympic gold medallist athlete, Brendan Brazier – the Ironman triathlete, Daniel Sturridge – premier league club Liverpool footballer, Serena and Venus Williams – the superstar tennis players and athletes, and many others.

Sensing the consumer shift to protein alternatives, major global meat producers are keen to stay in the game by participating in the new meats market. Tyson Foods in USA acquired a 5 percent share in the plant-based protein food manufacturer Beyond Meat. Similarly, the German meat packer company Rügenwalder Mühl and the Canadian Maple Leaf Foods are tailoring their marketing strategies to establish a strong platform in the plant-based proteins market (Strom, 2016).

A major component of the attractiveness of animal meat is its taste, smell, textural properties, fibrous structure, deliciousness and juicy mouth-feel – attributes stated by Australian Sydney residents (Bogueva et al., 2017). Using new meats' resemblance to these qualities can be a successful marketing strategy for a transition to healthier, environmentally better and morally higher diets.

The qualities of the new meats will continue to improve and their prices will become increasingly compatible. Any marketing and advertising campaigns will need to use this to reform and rebrand the consumer perceptions about food. However, there is a role for government and other institutions to play in supporting and facilitating these changes.

Against the ample evidence about the need to move towards healthier and environmentally respectful dietary patterns, the new meats alternatives are perfect novelties that must be supported as a trendy shift. Instead of lagging behind, government bodies should take an active stance and start developing and disseminating official dietary guidelines and recommendations, embedding health and sustainability objectives and creating policies fostering them (Fischer et al, 2016).

In addition to financial support for the new meats and removal of any funding benefiting the livestock sector (Hamilton, 2016; Di Croce et al. 2016), the government needs to engage in promoting the alternatives. In a similar way to dealing with tobacco and cigarettes, this should include freeing up the public advertising space from undesired messages and instigating social marketing of better alternatives. New meat options should be made available in public institutions, such as school canteens, hospitals and promoted in supermarkets, foodcourts and restaurants. Marketing strategies using the 4S model – sustainability, strength, self-confidence and sharing (Bogueva et al., 2017) can encourage transitioning to more sustainable diets.

WORLD HUNGER AND FOOD ALTERNATIVES

Although nearly half a billion people in the world identify themselves as vegetarians (Meat Atlas, 2014), the consumption of animal products continues to be strong in Western countries, including Australia, USA and Europe. Moreover, traditional diets are changing in places such as China and India exacerbating the seriousness of the climate change challenges (Myers & Kent, 2003; Vidal, 2013; Yu, 2015). Adding to this is the world's hunger problem of 1 billion people, among them 3 million children and 20 million people dying from starvation each year (Lappé & Collins, 2015). Global hunger will not be resolved by using the inefficient lengthened plant–to animal–to human food chains.

As seen in Figure 1, the losses of calories for global nutrition due to livestock production are enormous – 36 percent of the global cereal harvests (Schmid & Goldhofer, 2016) as well as 70 to 75 percent of the global soy harvests (Brack et al., 2016) are used for livestock. In 2016, 320 million tonnes of meat have been produced (FAO, 2016). According to Alexander et al. (2017), 1060 million tonnes of feed from crops plus 440 million tonnes of forage crops (e.g. alfalfa and forage maize) plus additional grass from grassland make up just 240 million tonnes of animal products in dry matter.

An average German person wastes about 400 kg of plant food just by eating meat. This is based on an average of 7 to 8 calories of plant-based feed to produce 1 calorie of meat (an estimate based on Smil, 2002 and Garnett, 2009). Milk and eggs are not even included in these figures. This waste of food for meat consumption alone is much higher than the annual 179 kg of wasted food per capita in the EU from private households, producers, supermarkets and gastronomy all together (European Commission, 2010)! The world produces more than enough to feed all humans on the planet Earth but not through inefficient food chains.

In response to the myriad of negative consequences triggered by livestock products, many are opting for plant-based alternatives (Market and Markets, 2016; Roy Morgan Research, 2016). This is also where the future of food lies and the quicker the transition, the better will be the outcomes for all.

CONCLUSION

The consumption of animal-based products is associated with serious impacts on human health, the natural environment and world hunger. The Stability/Energy Minimum hypothesis explains people's dominant eating behaviour as the one which conforms with the majority preferences within the society, circle of friends or at home and requires the least effort. A push towards more sustainable dietary choices needs to be facilitated by making plant-based options attractive in terms of flavours, textures, price, availability and varieties. By satisfying the five criteria related to taste, cost, health, shelf life and marketing, the alternatives to animal-based products can find their way into society and contribute to the creation of new more sustainable minimum energy conditions that encourage better health and environment related options.

As diets are expressed as a personal choice, the new meats based on fruit, vegetables, plants, TPV, cultured meat and other innovations can enrich the options available to the consumers who opt to exclude animal-based products from their dietary preferences. When wisely and properly marketed, these new meat food products will help shift the average diet and make it more sustainable. On a global scale this will free up a lot of waste associated with the current inefficient lengthened food chain, which feeds livestock first before feeding people, and allow world hunger to be eliminated. The future of food lies in many plant-based innovations as well as other options away from livestock products. Meat without livestock is the alternative we need to embrace if we are to dream for a brighter future.

ACKNOWLEDGMENT

The second and third authors acknowledge the contribution of an Australian Government Research Training Program Scholarship in supporting this research.

REFERENCES

Agence nationale de sécurité sanitaire de l'alimentation, de l'environnement et du travail (ANSES). (2017, January 24). *ANSES updates its food consumption guidelines for the French population*. French Agency for Food, Environmental and Occupational Health & Safety. Retrieved from https://www.anses.fr/en/content/anses-updates-its-food-consumption-guidelines-french-population

Aiking, H., & de Boer, J. (2006). Transition feasibility and implications for stakeholders. In H. Aiking, H., J. de Boer, & J. Vereijken (Eds.), Sustainable protein production and consumption: Pigs or peas? (pp. 193-215). Dordrecht, Netherlands: Springer. doi:10.1007/1-4020-4842-4_7

Alexander, P., Brown, C., Arneth, A., Finnigan, J., Moran, D., & Rounsevell, M. D. A. (2017). Losses, inefficiencies and waste in the global food system. *Agricultural Systems, 153*, 190–200. doi:10.1016/j.agsy.2017.01.014 PMID:28579671

Allied Market Research. (2016). *Meat substitute market by product type (tofu, tempeh, textured vegetable protein, quorn, seitan), source (soy, wheat, mycoprotein), category (frozen, refrigerated, shelf-stable): Global opportunity analysis and industry forecast, 2014 - 2020*. Retrieved from https://www.alliedmarketresearch.com/meat-substitute-market

Alternative Meat Co. (2017, January 12). *Dave Hughes addresses Australia*. Alternative Meat Co (AMC) Facebook Page. Retrieved https://www.facebook.com/altmeatco/videos/1856335437973845/

Apaiah, R. K. (2006). Methodology for chain design. In H. Aiking, J. de Boer, & J. Vereijken (Eds.), *Sustainable protein production and consumption: Pigs or peas?* (pp. 79–85). Dordrecht, Netherlands: Springer.

Balluch, M. (2009). *Widerstand in der Demokratie - ziviler Ungehorsam und konfrontative Kampagnen*. Vienna, Austria: Promedia Druck- und VerlagsgesmbH Wien.

Belvedere, M. (2016, August 1). *We tried the plant-based "impossible burger" that's backed by Bill Gates*. CNBC. Retrieved from http://www.cnbc.com/2016/07/29/impossible-burger-our-test-tube-meat-tastes-great.html

Blanchard, C. M., Courneya, K. S., & Stein, K. (2008). Cancer survivors' adherence to lifestyle behavior recommendations and associations with health-related quality of life: Results from the American Cancer Society's SCS-II. *Journal of Clinical Oncology, 26*(13), 2198–2204. doi:10.1200/JCO.2007.14.6217 PMID:18445845

Bogueva, D., Marinova, D., & Raphaely, T. (2017). Reducing meat consumption: The case for social marketing. *Asia Pacific Journal of Marketing and Logistics, 29*(3), 477–500. doi:10.1108/APJML-08-2016-0139

Bogueva, D., & Phau, I. (2016). Meat myths and marketing. In T. Raphaely & D. Marinova (Eds.), *Impact of meat consumption on health and environmental sustainability* (pp. 264–276). Hershey, PA: IGI Global. doi:10.4018/978-1-4666-9553-5.ch015

Brack, D., Glover, A., & Wellesley, L. (2016). *Agricultural commodity supply chains: Trade, consumption and deforestation.* London, UK: The Royal Institute of International Affairs, Chatham House.

de Boer, J., & Hoek, A. (2006). Social desirability: Consumer aspects. In H. Aiking, J. de Boer, & J. Vereijken (Eds.), *Sustainable protein production and consumption: Pigs or peas?* (pp. 99–127). Dordrecht, Netherlands: Springer. doi:10.1007/1-4020-4842-4_4

Deutsche Gesellschaft für Ernährung (DGE). (2017). Der Wissenschaft verpflichtet – Ihr Partner für Essen und Trinken (The science – Your partner for eating and drinking). Retrieved from https://www.dge.de

Di Croce, P., Lymbery, P., Dibb, S., Hameleers, R., Wates, J., & Renshaw, N. … Martin, F. (2016). Letter to the Commissioner for Agriculture and Rural Development, European Commission of 10 November 2016. Retrieved from https://www.foeeurope.org/sites/default/files/agriculture/2016/meat-letter-hogan.pdf

Elzerman, H. (2006). Substitution of meat by NPFs: Sensory properties and contextual factors. In H. Aiking, J. de Boer, & J. Vereijken (Eds.), *Sustainable protein production and consumption: Pigs or peas?* (pp. 116–123). Dordrecht, Netherlands: Springer.

European Commission. (2010). *Preparatory study on food waste across EU 27.* Retrieved from http://ec.europa.eu/environment/archives/eussd/pdf/bio_foodwaste_report.pdf

Fellet, M. (2015). A fresh take on fake meat. Can scientists deliver a meatless burger that tastes good and will not harm the planet? *ACS Central Science, 1*(7), 347–349. doi:10.1021/acscentsci.5b00307 PMID:27162992

Fischer, C., & Garnett, T. (2016). *Plates, pyramids and planets.* FAO and FCRN, University of Oxford. Retrieved from http://www.fao.org/3/a-i5640e.pdf

Food and Agriculture Organisation of the United Nations (FAO). (2016). Food outlook: Biannual report on global food markets. Retrieved from http://www.fao.org/3/a-i6198e.pdf

Garnett, T. (2009). Livestock-related greenhouse gas emissions: Impacts and options for policy makers. *Environmental Science & Policy, 12*(4), 491–503. doi:10.1016/j.envsci.2009.01.006

Gates, B. (2013, March 18). *Future of food.* The Gates Notes. Blog of Bill Gates. Retrieved from https://www.gatesnotes.com/About-Bill-Gates/Future-of-Food

Goodland, R. & Anhang, J. (2009). Livestock and climate change. *Worldwatch Institute Magazine,* November/December, 11-19.

Hamilton, J. (2016, December 7). *Common agricultural policy: Why is the EU pushing meat?* Honey Colony. Retrieved from https://www.honeycolony.com/article/common-agricultural-policy/

Harvard Medical School. (2016). *Becoming a vegetarian*. Harvard Health Publications. Retrieved from https://www.health.harvard.edu/staying-healthy/becoming-a-vegetarian

Herships, S. (2016, September 23). *A veggie burger that 'bleeds' might convince some carnivores to eat green*. Public Radio International "The World". Retrieved from https://www.pri.org/stories/2016-09-23/veggie-burger-bleeds-might-convince-some-carnivores-eat-green

Hoek, A. (2006). Substitution of meat by NPFs: Factors in consumer choice. In H. Aiking, J. de Boer, & J. Vereijken (Eds.), *Sustainable protein production and consumption: Pigs or peas?* (pp. 110–116). Dordrecht, Netherlands: Springer.

Hossain, A. (2016). Sustainable food consumption: A mission almost impossible because of the West. In T. Raphaely & D. Marinova (Eds.), *Impact of meat consumption on health and environmental sustainability* (pp. 255–263). Hershey, PA: IGI Global. doi:10.4018/978-1-4666-9553-5.ch014

Lappé, F. M., & Collins, J. (2015). *World hunger: Ten myths*. New York, NY: Grove Press.

Luca, N., & Suggs, S. (2010). Strategies for the social marketing mix: A systematic review. *Social Marketing Quarterly*, *16*(4), 122–149. doi:10.1080/15245004.2010.522767

Markets and Markets. (2016). *Meat substitutes market by type (tofu & tofu ingredients, tempeh, textured vegetable protein, seitan, quorn), source (soy-based, wheat-based, mycoprotein), category (frozen, refrigerated), and region – global forecast to 2022*. Markets and Markets. Retrieved from http://www.marketsandmarkets.com/Market-Reports/meat-substitutes-market-979.html

Meat Atlas. (2014). *Facts and figures about the animals we eat*. Berlin, Germany: Heinrich Böll Foundation and Brussels, Belgium: Friends of the Earth Europe. Retrieved from https://www.boell.de/sites/default/files/meat_atlas2014_kommentierbar.pdf

Merriam–Webster. (2017). *Meat*. Retrieved from https://www.merriam-webster.com/dictionary/meat

Molnár, P. J. (1989). A theoretical model to describe food quality. *Journal of Food Quality*, *12*(1), 1–11. doi:10.1111/j.1745-4557.1989.tb00305.x

Myers, N., & Kent, J. (2003). New consumers: The influence of affluence on the environment. *Proceedings of the National Academy of Sciences of the United States of America*, *100*(8), 4963–4968. doi:10.1073/pnas.0438061100 PMID:12672963

O'Kane, F. E. (2006). NPF Texture formation. In H. Aiking, J. de Boer, & J. Vereijken (Eds.), *Sustainable protein production and consumption: Pigs or peas?* (pp. 62–66). Dordrecht, Netherlands: Springer.

Pelligrini, M. (2014). *Extending shelf-life in protein products, naturally*. The Natural Provisioner. Retrieved from http://www.provisioneronline.com/articles/100955-extending-shelf-life-in-protein-products-naturally

Public Health England. (2017). *A quick guide to the government healthy eating recommendations*. Nutrition Advice Team, Public Health England. Retrieved from https://www.gov.uk/government/uploads/system/uploads/attachment_data/file/595133/A_quick_guide_to_govt_healthy_eating.pdf

Raphaely, T., & Marinova, D. (2014). Flexitarianism: A more moral dietary option. *International Journal of Sustainable Society*, *6*(1/2), 189–211. doi:10.1504/IJSSOC.2014.057846

Raphaely, T., & Marinova, D. (Eds.). (2016). *Impact of meat consumption on health and environmental sustainability*. Hershey, PA: IGI Global. doi:10.4018/978-1-4666-9553-5

Raphaely, T., Marinova, D., & Marinova, M. (2016). Antibiotics and the livestock sector. In T. Raphaely & D. Marinova (Eds.), *Impact of meat consumption on health and environmental sustainability* (pp. 178–200). Hershey, PA: IGI Global. doi:10.4018/978-1-4666-9553-5.ch009

Review on Antimicrobial Resistance. (2015). *Antimicrobials in agriculture and the environment: Reducing unnecessary use and waste*. Retrieved from https://amr-review.org/sites/default/files/Antimicrobials%20in%20agriculture%20and%20the%20environment%20-%20Reducing%20unnecessary%20use%20and%20waste.pdf

Roy Morgan Research. (2016). *The slow, but steady rise of Vegetarianism in Australia*. Retrieved from http://www.roymorgan.com/findings/vegetarianisms-slow-but-steady-rise-in-australia-201608151105

Ruiz, M. (2007). *Ausblick und Chancen des Vegetarismustrends im Lebensmittelhandel*. (Master thesis). Vienna, Austria: FH Corporate Governance and Management

Schmid, W., & Goldhofer, H. (2016). *Agrarmärkte 2016: 2 Getreide*. Retrieved from http://www.lfl. bayern.de/mam/cms07/iem/dateien/02_getreide__by_.pdf

Schmidinger, K. (2012). *Worldwide alternatives to animal derived foods – overview and evaluation models - solutions to global problems caused by livestock*. (Doctoral dissertation). Vienna, Austria: University of Natural Resources and Life Sciences.

Shen, A. (2013). Why we should stop obsessing over how expensive the world's first test-tube hamburger is. *ThinkProgress*. Retrieved from https://thinkprogress.org/why-we-should-stop-obsessing-over-how-expensive-the-worlds-first-test-tube-hamburger-is-c4e7011f52f4/

Shurtleff, W., & Aoyagi, A. (2014). History of meat alternatives (965CE to 2014): Extensively annotated bibliography and sourcebook. *Soyinfo Center*. Retrieved from http://www.soyinfocenter.com/pdf/179/MAL.pdf

Smil, V. (2002). Worldwide transformation of diets, burdens of meat production and opportunities for novel food proteins. *Enzyme and Microbial Technology*, *30*(3), 105–311. doi:10.1016/S0141-0229(01)00504-X

Springmann, M., Godfray, H. C. J., Rayner, M., & Scarborough, P. (2016). Analysis and valuation of the health and climate change cobenefits of dietary change. [PNAS]. *Proceedings of the National Academy of Sciences of the United States of America*, *113*(15), 4146–4151. doi:10.1073/pnas.1523119113 PMID:27001851

Steinfeld, H., Gerber, P., Wassenaar, T., Castel, V., Rosales, M., & de Haan, C. (2006). Livestock's long shadow: Environmental issues and options. Rome, Italy: Food and Agriculture Organization of the United Nations (FAO).

Strom, S. (2016, 10 October). Tyson Foods, a meat leader, invests in protein alternatives. *The New York Times*. Retrieved from https://www.nytimes.com/2016/10/11/business/tyson-foods-a-meat-leader-invests-in-protein-alternatives.html?_r=0

Sunder, K. (2016). Meet the world's smartest food scientist: GIUSEPPE. Biotechin Asia. Retrieved from https://biotechin.asia/2016/02/16/meet-the-worlds-smartest-food-scientist-guiseppe/

Swedish Research Council. (2008, May 30). New vegetarian food with several health benefits. *Science-Daily*. Retrieved from https://www.sciencedaily.com/releases/2008/05/080528095627.htm

Thackeray, R., & McCormack Brown, K. (2010). Creating successful price and placement strategies for social marketing. *Health Promotion Practice*, *11*(2), 166–168. doi:10.1177/1524839909360892 PMID:20400655

The Economist. (2017, 2 February). *The market for alternative-protein products*. Retrieved from https://www.economist.com/news/business/21716076-plant-based-meat-products-have-made-it-menus-and-supermarket-shelves-market

Vidal, J. (2013, 14 April). Climate change: How a warming world is a treat to our food supplies. *The Guardian*. Retrieved from https://www.theguardian.com/environment/2013/apr/13/climate-change-threat-food-supplies

Willemsen, F. (2006). Options for non-protein fractions. In H. Aiking, J. de Boer, & J. Vereijken (Eds.), *Sustainable protein production and consumption: Pigs or peas?* (pp. 86–91). Dordrecht, Netherlands: Springer.

Willemsen, F., & Apaiah, R. (2006). Combined chains. In H. Aiking, J. de Boer, & J. Vereijken (Eds.), *Sustainable protein production and consumption: Pigs or peas?* (pp. 166–175). Dordrecht, Netherlands: Springer.

Woods, B. (2015, 14 May). *Bill Gates bets on growing demand for sustainable foods*. CNBC.com. Retrieved from http://www.cnbc.com/2015/05/14/hampton-creek-and-impossible-foods-technology.html

Yu, X. (2015). Meat consumption in China and its impact on international food security: Status quo, trends, and policies. *Journal of Integrative Agriculture*, *14*(6), 989–994. doi:10.1016/S2095-3119(14)60983-7

KEY TERMS AND DEFINITIONS

Cultured Meat: Meat grown in vitro in laboratories which does not involve the slaughter of animals.

Meat Alternative: A substance with a high protein content used to replace animal flesh as food.

New Meat: Covers the entire spectrum of traditional and new food options which do not involve livestock.

Shelf Life: The recommended time for the sale of a food product.

Stability/Energy Minimum Hypothesis: A model which explains eating behaviour as a process conforming with the majority preferences in a society.

Textured Vegetable Protein (TVP): Dried vegetable matter with a high protein content by-product of extracting soybean oil used as a new meat in vegetarian and vegan food products.

World Hunger: Inefficient use and distribution of food resources, including feeding livestock instead of directly feeding people.

ENDNOTE

[1]   The terms soy and soya refer to the same bean – a legume type, with the preferred spelling in the USA being "soy" and in Europe – "soya". We have opted to use "soy" in this chapter; however, all products described here may also appear in the literature and on the market as "soya".

This research was previously published in the Handbook of Research on Social Marketing and Its Influence on Animal Origin Food Product Consumption edited by Diana Bogueva, Dora Marinova, and Talia Raphaely; pages 344-361, copyright year 2018 by Business Science Reference (an imprint of IGI Global).

Chapter 57
Application of the Dietary Processed Sulfur Supplementation for Enhancing Nutritional and Functional Properties of Meat Products

Chi-Ho Lee
Konkuk University, South Korea

ABSTRACT

In recent years, the consumer demands for healthier meat and meat products with reduced level of fat, cholesterol, decreased contents of sodium chloride and nitrite, improved composition of fatty acid profile and incorporated health enhancing ingredients are rapidly increasing worldwide and prevent the risk of diseases. This review focuses on strategies to investigate the changes in physical, physicochemical and microbial properties of meat and meat products in dietary processed sulfur fed animals. Overall, this review focuses on sulfur supplementation to pigs, growth performance of pigs and meat quality, enhancing the nutritional and functional values, shelf-life extension, improve sensory quality characteristics and health benefit etc. This review further discusses the current status, consumer acceptance, and market for functional foods from the global viewpoints. Future prospects for functional meat and meat products are also discussed.

INTRODUCTION

Meat and meat products are important sources for protein, fat, essential amino acids, minerals and vitamin and other nutrients (Biesalski, 2005). Pork meat is usually consumed than any other meat products in South Korea. In 2012, approximately, 50% of the total meat consumption was pork compared to 22% of beef meat and 28% of poultry meat. Meat consumption has increased from 17.8kg per person to 19.3 kg per person in 2010 (Ministry for Food, Agriculture, Forestry and Fisheries. 2011). Recently, there

DOI: 10.4018/978-1-7998-5354-1.ch057

has been a major shift in Korean consumer's preference for leaner and more functional meat. Especially, consumers become more concerned about nutrition and functional health that changed the consumption patterns of meat and meat products. The carcass and meat quality attributes could be affected by the differences in dietary components, such as fatty acids composition, genetic type, age, and other supplements including green tea, Korean ginseng, garlic etc. Limited scientific reports are available for the effects of the processed sulfur concentration of the diet on meat quality. Especially, garlic is an important spice which is inevitable in Korean food. Garlic contains plentiful di-allyl sulfide of pungent taste and is generally found in plant compounds that give certain distinguishable odors to onions, a green onion, leek, garlic (Stanley *et al.*, 1998). Garlic has been used by Koreans for major spices in ordinary diets. Sulfur has been used as a traditional healing material for infirm patients (Stanley *et al.*, The Miracle of MSM., a Berkley book/published by The Berkley Publishing Group, New York 10014). Recently, consumers prefer to the animal functional foods with low fat and high meat quality products rather than high saturated fatty acids containing meat products. The palatability of pork is positively associated with oleic acids of marbling fats (Kim *et al.*, 2015). Therefore, advanced technology needs to be considered for increasing the oleic acid, amino acids with umami, and water holding capacity with meat quality, and for decreasing the saturated fatty acids in pig performance and pork products.

Dry-cured ham was made of pork, solar salt, fresh air, and fermentation in Southern Europe 2000 years ago, and hind leg surface was rubbed with salt and other additives to remove moisture (Mikami *et al.*, . 2007). Drying typically took 6–12 months or more (Mikami *et al.*, 2007). Dry-cured ham reduces weight by about 18% during ripening periods (typically 20–35% for Spanish ham) and concentrates the unique taste and aroma (Mikami *et al.*, 2007). The unique aroma and flavor is produced by enzymatic action and chemical reactions that occur during the long ripening period (Mikami *et al.*, 2007).

Sulfur has four isotopes with atomic numbers of 16, 17, 18 and 20. Processed sulfur was made by heating and melting to material or light mineral, separated the upper liquid sulfur and cooled material. It usually contained selenium and tellurium (Lee *et al.*, 2010). In Chinese medicine, sulfur has effects on homeostasis, nerve paralysis, and cold hands and feet and promotes a stronger muscle skeletal system (Stanley *et al.*, 1998). Western medicine has used sulfur for local irritants, constipation, hemorrhoids and skin diseases. It was also used to treat for dysentery, cholera, and typhoid before the development of antibiotics as it inhibits the growth of pathogenic microorganisms (Stanley *et al.* 1998). However, sulfur is highly toxic, and it is necessary to process the sulfur to remove toxic property for use as a medicine. Sulfur can cause side effects if ingested by humans or animals (Lee *et al.*, 2010). Methyl sulfonyl methane is found *Allium hookeri*, garlic, and green onion. (Lee *et al.*, 2009). Sulfur is also a component of sulfuric amino acids, collagen, polysaccharides, glycoproteins, and glutathione.

This review was to investigate the changes in physical, physicochemical and microbial properties of carcass and meat products in dietary processed sulfur fed pigs.

EFFECTS OF THE PROCESSED SULFUR SUPPLEMENTATION ON THE GROWTH PERFORMANCE AND MEAT QUALITY IN PIGS

When weaning pigs and growing-finishing pigs take sulfur supplementation, two different level of 0.1% (T1), 0.3% (T2) processed sulfur was added to commercial feed (control) to study the effects on the productivity and meat quality of pigs (Ha Young Noh. 2014). The weight, daily gain, daily feed intake and feed efficiency of weaning pigs by taking processed sulfur supplementation showed no significant difference between the treatments. However, T1 and T2 in 1st week with reduced feed intake, tended to increase daily feed intake and improve feed efficiency compared to the control. In 2nd week, daily gain was lowered but did not show any significant difference compared to the treatments. In 4th week, T1 and T2 for weight and daily gain increased compared to the control and T1 for feed efficiency was highly improved. The addition of 0.1% processed sulfur supplementation could be used for weaning pigs as the appropriate level.

The results of weight, daily gain, daily feed intake and feed efficiency of growing-finishing pigs with processed sulfur supplementation showed no significant difference between the treatments. However, weight was increased in T1 and T2 during in the weaning and growing period. However, daily gain was lowered with processed sulfur supplementation. T1 was the highest as 33.4 kg/day/head in daily feed intake and T2 was the lowest. There was no significant difference in feed efficiency.

In hematological assay of growing-finishing pigs fed processed sulfur, most of the survey items did not show significant difference. However, total protein in T1(6.37 g/dl) was significantly higher than the control (5.73 g/dl) and T2(5.77 g/dl. T1 (2.67 g/dl) for globulin content had significantly higher than other treatments. T1 had higher HDL-Cholesterol concentration of 36.20 mg/dl which was higher than other treatments. T1 had the creatinine content of 2.03 mg/dl which was significantly lower than the control (2.30 mg/dl). T2contained the uric acid of 0.63 mg/dl and triglyceride of 32.20 mg/dl which were significantly lower than other treatments.

Analysis of blood fatty acids of growing-finishing pigs with processed sulfur supplementation represented that the control had higher total SFA (42.05%), while T2 had higher total MUFA (51.08%) and w6 (9.30%) than T1 and control. T2 was also the highest in total w3 fatty acid.

Carcass grade and characteristics for processed sulfur fed pigs indicated that the backfat thickness for T1 and T2 were 23.54 and 25.07 mm, respectively, which were higher than the control. The control did not have 1+A grade, whereas T1 and T2 had 9.8and 4.5%of 1+A grade in carcass, respectively. Thus, the addition of 0.1% processed sulfur supplementation might be suggested as an appropriate level in growing-finishing pigs for carcass grade.

There were no significant differences in moisture and crude protein contents among the treatments. T2 had relatively lower the crude fat content, heating loss, and expressible drip than the control and T1. The pH value of growing pigs was significantly lower in T2. Chromaticity of growing pigs showed no significant difference in brightness among the control and processed sulfur supplementation treatment, whereas growing pigs by taking processed sulfur supplementation had significantly higher red color intensity than the control. T2 had the lowest value of thiobarbituric acid reactive substances (TBARS) after 5 days storage compared to the control and T1. Amino acid composition of growing pigs showed no significant difference in total amino acid composition among the treatment, while the higher methionine and cysteine contents were found in growing pigs with processed sulfur supplementation. Fatty acid composition of growing pigs had no significant difference in saturated fatty acids among the treatment. However, T2 contained significantly lower saturated and higher total w3 fatty acids than the control and T1. Although T2 had lower marbling score than the control, T2 had higher aroma and juiciness scores than compared to the control and T1. It would suggest that the addition of 0.3% processed sulfur supplementation might be regarded as an appropriate level of the desirable nutritional and sensory propertiesfor growing pigs.

Sulfur Effects on the Carcass of Beef Cattle

The beef cattle NRC (2000) recommends 0.15% sulfur to support adequate growth of beef cattle. Sulfur is required for growth and metabolism of many ruminal bacteria, particularly cellulolytic bacteria (Spears et al., 1976). Additionally, S is needed as a component of the S amino acids methionine, cysteine, and cystine, as well as the B vitamins thiamine and biotin (NRC, 2000).

Processed Sulfur Effects on Broilers and Ducks

Processed sulfur-fed broilers gained weight with decreased saturated fatty acids (Park et al. 2010). Increased weight was also found in broiler when fed with dietary 0.2% sulfur supplementation (Shin et al. 2013). Sulfur feeding also decreased total fat content and undesirable odors, and increased texture property of meat (Park et al. 2003). The 0.15% Processed sulfur-fed broilers had more weight, increased gain weight and feed consumption compared to the control (Kim et al., 2013). Decreased crude fat, triglyceride, and abdominal fat contents were also found in sulfur fed broilers (Park et al., 2003; Wallis, 1999; Shin 2013). Processed sulfur fed ducks had higher polyunsaturated fatty acids than the control (Park et al., 1999)

Processed Sulfur Effects on Pork Meats

Few studies were available for the processed sulfur effects on carcass and meat quality in Korea. Lee et al (2009) informed that the physicochemical, meat color and texture properties of pork loin are not affected by Methyl Sulfonyl Methane (MSM) supplementation from comparison the quality characteristics of pork from finishing pigs fed different levels of MSM. Loughmiller et al., (1998) reported that dietary sulfur amino acids and methionine on growth performance and carcass characteristics of finishing gilts resulted in the reduction in body weight according to the increased dietary sulfur amino acids supplementation. Detoxified effect of processed sulfur has been proved by toxicity test with animal model (Kim et al 2006). Moreover, it was previously reported that feeding 0.1% processed sulfur fed pigs was efficient for growing performance (Jang et al. 2006). Recently, sulfur has been used to feed pigs in order to produce good quality of meat products (Cho et. al. 2015). Sulfur compounds are also known for high antioxidant activity to increase the shelf life of meat products (Cho et. al. 2015).

PROCESSED SULFUR EFFECTS ON FUNCTIONAL PROPERTIES OF DRY CURED HAM DURING STORAGE

Sulfur is the eighth most abundant element in all living organisms and is the major ingredientof essential amino acids, such as thiamine and biotin, being absorbed and utilized by the body (Kim et al., 2005). Processed Sulfur was made by heating and melting to material or light mineral to separate the upper liquid sulfur and obtained from the cooled material, which contain selenium and tellurium (Lee *et al.*, 2010). In Chinese medicine, sulfur has the effects on hemostasis, nerve paralysis, and cold hands and feet. It also promotes a stronger musculoskeletal system (Lee *et al.*, 2009). In western medicine, sulfur has been used for local irritants, constipation, hemorrhoids and skin diseases, and was also used to treat for dysentery, cholera, and typhoid before the development of antibiotics as it inhibits the growth of pathogenic microorganisms (Block, 1986, 1992; Kumar *et al.*, 1998). However, sulfur is known for highly toxic, and thus it is necessary for sulfur to remove toxic property being used as a proper medicine. Sulfur may cause side effects if ingested by humans or animals (Choi *et al.*, 2002; Park *et al.*, 2010; Barrenrine *et al.*, 1958; Bouchard *et al.*, 1973).Methyl sulfonyl methane is found in *Allium hookeri*, garlic, and green onion. (Son *et al.*, 2012). Sulfur is also the main component of sulfuric amino acids, collagen, polysaccharides, glycoproteins, and glutathione and is essential for the action of steroid hormones and various growth factors (Park *et al.*, 2010).

Proximate Analysis

Changes in physicochemical, microbiological and sensory properties of dry cured ham during storage in processed sulfur fcd pigs were investigated by Kim *et al.* (2014). Dry cured ham products were manufactured from processed sulfur (PS)-fed pigs according to the level of dietary PS. Three groups were used:CON, commercial basal dietary fed pigs; T1, 0.1% PS dietary fed pigs and T2, 0.3% PS dietary fed pigs. During the drying and ripening process, moisture content of CON, T1 and T2 significantly decreased from 71–73% to 50–55%, and crude protein, crude fat and ash contents significantly increased after 10 months storage. Moisture content in T2 was significantlyhigher than CON and crude fat content of T1 and T2 was significantly lower than that of CON. Lee et al (2009) and Li et al (2013) reported that feeding sulfur to pigs showed improve of water holding capacity and lower fat content in meat. In addition, a decrease in weight loss increased moisture content of dry cured ham during the drying and ripening period (Holden *et al.* 1998; Yeh & Liu, 2001). Therefore, the higher moisture content and reduced lipid level of T1 and T2 at 10 month seemed to be influenced by dietary sulfur supplement.

pH, Water Activity, and TBARS

pH values of dry cured ham in all groups increasedsignificantly at 4 months and remained stable during the ripening period.Previous studies indicated that lactic acid bacteria do not play an important role in dry cured ham preparation with salt added during storage (Molina *et al.* 1989; Jose *et al.* 2010). Initial pH value was not significantly different among CON, T1 and T2 groups. However, the pH of T1 and T2 was significantly lower than CON at 8 months. Several researches were investigated for increased pH in meat products during storage. Liberation of free amino acids, accumulation of ammonia or electrolyte changes during the ripening process can result in an increased pH value (Wardow *et al.* 1973; Hamm, 1974; Deymer & Vandekerckhove, 1979; Park *et al.* 1997).

Water activity of all dry cured ham significantly decreased from 0.99 to 0.92% during the drying and ripening period. The a_w of T2 was significantly higher than CON at 10 months. Dry cured hams made from processed sulfur-fed pigs may have increased lipid oxidation stability due to the negative relationship between a_w and lipid oxidation during the manufacture of dry cured meat products (Fanco *et al.* 2002; Lee *et al.* 2009).

TBA values for T1, T2 and CON significantly increased from 0.29 to 0.40 mg MDA/kg during processing. TBA values during the ripening of dry cured hams beyond 10 months were 0.29–0.44 mg MDA/kg (Cilla *et al.* 2006). A significant difference was observed between CON and sulfur-fed pigs (T1 and T2). Dietary sulfur-fed pigs showed increased antioxidant ability in dry cured ham. Glutathione is known as asulfur-containing protein that scavenges free radicals, and is synthesized throughout the trans-sulfuration pathway (Gulizar, 2004; Song *et al.* 2013; Martha & Iori, 2011). Changes in crude fat content and TBA values of all groups showed a positive relationship during storage (r = 0.56). Comparable results on lipid content and the level of lipid oxidation in meat products were also reported by Ismail *et al* (2009) and Veronica *et al* (2014).

VBN (Volatile Basic Nitrogen)

The value of VBN in CON, T1 and T2 groups increased significantly during the drying and ripening period. Previous studies indicated that some microbes have the ability to decompose proteins that generate volatile nitrogen compounds in meat products (Cilla *et al*. 2006; Darmadji *et al*. 1990). Other studies also reported that the concentration of free amino acids and peptides could increase during the ripening period, and free amino acids convert to biogenic amines during the ripening process (Virgili *et al*. 2007; Martuscelli *et al*. 2009). T1 and T2 had a significantly higher VBN value than CON at 4 and 10 months. A significant positive correlation was found between VBN and the level of dietary sulfur fed to pigs. Other studies indicated that sulfur-containing amino acids might be involved in the formation of cross-links or disulfide bonds between proteins (Marinaane *et al*. 2011; Stadman & Levine, 2003; Kim *et al*. 2000).

Microbial Counts during Ripening

A total aerobic bacterium of T2 was significantly lower than CON during storage. This could be attributed to the antimicrobial effect of sulfur. Antimicrobial activity of sulfur compounds has been studied by adding garlic to meat products (Yin & Cheng, 2003; Sallam *et al*., 2004). Total aerobic and lactic acid bacteria colonies of all groups increased significantly until 4 months, and then tended to decline during the drying and ripening period. A decrease in water activity of dry cured ham could inhibit the growth of microorganisms during ripening process. Furthermore, growth of lactic bacteria had progressed during the fermentation process, and adecrease in pH value of dry cured ham by lactic acids showed antioxidant ability (Egan, 1983; Lin & Yen, 1999). These tendencies were also observed by Jose *et al*. (2010) and Vilar *et al*. (2000).

Changes in Fatty Acids during the Storage

Fatty acid composition is important to the taste and flavor of dry cured ham (Pastorelli *et al*, 2003). Lipid degradation occurs during the drying and ripening period, and fat content and fatty acid composition affect the texture and appearance of dry cured ham (Ruiz-Carrascal *et al*. 2000; Seong *et al*. 2010). The most plentiful saturated fatty acids in dry cured ham were palmitic acid (23.18–24.24%), stearic acid (13.73–14.72%) and myristic acid (1.07–1.17%). T1 and T2 showed significantly lower concentrations of linoleic acid than CON. Many lipid oxidation products such as hexanal are formed from linoleic acid (Frankel 1984). Oleic acid concentrations in CON at the initial phase were significantly higher than T1 and T2. After fermentation, oleic acid of T1 and T2 was significantly higher than CON. Lunt and Smith (1991) reported that high oleic acid concentration improves the taste of meat and impacts positive sensory score. According to Ruiz *et al* (2000), high fat concentration in dry cured ham positively affects the ratio of oleic acid to unsaturated fatty acids. The saturated fatty acid of CON was significantly higher than T1 and T2, and PUFA of T1 and T2 was significantly higher than CON in raw meat. Cameron and Enser (1991) reported that an increase in the MUFA/PUFA ratio enhances the taste of meat. In this study, MUFA/PUFA of T1 and T2 was significantly higher than CON. The polyunsaturated fatty acid/ saturated fatty acid (PUFA/SFA ratio) in sulfur groups (0.35- 0.39) were significantly lower than CON

(0.43). One of the most important indicators for evaluating nutritional quality of meat products is the PUFA/SFA ratio. COMA (1984) recommended a PUFA/SFA ratio of 0.4–0.45.

Significant differences of Δ-9- desaturase (16) index among CON, T1 and T2 were not found in the state of raw meat. However, Δ-9- desaturase (18) index of T1 was significantly lower than that of the control and T2. Nevertheless, Δ-9- desaturase (16) index of T2 was significantly lower than that of the control group from dry cured loin, whereas Δ-9- desaturase (18) index of T1 and T2 was significantly higher than that of the control group. Pogge, Lonergan and Hansen (2014) exhibited that increasing the desaturase activity of beef was affected by dietary sulfur addition.

Change in Free Amino Acids during Storage

The concentration of free amino acids in T1, T2 and CON significantly increased during the drying and ripening period. Previous studies reported that free amino acid content is generated by proteolysis activity during storage (Toldra *et al.* 2000; Armenteros *et al.* 2012). Proteolysis activity is catalyzed by cathepsins and calpains, which affect the formation of flavor compounds and precursors (Seong *et al.* 2010; Careri *et al.* 1993). Total free amino acid content of T1 and T2 were significantly higher than CON. An increase in the amount of free amino acids was related to enhance sensory quality of meat products, such as attractive flavor and texture (Toldra *et al.* 1995). Due to the level of dietary processed sulfur, the methionine concentration of T1 and T2 was significantly higher than CON. Song *et al* (2013) found that high sulfur content in diet-fed pigs leads to higher methionine content than a normal diet-fed pig. In addition, methionine can be involved in the formation of glutathione, which is an antioxidant of sulfur-containing compounds (Gulizar 2004). Our results showed significant and negative correlations between methionine content and TBA value (r = −0.924) at 10 months. Glutamic acid (Glu) content of T2 was significantly higher than T1 and CON, and Glu and Asp content of T1 was significantly higher than CON.

Descriptive Sensory Test

Sensory attribute scores of dry cured ham after 10 months of processing showed that the redness of T1 was significantly higher than CON, while no difference was observed between T1 and T2. Brightness of T2 was significantly higher than CON. The color of meat products was affected by changes in pH value and the reaction of pigment enzyme activities with oxygen (Lawrie, 1985). Studies have indicated that sulfur-containing compounds such as furans and disulfides influence flavor characteristics (Donald *et al.* 1994; Yang *et al.* 2012). In this study, the off-odor score of CON was significantly higher than T1. Aroma score of T1 and T2 was higher than CON. However, there were no significant differences among groups. Meat flavor from sulfur-fed pigs could be improved by intramuscular fat content and oxidized products from lipids (Carrapiso *et al.* 2002; Ruiz *et al.* 2002; Lee *et al.* 2009). The juiciness score of T2 was significantly higher than CON. The bitterness of T1 was better than CON, and no significantdiffer-ence was observed between T2 and CON. Sweetness of T1 was significantly higher than CON, which suggests that the combination of Glu and Asp concentration in T1 could enhance umami taste of dry cured ham (Misako *et al.* 2002; Kenzo 2009).

CONCLUSION

Processed sulfur supplementation could improve economics for the livestock farms with increasing carcass weight, yield rate, and carcass grade, and enhancing the nutritional and functional values of meat. Long term supplementation with processed sulfur can be an effective means of an antioxidant in dry cured ham due to the reduction of lipid oxidation. Moreover, dietary processed sulfur could contribute to improve sensory quality characteristics with reducing the intensity of off odor and increasing palatability. Processed sulfur treatment might enhance proteolysis activity during storage by increasing free amino acids in dry cured ham made from processed sulfur fed pigs. Fatty acid composition of dry cured ham made from processed sulfur-fed pigs could be beneficial to health. Overall, this review demonstrates that sulfur supplementation to pigs can improve growth performance of pigs and meat quality of dry cured ham products with extended shelf-life during storage.

REFERENCES

Ahn, D. U., Olsonm, D. G., Chen, J. X., Wu, C., & Lee, J. I. (1998). Effect of muscle type packaging and irradiation on lipid oxidation volatile production, and color in raw pork patties. *Meat Science, 47*(1), 27–39. doi:10.1016/S0309-1740(97)00101-0 PMID:22063182

Bart, D. & Rex, G. H. (2002). Redox control of the transsulfuration and glutathione biosynthesis pathways. *Protein and Amino Acid Metabolism, 5,* 85-92.

Bartolmew, D. T., & Blumer, J. N. (1977). Microbial interactions in country-style hams. *Journal of Food Science, 42*(2), 498–502. doi:10.1111/j.1365-2621.1977.tb01531.x

Biesalski, H. K. (2005). Meat as a component of a healthy diet—Are there any risks or benefits if meat is avoided in the diet? *Meat Science, 70*(3), 509–524. doi:10.1016/j.meatsci.2004.07.017 PMID:22063749

Boles, J. A., Shand, P. J., Patience, J. F., McCurdy, A. R., & Schaefer, A. L. (1993). Acid base status of stress susceptible pigs affects sensory quality of loin roasts. *Journal of Food Science, 58*(6), 1254–1257. doi:10.1111/j.1365-2621.1993.tb06159.x

Brewer, M. S., Ikins, W. G., & Harbers, C. A. Z. (1992). TBA values, sensory characteristics, and volatiles in ground pork during long term frozen storage: Effects of packaging. *Journal of Food Science, 57*(3), 558–580. doi:10.1111/j.1365-2621.1992.tb08042.x

Cho, H. S., Park, W. J., Hong, G. E., Kim, J. H., Ju, M. G., & Lee, C. H. (2015). Antioxidant activity of Allium hookeri root extract and its effect on lipid stability of sulfur-fed pork patties. *Korean J. Food Sci. An., 35*(1), 32–40. PMID:26761799

Cho, J. H., Min, B. J., Kwon, O. S., Shon, K. S., Jin, Y. G., Kim, H. J., & Kim, I. H. (2005). Effect of MSM (Methyl Sulfonyl Methane) supplementation on growth performance and digestibility of CA and N in pigs. *Journal of Korean Soc. Food Sci. Nutr., 34*(3), 361–365. doi:10.3746/jkfn.2005.34.3.361

Cho, W. M., Yang, S. H., Lee, S. M., Jang, S. S., Kim, H. C., Hong, S. K., & Kim, H. S. (2012). Effects of different additives on the growth performance and carcass characteristics of Holstein steers. *Journal of Life Science, 22*(22), 61–166.

Choi, J. H., & Han, I. K. (1974). Effects of substitution of sodium on sodium sulphate for methionine on performance and nutrient metabolism of broiler chickens. *Korean Journal of Animal Sciences, 16*, 20–36.

Chung, T. K., & Baker, D. H. (1992). Efficiency of dietary methionine utilization by young pigs. *The Journal of Nutrition, 122*, 1862–1869. PMID:1512636

Drewnoski, M. E., Pogge, D. J., & Hanse, S. L. (2014). *Journal of Animal Science.* American Society of Animal Science. Retrieved from http://www.journalofanimalscience.org/content/early/2014/06/30/jas.2013-7242

Emery, R. S., Smith, C. K., & Huffman, C. F. (1957). Utilization of inorganic sulfate by rumen microorganisms. I. incorporation of inorganic sulfate into amino acids. APP. *Microbiol, 5*, 360–363. PMID:13488436

Folch, J., Lees, M., & Sloane-Stanley, G. H. (1957). A simple method for the isolation and purification of total lipids from animal tissue. *The Journal of Biological Chemistry, 226*, 497. PMID:13428781

Jang, H. D., Yoo, J. S., Chae, S. J., Park, S. I., Jung, J. C., & Kim, H. J. Kim & Seok, H. B. (2006). Effect of dietary methyl sulfonyl methane on growth performance and meat quality characteristics in growing finishing pigs. *Korean Journal of International Agriculture, 18*, 116–120.

Jung, D. H., & Jung, S. H. (2005). *Garlic Science, World science, Israel Goldberg, Functional Foods.* New York: Chapman & Hall.

Jung, K. H. (2004). *Effect of the processed sulfur on the growth performance, antivirus and meat quality in pigs.* Chonnam University.

Kerr, B. J., Weber, T. E., Ziemer, C. J., Spence, C., Cotta, M. A., & Whitehead, T. R. (2011). Effect of dietary inorganic sulfur level on growth performance, fecal composition, and measures of inflammation and sulfate-reducing bacteria in the intestine of growing pigs. *Journal of Animal Science, 89*(2), 426–437. doi:10.2527/jas.2010-3228 PMID:20952529

Kim, G. S., Jung, Y. R., Lee, N. J., Hong, S. H., Yu, J. H., Jeong, J. H., & Kang, J. K. (2006). The composition of the toxicity of processed sulfur with non processed sulfur in Sprague-Dawley rats. *J. Vet. Med. Biotechnol., 7*, 183–190.

Kim, J. H., Lee, H. R., Pyun, C. W., Hong, G. H., Kim, S. K., & Lee, C. H. (2015). Changes in physiochemical, microbiological and sensory properties of dry-cured ham in processed sulfur-fed pigs. *Journal of Food Processing and Preservation, 39*(6), 829–839. doi:10.1111/jfpp.12293

Kim, J. H., Pyun, C. W., Hong, G. H., Kim, S. K., Yang, C. Y., & Lee, C. H. (2014). Changes in physiochemical and microbiological properties of isoflavone-treated dry-cured sausage from sulfur-fed pork during storage. *Journal of Animal Sciences and Technology, 56*(1), 21. doi:10.1186/2055-0391-56-21 PMID:26290710

Lee, J., Lee, H. J., Park, J. D., Lee, S. K., Lee, S. I., Lim, H. D., ... Kim, E. C. (2008). Anti-cancer activity of highly purified sulfur in immortalized and malignant human oral keratinocytes. *Toxicology In Vitro, 22*(1), 87–95. doi:10.1016/j.tiv.2007.08.016 PMID:17920232

Lee, J. I., Min, H. K., Lee, J. W., Jeong, J. D., Ha, Y. J., Kwack, S. C., & Park, J. S. (2009). Changes in the quality of loin from pigs supplemented with dietary methyl sulfonyl methane during cold storage. *Korean J. Food Sci*, *2*(2), 229–237. doi:10.5851/kosfa.2009.29.2.229

Lee, J. S., Kwon, J. K., Han, S. H., An, I. J., Kim, S. J., Lee, S. H., ... Jung, J. Y. (2010). Toxicity study of detoxification sulfur at 3 months post-treatment in rats. *J F Hyg Safety*, *25*, 263–268.

Loughmiller, J. A., Nelssen, J. L., Goodband, R. D., Tokach, M. D., Titgemeyer, E. C., & Kim, I. H. (1998). Influence of dietary total sulfur amino acids and methionine on growth performance and carcass characteristics of finishing gilts. *Journal of Animal Science*, *76*(8), 2129–2137. PMID:9734863

Loughmiller, J. A., Tokach, M. D., Goodband, R. D., Nelssen, J. L., Titgemeyer, E. C., Kim, I. H., & Dritz, S. (1996). Dietary total sulfur amino acid requirement for optimal growth performance and carcass characteristics in finishing gilts. In *Kansas State University Swine Day. Report of Progress* (pp. 133–135). Kansas State University.

Mikami, M., Sekikawa, M., & Shimada, K. I. (2007). Non-heated meat products (Dry cured ham). *FFI Journal.*, *212*(7), 572–582.

Ministry for food, agriculture, forestry and fisheries. (2011). *Main statistic information for food, agriculture, forestry and fisheries*. Author.

Mortensen, J. Z., Schmidt, E. B., Nielsen, A. H., & Dyerberg, J. (1983). The effect of N-6 and N-3 polyunsaturated fatty acids on hemostasis, blood lipids and blood pressure. *Thrombosis and Haemostasis*, *50*, 543–546. PMID:6636033

Nimni, M. E., Han, B., & Cordoba, F. (2007). Are we getting enough sulfur in our diet. *Nutrition and Metabolism (Lond)*, *4*, 24.

Noh, H. Y. (2014). *Effects of the processed sulfur supplementation on the growth performance and meat quality in pigs*. Konkuk University.

Park, J. H., Ryu, M. S., Lee, Y. E., Song, G. S., & Ryu, K. S. (2003). A comparison of fattening performance, physic-chemical properties of breast meat, vaccine titers in cross bred meat type hybrid chicks fed sulfur. *Korean Journal of Poultry Science*, *30*, 211–217.

Pogge, D., & Hansen, S. L. (2012). Effect of vitamin C on performance and antioxidant capacity of cattle fed varying concentrations of dietary sulfur. *Animal Industry Report*, *658*, 21.

Rozenn, N. L., Irena, B. K., Dariush, M., Lewis, H. K., Russell, P. T., & David, S. S. (2003). N-3 Polyunsaturated fatty acids, fatal ischemic heart disease, and nonfatal myocardial infarction in older adults: The Cardiovascular health study. *The American Journal of Clinical Nutrition*, *77*, 319–325. PMID:12540389

SAS Institute. (2002). SAS User's Guide: Statistics. Cary, NC: SAS Institute Inc.

Shin, J. S., Kim, M. A., & Lee, S. H. (2013). Comparison of physiological changes in broiler chicken fed with dietary processed sulfur. *Korean Journal of Food Preservation.*, *20*(2), 278–283. doi:10.11002/kjfp.2013.20.2.278

Song, R., Chen, C., Wang, L., Johnston, J., Kerr, B. J., Weber, T. E., & Shurson, G. C. (2013). High sulfur content in corn dried distillers grains with soluble protects against oxidized lipids by increasing sulfur-containing antioxidants in nursery pigs. *Journal of Animal Science, 91*(6), 2715–2728. doi:10.2527/jas.2012-5350 PMID:23482577

Stanley W., Jacob, M. D., Ronald M., Lawrence, M.D. & Zucker, M. (1998). *The Miracle of MSM*. The Berkley Publishing Group.

Van Weerdn, E. J., & Schutte, J. B. (1976). Relation between methionine and inorganic sulphate in broiler rations. *Poultry Science, 55*(4), 1476–1748. doi:10.3382/ps.0551476 PMID:951375

Wallis, I. R. (1999). Dietary supplements of methionine increase breast meat yield and decrease abdominal fat in growing broiler chickens. *Australian Journal of Experimental Agriculture, 39*(2), 131–141. doi:10.1071/EA98130

Witte, V. C., Krause, G. F., & Bailey, M. E. (1970). A new extraction method for determining 2-thiobarbituric acid values of pork and beef during storage. *Journal of Food Science, 35*(5), 582–585. doi:10.1111/j.1365-2621.1970.tb04815.x

This research was previously published in Exploring the Nutrition and Health Benefits of Functional Foods edited by Hossain Uddin Shekhar, Zakir Hossain Howlader, and Yearul Kabir; pages 254-264, copyright year 2017 by Medical Information Science Reference (an imprint of IGI Global).

Chapter 58
Nutritional Benefits of Selected Plant–Based Proteins as Meat Alternatives

Seydi Yıkmış
https://orcid.org/0000-0001-8694-0658
Tekirdağ Namık Kemal University, Turkey

Ramazan Mert Atan
Bandırma Onyedi Eylül University, Turkey

Nursena Kağan
Tekirdağ Namık Kemal University, Turkey

Levent Gülüm
Abant İzzet Baysal University, Turkey

Harun Aksu
Istanbul University – Cerrahpaşa, Turkey

Mehmet Alpaslan
Tekirdağ Namık Kemal University, Turkey

ABSTRACT

Humans meet their nutritional requirements by consuming food, and our body uses naturally sufficient amounts of all necessary nutrients to maintain its functioning. Proteins form the basis of the human diet because they are necessary for immune responses, cell signals, muscle masses, and the repair of damaged cells. Animal and plant food products are the main protein sources in the human diet. Based on scientific evidence, proteins derived from animals recently started to be replaced by plant-based options as prefered proteins for a range of reasons. Consumption of non-meat protein sources being shown to be healthy and environmentally friendly is a major consideration. Plant-based protein is helping minimize high cholesterol, type 2 diabetes, high blood pressure, obesity, certain types of cancer, including colorectal, ovarian, and breast cancers, and a diet based on non-animal proteins could increase life expectancy and decrease greenhouse gases emissions from livestock as less resources are used for plant production. The chapter describes the nutritional benefits and current uses of nine non-animal protein sources and the health benefits arising from replacing animal protein.

DOI: 10.4018/978-1-7998-5354-1.ch058

INTRODUCTION

Nutrients play a crucial role in maintaining overall human health. Protein is the most important nutrient required for growth and development (Besler, Rakıcıoglu, Ayaz, Demirel Büyüktuncer, Özel, Samur Eroğlu, … & Yürük, 2015). The structure and function of our bodies, the regulations of cells, tissues and organs depend on proteins. Approximately 16% of the adult human body is composed of protein. As proteins in the body do not form storage depots, we need to get enough of them daily through a balanced diet. Proteins are long chains of amino acids, which are their building blocks created, formed and synthesised for our human body to function correctly. Although the properties of the amino acids vary between animal and plant sourced proteins, they both can supply the needed and recommended daily requirement for protein of 0.8 g/day, considered sufficient for almost all healthy adult individuals (Pasiakos, Agarwal, Lieberman, & Fulgoni, 2015).

Protein sources in a diet come from animal and vegetable sources (Lin, Lu, Kelly, Zhang, Zheng, & Miao, 2017). Common examples of animal protein sources are meat, poultry, fish and eggs, and common examples of plant–derived proteins are beans, lentil and soybean (Nehete, Bhambar, Narkhede, & Gawali, 2013). In the majority of industrialized countries, the main protein source of dietary protein is animal foods. However, increased consumption of red meat and processed meat along with other animal products has been shown to be associated with obesity, coronary heart disease, high blood pressure, cancer, elevated serum and urinary uric acid levels (Møller, Sluik, Ritz, Mikkilä, Raitakari, Hutri–Kähönen, … Raben, 2017). Because of the adverse effects of animal protein on health, vegetable protein sources seem to be a wise alternative in meeting proteins needs. Vegetable protein sources are increasingly being recommended because of their positive effects on health (Chen, Song, Chen, Ding, Peng, & Mao, 2016; Comerford & Pasin, 2016; Wu, Zeng, Huang, Li, Zhang, Ho, & Zheng, 2016). In order to provide human protein requirements, it is necessary to support the production of plant proteins which can replace the sources of animal protein (Comerford & Pasin, 2016). Vegetable proteins can meet the essential amino acids that people need (López, Galante, Robson, Boeris, & Spelzini, 2018). Such sources are known to provide greater saturation than animal protein sources because of their low energy content and high fibre content (Nielsen, Kristensen, Klingenberg, Ritz, Belza, Astrup, & Raben, 2018). It is known that consuming foods with high fibre content enhances insulin sensitivity and provides glycemic control (Moorthi, Vorland, & Hill Gallant, 2017). There is also evidence that the risk of cardiovascular diseases can be reduced by a flexitarian dietary model which involves the consumption of more vegetative proteins rather than a meat–rich diet (Richter, Skulas–Ray, Champagne, & Kris–Etherton, 2015).

This chapter presents an evaluation of the nutritional properties and the many human health advantages of nine important plant–derived proteins obtained from beans, soybean, chickpea, lentil, quinoa, buckwheat, chia, teff and spirulina in term of their physiological benefits. Amino acid composition, nutritional aspects, functional properties and their role in promoting good human health are examined. Although these plants are well-known, only recently nutritionists started drawing attention to them as superfoods and alternatives in meat replacement.

HEALTH BENEFITS AND DRAWBACKS OF PLANT AND MEAT CONSUMPTION

The health benefits and drawbacks of both plant and meat consumption are multifaceted and complicated. Evidentially meat production and overconsumption attract more negative health and environmental effects in contrast to the production and consumption of plants (Garnett, 2014; Raphaely & Marinova, 2016; Bogueva, Marinova, & Raphaely, 2017). Being central to our traditional dietary source of protein, meat tends to deliver all necessary amino–acids we need for our body to function properly in comparison with plant–based protein sources which may lack one or more essential amino acids. Meat is also a rich source of beneficial minerals and essential nutrients, B vitamins, iron and zinc; however, it can contain high amounts of saturated fat, claimed to link cholesterol to cardiovascular disease (Newby, 2009) and processed meats can be high in sodium and cancerogenic (WHO, 2015). Meat consumption and particularly red meat are associated with an increased risk of non–communicable diseases including cardiovascular, cancer, obesity and type 2 diabetes (Newby, 2009; Marsh, Zeuschner, & Saunders, 2016; 2018).

Compared to the meat–rich Western diet, from a nutritional perspective, plant–based diets are associated with health promotion and disease prevention. They contain nutrients and vitamins, unsaturated fatty acids and beneficial fibre. Eating a plant–based diet has been linked to lower risk of obesity and many chronic diseases, such as heart disease, type 2 diabetes (Satija, Bhupathiraju, Rimm, Spiegelman, Chiuve, Borgi,... Hu, 2016), inflammation and cancer (Mattisson, 2004). Plant–based diets are also associated with higher metabolic rates (Montalcini, De Bonis, Ferro, Carè, Mazza, Accattato, … Pujia, 2015). Additionally, eating little to no meat may increase your life expectancy, to have lower body weights compared to their meat–eating counterparts, and lower risk of obesity (Newby, 2009).

NINE PLANT–DERIVED PROTEINS

Protein obtained from plant–based sources plays a special role in vegetarian and plant–based diets. The nine plant–derived protein sources presented in this chapter are chosen particularly because of their highly valued nutritional properties and health advantages. They are more desirable than meat consumption because of their nutritional physiology discussed in this section. Quinoa is an important source of plant protein because it contains all essential amino acids. In quinoa, leucine and isoleucine branched-chain amino acids, also known as limiting amino acids, are present in significant amounts. The chia seed is known as a rich omega–3 source. It regulates blood sugar because of the high content of soluble fibre. Buckwheat has high biologically valuable protein with all essential amino acids. Quinoa and chia are alternatives for those with gluten sensitivity because they do not contain gluten. Dried beans, lentils, chickpeas, beans, kidney beans etc. are important protein and fibre sources, along with economic benefits. They are rich in calcium, iron, zinc, magnesium minerals, all B vitamins except B12 and vitamin E. Spirulina, an algae species of the blue–green algae, contains high amounts of β–carotene, B 12 vitamins and iron. According to the studies done, spirulina is an important antioxidant which reduces oxidative stress. Fatty seeds rich in unsaturated fatty acids also give diets diversity thanks to the protein and fibre they contain. Teff has an attractive nutritional profile because of the fact that most of the carbohydrates it contains are complex and gluten–free. It is also noted for its high iron, calcium and rich polyphenol content.

The overview in Table 1 presents the nine plants and their nutrient contents. All plants are discussed individually in the remainder of this section.

Table 1. Nutritional content of plant–based protein sources

Plant	Protein Content	Carbohydrate Content	Fat Content	Fibre Content
Quinoa (*Chenopodium quinoa Willd.*)	13.1–16.7%	58–68% starch and 5% sugar	2–9.5%	10%
Chia (*Salvia hispanica L.*)	15–25%	26–41%	30–33%	18–30%
Buckwheat (*Fagopyrum esculentum*)	12%	59–70% starch	1.7–4.0%	12.7–17.8%
Teff (*Eragrostis tef*)	8–11%	73%	23–32%	3–4.5%
Beans (*Phaseolus Vulgaris L.*)	20–30%	50–60%	2.5%	15–19%
Soybean	36.5%	30%	15.6%	9.3%
Lentils (*Lens Culinaris*)	23–27%	64–74%	2%	4–9%
Chickpea (*Ciger Arietinum*)	18–28%	50–70%	6–9%	10–20%
Spirulina	60–70%	8%	12%	14%

Quinoa (*Chenopodium Quinoa Willd.*)

The quinoa plant (*Chenopodium quinoa Willd.*) belongs to the family of Chenopodiaceae, which also includes spinach and beet. It is native to South America and has around 250 species all over the world. People who live in the Andes, especially in Peru and Bolivia, began to produce quinoa thousands of years ago by domesticating the wild species. In the local languages, the plant is called quinua and quinoa, especially in Bolivia, Peru, Ecuador, Argentina and Chile, while different names such as suphan, suba, jupha and dahue are also used. Although quinoa does not exhibit grain characteristics, it is considered to be a pseudo–grain and even a pseudo–seed because it does not belong to the Gramineae family (Abugoch James, 2009; Li & Zhu, 2018; Navruz–Varli & Sanlier, 2016).

Quinoa has a very good adaptation to different ecological agricultural conditions. It is a fertile plant that is resistant to moist soil and harvests at acceptable levels with 100–200 mm rainfall. It can grow at a relative humidity range of 40% –88% and withstands temperatures between –4 ° C and 38 ° C (Bojanic, 2011; Li & Zhu, 2018).

Similar to rice, the seeds are used for making soup where they absorb water and inflate; in grinding cereals for cookies, bread, biscuits, pasta, chips; bakery products are also produced, such as tortilla and flatbread (Navruz–Varli & Sanlier, 2016). In addition, quinoa is traditionally used in South America for making sweets, pastries, drinks and dry snacks (Bojanic, 2011). Quinoa seeds are fermented to make beer, used in the making of an alcoholic beverage called 'chicha' which is consumed in traditional ceremonies in South America (Vilcacundo & Hernández–Ledesma, 2017).

Nutritionally, quinoa is included in the whole grain category (Graf, Rojas–Silva, Rojo, Delatorre–Herrera, Baldeón, & Raskin, 2015). The quinoa seed is a source of starch, protein, dietary fibre, fat, minerals, polyphenols and vitamins (Li & Zhu, 2018). The superiority of quinoa compared to other cereals (such as rye, barley and oats) is due to its rich protein, lipid and ash content (Vilcacundo & Hernández–Ledesma, 2017). It contains 368 kcal energy per 100 g (Navruz–Varli & Sanlier, 2016).

The protein content of quinoa seeds (expressed as g/100 g of edible material) ranges from 13.1% to 16.7%. Quinoa's protein content is higher than the protein content of rice, barley, maize and rye, and is close to the protein content of wheat (Vilcacundo & Hernández–Ledesma, 2017). Similarly to animal–based products, it contains all essential amino acids. Quinoa is rich in histidine and lysine, essential amino acids found in many different cereals. The lysine amino acid aids in the formation of antibodies, enhances immunity, increases gastric function, assists in cell repair, participates in the metabolism of fatty acids, helps calcium absorption and transport, and slows or even prevents cancer metastasis with vitamin C (Bojanic, 2011). Preliminary studies on protein fractions show that the main proteins in quinoa seeds are albumin and globulin (about 77% of total proteins). The rest consists essentially of prolamins (Fischer, Wilckens, Jara, Aranda, Valdivia, Bustamante, … Obal, 2017). Quinoa protein is particularly well balanced in amino acid composition and does not contain gluten (Zhang, Li, Ma, Gao, Du, Han, … Qiao, 2017) which makes it a suitable food for celiac diet (Repo–Carrasco–Valencia & Serna, 2011).

Quinoa is an ideal energy source. Its seed's carbohydrates contain 58–68% starch and 5% sugar, which is released into the body slowly due to the high fibre content of 10% (Bojanic, 2011). Dietary fibre is essential for optimal digestive health and at the same time provides various functional benefits, such as facilitating satiety, reducing cholesterol and lipid absorption, regulating postprandial insulin response, converting endogenous cholesterol to bile acids, regulating intestinal microbiotics, gastrointestinal infection and reducing inflammation and severity.

Due to the quality and quantity of the lipid fraction, quinoa is considered an alternative oil seed. The fat content is between 2.0% and 9.5% and is rich in essential fatty acids such as linoleic and alpha–linolenic acids (Navruz–Varli & Sanlier, 2016). The essential fatty acids play an important role in brain development, insulin sensitivity, cardiovascular health, prostaglandin metabolism, immune, inflammation and membrane function (Graf, Rojas–Silva, Rojo, Delatorre–Herrera, Baldeón, & Raskin, 2015).

Quinoa helps to raise the good (high density lipoproteins or HDL) cholesterol in the body due to its omega 3 and omega 6 content and to lower the bad (high density lipoproteins – LDL) cholesterol (Bojanic, 2011). It is also rich in vitamins and minerals, especially calcium, phosphorus and iron (Bojanic, 2011).

In addition to its high nutritional value and its gluten–free properties, quinoa is reported to be beneficial to children, elderly, lactose intolerant persons and to consumers in high–risk groups such as anemia, diabetes, obesity, dyslipidemia and celiac disease (Vilcacundo & Hernández–Ledesma, 2017).

Chia (*Salvia Hispanica L.*)

Chia (*Salvia hispanica L.*) is a herbaceous plant that has been raised for centuries by ancient Mexican Aztecs, whose roots come from the Lamiaceae family, based on southern Mexico (Alican, 2017; de Campo, dos Santos, Costa, Paese, Guterres, Rios, de & Flôres, 2017; López, Galante, Robson, Boeris & Spelzini, 2018). It is grown in Argentina, Australia, Bolivia, Colombia, Guatemala, Mexico, Peru and Southeast Asia (Karim, Ashrafuzzaman, & Hossain, 2016).

The chia seed contains 15–25% protein, 30–33% fat, 26–41% carbohydrate, 18–30% high dietary fibre, 4–5% ash and 90–93% minerals, vitamins and dry substance. Because it contains high amounts of polyunsaturated fatty acids (w–3 and w–6) (60% alpha linolenic acid and 20% linoleic acid), it is an important source of essential fatty acids for the body (Alican, 2017). These two essential fatty acids make chia seed oil one of the healthiest oils with a more than 80% of the fatty acid composition (Timilsena, Vongsvivut, Adhikari, & Adhikari, 2017). Omega 3 fatty acids have strong anti–inflammatory properties, helping to reduce cardiovascular disease and blood pressure. It also reduces sleep deprivation and decreases the risk of depression (Giaretta, Lima, & Carpes, 2017). Chia seed has the highest content of omega–3 α–linolenic acid (C18: 3, ALA, up to 68%) when compared with flaxseed (50.6%), rapeseed

(8.1%), soybean (7.6%) and sunflower (estimated at 0.2%) and it is seen as a plant with a high antioxidant potential (Marineli, da S., Lenquiste, Moraes, & Maróstica, 2015).

Unlike many vegetable protein sources, chia seeds contain all essential amino acids, so they have a better protein quality than cereal and other fatty seeds (Caruso, Favati, Di Cairano, Galgano, Labella, Scarpa, & Condelli, 2018; López, Galante, Robson, Boeris, & Spelzini, 2018). Essential amino acids such as leucine, isoleucine and valine account for 42.2–42.9% of the total amount of amino acids in the chia seed. The chia seed is also rich in non–essential amino acids such as glutamic acid, arginine and aspartic acids. It is known that glutamic acid regulates the immunoregulatory response and enhances athletic performance; therefore, it is considered an important amino acid in the diet. Arginine is known to play a role in preventing heart disease (Timilsena, Adhikari, Barrow, & Adhikari, 2016).

Chia seeds are rich in dietary fibre, with a total content ranging from 34% to 50%, and the fibre content is higher than other grains such as flaxseed. Dietary fibre is known to have various biological effects such as delaying the release of glucose from foods and thus reducing postprandial glycosemia. These factors are certainly effective in reducing the incidence of diabetes and cardiovascular diseases (Menga, Amato, Phillips, Angelino, Morreale, & Fares, 2017). It has been reported that the intake of chia seeds significantly reduces serum triglycerides (TG) and low density lipoprotein (LDL) and increases high density lipoprotein (HDL) (Timilsena, Vongsvivut, Adhikari, & Adhikari, 2017).

Due to the diversity of phenolic compounds, chia seeds have excellent antioxidant capacity as well as antimicrobial activity and are also used against various pathological disorders such as atherosclerosis, brain dysfunction and cancer (Rahman, de Camargo, & Shahidi, 2017). Caffeic and rosmarinic acids are among the phenolic compounds currently identified in chia products and these acids prevent and play a role in different neurological disorders such as epilepsy (Oliveira–Alves, Vendramini–Costa, Betim Cazarin, Maróstica Júnior, Borges Ferreira, Silva, … Bronze, 2017).

Due to its nutritional value and chemical composition, the chia seed has been attributed different medical features and is considered as a new functional ingredient (Mesías, Holgado, Márquez–Ruiz, & Morales, 2016). For people on a plant-based diet, it can play an important role as an alternative to meat.

Buckwheat (*Fagopyrum Esculentum*)

Buckwheat is found in the pseudo–grain group of the genus Fagopyrum of the Polygonaceae family (Giménez–Bastida, Piskuła, & Zieliński, 2015; Zhu, 2016b). The most grown species are Fagopyrum esculentum and tartary karabuğday, commonly known as buckwheat (*Fagopyrum esculentum*). Tartary buckwheat is also known as bitter buckwheat because of the bitter taste found in the seeds and the high content of flavonoids (Zhu, 2016a). It is grown mostly in Asia (China, Bhutan, Nepal and India). Common buckwheat grows widely in Asia, Europe and America, while in low quantities it also grows in Europe (Luxembourg, Germany and Belgium) (Zhu, 2016b). Buckwheat has excellent ecological compatibility and can grow in harsh climatic conditions and unusual soil (Zhu, 2016b). Products made from buckwheat such as noodles, pancakes and cabbage are consumed in many countries, especially in China, Japan, Korea, Nepal, and also in European countries, such as Ukraine and Russia (Giménez–Bastida, Piskuła, & Zieliński, 2015; Sytar, Brestic, & Rai, 2013).

Buckwheat is a rich source of starch, protein, dietary fibre, vitamins (thiamine, riboflavin, pyridoxine), antioxidants and minerals as well as antioxidative substances such as rutin, quercetin, hyperin and catechin (Sun, Li, Hu, Zhou, Ji, Yu, … Luan, 2018). It is known for its wide flavonoid content characterized by health benefits such as lowering cholesterol, inhibiting tumors, regulating hypertension, controlling inflammation, carcinogenesis and regulating diabetes (Sytar, Brestic, & Rai, 2013).

The amount of protein in buckwheat is about 12% and is therefore similar to the protein content in wheat (Zhang, Zhou, Tang, Li, Tang, Shao, … Wu, 2012). Buckwheat protein has balanced amino acids and a high level of lysine, arginine in its aminoacid content delivering quality nutritional value (Sun et al., 2018). It has been reported that buckwheat protein has many unique physiological functions such as curing chronic diseases, lowering blood cholesterol, inhibiting breast cancer caused by 7,12–dimethylbenzene and gallstone inhibitor (Zhang, Zhou, Tang, Li, Tang, Shao, … Wu, 2012).

As in all cereals, the starch found in buckwheat most commonly contains 59–70% of the dry matter of buckwheat. The amount of resistant starch in buckwheat corn is between 7 and 37%, and the decrease in glycemic index is due to the increase in the amount of this resistant starch (Elif, 2017). The raw fibre concentration of buckwheat is very high, 12.7–17.8% (Zhang, Zhou, Tang, Li, Tang, Shao, … Wu, 2012). Dietary fibre contributes to physiological functions such as cholesterol and fat–stripping, reduction of blood glucose levels, prevention of constipation and regulation of colonic health (Zhu, Du, Li, & Li, 2014).

Unsaturated fatty acids constitute 80% of the total, with a total fat content of 40% of the buckwheat and 1.7–4.0%, polyunsaturated fatty acid (Elif, 2017). Compared to common buckwheat, the nutraceutical effect is higher in tartary buckwheat due to higher vitamin B content and antioxidants (Zhang, Li, Ma, Gao, Du, Han, … Qiao, 2017).

The buckwheat dietary fibre performs functions of cholesterol–lowering, antihypertensive effect, constipation and obesity–reducing effect (Sun, Li, Hu, Zhou, Ji, Yu, … Luan, 2018). It regulates bowel movements in the body. Buckwheat does not contain gluten and can be consumed on a celiac diet (Molinari, Costantini, Timperio, Lelli, Bonafaccia, Bonafaccia, & Merendino, 2017). It is also considered a prebiotic nutrient source because it contains lactic acid bacteria such as Bifidobacter and Lactobacillus. It is effective in protecting against radiation by increasing body resistance (Hande, 2015).

Teff (*Eragrostis Tef*)

Teff (*Eragrostis tef*) is a small tropical grain originating from Ethiopia, typically used for the production of traditionally fermented wheat flour, injera (Marti, Marengo, Bonomi, Casiraghi, Franzetti, Pagani, & Iametti, 2017). In Ethiopia and Eritrea, it is an important food product used for the production of traditional foods and drinks such as injera (food basement), kitta (unleavened bread) and tella (opaque beer). Teff granules do not contain gluten and have good potential to be formulated in many food and beverage products that can be used by celiac patients (Zhu, 2018).

Being a very adaptable plant, teff can be grown in changing environmental conditions such as drought and humidity (Zhu, 2018). Its seeds can survive for several years provided direct contact with moisture and sun is avoided. Compared to other common cereals, the teff seed is more resistant to attacks by harmful insects and other storage pests. Thus, it can be safely stored under conventional storage conditions without chemical protection (Gebremariam, Zarnkow, & Becker, 2012).

Teff varieties are defined according to the colors of the grains, flowers, flowering form and size of the plants. Different varieties are known as netch (white), qey (red/brown) and sergegna (mixed) according to the color of the beans and available in the market (Gebremariam, Zarnkow, & Becker, 2012). The grain mass (0.2–0.4 mg) is the smallest among carbohydrate–rich seeds (Gebremariam, Zarnkow, & Becker, 2012).

In recent years, teff has gained popularity in the world because of its quite attractive nutritional properties. Growing has been successfully adapted to other parts of the world, such as the US, India and Australia (Zhu, 2018).

As a result of its unique chemical composition and form of the whole grains, teff has been associated with a number of health benefits. For example, studies have shown that teff helps to prevent the incidence of malaria, anemia and diabetes by showing in vitro antioxidative activities, increasing the level of hemoglobin in the human body (Zhu, 2018).

It is also a very nutritious plant with 100 grams of raw teff containing 367 kcal of energy. Starch is the main component of the teff cereal and accounts for more than 70% of its dry weight (Zhu, 2018). Whole–grain teffin constitutes 9.8% of the dry weight of the dietary fibre (Zhu, 2018).

Teff is rich in carbohydrates, fibre and essential amino acids. It has a starch content of approximately 73%, making teff a starchy cereal, a protein content of 8–11% and a 3–4.5% fibre content (Baye, 2014). Teff contains a high amount of iron and has also higher contents of calcium, copper and zinc than other grains (Campo, del Arco, Urtasun, Oria, & Ferrer–Mairal, 2016). In the teff protein, the basic storage components are glutelin and albumin. The amino acid composition of teff flour is convenient and the teff protein is readily digestible compared to cereals, such as corn and sorghum, because it contains the most digestible types of major protein fractions such as albumin, glutelin and globulin. Teff grains are rich in unsaturated fatty acids – oleic acid 32.41%, and linoleic acid 23.83% (Gebremariam, Zarnkow, & Becker, 2012).

Recently, the teff Trolor [Eragrostis tef (zuccini.)] is used as a raw material for gluten–free alternatives. In addition, the presence of a nutritional property linked to essential amino acids, high mineral, polyphenol and dietary fibre content is the cause of this dissemination of the idea (Di Ghionno, Marconi, Sileoni, De Francesco, Perretti, 2017).

Beans (*Phaseolus Vulgaris L.*)

Beans are among the most consumed pulses in the world. Some of the most important consumers are: South America (9.3 kg/person/year), the Caribbean (9.1 kg/person/year), Central America (8.8 kg/person/year) and Central Africa (8.0 kg/person/year) (Luna–Vital, Mojica, González de Mejía, Mendoza, & Loarca–Piña, 2015). They are a source of energy for millions of people, especially in developing countries. Beans contain dietary fibre and are important dietary protein sources. They are a cheaper source of protein compared to foods of animal origin and can be added to different food formulations (Santiago–Ramos, Figueroa–Cárdenas, de, Véles–Medina, & Salazar, 2018).

Historically, beans have been an important component of the tropical and subtropical cuisine. It is the most important plant protein in the American and African continent, where animal proteins are limited due to economic, religious and cultural reasons. Besides, beans are closely related to the improvement of health. They have functional properties due to their chemical composition and are recommended for dietary treatment of diseases such as cardiovascular disease, diabetes mellitus, obesity and cancer (Oliveira, Mateó, dos Fioroto, Oliveira, de, & Naozuka, 2018). Beans contain 20–30% proteins, 2.5% fats and 50–60% carbohydrates (Hayat, Ahmad, Masud, Ahmed, & Bashir, 2014).

For the last decade, beans have been defined as nutraceutical foods due to bioactive compound contents, such as polyphenols, resistant starch, oligosaccharides, digestible fractions and bioactive peptides. Beans consist mainly of carbohydrates. The amount of protein is approximately 16–33% and is considered to be a good source of protein. In Central and South America, the amount of protein from bean consumption is about 5–6 g/person/day (Luna–Vital, Mojica, González de Mejía, Mendoza, & Loarca–Piña, 2015). In addition to the important nutritive value of beans, low levels of methionine and cysteine content and high resistance to proteolysis should not be overlooked (Carrasco–Castilla, Hernández–Álvarez, Jiménez–Martínez, Jacinto–Hernández, Alaiz, Girón–Calle, … Dávila–Ortiz, 2012).

Beans are the main sources of dietary fibre and contain 15–19% dietary fibre as raw (Ganesan & Xu, 2017). Per 100 grams of edible parts, beans have two to three times more fibre than other dietary sources. In recent years, the consumption of beans in developed countries has been replaced by other foods, and the proportion of fibre in people's diets has decreased. However, the resistant starch and the dietary fibre found in the bean paste have been associated with the protection of the digestive system of humans, particularly colon health. In addition, the beans are lower in the glycemic index due to the higher proportion of slower digestible starch in beans compared with carbohydrate–rich foods containing other dietary fibre. Thus, adding beans to foods and using them in the formulation of processed foods can reduce glycemic load and can bring significant advantages to human health (Los, Zielinski, Wojeicchowski, Nogueira, & Demiate, 2018).

After the beans are cooked, more than 70% of the copper and iron minerals are shown to be insoluble due to protein denaturation, polyphenols and phytate associations (Naozuka & Oliveira, 2012). Cooking, on the other hand, softens the food matrix and releases the substances bound to the protein, thus facilitating protein absorption. In addition, the heating of foods alters the natural factors which prevent mineral absorption, such as phytate and dietary fibre. For this reason, the positive effect of cooking on the chemical composition of the beans is evident (Oliveira, de, Mateó, dos, Fioroto, Oliveira, de, & Naozuka, 2018).

In most studies, beans are associated with improved health. It has been shown that diseases are positively affected by the reduction of risk of metabolic and cardiovascular disease, the decrease of serum cholesterol level and hyperglycemia, the prevention of colon, breast and prostate cancer by the non–nutritional substances in beans (Hall, Hillen, & Garden Robinson, 2017).

Soybean

Soybean (*Glycinemax*) is one of the most widely consumed legume products in the world (Vagadia, Vanga, & Raghavan, 2017). For centuries, soya has been grown in the eastern Asian countries as a crop. The ability to grow in a wide range of soil and climatic conditions makes it a versatile crop and one of the most commonly grown greasy seed products. In addition to the supply of vegetable oil for human consumption, soybean is one of the best sources of protein (Al Loman & Ju, 2017). Soy proteins are widely used to form foodstuffs with the goal of improving nutritional and functional qualities through a high protein level and a well–balanced amino acid composition (Vagadia, Vanga, & Raghavan, 2017). All essential amino acids found in animal proteins are also found in soy proteins. In addition, the nutritional value of soy protein equals animal protein with high biological value (Singh, Vij, & Hati, 2014). According to the United States Department of Agriculture's (USDA) nutrition database, soybean seeds contain approximately 36.5% protein, 19.9% lipid, 30% carbohydrate and 9.3% dietary fibre, 15.6% total saturated fatty acid, 57.7% total polyunsaturated fatty acid and 22.8% monounsaturated fatty acid (Vagadia, Vanga, & Raghavan, 2017).

Known locally as Bhatmala in Nepalese, soybean paste is traditionally used to prepare a variety of fermented and non–fermented recipes in Nepal, India and the Eastern Himalayan regions of Bhutan

(Tamang, 2015). Especially fermented soybean products have become an important part of the Korean diet, used daily in spices and consumed in side dishes and soups (Shin & Jeong, 2015).

Soybean consumption has increased over the last few years due to its positive effects on human health. It also serves as the main protein source for people who follow a vegan diet around the world. Commercial products derived from soya beans are very diverse: soybean sprouts and nuts, soybean flour, soy protein isolates and protein concentrates, soybean oil, soy milk, tofu, okara, tempeh, soy sauce, non–dairy desserts, soy sauce and textured meat products.

Soybean meal is an important source of phytochemicals such as isoflavones, phytosterols and lecithins. In addition, soluble fibres, saponins and polysaccharides can act collectively or through independent mechanisms to provide unique health benefits. For example, soy lecithins and saponins play a role in lipid metabolism; phytosterols and linolcic acid produce hypocholesterolemic effects and soy fibres have been shown to promote weight loss (Ramdath, Padhi, Sarfaraz, Renwick, & Duncan, 2017).

Epidemiological studies have shown that soybean meal consumption plays an important role in the prevention and treatment of a variety of chronic diseases including cardiovascular diseases, reduction of plasma cholesterol, protection against intestinal and kidney diseases and osteoporosis (Vagadia, Vanga, & Raghavan, 2017). Because it does not contain cholesterol, gluten, and lactose, it is a convenient food for vegetarians, people with lactose intolerance and milk allergies (Singh, Vij, & Hati, 2014).

Lentils (*Lens Culinaris*)

Lentils are the oldest grown crops among legumes. According to evidence from archaeological finds, their use dates back to 7500–6500 BC (Cokkizgin & Shtaya, 2013). Currently the annual lentil production is about 5 million tons, the largest production being in Western Canada (38%), followed by India (23%), Turkey (8%), Australia (7%) and USA (5%). More than 90% of the lentils produced in Canada, USA and Australia are exported to South East Asia, the Middle East and Africa (FAO, 2018).

Lentil are a rich source of protein containing a balanced amino acid profile, abundant low digestible carbohydrates and a variety of essential micronutrients. The nutritional content of 100 g of lentils is 2 g fat, 4–9 g dietary fibre, 23–27 g protein and 64–74 g carbohydrate (Chung, Liu, Hoover, Warkentin, & Vandenberg, 2008). There are 39.3 g of essential amino acids per 100 grams of protein in the lentil. The limiting amino acids in the lentil protein are sulfurized amino acids, tryptophan and threonine. For this reason, the consumption of lentil, rice, corn, potatoes and other root and tuber plants ensures that all necessary amino acids are met (Joshi, Timilsena, & Adhikari, 2017).

Similar to other legumes, lentils contain some anti–nutritional factors. Of these anti–nutritional factors, trypsin inhibitors inactivate key digestive enzymes. Tannins, another anti–nutritional factor, can alter protein bioavailability by complexing diet proteins to reduce digestibility of cholimetry (Nosworthy, Medina, Franczyk, Neufeld, Appah, Utioh, … House, 2018). However, studies have shown that culinary firing reduces the activity and concentration of anti–nutritional factors such as trypsin inhibitors, tannins and phytic acid (Hefnawy, 2011; Wang, Hatcher, Toews, & Gawalko, 2009). The reduction of the anti–nutritional factors increases the digestibility of the dietary protein and thus increases the bioavailability of the lentils (Nosworthy, Medina, Franczyk, Neufeld, Appah, Utioh, … House, 2018).

The lentil is a nutritious high medium energy pulp and contains various micronutrient ingredients, including 3.7–4.5 mg iron, 2.2–2.7 mg zinc, 22–34 µg selenium, 50–250 µg β–carotene and 216–290 µg folate (Siva, Thavarajah, Johnson, Duckett, Jesch, & Thavarajah, 2017). Unlike other grains, the lentil is very low in terms of phytic acid content (2.5–4.4 mg / g) linking iron and zinc, thus making these nutrients available (Thavarajah, Thavarajah, & Vandenberg, 2009).

Most carbohydrates found in lentils are starch and this starch refers to non–structural carbohydrates containing 47–52 g total starch in 100 g lentils. Lentil starch is composed of amylose (a few branched linear glucans) and amylopectin (a larger, highly branched molecule). The amylose ratio is higher than the amylopectin ratio, and the digestibility of the liquor is slower because of the character of the outermost layers of the crystallization grade or starch granule of amylose starch (Siva, Thavarajah, Johnson, Duckett, Jesch, & Thavarajah, 2017).

According to recent studies, lentils may be a good source of prebiotic carbohydrates. Total prebiotic carbohydrate concentrations indicate that more than 13 g of prebiotic can be provided by 100 g culinary portions (Johnson, Thavarajah, Combs, & Thavarajah, 2013). Prebiotics in the diet are defined as selectively fermented substances that cause specific changes in the gastrointestinal microbiotinin composition and/or activity, thus benefiting the host's health (Valcheva & Dieleman, 2016). These prebiotic carbohydrates in the lentils are associated with the hunger–toughness mechanism. They may decrease the rate and degree of starch digestibility and may lead to better management of body weight, decreased glycemic response and insulin resistance (Siva, Thavarajah, Johnson, Duckett, Jesch, & Thavarajah, 2017).

Chickpea (*Ciger Arietinum*)

Chickpea (*Cicer arietinum*) is the third most important species among legumes after soybeans and peas and the second most important legume grown in Asia, the Mediterranean regions, Australia, Canada, USA and Africa (Acharjee & Sarmah, 2013). It is one of the earliest grown vegetables and is thought to have originated in the Middle East about 7450 years ago (Roy, Boye, & Simpson, 2010). Worldwide, chickpeas are grown in 12 million hectares with 11 million tons produced. The South Asian region, including Iran, is the largest chickpea producer in the world and covers 76% of the total production (FAO, 2010).

There are two main species of chickpeas grown in the world – desi with smaller seeds and kabuli with larger seeds. The desi chickpea seed is dark, irregularly shaped and grown in semi–arid areas. Kabuli chickpeas (Garbanzo bean) have a light–colored seed coat, and are normally grown in temperate regions of the world (Roy, Boye, & Simpson, 2010).

Factors, such as climate, soil, nutrition, biotic and abiotic stress affect the nutritional composition of chickpeas. There are about 367 kcal per 100 g of chickpea seed. The composition of carbohydrate ranges from 50 to 70%. Generally, chickpeas contain more lipid (2–8%) and fibre (10–20%) compared to other legumes (Acharjee & Sarmah, 2013).

Chickpeas contain high quality protein. In addition, carbohydrates are a good source of vitamins (thiamine and niacin) and minerals (calcium, phosphorus, iron, magnesium and potassium). Their fat content is rich in linoleic base oil acidity. The quality of chickpea's protein is similar to soybean protein, but it contains eight essential amino acid residues.

Lysine, the limiting amino acid in grains, is found in the chickpea. Hence, when chickpeas are consumed together with cereals, they complement each other and provide balanced nutrition. Also, chickpeas contain vitamins such as vitamin B–complex, vitamin C, vitamin A and vitamin K, which are necessary for various metabolic pathways. Chickpea seeds are also a mineral-rich source for calcium, phosphorus, zinc and iron (Bar–El Dadon, Abbo, & Reifen, 2017).

Studies have reported that the amount of protein in chickpea varies between 18% and 28% and of fat between 6% and 9% (Alajaji & El–Adawy, 2006; Ghavidel & Prakash, 2006). Chickpeas are an important source of amino acids. However, they contain limited amounts of sulfur–containing amino acids. Accordingly, the content of methionine is 1.3–1.6% and the content of cysteine is 2.5–3.0% (Acharjee & Sarmah, 2013).

Chickpeas have some unwanted features. These are phenolic compounds that have long cooking times, contain enzyme inhibitors and phytates, form gas problems and must be removed for effective use (Milan–Carrillo, Valdez–Alarcon, Gutierrez–Dorado, Cárdenas–Valenzuela, Mora–Escobedo, Garzón–Tiznado, & Reyes–Moreno, 2007).

The consumption of chickpeas has been associated with the prevention of cardiovascular disease, the management of type 2 diabetes and lowering of LDL–cholesterol levels. While insoluble dietary fibre in chickpea is associated with a reduction in the incidence of colon cancer, it has been shown that soluble fibre has a beneficial effect on weight loss and weight management. They are used in stews, soups, salads and dips and can be processed into flour (Roy, Boye, & Simpson, 2010). Because chickpeas contain no gluten, they can provide excellent cooking characteristics in gluten–free cereal products (Shaabani, Yarmand, Kiani, & Emam–Djomeh, 2018).

Spirulina

Algae are photosynthetic organisms that convert light energy from the sun into chemical energy by photosynthesis and have a simple reproduction structure. Their biomass contains various compounds with diversified structures and functions. Algal biotechnology is divided into microalgae, macroalgae and cyanobacteria (Soni, Sudhakar, & Rana, 2017).

Spirulina was known in the past as filamentous spiral–shaped blue–green algae. Nowadays it is better known as photosynthetic bacteria (Arthrospira). This microorganism is regarded as an important food source for humans and the most popular microalgae, described by the World Health Organization as one of the world's most important superb foods (Deamici, Santos, & Costa, 2018).

It was first discovered in 1519 by the Spanish scientist Hernando Cortez who observed that spirulina was consumed by the Aztecs during a visit to Lake Texcoco in the Mexico Valley. Pierre Dangeard discovered spirulina's health benefits by observing that flamingos survived by consuming blue–green algae. The botanist Jean Leonard supported the findings of Dangeard and people soon began commercializing spirulina. It is a microalgae species that naturally grows in subtropical climates and saline lakes (Belay, Ota, Miyakawa, & Shimamatsu, 1993; Soni, Sudhakar, & Rana, 2017).

Spirulina is a concentrated food with antioxidants, phytotoxins, probiotics and nutraceuticals, which has a health–enhancing effect on people. It can quickly meet the various needs of people due to its nutritional composition. According to NASA and the European Space Agency, spirulina is one of the main things that can be consumed in long–term space missions. It is seen as "one of the best protein sources" (Soni, Sudhakar, & Rana, 2017).

Currently, spirulina is used in malnutrition treatment in many countries. According to the study on malnutrition treatment, the administering of spirulina at a dose of 10g/day improved the nutritional status of malnourished children in the intervention group compared to the control group – the malnutrition rate was 30% before spirulina and 20% after the spirulina intervention (Matondo, Takaisi, Nkuadiolandu, Kazadi Lukusa, & Aloni, 2016).

The two most important species of spirulina are Spirulina maxima and Spirulina platensis. Protein constitutes 60–70% of their content, and 47% of this protein contains all of the essential amino acids (Hannon, Gimpel, Tran, Rasala, & Mayfield, 2010). It also contains vitamins and minerals such as vitamin A, vitamin C, vitamin E, iron, calcium, chromium, copper, magnesium, manganese, phosphorus, potassium, sodium and zinc. Vitamin B12, which is not found in sufficient amounts in plant sources, is more than 4 times the amount found in raw liver. In addition, the content of iron is high and 20 times more than wheat. In addition, the content of β–carotene is unusually high and about 30 times higher than that of carrots (Soni, Sudhakar, & Rana, 2017).

Spirulina's main fatty acid is one of the best anti–inflammatories in the world because it is gamma–linolenic acid (GLA) with fat content of 12% and 14% fibre (Sathasivam Radhakrishnan, Hashem, & Abd–Allah, 2017). Anticancer, antioxidant and hepatoprotective agents have been shown in studies. Also, studies have shown that spirulina has a positive effect on cardiovascular diseases, hyperglycaemia, hyper-lipidemia, immunodeficiency, inflammatory processes and improves the immune system's resistance to various types of cancer as well as on the treatment of HIV and other viral diseases (Ovando, Carvalho, de, Vinícius de Melo Pereira, Jacques, Soccol, & Soccol, 2018). It is a functional food in the immune system that feeds the intestinal flora, including Lactobacillus and Bifidus (Sathasivam Radhakrishnan, Hashem, & Abd–Allah, 2017).

CONCLUSION

Proteins are the basis of the human diet because of their role for the repair of immune responses, cell signals, muscle masses and damaged cells. Animal and plant proteins are the main protein sources in human diet. Plant-derived proteins can meet all our protein needs with a balanced diet without the need to consume meat or other animal-based products. The benefits from proteins derived from plant–based sources compared with animal–based food sources are far–reaching and can protect against chronic disease, promote overall bodily health and can have positive health effects on preventing cardiovascular disease, diabetes, cancer, weight maintenance and other health risk factors.

REFERENCES

Abugoch James, L. E. (2009). Quinoa (Chenopodium quinoa Willd.): Composition, chemistry, nutritional, and functional properties. *Advances in Food and Nutrition Research, 58*, 1–31. doi:10.1016/S1043-4526(09)58001-1 PMID:19878856

Acharjee, S., & Sarmah, B. K. (2013). Biotechnologically generating 'super chickpea' for food and nutritional security. *Plant Science, 207*, 108–116. doi:10.1016/j.plantsci.2013.02.003 PMID:23602105

Al Loman, A., & Ju, L. K. (2017). Enzyme–based processing of soybean carbohydrate: Recent developments and future prospects. *Enzyme and Microbial Technology, 106*, 35–47. doi:10.1016/j.enzmictec.2017.06.013 PMID:28859808

Alajaji, S. A., & El–Adawy, T. A. (2006). Nutritional composition of chickpea (Cicer arietinum L.) as affected by microwave cooking and other traditional cooking methods. *Journal of Food Composition and Analysis, 19*(8), 806–812. doi:10.1016/j.jfca.2006.03.015

Alican, A. (2017). *Soğuk pres tekniği ile elde edilen chia tohumu atıklarının salata sosu üretiminde kullanılması*. Yıldız Teknik Üniversitesi.

Bar–El Dadon, S., Abbo, S., & Reifen, R. (2017). Leveraging traditional crops for better nutrition and health – The case of chickpea. *Trends in Food Science & Technology, 64*, 39–47. doi:10.1016/j.tifs.2017.04.002

Baye, K. (2014). *Teff: Nutrient composition and health benefits.* Ethiopia Strategy Support Program. Workig Paper 67. Retrieved from https://www.researchgate.net/profile/Kaleab_Baye2/publication/266316373_Teff_Nutrient_Composition_and_Health_Benefits/links/542c24320cf277d58e8b0b42.pdf

Belay, A., Ota, Y., Miyakawa, K., & Shimamatsu, H. (1993). Current knowledge on potential health benefits of Spirulina. *Journal of Applied Phycology, 5*(2), 235–241. doi:10.1007/BF00004024

Besler, T., Rakıcıoglu, N., Ayaz, A., Demirel Büyüktuncer, Z., Özel, G. H., Samur Eroğlu, G., . . . Yürük, A. (2015). *Türkiye'ye özgü besin ve beslenme rehberi.* Ankara. Retrieved from http://www.bdb.hacettepe.edu.tr/TOBR_kitap.pdf

Bogueva, D., Marinova, D., & Raphaely, T. (Eds.). (2018). Handbook of research on social marketing and its influence on animal origin food product consumption. Hershey, PA: IGI Global.

Bojanic, A. (2011). *La quinua : Cultivo milenario para contribuir a la seguridad alimentaria mundial.* Proinpa, 58. Food and Agriculture Organization of the United Nations.

Campo, E., del Arco, L., Urtasun, L., Oria, R., & Ferrer–Mairal, A. (2016). Impact of sourdough on sensory properties and consumers' preference of gluten–free breads enriched with teff flour. *Journal of Cereal Science, 67*, 75–82. doi:10.1016/j.jcs.2015.09.010

Carrasco–Castilla, J., Hernández–Álvarez, A. J., Jiménez–Martínez, C., Jacinto–Hernández, C., Alaiz, M., Girón–Calle, J., ... Dávila–Ortiz, G. (2012). Antioxidant and metal chelating activities of peptide fractions from phaseolin and bean protein hydrolysates. *Food Chemistry, 135*(3), 1789–1795. doi:10.1016/j.foodchem.2012.06.016 PMID:22953924

Caruso, M. C., Favati, F., Di Cairano, M., Galgano, F., Labella, R., Scarpa, T., & Condelli, N. (2018). Shelf–life evaluation and nutraceutical properties of chia seeds from a recent long–day flowering genotype cultivated in Mediterranean area. *Lebensmittel-Wissenschaft + Technologie, 87*, 400–405. doi:10.1016/j.lwt.2017.09.015

Chen, J.-H., Song, J., Chen, Y., Ding, Q., Peng, A., & Mao, L. (2016). The effect of vegan protein–based diets on metabolic parameters, expressions of adiponectin and its receptors in wistar rats. *Nutrients, 8*(10), 643. doi:10.3390/nu8100643 PMID:27763537

Chung, H.-J., Liu, Q., Hoover, R., Warkentin, T. D., & Vandenberg, B. (2008). In vitro starch digestibility, expected glycemic index, and thermal and pasting properties of flours from pea, lentil and chickpea cultivars. *Food Chemistry, 111*(2), 316–321. doi:10.1016/j.foodchem.2008.03.062 PMID:26047429

Cokkizgin, A., & Shtaya, M. J. Y. (2013). Lentil: Origin, cultivation techniques, utilization and advances in transformation. *Agricultural Science, 1*(1), 55–62. doi:10.12735/as.v1i1p55

Comerford, K. B., & Pasin, G. (2016). Emerging evidence for the importance of dietary protein source on glucoregulatory markers and type 2 diabetes: Different effects of dairy, meat, fish, egg, and plant protein foods. *Nutrients, 8*(8), 446. doi:10.3390/nu8080446 PMID:27455320 de Campo, C., dos Santos, P. P., Costa, T. M. H., Paese, K., Guterres, S. S., Rios, A. de O., & Flôres, S. H. (2017). Nanoencapsulation of chia seed oil with chia mucilage (Salvia hispanica L.) as wall material: Characterization and stability evaluation. *Food Chemistry, 234,* 1–9. doi:10.1016/j.foodchem.2017.04.153 PMID:28551210

Deamici, K. M., Santos, L. O., & Costa, J. A. V. (2018). Magnetic field action on outdoor and indoor cultures of Spirulina: Evaluation of growth, medium consumption and protein profile. *Bioresource Technology, 249,* 168–174. doi:10.1016/j.biortech.2017.09.185 PMID:29040851

Di Ghionno, L., Marconi, O., Sileoni, V., De Francesco, G., & Perretti, G. (2017). Brewing with prolyl endopeptidase from Aspergillus niger: The impact of enzymatic treatment on gluten levels, quality attributes and sensory profile. *International Journal of Food Science & Technology, 52*(6), 1367–1374. doi:10.1111/ijfs.13375

Elif, Ö. (2017). *Erişte üretiminde farklı oran ve kombinasyonlarda karabuğday, amarant ve kinoa unlarının kullanım imkanları.* Necmettin Erbakan Üniversitesi.

Fischer, S., Wilckens, R., Jara, J., Aranda, M., Valdivia, W., Bustamante, L., ... Obal, I. (2017). Protein and antioxidant composition of quinoa (Chenopodium quinoa Willd.) sprout from seeds submitted to water stress, salinity and light conditions. *Industrial Crops and Products, 107,* 558–564. doi:10.1016/j.indcrop.2017.04.035

Food and Agriculture Organization of the United Nations (FAO). (2010). *The state of addressing food insecurity in protracted crises.* Retrieved from http://www.fao.org/catalog/inter–e.htm

Food and Agriculture Organization of the United Nations (FAO). (2018). *Food and agriculture data.* Retrieved from http://www.fao.org/faostat/en/#home

Ganesan, K., & Xu, B. (2017). Polyphenol–rich dry common beans (Phaseolus vulgaris L.) and their health benefits. *International Journal of Molecular Sciences, 18*(11), 2331. doi:10.3390/ijms18112331 PMID:29113066

Garnett, T. (2014). *What is a sustainable healthy diet?* Food Climate Research Network. Retrieved from https://www.fcrn.org.uk/sites/default/files/fcrn_what_is_a_sustainable_healthy_diet_final.pdf

Gebremariam, M. M., Zarnkow, M., & Becker, T. (2012). Teff (Eragrostis tef) as a raw material for malting, brewing and manufacturing of gluten–free foods and beverages: A review. *Journal of Food Science and Technology, 51*(11), 2881–2895. doi:10.100713197-012-0745-5 PMID:26396284

Ghavidel, R. A., & Prakash, J. (2006). Effect of germination and dehulling on functional properties of legume flours. *Journal of the Science of Food and Agriculture, 86*(8), 1189–1195. doi:10.1002/jsfa.2460

Giaretta, D., Lima, V. A., & Carpes, S. T. (2017). (in press). Improvement of fatty acid profile in breads supplemented with Kinako flour and chia seed. *Innovative Food Science & Emerging Technologies.* doi:10.1016/j.ifset.2017.11.010

Giménez–Bastida, J. A., Piskuła, M., & Zieliński, H. (2015). Recent advances in development of gluten–free buckwheat products. *Trends in Food Science & Technology, 44*(1), 58–65. doi:10.1016/j.tifs.2015.02.013

Graf, B. L., Rojas–Silva, P., Rojo, L. E., Delatorre–Herrera, J., Baldeón, M. E., & Raskin, I. (2015). Innovations in health value and functional food development of quinoa (Chenopodium quinoa Willd.). *Comprehensive Reviews in Food Science and Food Safety, 14*(4), 431–445. doi:10.1111/1541-4337.12135 PMID:27453695

Hall, C., Hillen, C., & Garden Robinson, J. (2017). Composition, nutritional value, and health benefits of pulses. *Cereal Chemistry Journal, 94*(1), 11–31. doi:10.1094/CCHEM-03-16-0069-FI

Hande, A. (2015). *Hidrotermal işlemlerin karabuğday nişastasının fizikokimyasal özellikleri ve dirençli nişasta miktarı üzerindeki etkisi.* İstanbul Teknik Üniversitesi.

Hannon, M., Gimpel, J., Tran, M., Rasala, B., & Mayfield, S. (2010). Biofuels from algae: Challenges and potential. *Biofuels, 1*(5), 763–784. doi:10.4155/bfs.10.44 PMID:21833344

Hayat, I., Ahmad, A., Masud, T., Ahmed, A., & Bashir, S. (2014). Nutritional and health perspectives of beans (Phaseolus vulgaris L.): An overview. *Critical Reviews in Food Science and Nutrition, 54*(5), 580–592. doi:10.1080/10408398.2011.596639 PMID:24261533

Hefnawy, T. H. (2011). Effect of processing methods on nutritional composition and anti–nutritional factors in lentils (Lens culinaris). *Annals of Agricultural Science, 56*(2), 57–61. doi:10.1016/j.aoas.2011.07.001

Johnson, C. R., Thavarajah, D., Combs, G. F. Jr, & Thavarajah, P. (2013). Lentil (Lens culinaris L.): A prebiotic–rich whole food legume. *Food Research International, 51*(1), 107–113. doi:10.1016/j.foodres.2012.11.025

Joshi, M., Timilsena, Y., & Adhikari, B. (2017). Global production, processing and utilization of lentil: A review. *Journal of Integrative Agriculture, 16*(12), 2898–2913. doi:10.1016/S2095-3119(17)61793-3

Karim, M. M., Ashrafuzzaman, M., & Hossain, M. A. (2016). Effect of planting time on the growth and yield of chia (Salvia hispanica L.). *Asian Journal of Medical and Biological Research, 1*(3), 502. doi:10.3329/ajmbr.v1i3.26469

Li, G., & Zhu, F. (2018). Quinoa starch: Structure, properties, and applications. *Carbohydrate Polymers, 181*, 851–861. doi:10.1016/j.carbpol.2017.11.067 PMID:29254045

Lin, D., Lu, W., Kelly, A. L., Zhang, L., Zheng, B., & Miao, S. (2017). Interactions of vegetable proteins with other polymers: Structure–function relationships and applications in the food industry. *Trends in Food Science & Technology, 68*, 130–144. doi:10.1016/j.tifs.2017.08.006

López, D. N., Galante, M., Robson, M., Boeris, V., & Spelzini, D. (2018). Amaranth, quinoa and chia protein isolates: Physicochemical and structural properties. *International Journal of Biological Macromolecules, 109*, 152–159. doi:10.1016/j.ijbiomac.2017.12.080 PMID:29247732

Los, F. G. B., Zielinski, A. A. F., Wojeicchowski, J. P., Nogueira, A., & Demiate, I. M. (2018). Beans (Phaseolus vulgaris L.): Whole seeds with complex chemical composition. *Current Opinion in Food Science, 19*, 63–71. doi:10.1016/j.cofs.2018.01.010

Luna–Vital, D. A., Mojica, L., González de Mejía, E., Mendoza, S., & Loarca–Piña, G. (2015). Biological potential of protein hydrolysates and peptides from common bean (Phaseolus vulgaris L.): A review. *Food Research International, 76*, 39–50. doi:10.1016/j.foodres.2014.11.024

Marineli, R. da S., Lenquiste, S. A., Moraes, É. A., & Maróstica, M. R. Jr. (2015). Antioxidant potential of dietary chia seed and oil (Salvia hispanica L.) in diet–induced obese rats. *Food Research International*, *76*, 666–674. doi:10.1016/j.foodres.2015.07.039 PMID:28455051

Marsh, K., Zeuschner, C., & Saunders, A. (2016). Red meat and health: Evidence regarding red meat, health, and chronic disease risk. In T. Raphaely & D. Marinova (Eds.), *Impact of meat consumption on health and environmental sustainability* (pp. 131–177). Hershey, PA: IGI Global. doi:10.4018/978-1-4666-9553-5.ch008

Marsh, K., Zeuschner, C., & Saunders, A. (2018). The health impact of eating foods of animal origin: Evidence regarding animal foods, health, and disease risk. In D. Bogueva, D. Marinova, & T. Raphaely (Eds.), *Handbook of research on social marketing and its influence on animal origin food product consumption* (pp. 283–297). Hershey, PA: IGI Global. doi:10.4018/978-1-5225-4757-0.ch002

Marti, A., Marengo, M., Bonomi, F., Casiraghi, M. C., Franzetti, L., Pagani, M. A., & Iametti, S. (2017). Molecular features of fermented teff flour relate to its suitability for the production of enriched gluten–free bread. *Lebensmittel-Wissenschaft + Technologie*, *78*, 296–302. doi:10.1016/j.lwt.2016.12.042

Matondo, F. K., Takaisi, K., Nkuadiolandu, A. B., Kazadi Lukusa, A., & Aloni, M. N. (2016). Spirulina supplements improved the nutritional status of undernourished children quickly and significantly: Experience from Kisantu, the Democratic Republic of the Congo. *International Journal of Pediatrics*, *1296414*, 1–5. doi:10.1155/2016/1296414 PMID:27777589

Mattisson, I., Wirfält, E., Johansson, U., Gullberg, B., Olsson, H., & Berglund, G. (2004). Intakes of plant foods, fibre and fat and risk of breast cancer – a prospective study in the Malmö Diet and Cancer cohort. *British Journal of Cancer*, *90*(1), 122–127. doi:10.1038j.bjc.6601516 PMID:14710218

Menga, V., Amato, M., Phillips, T. D., Angelino, D., Morreale, F., & Fares, C. (2017). Gluten–free pasta incorporating chia (Salvia hispanica L.) as thickening agent: An approach to naturally improve the nutritional profile and the in vitro carbohydrate digestibility. *Food Chemistry*, *221*, 1954–1961. doi:10.1016/j.foodchem.2016.11.151 PMID:27979185

Mesías, M., Holgado, F., Márquez–Ruiz, G., & Morales, F. J. (2016). Risk/benefit considerations of a new formulation of wheat–based biscuit supplemented with different amounts of chia flour. *Lebensmittel-Wissenschaft + Technologie*, *73*, 528–535. doi:10.1016/j.lwt.2016.06.056

Milan–Carrillo, J., Valdez–Alarcon, C., Gutierrez–Dorado, R., Cárdenas–Valenzuela, O. G., Mora–Escobedo, R., Garzón–Tiznado, J. A., & Reyes–Moreno, C. (2007). Nutritional properties of quality protein maize and chickpea extruded based weaning food. *Plant Foods for Human Nutrition (Dordrecht, Netherlands)*, *62*(1), 31–37. doi:10.100711130-006-0039-z PMID:17243010

Molinari, R., Costantini, L., Timperio, A. M., Lelli, V., Bonafaccia, F., Bonafaccia, G., & Merendino, N. (2017). Tartary buckwheat malt as ingredient of gluten–free cookies. *Journal of Cereal Science*, *80*, 37–43. doi:10.1016/j.jcs.2017.11.011

Møller, G., Sluik, D., Ritz, C., Mikkilä, V., Raitakari, O. T., Hutri–Kähönen, N., ... Raben, A. (2017). A protein diet score, including plant and animal protein, investigating the association with HbA1c and eGFR–The PREVIEW Project. *Nutrients*, *9*(7), 763. doi:10.3390/nu9070763 PMID:28714926

Montalcini, T., De Bonis, D., Ferro, Y., Carè, I., Mazza, E., Accattato, F., ... Pujia, A. (2015). High vegetable fats intake is associated with high resting energy expenditure in vegetarians. *Nutrients*, *7*(7), 5933–5947. doi:10.3390/nu7075259 PMID:26193314

Moorthi, R. N., Vorland, C. J., & Hill Gallant, K. M. (2017). Diet and diabetic kidney disease: Plant versus animal protein. *Current Diabetes Reports*, *17*(3), 15. doi:10.100711892-017-0843-x PMID:28271467

Naozuka, J., & Oliveira, P. V. (2012). Cooking effects on iron and proteins content of beans (Phaseolus Vulgaris L.) by GF AAS and MALDI–TOF MS. *Journal of the Brazilian Chemical Society*, *23*(1), 156–162. doi:10.1590/S0103-50532012000100022

Navruz–Varli, S., & Sanlier, N. (2016). Nutritional and health benefits of quinoa (Chenopodium quinoa Willd.). *Journal of Cereal Science*, *69*, 371–376. doi:10.1016/j.jcs.2016.05.004

Nehete, J. Y., Bhambar, R. S., Narkhede, M. R., & Gawali, S. R. (2013). Natural proteins: Sources, isolation, characterization and applications. *Pharmacognosy Reviews*, *7*(14), 107–116. doi:10.4103/0973-7847.120508 PMID:24347918

Newby, P. K. (2009). Plant foods and plant-based diets: Protective against childhood obesity? *The American Journal of Clinical Nutrition*, *89*(5), 1572S–1587S. doi:10.3945/ajcn.2009.26736G

Nielsen, L. V., Kristensen, M. D., Klingenberg, L., Ritz, C., Belza, A., Astrup, A., & Raben, A. (2018). Protein from meat or vegetable sources in meals matched for fibre content has similar effects on subjective appetite sensations and energy intake – a randomized acute cross–over meal test study. *Nutrients*, *10*(1). doi:10.3390/nu10010096

Nosworthy, M. G., Medina, G., Franczyk, A. J., Neufeld, J., Appah, P., Utioh, A., ... House, J. D. (2018). Effect of processing on the in vitro and in vivo protein quality of red and green lentils (Lens culinaris). *Food Chemistry*, *240*, 588–593. doi:10.1016/j.foodchem.2017.07.129 PMID:28946315

Oliveira, A. P., de, & Mateó, B. (2018). Effect of cooking on the bioaccessibility of essential elements in different varieties of beans (Phaseolus vulgaris L.). *Journal of Food Composition and Analysis*, *67*, 135–140. doi:10.1016/j.jfca.2018.01.012

Oliveira–Alves, S. C., Vendramini–Costa, D. B., Betim Cazarin, C. B., Maróstica Júnior, M. R., Borges Ferreira, J. P., Silva, A. B., ... Bronze, M. R. (2017). Characterization of phenolic compounds in chia (Salvia hispanica L.) seeds, fibre flour and oil. *Food Chemistry*, *232*, 295–305. doi:10.1016/j.foodchem.2017.04.002 PMID:28490078

Ovando, C. A., de Carvalho, J. C., Vinícius de Melo Pereira, G., Jacques, P., Soccol, V. T., & Soccol, C. R. (2018). Functional properties and health benefits of bioactive peptides derived from Spirulina: A review. *Food Reviews International*, *34*(1), 34–51. doi:10.1080/87559129.2016.1210632

Pasiakos, S. M., Agarwal, S., Lieberman, H. R., & Fulgoni, V. L. III. (2015). Sources and amounts of animal, dairy, and plant protein intake of US adults in 2007–2010. *Nutrients*, *7*(8), 7058–7069. doi:10.3390/nu7085322 PMID:26308049

Rahman, M. J., de Camargo, A. C., & Shahidi, F. (2017). Phenolic and polyphenolic profiles of chia seeds and their in vitro biological activities. *Journal of Functional Foods*, *35*, 622–634. doi:10.1016/j.jff.2017.06.044

Ramdath, D., Padhi, E., Sarfaraz, S., Renwick, S., & Duncan, A. (2017). Beyond the cholesterol–lowering effect of soy protein: A review of the effects of dietary soy and its constituents on risk factors for cardiovascular disease. *Nutrients*, *9*(4), 324. doi:10.3390/nu9040324 PMID:28338639

Raphaely, T., & Marinova, D. (Eds.). (2016). *Impact of meat consumption on health and environmental sustainability*. Hershey, PA: IGI Global. doi:10.4018/978-1-4666-9553-5

Repo–Carrasco–Valencia, R. A.-M., & Serna, L. A. (2011). Quinoa (Chenopodium quinoa, Willd.) as a source of dietary fibre and other functional components. *Food Science and Technology (Campinas)*, *31*(1), 225–230. doi:10.1590/S0101-20612011000100035

Richter, C. K., Skulas–Ray, A. C., Champagne, C. M., & Kris–Etherton, P. M. (2015). Plant protein and animal proteins: Do they differentially affect cardiovascular disease risk? *Advances in Nutrition*, *6*(6), 712–728. doi:10.3945/an.115.009654 PMID:26567196

Roy, F., Boye, J. I., & Simpson, B. K. (2010). Bioactive proteins and peptides in pulse crops: Pea, chickpea and lentil. *Food Research International*, *43*(2), 432–442. doi:10.1016/j.foodres.2009.09.002

Santiago–Ramos, D., Figueroa–Cárdenas, J. de D., Véles–Medina, J. J., & Salazar, R. (2018). Physico-chemical properties of nixtamalized black bean (Phaseolus vulgaris L.) flours. *Food Chemistry*, *240*, 456–462. doi:10.1016/j.foodchem.2017.07.156 PMID:28946298

Sathasivam, R., Radhakrishnan, R., Hashem, A., & Abd–Allah, E. F. (2017). (in press). Microalgae metabolites: A rich source for food and medicine. *Saudi Journal of Biological Sciences*. doi:10.1016/j.sjbs.2017.11.003

Satija, A., Bhupathiraju, A. N., Rimm, E. B., Spiegelman, D., Chiuve, S. E., Borgi, L., ... Hu, F. B. (2016). Plant–based dietary patterns and incidence of type 2 diabetes in us men and women: Results from three prospective cohort studies. *PLoS Medicine*, *13*(6), e1002039. doi:10.1371/journal.pmed.1002039 PMID:27299701

Shaabani, S., Yarmand, M. S., Kiani, H., & Emam–Djomeh, Z. (2018). The effect of chickpea protein isolate in combination with transglutaminase and xanthan on the physical and rheological characteristics of gluten free muffins and batter based on millet flour. *Lebensmittel-Wissenschaft + Technologie*, *90*, 362–372. doi:10.1016/j.lwt.2017.12.023

Shin, D., & Jeong, D. (2015). Korean traditional fermented soybean products: Jang. *Journal of Ethnic Foods*, *2*(1), 2–7. doi:10.1016/j.jef.2015.02.002

Singh, B. P., Vij, S., & Hati, S. (2014). Functional significance of bioactive peptides derived from soybean. *Peptides*, *54*, 171–179. doi:10.1016/j.peptides.2014.01.022 PMID:24508378

Siva, N., Thavarajah, D., Johnson, C. R., Duckett, S., Jesch, E. D., & Thavarajah, P. (2017). Can lentil (Lens culinaris Medikus) reduce the risk of obesity? *Journal of Functional Foods*, *38*, 706–715. doi:10.1016/j.jff.2017.02.017

Soni, R. A., Sudhakar, K., & Rana, R. S. (2017). Spirulina – from growth to nutritional product: A review. *Trends in Food Science & Technology*, *69*, 157–171. doi:10.1016/j.tifs.2017.09.010

Sun, X., Li, W., Hu, Y., Zhou, X., Ji, M., Yu, D., ... Luan, G. (2018). Comparison of pregelatinization methods on physicochemical, functional and structural properties of tartary buckwheat flour and noodle quality. *Journal of Cereal Science*, *80*, 63–71. doi:10.1016/j.jcs.2018.01.016

Sytar, O., Brestic, M., & Rai, M. (2013). Possible ways of fagopyrin biosynthesis and production in buckwheat plants. *Fitoterapia*, *84*(1), 72–79. doi:10.1016/j.fitote.2012.10.008 PMID:23103298

Tamang, J. P. (2015). Naturally fermented ethnic soybean foods of India. *Journal of Ethnic Foods*, *2*(1), 8–17. doi:10.1016/j.jef.2015.02.003

Thavarajah, P., Thavarajah, D., & Vandenberg, A. (2009). Low phytic acid lentils (Lens culinaris L.): A potential solution for increased micronutrient bioavailability. *Journal of Agricultural and Food Chemistry*, *57*(19), 9044–9049. doi:10.1021/jf901636p PMID:19725537

Timilsena, Y. P., Adhikari, R., Barrow, C. J., & Adhikari, B. (2016). Physicochemical and functional properties of protein isolate produced from Australian chia seeds. *Food Chemistry*, *212*, 648–656. doi:10.1016/j.foodchem.2016.06.017 PMID:27374580

Timilsena, Y. P., Vongsvivut, J., Adhikari, R., & Adhikari, B. (2017). Physicochemical and thermal characteristics of Australian chia seed oil. *Food Chemistry*, *228*, 394–402. doi:10.1016/j.foodchem.2017.02.021 PMID:28317740

Vagadia, B. H., Vanga, S. K., & Raghavan, V. (2017). Inactivation methods of soybean trypsin inhibitor – A review. *Trends in Food Science & Technology*, *64*, 115–125. doi:10.1016/j.tifs.2017.02.003

Valcheva, R., & Dieleman, L. A. (2016). Prebiotics: Definition and protective mechanisms. *Best Practice & Research. Clinical Gastroenterology*, *30*(1), 27–37. doi:10.1016/j.bpg.2016.02.008 PMID:27048894

Vilcacundo, R., & Hernández–Ledesma, B. (2017). Nutritional and biological value of quinoa (Chenopodium quinoa Willd.). *Current Opinion in Food Science*, *14*, 1–6. doi:10.1016/j.cofs.2016.11.007

Wang, N., Hatcher, D. W., Toews, R., & Gawalko, E. J. (2009). Influence of cooking and dehulling on nutritional composition of several varieties of lentils (Lens culinaris). *Lebensmittel-Wissenschaft + Technologie*, *42*(4), 842–848. doi:10.1016/j.lwt.2008.10.007

World Health Organization (WHO). (2015). *Q&A on the carcinogenicity of the consumption of red meat and processed meat*. Retrieved from http://www.who.int/features/qa/cancer–red–meat/en/

Wu, J., Zeng, R., Huang, J., Li, X., Zhang, J., Ho, J. C.-M., & Zheng, Y. (2016). Dietary protein sources and incidence of breast cancer: A dose–response meta–analysis of prospective studies. *Nutrients*, *8*(11), 730. doi:10.3390/nu8110730 PMID:27869663

Zhang, L., Li, X., Ma, B., Gao, Q., Du, H., Han, Y., ... Qiao, Z. (2017). The tartary buckwheat genome provides insights into rutin biosynthesis and abiotic stress tolerance. *Molecular Plant*, *10*(9), 1224–1237. doi:10.1016/j.molp.2017.08.013 PMID:28866080

Zhang, Z. L., Zhou, M. L., Tang, Y., Li, F. L., Tang, Y. X., Shao, J. R., ... Wu, Y. M. (2012). Bioactive compounds in functional buckwheat food. *Food Research International, 49*(1), 389–395. doi:10.1016/j.foodres.2012.07.035

Zhu, F. (2016a). Buckwheat starch: Structures, properties, and applications. *Trends in Food Science & Technology, 49*, 121–135. doi:10.1016/j.tifs.2015.12.002

Zhu, F. (2016b). Chemical composition and health effects of Tartary buckwheat. *Food Chemistry, 203*, 231–245. doi:10.1016/j.foodchem.2016.02.050 PMID:26948610

Zhu, F. (2018). Chemical composition and food uses of teff (Eragrostis tef). *Food Chemistry, 239*, 402–415. doi:10.1016/j.foodchem.2017.06.101 PMID:28873585

Zhu, F., Du, B., Li, R., & Li, J. (2014). Effect of micronization technology on physicochemical and antioxidant properties of dietary fibre from buckwheat hulls. *Biocatalysis and Agricultural Biotechnology, 3*(3), 30–34. doi:10.1016/j.bcab.2013.12.009

ADDITIONAL READING

Abugoch James, L. E. (2009). Quinoa (Chenopodium quinoa Willd.): Composition, chemistry, nutritional, and functional properties. *Advances in Food and Nutrition Research, 58*, 1–31. doi:10.1016/S1043-4526(09)58001-1 PMID:19878856

Bar–El Dadon, S., Abbo, S., & Reifen, R. (2017). Leveraging traditional crops for better nutrition and health – The case of chickpea. *Trends in Food Science & Technology, 64*, 39–47. doi:10.1016/j.tifs.2017.04.002

Baye, K. (2014). *Teff: Nutrient composition and health benefits.* Ethiopia Strategy Support Program. Workig Paper 67. Retrieved from https://www.researchgate.net/profile/Kaleab_Baye2/publication/266316373_Teff_Nutrient_Composition_and_Health_Benefits/links/542c24320cf277d58e8b0b42.pdf

Caruso, M. C., Favati, F., Di Cairano, M., Galgano, F., Labella, R., Scarpa, T., & Condelli, N. (2018). Shelf–life evaluation and nutraceutical properties of chia seeds from a recent long–day flowering genotype cultivated in Mediterranean area. *Lebensmittel-Wissenschaft + Technologie, 87*, 400–405. doi:10.1016/j.lwt.2017.09.015

Cokkizgin, A., & Shtaya, M. J. Y. (2013). Lentil: Origin, cultivation techniques, utilization and advances in transformation. *Agricultural Science, 1*(1), 55–62. Retrieved from http://www.todayscience.org/AS/article/as.v1i1p55.pdf. doi:10.12735/as.v1i1p55

Hayat, I., Ahmad, A., Masud, T., Ahmed, A., & Bashir, S. (2014). Nutritional and health perspectives of beans (Phaseolus vulgaris L.): An overview. *Critical Reviews in Food Science and Nutrition, 54*(5), 580–592. doi:10.1080/10408398.2011.596639 PMID:24261533

Marsh, K., Zeuschner, C., & Saunders, A. (2018). The health impact of eating foods of animal origin: Evidence regarding animal foods, health, and disease risk. In D. Bogueva, D. Marinova, & T. Raphaely (Eds.), *Handbook of research on social marketing and its influence on animal origin food product consumption* (pp. 283–297). Hershey, PA: IGI Global. doi:10.4018/978-1-5225-4757-0.ch002

Ovando, C. A., de Carvalho, J. C., Vinícius de Melo Pereira, G., Jacques, P., Soccol, V. T., & Soccol, C. R. (2018). Functional properties and health benefits of bioactive peptides derived from Spirulina: A review. *Food Reviews International*, *34*(1), 34–51. doi:10.1080/87559129.2016.1210632

Ramdath, D., Padhi, E., Sarfaraz, S., Renwick, S., & Duncan, A. (2017). Beyond the cholesterol–lowering effect of soy protein: A review of the effects of dietary soy and its constituents on risk factors for cardiovascular disease. *Nutrients*, *9*(4), 324. doi:10.3390/nu9040324 PMID:28338639

Zhu, F. (2016a). Buckwheat starch: Structures, properties, and applications. *Trends in Food Science & Technology*, *49*, 121–135. doi:10.1016/j.tifs.2015.12.002

KEY TERMS AND DEFINITIONS

Beans: Edible, nutritious, widely grown seeds of various plants of the legume family, especially of the genus *Phaseolus*, usually oval or kidney-shaped.

Buckwheat: An edible plant (*Fagopyrum esculentum*) with high nutritional properties cultivated for its triangular grain-like seeds used as a food source.

Chia: An annual edible plant (*Salvia hispanica*) of the mint family, native to South America, and used for its nutritional values; its seeds are predominantly used as a food source.

Chickpea: A round yellowish edible seed (*Cicer arietinum*), a legume of the family *Fabaceae*, widely used as a pulse.

Lentils: A high-protein pulse, widely cultivated in Eurasian countries, an annual leguminous plant (*Lens culinaris*) with flattened edible seeds.

Nutritional Physiology: Deals with the study of nutrients, their role in the growth and health of different types of food and their effect on methabolism.

Plant-Derived Proteins: Foods obtained from plant sources, including vegetables, whole grains, nuts, seeds, legumes, and fruits, with no animal products.

Quinoa: A plant of the goosefoot family originally found in the Andes, where it is widely cultivated for its small, edible, starchy, ivory-colored seed, which is used as a food staple.

Soybean: Annual Asian legume (*Glycine max*) widely grown for its oil-rich proteinaceous seeds, for forage and soil improvement.

Spirulina: A biomass of cyanobacteria (blue-green algae) that can be consumed as food or nutritional supplement.

Teff: An African cereal native to Ethiopia, cultivated as a staple food crop, for flour and used for making traditional fermented breads.

This research was previously published in Environmental, Health, and Business Opportunities in the New Meat Alternatives Market edited by Diana Bogueva, Dora Marinova, Talia Raphaely, and Kurt Schmidinger; pages 62-83, copyright year 2019 by Business Science Reference (an imprint of IGI Global).

Chapter 59

Understanding Gender Identities and Food Preferences to Increase the Consumption of a Plant-Based Diet With Heuristics

Estela Seabra
The New School, USA

ABSTRACT

This chapter discerns existent food preferences and their correlation with women and men, and gender biases, in America. It then proposes a strategy to test the most efficient heuristics to nudge those more averse to a plant-based, sustainable diet. By understanding how negative biases can be reversed through the application of behavioral economics, the plant-based industry and American government can most effectively build marketing procedures to be employed in campaigns, menus, packaging, and media to portray sustainable diets as appealing for men and women, and important for environmental wellbeing. The study recognizes and navigates the irrationality of human preferences as actors in the food market. By accounting for gender norms, cultural roles, and subconscious behavior, it will effectively produce insight on the best heuristical approaches to cognitively orchestrate a wider acceptance, and consequent consumption, of plant-based foods.

INTRODUCTION

As the world's population climbs at a faster rate than ever before, global temperature levels mount with it. The emission of greenhouse gases produced directly and indirectly by individuals is the pivotal source for change, be that either positive or negative. Before the 1960's, society was not fully aware of the dire damage with which their overuse of finite resources and livelihoods could cause upon planet Earth. Since discovering that these overused resources, which are relied on for the majority of human

DOI: 10.4018/978-1-7998-5354-1.ch059

functions, are limited and being depleted, it became a global issue to minimize their use, and optimize energy efficiency. As a foundational phenomenon of global warming, greenhouse gases trap substances in the Earth's atmosphere, cause sea levels to rise, disrupt ecosystems, eradicates species of fauna and flora, and may render human existence in this planed infeasible.

Numerous attempts have been made to curb our intervention with nature, however many of the already proposed issues lack accountability for being much too broad in dimension, and consequently unlikely to be attainable on a daily basis for the average individual. Others view the tackling of the environmental degradation issue with a financial priority, as opposed to a behavioral one, and tend to overestimate the time of environmental consequences, underestimate their costs, and ignore countless externalities. In addition, classical behavioral insights overlook the human tendency for individuals to respond illogically, emotionally, or in a way that does not maximize their utility.

THEORETICAL BACKGROUND AND PURPOSE

It has been found by Pew Research Center that men who do not eat meat are perceived as approximately 40% less masculine than women. There are no hormonal imbalances, data or behavioral traits to support this observation. Moreover, it has been found that women are significantly more likely to try, adhere to and buy sustainably-produced foods, especially plant-based diets. It is theorized that strong ties between the public's perception of a vegan diet and sexism exist. This is likely the case due to media representation. If this is found to be true in the analysis, it will be crucial to identify potential instances of sexism and gender representations to understand the behavioral triggers they activate, and propose heuristic strategies to alter the outlook of a plant-based diet from one of "unmanliness", "fragility" and "undernutrition", to a more all-encompassing gender outlook that appeals to the participation of all people.

Moreover, beyond neutralizing the potential sexist cognitive biases revolving around veganism in the media, this proposal aims to suggest heuristic nudges to inspire and animate individuals towards a sustainable, plant-based diet as a symbol of personal empowerment based on responsibility and an interconnectedness with humanity. It may contribute to the goal of sustainable practices, illuminating the symbiotic nature of social circles and their environment. By harnessing behavioral pushes to perceive vegan diets as nutritionally complete, tasteful and empowering, public cognitive biases that hold no factual basis will become unfounded, unsustainable. Thus, individuals can be positively nudged to follow diet choices that benefit themselves, their peers, the ecosystem, and future lives. The study will discern the most effective heuristics, alone and in combination, focused on American target audiences, to create these nudges.

Research Question

How can heuristics most efficiently be used to nudge the American public to positively perceive vegan food and livelihoods, accounting for different gender preferences and gendered food biases?

Hypothesis

It is hypothesized that men and women will react differently to different heuristics. It is theorized that men will react more strongly to heuristics, colors, anchoring and such that reinforces their already existent, preconceived masculine ideals. Similarly, women will also strongly respond to heuristics that anchor veganism to feminine ideals. However, it is theorized that women, being less aversely biased to the vegan food industry, potentially due to its linkage with weight loss (a widespread archetype amongst US women), will also respond most strongly to heuristic use that reinforces vegan information, and the nutritional benefits of foods. Simultaneously, it is hypothesized that men will be more responsive to gustatory pleasure and lifestyle status than information.

Uses

By understanding the American female and male psyche regarding veganism, nudging procedures will be proposed to improve their public perceptions. Ultimately, the study's findings, when applied, can potentially curb consumer behavior. This will offer aid to appease part of the negative environmental externalities caused by the overuse of resources by the animal industry. Individuals will shift their internalized biases towards sustainable, vegan food without attributing disapproval due to unfounded, generalized ideas. Test results will allow the public to be heuristically targeted in their market actions, to find sustainable foods more appealing. It is intended that the results attained may be employed to generate positive public perceptions by the way of the lifestyle veganism may offer (wellbeing in the present and future), and create a superior status around it, to incite individuals to desire to be a part of it. Ideally, the heuristic procedures will be precise enough to be used across communities, socioeconomic dimensions, companies and industries, yet in a feasible, strategic manner intended for different audiences. Ultimately, target markets will be engaged to make choices occur multiple times each day, through food procurement and consumption.

Methodology

For the purpose of this study, conscious and subconscious actions and preferences, biases and mind triggers will be tested. This will allow for a more effective understanding of how average urban Americans respond in different ways, to preference architecture using varying heuristics. Because of the state of current urban and rural US food systems, industrialized food, which frequently contains animal by-products, is significantly cheaper than fresh foods. Thus, this questionnaire and study aims to target consumers with food security, availability, and enough disposable income to purchase food that may be costlier, but is sustainable.

The study will be carried out in three parts. Firstly, a questionnaire will determine the baseline gender norms an individual has, revolving around food. This will determine the consumption habits of the test subject, and how they are affected by social norms within their environment, which, as has been determined, greatly influence food psychology, preference and consumption.

A second questionnaire will then explicitly ask test subjects how they perceive people who follow a vegan diet, how they believe vegans are viewed and treated by civilization in different social instances, and how they believe eating less meat will influence their professional and social lives. It will also enquire how they feel about veganism, gustatory and nutritionally, how they consider current advertising and marketing (with a positive or negative bias, effectively or non-effectively), and how they believe the industry could better itself in marketing, identity and advertisement, to increase sales. In order to encourage test subjects to respond thoughtfully, the answers will be collected in written answers, with several lines to write on (anchoring subjects to write more), and also via phone polls (and recorded for tone, emotion and conversational purposes).

Furthermore, a prize will be offered to the most effective marketing strategy response for the last question, incentivizing subjects to propose advertising approaches that they truly believe will improve the attractiveness of the product. Lastly, the questionnaire will have a "tick the box" section. The questions will explicitly ask how the subject believes each heuristic (explained) can affect the sales, gustatory and nutritional perception, and public perception of different food products. For this series of questions, test subjects can explicitly mark "effective", "slightly effective", "no change", "slightly ineffective" or "ineffective". This section will be last in the questionnaire so as to prevent anchoring in the test subjects' minds when answering the primary questions. They will evaluate the explicit perceived effect of different heuristics on the packaging, branding and advertising of vegan food goods. For example, there will be e brief explanation of a heuristic, and the questionnaire will ask for the explicit perceived effect on the psyche of the consumer. This will tap into the conscious food preferences, which will complement the final part of the study – the implicit testing preferences.

Finally, the third portion of the study will analyze not-necessarily conscious biases of consumers. This protocol will place food products in supermarket isles, testing the customer response to heuristics mentioned in the introduction, one at each time, and measure the sales outcome. It will make use of one heuristic at each time, replacing the same product with the same packaging, except for the heuristic used, until all heuristics have been tested for the same products. Then, heuristics will be united in different combinations, to assess how different heuristics used together may boost psychological nudging when united with other behavioral nudges.

The products will vary in demographic, so as not to limit the study for the target market only of one food product (such as cookies, cereal or hamburger, to diverge the target audience and thus the information collected), but will be used on foods that may be traditionally vegan or not, so as to fairly test the general public response to a vegan option of a conventional food. Mid to high-end supermarkets will be proposed to be part of the study, because this is the general public with financial stability to be able to make the choice to potentially pay more for an organic, vegan, fair trade, sustainable product. The supermarkets will be offered the incentive of being able to benefit from the information obtained – learning more about their consumer audience, and how to target it effectively and increase their sales and profits. All goods will be tested throughout a year, to correct for temporal and seasonal preferences (such as thanksgiving turkey preferences, summer salad preferences, and so on).

Results

After analyzing the relationship between gender perceptions and how they interplay with sustainable plant-based diets in the methodology, recommendations that disseminate a positive mindset can be produced, available to all but specifically useful for sustainable food producers, governmental initiatives, restaurant owners, and any and all individuals/corporations interested in normalizing societal standards of eating sustainably. Suggestions will use key economics concepts to navigate public perceptions of sustainable diets. Behavioral economics' heuristics, color psychology, losses loom larger than gains, and other nudging to shift gender-related prospects within social norms will be tested and employed. By uniting behavioral economics with an environmental mission, the concluding strategy will generate more impact. Social perceptions of veganism (which is not the definition of a sustainable diet, but very much a key constituent of one) will be changed beside the current representation of plant-based diets and gender preferences tied to such diets.

By employing these guidelines in the modes described below, agents can behave in a more sustainable manner in the food production and consumption market, whether it be conscious or not. This study will ultimately orchestrate choice architecture to modify judgments and decision-making patterns in favor of a wider sustainable diet adoption.

Discussion

The heuristic concepts employed will target cognitive laziness, incorporating availability, representativeness, anchoring, paradox of choice, color theory, losses loom larger than gains, priming, reciprocity, familiarity and confirmation bias to architect consumers' gendered choices in the food industry. Cognitive biases will be targeted by using existing irrational patterns in judgment against the individual. Because, by nature, cognitive biases diverge from logic, individuals will ultimately be nudged differently between men and women, to make better food and environmental choices, be these choices conscious or involuntary. The results will be employed to ignite certain feelings, biases, perceptions and emotions in order to curb their food-choosing behaviors. Gender roles will be retained and observed, used in a way that paints veganism in a positive, empowering way for all genders in the final marketing strategy recommendations. The marketing protocol guide will also be used to reiterate the importance of adhering to a sustainable diet, after its gender preferences are dismantled/altered.

CONCLUSION

This study holds the possibility to change paradigms associated with sustainable diets being un-tasty, unmanly, nutritionally weak, and so forth. By making use of subconscious triggers within the human psyche, dietary nudging can foster a notion of interconnectedness now and in the future, behave in a more environmentally-conscious manner, and drop assumptions about gender constructs and diet choices, which are essentially unenlightened and lack reasoning. Among positive externalities is the potential of positive perceptions of veganism to promote health, by focusing on real, whole foods, as opposed to the current overconsumption of saturated animal fats and cholesterol, which is unsustainable to the environment. Moreover, broader acceptance of vegan foods through the marketing protocol produced may help develop a broader communal and individual awareness of what is positive and degrading to the environment, health, future generations, and nutritional information.

Lastly, this knowledge may externalize into more people understanding, becoming interested in improving other choices and behaviors in their lives to improve the environment. For example, it can induce individuals to become informed about "fair-trade" policies, and the benefits of local consumption. Should they adhere to these practices, they may boost the consumption of local or fair-trade foods, saving the businesses of many small agricultural workers, and empower them to cultivate an ethical food system. Lastly, actors will potentially promote animal welfare, through food consumption that is harmonious with practices deemed to return balance to the ecosystem around them. They may support and protect local communities, empower and protect workers, and improve the lives of their descendants in the future.

Limitations

This study will mostly be applicable to inelastic consumers, actors with food security and financial comfort, the resources to make assorted food choices, and access to pop culture and media advertisement. The ultimate aim is to expose which heuristics are most effective in targeting American mid/upper-class males' and females' biases against vegan foods, needed to dissolve to live more sustainably. Following this study, the use in the real world is to then use this consumer information for what is now a niche market, encouraging consumers to buy more vegan foods (and then consequently, the crowding-out effect of animal products to follow). This would expand the consumption of vegan foods, enlarge the vegan market, and thus create more availability, and representativeness, and normalization of vegan foods. Since the study has not yet been done, it cannot be discerned which heuristics work the most effectually to dissolve these gender-based assumptions against vegan foods. Only after understanding the nature of such negative perceptions may one distinguish where anti-vegan sentiments arise, from both men and women, which each stem from very different places during eating.

Secondly, behavioral triggers are by nature controversial, and may vary by year, with preference and diet trends, the change in price of complementary and substitute goods, and advances in knowledge or technology. While very powerful at times, marketing is also ethically questionable to use to modify behavior, and it would be necessary to make ethical use of the results amassed.

Finally, it would have been ideal to delve further into all the different measures of heuristics to develop the best behavioral understanding and strategy, fully testing all known nudging and perception-shifting tools. However, due to the length constraints of this study, if it were to do that cohesively, this entire study would only be able to accommodate one of the heuristics mentioned. An opportunity to be developed further in the future.

REFERENCES

Draft Concept Note: Commemoration of the 8th Africa Day for Food and Nutrition Security with Continental Symposium on Food Systems. (2017). Retrieved from www.nepad.org/resource/draftconcept-note-commemoration-8th-africa-day-food-and-nutrition-security-continental

GRACE Communications Foundation. (n.d.). *Why Buy Sustainable?* GRACE Communications Foundation. Retrieved from www.sustainabletable.org/943/why-buy-sustainable

Hardman, D. (2009). *Judgment and Decision Making: Psychological Perspectives*. Wiley-Blackwell.

Kahneman, D., Slovic, P., & Tversky, A. (1982). *Judgment Under Uncertainty: Heuristics and Biases*. Cambridge, UK: Cambridge University Press. doi:10.1017/CBO9780511809477

Sustainability. (2017, April 26). *The Nutrition Source*. Retrieved from www.hsph.harvard.edu/nutrition-source/sustainability/

Sustainable Table | Why Buy Sustainable? (n.d.). Retrieved from www.bing.com/cr?IG=9CAA4BD D276F4B0296D3B54B99C3B89E&CID=1134 A93065B065073EA8A2D2641F640F&rd=1&h=-r6WjqF3ltOZt9FzWVEo2Uz_UXf1M0-uAD1hcpICy_k&v=1&r=http://www.sustainabletable.org/943/why-buysustainable&p=DevEx.LB.1,5521.1

This research was previously published in Intergenerational Governance and Leadership in the Corporate World edited by Julia Margarete Puaschunder; pages 30-38, copyright year 2019 by Business Science Reference (an imprint of IGI Global).

Chapter 60
Lifelong Consumption of Plant-Based GM Foods:
Is It Safe?

Matthew Chidozie Ogwu
https://orcid.org/0000-0001-6054-1667
Seoul National University, South Korea

ABSTRACT

Genetically modified (GM) crops are cultivated in over 30 countries with their products and by-products imported by over 60 countries. This chapter seeks to highlight general concerns and potential lifelong effects of consuming GM plant-based food. The consumption of GM plant-based food is as risky as consuming conventional plant-based food. However, the alien genes in these products may be unstable leading to antinutritional and unintended short-term consequences. Due to the paucity of research, no long-term effects have been attributed to the lifelong consumption of these products. Nonetheless, possible lifelong health and socioeconomic effects may result from outcrossing of genes, increasing antibiotic resistance, development of new diseases, as well as potential effects on the environment and biodiversity. Biotechnology companies need to invest more in interdisciplinary research addressing the potential lifelong effects of these products. Although GM foods are safe for consumption, clarification of current risks and lifelong effects are required.

INTRODUCTION

Plants remain the central food resources for humans and other animals. However, there is increasing pressure on the resources to fulfil this basic need. Population growth, particularly in countries with developing economies, will result in a need to overexploit plant resources to increase food production (Ogwu et al., 2014; Delaney, 2015). Climate change might make economic crops unsuitable for cultivation in their centre of origins and diversity as these areas become increasingly threatened by drought, floods, spread of plant diseases and altered weather patterns (Thompson, 2017). More so, lifestyle changes continue to influence plant use patterns across the globe. For instance, Łuczaj et al. (2012), reported

DOI: 10.4018/978-1-7998-5354-1.ch060

significant changes in the contemporary use of wild food plants in parts of Europe due to the decline of plant knowledge, the disappearance of traditional methods of plant use, reduced availability of plants due to ecosystem changes, land access rights for foragers and intoxication hazards. Hence, even though global agricultural productivity has significantly improved, issues related to food security persist because of multidirectional issues (Lamichhane, 2014).

This chapter seeks to highlight general concerns pertaining to the consumption of genetically modified (GM) plant-based food products. The chapter will address it from an environment and health perspective. Short-term effects of consuming GM plant-based food are easily discernible but not the long-term effects, which may take years, decades or even a lifetime to appear (Murnaghan, 2018). The need to be vigilant and assess the potential risks of such unpredictable occurrences cannot be ignored (Butler and Reichhardt, 1999). GM plants and plant-based products are here to stay regardless of conflicting standpoints. In the sustainable future, which is a long-term global goal, these products might become indispensable. Therefore, so much needs to be done from the different players to make GM products more acceptable. The objective of this chapter is to promote the knowledge of GM plants and plant-based products, their lifelong health and environmental effects as well as to proffer salient recommendations to address pertinent issues. Through these contributions, this chapter will reduce existing fears as well as increase the knowledge, understanding and highlight practical gaps concerning the production and consumption of GM plants and plant-based products.

PUBLIC PERCEPTION OF THE NEEDS AND BENEFITS OF GM PLANTS

The need to achieve food security has led to the intensification of agriculture, which naturally interferes with natural ecological cycles. The agricultural sector contributes to the emission of environmentally dangerous chemicals like ammonia, methane, and nitrates (Zhu et al., 2006). GM plants held under cultivation has long been considered as a sustainable alternative to attain food self-sufficiency and sovereignty albeit controversial. The three pathways by which GM crops contribute to food security include increasing food production and availability, influencing food safety and quality as well as enhancing the economic and social situation of farmers, thereby influencing food accessibility (Qaim and Kouser, 2013). Hunger is a major threat to humanity and it affects an estimated more than 1 billion people many of whom live in developing countries (Delaney, 2015; Hefferon, 2016). It remains our moral obligation to feed the hungry billions. To this end, the GM crop movement has overseen enormous good but also presented significant adverse consequences and prompted controversies (Schlett and Beke, 2015).

GM is the application of gene technology to alter an organism's genome by combining genes from different organisms through recombinant DNA technology to produce a new or modified organism, which may be described as 'GM', 'genetically engineered' or 'transgenic' (Bawa and Anilakumar, 2013). This technology exploits gene variations, expressions and modifications to produce outstanding crops for human benefits. It is distinct from the production of clones, which culminates in genetically identical copies. This technology-based manipulation of living things began with microorganisms and then economic plants but have since expanded to include other organisms from diverse taxa. Insertion of defined foreign genes into the genome of bacteria, moulds, yeast, etc., has resulted in the creation of genetically modified organisms (GMOs). These GMOs or their by-products are primarily used for human food productions as well as in different industrial processes including the production of pharmaceuticals (Lisowska, 2011). Therefore, most GM foods stem mostly from plants, which have been GM to improve their yield, through the introduction of one or several resistant-components against plant pests, disease prevention or increased tolerance of herbicides and environmental extremes (Domingo, 2016).

The original aim of producing GM plants was to produce plant varieties that are fast-growing, disease and drought resistance, more nutritious and can out-compete weeds to maximize plant resources for food security. However, the pressure to feed the ever-increasing human population continues to drive the expansion of the limits of GM companies and GMOs. The potentials of this technology is limitless because of the possible manipulation of the processes and outcomes to serve other contemporary societal challenges besides food security with adverse implications on plant diversity and the environment. For instance, bananas that produce human vaccines against infectious diseases such as hepatitis B, fruit and nut trees that yield years earlier and plants that produce new plastics with unique properties (Bawa and Anilakumar, 2013). All these have succeeded in exacerbating the consequences of GM technology and public concerns. According to Frewer and Shepher (1995), these are manifested as an overall rejection of specific aspects of the technology, where public attitudes may be defined by a complex set of perceptions incorporating risk, benefit, control, and ethical concerns. Underlying this concern is that a large proportion of the public remains unaware of what a GM plant and plant-based product actually are or what advantages and disadvantages the technology has to offer (Key et al., 2008). This stem from the persistence of concerns related to environmental quality and human health risks since the introduction of the technology. As suggested by Qaim and Kouser (2013), GM products may have impacts on food quality, quantity, availability, nutrient composition, and household income. All of which may potentially lead to diverse psychological effects at the personal, family and community levels. In spite of the increase in available information on the potential toxic effects of GM foods and plants, concerns about their environment and health risks persist (Domingo, 2000; Domingo and Gomez, 2000; Domingo, 2007; Domingo, 2011; Domingo and Bordonaba, 2011; Domingo, 2016).

Recent concerns regarding the safety of GM plant-based foods from diverse groups including consumers and environmental non-governmental organizations (NGO) have led to social and political debates on the potential negative impacts of transgenic plants, with suggestions that all the related products should be subjected to long-term studies before approval for human consumption (Domingo and Bordonaba, 2011; Domingo, 2016). More than 20 years have passed since the approval of genetic modifications in food and the world is yet to fully come to terms with their success albeit increasing number of products. In the same vein, the declaration by the World Health Organization's (WHO) that these products should be subjected to risk assessments for human nutrition and health have not been systematically performed (Domingo, 2007; Magaña-Gómez and de la Barca, 2009). However, with an increasingly less productive environment affecting the yields of most major crops, the future is very promising for GM technologies to meet the future global needs for food, feed and fibre in a sustainable and responsible way (Oliver, 2014). GM plants for food use has the potential to offer benefits in agricultural practice, food quality, nutrition and health, but several aspects of GM technology still require further clarifications (The Royal Society, 2002) including areas under cultivation, risk assessment, and the level of uncertainty and unpredictability associated with each GM crop (Tsatsakis et al., 2017). In addition, the public is often uninformed or misinformed about most GMOs and their potential side effects (Twardowski and Małyska. 2015).

GM PLANTS AND GM PLANT-BASED FOOD AND PRODUCTS

There is a heavy burden on the world to eliminate food insecurity in all regions and technology seem to be the most plausible option. Plant breeders desire to develop plant varieties that express good agronomic qualities but through conventional breeding, there is little to no guarantee of obtaining any particular gene combination from millions of test crosses in search of desirable characters (Lamichhane, 2014). This shortcoming can be overcome through genetic engineering, which allows the direct transfer of one or just a few genes of interest between seemingly related or unrelated organisms to obtain the desired agronomic traits. Modern biotechnology has the potential to be a significant tool in fighting hunger as it is well positioned to address agricultural problems such as yield loss from insect infestation, competition with weeds, drought, etc. (Delaney, 2015). Hence, through modern biotechnology, GM plant and plant-based products are asexually and artificially produced when two or more alien genetic materials are added to the recombinant DNA technology or genetic engineering process to solve specific agricultural challenge.

Historically, the technology became popular in the twentieth century when the bacteria *Escherichia coli* was used to produce insulin in human diabetic patients. However, it was only after the discovery of Polymerase Chain Reaction technique, which allowed the amplification of target nucleic acid fragments, thus making it possible to copy or change DNA sequence that the technology could take on wider applications. Moreover, novel applications of recombinant DNA technology evolved alongside the development of genetic processes and biological variations, which made the production of important products possible (Shivanand and Noopur, 2010). In addition, there has been a generational trend aimed at making necessary techniques simpler and easier to perform. At that pace, plants with recognizable economic value became the subject of genetic modification with little to no consideration of their ethnobotany, diversity or environmental implications. The first attempts to genetically modify crops were undertaken in the 1980s on tobacco. However, the first GM food crops were FLAVR SAVR™ tomato that was engineered for delayed ripening and were subsequently commercialized in 1994 in the USA (Kok and Kuiper, 2003; Lisowska, 2011). The FLAVR SAVR™ tomato contained a foreign gene that prevented the breakdown of cell walls as the fruit ripened as well as for the fruits to remain firm after extended shipping and storage period (Schneider et al., 2017). Worldwide, over 148 million hectares of GM crops were cultivated in 2010 (ISAAA 2010). ISAAA (2012) reported that in 2012, GM crops were planted in 28 countries with developing countries accounting for a majority of the total GM harvest. From 1996 to 2014, 357 GM crops were approved and the global value of the GM crop market reached 35% of the global commercial seed market in 2014 albeit with different controversies (Lin and Pan, 2016). Each year the EU imports about 30 million tons of grain, soybeans, and maize, most of which are transgenic (Twardowski and Małyska. 2015).

In summary, GM crops are produced after identifying a trait of interest (in the same or different plant species), isolating that trait through comparative analysis (or via deletion, knock down, seed chipping process), inserting that trait into the genome of the test crop using gene gun or microorganism (commonly used ones are the bacteria *Agrobacterium tumefaciens* and *Bacillus thuringiensis*), and then propagating the GM crop (Figure 1). The newly produced plants containing genes from another organism are called "transgenic plant", "GM crop", "genetically engineered plants," or, more broadly, "genetically modified organisms" (Wieczorek, 2013, Magaña-Gómez and Calderón de la Barca, 2009).

Production of GM plant involves targeting the best genotypes based on phenotype for regeneration in tissue culture by exploiting the DNA transfer mechanisms of organisms like bacteria (Southgate et al., 1995; Powell, 2015; Bawa and Anilakumar, 2013). The main limiting steps are locating genes for

Figure 1. An overview of how GM crops are produced
Source: Pighin, 2003.

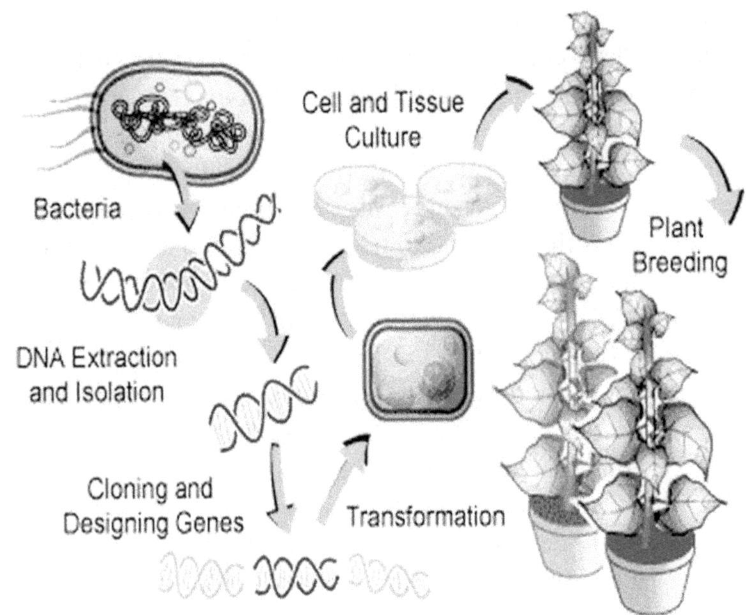

important traits (Bawa and Anilakumar, 2013). According to Schneider et al. (2017), GM plants are the outcome of moving genes from one organism to another causing the transferees' genetic makeup to be altered and the expression of hitherto unexpressed attributes like delayed-ripening in tomatoes, pest-resistant in squash and potato, herbicide-tolerance in cotton and soybean, etc. Through this process, major transgenic economic plants have been produced including tobacco, tomato, canola, alfalfa, cantaloupe, radicchio, papaya, flax, plum, wheat, apple, creeping bentgrass, sugar beet, maize, cotton, soybean, potato, squash, eggplants, strawberry, lettuce, rice, carrots, etc.

This procedure has raised health concerns through the use of selectable markers to identify transformed cells, transfer of extraneous DNA into the plant genome and the increased mutations in GM plants compared to non-GM counterparts due to tissue culture processes used in their production and the rearrangement of DNA around the insertion site of foreign genes (Key et al., 2008). Other considerations include antibiotic resistance, disease resistance, extreme weather resistance, early or delayed ripening, modified composition and herbicide resistance. Nonetheless, these crops find their way to our dining table, pharmaceutical and departmental stores through major biotechnology companies and their subsidiaries like Calgene, Monsanto, Asgrow, Zeneca and Peto. Different bodies like the Food and Drug Administration (in the USA) and European Food Safety Authority (of the European Union) regulate the production of GMO and their food or other products. Testing on GMOs in plant food can be done using molecular techniques like DNA microarrays or qPCR to screen for genetic elements like p35S, tNos, pat, or bar or event specific markers for the official GMOs like Mon810, Bt11, or GT73 (Bawa and Anilakumar, 2013). Hundreds of millions of people have knowingly or unknowingly used products derived from GM crops across the world for more than 15 years (Key et al., 2008).

When GM plants become mature, they are harvested either wholly or in parts and from it a variety of products (domestic and/or industrial) can be derived. Ready-to-eat plant-based food and/or food ingredients (materials) derived from plants whose genome has been modified through an artificial process is referred to as GM plant-based foods and GM plant-based products respectively. Some of these products include omega-3 supplements (Usher, 2017), vaccines (Phillips, 2008), industrial vegetable oil (European Chemicals Agency, 2012), fattening feed for farm animals (Grant, 2017), etc. The labelling of products with ingredients sourced from GM plant enables the identification of GM plant-based products (Wong, 2003; Carter and Gruere, 2003; Byrne et al., 2014). The review by Domingo and Bordonaba (2011) suggest that a huge research void exists for certain GM crops (especially cucumber, peas or tomatoes) while reporting that many research studies on certain GM crops (like maize and soybeans) implicate that they are as safe and nutritious as the respective conventional non-GM plant. Over 90% of biotechnology crops produced worldwide include just four plants: soybean, maize, rape and cotton (Lisowska, 2011). Most GM crops are commonly engineered to be resistant to the herbicide glyphosate that enables farmers to increase efficiency in eliminating weeds without harming their crops or with a natural insecticide to protect the yields of these crops against insect infestation, which is more environmentally friendly than using toxic sprays (Thompson, 2017). Most plants naturally perceive foreign organisms capable of causing infections but efficiency varies within and between species. Therefore, the proteins that identify an infection and activate defences can be moved between and within species using genetic modification to enable previously vulnerable crops to turn on their innate resistance mechanisms (Thompson, 2017). Recent advances in gene editing technology using CRISPR-Cas9 have also made it possible to rewrite plant genes so that they work for different sensing function.

Fernandez-Cornejo and Caswell (2006); Magaña-Gómez and Calderón de la Barca (2009); Lin and Pan (2016); Schneider et al. (2017) classified GM plants into one of four generations based on the objective of the introduced traits;

1. First-generation i.e. crops enhanced through the input of single traits to increase production, such as herbicide tolerance, better insect resistance, and tolerance to environmental stress. Most first-generation GM crops contain common transgene elements such as the cauliflower mosaic virus (CaMV), 35S promoter (CaMV35S-P), aminoglycoside 30 -phosphotransferase gene (nptII), phosphinothricin acetyltransferase gene (pat/bar), 5-enolpyruvylshikimate 3-phosphate (CP4-epsp) gene, nopaline synthase promoter (nos-P), and terminator (nos-T) (Lin and Pan, 2016).
2. Second-generation i.e. crops with added-value output through hybrid crosses between commercialized first-generation GM crops to increase consumer benefits, such as nutrient enhancement for animal feed.
3. Third-generation i.e. crops with increased resistant to abiotic stress with industrial roles including pharmaceuticals and biofuels. They are also called near-intragenic, or GM crops where the inserted transgenic.
4. The fourth generation i.e. these are true intragenic and cisgenic, which genuine host genes. Thus, fourth-generation GM crops/foods cannot be distinguished via their transgenic elements and can be identified by inspecting the specific order and insertion loci of its transgenes (Lin and Pan, 2016).

Seed producers are required to submit applications to USDA APHIS (United States Department of Agriculture Animal and Plant Health Inspection Service) for field-testing (Fernandez-Cornejo and Caswell 2006). Approvals are not easily granted but crops with most approvals include corn, cotton, tomatoes, soybeans, rapeseed/canola, potatoes, sugar beets, papaya, rice, squash, alfalfa, plum, rose, tobacco, flax, and chicory (USDA 2014). The percentage of products available in the market that contains at least one GM product is high. Approximately 60 – 70% of processed foods in the United States contain GM components (Ahmed 2002; Dahl, 2012; Schneider et al. 2017). More so, the use of GM plants has increased. For instance, Fernandez-Cornejo (2012) reported that the use of *Bacillus thuringiensis* corn has increased dramatically from its introduction in 1996 to about 15 per cent of total corn acreage in 2012, although those numbers have varied dramatically depending on the year. Recently, Bushey et al. (2014) opined that GM crops may contain newly expressed proteins that are described as ''intractable', which have properties that make it extremely difficult or impossible with current methods to express in heterologous systems; isolate, purify, or concentrate; quantify (due to low levels); demonstrate biological activity; or prove equivalency with plant proteins. Bushey et al concluded that their use and subsequent expression does not present any risk and gave the five classes of these intractable proteins as membrane proteins, signalling proteins, transcription factors, N-glycosylated proteins, and resistance proteins (R-proteins, plant pathogen recognition proteins that activate innate immune responses). Some of the contributions of GM crops and plant-based product include an increase in global agricultural production and farmer's income, reduced application of insecticides, herbicides and fertilizers, increased investment in agriculture, land management, and reduced GHG emission

LIFELONG EFFECTS OF CONSUMING GM PLANTS AND PLANT-BASED PRODUCTS

Lifelong experiences associated with the consumption of GM plants and plant-based products may be expressed in human (or animal) health as well as through lasting environmental changes. Although the issue remains unattractive to scientists and large GMO-based companies probably because of the potential outcomes. Whereas the possibility of short-term side effects of consuming GM crops has attracted attention from both scientific and public groups (Kok and Kuiper, 2003). Healthwise, these lifelong effects may include diseases or genetic predispositions with environment-specific interactions, which may result in physiological adaptations or disruptions with lifelong outcomes in learning, behaviour, as well as in emotional, physical and mental well-being. This is because constant experiences are built into our bodies, creating biological memories that shape development, for better or for worse. For instance, the elderly are most susceptible to new dietary experiences because they have an accumulated burden of chemical exposure over their lifetime hence, some of their body processes are shutting down as well as hormonal disruptions (Swanson, 2013). Moreover, Fontes et al. (2002) suggested some accumulated experience related to exposure of insect-resistant transgenic crops. In addition, the introduction of non-native GM plants in the ecosystems also pose potential long-term risks to the environment whose consequences may be difficult to predict from diverse standpoints (Tsatsakis et al., 2017). Kuiper et al (2001) argued that the consumption of non-GM crops might also result in similar side effects as those from GM crops. Nonetheless, it is worrisome that many potential short and long-term side effects remain undetected due to analysing focussed only on specific compounds or intermediates especially in relation to important nutritional and anti-nutritional pathways. Thereby giving rise to likely undetected lifelong effects.

The subsequent sections will focus on potential health and environmental lifelong effects from the consumption of GM plants and plant-based products.

1.   Potential Lifelong Health Effects of Consuming Plant-Based GM Products

The safety of plant-based GM foods for consumption has remained a hot topic and the rarity of research data in this regard may be a contributory factor. Health risks associated with GM foods fall into three main categories: toxins, allergens, and genetic hazards (Conner and Jacobs, 1999). The Royal Society (2002) without considering gene expression products, suggested that there is no evidence of intact gene transfer to humans (and animals) either from vector organisms used in GM plants in the gut or from foodstuffs, despite daily consumption of GM food. Thereby emphasizing that the risks associated with food and food products derived from this recombinant biotechnology are only similar to those for conventional foods (ISAAA, 2009). However, risks exist and may not have been properly defined neither are the consumers always made aware of whatever level of risk exist. Potential transfer of genes from GM plant-based foods are capable of inducing insertional mutagenesis resulting from gene integration due to the inserted genes and their expression products, secondary and pleiotropic effects of gene expression (Bawa and Anilakumar, 2013). More so, the proteins produced by the transgene may be toxic, which can result in additional allergic reactions and/or on the other hand, the production of complex multimeric proteins such as antibodies, which are not readily expressed by microbial systems (Key et al., 2008). These potential transgene protein activities were also acknowledged by USDA (2013) cited in Arya (2015) and could occur because the traits that are introduced into a particular plant are new to that plant but are often found naturally in other plants. The Royal Society (2002) supports this when they reported that the introduction of a new gene into a plant or a change in the expression of an existing gene might cause it to become allergenic, although, in principle, these might not be greater than those posed by conventionally derived crops. Swanson (2013) presented another scenario, wherein, the bacteria (vector) genes are not only potentially toxic but as in some cases, the transgenic herbicide-resistant plants are sprayed and absorb the poisons, which are later consumed and could cause infertility, birth defects, organ diseases as well as neurological, intestinal and immune-diseases. Although the author pointed out that correlation does not necessarily imply causation and there are now a host of other chemicals in our food and our environment.

Generally, food-related issues are known to have lifelong health and socio-psychological effects. For instance, because of food poisoning from microorganisms, kidney failure, chronic arthritis, gastrointestinal infections, Crohn's disease, brain and nerve damage, rheumatism, and death have developed. The safety of the vector used in producing GM plant-based food is a potential source of lifelong effects — such as the *Agrobacterium tumefaciens* vector (Butler and Reichhardt, 1999). Rats fed GM corn over a period of 90 days developed problems with their liver, kidneys, heart, blood cells, spleen and adrenal glands in a sex- and dose-dependent manner (de Vendômois et al., 2009). The authors also showed that rats fed with GM corn over a long period became increasingly infertile as well as developed mammary gland tumours and suggested that it may be due to the new pesticides specific to each GM corn. In the same way, broad unintended direct or indirect metabolic consequences of genetic modification cannot be excluded. Bawa and Anilakumar (2013) opined that many transgenes encode enzymes capable of altering biochemical pathways causing an increase or decrease in certain biochemical or enzyme substrate and a subsequent build-up of the enzymatic product that supports the latter point.

Furthermore, technological advancement in GM crop production have enabled the modification of traits that can affect the functional properties of the final product like the long-ripening tomatoes with favourable post-harvest characteristics suitable for processing the tomato into paste and oilseed crops with modified oil composition such as high oleic acid (more stable during frying) (Kok and Kuiper, 2003). Kok and Kuiper suggested that these modifications might be used to alleviate nutritional deficiencies such as vitamin A deficiency and/or anaemia in through consumption of 'Golden Rice' fortified with provitamin A and iron-fortified GM rice. Food allergies and severe allergic reactions (anaphylaxis) are caused by allergens, which are mostly proteins. The protein components of GM plants may be implicated in their functional properties because the introduction of a new gene into a plant, or a change in the expression of an existing gene, may cause that plant to become allergenic even though no evidence exists at present that GM foods cause any clinical manifestations of allergenicity (The Royal Society, 2002). The persistence of pesticide residues in GM food is a hot topic in Europe. A popular notion highlighted in Kok and Kuiper (2003) is that traditional crop plant varieties on which our livelihood depends are not elaborately tested for safety prior to their popular use, therefore this history of safe use can be used as a baseline for the safety assessment of new GM plant varieties derived from established plant lines. Although GM and conventional sources induce similar nutritional performance and growth, adverse microscopic and molecular effects of some GM foods in different organs or tissues have been reported to a certain extent (Magaña-Gómez and de la Barca, 2009; Domingo and Bordonaba, 2011). The norm is to *ab initio* compare GM outputs with cultivars but this approach is not sustainable. The principle of substantial equivalence is based on the notion that, "if a new food is found to be substantially equivalent in composition and nutritional characteristics to an existing food, it can be regarded as being as safe as the conventional food" (SOT, 2003). The application of the concept is not a safety assessment per se; rather it enables the identification of potential differences between the existing food and the new product, which should then be further investigated with respect to their toxicological impacts (Domingo and Bordonaba, 2011). Moreover, the concept of substantial equivalence was introduced with the aim of establishing a scientifically sound approach that would meet global acceptance but it emphasizes compositional analysis as a requirement for toxicological and nutritional studies (Kook and Kuiper, 2003). Such comparative analysis ignores the contribution of natural and artificial abiotic components that influence the expression of certain genes in both lines capable of causing lifelong or long-term health effects. More so, it is common knowledge that the principle fulfils local and national interest more than global considerations. New approaches have since evolved for food safety assessments of GM plant-based food like the European Thematic Network, Entransfood. The focus of Entransfood is on the different levels of the safety evaluation of GM food crops including:

- **DNA Level:** Based on sequence analysis of the insertion point of the gene fragment to identify any potential side effects through the interruption of regulatory or gene sequences.
- **Gene Expression Level:** Using microarrays techniques to monitor large-scale gene expression simultaneously.
- **Protein Level:** By monitoring shifts in protein levels using proteomic analysis of the tissues of interest.
- **Metabolite Level:** Direct analysis of secondary metabolites using gas and liquid chromatography (GC/LC) in combination with MS or nuclear magnetic resonance.

Kleter et al. (2005); Arya (2015) highlighted the possibility of horizontal gene transfer due to the absorption of DNA fragments by gut microflora or somatic cells lining the intestinal cell since the DNA from ingested food is not completely degraded by digestion and small fragments of DNA from GM foods have been found in different parts of the gastrointestinal tract. A comprehensive scientific evaluation of this problem is a colossal task because only about 1% of the naturally existing bacteria can be cultured and thus analysed. Already, GM crops with glyphosate have been implicated in different gastrointestinal disorders including irritable bowel syndrome, Celiac diseases and chronic constipation through interference with gut microflora and immune systems (Group, 2016). However, it is generally hypothesized that the uptake of GM DNA into the cells of the gastrointestinal tract will not have any biological consequences because they may be degraded in the cells. Recently, outcrossing have also been observed of genes from GM plants to traditional plants, related species and unrelated species. The insertion of a new gene may lead to an increase in the existing levels of anti-nutrients as well as interfere with the utilization of nutrients. Although humans have been ingesting CaMV and its 35S promoter in high amounts, no disease has been associated with it neither has it recombined with other viruses (Arya, 2015).

2. Potential Long-Term Environmental Effects of Plant-Based GM Products

Conventional agriculture and food production systems are environmentally costly, as it requires certain levels of environmental modification. Although GM plant production remains a possible pathway for humanity to achieve food security, it is a significant contributor to genetic erosion and reduction of plant gene pool and genetic diversity. The production of GM crops is not environmentally neutral rather it may have positive or negative impacts on the environment in the long and short-term albeit their detection remains challenging to measure economically and otherwise. Generally, the negative environmental impacts of GM crops result from their impacts on non-target species, increased weediness (combination of traits that make them as competitive as natural weeds), increase in soil toxin levels, exchange of genetic materials and selection for resistance among populations of the target pests (Fontes et al., 2002). Osawaru and Ogwu (2014) reported that global plant diversity and their ecological importance has not been sufficiently studied. Therefore, reducing this diversity through GM plant production may result in unpredictable environmental consequences including heightened vulnerability to climate change.

Environmental challenges of GM plant production only began to attract research attention long after the process has been established because it was earlier perceived to only pose ethical, health, biotechnology and bioengineering-related challenges. However, possible long-term environmental implications of GM plant production are expressed through direct impacts, indirect impacts and in science and governance (Figure 2) with evolutionary, ecological, epidemiological and environmental perspectives (Tsatsakis et al., 2017).

Gene transfer, trait effects on target and non-target species, wild plant changes through targeted and non-targeted invasiveness and genetic recombination of free DNA are considered as the direct environmental impacts whereas undesirable side-effects, evolution of new pests, diseases and weeds, environmental contamination and the global decline of biodiversity are indirect environmental impacts (Tutelyan, 2013; Tsatsakis et al., 2017). These broad challenges may be responsible for public anxiety, political activity, and regulations that have frustrated the resulting GM products (Regal, 1986). The dynamic requirement to establish societal policies and regulations make up the science and politics effects. According to Tsatsakis et al. (2017) the rapid expansion of GM-based technology and their applications, have led to altered agricultural, and food production practices posing multidimensional direct and indirect environmental implications through biodiversity and ecosystem gene flow and genetic recombination processes, function and services as well as evolution i.e. development of resistance in micro and macro-organisms. The science and politics dimension also include operational legal frameworks and environmental risk assessments of plant-based GM products. GM products environmental risk assessment deals with the potential long-term adverse effects resulting from interactions of GM components with populations, community, ecosystems and ecological resources. It does not focus on individuals rather it describes living and non-living groups by exposure potentials and characterizes the potential for adverse effects to

Figure 2. Dimensionality of the environmental implications of GM crops and plant-based products
Source. Adapted from Tsatsakis et al. (2017)

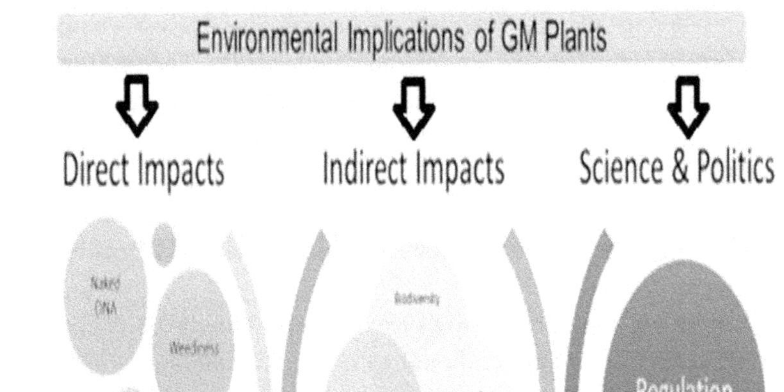

define uncertainties, generates response options to deal with the risks (Iyyanki and Manickam, 2017). The assessment has the assumption that with no risk on individual's life-history traits (i.e., feeding, survival, growth, reproduction) there will no environmental or ecosystem effects (Jager, 2016). With this approach, the lifelong environmental impact of plant-based GM products can be modelled. Risk assessments of the impacts of GM plants on the environment are conducted before they are approved for commercial use, as a core requirement of the biosafety regulatory frameworks (Fontes et al., 2002).

The lifelong risks from GM plant-based food and products have economic, environmental, social, ethical, and political dimensions. GM foods may reduce production costs and environmental degradation from pesticides and fertilizers but these costs are in turn passed on to the consumer through many other ways (Schneider et al., 2017). In addition, the toxic chemicals produced by GM crops result in a long-term challenge to the environment, non-target species as well as to the generation of the inherited plants with the potential of undesirable effects (Tsatsakis et al., 2017). The perceived benefits of this genetic engineering process include increased and sustainable crop production, natural resource conservation, to decrease nutrient runoff in the rivers, and to help meet the increasing world food demands using a limited amount of land (USDA, 2013; Arya, 2015' Tsatsakis et al., 2017).

Over thousands of years, farmers developed commercially viable plants with desirable traits, such as increased resistance to disease, larger fruit, and greater nutritional content with and without elaborate technological processes (Arya, 2015). The process was less environmentally costly compared to GM plant-based agricultural breeding but not sustainable enough to meet food needs. Post introduction of recombinant technology in the field of agriculture is synonymous with increased interest in the environmental impacts of food production practices. Traditional agricultural methods involve modification of plant genes to develop desirable traits but scientific breeders' selects for genes indirectly by selecting parent plants with the desirable traits; there is no direct control at the DNA level because the reorganization of the genetic material occurs in a random fashion (Arya, 2015). Moreover, recombinant DNA technology is used to change the plant's genome using the desired genetic trait that was identified, extracted and inserted in the plant. Lifelong environmental complication through the evolution of resistant pests and weeds termed superbugs and superweeds is a problem (Bawa and Anilakumar, 2013). Using the case of insect-resistant GM plants, Fontes et al. (2002) outlined the following environmental impacts, effects on individual natural enemies that may be beneficial to the environment and community, effects on non-target insect species that are directly susceptible to *Bt* toxin including bees, and persistence of insecticidal toxins produced by the plant in the soil environment. These environmental impacts persist beyond the growing season of the GM plant.

RECOMMENDATIONS AND CONCLUSION

Plant-based GM foods and products are leading the global fight to alleviate global food insecurity but questions about their long-term health and environmental suitability remains a militating factor. The use of fewer inputs including synthetic pesticides and herbicides to increase yield is an environmental gain that is clouded by the loss of biodiversity. Therefore, this paper joins voice with the call for more research to make GM plant-based products more acceptable through greater understanding of their long-term effects. Despite present gains and perceived safety of GM plant-based food products, the full range of economic, ecologic, environmental and epidemiologic potential can be reached after serious consideration is given to lifelong consequences of consuming the products. Although it is difficult to identify hazards that are fundamentally different from those that can occur in the short-term, in most cases, the long-term and cumulative hazards are the same as the short-term ones (Henry et al., 2006). Modelling potential long-term concerns after short and long-term consequences of consuming conventional (non-GM) plant food is a good starting point.

Scientists and biotechnology companies must engage with the public to ensure that potential concerns are debated rationally (Key et al., 2008). It is important to note that there is no epidemiological studies of the human population nor lifelong monitoring of farm animals and domestic pets in an attempt to correlate any ill health observed with the consumption of GM crops (Seralini et al., 2014). Lifelong studies of laboratory animals consuming GM plant-based feeds should be performed in contrast to what is currently obtainable from as little as two-year long tests. These life-long studies should be correlated with transgenerational, reproductive and endocrine research (Krimsky, 2015) as well as with environmental studies and impact assessments. However, with lifelong health effects, it is difficult to assess whether a single GM plant-based food is entirely responsible for observed effects. Therefore, this calls for a multi-dimensional and interdisciplinary approach. This can shape the future of businesses related to GM plant from product design to sale and eventual consumption. The popularity of a GM crop is commensurate with research investment regardless of clear policy regulations (Sánchez and León, 2016).

In addition, the global adoption of a standardized comparative safety risk assessment strategy and other toxicological and nutritional evaluations pertaining to GM technology, market, etc. is necessary (Kok and Kuiper, 2003). This may help allay some of the challenges associated with the current global imbalance in the acceptance of GM plant-based food and food product. Controversies should not be avoided rather they should be addressed with a resolve to innovate solutions where necessary. This could be in the form of an extended GM food safety evaluation based on the guidelines of OECD (1993; 1996), the

European Scientific Committee on Foodstuffs (1997), the United Nations Food and Agriculture Organisation [FAO]/WHO (1996; 2000; 2001; 2002), and Kuiper et al. (2001) summarized herein as comprising:

1. Molecular characterization of introduced genetic fragments especially those capable of producing new proteins and/or metabolites
2. Compositional analysis of plant parts correlated with key nutrients and anti-nutrients
3. Gene transfer potential
4. Allergenicity and toxicity assessment of the transgenes and their products
5. Estimated safety intake levels of the newly introduced proteins and their final products, including any altered constituent
6. Risk assessment of the transgene on the environment (especially on soil and biodiversity)

Also important is the adoption of a clear regulatory and assessment framework through environmental risk assessment, feed and feed approvals, product labelling, biosafety regulation and legislation, and research support in line with the recommendations of Sánchez and León (2016), which can be achieved through element-specific, construct-specific, and event-specific comprehensive detection of GM crops (Lin and Pan, 2016). The reason for existing gaps between public opinion and scientific evidence also needs to be clarified and balanced (Blancke et al., 2015).

According to the results of Entine and Wendel (2000) on the safety and environmental impacts of GM-foods, there is no short-term harm to humans or animals. This is a good basis for key players to support long-term studies. Biotechnology companies, international, national, regional and non-governmental organizations, should support and participate in the long-term investigations of the effects of GM plant-based foods. However, no country should be forced to adopt any GM plant-based food and food products without evidential support about their long-term health and environmental suitability.

Developing countries may be the future of sustainable market and development of GM products because they are the most stricken by food insecurities. However, the number of studies focused on the safety of GM plant-based food is limited, which may be responsible for their non-widespread acceptance in developing countries (Domingo and Bordonaba, 2011). In the same way, the existence of either financial or professional conflicts of interest is significantly associated with studies' showing favourable results for the GM foods (Diels et al., 2011), which does more harm than good to the reputation of GM plant-based food. Although strong public opposition to GMOs persists with resulting impacts on the development of national and international policies, GM crops continue to make valuable contributions towards the development of a sustainable type of agriculture (Blancke et al., 2015) by substantially increase productivity, quality, environmental sustainability and the nutritional content of crops (Sánchez and León, 2016).

Finally, labelling is an important tool, and knowing the ingredients of a product helps to decipher their risks and benefits. Hence, the European Union mandatory labelling of GMOs and GM products should be adopted globally.

REFERENCES

Ahmed, F. E. (2002). Detection of Genetically Modified Organisms in Foods. *Trends in Biotechnology, 20*(5), 215–223. doi:10.1016/S0167-7799(01)01920-5 PMID:11943377

Arya, D. (2015). *Genetically Modified Foods Benefits and Risks*. Massachusetts Medical Society. http://www.massmed.org/Patient-Care/Health-Topics/Nutrition-and-Physical-Activity/Genetically-Modified-Foods-(pdf)/

Bawa, A. S., & Anilakumar, K. R. (2013). Genetically modified foods: Safety, risks and public concerns - a review. *Journal of Food Science and Technology, 50*(6), 1035–1046. doi:10.100713197-012-0899-1 PMID:24426015

Blancke, S., Van Breusegem, F., De Jaeger, G., Braeckman, J., & Van Montagu, M. (2015). Fatal attraction: The intuitive appeal of GMO opposition. *Trends in Plant Science, 20*(7), 414–418. doi:10.1016/j.tplants.2015.03.011 PMID:25868652

Bushey, D. F., Bannon, G. A., Delaney, B. F., Graser, G., Hefford, M., Jiang, X., ... Harper, M. S. (2014). Characteristics and safety assessment of intractable proteins in genetically modified crops. *Regulatory Toxicology and Pharmacology, 69*(2), 154–170. doi:10.1016/j.yrtph.2014.03.003 PMID:24662477

Butler, D., & Reichhardt, T. (1999). Long-term effect of GM crops serves up food for thought. *Nature, 398*(6729), 651–653. doi:10.1038/19381 PMID:10227281

Byrne, P., Pendell, D., & Graff, G. (2014). *Labeling of Genetically Modified Foods. Food and Nutrition Series (Health). Colorado State University Extension.* Retrieved from https://extension.colostate.edu/docs/pubs/foodnut/09371.pdf

Carter, C.A., &. Gruere, G.P. (2003). Mandatory labeling of genetically modified foods: does it really provide consumer choice? *AgBioForum, 6*(1 and 2), 68 – 70.

Conner, A. J., & Jacobs, J. M. E. (1999). Genetic engineering of crops as potential source of genetic hazard in the human diet. *Mutation Research/Genetic Toxicology and Environmental Mutagenesis, 443*(1-2), 223–234. doi:10.1016/S1383-5742(99)00020-4 PMID:10415441

Dahl, R. (2012). To Label or Not to Label, Environmental Health Perspectives. *Environmental Health Perspectives, 120*(9), 359–361. Retrieved from http://ehp.niehs.nih.gov/wp-content/uploads/2012/09/ehp.120-a358.pdf PMID:23487845

de Vendômois, J. S., Roullier, F., Cellier, D., & Séralini, G. E. (2009). A Comparison of the Effects of Three GM Corn Varieties on Mammalian Health. *International Journal of Biological Sciences, 5*(7), 706–726. doi:10.7150/ijbs.5.706 PMID:20011136

Delaney, B. (2015). Safety assessment of foods from genetically modified crops in countries with developing economies. *Food and Chemical Toxicology, 86*, 132–143. doi:10.1016/j.fct.2015.10.001 PMID:26456807

Diels, J., Cunha, M., Manaia, C., Sabugosa-Madeira, B., & Silva, M. (2011). Association of financial or professional conflict of interest to research outcomes on health risks or nutritional assessment studies of genetically modified products. *Food Policy, 36*(2), 197–203. doi:10.1016/j.foodpol.2010.11.016

Domingo, J. L. (2000). Health risks of GM foods: Many opinions but few data. *Science, 288*(5472), 1748–1749. doi:10.1126cience.288.5472.1748 PMID:10877692

Domingo, J. L. (2007). Toxicity studies of genetically modified plants: A review of the published literature. *Critical Reviews in Food Science and Nutrition, 47*(8), 721–733. doi:10.1080/10408390601177670 PMID:17987446

Domingo, J. L. (2011). Human health effects of genetically modified (GM) plants: Risk and perception. *Human and Ecological Risk Assessment, 17*(3), 535–537. doi:10.1080/10807039.2011.571065

Domingo, J. L. (2016). Safety assessment of GM plants: An updated review of the scientific literature. *Food and Chemical Toxicology, 95*, 12–18. doi:10.1016/j.fct.2016.06.013 PMID:27317828

Domingo, J. L., & Bordonaba, J. G. (2011). A literature review on the safety assessment of genetically modified plants. *Environment International, 37*(4), 734–742. doi:10.1016/j.envint.2011.01.003 PMID:21296423

Domingo, J. L., & Gomez, M. (2000). Health risks of genetically modified foods: A literature review. *Revista Espanola de Salud Publica, 74*, 255–261. PMID:10918812

Entine, J., & Wendel, J. (2013). 2000+ Reasons Why GMOs Are Safe to Eat and Environmentally Sustainable. *Forbes*. Retrieved from http://www.forbes.com/sites/jonentine/2013/10/14/2000-reasons-why-gmos-are-safe-to-eat-and-environmentally-sustainable

European Chemicals Agency. (2012). *The status of industrial vegetable oils from genetically modified plants*. Retrieved from https://echa.europa.eu/documents/10162/22816103/the_status_of_industrial_vegetable_oils_from_genetically_modified_plants_expert_report_en.pdf/e6b0de1b-c9d5-4e07-8fc6-8f4dae318c55

European Union. (1997). EU 97/618/EC. Commission Recommendations 29 July 1997 concerning the scientific aspects and the presentation of information necessary to support applications for the placing on the market of novel foods and novel food ingredients and the preparation of initial assessment reports under Regulation EC 259/97 of the European Parliament and of the Council. *Official Journal of the European Communities*.

FAO/WHO. (1996). *Biotechnology and Food Safety. Report of a Joint*. FAO/WHO consultation, Rome, Italy, 1996. Retrieved from ftp://ftp.fao.org/es/esn/food/biotechnology.pdf

FAO/WHO. (2000). *Safety Aspects of Genetically Modified Foods of Plant Origin*. Report of a Joint FAO/WHO Expert Consultation on Foods Derived from Biotechnology, Geneva, Switzerland, 2000, Food and Agriculture Organisation of the United Nations, Rome. Retrieved from ftp://ftp.fao.org/es/esn/food/gmreport.pdf

FAO/WHO. (2001). *Allergenicity of Genetically Modified Foods. Report of a Joint FAO/WHO Expert Consultation on Foods Derived from Biotechnology*. Rome, 2001, Food and Agriculture Organisation of the United Nations, Rome. Retrieved from http://www.who.int/fsf/Documents/Biotech_Consult_Jan2001/report20.pdf

FAO/WHO. (2002). *Report of the Third Session of the Codex Ad Hoc Intergovernmental Task Force on Foods Derived from Biotechnology (ALINORM 01/34)*. Codex Ad Hoc Intergovernmental Task Force on Foods Derived from Biotechnology, Food and Agriculture Organisation of the United Nations, Rome. Retrieved from ftp://ftp.fao.org/codex/alinorm03/Al03_34e.pdf

Fernandez-Cornejo, J., & Caswell, M. (2006). The first Decade of Genetically Engineered Crops in the United States. *USDA ERS Economic Bulletin*. Retrieved from http://www.ers.usda.gov/publications/eib11/eib11.pdf

Fontes, E. M. G., Pires, C. S. S., Sujii, E. R., & Panizzi, A. R. (2002). The environmental effects of genetically modified crops resistant to insects. *Neotropical Entomology, 31*(4), 497–513. doi:10.1590/S1519-566X2002000400001

Frewer, L. J., & Shepherd, R. (1995). Ethical concerns and risk perceptions associated with different applications of genetic engineering: Interrelationships with the perceived need for regulation of the technology. *Agriculture and Human Values, 12*(1), 48–57. doi:10.1007/BF02218074

Grant, J. (2017). List of foods containing GMOs. *Live Strong*. Retrieved from https://www.livestrong.com/article/314824-list-of-foods-containing-gmos/

Group, E. (2016). GMO foods cause gut damage. *Global Healing Center*. Retrieved from https://www.globalhealingcenter.com/natural-health/gmo-foods-cause-gut-damage/

Hefferon, K.L. (2016*). Food Security of Genetically Modified Foods*. doi:10.1016/B978-0-08-100596-5.03532-0

Henry, C., Hugo, S., & Blackburn, J. (2006). Cumulative long-term effects of genetically modified (GM) crops on human/animal health and the environment: risk assessment methodologies. *European Union*. Retrieved from https://ec.europa.eu/food/sites/food/files/plant/docs/gmo_rep-stud_2006_report_lt-effects.pdf

International Service for the Acquisition of Agri-Biotech Applications. (2010). *Global Status of Commercialized Biotech/ GM crops: 2010. ISAAA Brief 42-2010: Executive Summary*. Retrieved from http://www.isaaa.org/resources/publications/briefs/42/executivesummary/default. asp

ISAAA. (2009). Pocket K No. 3: Are the food derived from GM crops safe? Retrieved from http://www.isaaa.org/resources/publications/pocketk/3/default.asp

ISAAA. (2012). *Annual report Executive Summary*. International Service for the Acquisition of Agribiotech Applications.

Iyyanki, V. M., & Manickam, V. (2017). Chapter Eight – Environmental Risk Assessment. In V. M. Iyyanki & V. Manickam (Eds.), *Environmental Management: Science and Engineering for Industry* (pp. 135–152). India: BS Publications. doi:10.1016/B978-0-12-811989-1.00008-7

Jager, T. (2016). Dynamic Modeling for Uptake and Effects of Chemicals. In J. Blasco, P. M. Chapman, O. Campana, & M. Hampel (Eds.), *Marine Ecotoxicology: Current Knowledge and Future Uses* (pp. 718–798). Academic Press. doi:10.1016/B978-0-12-803371-5.00003-5

Key, S., Ma, J. K. C., & Drake, P. M. W. (2008). Genetically modified plants and human health. *Journal of the Royal Society of Medicine, 101*(6), 290–298. doi:10.1258/jrsm.2008.070372 PMID:18515776

Kleter, G. A., Peijnenburg, A. A. C. M., & Aarts, H. J. M. (2005). Health Considerations Regarding Horizontal Transfer of Microbial Transgenes Present in Genetically Modified Crops. *Journal of Biomedicine & Biotechnology, 2005*(4), 326–352. doi:10.1155/JBB.2005.326 PMID:16489267

Kok, E. J., & Kuiper, H. A. (2003). Comparative safety assessment for biotech crops. *Trends in Biotechnology, 21*(10), 439–444. doi:10.1016/j.tibtech.2003.08.003 PMID:14512230

Krimsky, S. (2015). An illusory consensus behind GMO health assessment. *Science, Technology & Human Values, 1*, 32. doi:10.1177/0162243915598381

Kuiper, H. A., Kleter, G. A., Noteborn, H. P. J. M., & Kok, E. J. (2001). Assessment of the food safety issues related to genetically modified foods. *The Plant Journal, 27*(6), 503–528. doi:10.1046/j.1365-313X.2001.01119.x PMID:11576435

Lamichhane, S. A. (2014). Genetically Modified Foods-Solution for Food Security. *International Journal of Genetic Engineering and Biotechnology, 5*(1), 43–48.

Lin, C.-H., & Pan, T.-M. (2016). Perspectives on genetically modified crops and food detection. *Journal of Food and Drug Analysis, 24*(1), 1–8. doi:10.1016/j.jfda.2015.06.011 PMID:28911391

Lisowska, K. (2011). Genetically modified crops and food: Pros and cons. *Chemik, 65*, 1193–1203.

Łuczaj, L., Pieroni, A., Tardío, J., Pardo-de-Santayana, M., Sõukand, R., Svanberg, I., & Kalle, R. (2012). Wild food plant use in 21st century Europe: The disappearance of old traditions and the search for new cuisines involving wild edibles. *Acta Societatis Botanicorum Poloniae, 81*(4), 359–370. doi:10.5586/asbp.2012.031

Magaña-Gómez, J. A., & de la Barca, A. M. (2009). Risk assessment of genetically modified crops for nutrition and health. *Nutrition Reviews, 67*(1), 1–16. doi:10.1111/j.1753-4887.2008.00130.x PMID:19146501

Murnaghan, I. (2018). *The long-term effects of GM foods.* Retrieved from www.geneticallymodifiedfoods.co.uk/longterm-effects-gm-foods.html

OECD. (1993). *Safety Evaluation of Foods Derived by Modern Biotechnology: Concepts and Principles.* Organisation for Economic Co-operation and Development. Retrieved from http://www.oecd.org/pdf/M00034000/M00034525.pdf

OECD. (1996). *Food Safety Evaluation.* Paris: Organization for Economic Cooperation and Development.

Ogwu, M. C., Osawaru, M. E., & Ahana, C. M. (2014). Challenges in conserving and utilizing plant genetic resources (PGR). *International Journal of Genetics and Molecular Biology, 6*(2), 16–22. doi:10.5897/IJGMB2013.0083

Oliver, M. (2014). Why we need GMO crops in agriculture. *Missouri Medicine, 111*, 492–507. PMID:25665234

Osawaru, M. E., & Ogwu, M. C. (2014). Conservation and Utilization of Plant Genetic Resources. In: K. Omokhafe, & J. Odewale (Eds), *Proceedings of 38th Annual Conference of the Genetics Society of Nigeria.* (pp 105 -119). Nigeria: Empress Prints Nigeria Ltd.

Phillips, T. (2008). Genetically modified organisms (GMOs): Transgenic crops and recombinant DNA technology. *Nature Education, 1*(1), 213.

Pighin, J. (2003). Transgenic crops: how genetics is providing new ways to envision agriculture. *The Science Creative Quarterly*. Retrieved from http://www.scq.ubc.ca/transgenic-crops-how-genetics-is-providing-new-ways-to- envision-agriculture/

Powell, C. (2015). How to make a GMO. Retrieved from http://sitn.hms.harvard.edu/flash/2015/how-to-make-a-gmo/

Qaim, M., & Kouser, S. (2013). Genetically Modified Crops and Food Security. *PLoS One*, *8*(6), e64879. doi:10.1371/journal.pone.0064879 PMID:23755155

Regal, P. J. (1986). Models of genetically engineered organisms and their ecological impact. In H. A. Mooney & J. K. Drake (Eds.), *Ecology of Biological Invasions of North America and Hawaii* (pp. 111–129). New York: Springer. doi:10.1007/978-1-4612-4988-7_7

Sánchez, M. A., & León, G. (2016). Status of market, regulation and research of genetically modified crops in Chile. *New Biotechnology*, *33*(6), 815–823. doi:10.1016/j.nbt.2016.07.017 PMID:27474111

Schlett, A. & Beke, J. (2015). Food security and GMOS. *Studia Mundi – Economica, 2*(1), 94-102. doi:. doi:10.18531/Studia.Mundi.2015.02.01

Schneider, K. R., Schneider, R. G., & Richardson, S. (2017). *Genetically Modified Food. FSHN02-2 series Food Science and Human Nutrition Department*. UF/IFAS Extension.

Seralini, G. E., Mesnage, R., Defarge, N., & Spiroux de Vendômois, J. (2014). Conclusiveness of Toxicity Data and Double Standards. *Food and Chemical Toxicology*, *69*(7), 357–359. doi:10.1016/j.fct.2014.04.018 PMID:24747919

Shivanand, P., & Noopur, S. (2010). Recombinant DNA technology: Applications in the field of bio-technology and crime sciences. *International Journal of Pharmaceutical Sciences Review and Research*, *1*(1), 43–49.

SOT (Society of Toxicology). (2003). The safety of genetically modified foods produced through bio-technology. *Toxicological Sciences*, *71*(1), 2–8. doi:10.1093/toxsci/71.1.2 PMID:12520069

Southgate, E. M., Davey, M. R., Power, J. B., & Merchant, R. (1995). Factors affecting the genetic engineering of plants by microprojectile bombardment. *Biotechnology Advances*, *13*(4), 631–657. doi:10.1016/0734-9750(95)02008-X PMID:14536367

Swanson, N. L. (2013). *Genetically modified organisms and the deterioration of health in the United States*. Retrieved from https://people.csail.mit.edu/seneff/glyphosate/NancySwanson.pdf

The Royal Society. (2002). Genetically modified plants for food use and human health— an update. Policy document 4/02. Retrieved from https://royalsociety.org/~/media/royal_society_content/policy/publications/2002/9 960.pdf

Thompson, S. (2017). How GM crops can help us feed a fast-growing world. *The Conversation*. Retrieved from http://theconversation.com/how-gm-crops-can-help-us-to-feed-a-fast-growing-world-71112

Tsatsakis, A. M., Nawaz, M. A., Kouretas, D., Balias, G., Savolainen, K., Tutelyan, V. A., ... Chung, G. (2017). Environmental impacts of genetically modified plants: A review. *Environmental Research, 156*, 818–833. doi:10.1016/j.envres.2017.03.011 PMID:28347490

Tutelyan, V. A. (2013). *Safety Assessment and Control* (1st ed.). Academic Press. doi:10.1016/C2011-0-08818-X

Twardowski, T., & Małyska, A. (2015). Uninformed and disinformed society and the GMO market. *Trends in Biotechnology, 33*(1), 1–3. doi:10.1016/j.tibtech.2014.11.006 PMID:25528967

United States Department of Agriculture (USDA). (2014). *Genetically Engineered Crops in the United States, February 2014.*

USDA. (2013). *Biotechnology Frequently Asked Questions*. Retrieved from http://www.usda.gov/wps/portal/usda/usdahome?navid=AGRICULTURE&contentid=BiotechnologyFAQs.xml

Usher, S., Han, L., Haslam, R. P., Michaelson, L. V., Sturtevant, D., Aziz, M., ... Napier, J. A. (2017). Tailoring seed oil composition in the real world: Optimising omega-3 long chain polyunsaturated fatty acid accumulation in transgenic *Camelina sativa. Scientific Reports, 7*(1), 6570. doi:10.103841598-017-06838-0 PMID:28747792

Wieczorek, A. (2013). History of Agricultural Biotechnology: How Crop Development has Evolved. *Nature*. Retrieved from http://www.nature.com/scitable/knowledge/library/history-of-agricultural-biotechnology-how-crop-development-25885295

Wong, D. (2003). *Genetically Modified Food Labelling*. Hong Kong: Research and Library Services Division Legislative Council Secretariat. Retrieved from http://www.legco.gov.hk/yr02-03/english/sec/library/0203rp05e.pdf

Zhu, X., Van Wesenbeeck, L., & Van Ierland, E. C. (2006). Impacts of Novel Protein Foods on Sustainable Food Production and Consumption: Lifestyle Change and Environmental Policy. *Environmental and Resource Economics, 35*(1), 59–87. doi:10.100710640-006-9006-2

This research was previously published in Environmental Exposures and Human Health Challenges edited by Paraskevi Papadopoulou, Christina Marouli, and Anastasia Misseyanni; pages 158-176, copyright year 2019 by Medical Information Science Reference (an imprint of IGI Global).

Chapter 61
Nutritional Properties of Edible Insects

Anna K. Żołnierczyk
Wrocław University of Environmental and Life Sciences, Poland

ABSTRACT

Insects are the biggest animal group on earth. They constitute as much as 80% of the animal kingdom. Over 2000 species of insects are consumed in Central and South America, Africa, Asia, Australia, and New Zealand. Currently almost 1 billion people on this planet suffer from hunger, and we must strive to increase the efficiency of food production. One of the possible solutions is to use insects as a source of food. An important advantage of insect production is the high environmental safety compared to conventional livestock. Conventional animal husbandry is responsible for at least 18% of total greenhouse gas emissions and large consumption of drinking water. A much smaller amount of water is used to produce insect meat and insects require far less feed. Production of insect protein requires much less land and energy than the more widely consumed forms of animal protein. The nutritional usefulness of edible insects varies depending on the species, on the stage of development of the insect and the method of breeding and feeding. Insects have a high nutritional value. They are a rich source of protein which includes all eight essential amino acids (phenylalanine, isoleucine, leucine, lysine, methionine, threonine, tryptophan, and valine). Edible insects contain on average 10-30% of fat in dry matter and they are good source of edible oil which contains more than 50% of polyunsaturated fatty acids (PUFA) desirable for nutritional and health reasons. The average energy value of edible insects is about 400-500 kcal/100g of dry matter. Insects also contain a variety of water soluble or lipophilic vitamins and minerals. Their consumption can build a well-balanced diet. Insects can be regarded as safe, if properly managed and consumed, but international food regulations are needed.

INTRODUCTION

From the beginning of human existence on the Earth, most of the protein supplied with food was taken by hunting or fishing, but in many places collection of insects was necessary to allow to supplement nutritional deficiencies (Tosi & Daccordi, 1983). Insects are the biggest animal group on earth, they

DOI: 10.4018/978-1-7998-5354-1.ch061

constitute as much as 80% of the animal kingdom. It is estimated that over 2000 species of insects are consumed in almost 80% of the countries in the world (Wageningen University and Research, 2017). Eggs, larvae and adult forms of insects (Figure 1) are eaten as food in Central and South America, Africa, Asia, Australia and New Zealand.

Figure 1. Larvae of the mealworms Tenebrio molitor (left) and the adult form of the Jamaican field cricket Gryllus assimilis (right)
Photo credit: Tomasz Lewandowski

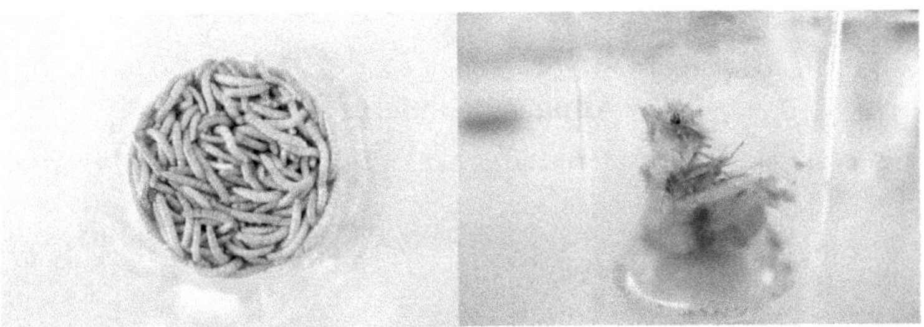

The taste and flavour of insects are very diverse (Payne, 2018). We can compare them to the ingredients we know and the ways of cooking are no different from the traditional ones. Also, insects can absorb the taste of the chosen seasoning with which they are fed. The total number of ethnic groups practicing entomophagy (from the Greek words ἔντομον éntomon meaning "insect" and φᾰγεῖν phagein meaning "to eat") exceeds 3000 (Ramos-Elorduy, 1998; MacEvilly, 2000). Entomophagy is not well accepted in western European populations but it is common in the world.

It is considered that eating insects may reduce the environmental risks (FAO, 2016). Insect breeding compared to livestock farms (pigs, cattle and poultry) releases six to ten times less ammonia (Oonincx, Kgomotso, & Letswiti, 2010). Conventional animal husbandry is responsible for at least 18% of greenhouse gas emissions and massive consumption of drinking water. Much smaller amounts of water are used to produce insect meat. Insects are able to derive their moisture demand from food. Also they require far less feed. For example, the production of 1 kg of live animal weight of crickets requires as little as 1.7 kg of feed (Collavo, Glew, Huang, Chuang, Bosse, & Paoletti, 2005). Typically, 1 kg of live animal weight in a conventional production system demands 2.5 kg of feed for chicken, 5 kg for pork and 10 kg for beef (Smil, 2002). Moreover, the production of insect protein takes much less land and energy than the more widely consumed forms of animal protein (Halloran, Hanboonsong, Roos, & Bruun, 2017; Oonincx & de Boer, 2012; Premalatha, Abbasi, Abbasi, & Abbasi, 2011). Edible insects can be grown at home, on small farms or large industrial facilities anywhere in the world. The interest in using insects for nutritional purposes is justified because (apart from nutritional qualities) insects are characterized by high survival capacity in various ecological conditions, short life cycle and high reproductive ability (DeFoliart, 1999; Illgner & Nel, 2000; Renault, Laparie, McCauley, & Bonte, 2018). However, it is first necessary to establish international food regulations regarding the safety of insect food products (Rumpold & Schluter, 2013a). Also, in countries where there is no tradition of eating insects, it takes time for people to get used to new possibilities.

The science of edible insects is a relatively new field of scientific research. Large-scale breeding is also a small percentage of the sources from which edible insects are obtained – for the most part they are collected in a natural environment. Insects are mainly material for animal feed. However, in recent years, there has been an increased interest in the subject of insects as a source of food, both among the scientific community and consumers. The global human population is growing by around 70 million people each year. If the growth rate continues, by 2050 the population will probably reach as much as 9 billion. To feed all these people, we will have to produce almost twice as much food as at present. This may be difficult to implement, because we are already using 70% of the agricultural land for cattle farming. Furthermore, we cause pollution of the environment and our activities lead to rapid climate changes, which adversely affect agricultural production. Considering the fact that currently almost 1 billion people on earth suffer from hunger, we must strive to increase the efficiency of food production (FAO, 2009). One of the possible solutions is to use insects as a source of food. Probably in the future, populations from developed countries will need to adapt to other sources of animal proteins because the traditional breeding of beef, poultry or pork will become insufficient.

NUTRITIONAL VALUE OF EDIBLE INSECTS

The nutritional usefulness of edible insects varies depending on the species and method of breeding and feeding. Even within the same species of insects, the composition of nutritional compounds changes depending on the stage of development of the insect.

As shown in Figure 2, the main component of the nutrient composition of insects represents protein. The average amount of protein contents in edible insects varies between 42% for beetles and grubs and 63% for crickets, grasshoppers and locusts (see Figure 2). Despite such a large difference, many species of insects can cover human demand for energy, protein or minerals.

Energy

The energy value of raw insects (see Table 1) is in the range of 89 kcal/100g for grasshopper (Cyrtacanthacris tatarica) to 1272 kcal/100g for green ant (Oecophylla smaragdina) (van Huis, 2013). The average energy value of edible insects is about 400–500 kcal/100g of dry matter (see Figure 3).

The energy value of edible insects is generally subject to a large variation which comes primarily from differences between developmental stages and depends mainly on the fat content. Insects in the early stages of development (larvae, pupae, maggots and grubs) are usually richer in energy compared to adults because they generally contain more fat whereas insects containing more protein have lower energy content. Such an information can be very useful for creating specific diets, for example for people who want to reduce the amount of fats in their food.

Protein

From a nutritional point of view, apart from the energy value, the most important aspect is the protein content in the diet. We are constantly hearing messages that protein should be the basis of our diet, because it is the building block of all cells and participates in important life processes. Due to the increasing cost of animal proteins, population growth, and increasing need for protein-rich options in the developed and less developed countries, alternative food sources are highly needed. Hence, insect consumption can help with food and feed insecurity and thus replace the conventional animal source in the future.

Figure 2. Average nutrient contents [%] (based on dry matter) of edible insects groups belonging to the same order
NFE – nitrogen-free extract, the fraction containing sugars and starches plus small amounts of other materials (Rumpold & Schluter, 2013a and b).

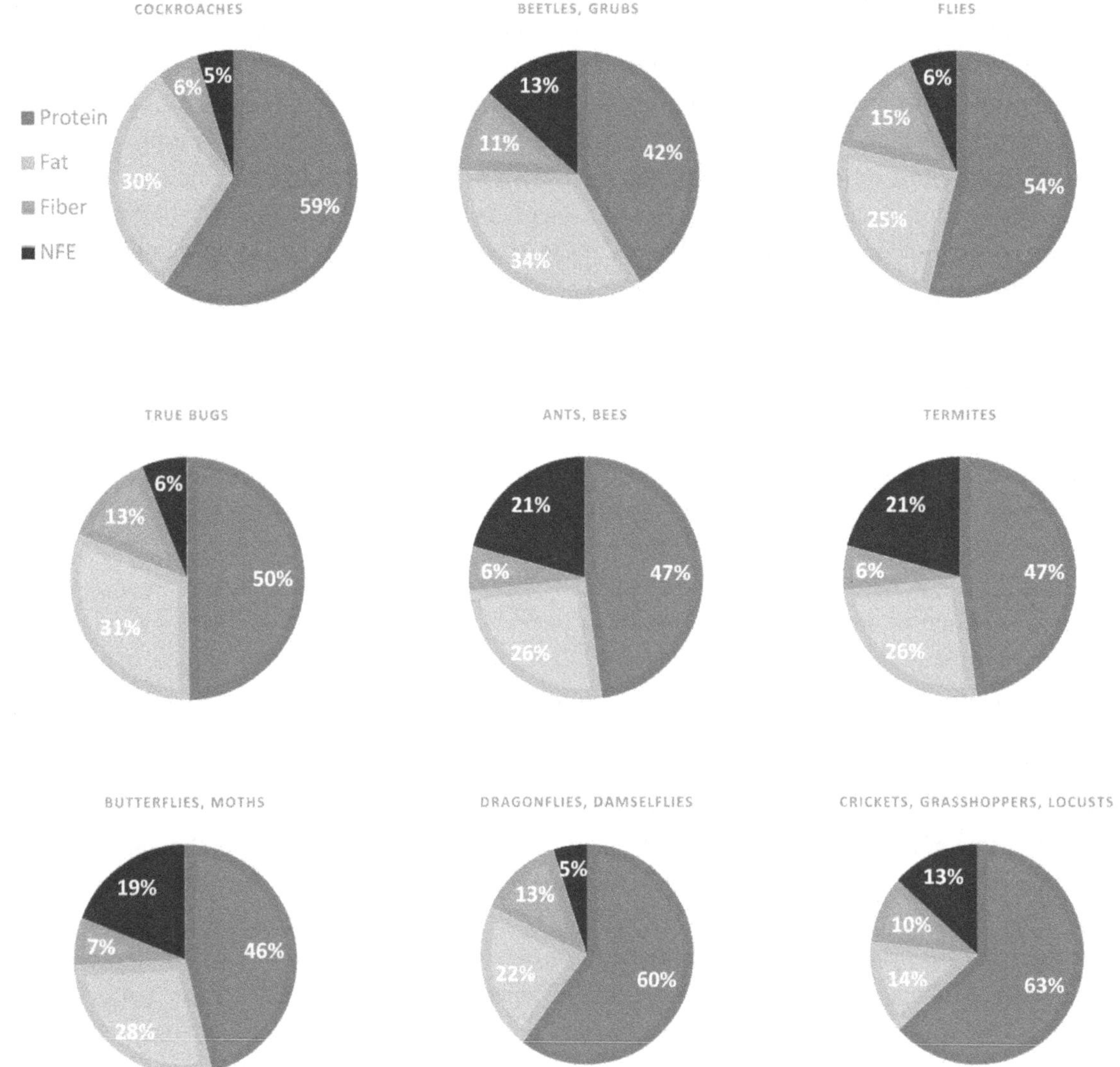

The findings from scientific research (see Table 2) show that insects are rich in protein (5–70%), while the protein content of boiled beef meat varies within the range of 11–27% (raw 19–26%), reptiles 11–27% and seafood 13–28%. The protein content of insects varies strongly by species. Also, the digestibility of protein from individual food products is diverse. For example, the digestibility of protein from egg white is 95–100%, dairy products 70–80%, vegetables and fruit 90–100% and meat about 65% (beef – 98%) while for insect protein it is from 76 to 96% (Ramos-Elorduy, Moreno, Prado, Perez, Otero, & de Guevara, 1997). For example, for dried, traditionally prepared mopane worms (caterpillars of the moth *Gonimbrasia belina*) the protein digestibility is 85.8% (Dreyer & Wehmeyer, 1982). Removal of chitin improves further the digestibility of insect protein (Finke, 2007). In wheat flour, there is about 10% of

Figure 3. Average energy value [kcal/100g of dry matter] for selected orders of insects (Rumpold & Schluter, 2013b)

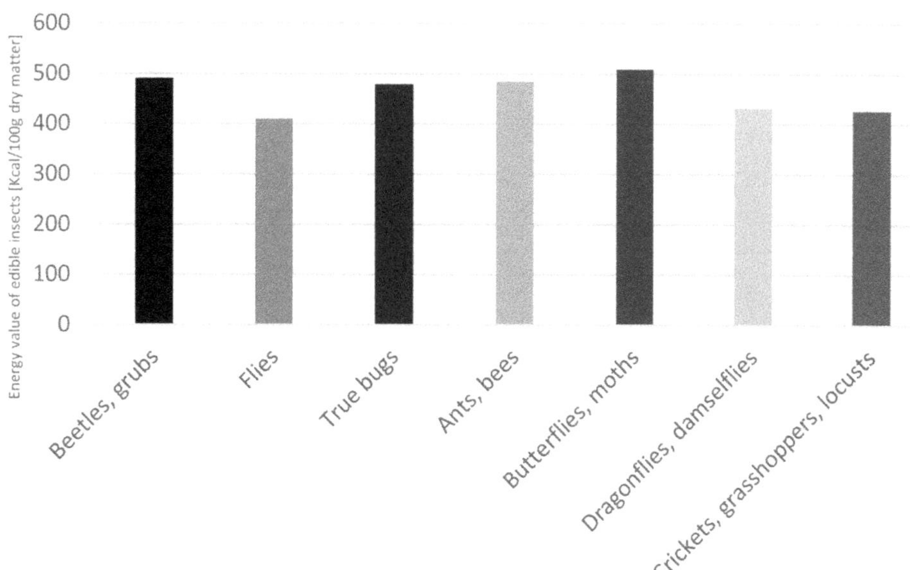

protein, which due to its vegetable origin, belongs to a deficient source of essential amino acids. In pasta, the protein content is about 5%. A flour made from crickets contains about 70% full-value protein and pasta made with just 10% cricket flour contains 14% of protein (which is more than the 13% protein in eggs). As protein sources, the nutritive value of edible insects is as good as that of other animals and plants or even better.

Protein content also depends on the feed. For example, reared grasshoppers that are fed with bran, have almost double the protein content of those fed on maize. Furthermore, the protein content of insects also depends on their metamorphosis stage (Ademolu, Idowu, & Olatunde, 2010): adults usually have higher protein content than instars (see Table 2).

However, it is not the amount of protein but the quality – the amino acid composition – that determines whether the food ration will be wholesome. A standard protein is one that contains all amino acids in quantities and proportions corresponding to human needs. Particularly important is the content of essential amino acids. The reference protein for adults is egg white but the key sources of proteins in human diets are often cereal proteins. They are low in lysine, tryptophan and threonine. In some insect species, these amino acids are very well represented (Bukkens, 2005). Insects offer a complete animal protein that includes all 8 essential amino acids (phenylalanine, isoleucine, leucine, lysine, methionine, threonine, tryptophan and valine) (see Table 3).

Comparing the average content of amino acids in the larvae of mealworm and beef (see Figure 4), tryptophan is found in insects and is not present in beef, four of the exogenous amino acids (isoleucine, leucine, lysine, and valine) are found in insects in a larger amount then in beef, threonine is in a comparable amount, and only two of the amino acids – phenylalanine and methionine, are present in insect larvae in lower amounts than in beef (about half as much) (USDA, 2012). The average amount of amino acids in edible insects is higher than that in beef (see Figure 4).

Table 1. Energy content [kcal/100g] based on dry matter or fresh weight for selected edible insects

Edible Insects		Stage	Energy Content [kcal/100g]	
Scientific Name	**Common Name**		**Based on Dry Matter**	**Based on Fresh Weight**
Tenebrio molitor	Yellow mealworm	Adult	380	139
Tenebrio molitor	Yellow mealworm	Pupae	550	-
Tenebrio molitor	Yellow mealworm	Larva	539.63–577.44	206
Zophobas morio	Zophobas	Larva	575	-
Bombyx mori	Domesticated silkworm	Larva	390	94
Macrotermes bellicosus	Termite	Adult	28–46	
Macrotermes subhyalinus	Termite/dried, flour	Adult	535	-
Locusta migratoria	Migratory locust	Adult	-	179
Cytracanthacris tatarica	Grasshopper	Adult	-	89
Acheta domesticus	House cricket	Adult	455	-
Melanoplus femurrubrum	Red-legged grasshopper	Adult	361	160
Oecophylla smaragdina	Green ant	Adult	-	1272
Atta mexicana	Leaf-cutter ant	Adult	555	404

Source of data: (Rumpold & Schluter, 2013b)

Eating foods which do not contain all essential amino acids requires a balanced diet and if not done properly can lead to health disorders. Based to their origin, we distinguish animal proteins and vegetable proteins. Animal protein which occurs in meat, fish, seafood, eggs, milk and dairy products (cheese, yoghurt and buttermilk) is a complete protein. Vegetable protein derived from vegetables, fruits, legumes, nuts, seeds and cereals is a source of incomplete protein (it does not contain all essential amino acids) with only a few exceptions. Animal protein has a higher nutritional value and through eating meat, fish, eggs and dairy products, it is easier to provide the body with the necessary dose of protein. Plant proteins contain less lysine, methionine, tryptophan and valine and people on a vegetarian or vegan diet need to balance their intake of a variety of foods. Although animal proteins are complete, the excess of animal products in the diet is not beneficial for human health. Animal products contain cholesterol and a lot of fat, so they can increase the risk of cardiovascular disease and obesity. There is growing interest in alternative protein sources to feed the increasing world population and insects represent one of the potential sources to exploit (Janssen, Vincken, van den Broek, Fogliano, & Lakemond, 2017).

Fiber

Edible insects contain a variable but significant amounts of fiber which ranges from several to several dozen percent (see Table 4). The exoskeleton of insects is made of chitin (the most common form of fiber in the body of insects). Fiber content is measured by crude fiber (CF), acid detergent fiber (ADF), and neutral detergent fiber (NDF) (Finke, 2002, 2007; Pennino, Dierenfeld, & Behler, 1991; Barker, Fitzpatrick, & Dierenfeld, 1998). For plant-based foods, the compositing of the various components of these fibers is well established: ADF is composed usually of cellulose and lignins while NDF is composed of cellulose, hemicellulose and lignin (Van Soest & Robertson, 1977). Insects contain significant

Table 2. Protein content in selected insect species and traditional food sources

Animal Group	Species and Common Name	Edible Product	Protein Content [g/100g fresh weight]
Insects	Locusts and grasshopppers (*Locusta migratoria, Acridium melanorhodon, Ruspolia differens*)	Larva	14–18
	Locusts and grasshopppers (*Locusta migratoria, Acridium melanorhodon, Ruspolia differens*)	Adult	13–28
	Chapulines – Mexico (*Sphenarium purpurascens*)	Adult	35–48
	Silkworm (*Bombyx mori*)	Larva	54–70
	Yellow mealworm (*Tenebrio molitor*)	Larva	14–25
	Crickets (*Gryllidae*)	Adult	8–25
	Termites (*Isoptera*)	Adult	13–28
	Cockroaches (*Blattodea*)	Adult	44–66
	Beetles (*Coleoptera*)	Adult	9–70
	Beetles (*Coleoptera*)	Larva/pupae	12–53
	Flies (*Diptera*)	Adult	36–56
	Flies (*Diptera*)	Larva/pupae	63–64
	Ants, bees (*Hymenoptera*)	Adult	5–66
	Ants, bees (*Hymenoptera*)	Larva/pupae	40–61
	High quality Cricket Flour (*Acheta domestica*)[a]	Adult	67.8
	Cricket protein pasta (*Acheta domestica*)[b]	Adult	14
Cattle		Beef (raw)	19–26
Reptiles (cooked)	Turtles (*Chelodina rugosa, Chelonia depressa*)	Flesh	25–27
		Intestine	18
		Heart	17–23
		Liver	11–27
Fish and seafoods (raw)	Finfish	Mackerel	16–28
		Tilapia	16–19
	Crustaceans (*Crustacea*)	Shrimp	13–27
		Lobster	17–19
	Molluscs (*Mollusca*)	Cuttlefish, squid	15–18

[a]http://www.bizarrefood.com/insect-bug-flour-powder (Accessed 13.04.2018)
[b]http://nutribug.com/product/cricket-protein-pasta/ (Accessed 13.04.2018)
Source of data: (Rumpold & Schluter, 2013b; Chen Feng, Zhang, & Chen, 2010)

amounts of both ADF and NDF; however the components that make up these fibers are unknown. Some authors have suggested that the fiber in insects represents chitin because chitin – linear polymer of b-(1-4) N-acetyl-D-glucosamine units, is similar structurally to cellulose – linear polymer of b-(1-4)-D-glucopyranose units (Barker, Fitzpatrick, & Dierenfeld, 1998). Chitin from insect exoskeletons acts in the human body like cellulose and because of this effect it is often called "animal fiber". It does not have a nutritional role in the human body as it is not digested like cellulose. The enzyme chitinase is found in human gastric juices (Paoletti, Norberto, Damini, & Musumeci, 2007), but it has been found that it may be inactive. Active chitinase response in the body dominates among people from tropical countries where the consumption of insects has a long-term tradition (Lee, Simpson, & Wilson, 2008). Chitin affects the work of the digestive system and the regulation of fat metabolism in the body. It reduces the appetite and inhibits the absorption of fats and sugars from the gastrointestinal tract, thus it lowers the calorie content of the diet. Chitin is used mainly in dietetics for the production of dietary supplements supporting slimming.

Lipids

Just like source of protein, insects can also be a rich source of fatty acids. Fats and carbohydrates are important nutritive elements in the human body. They are the main energy sources and fat is the most energetic ingredient of human food. Carbohydrates in insects are formed mainly by chitin. Insect fat is composed of 80% triacylglycerols and about 20% phospholipids. Fatty acid in triacylglycerols can either be saturated, unsaturated, or essential. The intake of fatty acid plays a key role in human health. Limiting the amount of saturated fatty acids (SFA) consumed in the diet may reduce the risk of cardiovascular disease. Edible insects contain on average 10 to 30% of fat in the dry matter (refer to Figure 2). Usually this is higher in the larval stages than in adults (Rumpold & Schluter, 2013a; Chen, Feng, Zhang, & Chen, 2010). Grubs and beetle larvae belong to the insects with the highest fat content. For example, the African palm weevil larvae in the early stage (*Rhynhophorus phoenicis*) contains about 70% fat, and adult rhinoceros beetles (*Oryctes rhinoceros*) contain only 0.7% fat (Rumpold & Schluter, 2013b). Termites are also a good source of fat with a fat content more than 30% in their bodies. The fat content of grasshoppers, crickets, locusts, flies and dragonflies is lower.

Figure 4. Average content of amino acids in selected edible insects and beef [mg/g dry matter protein] (Finke, 2002; Oonincx & Dierenfeld, 2012; Rumpold & Schluter, 2013b)

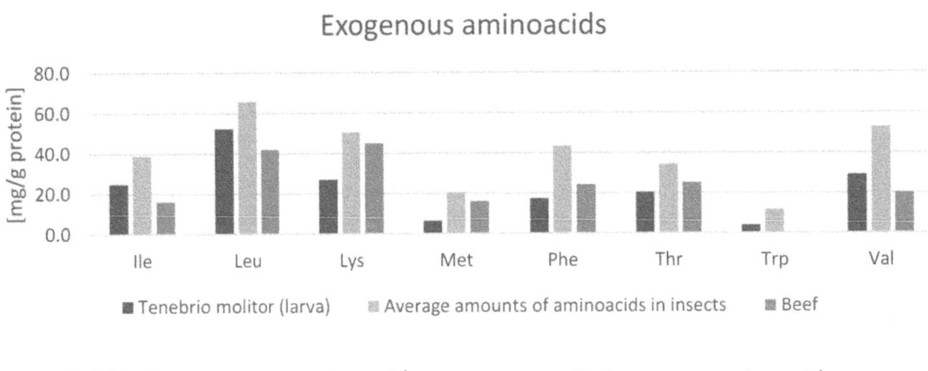

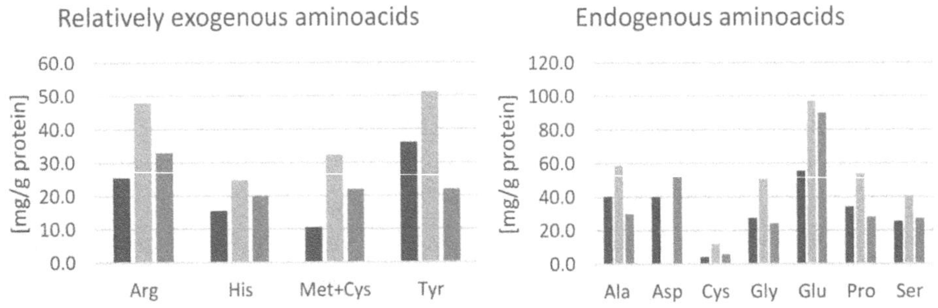

Table 3. Average amino acids content of selected edible insects

Group of Insects	Amino Acids																		
	His	Ile	Leu	Lys	Met	Cys	Met+Cys	Phe	Tyr	Phe+Tyr	Thr	Trp	Val	Arg	Ser	Pro	Ala	Gly	Glu
Cockroaches	19.4	29.9	56.4	48.0	29.8	11.6	41.4	30.6	62.3	92.9	34.6	6.0	53.8	41.5	41.9	65.0	56.6	58.7	99.7
Beetles, grubs	26.3	45.6	74.2	50.6	16.2	14.6	31.9	47.1	55.7	98.6	35.2	10.1	51.9	53.9	42.6	64.1	69.5	55.2	123.7
Flies	22.3	32.6	57.4	62.9	27.2	5.3	36.6	50.6	56.7	107.3	38.8	28.3	46.9	49.6	60	27.8	58.9	45.1	98.6
True bugs	15.7	31.5	49.8	28.0	21.7	12.9	32.2	34.4	38.7	63.8	29.9	10.3	44.3	24.9	10.3	-	26.4	16.4	23.7
Ants, bees	27.0	47.8	78.4	53.8	23.8	12.9	30.5	47.5	55.3	104.3	41.7	10.3	60.5	43.5	38.2	66.7	72.3	81.3	134.3
Termites	51.4	51.1	78.3	54.2	7.5	18.7	26.2	43.8	30.2	74.0	27.5	14.3	73.3	69.4	-	-	-	-	-
Butterflies, moths	23.7	40.4	62.7	57.7	22.1	12.2	34.7	46.3	49.1	95.8	40	11.2	54.1	46.9	48.34	44.9	48.9	43.8	103.4
Dragonflies, damselflies	21.2	39.6	74.8	53.9	19.3	12.8	29.8	46.6	61.5	100.3	35.8	8.1	50.3	53.6	41.9	53.9	77.4	54.0	94.5
Crickets, grasshoppers, locusts	15.0	30.0	59.0	45.0	16.0	6.0	22.0	-	-	30.0	23.0	6.0	39.0	-	-	-	-	-	-

His – histidine; Ile – isoleucine; Leu – leucine; Lys – lysine; Met – methionine; Cys – cysteine; Phe – phenylalanine; Tyr – tyrosine; Thr – threonine; Trp – tryptophan; Val – valine; Arg – arginine; Ser – serine; Pro – proline; Ala – alanine; Gly – glycine; Glu – glutamic acid.

Source of data: (Rumpold & Schluter, 2013b).

Table 4. Fiber content in selected insect species

Edible Insects		Stage	Fiber Content [% in Dry Matter]
Scientific Name	**Common Name**		
Locusta migratoria	African migratory locust	Nymph	27
Acheta domesticus	House cricket	Nymph	14.9–15.7
Acheta domesticus	House cricket	Adult	16.3–22
Gryllus assimilis	Jamaican field cricket	Nymph	8
Sphenarium purpurascens	Chapulines	Adult	4–11
Bombyx mori	Silkworm	Larva	5.9–6.4
Tenebrio molitor	Yellow mealworm	Larva	5–15
Tenebrio molitor	Yellow mealworm	Pupae	5.1
Tenebrio molitor	Yellow mealworm	Adult	20.2
Apis mellifera	Honey bee	Larva	1–1.3
Apis mellifera	Honey bee	Pupae	2.7–3
Apis mellifera	Honey bee	Adult	2–11

Source of data: (Chen, Feng, Zhang, & Chen, 2010; Rumpold & Schluter, 2013b; Kouřimská & Adámková, 2016)

Furthermore, insects are a good source of edible oil which contains more than 50% of polyunsaturated fatty acids (PUFA), mainly consisting of arachidonic, linolenic and linoleic acids desirable for nutritional and health reasons. The PUFA content of selected groups of edible insects is as high as about 30% (Figure 5). Oils extracted from several species of insects are rich in PUFA and often they contain the essential linoleic acid and α-linolenic acids which are very important for the proper development of children and infants (Womeni, Linder, Tiencheu, Mbiapo, Villeneuve, Fanni, & Parmentier, 2009). Adding essential fatty acids (EFA) to our daily diet is a great way to support human health. They support cardiovascular health, brain function and development, skin health, and offer many other benefits to our body. The composition of fatty acids in insects is promising – the content of linoleic acid, α-linolenic acids, omega-3 and omega-6 confirms that they can be successfully used in the diet as a source of unsaturated fatty acids (Womeni, Linder, Tiencheu, Mbiapo, Villeneuve, Fanni, & Parmentier, 2009).

Minerals

Vitamins and minerals are essential nutrients that our body needs in small amounts to work properly. Two kinds of minerals exist: macrominerals which the body needs in relatively larger amounts, namely calcium, phosphorus, magnesium, sodium, potassium, sulfur and chloride, and trace minerals required in small quantities, namely iron, zinc, manganese, copper, iodine, fluoride, cobalt and selenium. Most people should be able to get all the nutrients they need by eating a varied and balanced diet. We can find a variety of these minerals in fruits, vegetables, meat, and other foods. Minerals are necessary for three main reasons: building strong bones and teeth, controlling body fluids inside and outside the cells and turning the food we eat into energy. Essential minerals include calcium, iron, magnesium and potassium. It is difficult to refer to the content of micro- and macrominerals in edible insects in the context of the recommended daily intake because these values are set at different levels for various food products. In-

Figure 5. Average content [%] of the main groups of fatty acids in selected groups of edible insects
(Bukkens, 2005)
SFA – saturated fatty acids; MUFA – monounsaturated fatty acids; PUFA – polyunsaturated fatty acids

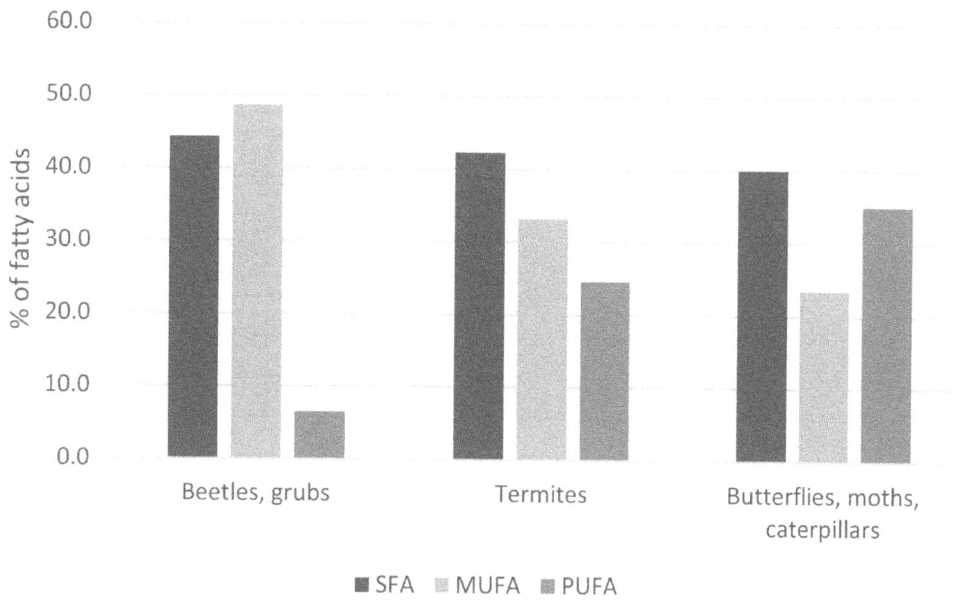

sects are rich in minerals and their content is higher than the content in the meat of slaughtered animals (Bukkens, 2005). For example, the concentration of iron in most insect species – 31–77 mg/100 g dry weight, is higher than in beef – 6mg/100g dry weight (Bukkens, 2005). The required amount of iron depends on its bioavailability, the consumer's age and sex. For example, this value is 9.1 mg per day for an adult male and 19.6 mg per day for an adult female. The content of iron, zinc and calcium are presented in Table 5. In the selected insects, the calcium content ranges from 32 in ants (*Onyoso mammon*) to 2010 in housefly larvae (*Musca domestica*) mg/100 g dry matter. The best absorbed calcium comes from milk and dairy products (the content of calcium in fat milk is about 120 and in various species of yellow cheese on average of 600 mg per 100 g of dry matter); however, many fruit and vegetables are also a good source of this macromineral.

Edible insects have the potential to provide specific micronutrients such as copper, iron, magnesium, manganese, phosphorous, selenium, and zinc. There are even suggestions that the consumption of insects could decrease some trace minerals deficiency in developing countries (Christensen, Orech, Mungai, Larsen, Friis, & Aagaard-Hansen, 2006).

Vitamins

Insects contain a variety of water soluble or lipophilic vitamins (Finke, 2002; Chen, Feng, Zhang, & Chen, 2010; Oonincx & Dierenfeld, 2012). Many species that have been analyzed contain only negligible amounts of these vitamins (Bukkens, 2005). The content of vitamins and minerals in wild edible insects is seasonal and in the case of farm bred species it can be controlled by properly selected feed.

Table 5. Content of calcium, iron and zinc in selected insects

Edible Insects			Content of Elements [mg/100g Dry Matter]		
Scientific Name	**Common Name**	**Stage**	**Ca**	**Fe**	**Zn**
Rhyncophorus phoenicis	African Palm Weevil	Larva	131	22.8	21.1
Tenebrio molitor	Yellow mealworm	Larva	45.8	5.46	12.5
Musca domestica	Housefly	Larva	2010	60.4	23.7
Bombyx mori	Silkworm	Larva	102.3	9.5	17.8
Onyoso mammon	Ant	Adult	32.6	17.7	11.1
Oyala	Termite	Adult	84.7	332	11.9
Ogawo	Termite	Adult	83	93.9	8.1
Agoro	Termite	Adult	132	161	14.3
Onjiri mammon	Cricket	Adult	341	1562	25.1
Average content of minerals [mg/g dry matter] in meat					
Beef			4-27	6	12.5
Pork			5-28	1.5	-
Poultry			5-14	1.2	-
Recommended nutrient intake [mg/day]					
Adult/male			750	9.1	4.2
Adult/female			750	19.6	3

Source of data: (Bukkens, 1997; FAO/WHO, 2001; Finke, 2002; Christensen, Orech, Mungai, Larsen, Friis, & Aagaard-Hansen, 2006; Hwangbo, 2009; Elemo, Elemo, Makinde, & Erukainure, 2011; Zielińska, Baraniak, Karaś, Rybczyńska, & Jakubczyk, 2015)

Table 6. Taste and smell of selected edible insects

Insect	Taste and Smell
Ants, termites	Sweet, nutty
Beetle larvae	Whole grain bread
Woodworm larvae	Fat meat
Dragonflies larvae, moths larvae	Fish
Cockroaches	Mushrooms
Bedbugs	Apples
Wasps	Pine
Maggots	Fried potatoes

Source of data: (Ramos-Elorduy, 1998)

Organoleptic Properties

Regardless of the content of nutrients, the culinary treatment determines the original value of food. Insects can be consumed immediately after catching, or after 1–3 days of starvation (Ramos-Elorduy, 1998). Depending on the species of insect and taste preferences, the insects can be fried, baked, grilled, cooked, marinated, smoked or dried. Organoleptic properties are an important criterion for the selection of the consumed insect and the process of its culinary treatment. The taste of insects is very diverse and can usually be compared with the taste of well-known dishes (see Table 6). In addition, if insects are fed with an intensely flavored feed, for example with cinnamon, they would have the taste of the feed used. The skeleton of adult forms of some insects (for example beetles) has a very big influence on the texture – the insects are crispy and fragile like crackers or crisps. Insects are more often consumed in the early stages of maturity as larvae as they contain less chitin, which can irritate the digestive system and therefore, they are a better digestible food (Pino-Moreno & Ramos-Elorduy, 2006).

Figure 6. Madagascar's cockroach (Gromphadorhina portentosa) grown at home fed with leftover meals
Photo: Tomasz Lewandowski

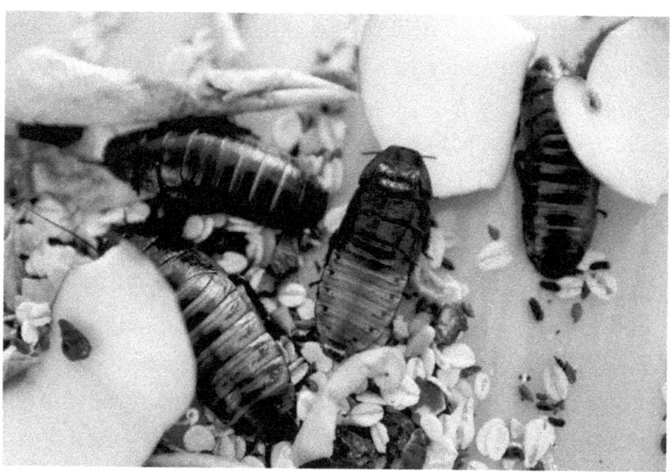

RISK FROM EATING INSECTS

Insects are considered as suitable alternatives to mainstream animal sources of food such as chicken, pork, beef and fish as well as an alternative feed. Because they are available in nature periodically (depending on the season and access to food), insect breeding can overcome their shortage (Yen, 2009, 2010; Sileshi & Kenis. 2010). Around the world, including in Europe, there are farms where insects are bred for animal feed and for human food. One of the important advantages of insect production is the high environmental safety compared to conventional livestock (Nakagaki & Defoliart, 1991).

Also, there are special devices on the market for home insect cultivation, for example mealworm larvae. The mealworms can be fed sustainably on vegetable scraps from the kitchen (Figure 6), because such waste can be used safely as animal feed (Fontenot, 1999).

Eating insects however could pose certain risks that must be taken into account. Such risk is expected to be comparable to other animal production systems (EFSA, 2015). There is need for further research to better assess the microbiological and chemical risks from insects destined as food and animal feed. Another risk associated with the consumption of insects is that some of them can contain naturally present toxic substances, such as cyanogenic glycosides (Zagrobelny, Dreon, Gomiero, Marcazzan, Glaring, Møller, & Paoletti, 2009). Moreover, eating insects can also cause allergies (EFSA, 2015). In China, there were over 1000 patients who suffered anaphylactic reactions after consuming silkworm pupa (Ji, Zhan, Chen, & Liu, 2008). A number of instances of allergic reactions to cochineal–biologically derived colorant obtained from the dried bodies of female cochineal insects (*Dactylopius coccus Costa/ Coccus cacti* L.), including anaphylaxis, have also been reported (Kagi, Wuthrich, & Johansson, 1994; DiCello, Myc, Baker, & Baldwin, 1999). Only a few cases of anaphylactic shock have been described following consumption of Mopane caterpillar (Kung, Fenemore, & Potter, 2011; Okezie, Kgomotso, & Letswiti, 2010).

The risk of food allergy after insect consumption needs further investigation and greater attention. Similar to other animal products, insects contain their gut microflora (Klunder, Wolkers-Rooijackers, Korpela, & Nout, 2012). This makes them susceptible to microbiological hazards if proper heat treatment or storage conditions are not applied. Edible insects need to be processed and stored with care to preserve microbiological safety, that is, to control the microflora inhabiting the body of insects (Cerritos & Cano-Santana, 2008). Therefore, further studies are needed to improve our knowledge of the microbiota thriving in insects with potential uses for food and feed production. More studies concerning the influence of the rearing conditions and processing on the associated microbiota of edible insects are also necessary (Garofalo, Osimani, Milanovic, Taccari, Cardinali, Aquilanti, … Clementi, 2017).

Parasites represent another potential hazard in relation to insect consumption. They could be present in edible insects and should be considered in the case of insects' consumption as food (Chai, Shin, Lee, & Rim, 2009). For example, particular attention should be paid to *Cryptosporidium parvum*, which is an important lethal agent for immunocompromised individuals (Graczyk, Knight, & Tamang, 2005). Chemical hazards in insects depend on their habitat and plant feed contamination and can be controlled by selected farming and dietary conditions. For example, crickets are able to introduce contaminants from solid waste into the food web by preying on discarded consumer products (Gaylor, Harvey, & Hale, 2012). Insects can be regarded as safe, if properly managed and consumed. Furthermore, international food regulations need to be established for food safety of insect products.

Figure 7. Chocolate with roasted larvae of the mealworms (Tenebrio molitor) made by members of the Student Scientific Circle of Molecular Cuisine, Faculty of Biotechnology and Food Science, Wroclaw University of Environmental and Life Sciences
Photo: Tomasz Lewandowski

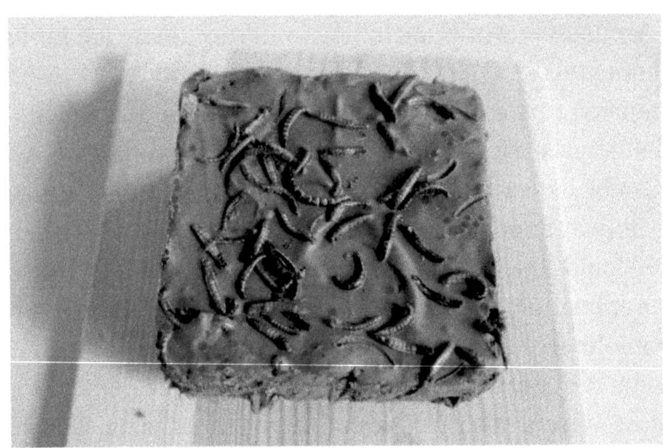

INTEREST IN EDIBLE INSECTS ON THE FOOD MARKET

Insect breeding carried out under controlled feeding conditions has resulted in the creation of new food products responding to market needs (Figure 7). The most popular are protein bars from mixtures of various species of insects as well as flour and pasta with the addition of ground crickets (University of California, Riverside, 2016). Currently, a wide range of protein rich powders/flours from insects is being produced. Insect flour can be used in a number of ways, for example, for energy bars, bread, pasta and much more. It can be used to increase the protein and nutrient content of any food. For example, 100 g of pasta with crickets delivers 14 g of protein and is also a good source of essential vitamins and minerals. Probably with the increase of consumer acceptance, the availability will increase not only in online stores but people will be able to buy insects in every supermarket. Some supermarkets are already announcing this (Borkhataria, 2017).

Nowadays an increasing number of restaurants around the world are introducing insects into their menu. An example is chocolate dessert with roasted ants (Figure 8). It was created as part of the realization of the educational project "Between Meadow and Forest" (Food Think Tank, 2014). A group of chefs, scientists and students from the Faculty of Biotechnology and Food Science of Wroclaw University of Environmental and Life Sciences, local farmers, photographers, filmmakers, sound engineers, artisans, architects, bartenders and baristas participated in the process. The essence of the project was to explore the richness of meadows and forest environments in terms of finding new sources of food and unfamiliar flavors and aromas.

Some of the world's best chefs, like Rene Redzepi from Noma (Copenhagen, Denmark) – ranked four times as the Best Restaurant in the World by Restaurant magazine, serve ants and promote insect food. The "Cook it Raw" project (Cook it Raw, 2015) created in 2009 at the climate summit in Copenhagen, invited chefs to cook dishes with minimal energy consumption, from what was available nearby. The

Figure 8. Chocolate dessert with roasted ants
Photo: Jędrzej Stelmaszek/Food Think Tank

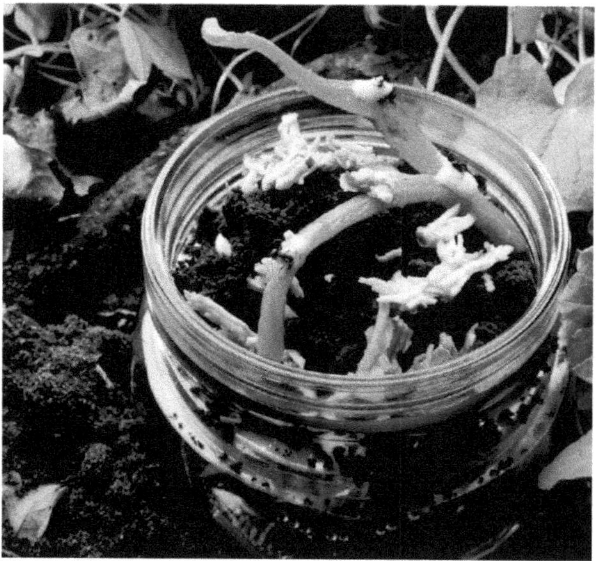

episode filmed in Poland in 2012 ended with a scene in which Rene Redzepi stood on a meadow with a grasshopper in his hand saying that this is our future, but we are not ready for it.

Although entomophagy is common in the world it is not yet accepted by western European populations. Popularization and information spreading about the advantages of eating insects could facilitate the integration of entomophagy in our feeding habits and behaviors (Megido, Sablon, Geuens, Brostaux, Alabi, Blecker, … Francis, 2014).

CONCLUSION

The existing research shows that insects have a high nutritional value, they are a rich source of protein and microelements (Banjo, Lawal, & Sangonuga, 2006). One of the important advantages of insect production is the reduced environmental impact compared to conventional livestock (Nakagaki & Defoliart, 1991). In addition, species such as crickets or mealworms contain many unsaturated fatty acids and vitamins. Their consumption can allow to build a well-balanced diet. Although some insects contain less protein than typical meat animal products, most of them also contain less fat, food products prepared from insects will have a lower energy value with the same nutritional value. The traditional use of insects as food is common in tropical countries but westerners should become more aware of the fact that their bias against insects as food has an adverse impact on the environmental health of the planet.

REFERENCES

Ademolu, K. O., Idowu, A. B., & Olatunde, G. O. (2010). Nutritional value assessment of variegated grasshopper, Zonocerus variegatus (L.) (Acridoidea: Pygomorphidae) during post-embryonic development. *African Entomology*, *18*(2), 360–364. doi:10.4001/003.018.0201

Banjo, A. D., Lawal, O. A., & Sangonuga, E. A. (2006). The nutritional value of fourteen species of edible insects in southern western Nigeria. *African Journal of Biotechnology*, *5*(3), 201–298. doi:10.5897/AJB05.250

Barker, D., Fitzpatrick, M. P., & Dierenfeld, E. S. (1998). Nutrient composition of selected whole invertebrates. *Zoo Biology*, *17*(2), 123–134. doi:10.1002/(SICI)1098-2361(1998)17:2<123::AID-ZOO7>3.0.CO;2-B

Borkhataria, C. (2017). Would you eat a burger made from insects? Mealworm-based food line set to hit grocery stores in Switzerland next week. *Daily Mail Australia*. Retrieved from https://www.dailymail.co.uk/sciencetech/article-4790414/Food-insects-sold-Swiss-supermarket.html

Bukkens, S. G. F. (1997). The nutritional value of edible insects. *Ecology of Food and Nutrition*, *36*(2-4), 287–319. doi:10.1080/03670244.1997.9991521

Bukkens, S. G. F. (2005). Insects in the human diet: Nutritional aspects. In M. G. Paoletti (Ed.), *Ecological implications of minilivestock: potential of insects, rodents, frogs and snails* (pp. 545–577). Enfield, NH: Science Publishers.

Cerritos, R., & Cano-Santana, Z. (2008). Harvesting grasshoppers Sphenarium purpurascens in Mexico for human consumption: A comparison with insecticidal control for managing pest outbreaks. *Crop Protection Journal*, *27*(3–5), 473–480. doi:10.1016/j.cropro.2007.08.001

Chai, J. Y., Shin, E. H., Lee, S. H., & Rim, H. J. (2009). Foodborne intestinal flukes in Southeast Asia. *Korean Journal of Parasitology*, *47*(Suppl), S69–S102. doi:10.3347/kjp.2009.47.S.S69 PMID:19885337

Chen, X., Feng, Y., Zhang, H., & Chen, Z. (2010). Review of the nutritive value of edible insects. In P. B. Durst, D. V. Johnson, R. N. Leslie & K. Shono (Eds), *Forest insects as food: Humans bite back* (pp. 85–92). Bangkok, Thailand: Food and Agriculture Organization of the United Nations. Retrieved from http://www.fao.org/docrep/012/i1380e/i1380e00.pdf

Christensen, D. L., Orech, F. O., Mungai, M. N., Larsen, T., Friis, H., & Aagaard-Hansen, J. (2006). Entomophagy among the Luo of Kenya: A potential mineral source? *International Journal of Food Sciences and Nutrition*, *57*(3–4), 198–203. doi:10.1080/09637480600738252 PMID:17127470

Collavo, A., Glew, R. H., Huang, Y.-S., Chuang, L. T., Bosse, R., & Paoletti, M. G. (2005). House crickets small-scale farming. In M. G. Paoletti (Ed.), *Ecological implications of minilivestock: potential of insects, rodents, frogs and snails* (pp. 519–544). Enfield, NH: Science Publishers.

Cook it raw. (2015). *Menu*. Retrieved from http://www.cookitraw.org/home/

DeFoliart, G. R. (1999). Insects as food: Why the Western attitude is important. *Annual Review of Entomology*, *44*(1), 21–50. doi:10.1146/annurev.ento.44.1.21 PMID:9990715

DiCello, M. C., Myc, A., Baker, J. R. Jr, & Baldwin, J. L. (1999). Anaphylaxis after ingestion of carmine colored foods: Two case reports and a review of the literature. *Allergy and Asthma Proceedings*, *20*(6), 377–382. doi:10.2500/108854199778251816 PMID:10624494

Dreyer, J. J., & Wehmeyer, A. S. (1982). On the nutritive value of Mopanie worms. *South African Journal of Science*, *78*, 33–35.

Elemo, B. O., Elemo, G. N., Makinde, M. A., & Erukainure, O. L. (2011). Chemical evaluation of African palm weevil, Rhychophorus phoenicis, larvae as a food source. *Journal of Insect Science*, *11*(146), 1–6. doi:10.1673/031.011.14601 PMID:22236060

European Food Safety Authority (EFSA). (2015). Risk profile related to production and consumption of insects as food and feed. *EFSA Journal*, *13*(10), 4257. doi:10.2903/j.efsa.2015.4257

Finke, M. D. (2002). Complete nutrient composition of selected invertebrates commonly fed to insectivores. *Zoo Biology*, *21*, 269–285. doi:10.1002/zoo.10031

Finke, M. D. (2007). Estimate of chitin in raw whole insects. *Zoo Biology*, *26*(2), 105–115. doi:10.1002/zoo.20123 PMID:19360565

Fontenot, J. P. (1999). Nutrient recycling: The North American experience — review. *Asian-Australasian Journal of Animal Sciences*, *12*(4), 642–650. doi:10.5713/ajas.1999.642

Food and Agriculture Organization of the United Nations (FAO). (2009). *How to feed the world in 2050?* Rome, Italy: FAO. Retrieved from http://www.fao.org/fileadmin/templates/wsfs/docs/expert_paper/How_to_Feed_the_World_in_2050.pdf

Food and Agriculture Organization of the United Nations (FAO). (2016). *The contribution of insects to food security, livelihoods and the enviroment*. Rome, Italy: FAO. Retrieved from http://www.fao.org/docrep/018/i3264e/i3264e00.pdf

Food and Agriculture Organization of the United Nations/World Health Organization (FAO/WHO). (2001). *Human vitamin and mineral requirements*. Rome, Italy: Food and Nutrition Division, FAO. Retrieved from http://www.fao.org/3/a-y2809e.pdf

Food Think Tank. (2014). *Between Meadow and Forest*. Retrieved from http://foodthinktank.pl/miedzylakaalasem (in Polish)

Garofalo, C., Osimani, A., Milanovic, V., Taccari, M., Cardinali, F., Aquilanti, L., ... Clementi, F. (2017). The microbiota of marketed processed edible insects as revealed by high-throughput sequencing. *Food Microbiology*, *62*, 15–22. doi:10.1016/j.fm.2016.09.012 PMID:27889142

Gaylor, M. O., Harvey, E., & Hale, R. C. (2012). House crickets can accumulate polybrominated diphenyl ethers (PBDEs) directly from polyurethane foam common in consumer products. *Chemosphere*, *86*(5), 500–505. doi:10.1016/j.chemosphere.2011.10.014 PMID:22071374

Graczyk, T. K., Knight, R., & Tamang, L. (2005). Mechanical transmission of human protozoan parasites by insects. *Clinical Microbiology Reviews*, *18*(1), 128–132. doi:10.1128/CMR.18.1.128-132.2005 PMID:15653822

Halloran, A., Hanboonsong, Y., Roos, N., & Bruun, S. (2017). Life cycle assessment of cricket farming in north-eastern Thailand. *Journal of Cleaner Production*, *156*, 83–94. doi:10.1016/j.jclepro.2017.04.017

Hwangbo, J., Hong, E. C., Jang, A., Kang, H. K., Oh, J. S., Kim, B. W., & Park, B. S. (2009). Utilization of house fly-maggots, a feed supplement in the production of broiler chickens. *Journal of Environmental Biology*, *30*, 609–614. PMID:20120505

Illgner, P., & Nel, E. (2000). The geography of edible insects in Sub-Saharan Africa: A study of the Mopane Caterpillar. *The Geographical Journal*, *166*(4), 336–351. doi:10.1111/j.1475-4959.2000.tb00035.x

Janssen, R. H., Vincken, J.-P., van den Broek, L. A. M., Fogliano, V., & Lakemond, C. M. M. (2017). Nitrogen-to-protein conversion factors for three edible insects: Tenebrio molitor, Alphitobius diaperinus, and Hermetia illucens. *Journal of Agricultural and Food Chemistry*, *65*(11), 2275–2278. doi:10.1021/acs.jafc.7b00471 PMID:28252948

Ji, K. M., Zhan, Z. K., Chen, J. J., & Liu, Z. G. (2008). Anaphylactic shock caused by silkworm pupa consumption in China. *Allergy*, *63*(10), 1405–1410. doi:10.1111/j.1398-9995.2008.01838.x PMID:18782121

Kagi, M. K., Wuthrich, B., & Johansson, S. G. (1994). Campari-orange anaphylaxis due to carmine allergy. *Lancet*, *344*(8914), 60–61. doi:10.1016/S0140-6736(94)91083-9 PMID:7912327

Klunder, H. C., Wolkers-Rooijackers, J., Korpela, J. M., & Nout, M. J. R. (2012). Microbiological aspects of processing and storage of edible insects. *Food Control*, *26*(2), 628–631. doi:10.1016/j.foodcont.2012.02.013

Kouřimská, L., & Adámková, A. (2016). Nutritional and sensory quality of edible insects. *NFS Journal*, *4*, 22–26. doi:10.1016/j.nfs.2016.07.001

Kung, S. J., Fenemore, B., & Potter, P. C. (2011). Anaphylaxis to mopane worms (Imbrasia belina). *Annals of Allergy, Asthma & Immunology, 106*(6), 538–540. doi:10.1016/j.anai.2011.02.003 PMID:21624756

Lee, K. P., Simpson, S. J., & Wilson, K. (2008). Dietary protein-quality influences melanization and immune function in an insect. *Functional Ecology, 22*(6), 1052–1061. doi:10.1111/j.1365-2435.2008.01459.x

Lefevre, M., Kris-Etherton, P. M., Zhao, G., & Tracy, R. P. (2004). Dietary fatty acids, hemostasis, and cardiovascular disease risk. *Journal of the Academy of Nutrition and Dietetics, 104*(3), 410–419. doi:10.1016/j.jada.2003.12.022 PMID:14993864

MacEvilly, C. (2000). Bugs in the system. *Nutrition Bulletin, 25*(4), 267–268. doi:10.1046/j.1467-3010.2000.00068.x

Megido, R. C., Sablon, L., Geuens, M., Brostaux, Y., Alabi, T., Blecker, C., ... Francis, F. (2014). Promising attitude for entomophagy development. *Journal of Sensory Studies, 29*(1), 14–20. doi:10.1111/joss.12077

Nakagaki, B. J., & Defoliart, G. R. (1991). Comparison of diets for mass-rearing Acheta domesticus (Orthoptera: Gryllidae) as a novelty food, and comparison of food conversion efficiency with values reported for livestock. *Journal of Economic Entomology, 84*(3), 891–896. doi:10.1093/jee/84.3.891

Okezie, O. A., Kgomotso, K. K., & Letswiti, M. M. (2010). Mopane worm allergy in a 36-year-old woman: A case report. *Journal of Medical Case Reports, 4*(1), 42. doi:10.1186/1752-1947-4-42 PMID:20205892

Oonincx, D. G., & Dierenfeld, E. S. (2012). An investigation into the chemical composition of alternative invertebrate prey. *Zoo Biology, 31*(1), 40–54. doi:10.1002/zoo.20382 PMID:21442652

Oonincx, D. G. A. B., & de Boer, I. J. M. (2012). Environmental impact of the production of mealworms as a protein source for humans – a life cycle assessment. *PLoS One, 7*(12), 51145. doi:10.1371/journal.pone.0051145 PMID:23284661

Oonincx, D. G. A. B., van Itterbeeck, J., Heetkamp, M. J. W., van den Brand, H., van Loon, J. J. A., & van Huis, A. (2010). An exploration on greenhouse gas and ammonia production by insect species suitable for animal or human comsumption. *PLoS One, 5*(12), e14445. doi:10.1371/journal.pone.0014445 PMID:21206900

Paoletti, M. G., Norberto, L., Damini, R., & Musumeci, S. (2007). Human gastric juice contains chitinase that can degrade chitin. *Annals of Nutrition & Metabolism, 51*(3), 244–251. doi:10.1159/000104144 PMID:17587796

Payne, C. (2018, January 18). Edible insects: Do insects actually taste any good? *BBC News.* Retrieved from: https://www.bbc.co.uk/news/world-42639877

Pennino, M., Dierenfeld, E. S., & Behler, J. L. (1991). Retinol, alpha-tocopherol and proximate nutrient composition of invertebrates used as feed. *International Zoo Yearbook, 30*(1), 143–149. doi:10.1111/j.1748-1090.1991.tb03477.x

Pino-Moreno, J. M., & Ramos-Elorduy, J. J. (2006). Algunos ejemplos de aprovechamiento comercial de varios insectos comestibles y medicinales. In E. Estrada, J. N. Romero, A. M. Equihua, C. L. Luna L., & J. L. A. Rosas (Eds.), Entomología mexicana (pp. 524-533). Mexico City, Mexico: Sociedad Mexicana de Entomología.

Premalatha, M., Abbasi, T., Abbasi, T., & Abbasi, S. A. (2011). Energy-efficient food production to reduce global warming and ecodegradation: The use of edible insects. *Renewable & Sustainable Energy Reviews, 15*(9), 4357–4360. doi:10.1016/j.rser.2011.07.115

Ramos-Elorduy, J. (1998). *Creepy crawly cuisine: The gourmet guide to edible insects*. Paris, France: Park Street Press.

Ramos-Elorduy, J., Moreno, J. M. P., Prado, E. E., Perez, M. A., Otero, J. L., & de Guevara, O. L. (1997). Nutritional value of edible insects from the state of Oaxaca, Mexico. *Journal of Food Composition Analisys, 10*(2), 142–157. doi:10.1006/jfca.1997.0530

Renault, D., Laparie, M., McCauley, S. J., & Bonte, D. (2018). Environmental adaptations, ecological filtering, and dispersal central to insect invasions. *Annual Review of Entomology, 63*(1), 345–368. doi:10.1146/annurev-ento-020117-043315 PMID:29029589

Rumpold, B. A., & Schluter, O. K. (2013a). Nutritional composition and safety aspects of edible insects. *Molecular Nutrition & Food Research, 57*(5), 802–823. doi:10.1002/mnfr.201200735 PMID:23471778

Rumpold, B. A., & Schluter, O. K. (2013b). Potential and challenges of insects as an innovative source for food and feed production Innovative. *Food Science and Emerging Technologies, 17*, 1–11. doi:10.1016/j.ifset.2012.11.005

Sileshi, G. W., & Kenis, M. (2010). Food security: Farming insects. *Science, 328*(5978), 568–568. doi:10.1126cience.328.5978.568-a PMID:20430996

Smil, V. (2002). Worldwide transformation of diets, burdens of meat production and opportunities for novel food proteins. *Enzyme and Microbial Technology, 30*(3), 305–311. doi:10.1016/S0141-0229(01)00504-X

Tosi, E., & Daccordi, M. (1983). Insetti commestibili. Slurp! *Nigrizia, 101*(6), 49–52.

United States Department of Agriculture (USDA). (2012). *The Pherobase: Database of pheromones and semiochemicals*. Retrieved from http://www.pherobase.com/

University of California, Riverside. (2016). *Entomophagy (Eating insects)*. San Diego, CA: Ceter for Invasive Species Research. Retrieved from http://cisr.ucr.edu/entomophagy.html

van Huis, A., Dicke, M., & van Loon, J. J. A. (2015). Insects to feed the world. *Journal of Insects as Food and Feed, 1*(1), 3–5. doi:10.3920/JIFF2015.x002

van Huis, A., Itterbeeck, J. V., Klunder, H., Mertens, E., Halloran, A., Muir, G., & Vantomme, P. (2013). *Edible insects: Future prospects for food and feed security*. Rome, Italy: Food and Agriculture Organisation of the United Nations. Retrieved from http://www.fao.org/docrep/018/i3253e/i3253e.pdf

Van Soest, P. J., & Robertson, J. B. (1977). What is fibre and fibre in food? *Nutrition Reviews, 35*(3), 12–22. doi:10.1111/j.1753-4887.1977.tb06532.x PMID:840446

Wageningen University and Research. (2017). *List of edible insects of the world (April 1, 2017)*. Retrieved from https://www.wur.nl/en/Expertise-Services/Chair-groups/Plant-Sciences/Laboratory-of-Entomology/Edible-insects/Worldwide-species-list.htm

Womeni, H. M., Linder, M., Tiencheu, B., Mbiapo, F. T., Villeneuve, P., Fanni, J., & Parmentier, M. (2009). Oils of insects and larvae consumed in Africa: Potential sources of polyunsaturated fatty acids. *OCL – Oleagineux, Corps Gras, Lipides, 16*(4), 230-235. Retrieved from https://www.ocl-journal.org/articles/ocl/abs/2009/04/ocl2009164p230/ocl2009164p230.html

Yen, A. L. (2009). Edible insects: Traditional knowledge or western phobia? *Entomological Research, 39*(5), 289–298. doi:10.1111/j.1748-5967.2009.00239.x

Yen, A. L. (2010). Edible insects and other invertebrates in Australia: future prospects. In P. B. Durst, D. V. Johnson, R. N. Leslie & K. Shono (Eds), *Forest insects as food: Humans bite back* (pp. 65–84). Bangkok, Thailand: Food and Agriculture Organization of the United Nations. Retrieved from http://www.fao.org/docrep/012/i1380e/i1380e00.pdf

Zagrobelny, M., Dreon, A. L., Gomiero, T., Marcazzan, G. L., Glaring, M. A., MøLler, B. L., & Paoletti, M. G. (2009). Toxic moths: Source of a truly safe delicacy. *Journal of Ethnobiology, 29*(1), 64–76. doi:10.2993/0278-0771-29.1.64

Zielińska, E., Baraniak, B., Karaś, M., Rybczyńska, K., & Jakubczyk, A. (2015). Selected species of edible insects as a source of nutrient composition. *Food Research International, 77*, 460–466. doi:10.1016/j.foodres.2015.09.008

ADDITIONAL READING

Borkhataria, C. (2017). *Would you eat a burger made from insects? Mealworm-based food line set to hit grocery stores in Switzerland next week.* Daily Mail Australia. Retrieved from https://www.dailymail.co.uk/sciencetech/article-4790414/Food-insects-sold-Swiss-supermarket.html

Bukkens, S. G. F. (1997). The nutritional value of edible insects. *Ecology of Food and Nutrition, 36*(2-4), 287–319. doi:10.1080/03670244.1997.9991521

Durst, P. B., Johnson, D. V., Leslie, R. N., & Shono, K. (Eds.). (2010). *Forest insects as food: Humans bite back.* Proceedings of a workshop on Asia-Pacific resources and their potential for development, Chiang Mai, Thailand, 19-21 February, 2008. Bangkok, Thailand: Food and Agriculture Organization of the United Nations. Retrieved from http://www.fao.org/docrep/012/i1380e/i1380e00.pdf

Food and Agriculture Organization of the United Nations (FAO). (2016). *The contribution of insects to food security, livelihoods and the enviroment.* Rome, Italy: FAO. Retrieved from http://www.fao.org/docrep/018/i3264e/i3264e00.pdf

Oonincx, D. G. A. B., van Itterbeeck, J., Heetkamp, M. J. W., van den Brand, H., van Loon, J. J. A., & van Huis, A. (2010). An exploration on greenhouse gas and ammonia production by insect species suitable for animal or human comsumption. *PLoS One, 5*(12), e14445. doi:10.1371/journal.pone.0014445 PMID:21206900

Paoletti, M. G. (Ed.). (2005). *Ecological implications of minilivestock: Potential of insects, rodents, frogs and snails.* Enfield, NH: Science Publishers. doi:10.1201/9781482294439

Ramos-Elorduy, J. (1998). *Creepy crawly cuisine: The gourmet guide to edible insects*. Paris, France: Park Street Press.

Rumpold, B. A., & Schluter, O. K. (2013b). Potential and challenges of insects as an innovative source for food and feed production Innovative. *Food Science and Emerging Technologies, 17*, 1–11. doi:10.1016/j.ifset.2012.11.005

Wageningen University and Research. (2017). List of edible insects of the world (April 1, 2017). Retrieved from https://www.wur.nl/en/Expertise-Services/Chair-groups/Plant-Sciences/Laboratory-of-Entomology/Edible-insects/Worldwide-species-list.htm

Zielińska, E., Baraniak, B., Karaś, M., Rybczyńska, K., & Jakubczyk, A. (2015). Selected species of edible insects as a source of nutrient composition. *Food Research International, 77*, 460–466. doi:10.1016/j.foodres.2015.09.008

KEY TERMS AND DEFINITIONS

Animal Protein: Protein is built from building blocks (amino acids); our bodies make amino acids from scratch, or by modifying others but a few amino acids (known as the essential amino acids) must come from food. Animal sources of protein tend to deliver all amino acids we need. Other protein sources, such as fruits, vegetables, grains, nuts and seeds, may lack one or more essential amino acids.

Conventional Livestock: Domesticated animals raised in an agricultural setting to produce meat, eggs, milk, leather, wool, and other products.

Diet: The sum of the food consumed by a person or another organism.

Edible Insects: Insects which can be consumed by humans.

Essential Fatty Acid (EFA): An unsaturated fatty acid that is essential to human health, but cannot be manufactured in the body; supplementation with EFAs could be useful as a treatment for certain neurological disorders.

European Food Safety Agency (EFSA): An organization which provides scientific advice and communications about existing and emerging risks associated with the food chain.

Energy Value/Content: The amount of energy available from an item of food when digested, mostly from carbohydrates and fats.

Entomophagy: From the Greek words ἔντομον *éntomon* – insect, and φᾰγεῖν *phagein* – to eat; the human use of insects as food.

Essential Amino Acid: An amino acid which is required for normal health and growth but cannot be synthesized *de novo* (from scratch) by the organism, and thus must be supplied in the diet.

Essential Nutrient: A nutrient required for normal body functioning which cannot be synthesized by the organism and must be provided by the diet.

Fatty Acids Profile: Percentage of fatty acids in food.

Fiber: Dietary material containing substances such as cellulose, lignin, and pectin, that are resistant to the action of digestive enzymes.

Food Allergy: An immune system reaction that occurs soon after eating a certain food; causes digestive problems, hives or swollen airways, in some people, a food allergy can cause severe symptoms or even a life-threatening reaction known as anaphylaxis.

Food and Agriculture Organization of the United Nations (FAO): A specialized agency of the United Nations which leads international efforts to defeat hunger.

Greenhouse Gas: Gas that contributes to the greenhouse effect by absorbing infrared radiation (for example carbon dioxide and chlorofluorocarbons).

Insect Farming: The practice of raising insects as livestock. Insect farming in a closed or indoor environment is an important means for making food available continuously year-round.

Insect Protein: A new source for animal feed and food; as protein sources, the nutritive value of edible insects is as good as other animals (or plants) or even better.

Macrominerals: A number of minerals, such as calcium, phosphorus, magnesium, sodium, potassium, chloride, and sulfurase, which are needed in large amounts to maintain the proper functioning of an organism.

Monounsaturated Fatty Acids (MUFAs): Acids with one double bond in the fatty acid chain, the remaining carbon atoms are bound by single bond.

Nutrient Content: A source of nourishment, especially a nourishing ingredient in a food.

Nutritive Value: The contribution of a food to the nutrient content of the diet. This value depends on the quantity of the food which is digested and absorbed and the amounts of the essential nutrients (protein, fat, carbohydrate, minerals, vitamins) which it contains.

Organoleptic Properties: The aspects of food that an individual experiences via the senses—including taste, sight (color), smell, and touch (texture).

Polyunsaturated Fatty Acids (PUFAs): Fatty acids with two or more double bonds between the carbon atoms.

Protein Bars: Lower in carb, vitamins, and dietary minerals and significantly higher in protein than other bars; they are mainly used by athletes for muscle building.

Saturated Fatty Acids (SFAs): Fatty acids in which all carbon atoms in the hydrocarbon chain are joined by single bonds. They exist mostly as components of fats (triglycerides) or other lipids of animal origin; a diet high in saturated fatty acids may contribute to a high blood cholesterol level.

Trace Minerals: Essential minerals, such as iron, zinc, selenium, fluoride, chromium, copper, iodine, manganese, and molybdenum, which help the body perform regulatory and structural functions.

Vitamins: A group of organic compounds which are essential for normal growth and nutrition and are required in small quantities in the diet because they cannot be synthesized by the body; they have diverse biochemical functions.

World Health Organization (WHO): An international organization whose primary role is to direct international health within the United Nations' system and to lead partners in global health responses.

This research was previously published in Environmental, Health, and Business Opportunities in the New Meat Alternatives Market edited by Diana Bogueva, Dora Marinova, Talia Raphaely, and Kurt Schmidinger; pages 143-165, copyright year 2019 by Business Science Reference (an imprint of IGI Global).

Chapter 62

The Nutritional and Health Potential of Blackjack (Bidens pilosa l.):
A Review – Promoting the Use of Blackjack for Food

Rose Mujila Mboya

Independent Researcher, Pietermaritzburg, South Africa

ABSTRACT

Blackjack (bidens pilosa l.) grows naturally as a perennial herb across the world, especially in tropical regions, and it is used in many parts of the world for treating illnesses such as diarrhea, indigestion, wounds, and respiratory infections. Blackjack's agricultural and pharmaceutical benefits have been well studied by scientists, following which several suggestions for using it as a source of supplements and alternative antibiotics have been made. Moreover, blackjack is edible but very much underutilized for food purposes. In this article, the author reviews the advantages and disadvantages of blackjack and argues for the deliberation of promoting its use for food.

INTRODUCTION

Blackjack (Bidens pilosa L) is a widespread plant said to have its origin in tropical America. It is currently recognized as an invasive weed and a threat to natural vegetation in many countries (Arthur, Naidoo & Coopoosamy 2012), requiring serious preventative measures. It is therefore mostly destroyed and wasted. However, blackjack is well recognized for its curative characteristics in many parts of the world, thus used to treat illnesses such as respiratory infections, wounds, dysentery, diarrhoea and indigestion (Arthur et al., 2012). It is also consumed in some parts of the world, especially when other vegetables are scarce (Lusweti, Wabuyele, Ssegawa & Mauremootoo, 2011). In general, blackjack is greatly underutilized as a food source. It's occurrence as a weed or wild plant would naturally create negative perceptions with

DOI: 10.4018/978-1-7998-5354-1.ch062

regard to its consumption regardless of its benefits. The fact that it is consumed in some communities only when other vegetables are scarce implies that blackjack is not a preferred food.

Although its nutritional benefits have been studied, they have not been reported as much as its pharmaceutical and agricultural benefits. Considering the minimal labour required to grow blackjack together with its potentially significant nutritional benefits, in this paper, the author argues for the domestication of the blackjack plant and the deliberation of its use for food. The main objective for this paper was to review the advantages and disadvantages of blackjack and argue for its promotion for use as food based on its nutritional benefits and its potential for combating micronutrient deficiencies and chronic diseases.

BACKGROUND

Blackjack (Figure 1) falls under the following taxonomic tree (Bartolome, Villaseñor & Yang, 2013):

Figure 1. Blackjack (Bidens pilosa L.)

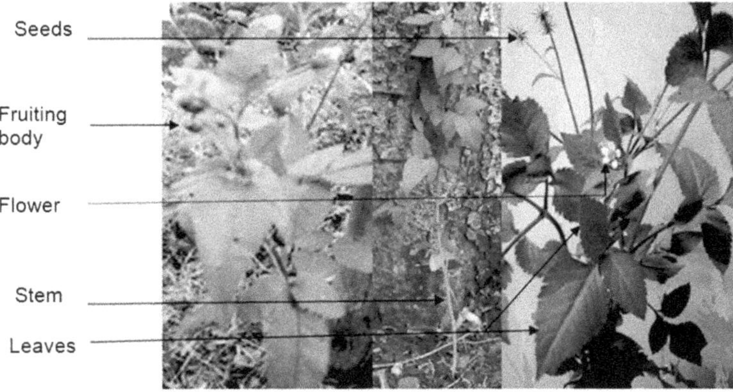

Taxonomic Tree

Kingdom: *Plantae*
Subkingdom: *Tracheobionta*
Phylum: *Spermatophyta*
Subphylum: *Angiospermae*
Class: *Magnoliopsida*
Order: *Asterales*
Family: *Asteraceae*
Genus: *Bidens*
Species: *Bidens pilosa*

Characteristics, Favourable Conditions, Growth and Dispersion

Blackjack is said to grow in all seasons in the tropics, most actively in the warmer and wetter parts of the seasons (Holm, Plucknett, Pancho & Herberger, 1977). It is highly resistant to harsh climatic conditions such as drought and cold and it may have a life cycle of 150-360 days. Each blackjack plant has the capacity to produce more than 30000 highly viable seeds. Thus it is possible for blackjack to produce three to four generations per year (Mitich, 1994). Also, blackjack's seeds are light and spikey, thus they can readily attach to animal skin, machinery or clothing, and in so doing are easily dispersed.

Furthermore, blackjack's seeds germinate on the soil surface or in shallow soil of 1 - 4 cm depth and at greater depths they remain viable in the soil for many years (Chivinge, 1996). Tilled land, moisture and temperatures at 20, 25 and 30°C arc known to favour germination, with 25°C being the most favourable temperature at which 70% of seeds were reported to germinate (Chivinge, 1996). The ease with which blackjack is dispersed, and its capacity to produce huge quantities of highly viable seeds provide capacity for blackjack to grow profusely (Figure 2) and to be available throughout the year.

Figure 2. Blackjack colony

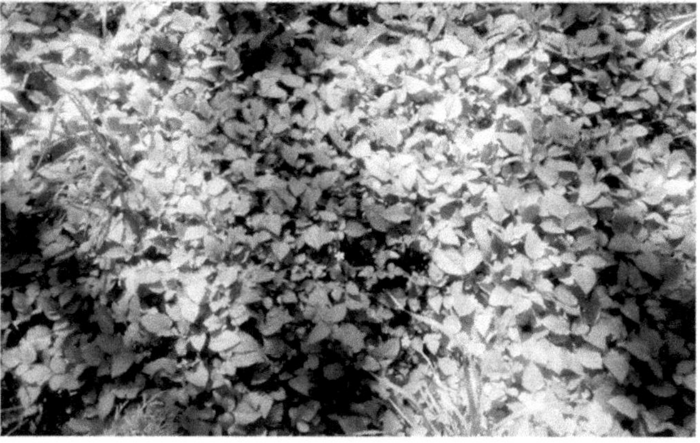

METHODOLOGY

Desk top research on literature was conducted to investigate the known uses, benefits and disadvantages of blackjack. To further understand the suitability of blackjack for use as food, seventeen individuals, twelve of whom were familiar with using blackjack for food were selected using convenience sampling and interviewed using telephone interviews. They included two nurses and five medical doctors working in South Africa, three individuals from Tanzania, three from Zimbabwe, two from Malawi and two from Zambia. It is worth noting the fact that since very few people seem to use blackjack for food, it was impossible to obtain a large sample for interviews.

Participants who consume blackjack were interviewed with regard to the length of time for which they had used blackjack for food and whether they or any other person they knew had ever fallen ill due to eating blackjack. The nurses and medical doctors were specifically interviewed with regard to having heard of or having attended to patients seeking medical attention after falling sick due to eating blackjack. This information was regarded as necessary for providing evidence of any negative health effects that might be incurred due to the consumption of blackjack.

ADVANTAGES AND DISADVANTAGES OF BLACKJACK

Several advantages and disadvantages attributed to blackjack are reviewed in this section.

Disadvantages

Being an Aggressive Weed

Blackjack's tendency to grow profusely (Figure 2) is detrimental to crops as it would lead to large amounts of nutrients that should otherwise be utilized by crops being lost to it, leading to a reduction in crop yield. In Argentina, a density of one blackjack plant per meter of soya bean field caused 9.4% of bean yield loss and densities higher than eight blackjack plants per meter of soya bean field caused a 43% soya bean loss (Arce, Robinet, Mansilla de Andrada, Guillén & Dfazy, 1995). Up to 80% of sugarcane growth suppression was reported at Sambaru, Okinawa, Japan (Ishimune et al., 1986). Blackjack's potential for significant proliferation can lead to alarming amounts of crop yield loss. In part, this explains why blackjack is regarded as a problematic weed requiring serious preventative action.

A Host to Many Pathogens

Viruses such as the Tomato Spotted Virus which causes disease to fruits and vegetables as well the Bidens Mottle Virus which attacks lettuce and endive were reported to be hosted by blackjack (Purciful, Christie, Zitter & Bassett, 1971). Blackjack was also reported to host several fungal species including *Cladisporium, Penicillium, Aspergillus, Fusarium, Trychoderma* and *Botrytis* (Prete, Nunes Júnior & Menten, 1984. Furthermore, blackjack was also reported to be a host for *Orobanche ramosa*, a phanerogamous parasite and moths, such as those belonging to the family *Noctuidae*, a coffee-foliage feeding moth, thus aiding their spread (Torres, 1986; Bardner & Mathenge, 1974). It similarly attracts other types of insects such as *Empyreuma pugione*, a wasp-like moth (Adams & Goss, 1978). Pathogens that are hosted by blackjack pose a threat to the health and productivity of the other food plants in the fields where blackjack is a weed, and to the extent to which they are safe for consumption.

Capacity to Promote Cancer of the Throat

In KwaZulu-Natal, South Africa, Arthur et al. (2012) reported that the consumption of blackjack leaves promotes the development of cancer of the throat, but no empirical evidence was provided to support this claim. However, blackjack is a host to pathogenic fungi, among them *Aspergillus* and *Fusarium* species, which are known to cause cancer of the throat (Pitt, 2000; Bayman & Baker, 2006; Bennet & Klich, 2003, as cited by Mboya, Tongoona, Yobo, Derera & Langyintuo, 2011). It is therefore possible that cancer of the throat which was associated with the consumption of blackjack in KwaZulu-Natal was caused by the pathogenic fungi hosted by blackjack rather than being caused by the plant itself.

Capacity to Inhibit Useful Bacteria

Blackjack was found to have inhibiting characteristics on *Bacillus pumilus* and *Bacillus subtilis* (Bartolome et al., 2013). *Bacillus subtilis* is among the several *Bacillus* species that have been used as probiotic supplements in both animals and humans and they are regarded as safe (Cutting, 2011; Sumi, Yang, Yeo & Hahm, 2015). Also, several antimicrobial peptides such as *bacitracin, iturin, fengicin*, and *lactosporin* produced by *Bacillus* species, have been proven to have antibacterial, antifungal, antiviral and antitumor characteristics (Sumi et al., 2015). Thus they promote plant, animal and human health. Unlike conventional antibiotics, antimicrobial peptides kill microbes through generating membrane pores, thus making it hard for the microbes to develop resistance against them and are therefore regarded as having potential for combating antibiotic resistance ((Sang & Blecha, 2008; Sumi et al., 2015). The tendency for blackjack to inhibit *Bacillus subtilis* and *Bacillus pumilus* is therefore a disadvantage as it hinders the beneficial functioning of the latter.

The Nutritional Content of Blackjack

Blackjack has been reported to contain several nutrients, some of them having antioxidant characteristics.

The Macronutrient Content of Blackjack

In studies conducted by Odhav, Beekrumb, Akulaa & Baijnath (2006); Food and Agricultural Organization of the United Nations (FAO, 1997), as cited by Bartolome et al. (2013) and Alikwe, Ohimain & Omotosho (2014) nutrients shown in Table 1 were detected per 100 g of blackjack. Except for carbohydrates, quantities of macronutrients reported by Alikwe et al. (2014) per 100 g of blackjack are much higher than the quantities of macronutrients reported by Odhav et al. (2006) and FAO (1997), as cited by Bartolome et al. (2013).

In part the difference in the quantities of macronutrients reported can be explained in that as opposed to Odhav et al. (2006) and FAO's studies, dry leaves were used in the study by Alikwe et al. (2014), which implies that there was a higher mass per 100 g of dried blackjack leaves compared to the amount per 100 g of fresh blackjack leaves.

Amino Acids Detected in Blackjack

Alikwe et al. (2014) detected five amino acids in blackjack, namely methionine, lysine, alanine, cysteine and tryptophan. Amino acids are the building blocks of all protein and are intermediates in various metabolic pathways. They are important for the synthesis of a wide range of biologically important substances including nucleotides, peptide hormones, enzymes and neurotransmitters (Mohanty et al., 2014). Nine essential and 11 non-essential amino acids exist. The former cannot be synthesized by our bodies, therefore they have to be obtained from food, whereas the latter can be made by our bodies using the essential amino acids. The fact that blackjack was found to consist of five essential amino acids implies that although it has the potential for being a source of protein, it does not contain all essential amino acids (Woolf, Fu & Basu, 2011). Therefore, like the other plant foods, blackjack would be unable to supply all the protein the body needs by itself. The consumption of a plant alongside other complementary plant foods was found to enhance the quality of protein consumed (Woolf et al., 2011). Therefore edible

Table 1. Nutrients reported per100 g of blackjack

Study by Odhav et al., 2006 (Fresh Leaves Used)		Study by FAO, as cited by Bartolome et al., 2013 (Fresh Leaves Used)	Study by Alikwe et al., 2014 (Dry Leaves Used)
Protein	5.0 g	3.8 g	15.86 g
Fat	0.6 g	0.5 g	7.49 g
Carbohydrate	8.4 g	8.4 g	-
Fibre	2.9 g	3.9 g	18.13 g
Micronutrients per 100 g of Dry Leaves			
Calcium	1354.0 mg	111.0 mg	0.39 mg
Phosphorus	504.0 mg	39.0 mg	0.31 mg
Sodium	290.0 mg	-	0.54 mg
Manganese	21.0 mg	-	2.2 mg
Copper	10.0 mg	-	1.26 mg
Zinc	22.0 mg	-	4.53 mg
Magnesium	658.0 mg	-	0.23 mg
Iron	17.0 mg	2.3 µg	78.9 mg

plants that are rich in amino acids such as blackjack should be eaten along with other complementary foods such as cereals and nuts in order to improve the quality of protein.

Micronutrient Content in Blackjack

Blackjack was found to have great potential for providing the recommended daily intake (RDI) of micronutrients, and in so doing, making a contribution towards fighting against micronutrient deficiency, also known as hidden hunger. In pregnant women, hidden hunger can cause low birth rate, high mortality rate and impaired mental development. Stunting, reduced mental capacity, reduced learning capacity and increased frequency of infection are among the problems that hidden hunger can cause in children (Beiley, West & Black, 2015). Likewise, in adults hidden hunger leads to malnutrition and increased risk of chronic diseases (Beiley et al., 2015). This can further lead to reduced productivity and poor socio-economic status of the affected individuals. In senior adults, many age- related health challenges are associated with hidden hunger (Hoffmann, 2017).

Odhav et al. (2006) reported much higher amounts of micronutrients with the exception of iron, which was reported in far greater amounts in the study conducted by Alikwe et al. (2014). Minute amounts of iron (2.8 µg/100g) were reported in the findings sourced from FAO (Bartolome et al., 2013). These findings also imply that the variations in the reported quantities of specific nutrients, especially micronutrients per specific weight of blackjack, are not really determined by the dry or fresh statuses of samples used.

Variations with regard to blackjack's vitamin content were also noted. Fober, Delofse, Van Jaarsveld, Wenhold & Van Rensburg (2010) reported finding 428 µg RAE (vitamin A) of beta carotene per 100 g of blackjack, whereas Wolmarans, Danster, Dalton, Schonfeld & Rossouuw (2010) detected 983 µgRAE (vitamin A) beta carotene from the same weight of blackjack. Similarly, Agea et al. (2014) reported finding 74 mg of vitamin C per 100 g of fresh blackjack leaves, whereas Abidemi (2013) detected 16 mg of vitamin C per 100 g of the former.

Mzengezera et al. (2014) reported that vitamin C constituted an estimate of 5% out of 5 g of blackjack dry matter. Calculating from these numeric figures, 5 g of dry blackjack matter would contain 0.25 g of vitamin C, and 1 g of dry blackjack matter would contain 0.05 g of vitamin C. Therefore, 100 g of blackjack dry matter would contain 5 g of vitamin C. The huge amount of vitamin C reported in dry blackjack matter by Mzengezera et al. (2014) raise questions with regard to the accuracy of the methods used in the study. Vitamin C is sensitive to heat, thus, like other vitamins it is easily destroyed by heat (Njoku, Ayuk & Okoye, 2011). The process of obtaining dry blackjack matter in the research reported by Mzengerera et al. (2014) involved drying fresh blackjack samples at 105 °C for six hours. Considering the high temperature used to dry the samples and the time spent drying them, one would expect very small amounts of vitamin C to be detected in the dry matter.

The variations in the reported blackjack's nutrient content make it impossible to determine common amounts of specific nutrients that can be obtained per weight of blackjack and also raise the following questions: Could the variations be the result of different types of nutrients in the soil where blackjack was harvested, the different climatic conditions of the places it grew in or the degree of accuracy of the analytical methods used? More research is required to find answers to these questions.

The Contribution Blackjack Can Make Towards Meeting Recommended Intakes of Vitamin E

Although Modi et al. (2006) recorded that blackjack was rich in vitamin E, reports on quantities of vitamin E per weight of blackjack were not found, implying that this nutrient has hardly been studied in blackjack. Consequently, in Table 2 vitamin E has been excluded from the review of the estimated contribution which 100 g of blackjack can make towards the dietary intake of vitamins found in this plant.

Apart from primarily functioning as an antioxidant, vitamin E also promotes muscle membranes repair and enhances the immune system (Labazi, McNeil & Kurtz, 2015, as cited by Raedestorff, Wyss, Calder, Weber & Eggersdorfer, 2015; Rizvi et al., 2014). The proper functioning of vitamin E is said to be highly dependent on vitamin C, B_3, Selenium, and glutathione (Rizvi et al., 2014). This implies that maximum functioning of vitamin E can only be realized where food is rich in all of the indicated nutrients. Blackjack also consists of vitamin C. However, no empirical evidence is available to affirm that blackjack consists of vitamin B_3, Selenium, and glutathione as well. This suggests that for vitamin E in blackjack to be fully utilized by the body, blackjack should be consumed alongside foods rich in vitamin B_3, Selenium, and glutathione.

The Extent of Contribution Blackjack Can Make Towards Meeting Recommended Intakes of Vitamin A and C

The contribution which 100 g of blackjack can make towards the recommended dietary intake (RDI) of vitamin A and vitamin C, based on the quantities of these vitamins detected per 100 g of blackjack by Fober et al. (2010), Wolmarans et al. (2010), Abidemi (2013) and Agea et al. (2014) are shown in Table 2.

Vitamin A is important for regulating the immune function, supporting the normal functioning of the visual system, the production of red blood cells, maintenance of cell function, cell differentiation, reproduction, protein synthesis, growth and development as well as maintaining healthy skeletal and soft tissue, skin, teeth and mucous membranes (Mayo-Wilson, Imdad, Marshall, Yakoob & Bhutta, 2011; Arigony et al., 2013). Vitamin A deficiency increases the vulnerability to several diseases, and can further lead to blindness and death especially in children (WHO, 2017). An estimate of 250 million pre-school children suffer from vitamin A deficiency worldwide, and an estimate of 250,000 - 500,000 vitamin A deficient children die each year, half of them dying within 12 months of losing their sight (WHO, 2017).

All or up to double the amount of vitamin A required by infants can be obtained from 100 g of blackjack depending on the obtainable quantities per weight of blackjack (Table 2). This also implies that by consuming 100 g of blackjack per day, breastfeeding mothers could be able to meet the dietary requirements of vitamin A for both, themselves and their babies. Likewise, all or up to three times the required amounts of vitamin A required by young children aged 1.1 - 8 years could be obtained from 100 g of blackjack. Also, 100 g of blackjack could provide 32% - 98% of vitamin A required by expectant mothers. It is therefore evident that blackjack has enormous potential to enhance the nutrition and health of expectant mothers, infants and young children and to prevent diseases and deaths associated with vitamin A deficiency.

Male children and male adults could also obtain 71% or more and 61% or more than their required amounts of vitamin A, respectively, from 100 g of blackjack. Likewise, 100 g of blackjack could provide 71% to more than the required amounts of vitamin A for female children aged 9 - 13 years. Female children aged 14 -18 years as well as female adults could obtain more than their recommended daily amounts of vitamin A from 100 g of blackjack.

Table 2. Estimated percentage blackjack can contribute towards RDIs by age Source of RDI of vitamins A and C by age: FDA, 2016

	Age (Years)	RDI of Vitamin A (µg/day)	% 428 µgRAE/100 g of Blackjack Can Contribute Towards RDI of vit. A	% 983 µgRAE/100 g of Blackjack Can Contribute Towards RDI of vit. A	RDI of Vitamin C (mg/day)	% 74 mg/100 g of Blackjack Can Contribute Towards RDI (vit. C)	% 16 mg/100 g of Blackjack Can Contribute Towards RDI (vit. C)
Infants	0 – 0.5	400	107.0	245.8	40	185	40
	0. 6 - 1	500	85.6	196.6	50	148.0	32
Little children	1.1 - 3	300	142.7	327.7	15	493.3	106.7
	4 - 8	400	107.0	245.8	25	296.0	64.0
Males	9 - 13	600	71.3	163.8	45	164.4	35.6
	14 - 18	900	47.6	109.2	75	98.7	21.3
	19 – 70 and >70	900	47.6	109.2	90	82.2	17.8
Females	9 - 13	600	71.3	163.8	45	164.4	35.6
	14 - 18	700	61.1	140.4	65	113.8	24.6
	19 – 70 and > 70	700	61.1	140.4	75	98.7	21.3
Expectant mothers	14 -18	1200	35.7	81.9	115	64.3	13.9
	19 - 30	1000	42.8	98.3	120	61.7	13.3
	31 - 50	1300	32.9	75.6	120	61.7	13.3

With regard to vitamin C, 100 g of blackjack have been shown to have the capacity to provide up to four times the required RDI for children aged 1 - 8 years, up to 99% of RDI for male children aged 14 - 18 years, and far greater amounts than the RDI for female children aged 9 - 18 years. Males and females aged 19 - 70 years and above could obtain up to 82% and 99% of their recommended daily amounts of vitamin C, respectively, from 100 g of blackjack, whereas expectant mothers could obtain up to 64% of their RDI.

Vitamin C is known to be involved in the maintenance of several body functions, such as the formation of collagen (Naidu, 2003). Collagen is the most abundant protein in our bodies, found in muscles, ligaments, bones, skin, blood vessels, tendons, cartilage, teeth, heart valves, intervertebral discs, cornea, and eye lens (Cescon, Gattazzo, Che & Bonaldo, 2015; Hauser & Dolan, 2011; Naidu, 2003). Other functions of vitamin C include promoting the healing of wounds, the transformation of cholesterol into bile acids, thus prevents the accumulation of cholesterol in the liver as well as the formation of gall-stones (Naidu, 2003). Vitamin C is also necessary for the synthesis of carnitine, required for transport and transfer of fatty acids to mitochondria where it can be used for energy production (Figueroa-Méndez & Rivas-Arancibia, 2015).

Furthermore, vitamin C acts as co-factor in several enzymatic activities and it helps the body to fight against viruses that cause colds and flu (Naidu, 2003). It is also necessary for the activation of folic acid and the conversion of tryptophan to serotine, a neurotransmitter (Figueroa-Méndez & Rivas-Arancibia, 2015). In addition, vitamin C promotes the bioavailability and absorption of iron from non-heme sources (Chambial, Dwivedi, Shukla & Sharma, 2013), and thus promotes the formation of red blood cells and prevents anaemia. Due to being rich in vitamin C, blackjack can make a significant contribution towards enhancing the functions vitamin C.

Vitamins C, E and A are also known to have antioxidant functions (Chambial, Dwivedi, Shukla & Sharma, 2013; Arigony et al., 2013; Chow & Chow-Johnson, 2013; Rizvi et al., 2014). Antioxidants inhibit some of the damage caused by free radicals, also known as reactive oxygen species (ROS) and reactive nitrogen species (RNS) that damage cells (Nimse & Pal, 2015). Free radicals may occur in the body as by-products of normal metabolism of oxygen (Ozcan & Ogun, 2015) and other factors such as prolonged exposure to radiation, age, enzyme activity as well as prolonged use of chemicals and drugs (Nimse & Pal, 2015). ROS and RNS cause chain reactions that lead to cell damage.

Also, the build- up of ROS and RNS cause oxidative stress, which in turn modifies the cellular components of the body (Kim & Byzova, 2014). Consequently this further promotes aging and the development of various health conditions such as cancer and coronary heart disease. Common ROS are superoxide radical (O^{2-}), hydroxyl radical (OH^-), peroxyl radical (ROO), alcoxyl radical (RO), ozone (hypochlorous acid (HOCl), singlet oxygen ($^1O_2$), hydrogen peroxide (H_2O_2) and hypochlorous acid (O_3), whereas common RNS include nitric oxide (NO), peroxynitrite ($ONOO^-$), nitrite (NO_2^-), nitrate (NO_3^-), and nitrogen dioxide (NO_2) (Ozcan & Ogun, 2015). Some of the reactive species such as hydrogen peroxide and nitrogen dioxide are non-radicals, but they are either oxidizing agents or easily converted into radicals.

Antioxidants are particularly important as they inhibit the oxidation of other molecules and terminate chain reactions caused by free radicals, thus delaying or preventing cellular damage (Nimse & Pal, 2015). Antioxidants' activity helps to inhibit cardiovascular diseases, type 2 diabetes and the growth of cancer cells, and prevents anaemia which can occur as a consequence of oxidative damage of red blood cells.

In 2012, it was reported that 14.1 million cancer cases and 8.2 million deaths due to cancer alone occurred worldwide (Torre, et al., 2012). Likewise, the World Health Organization (WHO) reported that 1.5 million deaths due to diabetes and 142 million diabetes cases among adults occurred globally in 2012 and 2014, respectively. In 2014, Sant-Rayri (2014) reported that 32.9% of the global population was suffering from anaemia, whereas 422.7 cases of cardiovascular diseases and 17.9 million deaths due to cardiovascular diseases were reported globally in 2015 (Roth et al., 2015). The indicated diseases are costly and have negative implications on economic participation. It is therefore necessary to prioritize preventative methods against these diseases. This includes encouraging people to eat plant foods that are rich in antioxidants such as blackjack.

Although antioxidants are often made available in the form of supplements, they are quite expensive, and may have side effects when taken for a long time. The consumption of plant foods rich in antioxidants, among them blackjack, provides a safer alternative way of obtaining antioxidants. This argument is based on the understanding that unlike supplements, antioxidants in plant foods are consumed in their natural form alongside the other food components.

Other Compounds of Biological Importance Detected in Blackjack

Apart from vitamins, minerals and amino acids, blackjack was reported to contain several other compounds which have potential to provide clinically proven health benefits (Deba, Xuan, Yasudi & Tawata, 2008). They include triterpenes, caffeic acid, flavonoids, tannins, polyacetylenes, essential oils and organic acid. The biological importance of these compounds is further reviewed as follows:

Triterpenes

Triterpenes are a structurally diverse group of natural compounds widely found in plant leaves, fruits, roots and barks of stems (Nazaruk & Borzym-Kluczyk, 2015). Some triterpenes such as sterols are known to have anticarcinogenic, antioxidant, antiviral, anti-inflammatory and insecticidal properties (Laszczyk, 2009; Ramachandran & Prasad, 2008; Baltina et al., 2003; Doughari, 2012). Triterpenes were also found to have curative properties against diabetes type 2 and they can regulate body weight, total cholesterol and triglycerides in the body (Nazaruk & Borzym-Kluczyk, 2015).

Flavonoids

Flavonoids are a diverse group of polyphenolic phytochemicals consisting of more than 9,000 types with distinct benefits and food source (Kumar & Panday, 2013). Together with carotenoids they are responsible for the colours in fruits and vegetables, for taste, for the prevention of fat oxidation and the protection of vitamins and enzymes (Yao, Jiang & Shi, 2004). Furthermore, flavonoids are soluble in water and they have powerful antioxidants, anti-inflammatory, antiallergic, antiproliferation, anti-human immunodeficiency virus functions as well as immune boosting benefits (Yao et al., 2004; Xiao et al., 2011). Due to their antioxidant functions, flavonoids have also been acknowledged as having preventative characteristic against cardiovascular diseases, cancer, type 2 diabetes and neurodegenerative diseases (Yao et al., 2004).

Caffeic Acid

Caffeic acid is a class of phenolic phytochemicals known to be soluble in water and to have antioxidant, anticancer, anti-inflammatory as well as antiviral characteristics (Doughari, 2012). Due to its antioxidant functions it also exhibit preventative properties against diabetes, aging, neurodegenerative disease, cardiovascular diseases and reduce exercise related fatigue. Like other phenols, caffeic acid occurs as natural colour pigments responsible for the colour of fruits and vegetables and is soluble in water.

Essential Oils

In the study conducted by Deba et al. (2008), at least 40 essential oils were extracted from fresh leaves and roots of blackjack. Essential oils are highly complex, naturally occurring, volatile, fragrant compounds synthesized by plants as secondary metabolites (Ayaz et al., 2017). The chemical composition of essential oils differs from one another, hence the distinct characteristic flavour and odour (Firn, 2010).

In general, essential oils are known to have antibacterial, antiviral, antioxidant and antidiabetic functions (Inouye, Takizawa & Yamaguchi, 2001; Tanu & Harpreet, 2016; Tanu & Harpreet, 2016), thus they are used in medicine. They are also used in perfumes, food flavourings, and aromatherapy for promotion of relaxation and sleep, relief of pain, and management of alzheimer and dementia (Ayaz et al., 2017).

Tannins

Like essential oils, tannins are another group of naturally occurring phytochemicals known to have antioxidant, antibacterial, antiseptic and therapeutic functions (Ghosh, 2015). They therefore have the potential to be anticancer, antidiabetic, anti-cardiovascular diseases and antidiarrhoeal (Doughari, 2012).

Organic Acids

Organic acids are a group of chemicals known as organic carboxylic acid of the general structure R-COOH (Khan & Iqbal, 2016). They include simple mono-carboxylic acids such as formic, acetic, propionic and butyric acids as well as carboxylic acids which have a hydroxyl group such as lactic, malic, tartaric and citric acids or short-chain carboxylic acids containing double bonds like fumaric and sorbic acids (Shahidi, Maziar & Delaram, 2014). Organic acids were found to have antibacterial characteristics as well as the capacity to boost the immune system and to enhance the digestibility of nutrients in feed for poultry (Khan & Iqbal, 2016).

Polyacetylenes

Polyacetylenes are another group of secondary phytochemicals' metabolites. Some polyacetylenes are said to be neurotoxic when consumed in high concentrations (Christensen & Brandt, 2006). Their neurotoxicity activity was demonstrated by injecting high doses of the metabolites into mice, but no poisoning of mammals from consumption of natural sources has been reported. Furthermore, some polyacetylenes were found to have antifungal, anticancer, anti-inflammatory and antibacterial functions (Christensen & Brandt, 2006). This implies that plant foods rich in polyacetylenes, such as blackjack, promote health rather than suppress it.

ANTIFUNGAL PROPERTIES AGAINST SEVERAL PATHOGENIC FUNGI

Blackjack was found to have significant antifungal activities against several fungi species including *Sporobolomyces salmonicolor, Succharomyces cerevisiae, Candida albicans, Penicillium notatum, Penicillium avellanea, Fusarium oxysporum, Aspergillus terreus, Fusarium solani, Corticum rolfsii* and *Aspergillus niger* (Abdou et al., 2010; Deba et al. 2008; Ashafa & Afloyan 2009). Abdou et al (2010) reported the antifungal activity of essential oils from blackjack's flowers, whereas Deba et al. (2008) as well as Ashafa & Afloyan (2009) reported the antifungal activity of essential oils from both its flowers and roots. Abdou et al. (2010) also argued that the antifungal activity of blackjack was possibly a consequence of the activity of endophytes that attack it rather than the blackjack plant itself. The argument by Abdou et al. (2010) was based on the idea that the endophytes' activity leads to blackjack building immunity against them, consequently developing and enhancing antifungal characteristics. However, contrary to the argument by Abdou et al. (2010), Firn (2010) indicated that essential oils naturally consist of hundreds of chemical components each, responsible for the characteristics of the essential oils. In a study carried out by Kurita et al. (1981), 40 chemical components of essential oils were confirmed to have antifungal activity. It therefore seems that the antifungal activity of blackjack occurs naturally as a result of the components in its essential oils rather than anything else.

Although blackjack is said to have capacity to host certain types of fungi, it also have the capacity to inhibit the growth of several species of fungi depending on the concentration of the essential oils or root extracts used. In general, 80% to 100% of fungal growth inhibition was observed, the latter being specifically observed on *Penicillium notatum* (Abdou et al., 2010; Ashafa & Afolayan, 2009). Best results were observed when using higher concentrations of the plant extracts rather than less concentrated ones and when using extracts from flowers, rather than leaves and roots.

Pathogenic fungi, amongst them *Fusarium, Aspergillus* and *Penicillium* species have been associated not only with massive grain losses, but also with serious diseases such as cancer of the throat, kidney failure as well as liver damage (Pitt, 2000; Bayman & Baker, 2006; Bennet & Klich, 2003, as cited by Mboya et al., 2011). Blackjack is therefore an interesting plant with potential to offer affordable possibilities for poor farmers in Africa and other developing countries to protect crops from *Penicillium notatum, Penicillium avellanea, Fusarium oxysporum, Aspergillus terreus* and *Aspergillus niger*, thus preventing diseases that could otherwise result as a consequence of the consumption of the indicated fungi in food.

Antibacterial Properties

Essential oils from blackjack were found to have strong inhibiting characteristics on harmful bacteria, specifically *Micrococcus flavus, Bacillus cereus* and *Escherichia coli* (Abdou et al., 2010). Stronger inhibition capacity on *E. coli* was observed from essential oils extracted from flowers by Abdou et al. (2018) rather than from other parts of the plant, whereas Singh, Passsari, Singh, Singh, Kumar, Subbarayan, Kumar (2017) detected its highest inhibition from leaf extracts.

Other bacteria against which blackjack's extracts activity was observed include *Klebsilla pneumonia, Micrococcus kristinae, Pseudomonas aeruginosa, Staphylococcus aureus, Sraphylococcus epidermidis, Serratia marcescens, Shigella flexneri, Streptococcus faecalis, Enterococcus faecalis, Candida albicans* and *Helicobacter pylori* (Bartolome et al., 2013; Mabeku, Bille& Nguepi, 2016). Blackjack is therefore an important plant offering affordable possibilities of fighting against several harmful bacteria.

Antimalarial Activity

Conventional antibiotics generally target metabolic enzymes (Sumi et al., 2015). Over the years, the use of conventional chemical drugs against pathogens such plasmodium parasites known for causing malaria has resulted in drug-resistant mutants (Bartolome et al., 2013). A study conducted by Kumari et al. (2009, as cited by Bartolome et al., 2013) confirmed the antimalarial activity of the leaf and aerial extracts of blackjack extracts against *Plasmodium falciparum* NF54 and FCR-3 strains, respectively. Blackjack is therefore considered to have the potential to provide an effective, alternative treatment against malaria, and could be the solution to drug resistant *Plasmodium* mutants.

As also rightly argued by Deba (2008), due to its antioxidant characteristics and its capacity to inhibit pathogens, blackjack has great potential for providing significant benefits to the food and pharmaceutical industries. However, its use in the pharmaceutical industries implies that drugs should be made from it, which requires the use of costly technologies and would involve middle persons before the drugs could reach consumers, ultimately making the drugs expensive, and thus not easily accessible by poor communities.

Other Benefits of Blackjack

Requires Minimal Human Labour

Blackjack grows naturally as a wild plant (Marc, 2013). Therefore very little human effort is required to cultivate it. This implies that blackjack could be an important plant especially among poor farmers in Africa who often fail to afford the high expenses of farming. The deliberate production of blackjack could help to cut costs related to vegetable production among poor farmers.

Capacity to Produce Huge Amounts of Harvest Per Unit of Land

Blackjack is also highly beneficial especially where land is scarce. Where it is grown deliberately, it would provide large amounts of harvests from small pieces of land, in turn making it possible to access huge quantities of the nutrients and other bioactive compounds contained in it, merely from gardens. Blackjack is therefore an important plant that should be deliberately cultivated, especially where land is scarce.

Cultivating blackjack could also provide opportunities for residents in urban areas to produce vegetables without altering the urban landscape because apart from blackjack plants being short, harvesting them before they reach maturity would ensure that they do not grow to exceed the desired height.

IS BLACKJACK THE ANSWER FOR SUB-SAHARAN AFRICA?

It was estimated that the prevalence of undernourishment in sub-Saharan Africa rose from 20.6% in 2010 to 22.7% in 2016; whereas in Asia and the Pacific region it dropped from 13.4% in 2010 to 11.7% in 2016 (FAO. 2017a; FAO, 2017b). In general, FAO's (2017a) report has shown that regardless of the effort to curb it, undernourishment, is still most prevalent in sub-Saharan Africa compared to the rest of the world, affecting 224.3 million of people. The rise in the prevalence of undernourishment has been observed in all sub-Saharan Africa regions (Table 3). This has been attributed to adverse climatic conditions followed by conflicts. Blackjack's characteristics, specifically being highly resistant to adverse conditions, being able to grow prolifically, having the capacity to be available throughout the year and requiring scanty human labour create potential for it to be an important source of food in areas that are prone to adverse climatic conditions and conflicts. By deliberately growing it, the availability of food nutrients in all climatic conditions even where constant human labour is not guaranteed could be ensured.

Table 3. The prevalence of undernourishment in sub-Saharan Africa regions (2010 and 2016) Source: FAO, 2017a

Region	2010 (%)	2016 (%)
Western Africa	10	11.5
Central Africa region	23.8	25.8
Eastern Africa	30.9	33.9
Southern Africa	6.7	8.0

However, there seems to be stigma attached to the consumption of blackjack leading to its underutilization for food. In some places such as in the context of the community where the author comes from, when asking community members if they could consume blackjack, the author came across responses such as: "oh, that is food for rabbits and we are not rabbits", "we are not that hungry", "am I that poor?", and "we have plenty of vegetables, why would we eat weeds?" These responses show a negative attitude towards blackjack. To access all the benefits that blackjack has to offer, the deliberate and sustained promotion of its consumption is essential.

Findings From Interviews

The 12 participants that were familiar with using blackjack for food had been using it for food for a range of 7 to 47 years (Table 4). The majority (83.3%) of them had been consuming blackjack for more than twenty years, one had been consuming it for 10 years and only two had been consuming it for fewer than 10 years. None of them had ever fallen ill or knew someone who had ever fallen ill due to consuming blackjack, and none of them was suffering or had ever suffered from cancer of the throat.

Furthermore, the two nurses had been working in the medical profession for about 28 years each, whereas the five medical doctors had been in the medical profession for 9 - 15 years. Unlike the nurses, the medical doctors were unaware that blackjack is edible. However, both the nurses and the medical doctors had never heard of or attended to any patient who sought medical help after falling sick due to consuming blackjack

Participants used blackjack's young tender leaves in the same manner that common leafy vegetables such as spinach are used and consumed it alongside a cereal grain dish. Sometimes participants added ground peanuts to blackjack to improve its taste. The consumption of blackjack to complement cereal grain dishes and the addition of ground peanuts to blackjack are commendable because such practices have been shown to improve the quality of plant protein (Woolf et al., 2011).

Table 4. Number of years during which participants had been consuming blackjack

Participant's ID Number	Number of Years Participant Had Been Consuming Blackjack	Participant's Nationality
1	47	Malawian
2	47	Malawian
3	40	Zambian
4	47	Malawian
5	30	Zimbabwean
6	40	Zimbabwean
7	25	Zambian
8	28	Zambian
9	10	Tanzanian
10	7	Tanzanian
11	7	Tanzanian
12	30	Zimbabwean
13	0	South African
14	0	South African
15	0	South African
16	0	South African
17	0	South African

DISCUSSION

The Capacity of Blackjack to Cause Massive Crop Losses

The capacity of blackjack to cause huge crop losses is of much concern and calls for effective methods to control it. Currently, no specific method is exclusive for preventing the growth and development of blackjack in the fields. However, methods that are used for controlling weeds are applicable for controlling blackjack as well. They include the following:

- **Frequent mowing or hoeing to eliminate unwanted plants:** Constant inspection of the fields and uprooting blackjack plants before they grow to maturity would hinder the development of new seeds and ultimately their dispersion, thus can help to ensure that fields are free from blackjack. In turn, this will protect crops from losing nutrients to blackjack;
- **Intercropping:** In Nicaragua, maize-bean intercropping was found to suppress the growth of blackjack where the density of the intercropped plants was high (Solomon, 1990). Nevertheless, it is not clear as to whether this method works for other crops apart from maize and beans;
- **Soil solarisation prior to planting:** Soil solarisation involves covering the soil with plastic films such that heat from the sun accumulates and creates hot temperatures capable of killing pathogens in the covered area (Scopa & Dumontet, 2007). This was found to be effective in killing blackjack plants as well;

- **Traditional methods such as Applying large quantities of sorghum straw:** The application of four tonnes of sorghum straw per hectare of land was found to reduce the development and growth of blackjack by 59% (Głab, Sowiński, Bough & Dayan, 2017). However, this method dependent on the availability of sorghum straw, and thus it is limited to places where sorghum is grown;
- **Using conventional methods:** Anti-weed chemicals are commonly used to largely eliminate or control the development and growth of weeds (McErlich, 2013). This method is applicable for preventing the development and growth of blackjack as well.

The Need to Ensure Blackjack Is Free From Pathogens

The capacity for blackjack to host pathogens implies that there is a need to ensure that it is free from pathogens because pathogens could put consumers at risk of ill health. The application of conventional pesticides prior to planting or at different stages of cultivation are used to ensure that fields are free from pathogens are common (Walia, Mehta, Guleria, Chauhan & Shirkot, 2014; Van Zwieten, Merrington, Rust, Kingston & Walker, 2014; Nicolopoulou-Stamati, Maipas, Kotampasi, Stamatis & Hens, 2016). However, the understanding that pesticides have serious negative effects on the health of the soil and plant food consumers, both humans and animals is widely acknowledged, following which many food consumers have expressed preference of foods that are produced without the use of pesticides (McErlich, 2013). Interestingly, concentrated extracts from blackjack, especially from its flowers were reported to have immense inhibiting characteristics towards pathogenic species (Abdou et al., 2010; Ashafa & Afloyan, 2009; Deba et al., 2008). More research is required to explore the possibility of using concentrated blackjack extracts as an alternative, safe way of keeping fields and crops, including blackjack plants, free from pathogens.

In addition, although blackjack has the capacity to inhibit the functioning of *Bacillus pumilus* and *Bacillus substilis*, which are said to promote both human and animal health through their antibacterial, antifungal, antiviral and antitumor characteristics is of concern, blackjack has been reported to exhibit the same characteristics. These are being antibacterial, antifungal, antiviral and antitumor. Therefore, blackjack should have the potential to be used as an alternative to both *Bacillus pumilus* and *Bacillus substilis* where necessary.

The Importance of the Nutrition and Health Benefits of Blackjack

Lastly, due to the many nutrients contained in it, blackjack has enormous potential to enhance nutrition and health of consumers. The use of blackjack for food could ensure that its nutrients and health benefits are easily accessible to all, which is important, especially in the developing countries, as it would tremendously help to prevent and fight against hidden hunger.

Also, due to its antioxidant characteristics, blackjack has great potential for combating chronic diseases such as diabetes and cancer. Its long-term use in mice was found to decrease lipid accumulation and the size of adipose tissues, and increase lean tissue content (Liang, Yang, Lin, Chang & Yang, 2016), implying that it can help to combat obesity. Its antiviral, antibacterial and antifungal characteristics also add to its capacity to combat diseases caused by viruses, bacteria and fungi. The consumption of blackjack is therefore necessary, especially in communities which are prone to micro nutrient deficiency and chronic diseases.

Toxicology

Although Arthur et al. (2012) claimed that blackjack is toxic, there is no empirical evidence to confirm this claim. The fact that individuals that were interviewed for this study had been using blackjack for many years and had never experienced any negative health effects from it also supports the argument that blackjack is non-toxic. Furthermore, if blackjack plants were toxic, the nurses and the medical doctors interviewed would have come across or at least they would have heard of patients who sought medical help due to getting sick after consuming blackjack.

The non-toxic characteristic of blackjack was also confirmed by a study by Shandukani, Shidino, Masoko & Moganedi (2018), who found that blackjack was non-toxic against muscle cells but effective against bacteria. Long term use of blackjack was also found to increase lean tissue, to reduce lipid accumulation and increase lean tissue (Liang, Yang, Lin, Chang & Yang (2016). Other health benefits of blackjack include its capacity to improve blood homeostasis and ß -cell function in men (Lai, Chen Huang, Kuo, Chang, Chiang,::: Chang (2015). These findings show that blackjack is beneficial rather than detrimental to health.

CONCLUSION

Blackjack is a plant food with significant health benefits. This review has demonstrated that apart from its agricultural and pharmaceutical importance, blackjack has immense nutritional importance which has not been given adequate attention. Its deliberate consumption could help to alleviate hidden hunger and prevent associated diseases. This review has also shown that blackjack has several characteristics of concern which can directly or indirectly affect crop yield in a negative way. However, most of these characteristics can be controlled. Constant inspection of the fields and uprooting of blackjack plants while they are still very young as well as deliberately planting blackjack away from the other crops will ensure that blackjack does not grow or flourish in the fields or near the other crops. In turn this will protect crops from losing nutrients to blackjack and to pathogens that might be hosted by blackjack.

It is therefore recommended that the deliberate cultivation and consumption of blackjack as well as new food products development using blackjack should be promoted, especially among communities that are most hit by micronutrient deficiency, malaria and chronic diseases such as diabetes and cancer. In addition, more research should be conducted to establish quantities of nutrients and other chemical compounds of biological importance that can be obtained per specific weight of blackjack. This is necessary for determining quantities of blackjack that should be consumed per day to ensure that nutrients and other chemical compounds of biological importance are consumed within acceptable limits.

LIMITATIONS

This research was mostly based on the review of available literature. The small sample size for the interviews conducted is inadequate for making definite conclusions regarding the extent to which blackjack is safe for use as food.

WAY FORWARD

There is a need to conduct more research on the nutritional and health potential of blackjack using samples from different soils and climatic conditions, and to include a larger number of participants who use blackjack for food as well as medical doctors from different countries. There is also a need to conduct more studies on the cancer related to pathogens that blackjack hosts. The author looks forward to engaging in conducting these studies in the near future.

REFERENCES

Abdou, R., Scherlach, K., Dahse, H., Sathler, L., Hetwek, C., & Botryorhodines, A. D. (2010). Antifungal and cytotoxic pepsidone from *Botryosphaeria rhodina*, an endophyte of the medicinal plant *Bidens pilosa*. *Phytochemistry*, *71*, 110–116. doi:10.1016/j.phytochem.2009.09.024 PMID:19913264

Abidemi, O. O. (2013). Proximate composition and vitamin levels of seven medicinal plants. *International Journal of Engineering Science Invention*, *2*(5), 47–50.

Adams, R. M., & Goss, G. J. (1978). *Empyreuma pugione* L. (Lepidoptera: Ctenuchidae) - a new U.S. introduction. *The Florida Entomologist*, *61*(4), 250. doi:10.2307/3494219

Agea, G. J., Kimondo, J. M., Woiso, D. A., Okia, C. A., Obaa, B. B., Isubikalu, P., & Teklehaimanot, Z. (2014). Proximate composition, vitamin C and Beta- carotene contents of fifteen selected leafy wild and semi-wild food plants (WSWFPs) from Bunyororo - Kitara kingdom, Uganda. *Journal of Natural Products and Plant Resources*, *4*(3), 1–12.

Alikwe, P. C. N., Ohimain, E. I., & Omotosho, S. M. (2014). Evaluation of the proximate, mineral, phytochemical and amino acid composition of *Bidens pilosa* as potential feed/feed additive for non-ruminant livestock. *Animal and Veterinary Sciences*, *2*(2), 18–21. doi:10.11648/j.avs.20140202.11

Arce, O. E., Robinet, H. A., Mansilla de Andrada, N., Dfazy, B. E., & Guillén, S. (1995). *Determinación de pérdidas de cultivo de soja (Glycine max) por competencia de saetilla (Bidens subalternans) en el noroeste de la provincia de Tucumán-Argentina*. Res·menes XII Congreso Latinoamericano de Malezas, Montevideo, Uruguay.

Arigony, A. L. V., Oliveira, I. M., Machado, M., Bordin, D. L., Bergter, L., Prá, D., & Henriques, J. A. P. (2013). The influence of micronutrients in cell culture: A reflection on viability and genomic stability. *BioMed Research International*, *2013*, 1–22. doi:10.1155/2013/597282 PMID:23781504

Arthur, G. D., Naidoo, K. K., & Coopoosamy, R. M. (2012). *Bidens pilosa* L.: Agricultural and pharmaceutical importance. *Journal of Medicinal Plants Research*, *6*(17), 3282–3287. doi:10.5897/JMPR12.195

Ashafa, A. O. T., & Afloyan, A. J. (2009). Screening the root extracts from *Biden pilosa* L. var. radiata (Asteraceae) for antimicrobial potentials. *Journal of Medicinal Plants Research*, *3*(8), 568–572.

Ayaz, M., Sadiq, A., Junaid, M., Ullah, F., Subhan, F., & Ahmed, J. (2017). Neuroprotective and anti-aging potentials of essential oils from aromatic and medicinal plants. *Frontiers in Aging Neuroscience*, *9*(168), 1–16. PMID:28611658

Bailey, R. L., West, K. P. Jr, & Black, R. E. (2015). The epidemiology of global micronutrient deficiencies. *Annals of Nutrition & Metabolism, 66*(2), 22–33. doi:10.1159/000371618 PMID:26045325

Baltina, L. A., Flekhter, O. B., Nigmatullina, L. R., Boreko, E. I., Pavlova, N. I., Nikolaeva, S. N., & Tolstikov, G. A. (2003). Lupane triterpenes and derivatives with antiviral activity. *Bioorganic & Medicinal Chemistry Letters, 13*(20), 3549–3552. doi:10.1016/S0960-894X(03)00714-5 PMID:14505668

Bardner, R., & Mathenge, W. M. (2015). First record of *Phytometra orichalcea* (F.) (Lepidoptera: Noctuidae) feeding on coffee foliage. *East African Agricultural and Forestry Journal, 40*(2), 214. doi:10.1080/00128325.1974.11662735

Bartolome, A. P., Villaseñor, I. M., & Yang, W. (2013). *Bidens pilosa* L. (Asteraceae): Botanical properties, traditional uses, phytochemistry, and pharmacology. *Evidence-Based Complementary and Alternative Medicine, 2013*, 1–50. doi:10.1155/2013/340215 PMID:23935661

CABI. (2017). *Invasive Species Compendium. Datasheets, maps, images, abstracts and full text on invasive species of the world.* Retrieved from https://www.cabi.org/isc/datasheet/9148

Cescon, M., Gattazzo, F., Chen, P., & Bonaldo, P. (2015). *Collagen VI at a glance.* Journal.

Chambial, S., Dwivedi, S., Shukla, K. K., & Sharma, P. (2013). Vitamin C in disease prevention and cure: An overview. *Indian Journal of Clinical Biochemistry, 28*(4), 314–328. doi:10.100712291-013-0375-3 PMID:24426232

Chivinge, O. A. (1996). Studies on the germination and seedling emergence of Bidens pilosa and its response to fertilizer application. *Transactions of the Zimbabwe Scientific Association, 70*, 1–5.

Chow, C. K., & Chow-Johnson, H. S. (2013). Antioxidant function and health. *The Open Nutrition Journal, 7*(1), 1–6. doi:10.2174/1874288201307010001

Christensen, L. P., & Brandt, K. (2006). Bioactive polyacetylenes in food plants of the Apiaceae family: Occurrence, bioactivity and analysis. *Journal of Pharmaceutical and Biomedical Analysis, 41*(3), 683–693. doi:10.1016/j.jpba.2006.01.057 PMID:16520011

Cutting, S. M. (2011). Bacillus probiotics. *Food Microbiology, 28*(2), 214–220. doi:10.1016/j.fm.2010.03.007 PMID:21315976

De Almeida, P. D. O., Boleti, A. P. A., Rüdiger, A. L., Lourenço, G. A., Da Veiga, F. V. Jr, & Lima, E. S. (2015). Anti-inflammatory activity of triterpenes isolated from Protium paniculatum oil-resins. *Evidence-Based Complementary and Alternative Medicine.* PMID:27034686

Deba, F., Xuan, T. D., Yasudi, M., & Tawata, S. (2008). Chemical compsition and anioxidant, antibacterial, and antifungal activities of the essential oils form *Bidens pilosa* Linn. Varr. Radiata. *Food Control, 19*(4), 346–352. doi:10.1016/j.foodcont.2007.04.011

Doughari, J. H. (2012). Phytochemicals: Extraction methods, basic structures and mode of action as potential chemotherapeutic agents. In V. Rao (Ed.), *Phytochemicals - A Global Perspective of Their Role in Nutrition and Health (pp. 1 - 32).* Rijeka, Shanghai: InTech.

FAO. (2017a). *Regional Overview of Food Security and Nutrition. The food security and nutrition –conflict nexus: building resilience for food security, nutrition and peace.* Accra: FAO.

FAO. (2017b). *Asia and the Pacific. In Regional overview of food security and nutrition. Investing in food systems for better nutrition.* Bangkok: FAO.

FDA. (2016). *Frequently asked questions for industry on nutrition facts labelling requirements.* Retrieved from https://www.fda.gov/downloads/Food/GuidanceRegulation/GuidanceDocumentsRegulatoryInformation/LabelingNutrition/UCM513817

Figueroa-Méndez, R., & Rivas-Arancibia, S. (2015). Vitamin C in health and disease: Its role in the metabolism of cells and redox state in the brain. *Frontiers in Physiology, 6*(397), 1–11. PMID:26779027

Firn, R. (2010). *Nature's chemicals.* Oxford, UK: Oxford University Press.

Fober, M., Delofse, A., Van Jaarsveld, P. J., Wenhold, F. A. M., & Van Rensburg, W. S. (2010). African leafy vegetables consumed by households in the Limpopo and KwaZulu-Natal provinces in South Africa. *Journal of clinical nutrition, 23*(1), 30–38.

Ghosh, D. (2015). Tannins from foods to combat diseases. *International Journal of Pharma Research & Review, 4*(5), 40–44.

Hauser, R. A., & Dolan, E. E. (2011). Ligaments injury and healing: An overview of current clinical concepts. *Journal of Prolotherapy, 3*(4), 836–846.

Hoffman, J. R., & Falvo, M. J. (2004). Protein - which is best? *Journal of Sports Science & Medicine, 3*, 118–130. PMID:24482589

Hoffmann, R. (2017). Micronutrient deficiencies in the elderlies - could ready meals be part of the solution? *Journal of Nutritional Science, 6*, e2. doi:10.1017/jns.2016.42 PMID:28620477

Holm, L. G., Plucknett, D. L., Pancho, J. V., & Herberger, J. P. (1977). *The world's worst weeds. Distribution and biology.* Honolulu, HI: University Press of Hawaii.

Inouye, S., Takizawa, T., & Yamaguchi, H. (2001). Antibacterial activity of essential oils and their major constituency against respiratory tract pathogens by gaseous contact. *The Journal of Antimicrobial Chemotherapy, 47*(5), 565–573. doi:10.1093/jac/47.5.565 PMID:11328766

Ishimine, Y., Nakama, M., & Matsumoto, S. (1987). Allelopathic potential of *Paspalum urvillei* STEUD, *Bidens pilosa* L. var. radiata SCHERFF, and *Stellaria aquatica* SCOP, dominant weeds in sugarcane fields in the Ryukyu Islands. *Weed Research, Japan, 32*(4), 274–281.

Khan, S. H., & Iqbal, J. (2016). Recent advances in the role of organic acids in poultry nutrition. *Journal of Applied Animal Research, 44*(1), 359–369. doi:10.1080/09712119.2015.1079527

Kim, Y. W., & Byzova, T. V. (2014). Oxidative stress in angiogenesis and vascular disease. *Blood, 123*(5), 625–631. doi:10.1182/blood-2013-09-512749 PMID:24300855

Kumari, P., Misra, K., Sisodia, B.S., Faridi, U., Srivastava, S., Luqman, S., &Kumar, J. K. (2009). A promising anticancer and antimalarial component from the leaves of *Bidens pilosa. Planta Medica Journal, 75*(1), 59–61. doi:10.1055-0028-1088362 PMID:19031368

Kumar, S., & Panday, A. K. (2013). Chemistry and biological activities of flavonoids: An overview. *The Scientific World Journal*, 1–16. PMID:24470791

Kurita, N., Miyaji, M., Kurane, R., & Takahara, Y. (1981). Antifungal activity of components of essential oils. *Agricultural and Biological Chemistry*, *45*(4), 945–952.

Laszczyk, M. N. (2009). Pentacyclic triterpenes of the lupane, oleanane and ursane group as tools in cancer therapy. *Planta Medica*, *75*(15), 1549–1560. doi:10.1055-0029-1186102 PMID:19742422

Liang, Y., Yang, M., Lin, C., Chang, C., & Yang, W. (2016). *Bidens pilosa* formulation improves blood homeostasis and ß -cell function in men: A pilot study. *Evidence-Based Complementary and Alternative Medicine*, *2015*, 832314.

Lusweli, A., Wabuyele, E., Ssegawa, P., & Mauremootoo, J. (2011). *Bidens pilosa (Blackjack). BioNET-EAFRINET keys and fact sheets*. Retrieved from http://keys.lucidcentral.org/keys/v3/eafrinet/weeds/key/weeds/Media/Html/Bidens_pilosa_(Blackjack).htm

Mabeku, L. K., Bille, B. E., & Nguepi, E. (2016). InVitro and inVivo anti-Helicobacter activities of Eryngium foetidum (Apiaceae), Bidens pilosa (Asteraceae), and Galinsoga ciliata (Asteraceae) against Helicobacter pylori. *BioMed Research International*, *2016*, 2171032. PMID:27631003

Mboya, R., Tongoona, P., Yobo, K. S., Derera, J., & Langyintuo, A. (2011). The quality of maize stored using roof and sack storage methods in Katumba ward, Rungwe district, Tanzania: Implications on household food security. *Journal of Stored Products and Postharvest Research*, *2*(9), 189–199.

McErlic, A. F., & Boydstone, R. A. (2013). *Current state of weed management in organic and conventional cropping systems*. Lincoln, NE: University of Nebraska.

Mitich, L. W. (1984). Beggarticks. *Weed Technology*, *8*(1), 172–175. doi:10.1017/S0890037X00039403

Modi, M., Modi, A. T., & Hendricks, S. (2006). Potential role for wild vegetables in household food security: A preliminary case study in Kwazulu-Natal, South Africa. *African Journal of Food, Agriculture, Nutrition and Development*, *6*(1), 1–13. doi:10.4314/ajfand.v6i1.19167

Mohanty, B., Mahanty, A., Ganguly, S., Sankar, T. V., Chakraborty, K., Rangasamy, A., & Sharma, A. P. (2014). Amino acid compositions of 27 food fishes and their importance in clinical nutrition. *Journal of Amino Acids*, *269797*, 1–7. doi:10.1155/2014/269797 PMID:25379285

Mzengereza, K., Msiska, O.V., Kapute, F., Kang'ombe, J., Singini, W. & Kamangira, A. (2014). Nutritional value of locally available plants with potential for diets of *Tilapia Rendalli* in pond aquaculture in Nkhata Bay, Malawi. *Journal of Aquaculture Research & Development*, *5*(6), 1 - 6.

Naidu, K. A. (2003). Vitamin C in human health and disease is still a mystery? An overview. *Nutrition Journal*, *2*(7), 1–10. PMID:14498993

Nazaruk, J., & Borzym-Kluczyk, M. (2015). The role of triterpenes in the management of diabetes mellitus and its complications. *Phytochemicals Review*, *14*(4), 675–690. doi:10.100711101-014-9369-x PMID:26213526

Nicolopoulou-Stamati, P, Maipas, S., Kotampasi, C., Stamatis, P. & Hens, L., 2016. *Chemical pesticides and human health: The urgent need for a new concept in Agriculture*. PMID. (27486573)

Nimse, S. B., & Pal, D. (2015). Free radicals, natural antioxidants, and their reaction mechanisms. *Royal Society of Chemistry, 5*, 27986–28006.

Njoku, P. C., Ayuk, A. A., & Okoye, C. V. (2011). Temperature effects on vitamin C content in citrus fruits. *Pakistan Journal of Nutrition, 10*(12), 1168–1169. doi:10.3923/pjn.2011.1168.1169

Odhav, B., Beekrumb, S., Akulaa, U., & Baijnath, H. (2006). Preliminary assessment of nutritional value of traditional leafy vegetables in KwaZulu-Natal, South Africa. *Journal of Food Composition and Analysis, 20*(5), 430–435. doi:10.1016/j.jfca.2006.04.015

Ozcan, A., & Ogun, M. (2015). Biochemistry of reactive oxygen and nitrogen species. In S. J. T. Gowder (Ed.), *Basic Principles and Clinical Significance of Oxidative Stress (pp. 37 - 58).* Shanghai: INTECH. doi:10.5772/61193

Prete, C. E. C., Nunes Júnior, J., & Menten, J. O. M. (1984). Fungi associated with weed seeds. *Summa Phytopathologica, 10*(3/4), 260–267.

Purciful, D. E., Christie, S. R., Zitter, T. A., & Bassett, M. J. (1971). Natural infection of lettuce and endive by Bidens mottle virus. *Plant Disease Reporter, 55*, 1061–1063.

Raederstorff, D., Wyss, A., Calder, P. C., Weber, P., & Eggersdorfer, M. (2015). Vitamin E function and requirements in relation to PUFA. *British Journal of Nutrition, 114*(08), 1113–1122. doi:10.1017/S000711451500272X PMID:26291567

Ramachandran, S., & Prasad, N. R. (2008). Effect of ursolic acid, a triterpenoid antioxidant, on ultraviolet-B radiation-induced cytotoxicity, lipid peroxidation and DNA damage in human lymphocytes. *Chemico-Biological Interactions Journal, 176*(2-3), 99–107. doi:10.1016/j.cbi.2008.08.010 PMID:18793624

Rizvi, S., Raza, S. T., Ahmed, F., Ahmad, A., Abbas, S., & Mahdi, F. (2014). The Role of vitamin E in human health and some diseases. *Sultan Qaboos University Medical Journal, 14*(2), 157–165. PMID:24790736

Roth, G. A., Johnson, C., Abajobir, A., Abd-Allah, A., Abera, S. F., & Abyu, G. (2017). Global, regional and national burden of cardiovascular disease for 10 causes, 1990 - 2015. *Journal of the American College of Cardiology, 7*(1), 26–28. PMID:28527667

Sang, Y., & Blecha, F. (2008). Antimicrobial peptides and bacteriocins: Alternatives to traditional antibiotics. *Animal Health Research Reviews, 9*(2), 227–235. doi:10.1017/S1466252308001497 PMID:18983725

Sant-Rayri, P. (2014). Anaemia: A comprehensive global estimate. *Blood, 123*, 661–612.

Shahidi, S., Maziar, Y., & Delaram, N. Z. (2014). Influence of dietary organic acids supplementation on reproductive performance of freshwater Angelfish (Pterophyllum scalare). *Global Veterinaria, 13*, 373–377.

Shandukani, P. D., Tshidino, S. C., Masoko, P., & Moganedi, K. M. (2018). Antibacterial activity and in situ efficacy of Bidens pilosa Linn and Dichrostachys cinerea Wight et Arn extracts against common diarrhoea-causing waterborne bacteria. *BMC Complementary and Alternative Medicine, 18*(1), 171. doi:10.118612906-018-2230-9 PMID:29859076

Singh, G., Passsari, A. K., Singh, P., Leo, V. V., Subbarayan, S., Kumar, N. S., ... Kumar, N. S. (2017). Pharmacological potential of *Bidens pilosa* L. and determination of bioactive compounds using UHPLC-QqQ $_{LIT}$-MS/MS and GC/MS. *BMC Complementary and Alternative Medicine, 17*(1), 492. doi:10.118612906-017-2000-0 PMID:29145848

Sumi, C. D., Yang, B. Y., Yeo, I., & Hahm, Y. T. (2015). Antimicrobial peptides of the genus Bacillus: A new era for antibiotics. *Journal of Microbiology (Seoul, Korea), 61*, 93–103. PMID:25629960

Tanu, B., & Harpreet, K. (2016). Benefits of essential oil. *Journal of Chemical and Pharmaceutical Research, 8*(6), 143–149.

Torre, L. A., Siegel, R. L., Ward, E. M., & Jamal, A. (2016). Global cancer incidence and mortality rates and trends-An update. *Cancer Epidemiology, Biomarkers & Prevention, 25*(1), 16–27. doi:10.1158/1055-9965.EPI-15-0578 PMID:26667886

Torres, R. (1986). Orobanche ramosa, phanerogamous parasite. Host plant species. Ciencia y Tecnica en la Agricultura. *Tabaco, 9*(1), 7–17.

Van Zwieten, L., Merrington, G., Rust, J., Kingston, T., & Walker, B. (2014). *Fungicides and soil health: Challenges for the industry*. Academic Press.

Walia, A., Mehta, P., Guleria, S., Chauhan, A., & Shirkot, C. K. (2014). Impact of fungicide macoseb at different application rates on soil microbial populations, soil biological processes and enzymatic activities in soil. *The Scientific World Journal*.

WHO. (2017). *Nutrition; nutrition health topics*. Retrieved from https://www.who.int/nutrition/topics/val/en

WHO. (2017). *World malaria report, 2016 summary*. Geneva: WHO.

Wolmarans, P., Danster, N., Dalton, A., Rossouuw, K., & Schonfeld, H. (2010). *Condensed food composition tables for South Africa*. Cape Town: Medical Research Council.

Woolf, P. J., Fu, L. L., & Basu, A. (2011). vProtein: Identifying optimal amino acid complements from plant-based foods. *PLoS One, 6*(4), e18836. doi:10.1371/journal.pone.0018836 PMID:21526128

Xiao, Z. P., Peng, Z. Y., Peng, M. J., Yan, W. B., Ouyang, Y. Z., & Zhu, H. L. (2011). Flavonoids health benefits and their molecular mechanism. *Mini-Reviews in Medicinal Chemistry, 11*(2), 169–177. doi:10.2174/138955711794519546 PMID:21222576

Yao, L. H., Jiang, Y. M., Shi, J., Tom'as-Barber'an, F. A., Datta, N., Singanusong, R., & Chen, S. S. (2004). Flavonoids in food and their health benefits. *Plant Foods for Human Nutrition (Dordrecht, Netherlands), 59*(3), 113–122. doi:10.100711130-004-0049-7 PMID:15678717

Yooussef, M. M., Pham, Q., Achar, P. N., & Sreenivasa, M. Y. (2016). Antifungal activity of essential oils on Aspergillus parasiticus isolated from peanuts. *Journal of Plant Protection Research, 15*(2), 139–142. doi:10.1515/jppr-2016-0021

This research was previously published in the International Journal of Applied Research on Public Health Management (IJARPHM), 4(1); edited by Qiang (Shawn) Cheng and Joseph Tan; pages 47-66, copyright year 2019 by IGI Publishing (an imprint of IGI Global).

Chapter 63
Special Legume–Based Food as a Solution to Food and Nutrition Insecurity Problem in the Arctic

Anna Veber

https://orcid.org/0000-0003-0715-0426
Omsk State Agrarian University, Russia

Svetlana Leonova
Bashkir State Agrarian University, Russia

Nina Kazydub
Omsk State Agrarian University, Russia

Inna Simakova
Saratov State Agrarian University, Russia

Liudmila Nadtochii
ITMO University, Russia

ABSTRACT

Amid the progressing growth in the world's population, changing climate conditions, and increasing demand, food production transforms to ensure food security for the mankind. On the national level, the concept of food security is defined as an economic and agro-industrial capacity of a country, which allows the people consuming environmentally friendly and healthy food products on a continuing basis, at reasonable prices, and above the scientifically based nutrition threshold. In circumpolar territories, the people are especially vulnerable to food and nutrition insecurity due to a number of reasons, including severe climate, underdevelopment of local agricultural production, heavy reliance on imported food, higher nutrition requirements, among others. This chapter discusses the potential of legume-based food products to contribute to the improvement of food and nutrition security in northern communities.

DOI: 10.4018/978-1-7998-5354-1.ch063

INTRODUCTION

Over the past few years, the Arctic has become firmly entrenched in the geopolitical interests of not only the Arctic countries, such as Russia, the United States, Canada, Denmark, Norway, and Iceland, but also the states located far from this region, i.e. China, Japan, and the Republic of Korea, and also a number of international organizations that had not previously participated in the Arctic affairs – North Atlantic Treaty Organization (NATO) and the European Union (EU). The countries which have not been actively involved into the Arctic-related issues so far also took an interest in the development, exploration, and governance of the North. The strengthening of geopolitical, economic, military, and political interest to the northern parts of the planet is related to new opportunities offered by the development of transport routes (Northern Sea Route (NSR)), exploration of natural resources, and other factors. Nordic countries, which possess circumpolar territories, are getting increasingly concerned in the security-related issues: not military defense only, but also climate change, environmental protection, biodiversity, and food production.

Food provision is the most important basis for life support and healthy life in the harsh climate conditions of the Arctic. Food production and nutrition security are the crucial issues of national security in all Nordic countries. The study considers historical, archival, and statistical data, academic papers, and reports, as well as national and international legislation and regulations in the sphere of food and nutrition security issues in circumpolar territories.

According to the Food Security Doctrine of the Russian Federation (President of the Russian Federation, 2010), the main criteria of food security are well-balanced consumption rates of food products, economic and factual affordability, and food independence.

The authors propose the development of the specialized products with different functional orientation for mass consumption and a predetermined level of protein content, as well as essential food components, in particular, macro- and microelements and fibers based on the raw materials of animal origin with the addition of plant ingredients.

BACKGROUND

The issue of food security is especially relevant in the Arctic zone of Russia, the biggest and the most sparsely-inhabited circumpolar territory in the North, where settlements are extremely remote from the mainland, almost isolated during long winter, and thus critically dependent on the stable supply of high-nutritious food. The relevancy of the issue is confirmed by the high level of attention paid to the development of food production and ensurance of food security in the High North by the Russian government, research institutions, and non-governmental organizations.

Establishment of food and nutrition security in the Arctic should be considered not only in the view of expenses. It is a composition of many factors, including the contamination of food products by various kinds of xenobiotics, geography, climate change effects, lack of the advanced infrastructure, various economic issues, and other factors (Inuit Circumpolar Council, 2012; Rautio et al., 2015). Numerous studies in the sphere of food supply in the Arctic have all arrived at common conclusion: the principal priority in the establishment of a food supply system in circumpolar territories is the development of a sociological form of food supply system based on the import of the majority of food and agricultural products (Polbitsyn, Drokin, & Zhuravlev, 2012).

According to Ivanov and Ivanova (2017), the rationale and necessity of food provision of people inhabiting the circumpolar territories are determined by the following factors:

- Extreme climatic conditions;
- Demographic factors (small and sparsely located communities);
- Existing consumption rate and the one recommended by international standards;
- Relation between permanently residing and recruited population;
- Domestic agricultural output;
- Seasonal limitations of the food supply.

For the well-being of the northern population, reinforcement of peoples' health, improvement of peoples' physical and intellectual capacity, and the enhancement of the resistance to various Arctic-specific deceases, the issue of food security must be addressed with the consideration of the relevant standard physiological needs of different social groups in energy and basic nutrients (Table 1, Table 2). Knowledge of the physiologically balanced diet as well as the rational and functional alimentation and practically proven vital principles included in the US National Strategy, or the Harvard Pyramid proposed by Willett (2005) must also be taken into account.

According to the data in Table 1 and Table 2, for people working under the conditions of the Arctic, energy expenditure is higher by 15%, as well as the requirements for proteins, fats, and carbohydrates compared to other climatic zones.

The authors share the point of view of Eganyan (2013) that one of the fundamental foundations of the formation of human health is the nutritional factor. In the diet of the northern people, all three basic principles of rational nutrition are violated: energy balance, balance in basic nutrients, proteins, fats, carbohydrates, vitamins, minerals, and diet.

In the Arctic conditions, life is characterized by a common type of nutrition. The studies carried out at the Alimentation Centre of the Science and Research Institute of the North Eastern Federal University named after professor Ammosov (Irkutsk, Russia) and the data collected by Panin (2010a, 2010b) and Sevostyanova (2013) have shown a protein-lipid-based type of nutrition to be common for the indigenous peoples in the High North. In the Arctic zone of Russia, despite its geographical extent and the diversity of indigenous societies, people commonly under-consume food products containing vegetal and animal proteins and fibers, as well as cereals, but overconsume sugar-containing foods. Malnutrition due to an inadequate consumption of nutrients, especially, vitamins, macro- and microelements, is observed throughout the Russian Arctic.

A decrease in the consumption of proteins by 13% and fats by 18% has been observed in the daily intake, whereas the share of carbohydrates has increased by 65%. As a result, the type of nutrition has shifted to the carbohydrate-lipid-based one with the underconsumption of fibers, vitamins, and minerals, and overconsumption of refined products (Rautio et al., 2015).

In the last decade, the actual nutrition of the population is defined as substandard. The short-lasting physical stress along with the low temperature, tough economic and social situation, restricted delivery of food products, lack of the required stock supplies in the region bring about the changes in the structure of food ration, particularly, a deficit of C vitamin and B-group vitamins, as well as macro- and microelements (calcium, potassium, magnesium, fluoride, selenium, and iodine). The deficit results in the emergence of chronic diseases spurred by the wrong lifestyle and misuse of social toxins.

Table 1. Standard physiological requirements in energy and basic nutrients for males

Nutrient (daily)	Physical activity groups (Physical activity coefficient)															>60
	I (1.4)			II (1.6)			III (1.9)			IV (2.2)			V (2.5)			
	Age groups															
	18-29	30-39	40-59	18-29	30-39	40-59	18-29	30-39	40-59	18-29	30-39	40-59	18-29	30-39	40-59	
Energy and macronutrients																
Energy, kcal	2,450	2,300	2,100	2,800	2,650	2,500	3,300	3,150	2,950	3,850	3,600	3,400	4,200	3,950	3,750	230
Proteins, g	72.0	68.0	65.0	80.0	77.0	72.0	94.0	89.0	84.0	108.0	102.0	96.0	117.0	111.0	104.0	68.0
including animal proteins, g	36.0	34.0	32.5	40.0	38.5	36.0	47.0	44.5	42.0	54.0	51.0	48.0	58.5	55.5	52.0	34.0
Proteins, % of kcal	12.0	12.0	12.0	12.0	12.0	12.0	11.0	11.0	11.0	11.0	11.0	11.0	11.0	11.0	11.0	12.0
Fat, g	81.0	77.0	70.0	93.0	88.0	83.0	110.0	105.0	98.0	128.0	120.0	113.0	154.0	144.0	137.0	77.0
Fat, % of kcal	30.0	30.0	30.0	30.0	30.0	30.0	30.0	30.0	30.0	30.0	30.0	30.0	33.0	33.0	33.0	30.0
MUFA*, % of kcal	10.0	10.0	10.0	10.0	10.0	10.0	10.0	10.0	10.0	10.0	10.0	10.0	10.0	10.0	10.0	10.0
PUFA*, % of kcal	6-10	6-10	6-10	6-10	6-10	6-10	6-10	6-10	6-10	6-10	6-10	6-10	6-10	6-10	6-10	6-10
Omega-6, % of kcal	5-8	5-8	5-8	5-8	5-8	5-8	5-8	5-8	5-8	5-8	5-8	5-8	5-8	5-8	5-8	5-8
Omega-3, % of kcal	1-2	1-2	1-2	1-2	1-2	1-2	1-2	1-2	1-2	1-2	1-2	1-2	1-2	1-2	1-2	1-2
Phospholipids, g	5-7	5-7	5-7	5-7	5-7	5-7	5-7	5-7	5-7	5-7	5-7	5-7	5-7	5-7	5-7	5-7
Carbohydrates, g	358.0	335.0	303.0	411.0	387.0	366.0	484.0	462.0	432.0	566.0	528.0	499.0	586.0	550.0	524.0	335.0
Sugars, % of kcal	<10.0	<10.0	<10.0	<10.0	<10.0	<10.0	<10.0	<10.0	<10.0	<10.0	<10.0	<10.0	<10.0	<10.0	<10.0	<10.0
Fibers, g	20.0	20.0	20.0	20.0	20.0	20.0	20.0	20.0	20.0	20.0	20.0	20.0	20.0	20.0	20.0	20.0
Vitamins																
C, mg	90.0	90.0	90.0	90.0	90.0	90.0	90.0	90.0	90.0	90.0	90.0	90.0	90.0	90.0	90.0	90.0
B_1, mg	1.5	1.5	1.5	1.5	1.5	1.5	1.5	1.5	1.5	1.5	1.5	1.5	1.5	1.5	1.5	1.5
B_2, mg	1.8	1.8	1.8	1.8	1.8	1.8	1.8	1.8	1.8	1.8	1.8	1.8	1.8	1.8	1.8	1.8
B_6, mg	2.0	2.0	2.0	2.0	2.0	2.0	2.0	2.0	2.0	2.0	2.0	2.0	2.0	2.0	2.0	2.0
Niacin, mg	20.0	20.0	20.0	20.0	20.0	20.0	20.0	20.0	20.0	20.0	20.0	20.0	20.0	20.0	20.0	20.0
B_{12}, µg	3.0	3.0	3.0	3.0	3.0	3.0	3.0	3.0	3.0	3.0	3.0	3.0	3.0	3.0	3.0	3.0
Folates, µg	400.0	400.0	400.0	400.0	400.0	400.0	400.0	400.0	400.0	400.0	400.0	400.0	400.0	400.0	400.0	400.0

continues on following page

Table 1. Continued

Nutrient (daily)	Physical activity groups (Physical activity coefficient)															>60
	I (1.4)			II (1.6)			III (1.9)			IV (2.2)			V (2.5)			
	Age groups															
	18-29	30-39	40-59	18-29	30-39	40-59	18-29	30-39	40-59	18-29	30-39	40-59	18-29	30-39	40-59	
Pantothenic acid, mg	5.0	5.0	5.0	5.0	5.0	5.0	5.0	5.0	5.0	5.0	5.0	5.0	5.0	5.0	5.0	5.0
Biotin, µg	50.0	50.0	50.0	50.0	50.0	50.0	50.0	50.0	50.0	50.0	50.0	50.0	50.0	50.0	50.0	50.0
A, µg RE*	900.0	900.0	900.0	900.0	900.0	900.0	900.0	900.0	900.0	900.0	900.0	900.0	900.0	900.0	900.0	900.0
Beta-carotene, mg	5.0	5.0	5.0	5.0	5.0	5.0	5.0	5.0	5.0	5.0	5.0	5.0	5.0	5.0	5.0	5.0
E, mg TE*	15.0	15.0	15.0	15.0	15.0	15.0	15.0	15.0	15.0	15.0	15.0	15.0	15.0	15.0	15.0	15.0
D, µg	10.0	10.0	10.0	10.0	10.0	10.0	10.0	10.0	10.0	10.0	10.0	10.0	10.0	10.0	10.0	15.0
K, µg	120.0	120.0	120.0	120.0	120.0	120.0	120.0	120.0	120.0	120.0	120.0	120.0	120.0	120.0	120.0	120.0
Minerals																
Calcium, mg	1,000	1,000	1,000	1,000	1,000	1,000	1,000	1,000	1,000	1,000	1,000	1,000	1,000	1,000	1,000	1,200
Phosphor, mg	800.0	800.0	800.0	800.0	800.0	800.0	800.0	800.0	800.0	800.0	800.0	800.0	800.0	800.0	800.0	800.0
Magnesium, mg	400.0	400.0	400.0	400.0	400.0	400.0	400.0	400.0	400.0	400.0	400.0	400.0	400.0	400.0	400.0	400.0
Potassium, mg	2,500	2,500	2,500	2,500	2,500	2,500	2,500	2,500	2,500	2,500	2,500	2,500	2,500	2,500	2,500	2,500
Sodium, mg	1,300	1,300	1,300	1,300	1,300	1,300	1,300	1,300	1,300	1,300	1,300	1,300	1,300	1,300	1,300	1,300
Chloride, mg	2,300	2,300	2,300	2,300	2,300	2,300	2,300	2,300	2,300	2,300	2,300	2,300	2,300	2,300	2,300	2,300
Iron, mg	10.0	10.0	10.0	10.0	10.0	10.0	10.0	10.0	10.0	10.0	10.0	10.0	10.0	10.0	10.0	10.0
Zinc, mg	12.0	12.0	12.0	12.0	12.0	12.0	12.0	12.0	12.0	12.0	12.0	12.0	12.0	12.0	12.0	12.0
Iodine, µg	150.0	150.0	150.0	150.0	150.0	150.0	150.0	150.0	150.0	150.0	150.0	150.0	150.0	150.0	150.0	150.0
Copper, mg	1.0	1.0	1.0	1.0	1.0	1.0	1.0	1.0	1.0	1.0	1.0	1.0	1.0	1.0	1.0	1.0
Manganese, mg	2.0	2.0	2.0	2.0	2.0	2.0	2.0	2.0	2.0	2.0	2.0	2.0	2.0	2.0	2.0	2.0
Selenium, µg	70.0	70.0	70.0	70.0	70.0	70.0	70.0	70.0	70.0	70.0	70.0	70.0	70.0	70.0	70.0	70.0
Chrome, µg	50.0	50.0	50.0	50.0	50.0	50.0	50.0	50.0	50.0	50.0	50.0	50.0	50.0	50.0	50.0	50.0
Molybdenum, µg	70.0	70.0	70.0	70.0	70.0	70.0	70.0	70.0	70.0	70.0	70.0	70.0	70.0	70.0	70.0	70.0
Fluorine, mg	4.0	4.0	4.0	4.0	4.0	4.0	4.0	4.0	4.0	4.0	4.0	4.0	4.0	4.0	4.0	4.0

Note: MUFA – monounsaturated fatty acid; PUFA – polyunsaturated fatty acid; RE – retinol equivalent; TE – tocopherol equivalent
Source: Government of the Russian Federation (2008)

Table 2. Standard physiological requirements in energy and basic nutrients for females

	Physical activity groups (Physical activity coefficient)												>60
	I (1.4)			II (1.6)			III (1.9)			IV (2.2)			
	Age groups												
	18-29	30-39	40-59	18-29	30-39	40-59	18-29	30-39	40-59	18-29	30-39	40-59	
Energy and macronutrients													
Energy, kcal	2,000	1,900	1,800	2,200	2,150	2,100	2,600	2,550	2,500	3,050	2,950	2,850	1,975
Proteins, g	61.0	59.0	58.0	66.0	65.0	63.0	76.0	74.0	72.0	87.0	84.0	82.0	61.0
including animal proteins, g	30.5	29.5	29.0	33.0	32.5	31.5	38.0	37.0	36.0	43.5	42.0	41.0	30.5
Proteins, % of kcal	12.0	12.0	12.0	12.0	12.0	12.0	12.0	12.0	12.0	12.0	12.0	12.0	12.0
Fat, g	67.0	63.0	60.0	73.0	72.0	70.0	87.0	85.0	83.0	102.0	98.0	95.0	66.0
Fat, % of kcal	30.0	30.0	30.0	30.0	30.0	30.0	30.0	30.0	30.0	30.0	30.0	30.0	30.0
MUFA*, % of kcal	10.0	10.0	10.0	10.0	10.0	10.0	10.0	10.0	10.0	10.0	10.0	10.0	10.0
PUFA*, % of kcal	6-10	6-10	6-10	6-10	6-10	6-10	6-10	6-10	6-10	6-10	6-10	6-10	6-10
Omega-6, % of kcal	5-8	5-8	5-8	5-8	5-8	5-8	5-8	5-8	5-8	5-8	5-8	5-8	5-8
Omega-3, % of kcal	1-2	1-2	1-2	1-2	1-2	1-2	1-2	1-2	1-2	1-2	1-2	1-2	1-2
Phospholipids, g	5-7	5-7	5-7	5-7	5-7	5-7	5-7	5-7	5-7	5-7	5-7	5-7	5-7
Carbohydrates, g	289.0	274.0	257.0	318.0	311.0	305.0	378.0	372.0	366.0	462.0	432.0	417.0	284.0
Sugars, % of kcal	<10.0	<10.0	<10.0	<10.0	<10.0	<10.0	<10.0	<10.0	<10.0	<10.0	<10.0	<10.0	<10.0
Fibers, g	20.0	20.0	20.0	20.0	20.0	20.0	20.0	20.0	20.0	20.0	20.0	20.0	20.0
Vitamins													
C, mg	90.0	90.0	90.0	90.0	90.0	90.0	90.0	90.0	90.0	90.0	90.0	90.0	90.0
B_1, mg	1.5	1.5	1.5	1.5	1.5	1.5	1.5	1.5	1.5	1.5	1.5	1.5	1.5
B_2, mg	1.8	1.8	1.8	1.8	1.8	1.8	1.8	1.8	1.8	1.8	1.8	1.8	1.8
B_6, mg	2.0	2.0	2.0	2.0	2.0	2.0	2.0	2.0	2.0	2.0	2.0	2.0	2.0
Niacin, mg	20.0	20.0	20.0	20.0	20.0	20.0	20.0	20.0	20.0	20.0	20.0	20.0	20.0
B_{12}, µg	3.0	3.0	3.0	3.0	3.0	3.0	3.0	3.0	3.0	3.0	3.0	3.0	3.0
Folates, µg	400.0	400.0	400.0	400.0	400.0	400.0	400.0	400.0	400.0	400.0	400.0	400.0	400.0
Pantothenic acid, mg	5.0	5.0	5.0	5.0	5.0	5.0	5.0	5.0	5.0	5.0	5.0	5.0	5.0

continues on following page

Table 1. Continued

	Physical activity groups (Physical activity coefficient)												>60
	I (1.4)			II (1.6)			III (1.9)			IV (2.2)			
	Age groups												
	18-29	30-39	40-59	18-29	30-39	40-59	18-29	30-39	40-59	18-29	30-39	40-59	
Biotin, µg	50.0	50.0	50.0	50.0	50.0	50.0	50.0	50.0	50.0	50.0	50.0	50.0	50.0
A, µg RE*	900.0	900.0	900.0	900.0	900.0	900.0	900.0	900.0	900.0	900.0	900.0	900.0	900.0
Beta-carotene, mg	5.0	5.0	5.0	5.0	5.0	5.0	5.0	5.0	5.0	5.0	5.0	5.0	5.0
E, mg TE*	15.0	15.0	15.0	15.0	15.0	15.0	15.0	15.0	15.0	15.0	15.0	15.0	15.0
D, µg	10.0	10.0	10.0	10.0	10.0	10.0	10.0	10.0	10.0	10.0	10.0	10.0	15.0
K, µg	120.0	120.0	120.0	120.0	120.0	120.0	120.0	120.0	120.0	120.0	120.0	120.0	120.0
Minerals													
Calcium, mg	1,000	1,000	1,000	1,000	1,000	1,000	1,000	1,000	1,000	1,000	1,000	1,000	1,200
Phosphor, mg	800.0	800.0	800.0	800.0	800.0	800.0	800.0	800.0	800.0	800.0	800.0	800.0	800.0
Magnesium, mg	400.0	400.0	400.0	400.0	400.0	400.0	400.0	400.0	400.0	400.0	400.0	400.0	400.0
Potassium, mg	2,500	2,500	2,500	2,500	2,500	2,500	2,500	2,500	2,500	2,500	2,500	2,500	2,500
Sodium, mg	1,300	1,300	1,300	1,300	1,300	1,300	1,300	1,300	1,300	1,300	1,300	1,300	1,300
Chloride, mg	2,300	2,300	2,300	2,300	2,300	2,300	2,300	2,300	2,300	2,300	2,300	2,300	2,300
Iron, mg	18.0	18.0	18.0	18.0	18.0	18.0	18.0	18.0	18.0	18.0	18.0	18.0	18.0
Zinc, mg	12.0	12.0	12.0	12.0	12.0	12.0	12.0	12.0	12.0	12.0	12.0	12.0	12.0
Iodine, µg	150.0	150.0	150.0	150.0	150.0	150.0	150.0	150.0	150.0	150.0	150.0	150.0	150.0
Copper, mg	1.0	1.0	1.0	1.0	1.0	1.0	1.0	1.0	1.0	1.0	1.0	1.0	1.0
Manganese, mg	2.0	2.0	2.0	2.0	2.0	2.0	2.0	2.0	2.0	2.0	2.0	2.0	2.0
Selenium, µg	55.0	55.0	55.0	55.0	55.0	55.0	55.0	55.0	55.0	55.0	55.0	55.0	55.0
Chrome, µg	50.0	50.0	50.0	50.0	50.0	50.0	50.0	50.0	50.0	50.0	50.0	50.0	50.0
Molybdenum, µg	70.0	70.0	70.0	70.0	70.0	70.0	70.0	70.0	70.0	70.0	70.0	70.0	70.0
Fluorine, mg	4.0	4.0	4.0	4.0	4.0	4.0	4.0	4.0	4.0	4.0	4.0	4.0	4.0

Note: MUFA – monounsaturated fatty acid; PUFA – polyunsaturated fatty acid; RE – retinol equivalent; TE – tocopherol equivalent

Source: Government of the Russian Federation (2008)

Dairy products are one of the major kinds of food vitally important for the people living in the North. Lactase deficiency (hypolactasia) causes severe diseases caused by a decrease in the lactase, an enzyme which is needed for a proper digestion of lactose. To prevent and treat gastroenterological diseases of people suffering from lactase deficiency, food ration should include lactose-free products.

According to AllergyFree (n.d.), the problem of lactose intolerance varies in different regions and is correlated to climate zones: the closer the area to the equator, the higher the percentage of population suffering from this unpleasant reaction. For example, people intolerant to lactose comprise 11% of the population in Northwest Russia, 33-34% in the Urals, 45% in the South of Russia, and 45% in the Far East of Russia. In general, about 16-18% of the adult population in Russia suffers from such unwanted reaction to dairy products as lactose intolerance.

People living in Northern Europe, North America, and Australia demonstrate the lowest liability to the disease: from 5% in the UK to 17% in Finland and northern parts of France. On the contrary, 50% of the population in South America and Africa and even 100% of the population in some countries of Asia are lactose intolerant (Lomer, Parkes, & Sanderson, 2008). Currently, the food industry provides a small volume of such products.

MAIN FOCUS OF THE CHAPTER

Several integrated programs, in particular, the State Program "Socio-Economic Development of the Arctic and Northern Districts of the Republic of Sakha (Yakutia) for 2014-2017 and the Period till 2020" (Government of the Republic of Sakha (Yakutia), 2014), have been development and introduced in Russia to achieve the optimal balance between the structure of the industrial production and spatial organization of the economy in the Russian Arctic. The program module "Modernization of the Conventional Industries of the North and Development of Food Processing Industry" sets the major objectives of such development:

- Satisfaction of the need for high-quality fermented milk products;
- Production of dairy products out of the liquid and powdered milk;
- Production of non-durable bread and flour-based confectionery products;
- Increase of food output by means of the modernization of production facilities, development of the infrastructure and logistics services, which taken together can allow an increase in the capacities for the conservation of raw materials and finished products.

Taking into account the above-mentioned priority objectives, the development of a local dairy and meat husbandry, swine and poultry breeding, horticulture, fodder production, fur farming, and flax breeding are undoubtedly crucial in the Arctic. Nevertheless, self-sufficiency of the region in high-nutritious food is possible only by means of those raw materials and finished products produced with an involvement of high bioclimatic potential and effective use of land and human resources (Table 3).

The analysis of the natural resource potential of the Arctic and the current state of crop areas and cattle population shows that the decrease of the dependence of the circumpolar and sub-Arctic regions on food imports, decrease in the supply and delivery costs, as well as the increase of the quality of food products are all possible by means of the collaboration with other regions, those with more fertile soils and better vegetation conditions. For the Russian part of the Arctic, one of the potential regions of such type is Omskaya Oblast.

Table 3. Areas under crops and cattle population in selected Arctic and sub-Arctic territories of Russia

Territories	Cereal and leguminous crops (wheat, rye, barley, millet, triticale), ha	Legumes (linen, soy, colza), ha	Cattle population, thousands of animals
Far Eastern Federal District, total	353.3	0.6	173.2
Republic of Sakha (Yakutia)	12.5	0.0	81.5
Kamchatsky Krai	0.2	0.0	3.8
Primorsky Krai	105.5	0.2	29.6
Khabarovsky Krai	9.4	0.0	10.1
Amurskaya Oblast	218.4	0.0	36.1
Jewish Autonomous Region	7.3	0.4	3.5

Source: Federal Service for State Statistics of the Russian Federation (2016)

Exploration

Located in Southwest Siberia, Omskaya Oblast has favorable conditions for the cultivation of leguminous crops, which provide high yields within a short period. Leguminous crops are a substantial part of food production of vegetable origin due to their unique biochemical composition, characterized by a high content of proteins. In 2010, Russia's total area under all types of leguminous crops, including peas, vetch, beans, lupine, lentil, chickpeas, peavine, and favas, amounted to 1,305,000 ha, while in 2015, it increased up to 1,989,000 ha.

Species of Beans Cultivated in Omskaya Oblast

In Russia, the most popular and valuable leguminous crops are beans, chickpeas, peas, soybeans, and lentil. Cultivation of beans for the food industry is carried out in Omskaya Oblast and other territories of Russia. In particular, highly productive species of beans have been cultivated at Omsk State Agrarian University (OSAU) (Department of Agronomy, Plant Breeding, and Seed Studies) under the supervision of Professor Nina Kazydub (Table 4).

Table 4. Standard characteristics of beans for dry consumption

Species	Shape, dimension	Linear dimensions (length / width / thickness), mm	Color
Lukeriya	Long-cylindrical, slightly arcuate with round edges	11.0 / 7.0 / 5.0	Black
Omichka	Long-cylindrical, slightly arcuate with round edges	11.0 / 6.0 / 5.0	White
Sizaya	Long-cylindrical, slightly arcuate with round edges	11.0 / 7.0 / 6.0	Blue-grey
Olivkovaya	Long-cylindrical, slightly arcuate with round edges	12.0 / 7.0 / 6.8	Olive green
Nerussa standard	White elliptical seeds, white hilum	8.0 / 6.0 / 5.0	White

Source: Authors' development

The seeds of the five species comply with the Interstate Standard "Grain. Methods for Determination of Odour and Colour" (Government of the Russian Federation, 1991). As for the linear dimensions, the organoleptic characteristics of the species cultivated at OSAU are consistently above the standard. Olivkovaya, Sizaya, and Lukeriya species are bigger than Omichka species. They have a bright color which intensity fades during the hydromechanical and hydrothermal processing. For Omichka species, color stability before and after the hydrothermal processing is originally white (Figure 1).

Figure 1. Species of beans
Source: Authors' development

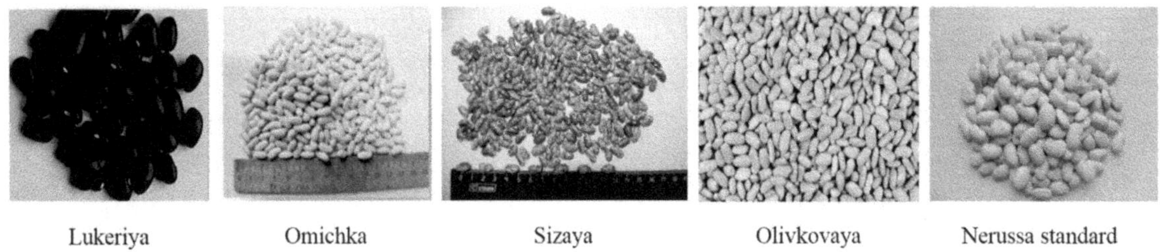

In order to use the species of beans as raw material for the production of complex food products, the security characteristics regulated by the technical regulation of the Customs Union "On Grain Safety" (Customs Union Commission, 2011) were evaluated. In the examined samples, the content of toxic elements did not exceed the allowed level of safety. In particular, mycotoxins were not detected, while the content of pesticides was half as high as the allowed standard.

The comparative analysis of the agronomic characteristics of the species cultivated at OSAU with the standard Nerussa species has demonstrated that those cultivated in Omsk have rather thousand kernel weight (TKW) (362.0-494.0 g) and kernel weight (21.1-28.7 g). The higher the kernel weight the higher the weight in each volume unit, subsequently, the higher the content of useful substances. Under different conditions of the species, it is possible to obtain the higher output of seeds and, as a result, higher output of functional products.

During the hydrothermal processing of Olivkovaya, Sizaya, and Lukeriya species, there are observed a change in color of the aqueous solution and decrease in the color intensity of the seed coat of the beans which characterizes the color of the seeds. Omichka species is characterized by color stability. All varieties can be classified as part of the first group of cooking property (excellent). For some samples, this characteristic ranged from 57 min to 61 min. The organoleptic evaluation of the cook legumes (National Standard of the Russian Federation #53104-2008 "Public Catering Service. Method of Sensory Evaluation of Catering Products Quality (Government of the Russian Federation, 2010)) has demonstrated that Nerussa species is tastier when cooked. This species can be used in cooking culinary dishes, whereas Omichka and Lukeriya species do not possess a pronounced specific bean flavor. The use of the protein-carbohydrate complexes of these varieties as additives of vegetable origin do not significantly change the flavor of food products.

The results of the determination of the content of basic nutrients, macro- and microelements, and proteins (Table 5) are in line with the recent data from other studies. In particular, Balja (2016) detected an increased phytochemical potential of beans for dry consumption, but the content of proteins in the

Table 5. Characteristics of the species cultivated at OSAU regarding the chemical content of kernel in 2015-2017

Bean species	Average content				
	Zinc, mg/kg	Weight ratio of proteins, %	Iodine, mg/kg	Weight ratio of calcium, %	Iron, mg/kg
Lukeriya	20.90	23.38	0.23	0.03	57.00
Omichka	36.60	25.19	0.19	0.03	80.00
Sizaya	24.30	24.06	0.19	0.05	54.00
Olivkovaya	28.10	23.13	0.21	0.08	41.00
Nerussa standard	30.90	22.59	0.10	0.02	45.00

Source: Authors' development

species varied from 20.81% to 22.03%, while in the species cultivated at OSAU it ranges from 23.13% to 25.19% and exceeds the Nerussa standard (22.59%).

The content of zinc in the bean samples ranges from 20.9 mg/kg to 36.6 mg/kg, which is significantly above the Nerussa standard. The average content of iron (41.0-80.0 mg/kg) also exceeds the standard. The content of iodine is over two times as high compared to the Nerussa standard and ranges from 0.19 mg/kg to 0.23 mg/kg. Omichka and Lukeriya species possess a more stable content of proteins and microelements in their seeds (Federal Centre of Quality and Safety Assurance for Grain and Grain Products, 2016). The species are also characterized by a relatively high ash content of fibers, ranging from 3.1% to 3.9% (2.8% in Nerussa standard). The presence of fibers confirms the utility of using beans as an ingredient of products with a complex raw material composition not containing such substances. The protein content index was the highest for Omichka species.

All the above-mentioned characteristics summarize the nutritious value of beans for dry consumption as a raw material, as well as the possibility of predicting the technological properties of products aimed at the nutrition of people living in the North, where a deficit of different micronutrients reaches 100%.

Bean proteins contain irreplaceable amino acids, thus they are characterized by a high biological value. The determination of the amino acid content was carried out for Omichka and Lukeriya species, the more promising ones for the utilization in the Arctic conditions due to the enhanced alimentary value compared to the Nerussa standard. The analysis was conducted on Knauer Smartline 5000 chromatograph by means of high-performance liquid chromatography (HPLC) by the method of reversed phase chromatography on the column Diasphere 110 C18, 5μm, 2*150 mm with a pre-column modification of amino acids with 6-aminoquinoline-n-hydroxy-succinimidyl carbamate following the Waters WAT 052880 method. Photometrical detection for λ 248 nm. Injection volume 20 μl. The amino acid content was detected in relation to the peak areas in the sample (Figure 2) and the standard (Figure 3).

All species contain all irreplaceable amino acids but in different volumes (Table 6). In particular, Omichka distinguishes for the high content of amino acid. The share of irreplaceable amino acids in proteins in white bean species amounts to 42% for Omichka and 45% for the standard species, which can condition high biological value.

In order to make more consistent conclusions about the biological value of species, the amino acid score and protein digestibility-corrected amino acid score (PDCAAS) should be determined. The products containing high-quality proteins with PDCAAS = 1.0 are considered appropriate in terms of the supply of an intended ratio of daily protein intake (Table 7).

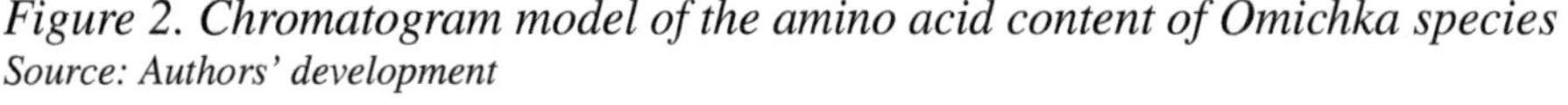

Figure 2. Chromatogram model of the amino acid content of Omichka species
Source: Authors' development

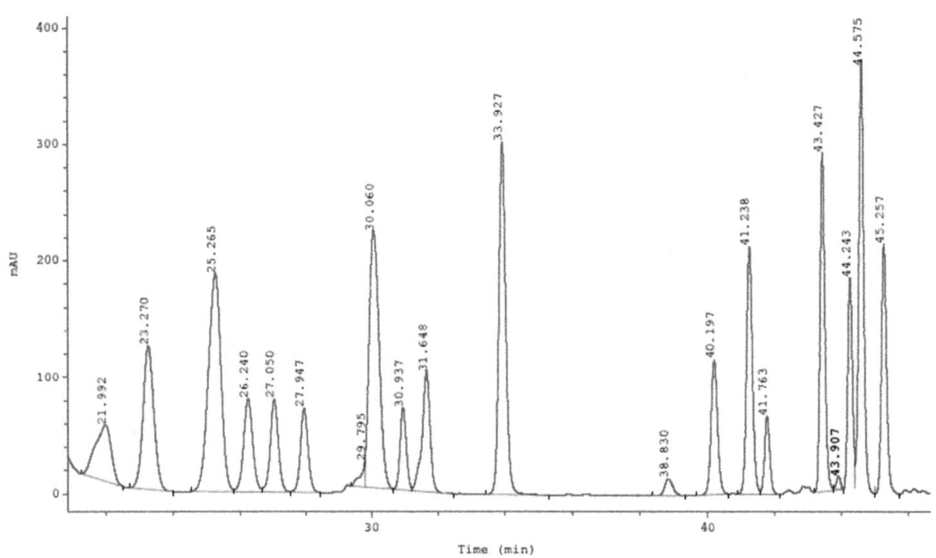

Figure 3. Chromatogram model of amino acid standard
Source: Authors' development

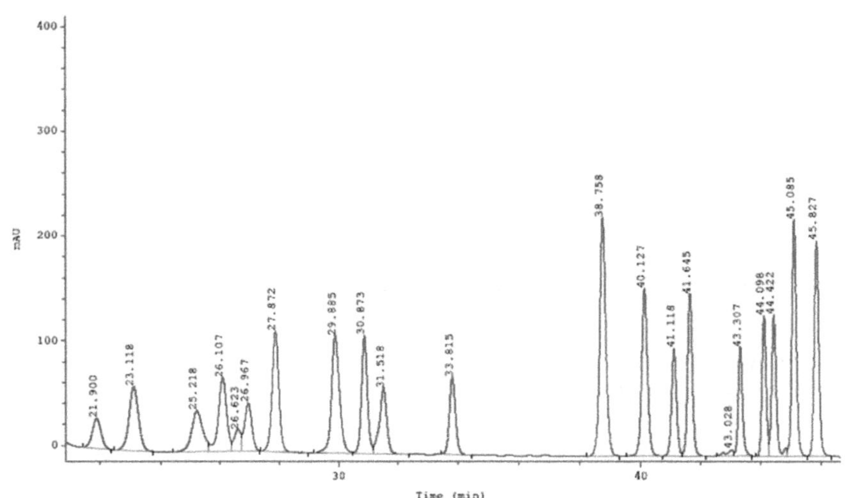

For Omichka and Lukeriya, the limiting amino acid is isoleucine, whereas that for Nerussa standard is methionine+cysteine. The PDCAAS is closer to one for Omichka and Lukeriya species, while only 0.45 for Nerussa standard, which demonstrates the low biological value of proteins. On the contrary, the species distinguish themselves for their higher indexes as regards the limiting amino acids and PD-CAAS coefficient. It allows concluding that proteins in the species are closer to the appropriate protein content and possess a high nutritious value (Federal Centre of Quality and Safety Assurance for Grain and Grain Products, 2016).

Table 6. Content indexes of mass concentration of amino acids, g/100g of dry substances

Amino acids	Bean species		
	Omichka	Lukeriya	Nerussa standard
Aspartic acid	3.06	2.16	1.46
Serine	1.49	1.30	1.37
Glutamic acid	4.56	3.85	3.77
Glycine	0.95	0.80	0.92
Histidine	0.72	0.62	0.63
Threonine	1.03	0.91	1.10
Arginine	1.27	0.97	1.14
Alanine	0.90	0.80	0.93
Proline	0.76	0.53	0.61
Cysteine	0.09	0.10	0.07
Tyrosine	0.83	0.69	0.72
Valine	1.16	0.97	1.11
Methionine	0.87	0.87	0.23
Lysine	1.75	1.60	1.88
Tryptophan	0.29	0.26	0.27
Isoleucine	0.89	0.75	0.89
Leucine	1.80	1.54	1.80
Phenylalanine	1.39	1.14	1.39
Total amino acids	23.81	19.86	19.42
Total ratio of irreplaceable amino acids in proteins, %	42.00	37.00	45.00

Source: Authors' development

Table 7. Amino acid scores of the species

Index	Amino acid score as related to the ideal proteins, %		
	Omichka	Lukeriya	Nerussa standard
Threonine	107.70	96.40	131.00
Valine	97.10	82.20	105.70
Methionine+cysteine	114.80	105.30	40.80
Lysine	133.10	123.30	162.80
Tryptophan	121.30	110.20	128.60
Isoleucine	93.10	79.40	106.00
Leucine	107.60	93.20	122.40
Phenylalanine+Tyrosine	154.80	129.20	167.50
PDCAAS	0.86	0.77	0.45

Source: Authors' development

Usage of Bean Seeds and Processed Products for Nutrition Purposes

In the Arctic, provision of people with high-quality food products of domestic origin is possible by means of the diversification of supply. In order to decrease the dreary diet, improve its completeness, increase the share of traditional food in the consumption, and introduce new products with sufficient content of C, B, A, and D vitamins, macro- and microelements (calcium, potassium, magnesium, fluorine, iodine, selenium), and fibers, it is necessary to utilize the alternative sources of nutritious and biologically active substances.

Leonova, Nuretdinova, and Fazylov (2015), Sergeeva, Simonenkova, and Mamaev (2016), Ziarno, Weber, Kazydub, & Leonova (2016), and Balja (2016) have confirmed the efficiency of using leguminous raw materials and additives of vegetable origin not only to increase the quality and nutritious value of the diets, but also to supply the economy with raw materials. Kleiman (2006) proposes the usage of millet, milo, lentils, brown rice, corn, wheat, Azuki beans, black gram, seeds, nuts, barley, soy, and other vegetable crops as cereal and leguminous raw materials for the production of alimentary products which accelerate or block endopathic factors totally, or for some basic products.

Studies on the usage of beans in dairy production and the possibility of mixing them with other ingredients, as well as the study of the consumption properties of final products are also significant. In general, more emphasis has been given soy since its derivatives have received a wide application in food production. However, the attention should be paid to beans, a leguminous crop traditionally cultivated in Russia.

Ma and Boye (2015) demonstrated the necessity of further study of the usage of beans (Phaseolus spp.), peas (Pisum sativum L.), chickpeas (Cicer arietinum L.), and lentils (Lens culinaris Medik.), as well as oil crops such as soy (Glycine max (L.) Merr.) and peanuts (Arachis hypogaea L.) to optimize the quality of the final product.

Application of Nature-Like Technologies in the Production of Complex Food Products

Nature-like technologies were first defined at the 70th session of the United Nations General Assembly. Boye and Arcand (2013) confirmed the utility of nature-like technologies by analyzing the data on the insufficiency of food products for almost three billion people, insufficient intake of proteins/calories for almost 800 million people, iron deficiency for almost two billion people, and the misuse of land and water resources. Amid such insufficient availability of food and intake of nutritious elements, 30-35% of food produced globally is wasted. As an example of the application of nature-like technologies in food production, the authors have elaborated a scheme for the utilization of beans cultivated at the OSAU for dry consumption as raw material (Figure 4). In its implementation, the scheme follows the principles and regularities laid down by nature.

The technologies used in the products meet all the requirements of nature-like technologies. Chemical substances are not applied. The final product is produced by the implementation of biotechnological methods of natural fermentation of raw materials. Processing of the species cultivated at the OSAU uses both the final product and production waste. Omichka species is particularly recommended for the production of bean paste, vegetable dispersion, and derived products due to its organoleptic characteristics and white color. Black kernels of Lukeriya species are recommended for the production of the finely dispersed vegetable component which can be used in dairy production and bread making, as well as in the production of other products.

Figure 4. Scheme for the processing of bean kernels with the implementation of nature-like technologies
Source: Authors' development

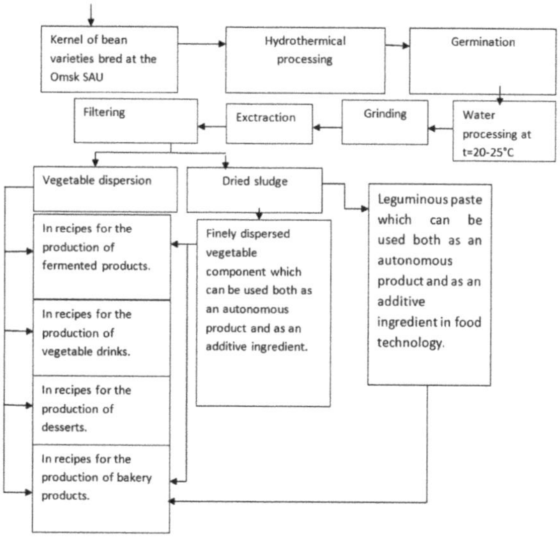

Production of Lactose-Free Products

Despite a substantial number of studies of the properties of beans and derived products, most of them regard beans as an ingredient used in the production of processed meat, flour, and confectionery products. The studies related to the use of beans in dairy production and the possibility of mixing them with other ingredients, as well as the studies of the consumer properties of final products, are inconspicuous (Mecha, Figueira, Vaz Patto, & Bronze, 2015). Due to the narrow variety of food products appropriate for the people suffering from lactose deficiency, the development of lactose-free product technologies is one of the priorities of food production.

Technology of Food Dispersion of Bean Kernels

Vegetable dispersion of bean kernels ("vegetable milk") is a part of the so-called Health & Wellness product range. The market for such kind of products, including vegetable drinks, increases by 6-8% annually in America, Europe, and Asia. The developed natural food product imitates the properties of a natural dairy product, fulfills the deficiency of essential nutrients necessary for the body, and is an important part in the program of activities aimed at creating a healthy lifestyle which is principally necessary for the population of the Arctic region.

Biotechnological methods of natural fermentation during germination, which promote the improvement of the organoleptic properties (to some extent, eliminate unpleasant bean flavor and odor), increase the digestibility and biological activity of raw materials were used to obtain a vegetable dispersion from bean kernels. A soaked grain is placed in a sprouting device additionally equipped with an ultrasonic steam generator. During the germination of seeds, a sprout is formed, the length of which increases in proportion to the duration of germination. The grains are germinated for 14-21 hours until the length of a sprout reaches at least 3-7 mm (Federal Service for Intellectual Property, 2015a). The germinated grain is enriched with B, C, and E vitamins. The concentration of the elements necessary for the body (Zn, Fe, Ca, P, Mg, etc.) increases. Nutrients become more accessible to the effects of the digestive enzymes. The nutritional value increases due to the saccharification of starches; the content of soluble nitrogenous compounds increases. There is a redistribution of the relative concentration of individual amino acids. At the same time, the content of proteins, lipids, and carbohydrates consumed in the processes associated with the formation and development of the plant embryo is reduced. The maximum accumulation of vitamin C occurs. A similar effect was obtained with the germination of seeds of dicotyledonous soy plants (Grace, Sogo, James, & Olanike, 2015).

Relf (n.d.) has confirmed the prospects of using sprouted legumes in food production. Germinated bean grains are washed in the water (20-25°C). Washing both ensures the preservation of biologically active substances and prevents infection with Escherichia coli and Salmonella. Germinated grains are crushed, subjected to the extraction at a grain-to-water ratio of 1:5-1:6 at a temperature of $80 \pm 5°C$ during 10-15 minutes, and then filtered through a sieve (0.2 mm holes).

A comparative analysis of the obtained bean dispersion with cow milk and other dispersions of vegetable origin is presented in Table 8.

Table 8. Physicochemical indicators of vegetable dispersions and cow milk

Definition	Testing	Vegetable dispersions			
	Cow milk	Oat dispersion	Soy dispersion	Bean dispersion	Coconut dispersion
Mass ratio of proteins, %	2.8 ± 0.2	1.0 ± 0.2	2.6 ± 0.2	3.0 ± 0.2	0.1 ± 0.2
Mass ratio of fats, %	2.5 ± 0.05	1.0 ± 0.2	1.8 ± 0.2	1.2 ± 0.2	0.9 ± 0.2
Mass ratio of carbohydrates, %	4.5 ± 0.2	6.0 ± 0.2	1.8 ± 0.2	2.0 ± 0.2	2.5 ± 0.2
Mass ratio of fibers, %	-	0.9	0.7	0.9	0.1
pH	6.8 ± 0.2	6.7 ± 0.2	6.6 ± 0.2	6.7 ± 0.2	6.8 ± 0.2

Source: Authors' development

The bean dispersion has a high protein content amounting to $3.0 \pm 0.2\%$ if compared to other vegetable dispersions. This confirms the assumption about the hydrolysability of bean proteins. The bean dispersion also has a relatively low content of total carbohydrates, fats, but a sufficient content of fibers.

Development of Complex Raw Material Products Using Vegetable Dispersion

Further studies were aimed at the possibility of using the bean dispersion in the technology of products of mixed raw material composition. The authors have used an example of an ice cream, a complex multi-component system containing various ingredients. However, most of those ingredients are of animal origin. In the Arctic, despite the harsh climate conditions some people follow a strict vegetarian diet. Those who suffer from allergy are mostly children who cannot consume dairy products. A recipe for an ice cream that does not contain ingredients of animal origin (eggs and milk) has been developed. Instead, it contains vegetable fat (coconut oil) and bean dispersion (Omichka species), coconut in the form of coconut water, pre-activated biomass of bifidobacteria, lyophilized according to the standard, and other nutritional additives. The production of "Fa-sol" ("bean" in Russian) ice-cream is carried out in accordance with the elaborated technological regimes. The final product possesses high organoleptic characteristics, i.e. dense, homogeneous consistency, without perceptible lumps of fat and ice crystals, pleasant moderately sour-sweet taste, slight aftertaste, and slightly expressed coconut aroma. It possesses the following characteristics: moisture content 71.0%, protein content at least 3.5%, fat content at least 4.5%, reduced energy value 114.5 kcal. The number of viable cells of probiotic cultures (CFU) in the product is at least 1.2×10^6 CFU/g at the expiration date, which indicates the high probiotic properties of the product. The product possesses high organoleptic characteristics if compared to ice cream made from rice, soy, or coconut milk (Federal Centre of Quality and Safety Assurance for Grain and Grain Products, 2018).

Technology of Finely Divided Roasted Product

In order to obtain an optimal technology for the production of a finely-divided roasted product with pleasant smell, light brown color, high content of water-soluble substances that guarantee good absorption of the product, humidity of 15-16%, intended for both direct use as food or as a component in dairy and bakery industry, the authors propose the usage of bean grains of Lukeriya and Omichka species sprouted using the above-described technology during 14-21 hours. At the end of germination, drying to a moisture content of 17.5% is carried out, and then the grain is roasted at a temperature of 80-100°C. The product readiness is determined by its organoleptic characteristics: a grain becomes light and crisp and reduces the mass ratio of moisture to a value of 15-16%. The roasted bean grains are cooled to a temperature of 18-20°C and ground to a particle size of 0.3-0.5 mm (sieves 7-12).

As regards the organoleptic characteristics, the final product has a color similar to the original color of a grain of the particular species (from cream to black) and light bean flavor and smell. Physicochemical parameters are presented in Table 9.

Table 9. Physicochemical characteristics of the finely divided roasted product

Description	Index value (normalized)
Humidity, % (max.)	15.0-16.0
Falling-number, s (max.)	120.0
Grinding coarseness	
Residue on a sieve, % (max.)	5, sieve 10 PA-220

Source: Authors' development based on Federal Service for Intellectual Property (2015b)

Yoghurt Technology Using the Finely Divided Roasted Product

The product obtained in an above-described way was used to produce a yoghurt-type fermented dairy product from cow milk according to the developed technology. A comparative analysis of the nutritional value of a yoghurt-type fermented dairy product with the addition of 3-5% of the bean component (Table 10) demonstrated the high nutritional value compared to the control sample. The thus-obtained product possessed high organoleptic properties, had a pleasant sour-milk smell and taste and a gentle consistency.

Table 10. Physicochemical characteristics of the yoghurt-type fermented dairy product with the addition of the finely divided roasted product

Product	Mass ratio, %			Energy value per 100 g	
	Fats	Proteins	Dry substances	kcal	kJ
Control sample (cow milk yoghurt)	2.5	4.2	12.2	72.65	316.73
Experiment 1: a component obtained from Lukeriya species beans	2.5	7.2	13.9	90.33	378.18
Experiment 2: a component obtained from Omichka species beans	2.5	7.9	15.7	90.33	378.18
Experiment 3: a component obtained from a 1:1 mix of Lukeriya and Omichka species	2.5	7.5	14.5	90.33	378.18

Source: Authors' development based on Federal Service for Intellectual Property (2015c)

Taking into account that the daily intake for men aged 40-59 with a coefficient of physical activity 1 and for women aged 40-59 with a coefficient of physical activity 2 amounts to 2,110 kcal, it can be concluded that the use of yoghurt-type fermented dairy products with the finely-divided roasted component allows to fulfil the daily energy norm percentage by 4.28%, while a traditional product by 3.44%. Given that the daily intake of proteins for men of the same age and activity coefficient amount to 65.0 and for women to 63.0, the use of yoghurt-type fermented dairy products with the addition of the finely-divided roasted component allows to fulfil the daily protein intake by 15% on average, while the use of a traditional product by 6.46%.

Use of Bean Kernels in the Hummus Paste Technology

For the nutrition of the population in the Arctic region, the authors propose using the Hummus paste made from the beans of the OSAU species. Hummus is a traditional dish in some of the countries of Europe and the Middle East. The introduction of this product into the diet of the people in the Arctic allows reducing the lack of amino acids, vitamin B, and micro and macro elements. Due to the use of natural ingredients with increased phytochemical potential, the shelf life of Hummus bean paste in hermetically sealed packaging is below 100 days at a temperature below -18°C. The protein content in the product is above 8.0%, the fat content is above 20.8%, the energy value amounts to 269 kcal. This product can be used both as an independent dish and as an ingredient.

SOLUTIONS AND RECOMMENDATIONS

Given the actual state of the level and quality of food, different nutritional groups and strata of the population, local climate and economic conditions in the Arctic, the integrated study allows recommending the OSAU bean species for food production and nutrition of the people due to the high yielding capacity, enhanced quality in the technical phase of ripeness, the highest content of micro and macro elements, proteins and other biologically active substances. The beans may be produced in Southwest Siberia, particularly, in Omskaya Oblast, and then supplied to the northern parts of Russia. The developed products are similar to the dairy ones according to some parameters of their chemical composition. The use of bean processing products of the OSAU species allows an expansion in the range of competitive products intended for the Arctic conditions due to their high nutritional and biological values.

FUTURE RESEARCH DIRECTIONS

In the future, research in this direction will be aimed at expanding the range of food products from vegetable raw materials for urban residents and indigenous peoples. The development of cascade processing local environmentally-friendly raw materials on the example of bean grains and chia seed with the utilization of nature-like technologies is planned. The implementation of the approach should be studied in the specific climate and vegetation conditions of other Nordic countries. In general, it is expected that the use of nature-like technologies in the North will allow satisfying the existing demand in the basic food products, as well as supplying healthy and high-nutritious food and agricultural products to the circumpolar territories of Nordic countries.

CONCLUSION

Given the peculiarities of the economic and geographical situation in the Arctic, actual level of food prices, solvent consumer demand, level of monetary incomes, and the volume of locally produced food, food security can be recognized as unsatisfactory. Food products of vegetable origin may be imported from other regions of Russia to improve food security in the North. The establishment of the enterprises for processing, storing, and distribution of food products along with the formation of rear food bases in adjacent favorable agricultural areas are required to ensure the physical and economic accessibility of socially significant products for the residents of the North. Those activities will eliminate the dependence of the circumpolar territories on the imports, reduce losses, and improve the quality of food products. This study makes it possible to recommend to deliver the OSAU varieties of vegetable beans due to their high yield, quality in the technical ripeness phase, content of micro- and macro-elements, protein, and other biologically active substances. Complex research have made it possible to establish differences in the chemical composition of the selected varieties as compared to the variety of the standard and to develop technological methods for its processing into food products. The proposed nature-friendly scheme does not violate the environment because of the implementation of the waste-free re-cultivation technologies and the omission of genetically modified food products and components that use synthesized biologically active components. A range of products, which is balanced in terms of nutritional and biological value and contributes to the improvement of the feeding system in the Arctic, has been developed. The studies have demonstrated that, when using Omichka species, the products allow supplying the human body with the following essential amino acids: threonine, methionine + cysteine, lysine, tryptophan, leucine, phenylalanine + tyrosine. Lukeriya species supplies amino acids such as methionine + cysteine, lysine, tryptophan, phenylalanine + tyrosine. The products produced with the use of those species have the high content of iodine, calcium, iron, zinc, and other important micro and macro elements, as well as fibers.

REFERENCES

AllergyFree. (n.d.). *Lactase Deficiency.* Retrieved July 30, 2018, from http://www.allergyfree.ru/category/info/type.html

Balja, L. (2016). Determination of Chemical Composition and Quality Characteristics of the Grain Bean White. *Grain Products and Mixed Fodder's, 61*(1), 17–20.

Boye, J., & Arcand, Y. (2013). Current Trends in Green Technologies in Food Production and Processing. *Food Engineering Reviews, 5*(1), 11–17. doi:10.100712393-012-9062-z

Customs Union Commission. (2011). *Technical Regulation of the Customs Union 015/2011 "On Grain Safety".* Retrieved July 3, 2018, from http://docs.cntd.ru/document/902320395

Eganyan, R. (2013). Nutritional Characteristics in Dwellers of the Far North of Russia (A Review of Literature). *Preventive Medicine, 16*(5), 41–47.

Federal Centre of Quality and Safety Assurance for Grain and Grain Products. (2016). *Test Protocol #1662, 18/10/2016.* Moscow: Federal Centre of Quality and Safety Assurance for Grain and Grain Products.

Federal Centre of Quality and Safety Assurance for Grain and Grain Products. (2018). *Test Protocol #B-3820, 09/06/2018.* Moscow: Federal Centre of Quality and Safety Assurance for Grain and Grain Products.

Federal Service for Intellectual Property. (2015a). *Patent #160896 "Device for Plant Growing".* Retrieved July 30, 2018, from http://xn--90ax2c.xn--p1ai/catalog/000224_000128_0000160896_20160410_U1_RU/viewer/

Federal Service for Intellectual Property. (2015b). *Patent #2599569 "Functional Alimentary Product from Sprouted Kernels".* Retrieved July 30, 2018, from http://xn--90ax2c.xn--p1ai/catalog/000224_000128_0002599569_20161010_C1_RU/viewer/

Federal Service for Intellectual Property. (2015c). *Patent #2616864 "Process for Producing Fermented Milk Drink".* Retrieved July 30, 2018, from http://www.findpatent.ru/patent/261/2616864.html

Federal Service for State Statistics of the Russian Federation. (2016). *Preliminary Results of the All-Russian Agricultural Census for 2016.* Retrieved July 3, 2018, from http://www.gks.ru/free_doc/new_site/business/sx/vsxp2016/VSHP-2016.pdf

Food and Agriculture Organization of the United Nations. (n.d.). *International Food Standards.* Retrieved July 30, 2018, from http://www.fao.org/fao-who-codexalimentarius/codex-texts/list-standards/en/

Government of the Republic of Sakha (Yakutia). (2014). *Decree #251 from August 15, 2014, "On the Integrated Program of the Republic of Sakha (Yakutia) "Socio-Economic Development of the Arctic and Northern Districts of the Republic of Sakha (Yakutia) for 2014-2017 and the Period till 2020"".* Retrieved July 3, 2018, from http://docs.cntd.ru/document/432880477

Government of the Russian Federation. (1991). *Interstate Standard "Grain. Methods for Determination of Odour and Colour".* Retrieved July 30, 2018, from http://docs.cntd.ru/document/1200024311

Government of the Russian Federation. (2008). *Methodical Recommendations #2.3.1.2432-08 "Normative of Physiological Needs in Energy and Nutritious Elements for Various Groups of Population in the Russian Federation"*. Retrieved July 3, 2018, from http://base.garant.ru/2168105/

Government of the Russian Federation. (2010). *National Standard of the Russian Federation #53104-2008 "Public Catering Service. Method of Sensory Evaluation of Catering Products Quality"*. Retrieved July 30, 2018, from http://docs.cntd.ru/document/1200069392

Grace, O., Sogo, J., James, A., & Olanike, O. (2015). Effect of the Germination Process on Some Anti-Nutritional Factors, Proximate Composition, Mineral and Vitamin Contents of Soybean. *Journal of Chemical and Pharmaceutical Research, 11*(7), 494–498.

Inuit Circumpolar Council. (2012). *Food Security across the Arctic*. Retrieved July 3, 2018, from http://www.inuitcircumpolar.com/uploads/3/0/5/4/30542564/icc_food_security_across_the_arctic_may_2012.pdf

Ivanov, V., & Ivanova, E. (2017). Arctic Specifics of Food Supply and Development of Agriculture in the European North-East of Russia. *The Arctic: Ecology and Economics, 26*(2), 117–130.

Kleiman, J. (2006). *Patent #10/133935 "Method of Preparing Nutritional Legume Product"*. US 7022369 B1. A23L1/20.

Leonova, S., Nuretdinova, O., & Fazylov, M. (2015). Technology of Receiving of National Cereal Product from Germinated Grain of Oats with Addition of Apples. *Khleboprodukty, 9*, 52–53.

Lomer, M. C., Parkes, G. S., & Sanderson, J. D. (2008). Review Article: Lactose Intolerance in Clinical Practice: Myths and Realities. *Alimentary Pharmacology & Therapeutics, 27*(2), 93–103. doi:10.1111/j.1365-2036.2007.03557.x PMID:17956597

Ma, Z., & Boye, J. I. (2015). Legumes: An Emerging Source of Ingredients for Health and Wellness Foods and Their Potential for Application in Various Products. *The Journal of the International Legume Society, 9*, 7–9.

Mecha, E., Figueira, M. E., Vaz Patto, C., & Bronze, M. R. (2015). Common Bean (Phaseolus Vulgaris L.): Underexplored Attributes for Food Development. *The Journal of the International Legume Society, 9*, 28–30.

Panin, L. (2010a). Homeostasis and Problems of Circumpolar Health (Methodological Aspects of Adaptation). *Bulletin of the Siberian Branch of the Russian Academy of Medical Sciences, 30*(3), 6–11.

Panin, L. (2010b). Man in Extreme Conditions in the Arctic. *Bulletin of the Siberian Branch of the Russian Academy of Medical Sciences, 30*(3), 92–98.

Polbitsyn, S., Drokin, V., & Zhuravlev, A. (2012). Strategic Priorities in the Formation of a Food Supply System in the Northern, Polar, and Arctic Territories. *Management of Economic Systems, 47*(11). Retrieved July 3, 2018, from http://uecs.ru/uecs47-472012/item/1636-2012-

President of the Russian Federation. (2010). *Food Security Doctrine of the Russian Federation*. Retrieved July 30, 2018, from http://old.mcx.ru/documents/document/v7_show/37135.133.htm

Rautio, A., Piippo, S., Pongracz, E., Golubeva, E., Soloviev, A., & Grini, I. S. … Helgesen, H. (2015). *Healthy Living, Nutrition and Food Waste in the Barents Region*. Retrieved July 3, 2018, from http://www.oulu.fi/sites/default/files/108/REPORT_Lifestyle.pdf

Relf, D. (n.d.). *Sprouting Seeds for Food*. Retrieved July 3, 2018, from http://pubs.ext.vt.edu/content/dam/pubs_ext_vt_edu/426/426-419/426-419_pdf.pdf

Sergeeva, E., Simonenkova, A., & Mamaev, A. (2016). *Compound Products with the Usage of Lentil Dispersion*. Saarbrucken: LAP Lambert Academic Publishing.

Sevostyanova, Y. (2013). Some Features of Human Lipid and Carbohydrate Metabolism in the North. *Bulletin of Siberian Medicine*, *12*(1), 93–100.

Willett, W. C. (2005). *Eat, Drink, and Be Healthy: The Harvard Medical School Guide to Healthy Eating*. Boston, MA: Harvard Medical School.

Ziarno, M., Weber, A., Kazydub, N., & Leonova, S. (2016). Investigation of Possibility of Fruit-Bean Mixture Use in Production of Fermented Dairy Food. In *Proceedings of the First International Forum "Leguminous Crops – Developing Direction in Russia"*. Omsk: KAN Polygraphic Center.

ADDITIONAL READING

Government of the Russian Federation. (2010). *Decree #1873 from October 25, 2010, "Foundations of the State Policy of the Russian Federation in the Sphere of Healthy Nutrition of the Population for a Period till 2020"*. Retrieved July 3, 2018, from https://www.gnicpm.ru/UserFiles/osnovi_zdor_pitania_do_2020.pdf

Government of the Russian Federation. (2012). *Decree #717 from July 14, 2012, "On the State Program of the Development of Agricultural Production and Regulation of the Markets of Agricultural Products, Raw Materials, and Food for a Period of 2013-2020"*. Retrieved July 3, 2018, from http://base.garant.ru/70210644/

Government of the Russian Federation. (2016). *Decree #1378 from June 30, 2016, "Strategy of Development of Food and Food Processing Industry in the Russian Federation for a Period till 2020"*. Retrieved July 3, 2018, from http://static.government.ru/media/files/65bZISIOP6bA0VSJ67GnnpKIhhoHhxgP.pdf

Larionov, V. (2015). Food Security in Russia. *Food Policy and Security*, *2*(1), 47–58.

Ministry of Health of the Russian Federation. (2016). *Order #614 from August 19, 2016, "On the Approval of the Recommendations on the Normative of the Rational Consumption of Food Products According to the Modern Requirements of Healthy Nutrition"*. Retrieved July 3, 2018, from http://www.garant.ru/products/ipo/prime/doc/71385784/

Nikitenko, M., & Trofimova, I. (2016). Food Security in the Arctic Territories of the Russian Federation. *Society: Politics, Economics. Law*, *9*, 33–37.

Nuttall, M., Berkes, F., Forbes, B., Kofinas, G., Vlassova, T., & Wenzel, G. (2015). *Hunting, Herding, Fishing, and Gathering: Indigenous Peoples and Renewable Resource Use in the Arctic*. Retrieved July 3, 2018, from https://www.researchgate.net/publication/242274643_Hunting_Herding_Fishing_and_Gathering_Indigenous_Peoples_and_Renewable_Resource_Use_in_the_Arctic

President of the Russian Federation. (2014). *Decree #286 from May 2, 2014, "On Land Territories of the Arctic Zone of the Russian Federation"*. Retrieved July 3, 2018, from http://www.kremlin.ru/acts/bank/38377

President of the Russian Federation. (n.d.). *Draft of the Decree "On the Introduction of Changes to the Food Security Doctrine of the Russian Federation Approved by the Decree of the President of the Russian Federation #120 from January 30, 2010"*. Retrieved July 3, 2018, from http://www.garant.ru/products/ipo/prime/doc/56641501/

Tatarkin, A., Zakharchuk, E., & Loginov, V. (2015). The Modern Paradigm of Development of the Arctic Zone of the Russian Federation. *The Arctic: Ecology and Economics*, *18*(2), 4–13.

KEY TERMS AND DEFINITIONS

Beans: A leguminous plant.

Energy Value: The amount of energy in kilocalories released from the food products in the human body to ensure its physiological functions.

Macronutrients: The food substances (proteins, fats, and carbohydrates) necessary for plastic, energetic, and other needs a body in the quantities measured in grams.

Micronutrients: The food substances (vitamins, minerals, and microelements) contained in food in very small quantities – milligrams or micrograms. They are not sources of energy, yet they are involved in the assimilation of food, regulation of functions, implementation of growth processes, and adaptation and development of an organism.

Nutrients: The constituent parts of food products that are used by the body as energy sources, sources or predecessors of substrates for the creation, growth, and renewal of organs and tissues, the formation of physiologically active substances involved in the regulation of life processes, and that determine the nutritional value of food products.

Nutritional Value of a Product: A set of properties of the food product, in the presence of which a person's physiological needs in the necessary substances and energy are met.

This research was previously published in the Handbook of Research on International Collaboration, Economic Development, and Sustainability in the Arctic edited by Vasilii Erokhin, Tianming Gao, and Xiuhua Zhang; pages 570-592, copyright year 2019 by Business Science Reference (an imprint of IGI Global).

Chapter 64
Soybeans Consumption and Production in China:
Sustainability Perspective

Xiumei Guo
Curtin University, Australia

Xiaoling Shao
Nanjing Audit University, China

Shagufta M. Trishna
Curtin University, Australia

Dora Marinova
https://orcid.org/0000-0001-5125-8878
Curtin University, Australia

Amzad Hossain
Curtin University, Australia & Rajshahi University, Bangladesh

ABSTRACT

China is the world's top consumer and largest importer of soybeans used as human food and livestock feed. Since the 1980s, China's meat consumption has been growing despite this being an inefficient way of feeding the world's largest population. It diverts resources which can be used directly for human consumption. If the Chinese people were to maintain or expand their high consumption of soybean-based foods instead of switching to a meat-rich diet, greenhouse gas emissions would be reduced, and natural resource use improved. This chapter examines the trends in soy consumption and production in China and explores people's dietary preferences for soybeans, including concerns about the import of genetically modified soybeans. Without diverting soybeans to animal feed, the demand for them will decrease and will make China more self-sufficient. This study also provides educational guidance about the health benefits of plant-based foods and environmental damage associated with high consumption of animal-based products.

DOI: 10.4018/978-1-7998-5354-1.ch064

INTRODUCTION

It is well known that China is not able to produce enough soybeans for processing to meet the growing demands for human soybean-based food and animal feed for livestock. With the increasing household incomes of the Chinese people, their demand for meat and other animal-based foods is also growing. Foods that were once considered unaffordable or foreign are now part of the transition to more western style dietary habits (Ma Verkuil, Reinbach, & Meinert, 2017).

Although pork continues to be the dominate animal protein, there is surging interest in beef and poultry with China's total and per capita meat consumption on the rise since the 1980s (Nam, Jo, & Lee, 2010). Meat production reached 86.45 million tonnes in 2014 and annual meat consumption was 61.82 kg per person per year in 2013 (Ritchie & Roser, 2018). In 2014, the number of livestock animals raised for human consumption in China included 480 million pigs, 114 million cattle and 5.58 billion poultry compared to respectively 326 million, 52 million and 1.18 billion in 1980 (Ritchie & Roser, 2018).

Since the discovery by animal nutritionists that combined with grain, soybean can be used very efficiently as feed for livestock and poultry to boost the production of animal protein, soybeans have been consistently given to farm animals (Brown, 2011). As China's appetite for animal-based products, such as meat and milk grew, so did the conversion of soybeans to animal meal (Brown, 2011). According to Brown from the Earth Policy Institute (2011, p. 95), "since half of the world's pigs are in China, the lion's share of soy use is in pig feed. Its fast-growing poultry industry is also dependent on soybean meal".

This is in sharp contrast with the traditional use of soy which was domesticated as a garden plant by Chinese farmers around 1100 BC (NC Soybean Producers Association, 2014). The legume plant was named "miracle crop" because of its versatile properties and its ability to produce oil and other byproducts suitable for human consumption, such as tofu and soy drinks (U.S. Soybean Export Council, 2006). More recently, soybeans have been grown commercially all around the world for animal feed. In this day and age, "[s]oybean oil is the most widely used edible oil in the world and soybean meal is the leading protein and energy source for animal feeds" (U.S. Soybean Export Council, 2006, p. 4). Soy is also used in cosmetics, pharmaceutical, manufacturing and other industries, as a lubricant, in inks, paints and varnishes as well as biofuel.

The list of applications is long, but nowhere is soy as wanted as it has been as animal feed. This has led to land clearing and conversion to grow soy in some of the most important from a biodiversity point of view places, such as the rainforests of the Amazon (Brügger, Marinova, & Raphaely, 2016). The conflict between the use of soybeans as food and feed on a limited planet has escalated to enormous proportions and China (together with all other high-meat consuming countries) is contributing to large scale deforestation, greenhouse gas emissions, biodiversity loss and inefficient ways for feeding the human population (Schmidinger, Bogueva, & Marinova, 2018). Instead of being used for feeding people directly, soybeans are prepared as animal meal and fed to livestock. In the case of pork – the most popular meat choice in China, 11 calories are fed to the animal to produce 1 calorie for human consumption (Eshel, Shepon, Makov, & Milo, 2014). The respective figures for beef are 38 and for poultry 9 (Eshel, Shepon, Makov, & Milo, 2014).

A solution to the global demand for soy has been through genetic engineering and the development of genetically modifies (GM) versions of soybeans. More than 90% of the soy planted in the US is genetically engineered with the assertions that this helps increase yields and reduce the use of pesticides (Brookes & Barfoot, 2017). However, some disagree with such a view (e.g. Satheesh, 2012) and are of the opinion that GM seeds have not delivered better performance than conventional soy. There are also serious concerns raised about the ethics, risks and impacts (often unknown) on human wellbeing and the health of the planet from GM crops. Such concerns are widely spread across the globe (Bawa & Anilakumar, 2013; Bodnar, 2018) and this is an area with a large gap between public perception and scientific position – 88% of scientists believe that it is safe to eat GM crops while only 37% of the general public are of the same opinion (Funk & Rainie, 2016). These concerns are particularly valid for China as the country currently imports large amounts of soybeans to be used as animal feed and human food, including from USA and Brazil where GM seeds are allowed.

Although in the last few decades China has experienced a growing human consumption of soybeans, the direct use for food products, such as tofu, soy drinks and soy sauce, remains low. It has increased from 10% of the crop used directly as food products in 2010 (Brown, 2011) to 14% in 2017 (China Industrial Information Network, 2018). The remaining 86% are used as pressed oil and animal feed. It is well established that plants and soy in particular are more environmentally friendly than meat production and generate lower greenhouse gas emissions, less pollution and have less requirements for land (Raphaely & Marinova, 2016). Research also shows that soy food products are recognized as the best protein alternatives to meat as they contain a complete set of essential amino acids (Marsall & Marinova, 2019). Therefore, promoting soybeans-based food consumption in China – the country with the world's largest population, becomes an urgent task when tackling environmental issues locally and globally.

This chapter elaborates on the issue about soy production and consumption in China making the argument that if soy is used for direct human consumption with a shift to nutritious and healthy plant-based food options, there will be much less need for this versatile crop to grown in the current excessive amounts. Hence, there will also be no need for genetic engineering and genetic modifications to artificially increase the already healthy yield capacities of this miracle crop. The chapter examines first China's soybean production and trade. Then it analyses the actual soybean consumption in the country, including presenting an overview of some soy-based meat alternatives. It finally makes policy recommendations to encourage behavior changes away from high meat consumption which will be beneficial for China from a human health as well as planetary wellbeing point of view, and given this country's population size such a transition will be advantageous for the entire globe.

The study aims to improve Chinese consumers' awareness of considering the environment when making decisions about what to choose to eat and encourages soybean consumption, with less meat intake, in order to achieve the decoupling between food consumption and production and the environmental damage, simultaneously maintaining better health. In addition, this study highlights the importance of social marketing and policy interventions in encouraging healthy food consumption to maintain the sustainability of modern society.

SOYBEANS PRODUCTION AND TRADE IN CHINA

China has a long history of soybeans production, which has been playing an essential role in poverty reduction by providing plant protein resources and a healthy edible vegetable oil for Chinese people. Planting soybeans domestically in rural areas of the country has contributed significantly to agricultural sustainability. With soybean being a legume, it transfers the atmospheric nitrogen into the soil and does not require as much fertiliser while improving the fertility of the land. The Rhizobia bacteria which infects the roots of all legumes, supplies enough nitrogen to the plant from the air and also helps with nitrogen fixing of the soil (Mosaic Company, 2018). Farmers learn to rotate the crops, maintain the nitrogen cycle and reduce the need to use fertilisers with soybeans fixing naturally and biologically the soil's fertility. In temperate and tropical climates, atmospheric nitrogen transfer to the soil through the symbiotic association between the Rhizobia bacteria and the legume plants, including soybeans, represents a renewable source for fixing soil fertility even for arid and semi-arid lands (Zahran, 1999). The Chinese government is keen to promote sustainable soybeans production for optimizing the planting structure and balancing the supply and demands of soybeans with other agricultural crops (Ministry of Agriculture and Rural Affairs of the People's Republic of China, 2016).

Due to population growth, industrialisation and fast urbanisation, China's planting areas for soybeans have been generally decreasing in the past 20 years (see Figure 1). The amount of land for soybean planting peaked in the years 2004 and 2005 to over 9.5 million hectares but in recent years has been lower at around 6.5 million hectares. Although total soybeans output per hectare has remained relatively stable since 2011 (see Figure 2) due to improved agricultural technology, planting innovation or favourable weather conditions (FAO, 2016), the overall production has decreased because of the shrinking amount of available land.

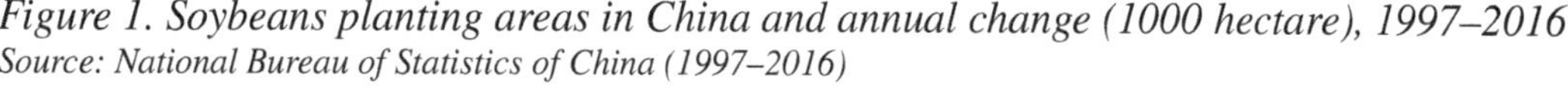

Figure 1. Soybeans planting areas in China and annual change (1000 hectare), 1997–2016
Source: National Bureau of Statistics of China (1997–2016)

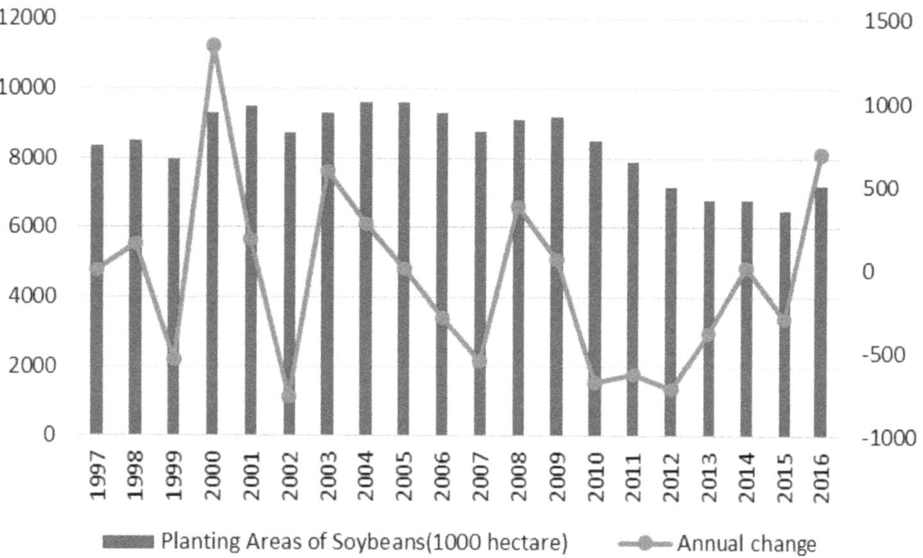

In 2016, the planting area for soybeans started to increase after six years of decrease. It is expected that China will continue to restoratively increase its soybeans planting areas in 2018 at an 1.1% annual growth rate towards achieving a total output of 15 million tonnes (Xinhua, 2018). In 2017, the total soybeans production was already 14.3 million tonnes (Wang, 2018). The domestic sources of soybeans outputs were mainly from the traditional agricultural provinces – Heilongjiang (41%), Anhui (11%), Inner Mongolia, Henan and others. As a matter of priority, the Chinese Government is encouraging farmers to continue to increase the land areas available to grow soy in order to reduce the country's current reliance on imports (Wang, 2018).

Figure 2. Total production of soybeans (10 thousand tonnes) and soybeans output per hectare (kg) in China, 1997–2016
Source: National Bureau of Statistics of China (1997-2016)

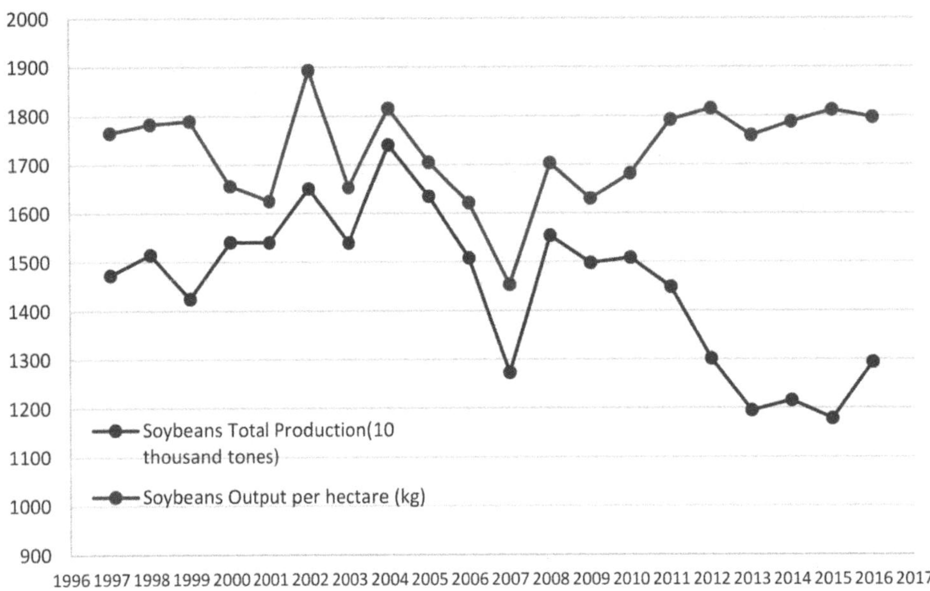

This however will not be enough for the current demand for soy products. Since 1994, China has been a net importer of soybeans and due to the large trade volumes, it has been the top soybeans importer in the world since 2013 (The Statistics Portal, 2018). China's gradually growing imports of soybeans (see Figure 3) reached over 83 million tonnes in 2016 followed by a further drastic 14.8% increase to 95.5 million tonnes in 2018 (Wang, 2018).

Due to this continuous demand for soybeans products, including for human consumption and as animal feed, the soybean import is likely to be maintained at a high level (Central People's Government of the People's Republic of China, 2018b). The shortage of land availability for soybeans planting means that with the current consumption patterns China will continue to depend on imports from foreign countries for the supply of this valuable commodity for domestic use. In 2017, 87% of all domestically consumed soybeans were imported (Wang, 2018) and China in fact accounts for two-thirds of the global imports (Sheldon, 2018). A lot of the imported soy comes from the two major players on the global market – USA and Brazil (Sheldon, 2018). The two countries are the world's largest producers of soybeans and essentially dominate the global market. In 2017, Brazil supplied half (namely 53%) of China's soybeans imports whilst another third (namely 34%) came from USA (Wang, 2018). These two countries are also the world's largest producers of genetically modified crops (Reuters, 2018a), including a lot of the soybeans exported to China.

In 2018, the China Agriculture Outlook Report 2016-2025 issued by the Ministry of Agriculture emphasized the need for China to focus on steady growth in its soybeans production. However, given the limited area available for cultivation and the large scale of demand from a growing population and fast-expanding livestock sector, it will be very challenging for China to achieve self-sufficiency in soybean production. Therefore, imported soybeans will continue to be in large demand as a supply channel in the future (Food Business Net, 2016). Together with this, the concerns about GM crops will also remain.

Figure 3. Soybeans export and import and the net import in China, 1980–2016
Source: National Bureau of Statistics of China (1997-2016)

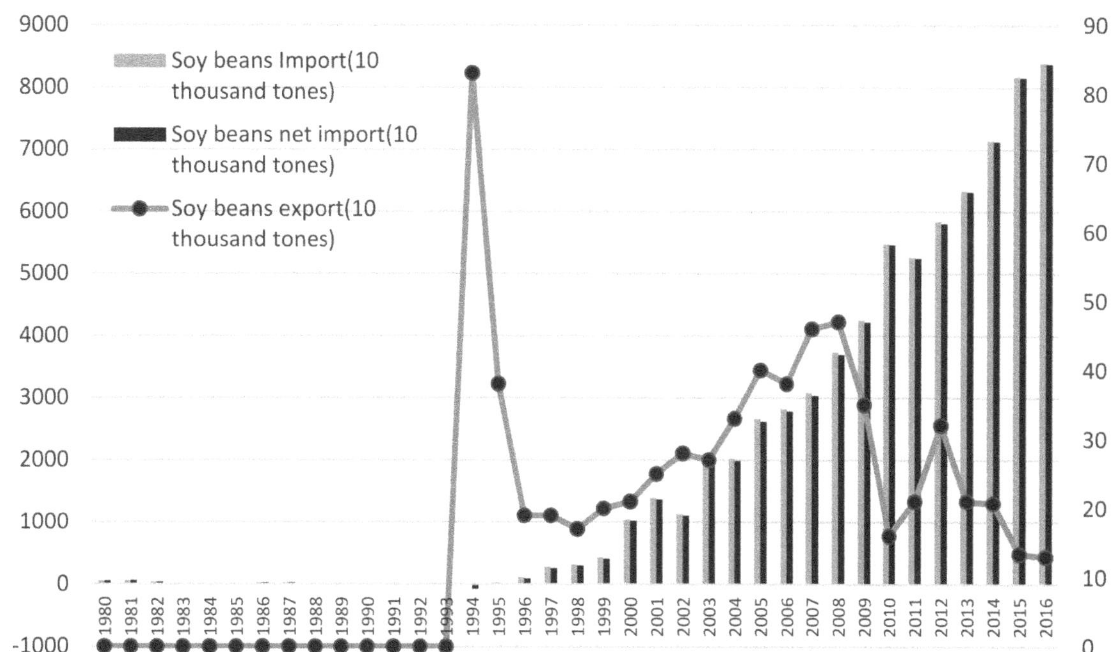

SOYBEANS CONSUMPTION IN CHINA

Until mid-20th century China was the largest soybean producer in the world (Jamet & Chaumet, 2016). Since then, China has become the world's largest consumer of soybeans and this consumption is continuously increasing. According to the National Agricultural Market Research Centre of the Agricultural University of China (2018), China's soybeans consumption grew over 4% in 2017. The Chinese customs data report even higher growth of more than 14% for both domestic supply and imports of soybeans (Wang, 2018). These recent changes are driven by growing domestic demand which is shifting not only in volumes but also in nature.

Overview

China has a long history of plantation and consumption of soybeans. The consumption volume was relatively stable before 1984 at around 800 tonnes from which 70% were consumed as human food products, 20% as pressed products, such as soy oil and animal meals, and the remaining 10% were used directly as animal feed, seeds and loss in the agricultural system. After 1985, the amount of pressed products, including animal meals, increased significantly between 28% and 45%, while the use for human food products decreased to 50%–60%. This trend continued in the 1990s and 2000s. At the moment, the pressed products, including animal meals, dominate China's domestic consumption at 83% while direct human food consumption is at 14% and direct animal feed at 2% (China Industrial Information Network, 2018). Seeds for re-planting represent only 0.8% of the soybean consumption and the loss in the system is low at 0.2%.

Soybeans for Animal Consumption

It is very important to unpack the pressed oil category as it combines products destined for industrial use and animal feed. In 2017, 80% of the pressed soybeans (or 66.4% of the total consumed soybeans) were used to manufacture animal soybean meals (China Industrial Information Network, 2018). Together with the 2% directly used as feed, this means that more than two-thirds of the soybeans consumed in China, namely 68.4%, are used to feed livestock animals (see Figure 4). China's pig, cattle and poultry livestock are fed mainly from soybean meals, which has intensified both, the demand and consumption of soybeans. This is not surprising given the high numbers of these animals raised for human consumption (see Figure 5).

Figure 4. Soybeans use in China [%], 2017
Source of data: China Industries Information Net (2018)

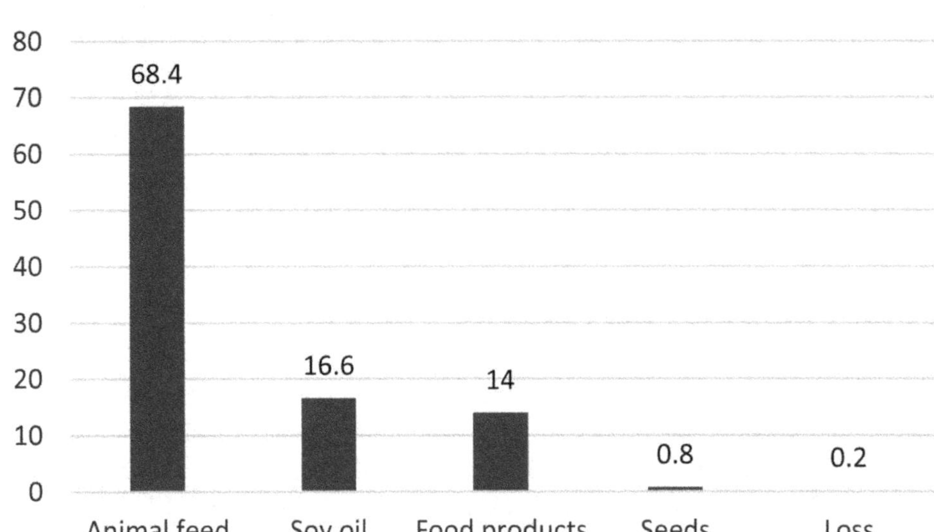

Soybeans for Human Consumption

Figure 6 presents the versatility of uses of the soybeans. Direct food products and soy oil represent less than a third (namely 30.6%) of the total soybean consumption despite the myriad of uses (see Figure 4). Of particular interest because of their nutritional value are the bean products (the middle column of Figure 6) for direct human intake which in 2017 were only 14% of the total soybean consumption in China. From the category of fat products, soybean oil can be used for cooking and is sold at a reasonable price.

The other soybean products have many specialised applications within and outside the food industry. For example, from the group of deeply processed soybeans products, soy lecithin which supports the development of the human nervous system is widely used in the confectionery food industry as well as for medicines, paper and in the leather industries.

Figure 5a. Cattle livestock counts (heads) in China, 1961–2014
Source: Ritchie & Roser (2018)

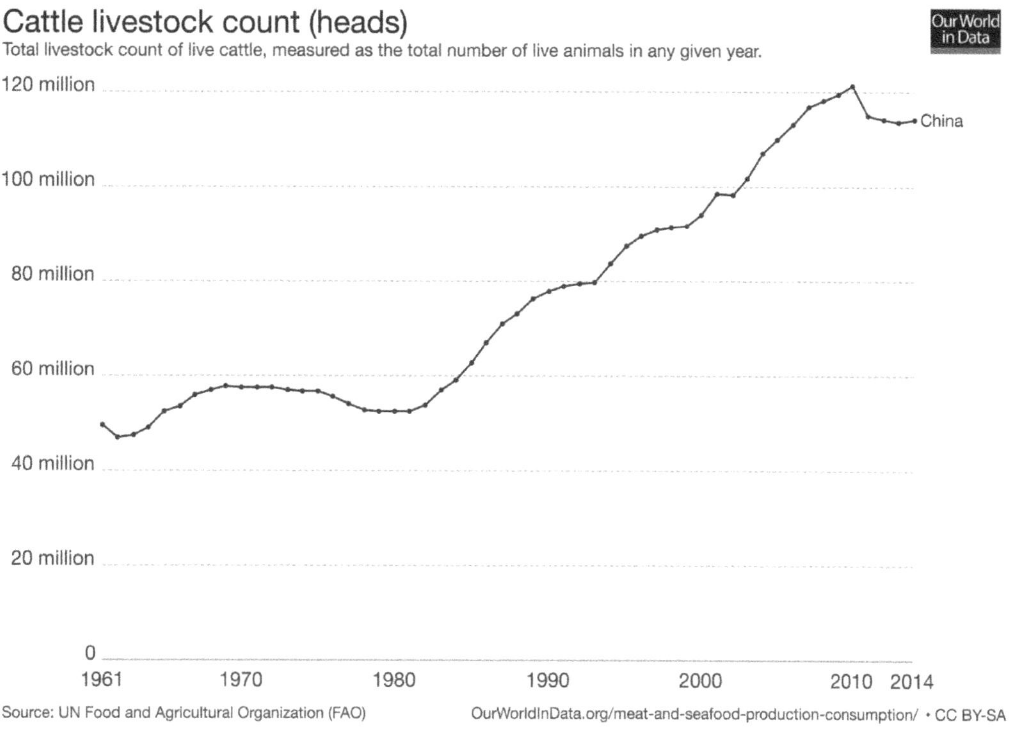

Figure 5b. Pig livestock counts (heads) in China, 1961–2014
Source: Ritchie & Roser (2018)

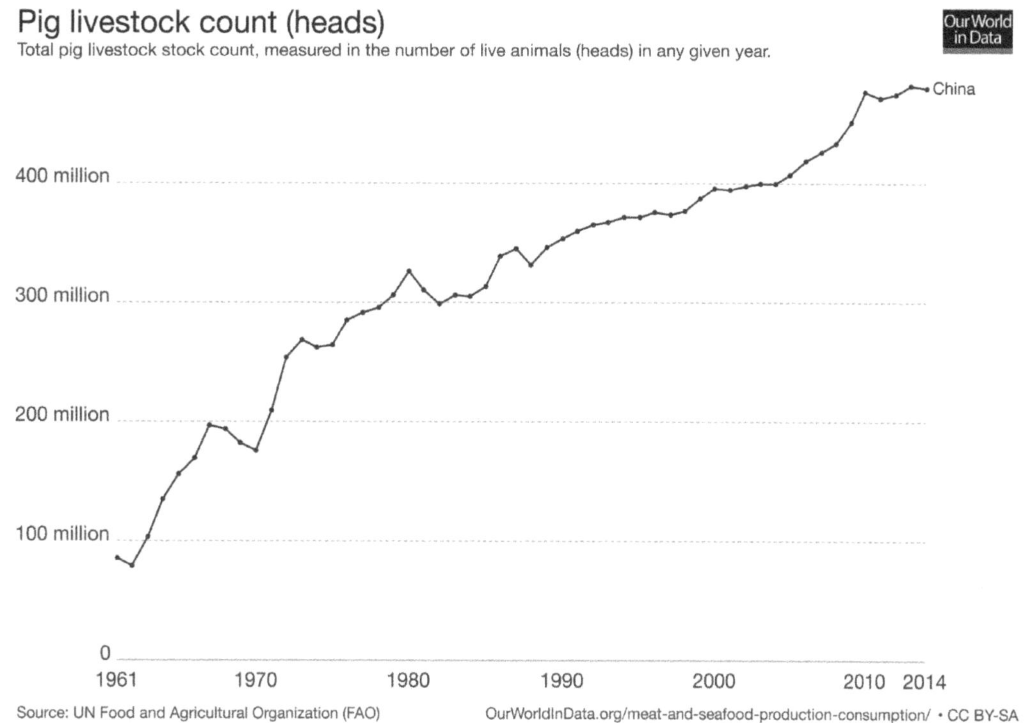

Figure 5c. Poultry livestock counts (heads) in China, 1961–2014
Source: Ritchie & Roser (2018)

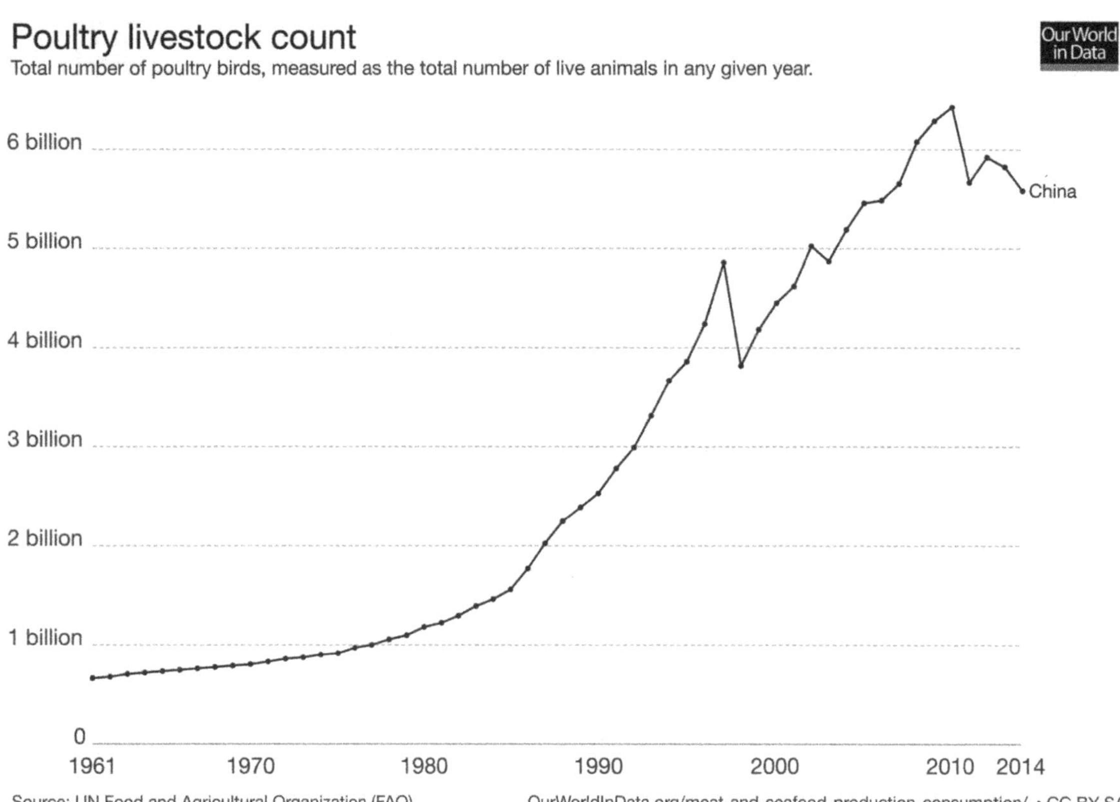

The soybean products include non-fermented varieties, such as tofu (including water tofu and dried tofu), yuba (referred also as tofu skin or bean curd sheet), soymilk and others, and fermented varieties, such as fermented bean curd, stinky tofu, bean paste, soy sauce etc. Other bean products cover bean sprouts, fried soy products, smoked soy products, frozen soy products, soy flour etc. The soy flour can be used to make a variety of foods, including baby foods. All bean products contain the nine essential amino acids and are complete high-content proteins which can replace meat and other animal-based products.

In the past, the bean products were widely used in traditional recipes and typical Chinese dishes; however, in more recent years with the country's fast economic growth leading to increasing household incomes, there has also been a dietary shift towards increasing demand and intake of animal products. The liberation of trade since the 1978 open door economic policy, allowed imports of soybeans which fuelled their use as animal feed. Previously, China did not have enough feed to support large livestock production, but the soybean imports allowed this sector to expand (Jamet & Chaumet, 2016). Increased supply of domestic meat – coupled also with meat imports, also as a result from trade liberalisation (Guo, Raphaely, & Marinova, 2016), resulted in a fast expansion of the place of animal proteins in the Chinese dietary preferences (see Figure 7). The humble soybean, the miracle crop, caused a dietary revolution that affects not only the Chinese population but also all populations on this planet.

Figure 6. Use of soybeans in China
Source: The Authors.

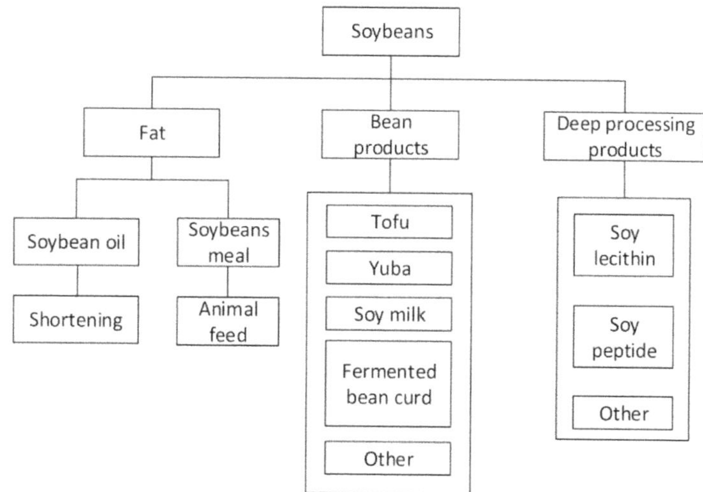

Figure 7. Per capita meat supply in China [kg], 1961–2013
Source: Ritchie & Roser (2018)

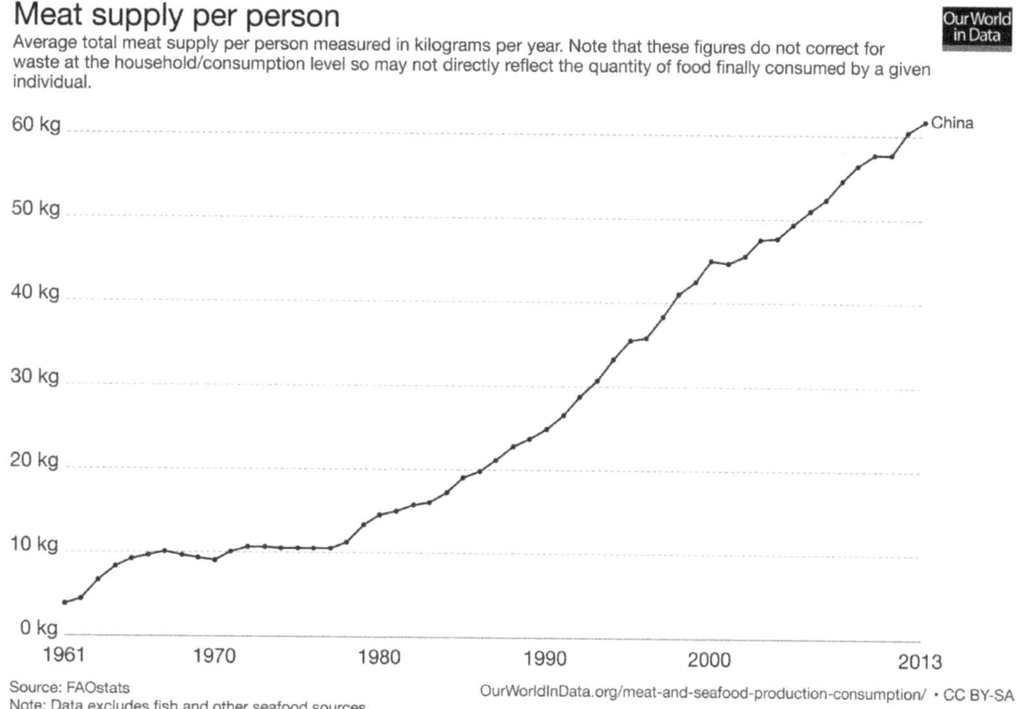

Dietary Changes

There is ample research evidence demonstrating the positive role of plant-based foods (e.g. Raphaely & Marinova, 2016; Craig, 2018), and particularly soybeans intake (Barret, 2006), in the human diet. Furthermore, there is convincing evidence about the negative impacts of excessive meat consumption on human health, including in the case of China (Campbell & Campbell, 2006). However, China has been on a dietary trend of increased meat consumption (see Figure 7) with the westernisation of diets spreading not just in urban centres but also to rural people (see Figure 8). Although the direct consumption of soybeans products has increased recently, this was accompanied with higher increases in the consumption of meat-based foods. This is fuelling the demand for soybeans, establishing a strong dependence on imports and with it, creating concerns about GM products.

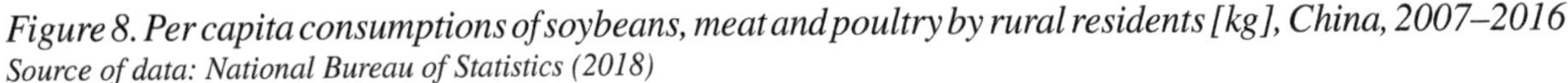

Figure 8. Per capita consumptions of soybeans, meat and poultry by rural residents [kg], China, 2007–2016
Source of data: National Bureau of Statistics (2018)

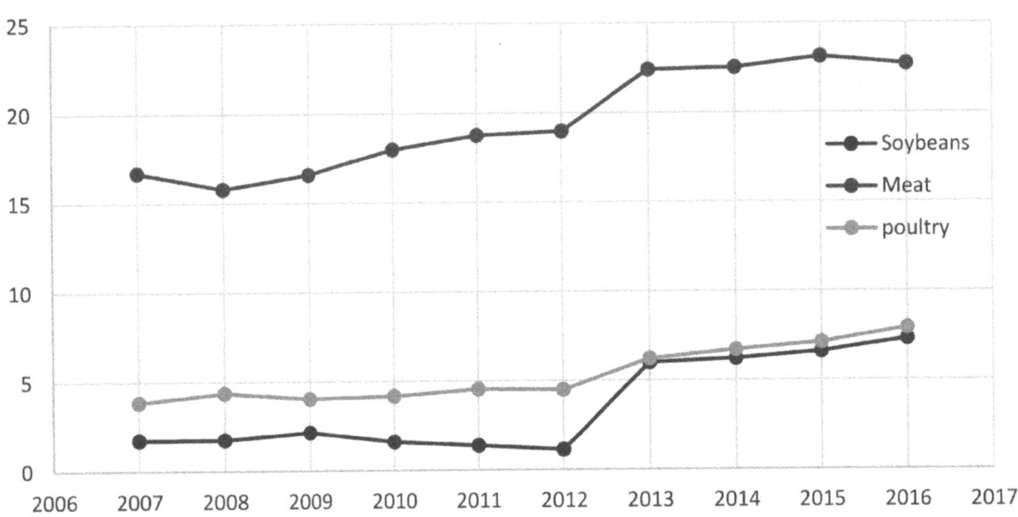

The response from the Chinese Government has been two-pronged. On the one hand, farmers are encouraged to grow more soybeans which should play the leading role in domestic food consumption (China Economy Net, 2018). The aim is to make sure that at least the domestic human consumption is self-sufficient. On the other hand, China's latest dietary guidelines are recommending significant cut in the current levels of meat consumption in line with other reputable international health bodies. They are calling for an intake of 40 g to 75 g of meat per day and overall halving of the country's current meat consumption (Froggatt & Wellesley, 2016). This will also reduce the environmental and climate change pressure caused by the country's large livestock sector – a move, strongly supported by the global community (Milman & Leavenworth, 2016).

With China having the largest meat consumption in the world, a replacement of animal-based proteins with soybeans will reduce greenhouse gas emissions, improve land use, reduce competition for water and contribute towards better health outcomes (Aleksandrowicz, Green, Joy, Smith, & Haines, 2016). Soybean products are essentially meat replacement alternatives with a much smaller environmental impact.

Halving meat consumption in China will also pave the way to restoring the traditional beauty of soy-based products as a healthy dietary choice. It will allow China to lead a global transformation along the lines of those initiated by international non-government organisations, such as Greenpeace (2018). This will further reduce the pressure on imports and the global demand for ever-increasing yields of soybeans. Even if GM soy is to be shown to be harmless in the long run, the opportunity to take a more precautionary approach in preserving and cultivating a diversity of local strains will be beneficial for biodiversity conservation.

POLICY IMPLICATIONS

There is always need for future research to find out people's reaction to the strong messages about reducing meat consumption in China. Dietary behavioural changes are easy as an avenue to pursue because they do not require large investment in technology. They are however very difficult to implement as they often go against the zones of comfort or habit that we all have. Smart strategies are required to shift people's perceptions and encourage them to implement personal changes with multiple individual and societal co-benefits. Below is a list of suggestions for policy interventions which can target more sustainable food consumption in China.

Promote Consumption of Local Soybean Products

With Chinese people being concerned about the imported genetically modified soybeans, particularly those from the US and Brazil, it is important to promote the consumption of local soybean products as healthy and tasty meat alternatives. Given that local soybeans are believed not to be genetically modified, this will reduce the anxiety about soybean foods. Indirectly it will also send the message that human health is a priority for the government while global scientists cooperate to solve the puzzle around GM foods.

Promote the Health Benefits of Soybeans Consumption

At this moment in time, the Western world is rediscovering the health benefits of soybeans and their nutritional values associated with high content of complete proteins and low cholesterol (The Dutch Soy Coalition, 2008). The Chinese doctors often recommend patients with obesity and high risk of type 2 diabetes, heart disease and high blood pressure, to eat tofu. Such recommendations should be given to everybody as a preventative measure.

Barriers of people to consume soybeans include unclear information, particularly the source of the soybeans beans (Wong & Chan, 2016), nutritional values and benefits. Possible interventions can include getting people familiar with soy-based products, such as soy milk. According to Ahenkora et al. (2012, p. 188), "acceptability is influenced by the degree of familiarity with soymilk and high satisfaction derived from exposure influenced consumer intention to purchase". There should also be ways to communicate the latest research results about the effects of soybeans consumptions on humans, for example, in reducing cancer incidents and mortality (Lu, Pan, Ye, Duan, Xu, Yin ... Zhang, 2017), improving metabolic diseases and cardiovascular health (Liu, Ho, Hao, Chen, Woo, Wong, ... Ling, 2016).

Subsidies to Soybean Farmers

China implemented an urgent campaign to increase soybeans output (Reuters, 2018b). The government encourages Chinese citizens to consume soybeans as food through implementing a structural reform on the agricultural supply side and accelerating soybeans planting (Soybeans Association of Heilongjiang Province, 2018). To maximize growers' economic profits, the government also provides subsidies to the soybeans planting farmers and it guarantees higher floor prices for the government purchasing of soybeans (Yoon, 2018). Through agricultural innovation and technology, the outputs can be improved and the quality of soybeans increased which is beneficial to the oil yield. For example, farmers in China's north-eastern provinces were offered higher subsidies for growing soybean than for corn directing their choice of crops (Reuters, 2018c).

Media Influence

The media can be used to encourage the consumption of soybeans products (AIC Technology, 2017) by providing educational materials and well-balanced perspectives on the qualities of soy products, including baby food. According to the medium and long-term planning outline for China's food and nutrition development 2011–2020, by 2020, China's per capita soybean consumption should reach 13 kg. The media can influence the uptake of soybean products by offering a platform for advertising quality and brand competition to provide excellent products, services and consumer experiences.

Social Marking

According to Firestone et al. (2017), social marketing is playing an important role in improving health on a global scale where the benefits are for the greater good. Bogueva et al. (2018) specifically examined social marketing opportunities for reduction in meat consumption. For example, Sun et al. (2007) described the success social marketing has already had in Guizhou, China for the use of iron-fortified soy sauce in enhancing women's knowledge, attitudes, perceptions about benefits and barriers, willingness to buy, and consumption.

Soybeans products and technology exhibitions are held frequently and are an ideal opportunity for social marketing. For example, the Eighth China International Exhibition of Soyfood Processing Technology and Equipment (2018) was held in Shanghai in 2018. During the event, there were many activities conducted, such as the annual soybeans enterprises conference, soybeans food festival, soybeans food tasting, local soybeans products exhibition and soybeans processing technology and innovation exhibits.

Investment in Research and Development

There is a need to provide more variety and new products on the market. Investment in research and development at a company level can deliver such innovative quality products in response to the needs of different customer groups. China's soybean food processing technology and equipment also need to adapt to the increasing consumer demands for soy products with good and strong technical support for the soybean food production enterprises.

CONCLUSION

Irrespective as to where one sits within the current debate surrounding GM soybeans and their impacts on the ecosystems of the planet, public health needs to be protected and environmental harm avoided (Maghari & Ardekani, 2011). An easier alternative to achieve this is to divert the inefficiently used feed calories into direct human nutrition. The current and increasing consumption of soybeans as animal feed can be circumvented by influencing human diets towards decreased intake of animal products and taking advantage of the numerous benefits plant-based diets have.

In 2017, China's domestic soybeans consumption was over 1.1 billion tonnes with 68.4% of this amount used as animal feed. This is an inefficient use of resources as well as a pathway which leads to economic dependence on imports. Encouraging people to consume directly more soy-based products, such as tofu, yuba and soy milk, is beneficial for their personal health, offers environmental co-benefits and allows to build a self-reliant domestic market for human consumption. Rather than succumb to the westernisation of the Chinese diet, China should focus its efforts on achieving the goal of halving the current levels of meat production. The miracle soy crop has a special place in this process.

REFERENCES

Ahenkora, K., Arthur, K., & Banahene, S. (2012). Marketing strategy for soybean products: Familiarity breeds content. *International Journal of Marketing Studies*, *4*(3), 186–189. doi:10.5539/ijms.v4n3p186

Aleksandrowicz, L., Green, R., Joy, E. J. M., Smith, P., & Haines, A. (2016). The impacts of dietary change on greenhouse gas emissions, land use, water use, and health: A systematic review. *PLoS One*, *11*(11), e0165797. doi:10.1371/journal.pone.0165797 PMID:27812156

Barret, J. R. (2006). The Science of soy: What do we really know? *Environmental Health Perspectives*, *114*(6), A352–A358. Retrieved from https://ehp.niehs.nih.gov/doi/pdf/10.1289/ehp.114-a352 PMID:16759972

Bawa, A. S., & Anilakumar, K. R. (2013). Genetically modified foods: Safety, risks and public concerns – a review. *Journal of Food Science and Technology*, *50*(6), 1035–1046. doi:10.100713197-012-0899-1 PMID:24426015

Bodnar, A. (2018). The scary truth behind fear of GMOs. *Biology Fortified*. Retrieved September 12, 2018 from https://www.biofortified.org/2018/02/scary-truth-gmo-fear/

Bogueva, D., Marinova, D., & Raphaely, T. (Eds.). (2018). *Handbook of research on social marketing and its influence on animal origin food product consumption*. Hershey, PA: IGI Global. doi:10.4018/978-1-5225-4757-0

Brookes, G., & Barfoot, P. (2017). Farm income and production impacts of using GM crop technology 1996–2015. *Biotechnology in Agriculture and the Food Chain*, *8*(3), 156–193. doi:10.1080/21645698.2017.1317919 PMID:28481684

Brown, L. R. (2011). *Full planet, empty plates: The new geopolitics of food scarcity. Earth Policy Institute*. New York, NY: W. W. Norton & Company.

Brügger, P., Marinova, D., & Raphaely, T. (2016). Animal production and consumption: an ethical educational approach. In T. Raphaely & D. Marinova (Eds.), *Impact of meat consumption on health and environmental sustainability* (pp. 295–312). Hershey, PA: IGI Global. doi:10.4018/978-1-4666-9553-5.ch017

Campbell, T. C., & Campbell, T. M. (2006). *The China Study: The most comprehensive study of nutrition ever conducted and the startling implications for diet, weight loss and long-term health*. Dallas, TX: Benbella Books.

Central People's Government of the People's Republic of China. (2018b). *Domestic soybeans should give full play to food consumption advantages.* Retrieved September 13, 2018 from http://www.gov.cn/zhengce/2018-05/21/content_5292362.htm

Central People's Government of the People's Republic of China. (2018b). *Figure: The report about China's agricultural forecast shows that China's soybeans planting areas will be restoratively increasing in 2018.* Retrieved September 13, 2018 from http://www.gov.cn/xinwen/2018-04/20/content_5284607.htm

China Economy Net. (2018) *Domestic soybeans should play a leading role in food consumption. This year's output may hit a new high in 10 years.* Retrieved September 13, 2018 from http://www.ce.cn/cysc/sp/info/201805/21/t20180521_29192313.shtml

China Industrial Information Network. (2018). *Analysis on China's soybeans' production and consumption in 2018 including export and import.* Retrieved September 13, 2018 from http://www.chyxx.com/industry/201805/638760.html

Craig. (Ed.). (2018). *Vegetarian nutrition and wellness*. Boca Raton, FL: CRC Press.

Eighth China International Exhibition of Soyfood Processing Technology and Equipment. (2018). *Exhibition network.* Soy Products Professional Association of the National Food Industry Association of China. Retrieved September 13, 2018 from http://www.onezh.com/web/index_54336.html

Eshel, G., Shepon, A., Makov, T., & Milo, R. (2014). Land, irrigation water, greenhouse gas, and reactive nitrogen burdens of meat, eggs, and dairy production in the United States. *Proceedings of the National Academy of Sciences of the United States of America, 111*(33), 11996–12001. doi:10.1073/pnas.1402183111 PMID:25049416

Firestone, R., Rowe, C. J., Modi, S. N., & Sievers, D. (2017). The effectiveness of social marketing in global health: A systematic review. *Health Policy and Planning, 32*(1), 110–124. doi:10.1093/heapol/czw088 PMID:27476502

Food and Agriculture Organization of the United Nations (FAO). (2016). *The state of food and agriculture: Climate change, agriculture and food security.* Rome, Italy: FAO. Retrieved September 13, 2018 from http://www.fao.org/3/a-i6030e.pdf

Food Business Net. (2016). *China's soybeans consumption reached to about 100 million tones, with 80% imported, what are they use for?* Retrieved September 13, 2018 from http://news.21food.cn/33/2772440.htmlhttp://news.21food.cn/33/2772440.html

Froggatt, A., & Wellesley, L. (2016). *China shows way with new diet guidelines on meat.* Chatham House. Retrieved September 13, 2018 from https://www.chathamhouse.org/expert/comment/china-shows-way-new-diet-guidelines-meat

Funk, C., & Rainie, L. (2016). *Public and scientists' views on science and society.* Pew Research Centre Internet & Technology. Retrieved September 13, 2018 from http://www.pewinternet.org/2015/01/29/public-and-scientists-views-on-science-and-society/

Greenpeace. (2018). *Less is more: Reducing meat and dairy for a healthier life and planet.* Scientific background of the Greenpeace vision of the meat and dairy system towards 2050. Retrieved from https://storage.googleapis.com/p4-production-content/international/wp-content/uploads/2018/03/6942c0e6-longer-scientific-background.pdf

Guo, X., Raphaely, T., & Marinova, D. (2016). China's growing meat demands, implications for sustainability. In T. Raphaely & D. Marinova (Eds.), *Impact of meat consumption on health and sustainability* (pp. 221–233). Hershey, PA: IGI Global. doi:10.4018/978-1-4666-9553-5.ch011

Jamet, J. P., & Chaumet, J. M. (2016). Soybean in China: Adapting to the liberalization. *OCL (Oilseeds & Fats, Crops and Lipids), 23*(6), D604. doi:10.1051/ocl/2016044

Liu, Z., Ho, S., Hao, Y., Chen, Y., Woo, J., Wong, S. Y., ... Ling, W. (2016). Randomised controlled trial of effect of whole soy replacement diet on features of metabolic syndrome in postmenopausal women: Study protocol. *BMJ Open, 6*(9), e012741. doi:10.1136/bmjopen-2016-012741 PMID:27678545

Lu, D., Pan, C., Ye, C., Duan, H., Xu, F., Yin, L., … Zhang, S. (2017). Meta-analysis of soy consumption and gastrointestinal cancer risk. *Nature Scientific Reports, 7*, 4048. Retrieved September 13, 2018 from https://www.nature.com/articles/s41598-017-03692-y

Ma, X. Q., Verkuil, J. M., Reinbach, H. C., & Meinert, L. (2017). Which product characteristics are preferred by Chinese consumers when choosing pork? A conjoint analysis on perceived quality of selected pork attributes. *Food Science & Nutrition, 5*(3), 770–775. doi:10.1002/fsn3.457 PMID:28572967

Maghari, B. M., & Ardekani, A. M. (2011). Genetically modified foods and social concerns. *Avicenna Journal of Medical Biotechnology, 3*(3), 109–117. PMID:23408723

Marsall, P., & Marinova, D. (2019). Health benefits of eating more plant foods and less meat. In D. Bogueva, D. Marinova, T. Raphaely, & K. Schmidinger (Eds.), Environmental, health and business opportunities in the new meat alternatives market. Hershey, PA: IGI Global.

Milman, O., & Leavenworth, S. (2016). China's plan to cut meat consumption by 50% cheered by climate campaigners: New dietary guidelines could reduce greenhouse gas emissions by 1bn tonnes by 2030, and could lessen country's problems with obesity and diabetes. *The Guardian.* Retrieved September 13, 2018 https://www.theguardian.com/world/2016/jun/20/chinas-meat-consumption-climate-change

Ministry of Agriculture and Rural Affairs of the People's Republic of China. (2016). *Ministry of Agriculture's guide on promotion of soybeans' production.* Retrieved September 13, 2018 from http://www.moa.gov.cn/govpublic/ZZYGLS/201604/t20160412_5091357.htm

Mosaic Company. (2018). *Crop nutrition: Nitrogen*. Retrieved September 12, 2018 from https://www.cropnutrition.com/efu-nitrogen

Nam, K. C., Jo, C., & Lee, M. (2010). Meat products and consumption culture in the East. *Meat Science*, *86*(1), 95–102. doi:10.1016/j.meatsci.2010.04.026 PMID:20510536

National Agricultural Market Research Centre of the Agricultural University of China. (2018). *China's soybeans consumption grew over 4%*. Retrieved September 13, 2018 from http://finance.sina.com.cn/money/future/agri/2018-02-02/doc-ifyremfz3770325.shtml

National Bureau of Statistics. (2018). *Rural residents' per capita consumptions of soybeans, meat and poultry*. Retrieved September 13, 2018 from http://www.stats.gov.cn

National Bureau of Statistics of China. (1997–2016). *China statistical yearbook*. Retrieved September 13, 2018 from http://www.stats.gov.cn/english/statisticaldata/annualdata/

North Carolina (NC) Soybean Producers Association. (2014). *History of soybean*. Retrieved September 12, 2018 from http://ncsoy.org/media-resources/history-of-soybeans/

Raphaely, T., & Marinova, D. (Eds.). (2016). *Impact of meat consumption on health and environmental sustainability*. Hershey, PA: IGI Global. doi:10.4018/978-1-4666-9553-5

Reuters. (2018a). *Brazil boasts world's second largest genetically modified crop area: ISAAA. Environment*. Retrieved September 13, 2018 from https://www.reuters.com/article/us-brazil-gmo/brazil-boasts-worlds-second-largest-genetically-modified-crop-area-isaaa-idUSKBN1JN1KW

Reuters. (2018b). *CORRECTED-China launches "emergency" campaign to boost soy output*. Retrieved September 13, 2018 from https://www.reuters.com/article/china-soybeans/china-launches-emergency-campaign-to-boost-soy-output-idUSL3N1SA32I

Reuters. (2018c). *China grants more subsidies to soy farmers as it cuts corn stocks*. Retrieved September 13, 2018 from https://www.reuters.com/article/us-china-agriculture-subsidies/china-grants-more-subsidies-to-soy-farmers-as-it-cuts-corn-stocks-idUSKCN1HA176

Ritchie, H., & Roser, M. (2018). *Meat and seafood production & consumption*. Our World in Data. Retrieved September 12, 2018 from https://ourworldindata.org/meat-and-seafood-production-consumption

Satheesh, P. V. (2012). Genetically engineered promises & farming realities. In D. Bollier & S. Helfrich (Eds.), *The wealth of the commons: A world beyond market and state* (pp. 141–146). Amherst, MA: The Common Strategies Group.

Schmidinger, K., Bogueva, D., & Marinova, D. (2018). New meat without livestock. In D. Bogueva, D. Marinova, & T. Raphaely (Eds.), *Handbook of research on social marketing and its influence on animal origin food product consumption* (pp. 344–361). Hershey, PA: IGI Global. doi:10.4018/978-1-5225-4757-0.ch023

Sheldon, I. (2018). Why China's soybean tariffs matter. *The Conversation*. Retrieved September 13, 2018 from http://theconversation.com/why-chinas-soybean-tariffs-matter-94476

Soybeans Association of Heilongjiang Province. (2018). Document No. 1 of the Central Committee in 2017: Several suggestions on deepening the structural reform of the supply side of agriculture and accelerating the cultivation of new momentum of agricultural and rural development. *Economy Daily*. Retrieved September 13, 2018 from http://www.chinasoy.com.cn/Page_Views/AllView.aspx?ID=2716 &cateorgy=%e7%89%b9%e5%88%ab%e5%85%b3%e6%b3%a8

Sun, X., Guo, Y., Wang, S., & Sun, J. (2007). Social marketing improved the consumption of iron-fortified soy sauce among women in China. *Journal of Nutrition Education and Behavior, 39*(6), 302–310. doi:10.1016/j.jneb.2007.03.090 PMID:17996625

Technology, A. I. C. (2017). *How to create a powerful social media strategy for food products*. Retrieved September 13, 2018 from https://aictechnologies.com.au/2017/05/23/selling-food-products-social-media/

The Dutch Soy Coalition. (2006). *Soy: Big business, big responsibility. Addressing the social- and environmental impact of the soy value chain*. Retrieved September 13, 2018 from http://www.bothends. org/uploaded_files/document/2006_Soy_big_business.pdf

The Statistics Portal. (2018). *Import volume of soybeans worldwide from 2013/14 to 2017/18, by country (in million metric tons)*. Statista. Retrieved September 13, 2018 from https://www.statista.com/statistics/612422/soybeans-import-volume-worldwide-by-country/

U.S. Soybean Export Council. (2006). *U.S. Soy: International Buyers' Guide*. Retrieved September 12, 2018 from https://ussec.org/wp-content/uploads/2015/10/buyers-guide.pdf

Wang, O. (2018). *China orders farmers to grow more soybeans despite deal to buy more produce from US: Officials have ordered farmers to grow more soybeans even though Donald Trump has claimed China will buy 'as much as our farmers can produce'*. US–China Trade Wars. South China Morning Post. Retrieved September 13, 2018 from https://www.scmp.com/news/china/economy/article/2147296/china-orders-farmers-grow-more-soybeans-despite-deal-buy-more

Wong, A. Y., & Chan, A. W. (2016). Genetically modified foods in China and the United States: A primer of regulation and intellectual property protection. *Food Science and Human Wellness, 5*(3), 124–140. doi:10.1016/j.fshw.2016.03.002

Xinhua. (2018). China soybean production forecast to recover. *China Daily*. Retrieved September 13, 2018 from http://www.chinadaily.com.cn/a/201804/23/WS5add59d9a3105cdcf6519e50.html

Yoon, E. (2018). *How China is working hard to be less reliant on US farmers*. Retrieved September 13, 2018 from https://www.cnbc.com/2018/05/11/china-looking-to-rely-less-on-us-for-soybeans.html

Zahran, H. H. (1999). *Rhizobium*-legume symbiosis and nitrogen fixation under severe conditions and in an arid climate. *Microbiology and Molecular Biology Reviews, 63*(4), 968–989. PMID:10585971

ADDITIONAL READING

Aleksandrowicz, L., Green, R., Joy, E. J. M., Smith, P., & Haines, A. (2016). The impacts of dietary change on greenhouse gas emissions, land use, water use, and health: A systematic review. *PLoS One*, *11*(11), e0165797. doi:10.1371/journal.pone.0165797 PMID:27812156

Bawa, A. S., & Anilakumar, K. R. (2013). Genetically modified foods: Safety, risks and public concerns – a review. *Journal of Food Science and Technology*, *50*(6), 1035–1046. doi:10.100713197-012-0899-1 PMID:24426015

Funk, C., & Rainie, L. (2016). *Public and scientists' views on science and society.* Pew Research Centre Internet & Technology. Retrieved September 13, 2018 from http://www.pewinternet.org/2015/01/29/public-and-scientists-views-on-science-and-society/

Greenpeace (2018). *Less is more: Reducing meat and dairy for a healthier life and planet.* Scientific background of the Greenpeace vision of the meat and dairy system towards 2050. Retrieved from https://storage.googleapis.com/p4-production-content/international/wp-content/uploads/2018/03/6942c0e6-longer-scientific-background.pdf

Jamet, J. P., & Chaumet, J. M. (2016). Soybean in China: Adapting to the liberalization, *OCL (Oilseeds & Fats, Crops and Lipids), 23*(6), D604. doi:10.1051/ocl/2016044

Maghari, B. M., & Ardekani, A. M. (2011). Genetically modified foods and social concerns. *Avicenna Journal of Medical Biotechnology, 3*(3), 109–117. PMID:23408723

Ritchie, H., & Roser, M. (2018). *Meat and seafood production & consumption.* Our World in Data. Retrieved September 12, 2018 from https://ourworldindata.org/meat-and-seafood-production-consumption

Schmidinger, K., Bogueva, D., & Marinova, D. (2018). New meat without livestock. In D. Bogueva, D. Marinova, & T. Raphaely (Eds.), *Handbook of research on social marketing and its influence on animal origin food product consumption* (pp. 344–361). Hershey, PA: IGI Global. doi:10.4018/978-1-5225-4757-0.ch023

Sheldon, I. (2018). *Why China's soybean tariffs matter.* The Conversation. Retrieved September 13, 2018 from http://theconversation.com/why-chinas-soybean-tariffs-matter-94476

Zahran, H. H. (1999). *Rhizobium*-legume symbiosis and nitrogen fixation under severe conditions and in an arid climate. *Microbiology and Molecular Biology Reviews, 63*(4), 968–989. PMID:10585971

KEY TERMS AND DEFINITIONS

Fermented: A food which has been through the process of fermentation, that is, chemical breakdown of its substance by bacteria, yeast, or other microorganisms.

Genetically Modified (GM): (Also genetically engineered). Applied to food crops and organisms whose genetic material, namely deoxyribonucleic acid (DNA) has been altered in a way that does not occur in nature.

Import: Goods or commodities brought into a country across its borders.

Protein: An organic substance – polymer chains of amino acids, considered an essential nutrient for the human body; there are 20 types of amino acids representing the building blocks for the human proteins – 11 are non-essential which can be synthesized by the human organism and 9 are essential which need to be provided by food.

Social Marketing: Marketing which aims at inducing a behavioral change and maintaining such behavior for the greater social good, including benefits for the individual and society as a whole.

Soy: (Also soybean and soya). A legume plant native to East Asia with a high content of complete protein and beneficial nutritional value.

Soybean Meal: A product prepared from soybeans to be used in animal feed as a source of protein; very often soybean meal is made from the residue after the oil from the soybean has been extracted.

Trade Liberalization: Removal of barriers or other restrictions to the free movement of goods and commodities between countries.

Tofu: Soy bean curd often used as a meat alternative; it is very popular in Asian countries, such as China and Japan, and more recently has started to also be included in a western type of diet.

Yuba: (Also tofu skin, bean curd skin, bean curd sheet or bean curd robe). A food product made from soybeans during the boiling of soy milk; the thin skin formed at the top of the boiling pan is collected and dried in sheets which can be used as wraps.

This research was previously published in Environmental, Health, and Business Opportunities in the New Meat Alternatives Market edited by Diana Bogueva, Dora Marinova, Talia Raphaely, and Kurt Schmidinger; pages 124-142, copyright year 2019 by Business Science Reference (an imprint of IGI Global).

Chapter 65
The Potential of Traditional Leafy Vegetables for Improving Food Security in Africa

Praxedis Dube
Wageningen University, The Netherlands

Wim J. M. Heijman
Wageningen University, The Netherlands

Rico Ihle
Wageningen University, The Netherlands

Justus Ochieng
World Vegetable Center, Eastern and Southern Africa, Tanzania

ABSTRACT

Feeding the quickly growing population in Africa remains a global challenge. As the demand for food increases, climate change, on the other hand, poses more challenges to agricultural productivity, implying that the provision of sufficient quantities and qualities of food is threatened. Traditional leafy vegetables (TLVs) in Africa are resilient to adverse weather conditions and are naturally rich in nutrients including vitamins A & C, iron, protein and other micronutrients. The objective of this chapter is to assess the potential of TLVs improving food security in Africa. TLVs represent a robust local source of food, their consumption is crucial in complementing Africa's diet with micronutrients. TLVs have therefore the potential to play a major role in improving food security and facilitating food sovereignty. Research on seeds, developing seed systems, coupled by preparing and processing methods to TLV products like cakes or flour is needed to increase their consumption, particularly among the young, elite and urban dwellers.

DOI: 10.4018/978-1-7998-5354-1.ch065

INTRODUCTION

Feeding the quickly growing population in Africa remains a worldwide challenge. Globally, close to a billion people are hunger stricken (Food and Agriculture Organization of the United Nations [FAO], 2015) and approximately one-third of them live in Africa (Sasson, 2012). As the demand for food increases, climate change, on the other hand, poses challenges to domestic food production in Africa, implying that the provision of sufficient quantities of food of the necessary quality is threatened. A lack of sufficient quantities of sufficiently diversified food compromises human health, resulting in an increase in the risk of contracting diseases related to malnutrition, which affect one in every four people (FAO, 2015). Figure 1 illustrates the prevalence of hunger and the distribution of the undernourished population across Africa. The map reveals substantial differences between African regions. Sub-Saharan Africa is the most severely affected by the prevalence of hunger and undernourishment.

Figure 1. Hunger and undernourishment persistence in Africa in 2015
Source: FAO, 2015

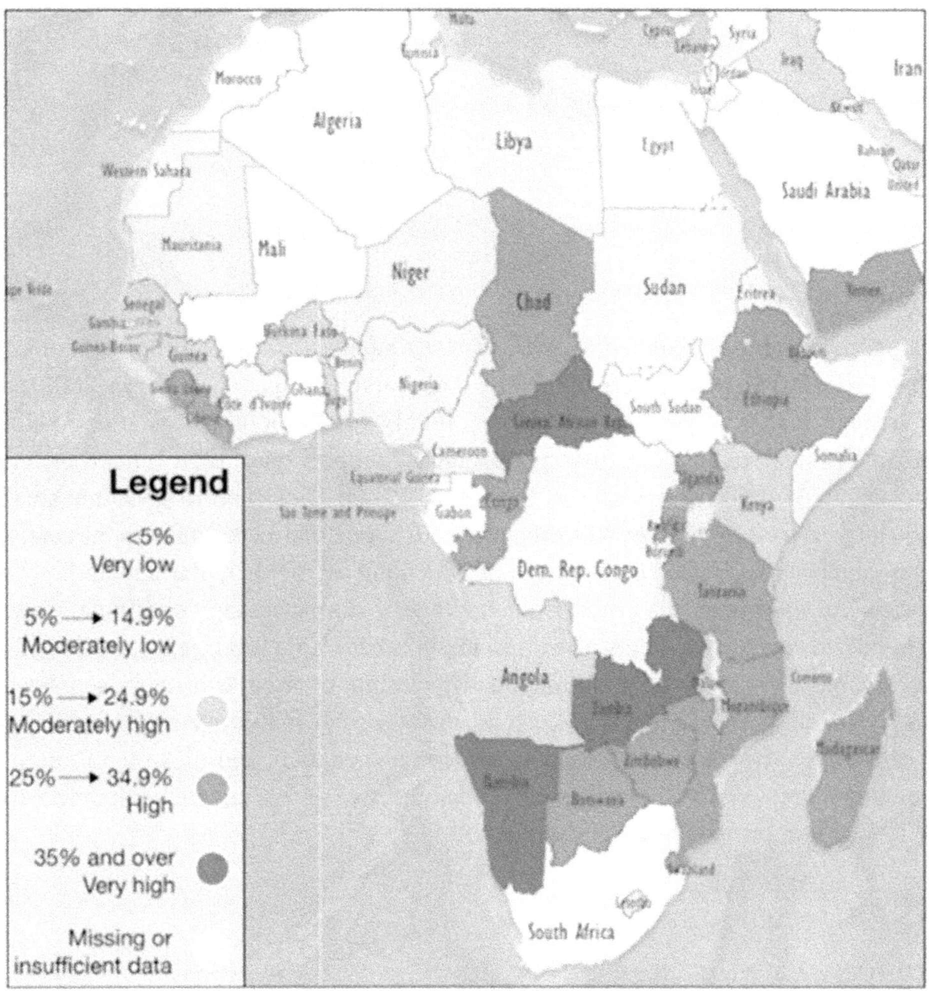

In contrast, Northern Africa accounts for 1% of the undernourished population, as depicted in Figure 2.

Figure 2. Prevalence percentage of undernourishment in Africa in 2014-2016
Source: Authors based on FAO, 2015

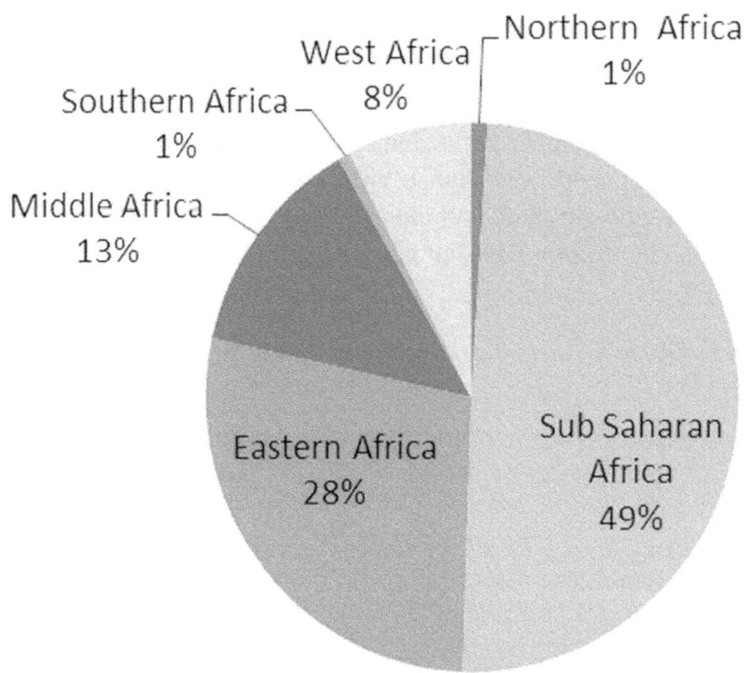

The differences in undernourishment in Africa are attributed to price volatility, an exploding population, droughts (FAO, 2015), poor governance (Ihle, von Cramon-Taubadel, & Zorya, 2009) and political instability (Veninga & Ihle, in press). For instance, highly volatile food prices affect mainly the poor people in urban and rural areas, since they spend a higher proportion of their limited incomes on their food needs (Luckmann, Ihle, Kleinwechter, & Grethe, 2014). They tend to consume smaller quantities less frequently as well as cheaper and less nutritious foods that lack vitamins, minerals, and other essential micronutrients, e.g. zinc or iron, both of which are required by the human body for healthy growth. This leads to widespread undernourishment. Vegetables, particularly traditional leafy vegetables (TLVs) might provide dietary elements often missing in other staple foods, e.g. cereals and root foods, which are affordable also for the poor population. They might be used as primary sources of minerals because they are naturally rich in nutrients such as iron and other micronutrients that are important for a human's well-being. They have also the potential to balance diets and make them more healthy as they also include vitamins A and C, and proteins. The objective of this chapter is therefore to assess the potential of TLVs for improving food security in Africa.

BACKGROUND

The Current Status of Agriculture in Africa

Agriculture contributes significantly to Africa's economy. It is responsible for a relatively large share of the economy in terms of labor force. It accounts for 70% of jobs, contributes 33% of the gross domestic product, and generates 40% of the total export earnings in Africa (Otsuka, Larson, & Hazell, 2013). Africa faces the challenge of low food productivity due to a number of factors, including poor uptake of modern technologies, and high incidences of poverty culminating in the prevalence of an undernourished population among others. At the United Nations Sustainable Development Summit on September 25, 2015, world leaders adopted the Sustainable Development Goals (SDGs) to end poverty, fight inequality and injustice, and tackle climate change by 2030 (United Nations Development Programme [UNDP], 2016).

The modern technologies have resulted in the replacement of TLVs with the conventional vegetable varieties such as rape, cabbages etc. However, these exotic vegetables usually grow in high-altitude areas with a cool climate and require modernized technologies, like irrigation which is far beyond the reach of many smallholder farmers in Africa. In the humid lowland areas of West Africa, the arid areas of Namibia and Botswana, in the blistering heart of Kalahari, in hot dry regions in other parts of the continent, the exotic vegetables cannot grow well, but TLVs can grow (Schippers, 2000) allowing for the effective use of non-productive areas.

Traditional Leafy Vegetables in Africa

TLVs are plants which originate from the African continent and have a century-long history of cultivation and domestication subject to regional agro-climatic conditions (Ambrose-Oji, 2009). They are often more resilient to adverse weather conditions and withstand better unpredictable weather changes than varieties of staple crops and vegetables bred in industrialized countries, fitting very well to bioregional foods.

TLVs are naturally important to many people in Africa due to their inherent nutrient content and a vast range of phytochemicals (Yang & Keding, 2009). Generally, TLVs are more nutritious than commonly known exotic vegetables. Commonly consumed vegetables across Africa include Amaranth (*Amaranthus spp.*), Okra (*Abelmoschus esculentus*), Spider flower (*Cleome gynandra*), Pumpkin leaves (*Cucurbita spp.*), Cowpea leaves (*Vigna unguiculata*), Black jack (*Bidens pilosa*), Sweet potato leaves (*Ipomoea batatas*), Nightshade (*Solanum spp.*), Moringa (*Moringa oleifira*), African eggplant (*Solanum spp.*), Baobab leaves (*Adonsonia digitata*), Jute (*Corchorus olitorius*), and Cassava leaves (*Manihot esculentum*).

Table 1 shows laboratory results on the nutritional contents of TLVs found by the World Vegetable Center, TLVs have substantial amounts of micronutrients, vitamins, and minerals which are essential for a balanced and healthy diet. These vegetables often have higher amounts of nutrients than vegetables which are traditionally grown on other continents such as tomatoes and cabbage. For example, Moringa provides the highest quantity of micronutrients among the most used TLVs. TLVs are generally rich in vitamins A, C and E, zinc, calcium, iron, and antioxidants (Yang & Keding, 2009). In comparison, TLVs have higher nutrient amounts than other vegetables such as tomatoes and cabbages, Table 1.

Some TLVs can be produced or collected from forests or fallow lands. In Eastern and Western Africa, TLVs production is commercial in both urban and peri-urban areas (Weinberger & Pichop, 2009). Most farmers producing TLVs sell about 50% of the produce through different market channels, and the remainder is consumed within households. Table 2 shows that the total volume of TLVs produced by

Table 1. Micronutrient content of common TLVs

Micronutrient	Range	Vegetable type				
		Tomato	Cabbage	Moringa	Amaranth	Sweet potato leaf
β- Carotene, mg	0.0 – 22	0.40	0.00	15.28	9.23	6.82
Vit C, mg	1.1 – 353	19	22	459	113	81
Vit E, mg	0.0 – 71	1.16	0.05	25.25	3.44	4.69
Iron, mg	0.2 – 26	0.54	0.30	10.09	5.54	1.88
Folates, mg	2.8 – 175	5	ND	93	78	39
Antioxidant activity, TE	0.6 – 82,000	323	496	2,858	394	870

Note: ND = Not Done
Source: Ojiewo, Tenkouano, Oluoch, & Yang, 2010

seven countries was 9,300 tons/year (Weinberger & Pichop, 2009). The quantity is relatively small given that it is produced by seven countries. The total volume was largest in Eastern Africa, followed by Western Africa. The production of TLVs in these three parts of Africa is driven by generating extra income and home consumption, among others (Weinberger & Pichop, 2009). Given their nutritional potential, promotion campaigns such as road and cook shows, nutritional awareness and educational programs in hospitals, schools and markets have been used, for example in Tanzania to increase consumption of traditional vegetables by rural and urban consumers (Ochieng et al., 2016).

Table 2. Total TLVs production by African regions in 2016

Region (countries)	Total volume (tons)
Eastern Africa (Kenya, Tanzania, and Uganda)	6,900
Western Africa (Senegal, Benin, and Côte d'Ivoire)	2,400
Southern Africa (South Africa)	27
Total volume	9,327

Source: Authors based on IndigenoVeg survey data (Weinberger & Pichop, 2009)

The quantities consumed per day vary across the African regions. For instance, in Southern Africa, 29–41 kg/year are consumed by South Africans/households depending on the location (rural or urban dwellers, with the latter consuming less) (Yang & Keding, 2009). A study of the TLVs consumption in seven countries of Africa showed that Tanzania consumed largest quantities of TLVs/capita/day, while Senegal consumed the least, as shown in Figure 3. On average, Eastern African countries consumed larger quantities, indicating the importance of nutrition awareness.

Over the last two decades in the context of the realization of the limitations of the Green Revolution, the national food programs and strategies, and the effects of climate change, researchers realized a need for a paradigm shift to look at underutilized plants such as TLVs. These neglected species have begun to attract considerable interest due to their multiple underexploited benefits in terms of nutritional value,

Figure 3. TLVs per capita per day (grams) by country
Source: Authors based on IndigenoVeg consortium data (Weinberger & Pichop, 2009)

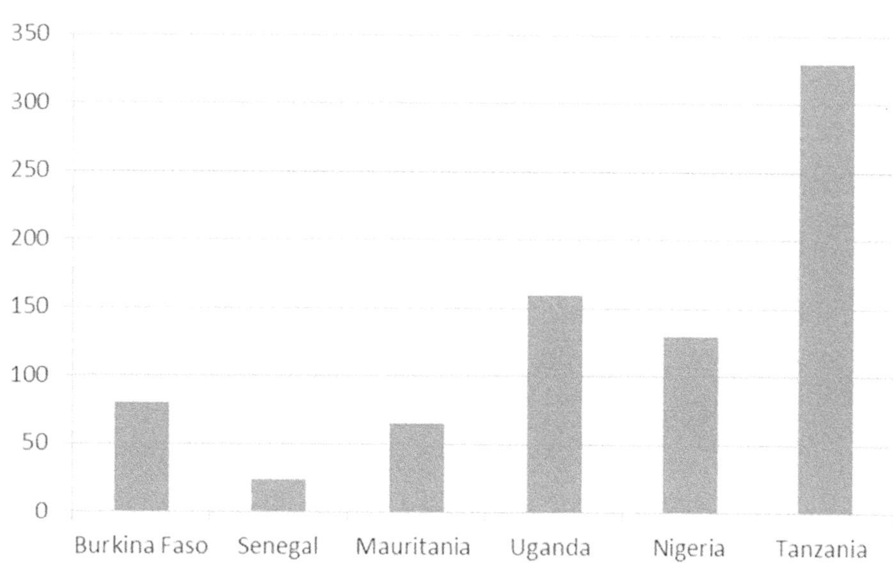

food security, income generation, medicinal value, and suitability for low input systems and for marginal environments (Shackleton, Pasquini, & Drescher, 2009). The interest in the underutilized species for research and development came during the late 1980s. For example, there was the establishment of the International Centre for Underutilised Crops in 1988, the Plant Resources of Tropical Africa in 2000, the Global Facilitation Unit of Underutilised Species in 2002, Consultative Group on International Agricultural Research in 2005 and the inclusion of indigenous vegetables for biodiversity, healthy diet and marketing opportunities as one of the World Vegetables Centre's strategic programme directions in 2002 (Shackleton et al., 2009). All these strategies aimed at increasing the use of the underutilized crop species such as TLVs to retard biodiversity losses, increase community-driven rural development, exploit the nutritional value, food security, income generation, and medicinal value and make marginal lands more productive.

Recent milestones in TLVs production and consumption include a significant growth of interest in re-activating traditional food and a reversal of an earlier decline in farming of indigenous crops that this food is based upon. Scientists in Africa and elsewhere have been engaged in research to develop TLVs in order to tap into their health benefits (Cernansky, 2015). These researches have created new opportunities for TLVs in many countries. A study on TLVs production has shown that Kenyan farmers have increased the TLVs production area by 25% between 2011 and 2013 (Cernansky, 2015). Also, the number of bunches sold in Kenya have been increasing rapidly, estimated at 164%, as depicted in Figure 4. The TLVs have gained a commercial status in large cities like Nairobi (Irungu, Mburu, Maundu, Grum, & Hoeschle-Zeledon, 2011). Some TLVs, e.g. African nightshade, have gained 32% in the total Nairobi vegetable markets share (Irungu et al., 2011) and 11% in Tanzania. The World Vegetable Center is currently budgeting annually around $20 million on TLVs research (Cernansky, 2015).

Figure 4. Supply trends of TLVs in Nairobi markets
Source: Authors based on Irungu et al., 2011

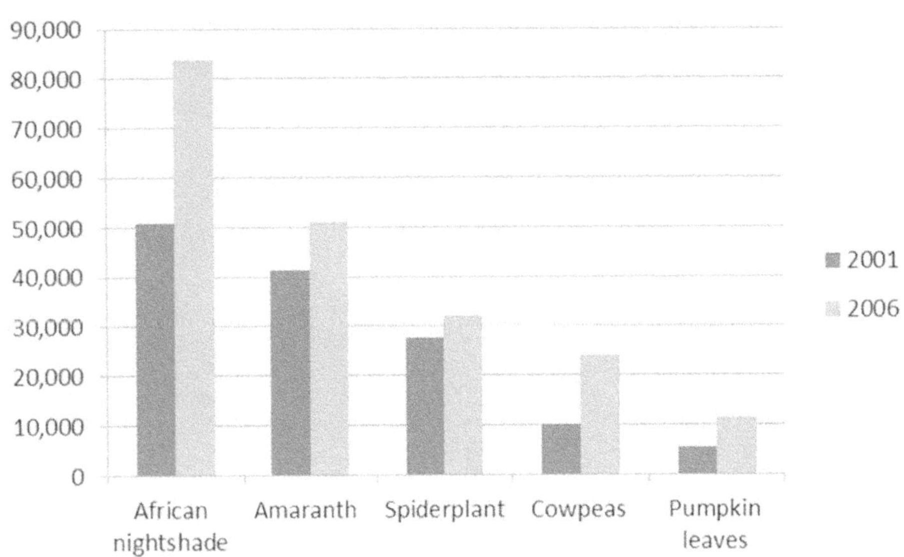

MAIN FOCUS OF THE CHAPTER

Current Status of Traditional Leafy Vegetables in Africa

TLVs play significant roles in the livelihoods of people along the supply chain in Africa. They contribute approximately 13%, 35%, and 30% of the smallholders' income in Tanzania, Malawi, and Mozambique, respectively (Chagomoka, Afari-Sefa, & Pitoro, 2014; Weinberger & Msuya, 2004), 29% to 76% in Uganda, Côte d'Ivoire, Kenya, Tanzania, Senegal, South Africa, and Benin (Weinberger & Pichop, 2009). Figure 5 depicts the share TLVs farmer receive of the consumer selling price. The data shows substantial differences between African countries. Higher shares are realized in South Africa and Benin. The differences in shares can be partially explained by prices. For example, a farmer in South Africa realizes better shares due to the price difference per kilogram of cowpea leaves selling at $3.20 for South Africa compared to $0.22 for Tanzania (Weinberger & Pichop, 2009).

A market study conducted in seven countries within Africa in 2009 shows the total volume and total turnover for the three most important TLVs traded at retail levels, as depicted in Figure 6. This study established that TLVs are relatively high-value crops generating a total turnover of $5.5 million (Weinberger & Pichop, 2009). Assuming the same turnover being produced by 53 African countries, calculated, would yield approximately $50 million generated by TLV supply chain markets.

Kenya shows the highest volume traded for the three most important TLVs, almost thrice the volume traded in Senegal yet with the total turnover lower than that of Senegal. South Africa exhibits the least total volume traded, but its total turnover is higher than that of Côte d'Ivoire. For the rest of the countries included in this data, only Senegal and South Africa have a total turnover higher than the total volume traded. These differences can be partially explained by the difference in selling prices ($/kg) at retailers between these countries. For example, cowpea leaves selling per kilogram at $3.64 and $3.20 in Senegal and South Africa, respectively, compared to $0.30, $0.45, $0.30, $0.22 for Benin, Kenya, Uganda, and Tanzania, respectively (Weinberger & Pichop, 2009).

For TLVs, the trader and retailer share contribution at consumer selling point is the lowest in Benin at 24% and in South Africa at 30%. It is the highest in Uganda (71%), Côte d'Ivoire (62%), and Tanzania (around 55%) (Weinberger & Pichop, 2009). These differences can be partly explained by the share that is allocated to the farmers, e.g. the share received by farmers is relatively higher in Benin and South Africa, as shown in Figure 5.

Figure 5. TLVs farmers' percentage share in consumer selling price
Source: Authors based on Weinberger & Msuya, 2004; Weinberger & Pichop, 2009; Chagomoka et al., 2014

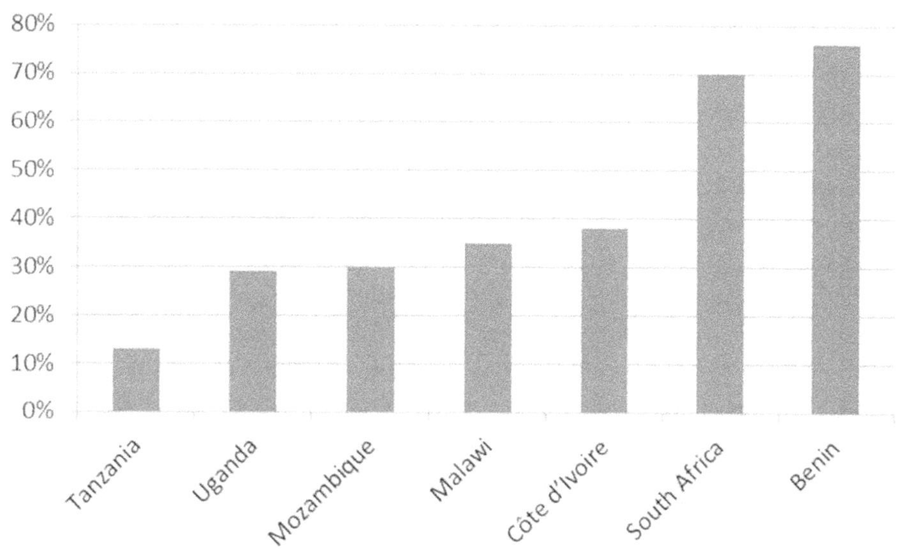

Figure 6. Total volume and total turnover for TLVs traded at retail/ country
Source: Authors based on IndigenoVeg survey data (Weinberger & Pichop, 2009)

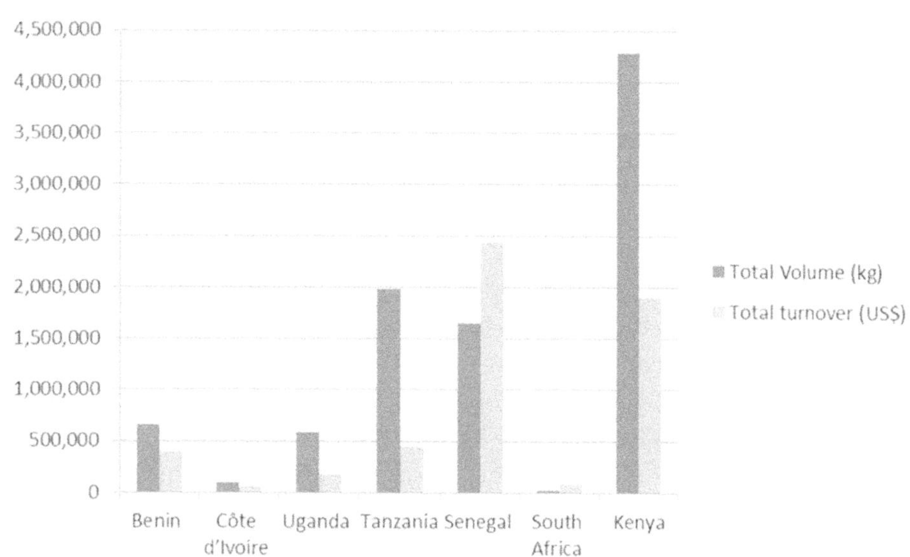

Supply Chains of Traditional Leafy Vegetables

The authors assessed the role of TLVs in small-scale farmers' diets and incomes, the survey was conducted in five provinces of Zimbabwe (Mashonaland East, West and Central, Harare, Manicaland). The respondents were chosen using the snowball technique, starting with the seed production and supply segment upstream to traders, gathering data from five key informants within each segment. The authors developed question guides to help consistent data collection and interview technique at each segment. The information collected included crop management, marketing of the produce and information, among others. The content of this chapter is partly based on the results obtained from the survey.

The TLV supply chain is very short, due to high perishability. During the harvesting process, farmers normally place TLVs under the shade and at times sprinkle water on the vegetables. In Zimbabwe, farmers or intermediates pack TLVs in jute bags and then transport the product to the markets. Some bags are packed in big lorries or placed on top of the commuter buses and tied by a rope to avoid falling. Transportation is done during the evening when temperatures are low. Unfortunately, there is no appropriate storage during transportation and at the marketplaces, which can result in reduced shelf life of vegetables. To avoid losses through spoilages, the producers and traders are forced to bring or buy the TLVs in small enough quantities such that they can be sold within a day or two.

The producers minimize the transactional costs and losses due to high perishability by taking the TLVs directly to the markets. In such cases, it may be worthwhile for the producers to have market information before taking the TLVs to the markets. Alternatively, the producers sell their TLVs to intermediates moving around their farm gates and sourcing the vegetables. In that way, the producers would reduce transport costs and other costs that can be incurred, i.e. high market fees. For example, in Harare, the farmer is charged $10 per day, which means that if the farmer has unsold TLVs, the farmer either has to pay another $10 for the following day, is forced to dump the remaining product or give it away for free.

Figure 7 depicts an example of the movement of TLV seed and vegetables from the areas of production to markets. The TLV seeds are primarily produced, sold and exchanged locally, with many people deriving their incomes and livelihoods through various activities carried along the supply chain, thus having the potential for facilitating the attainment of the current imperative to foster food and seed sovereignty and strengthen various of their components. Since their production is local, farmers have control over seeds and the resulting vegetables can then be quickly supplied to consumers, supporting domestic marketing structures in developing countries. This chain supports the flow of purchasing power from more affluent urban regions to rural areas, as depicted in Figure 7.

The highly perishable nature of TLVs makes them unsuitable for long-distance transport. This statement is true across Africa. These vegetables are sold to neighboring urban areas and locals and in small quantities in processed form are exported to neighboring countries. For example for Zimbabwe, Botswana and South Africa are importers. Most of the production areas are near urban areas, while there exist others that are located more than 100 km away from the urban areas. In Zimbabwe, locations, where the authors collected data, are around 100 km away from the major markets, translating to an average of three to four hours to reach the market using public transport. In Kenya, the TLV production areas are near Nairobi, whereas others are more than 100 km away and other retailers had to walk 15 km daily for fresh TLVs (Nekesa & Meso, 1997). In Zambia, Lusaka supermarkets source their TLVs from local farmers in the peri-urban areas. In Uganda, the average distance traveled and time used to travel in order to sell the TLVs is not large. It rarely takes more than an hour and the traveling distance is around 14

Figure 7. TLVs seed production regions and markets in Zimbabwe
Source: Authors

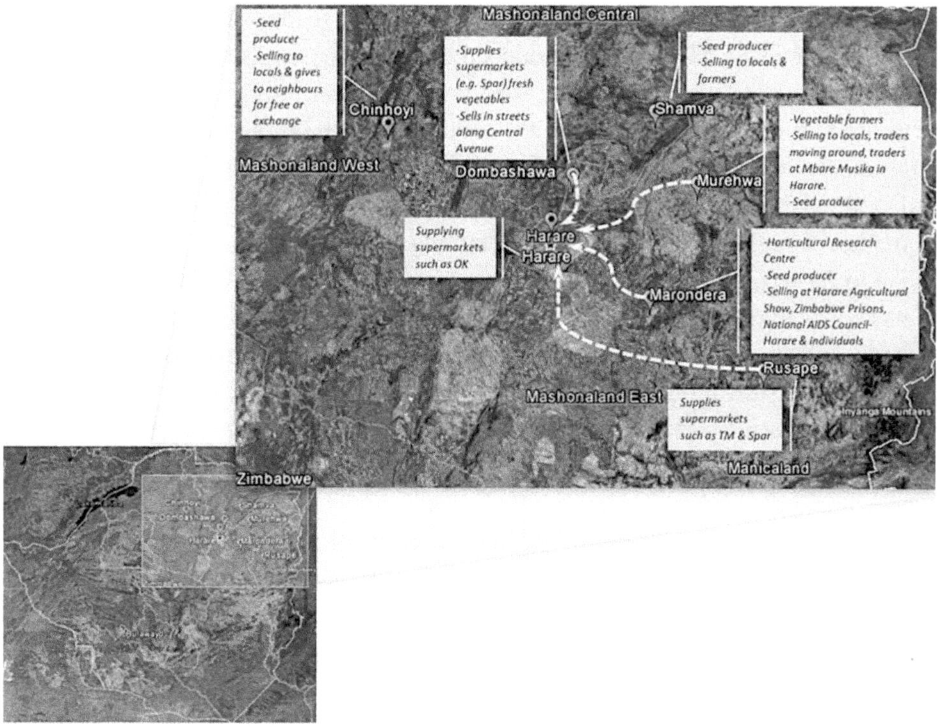

km (Weinberger & Pichop, 2009). TLVs are very perishable and there is a need to produce them near or at the point of use.

In the community, the TLVs are sold at various market outlets, including at farm gates, on the side of the road and door-to-door. In this scenario, the traders are producers as well, as they sell their TLVs directly to consumers and to some intermediaries. Some of the intermediaries visit various farm gates, purchase the TLVs, transport them to the markets and eventually sell them to the consumers. It is mainly men who do the purchasing. In case the TLVs are not bought, in the case of Zimbabwe, the producers would process them and sell them later, some would be consumed in their households.

Women play significant roles in the TLV supply chain as producers, processors, and marketers (Weinberger & Pichop, 2009). In Uganda, men mainly act as intermediaries, as they move around to buy TLVs from producers (mostly women) and transport them to markets. In the markets, women buy them from the intermediaries and then sell these vegetables to the public. Women are, therefore, economically empowered as they are able to pay fees for their children and provide food their households.

Vegetable Varieties, Seed Production, and Farming Characteristics

Many TLV types are produced within homesteads, sold in local markets, exchanged as seeds or sold in the local markets, fostering localized developments. Despite their high potential in offering better opportunities for gender oriented developments, transforming the rural livelihoods through localized markets and addressing food insecurity problems, there are many challenges persisting along the supply chain.

The availability of seed and undeveloped seed systems, depriving farmers' access to high-quality seed of preferred varieties. More so, with the supplies of vegetables now getting into big cities (increased demand for vegetables), this translates to increased demand for seed as well.

In Eastern Africa, mostly, TLV seed is produced by farmers. Seed stockists buy this seed and then sell it to many emerging TLV farmers. These seed producers are registered with renowned companies and are able to produce certified seed, giving the seed a commercial market value. They are capable of producing high-quality seed with the supervision of big seed companies. More so, the TLV seed markets are organized well, enabling seed producers to realize profits and incentivise. The farmers are assured of the ready markets and they know well before planting the types of TLVs preferred by their targeted markets. Unlike in Eastern Africa, Southern Africa, Western Africa and Central Africa, the production of TLV seed has not been formalized. There, no commercial seed company has shown interest in venturing into the seed production and marketing sector. One example where this has happened is Cameroon. Various international organizations funded the training and production of TLV seed, aiming at improving seed availability to farmers through the involvement of local seed companies in Eastern Africa and a few in Southern Africa. The top five selected for increased production, consumption and marketing include cowpea, amaranth, nightshade, spider flower, and African eggplant.

In Zimbabwe, TLV seed is produced by a government institute under the Department of Research & Specialist Services (Horticultural Research Centre) and by farmers dotted around the country. The most common TLV seed produced include spider flower, cowpea, amaranth, black jack, okra, tsunga, and pumpkin, with the most traded being spider flower and pumpkin seed. Similarly, findings by Chagomoka et al. (2014) revealed that TLV seed produced in Malawi included Ethiopian mustard, okra, pumpkin, and African eggplant. In Mozambique, the same authors found that most TLV farmers use returned seed, with some of the seed imported from Tanzania. The seed is usually packed in a plastic bag or plastic coated paper. In Zimbabwe, three main sections of TLV seed production were found, notably, the low section (subsistence farmer without knowledge of seed production), the middle section (commercialized farmer with relatively basic knowledge of seed production) or high section (commercialized seed producing company i.e. Horticultural Research Centre). The seed from the high section was more expensive than other seed sections, costing $50 per kilogram. The seed is marketed to different channels: to neighbors, at agricultural shows, and to various organizations promoting the use of TLVs for nutrition and health benefits.

The farmers generally measure out the seed in tablespoonfuls or pet coke cola leads. A tablespoonful is estimated to weigh approximately 15 grams and a pet coke cola lead is approximately 2 grams, marketed at $2.00 and $0.50 respectively or $50 per kilogram in Zimbabwe markets and $1.80 per 25g of amaranth seed in Kenya markets (Mumbi et al., 2006). When these seed weights and prices were calculated and estimated per hectare of spider flower and amaranth for one season, the gross income presented in Table 3 are derived. In comparison, spider flower seed's gross margin is higher than that of amaranth seed, valued at $6,500/hectare. The gross margin for farmers in the production of TLVs vegetables varies due to the TLV type. The least gross margin is obtained from cowpeas with $2,426. Nevertheless, in Zimbabwe, the TLV seed is rarely packaged, labeled and traded directly to the public without hiring the chain of people or companies to market the seed. Seed produced is sold locally to neighbors, friends, and relatives or nearby urban areas. The transactions are mostly based on the cash market.

Table 3. Seasonal and annual gross margin analysis for TLV seed and TLVs ($)

Category	TLV grown	Country	Production cost	Gross income	Gross margins
Seed (per ha and season)	Spider flower	Zimbabwe	1,000	7,500	6,500
Seed (per ha and season)	Amaranth	Kenya	185	3,145	2,960
Vegetables (0.1 per ha/ year)	Amaranth	Kenya	1,142	5,714	4,571
Vegetables (0.1 per ha/ year)	Cowpea	Kenya	1,306	3,733	2,426
Vegetables (0.1 per ha/ year)	Nightshade	Kenya	1,633	4,666	3,033

Source: Authors and Mumbi et al., 2006

Production of Traditional Leafy Vegetables

Similar to countries in Eastern and Western Africa, the production of TLVs can be commercialized in Zimbabwe, in particular areas close to major cities. For example, a Zimbabwean farmer who produces and sells the TLVs throughout the year as opposed to seasonally gets better prices when the market supplies are low, while also taking advantage of the fast moving of the TLVs when incoming supplies dwindle. The spider flower fetches the highest price and sells fastest. TLVs winter production is mainly carried along major rivers in some parts of Zimbabwe (Mpala, Dlamini, & Sibanda, 2013), concentrated in irrigation schemes during the dry seasons and in rural areas during the summer season. Most of the TLVs produced are consumed domestically, either by households or through local markets in nearby urban areas. Similarly, the production and marketing of TLVs has been increasing and becoming increasingly commercialized in Kenya, particularly within Nairobi and the peri-urban areas (Irungu et al., 2011). Women participation in the TLVs supply chain is constantly high in Kenya, Benin and South Africa (Table 4). Female participation in TLV production tends to be lowest to other levels of the supply chain. Table 4 shows that it is especially low in Côte d'Ivoire and Senegal.

However, production of TLVs is hindered by unavailability of certified or high-quality seed coupled with the underdeveloped seed systems. The underdeveloped seed systems limit the seed movement, subsequently, limits the farmers' variety of choices.

Table 4. Share of women along the TLVs supply chain across countries (%)

Category	Country						
	Benin	Côte d'Ivoire	Senegal	Kenya	Tanzania	Uganda	South Africa
Farmers	40	16	14	59	34	37	65
Intermediaries	78	100	26	95	75	69	unknown
Retailers	100	100	58	86	58	68	86

Source: Weinberger & Pichop, 2009

Processing of Traditional Leafy Vegetables

Processing and packaging is a way of minimizing spoilage of TLVs due to their high perishability. During the periods when the TLVs are abundant in the markets and in gardens, TLVs are partly processed for future use in the dry season or for distant marketing (Mpala et al., 2013). In Zimbabwe, 97% of the TLV farmers process parts of the vegetables harvested (Mpala et al., 2013), in Uganda 1.2%, in Côte d'Ivoire 9.3%, in Kenya 2.1%, in Senegal 0.8%, and in South Africa 10.3% (Weinberger & Pichop, 2009). Similarly, Chagomoka et al. (2014) note that TLVs are processed prior to selling as a way of minimizing quantity and quality losses. Only 12% of retailers in Malawi and 6% of retailers in Mozambique process the TLVs prior to selling. About 50% of the households in South Africa preserve vegetables for both selling and own consumption.

There are various methods of processing, including; sun-drying without any pre-treatment, blanching and sun-drying and blanching then freezing (Bioversity International, n.d.). Sun-drying without any pre-treatment method is the most preferred among the commonly preserving methods (Mpala et al., 2013). In Zimbabwe, cowpea tender leaves are harvested, boiled, and dried in direct sunlight. They are twisted by rolling them between the pumps. The processing varies across the nations, regions, and cultures. For example, in Malawi cowpea leaves are processed by sun-drying and/or blanching (Chagomoka et al., 2014), but not twisting. The pumpkin leaves are sold fresh across Africa. Except in some countries in Southern African, including Zimbabwe, they are traded in their dried form. They are dried without cooking and normally their flowers are added.

In Zimbabwe, drying is generally done in a semi-closed cabinet that protects the processed vegetables from fine dust particles that may settle on it in order to avoid making them gritty. Quality attributes such as twisted and dried for cowpea, the absence of pathogens, i.e. dried without visible moulds, and neatly packaged with the labels showing shelf life, net weight and processors' details are mandatory. The concerns arise especially if the quality attributes are not met. This can result in negative perceptions among some urban dwellers and educated elite in response to their fear for their health. The worries related to the health risks were highlighted in the World Vegetable Center (2006) report on determination knowledge and use of TLVs by the elite urban dwellers. The average to middle-income earners consumed little in fear of risking their health.

Marketing Channels of Traditional Leafy Vegetables

Trading TLVs in Kenya dates back to the 1960s (Irungu et al., 2011). The trade of TLVs is highly specialized, as is the consumption. Nairobi has ten large markets, which sell TLVs in larger amounts. These markets are located in residential places and serve the surrounding consumers. Supermarkets and green grocery stores serve the affluent minority who have limited time to visit some of the city council markets, such as Harare and Nairobi City Council markets. In addition, there are several evening traders along the streets who target the people coming from work.

Similarities in trading of TLVs can be found across African regions. In Zimbabwe, the authors noted that three-quarters of traders interviewed purchased the TLVs from farmers moving around the market looking to sell to traders they know. While supermarkets in both Kenya and Zimbabwe buy directly from individuals, groups or processors. In comparison, Zimbabwean supermarkets mainly sell dried TLVs with the exception of pumpkin, spider plant, and amaranth leaves, while Kenyan supermarkets sell fresh TLVs.

The traders purchase a bundle of TLVs or two cups of dried TLVs for $0.50. A standard cup consists of around 60 g. The traders split the bundle into two and each is sold to consumers at $0.50. In Zimbabwe, a sachet weighing approximately 80 g sells for $2.00 in the green grocery, while a range of $2.00 to $2.35, depending on the TLVs type, for 60 g is sold in supermarkets. Similarly, in Kenya, the wholesaler buys a bundle of TLVs for KES2 ($0.04), splits the bundle into two and sells each for KES2 to the retailer. In turn, the retailer further splits the bundle before selling it to the consumer (Nekesa & Meso, 1997). In Zambia, a bundle of TLVs weighing 500 g is sold between 500 and 800 Zambian Kwacha ($0.25 – $0.30). The profit made on TLV sales is over 100% in Zimbabwe (Mpala et al., 2013), 33% in Tanzania, and over 75% in Kenya (Nekesa & Meso, 1997).

The major TLV dominate marketing channels across Africa, including city council markets, supermarkets, greengroceries, open markets and roadside, as reported by Irungu et al. (2011) and Schippers (2000). Table 5 shows some of the most popular TLVs consumed and found most tradeable in African regions. The types of TLVs popularly consumed and found most tradeable vary substantially by region, except for amaranth. Amaranth is sold fresh in all cities (Maundu, Achigan-Dako, & Morimoto, 2009). Contrary, spider flower is sold in the fresh or dried form in the Southern Africa region. These variations can be explained by different attributes, including cultural backgrounds, geographical location, and diversity. In comparison, in Western Africa, baobab leaves are some of the most popular TLVs consumed, whereas black jack is the most commonly consumed TLVs in the Southern African region. Northern Africa, due to its climate conditions, a few types of TLVs exist in the region.

Table 5. Some of the most popular TLVs consumed and traded in Africa

Region	Popular TLVs	Tradeable TLVs
Southern Africa	Amaranth, Okra, Spider flower, Pumpkin leaves, Cowpea leaves, Black jack, Sweet potato leaves	Spider flower, amaranth, black jack, cowpeas and pumpkin leaves, okra, African eggplant, amaranth, jute mallow, Ethiopian mustard, and wild cucumber
Eastern Africa	Amaranth, Cowpea vegetables, Pumpkin vegetables, Corchorus, Nightshade, Spider flower, Sweet potato leaves, Moringa	African nightshade, amaranth, Spider flower cowpea leaves, crotalaria, okra, Ethiopian kales, Ethiopian mustard, sweet potato leaves, cassava leaves
Western Africa	Amaranth, African eggplant, Corchorus, Okra, Sweet potato leaves, Cowpea leaves, Baobab leaves, Spider flower, Moringa,	Sweet potato leaves, African nightshade, cassava leaves, pumpkin leaves, jute, Amaranth
Central Africa	Amaranth, Pumpkin leaves, Sweet potato leaves, Okra, Jute, Spider flower, Cassava leaves	Moringa, jute, hibiscus, okra, amaranth, cowpea leaves

Source: Authors; Nekesa & Meso, 1997; Maundu et al., 2009; Irungu et al., 2011; Chagomoka et al., 2014

Challenges in Realising the Economic Potential of TLVs

TLVs have for decades not been recognized as a potential contributor to food and nutrition security by policy makers (Schippers, 2000). Only recently, TLVs have become important food crops and have attracted international spotlight because of their potential for human nutrition by providing essential micronutrients, phytochemicals, and antioxidants for achieving a balanced diet. The realization of their potential is subject to a number of challenges persisting along the TLV supply chain. Major challenges include the unavailability of quality-certified seed to enhance productivity, undeveloped seed systems depriving farmers' choices of varieties, limited preservation methods given their high perishability, resulting in poor quality, processed products, and negative perceptions among some of the young generation, educated elite, and urban dwellers.

Results from a study conducted by Weinberger & Pichop (2009) in three regions of Africa (Eastern, Southern, and Western), show that the median and inter-quartile range for urban areas dedicated to vegetable production is larger in Nairobi and Kisumu, for peri-urban areas of Cotonou, Durban, Lokossa, and Shoshangwe, reflecting increased demand of TLVs in the urban areas in Kenya (Figure 8 and Figure 9).

Figure 8. Cultivated areas in urban and peri-urban for six cities
Notes: Median values and interquartile ranges are displayed
Source: Weinberger & Pichop, 2009

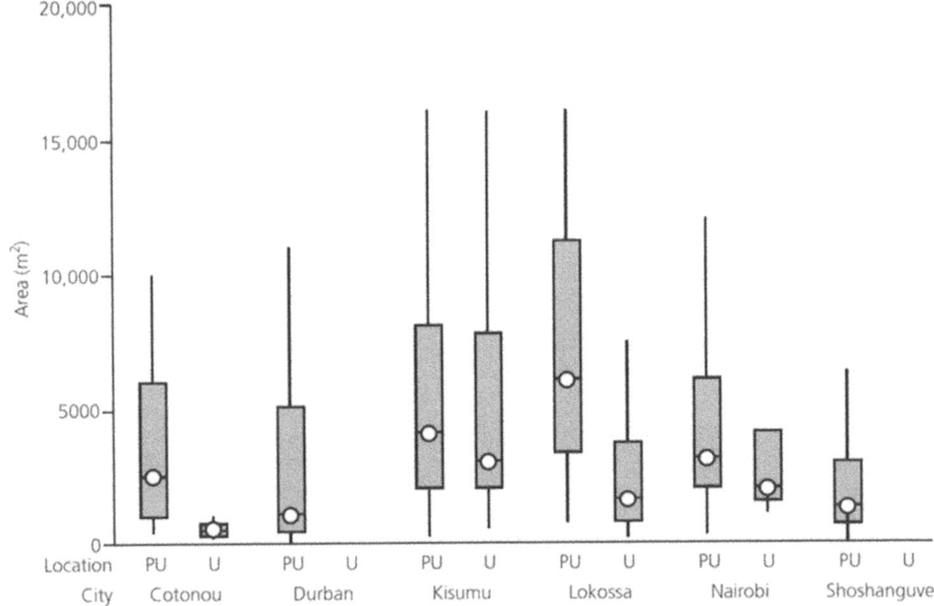

If the quality of TLV seed would be improved and become more homogenous, farmers might additionally benefit by having fewer expenditures for the seed and eventually get higher yields. However, this potential of increased earnings depends on the structure of the value chain, number of actors and their market power, and the value added at its various value chain nodes. The more diverse and immediate the marketing possibilities of the farmers are, the higher their benefits can be. The potential socio-economic and societal benefits of investing in the improvement of TLV seed quality by eventually incorporating TLV seed into the formal seed market crucially depends on the potential contributions which these indigenous food products can have towards the income of the stakeholders in the value chain on the one hand and the benefits for food security and the healthy nutrition of the consumers on the other. Most commercial seed companies consider the TLV seed production as uneconomic. Across Africa, TLV seed is marketed informally, with less than 10% of seed planted being purchased from the formal markets. Few seed companies have committed themselves to the TLV seed production, for

Figure 9. Vegetable production in urban and peri-urban areas of six major African cities
Notes: Median values and interquartile ranges are displayed
Source: Weinberger & Pichop, 2009

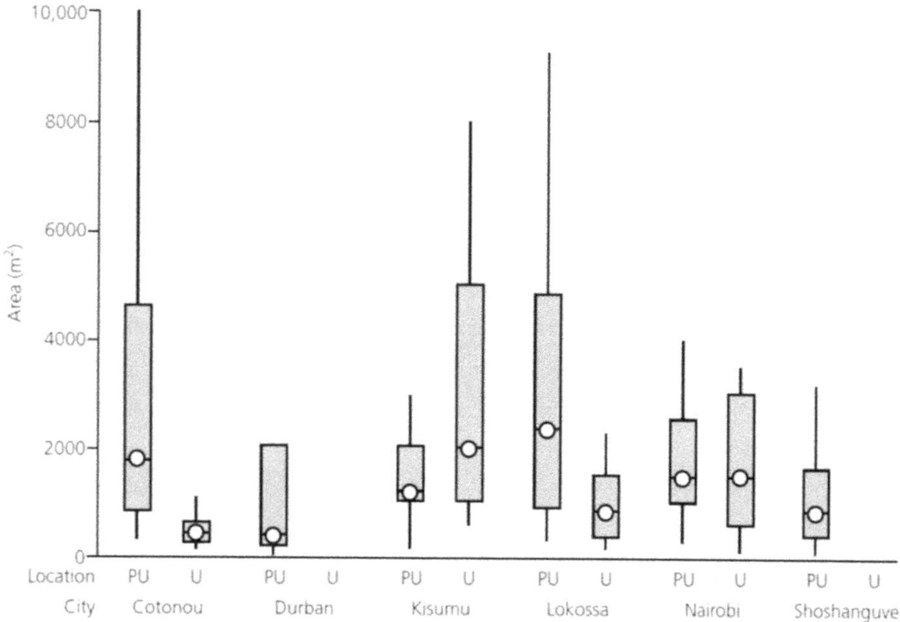

example in Kenya and Tanzania farmers have benefited from the involvement of big seed companies with many of them changing from using own farm-saved seed to certified seed. Switching from own saved to certified seed increased the farmers market gross value by 213% between the period of 2001 and 2006 (Irungu et al., 2011).

During the period of vegetable shortages, particularly during the dry seasons throughout the year, dried and processed TLVs become very important in household food security. Their abundance normally coincides with the peak of the rain season, making it difficult to preserve them well and for larger quantities to be marketed throughout the relish gap. TLVs, like some of the modernized horticultural crops, are highly perishable. They are produced by resource-poor rural sectors, who cannot afford the modernized preservation methods like refrigerating. The production of TLVs is relatively low especially during the dry seasons, meaning that the TLV market niche during this period can only be filled by the farmers using an irrigation mechanism. However, the quality of the processed TLVs is poor in some cases, can result in negative perceptions by the young generation, elite, and urban dwellers.

If the quality of the processed TLVs improves through preserving and turning them into products like cakes or flour, such products could increase the TLVs consumption by the young, elite, and urban dwellers. Also, the creation of awareness for the preparation or cooking of TLVs through cooking recipes can effectively and positively increase their consumption, particularly among the young, elite, and urban dwellers. Although the TLVs have the potential to facilitate the current imperative to foster food sovereignty and strengthen various of its components, this potential is not realized because they are classified as minor crops.

SOLUTIONS AND RECOMMENDATIONS

The availability of certified quality seeds coupled with the developed seed systems will enhance the production of TLVs. For example, Asfaw, Shiferaw, Simtowe, and Lipper (2012) reported better incomes were realized by smallholder farmers who adopted improved or certified seed varieties. The authors recommend the international organization such as the World Vegetable Center, already working in Eastern Africa to extend working with other countries in Southern and Western Africa to ensure quality seed production and develop TLV seed systems.

Different recipes and preparation methods that are passed through generations have also been promoted in Tanzania and should be scaled out in other countries in the continent to create awareness among the elite, young, and urban dwellers. For example, the World Vegetable Center is promoting consumption of TLVs and processing them into other products such as cakes and flour (Ochieng et al., 2016). The authors recommend an increase in production and processing of traditional leafy vegetables to enhance their consumption by the elite groups and children.

The Potential of TLVs to Improve Food and Nutrition Security

TLVs contribute significantly to food security in the dry regions of Zimbabwe, as they are consumed by more than 60% of the households in these regions (Mpala et al., 2013); about 21% and 30% of the produced indigenous vegetables are consumed at home in Malawi and Mozambique (Chagomoka et al., 2014). TLVs account for about 80% of the total food use during winter in South Africa. Another key important issue regarding food security: the cash obtained from selling TLVs contributes significantly to food security at the household level, as it can be used to buy other food related items. In Zimbabwe, the rural poor people rely on TLVs for a period of nine months (five months of the rainy season and four of the dry months). They are prime sources of minerals and are naturally rich in nutrients, i.e. iron, protein, vitamins, and other micronutrients needed by the human body for healthy growth. They have the potential to help address micronutrient deficiency problems in many African countries.

Some TLVs have relatively high levels of nutrients, e.g. cleome and cowpea leaves contain more than 4 g (4.5 g and 4.4 g, respectively) of protein and 275 mg and 186 mg of calcium, respectively, while sweet potato and cleome have 3.9 mg and 2.2 mg of iron, respectively, and cowpea leaves and cleome have 75 mg and 113 mg of Vitamin C, respectively per 100 g edible portion (Yang & Keding, 2009). If incorporated in the daily diets of people in Africa, this new diet can be a key step in reducing malnutrition and food security problems faced by the continent. Most of the nutrients found in TLVs are very important, especially for the poor population who consumes mostly staples and tubers with little or no meat. Khoury et al. (2014) reported a global change in the dietary patterns, people are consuming calories, protein and fat, relying increasingly on wheat, maize, and soybeans, along with meat and dairy products, showing increasingly shift towards monotonous and homogeneous diets. TLVs can serve both purposes, as vegetables and as a supplement to starchy foods, as some TLVs, such as sweet potato and cassava roots, provide much-needed energy as well, break the increasingly relying on monotonous diets.

TLVs are produced locally; farmers have control over seed and they can be quickly supplied to consumers, which ultimately supports domestic marketing structures in developing countries. Their marketing supports the flow of purchasing power from more affluent urban regions to rural areas. The development of TLV markets within African cities and other major urban centers could be considered a milestone in the re-introduction of underutilized local food crops for food security, food sovereignty, on-farm biodiversity conservation as well as halting biodiversity losses alluded to in SDG 15. Precious genetic variability of these domesticated plants, traditional foods and farming customs in developing countries can be preserved. From an agronomic perspective, TLVs might yield general beneficial effects for the cropping pattern and for fighting crop diseases.

Potential Socio-Economic Benefits for National Food Supply Chains

TLVs do not have high needs in terms of farming practices, production inputs, and weather conditions as they produce seed under the tropical condition, unlike the exotic vegetables. This opens up the potential for farmers to easily expand TLVs production and obtain higher incomes through increased marketing of TLV seed and of TLVs. TLVs, therefore, possess a substantial potential for sustainably improving the livelihoods of the poor rural population and provision of food for the poor urban dwellers.

The contribution of TLVs to household incomes have been reported to be higher than 20% in Malawi and Mozambique (Chagomoka et al., 2014). Besides income benefits, the production and trading of TLVs have been associated with women. In Zimbabwe and Kenya, the majority of the TLV traders and producers were women (60% and 65% of the sample, respectively). This proportion confirms the trend shown in other reports. Mpala et al. (2013) reported that most TLV traders are women. Women are predominant in the production and marketing of TLVs, accounting for 57% and 95%, respectively. Meaning that the women are empowered and therefore financially independent, consequently reducing their vulnerability. The incomes earned is very important, as it can be used for buying food for their families, provide housing and secure health care for the families among others (Schippers, 2000).

Potential Socio-Economic Benefits for Rural Areas

Only in the late 1990s health institutions increased awareness designed to reduce the diseases of the affluent (i.e. diabetes, high blood pressure, and ulcers, among others) (Irungu et al., 2011). These ailments were predominantly associated with people dwelling in urban areas because of their unhealthy food consumption pattern. Whereas for their counterparts in rural areas, many diseases caused by food insecurity (such as malnutrition) have been associated with an unbalanced diet. But note that other patients who suffer from HIV/AIDS could benefit from TLVs, as they are said to mitigate this type of ailment (Irungu et al., 2011).

For years, the rural people valued the TLVs for food security as well as medicinal, social, cultural, and income-generating item (Mpala et al., 2013). TLVs are important sources of essential macro- and micro-nutrients, hence their potential to reduce diseases of the affluent and diseases resulting from food insecurity. They are also important dietary components which are used to prepare sauces and relishes that accompany carbohydrate staples. Beyond their fundamental subsistence use, TLVs have the potential to address some of the Sustainable Development Goals (SDGs) that pertain to poverty, health, food and nutrition security in Africa.

Moreover, TLVs represent an inexpensive food of high and beneficial nutrient content (Schippers, 2000). With TLVs, a one-sided nutrition, especially for the poorer parts of the population, can be avoided by boosting this kind of crop production. In urban markets, TLVs command relatively better prices than the exotic vegetables and can be effectively produced by rural resource-limited farmers, hence the potential to foster rural development.

The Potential of Traditional Leafy Vegetables to Contribute to the Sustainable Development Goals

Recent food price volatility has resulted in poverty and food insecurity in many developing countries, in particular, Africa. The leaders from various countries created the MDGs to address some of the challenges, including poverty reduction and food insecurity problems. Several countries managed to reduce the number of the population deemed poor by half. Following the successful implementation of the MDGs, the leaders of various countries created a new set of goals "Sustainable Development Goals", aimed to end poverty and hunger by 2030.

TLVs have high nutritional values that can overcome malnutrition problems faced by Africa that still persist due to the lack of diversified diets. The consumption of TLVs has potential health benefits because they are rich in naturally inherent nutrients. TLVs can, therefore, contribute to the SDG 3 aimed at maintaining good health. These vegetables are resilient to adverse conditions prevailing in Africa. They can, therefore, provide food for many people across the continent, a trait making them excellent contributors to SDGs 1 and 2.

TLVs help smallholder farmers to diversify their limited income sources and provide an important source of employment in rural areas. TLVs command relatively high prices on the markets, giving them the potential to relieve rural poverty, in particular, for the vulnerable group, females. In most parts of Africa, TLVs are regarded as women crops, therefore, supporting their production and use can go a long way in the economic empowering of women, which in turn reduces the vulnerability of women and addresses gender inequality, as enshrined in SDG 5. Traditionally, African women are responsible for household food availability, preparation, and preservation. Women's involvement in the TLVs marketing is significantly high. Indigenoveg survey in Weinberger & Pichop (2009) reported that women play a central role in the production, peddling, and marketing of TLVs. They, therefore, offer a convenient pillar for lifting the women higher. Women dominate 100% in the retail markets and middle actors in Cote d'Ivoire, 68% in Uganda, 90% in Kenya, 65% in Tanzania, and 80% in South Africa (Indigenoveg in Weinberger and Pichop (2009)). These vegetables, therefore, form a crucial part of the female existence. TLVs have the potential to transform Africa's economy due to the high turnover and its effect on the income of women, as they play significant roles in the production and marketing of TLVs across Africa.

Currently, some countries are supplementing the vegetable demand shortfalls through importing vegetables from neighboring countries. For example, it is worth mentioning that Botswana and Zimbabwe have an import/export relationship. The local broadcasting company in Zimbabwe reported that Zimbabwe has spent more than $15 million in importing vegetables and citrus commodities in the first two months of 2016. Similarly, vegetables in Botswana are mostly imported from the neighboring South Africa. Thus, the limited foreign exchange is used to purchase products which could be supplied locally. The promotion of production, marketing, and consumption of TLVs enhances local markets, curbing the externalization of much needed foreign currency. It would also reduce enrichment of the richer nations enshrined in SDG number 10.

Nevertheless, TLVs can contribute to the environment through the reduction of biodiversity loss, enshrined in SDG 15. Some of the TLVs types, like the cowpea, can easily adapt to poor soils, making them useful staple crops for marginalized areas. They can be incorporated in the production of crops by farmers living in areas marked by water scarcity and prone to hot temperatures caused by climatic change. In addition, some TLVs are deep rooted, hence they help to stabilize the soils. They also grow faster and provide canopy cover to the soil, reducing soil erosions and loss of soil moisture.

TLVs, therefore, have the potential to contribute to the Sustainable Development Goals 1, 2, 3, 5, 10, 12,13, and 15 (UNDP, 2016). Biodiversity loss reduction, good health maintenance, and the reduction of poverty and hunger can be strongly achieved through activities and policies promoting the production and use of TLVs. They are traded locally, supporting purchasing power from more affluent urban regions to rural areas and involve women command in the supply chain. Many people derive their income from various activities along the supply chain. They are sources of micronutrients required by the human body, food sources during crop failures. African national food and health policies should spearhead the production as well as promote their consumption to help address food insecurity and micronutrient deficiency problems in Africa. The national programs are key in the implementation of such policies. A good example is the Malawi agricultural input program, from which the country succeeded in feeding its people in a short period of time. The Green Revolution in India also transformed the agriculture; the country produced a surplus and ended up exporting food.

FUTURE RESEARCH DIRECTIONS

The outcome of our chapter noted that relatively few countries in Africa have soundly developed TLV seed systems and supply chains, that incentivize the actors along the TLV chains, resulting in the limited investment towards research. If the quality of TLV seed and distribution would be improved, then actors might benefit, realizing that more profits can also attract investors and researchers. Such successes can only be realized if Africa regions work collectively to improve the seed systems and supply chains. In particular, countries which already have seed policies in place should collaborate with the ones lagging behind, in order to improve the quality and accessibility of good quality seed by TLVs farmers. More research on determining the quality of TLV seed would contribute to the availability of high-quality seed on the markets. Equally important, researches aimed at understanding how the TLV supply chains are organized, improved seed distribution channels considering TLVs are increasingly marketed in cities across Africa. Such researches could provide the basis of improved TLVs supplies across Africa.

There is still a lack of knowledge about the methods of preserving and drying TLVs. The presence of contaminants, like moulds or gritty-due fine sands, make TLVs at times unpalatable, due to abnormal smells. Much more attention needs to be given to improving the drying, preserving, and processing of the TLVs into products. Some TLV products such as cakes or flour may attract the elite and urban dwellers to consume them. Besides, more effort needs to be channeled towards how to prepare or cook these vegetables. Most of the elite and urban dwellers lack the knowledge on how to prepare TLVs. Preparation or cooking of TLVs awareness creation through cooking recipes may effectively and positively increase their consumption, especially by the elite and urban dwellers. Research on post-harvest practices is needed.

CONCLUSION

This chapter demonstrates the potential importance of TLVs in transforming the consumers' health and increasing farmers' incomes, particularly women as well as contributing to food security and the economies of African countries. TLVs have increasingly become crops of economic importance and their production cannot only feed an increasing and undernourished population but also make people living in the marginalized areas more productive, given that TLVs grow well even in such stressful environments. Besides offering a greater opportunity to utilize the marginal areas, these vegetables help in diversification of the food basket and breaks the monotonous diets, which is commonly missing in the daily diets of many households in Africa.

There is minimal attention channeled towards these vegetables, yet they could quickly contribute a reduction of the environmental biodiversity losses as well as contributing to a better food and nutrition security. In addition, relative to other field crops like maize, a conventional bred exotic vegetable, TLVs have received little attention in terms of research and funding from governments and international organizations. Just a few countries have put in place policies on TLV seed production, marketing, and distribution.

Nevertheless, TLVs are now getting into the cities, showing an increase in demand for both vegetables and seed. The TLV seed systems in Africa are undeveloped, depriving the farmers of a variety of vegetables, as seed cannot be moved from one region to another. Commercial seed companies also shun the multiplication of TLV seed because they are considered to be less economically viable.

The seasonality and high perishability of these vegetables reduce their potential to be an important tool for addressing food and nutrition insecurity in Africa. In some countries, the urban dwellers and elite consumers still have negative perceptions of TLVs, considering them as food for poor people. Researchers need to prepare tasty and appetizing TLV dishes that can entice the young generation to consume them as well as promote consumer awareness campaigns concerning the nutritional benefits of eating TLVs.

The supply chains of TLVs is not organized in many countries with exception of Kenya and Tanzania where farmers are benefiting from organized markets. In these countries, TLVs production and marketing has been transformed to be commercial and small-scale business entities and changing the livelihoods of many households. For example, in Kenya seed farmers under contract jointly produce seed of various TLV type with a total gross income of half a million US$ with farmers earning on average almost $5,000.

The women involvement in all activities along the TLV supply chain reduces women vulnerability and increases the women empowerment potential. TLVs have the potential to contribute to a number of SDGs, as they are traded locally, their consumption supports purchasing power from more affluent urban regions to rural areas, their market involves women command in the supply chain, their production, marketing and selling involve many people deriving their income through various activities along the supply chain, they are resources of micronutrients required by human body, they can be considered as an option for food during crop failures and their increase in production and consumption will reduce biodiversity.

Smallholder farmers particularly, women who engage in production and marketing TLV, would be more financially empowered. However, the upscaling of these national successes to the entire Africa will be challenging because of the different national perceptions among policy makers.

REFERENCES

Ambrose-Oji, B. (2009). Urban Food Systems and African Indigenous Vegetables: Defining the Spaces and Places for African Indigenous Vegetables in Urban and Peri-Urban Agriculture. In C. M. Shackleton, M. W. Pasquini, & A. W. Drescher (Eds.), *African Indigenous Vegetables in Urban Agriculture* (pp. 1–33). London: Earthscan.

Asfaw, S., Shiferaw, B., Simtowe, F., & Lipper, L. (2012). Impact of Modern Agricultural Technologies on Smallholder Welfare: Evidence from Tanzania and Ethiopia. *Food Policy*, *37*(3), 283–295. doi:10.1016/j.foodpol.2012.02.013

Bioversity International. (n.d.). *Nutritious Underutilized Species.* Retrieved February 15, 2017, from http://www.bioversityinternational.org//Nutritious_underutilized_species_-_Amaranth_1682.pdf

Cernansky, R. (2015). Super Vegetables Long Overlooked in Parts of Africa, Indigenous Greens Are Now Capturing Attention for their Nutritional and Environmental Benefits. *Nature*, *522*, 146–148. doi:10.1038/522146a PMID:26062494

Chagomoka, T., Afari-Sefa, V., & Pitoro, R. (2014). Value Chain Analysis of Traditional Vegetables from Malawi and Mozambique. *International Food and Agribusiness Management Review*, *17*(4), 59–86.

Food and Agriculture Organization of the United Nations. (2015). *The State of Food Insecurity in the World 2015. Meeting the 2015 International Hunger Targets: Taking Stock of Uneven Progress.* Rome: Food and Agriculture Organization of the United Nations.

Ihle, R., von Cramon-Taubadel, S., & Zorya, S. (2009). Markov-switching Estimation of Spatial Maize Price Transmission Processes between Tanzania and Kenya. *American Journal of Agricultural Economics*, *91*(5), 1432–1439. doi:10.1111/j.1467-8276.2009.01360.x

Irungu, C., Mburu, J., Maundu, P., Grum, M., & Hoeschle-Zeledon, I. (2011). The Effect of Market Development On-farm Conservation of Diversity of African Leafy Vegetables around Nairobi. *International Journal of Humanities and Social Science*, *8*(1), 198–207.

Khoury, C. K., Bjorkmanc, A. D., Dempewolfd, H., Ramirez-Villegasa, J., Guarinof, L., Jarvisa, A., ... Struik, P. C. (2014). Increasing Homogeneity in Global Food Supplies and the Implications for Food Security. *Sustainability Science Agricultural Sciences*, *111*(11), 4001–4006. PMID:24591623

Luckmann, J., Ihle, R., Kleinwechter, U., & Grethe, H. (2014). World Market Integration of Vietnamese Rice Markets during the 2008 Food Price Crisis. *Food Security. The Science. Sociology and Economics of Food Production and Access to Food*, *6*(6), 1–17.

Maundu, P., Achigan-Dako, E., & Morimoto, Y. (2009). Biodiversity of African Vegetables. In C. M. Shackleton, M. W. Pasquini, & A. W. Drescher (Eds.), *African Indigenous Vegetables in Urban Agriculture* (pp. 65–104). London: Earthscan.

Mpala, C., Dlamini, M., & Sibanda, P. (2013). The Accessibility, Utilisation and Role of Indigenous Traditional Vegetables in Household Food Security in Rural Hwange District. *International Open & Distance Learning Journal International Research Conference Special Edition*, *3*(1), 40–48.

Mumbi, K., Karanja, N., Njenga, M., Kamore, M., Achieng, C., & Ngeli, P. (2006). *Investigative Market Research: Viable Market Opportunities and Threats for Urban and Peri-Urban Farmers, Farm Concern International.* Nairobi: Urban Harvest and International Potato Centre.

Nekesa, P., & Meso, B. (1997). Traditional African Vegetables in Kenya: Production, Marketing and Utilization. In *Proceedings of the IPGRI International Workshop on Genetic Resources of Traditional Vegetables in Africa: Conservation and Use.* Rome: International Plant Genetic Resources Institute.

Ochieng, J., Afari-Sefa, V., Karanja, D., Kessy, R., Rajendran, S., & Samali, S. (2016). How Promoting Consumption of Traditional African Vegetables Affects Household Nutrition Security in Tanzania. *Renewable Agriculture and Food Systems*, 1–11. doi:10.1017/S1742170516000508

Ojiewo, C., Tenkouano, A., Oluoch, M., & Yang, R. (2010). The Role of AVRDC – the World Vegetable Centre in Vegetable Value Chains. *African Journal of Horticultural Science*, 3, 1–23.

Otsuka, K., Larson, D. F., & Hazell, P. B. R. (2013). An Overview. In K. Otsuka & D. F. Larson (Eds.), *An African Green Revolution. Finding Ways to Boost Productivity of Small Farms* (pp. 1–14). Amsterdam: Springer. doi:10.1007/978-94-007-5760-8_1

Sasson, A. (2012). Food Security for Africa: An Urgent Global Challenge. *Agriculture & Food Security*, 2(1), 1–16.

Schippers, R. R. (2000). *African Indigenous Vegetables. An Overview of the Cultivated Species*. Chatham: Natural Resources Institute/ACP-EU Technical Centre of Agricultural and Rural Cooperation Book.

Shackleton, C. M., Pasquini, M. W., & Drescher, A. W. (Eds.). (2009). *African Indigenous Vegetables in Urban Agriculture*. London: Earthscan.

United Nations Development Programme. (2016). *Support to the Implementation of the 2030 Agenda for Sustainable Development*. Retrieved July 27, 2016, from http://www.undp.org/content/undp/en/home/librarypage/sustainable-development-goals/undp-support-to-the-implementation-of-the-2030-agenda/

Veninga, W., & Ihle, R. (in press). Import Vulnerability in the Middle East: Effects of the Arab Spring on Egyptian Wheat Trade. *Food Security: The Science, Sociology and Economics of Food Production and Access to Food*.

Weinberger, K., & Msuya, J. (2004). *Indigenous Vegetables in Tanzania- Significance and Prospects*. Shanhua: AVRDC – The World Vegetable Center.

Weinberger, K., & Pichop, G. N. (2009). Marketing of African Indigenous Vegetables along Urban and Peri-Urban Supply Chains in Sub-Saharan Africa. In C. M. Shackleton, M. W. Pasquini, & A. W. Drescher (Eds.), *African Indigenous Vegetables in Urban Agriculture* (pp. 225–244). London: Earthscan.

World Vegetable Center. (2006). *Empowering Small Scale and Women Farmers through Sustainable Production, Seed Supply and Marketing of African Indigenous Vegetables in Eastern Africa*. Bangkok: AVRDC – The World Vegetable Center and Family Concern.

Yang, R., & Keding, G. B. (2009). Nutritional Contributions of Important African Indigenous Vegetables. In C. M. Shackleton, M. W. Pasquini, & A. W. Drescher (Eds.), *African Indigenous Vegetables in Urban Agriculture* (pp. 105–143). London: Earthscan.

ADDITIONAL READING

Afari-Sefa, V., Rajendran, S., Kessy, R. F., Karanja, D. K., Musebe, R., Samali, S., & Makaranga, M. (2016). Impact of Nutritional Perceptions of Traditional African Vegetables on Farm Household Production Decisions: A Case Study of Smallholders in Tanzania. *Experimental Agriculture*, *52*(2), 300–313. doi:10.1017/S0014479715000101

Afari-Sefa, V., Tenkouano, A., Ojiewo, C.O., Keatinge, J.D.H., & Hughes, J.d'A. (2012). Vegetable Breeding in Africa: Constraints, Complexity and Contributions toward Achieving Food and Nutritional Security. Food Security: *The Science. Sociology and Economics of Food Production and Access to Food*, *4*(1), 115–127.

Durst, P., & Bayasgalanbat, N. (Eds.). (2014). *Promotion of Underutilized Indigenous Food Resources for Food Security and Nutrition in Asia and the Pacific*. Bangkok: Food and Agriculture Organization of the United Nations, Regional Office for Asia and the Pacific.

KEY TERMS AND DEFINITIONS

Gross Margin Analysis: An analysis conducted between the revenue and the cost of producing TLVs, in our case per hectare per season.

Marketing Channels: A set of activities that necessitate the movement of the produced TLVs to the end user, i.e. the consumer.

Processors: Dehydrating the fresh vegetables from a perishable form into one that encourages a long shelf-life and thereby allows later usage.

Supply Chain: A sequential process involved in the TLVs production to the distribution of the produce. The supply chain for TLVs is relatively short because of the high perishability of the vegetables.

Sustainable Development Goals: Goals that aim at transforming our world through ending poverty and hunger, thereby achieving food security and improving nutrition and promoting sustainable agriculture.

Traders: Persons who engage in the buying and selling TLVs.

Traditional Leafy Vegetables: Plants which originate on the African continent and have a century-long history of cultivation and domestication subject to regional agro-climatic conditions.

Traditional Leafy Vegetables Producers: Farmers that grow the TLVs.

Chapter 66
Veganism in the Bhagwad Gita

Pratyush Ranjan
G. M. University, India

Sanskruti Pujari
G. M. University, India

ABSTRACT

This chapter will start by giving a brief description about the most contextually relevant portions of the Bhagwad Gita (the Song of the Spirit) and go on to establish its stark opposition to egoism in general and anthropocentrism, in particular, which is responsible for most of the global problems in the age of the Anthropocene. It contends that anthropocentrism (including speciesism) is guilty for the globalized industry of animal agriculture that is responsible for large-scale suffering and various major global problems. It then seeks directions from the Gita on the appropriate principled responses to the industry, including that of changing dietary habits towards plant-based sources, before finally exploring whether the Gita would promote veganism.

INTRODUCING BHAGWAD GITA

The Plot

To a beginner, the *Bhagwad Gita* is a classical treatise involving a dialectical exchange between Arjuna-the warrior, and, Krishna- the enlightened charioteer, in the midst of the two fraternal armies of Pandavas (Arjuna's side) and Kauravas, during the fabled Mahabharata War, dated to ancient times, having possibly been fought in Kurukshetra, in present-day northern India. According to the laws and ethics of that space and age, the Pandavas are considered to be more righteous, and the war becomes an unavoidable instrument of the last resort to uphold righteousness- or a *Dharma Yuddha*. Arjuna happens to develop cold feet, deeply enmeshed in the technicalities of *jus ad bellum* and *just in bello*, that is- whether and how to undertake a war that would involve the wanton massacre of one's kith and kin, would involve utter uncertainties and travails, during and after it is over, having possible ramifications on the established political order, on social and economic stability, and would raise ethical and moral questions that mainly

DOI: 10.4018/978-1-7998-5354-1.ch066

the victors would be liable to account for. Krishna, having royal as well as divine roots, being a paragon of intellectual and spiritual knowledge, comes to the rescue of Arjuna, and, engages in a dialogue, to inform the warrior of his necessary duties, of the knowledge of the absolute (and of the temporary), and the need to perform the action with utter altruism and devotion. The dialogue starts with a discussion, with both sides engaging dialectically in propositions, rebuttals and clarifications, and ends with Arjuna professing absolute devotion to Krishna and the willingness to contribute proactively in the war, after the latter had unfolded the laws of the universe, having proven how the war was indeed just, and after having revealed his *Vishwaroopam Avatar*- the personification of the universal and eternal truth.

The *Gita* (in short) may have different hermeneutical versions, based on the interpreter. A very narrow interpretation may conceive of it as a mere exposition of the virtues of warfare and of violence. However, if the lenses are sufficiently zoomed out, and the symbolisms and metaphors of characters and situations suitably read it could serve as a compass to any shipwrecked sailor to find the appropriate shore. This paper will embark on the endeavor to interpret the text selectively- in parts, and in a way that appear relevant with respect to the undertaken context of the global situation.

The paper neither claims nor disputes the scientific historicity of the events or the factuality of the characters that have been recorded in the popular versions of the texts, which would have undergone substantial additions and subtractions, through the generations, and, in the written and memorized forms are (in most probabilities) the works of error-prone humans- constrained by the knowledge of their respective ages. This paper only aims to very strategically extract some timeless and universally-relevant wisdom, purposefully in accordance with the requirements of these times in mind, while adopting as scientific an interpretation as is possible and necessary. It looks at the *Gita* as a philosophical masterpiece that can artfully be referred to as a great guide by anyone who is in need of moral and spiritual direction. Kindly bear with the issues of transliteration and of translation of complex concepts, which bear different spellings and interpretations in different sources of literature.

The Characterization and Symbolic Analysis

The Battlefield

The *Kshetra,* or the field of action which symbolizes the bivouac of life full of struggles and conflicts all around. It's an atmosphere of quandary which forces the mind to seek answers to little known questions. The great *Dharma Yuddha* is the perfect ambience which puts ample pressure on the great warrior Arjuna and sends him into a perplexed state of mind where he starts questioning his ethics. An ordinary individual may also come across such a perplexing situation in life and face a similar dilemma. The *Gita* can therefore be called a timeless classic that is relevant in every time and age.

The Chariot

The chariot symbolizes the mortal body which is driven by the mind or consciousness that is the charioteer. The five horses stand for the five sense organs (*indriyas)* that are controlled by the reins of the mind (*manas*). The passenger is the *Jivatma* or the individual soul guided by the charioteer. The ultimate destination of this journey is self-realization and *moksha* (salvation).

Arjuna

The hamartia (tragic flaw) of this particular character is his lack of effective reason in the face of impending chaos. Arjuna, in this day and age can be anyone or anything who/which is in a state of dilemma or moral conflict (including today's corporate institutions, nation states, societies and even the world morality, and so on) and is in dire need of enlightenment and compass. Arjuna is emotional, sentimental, disillusioned and moreover purposelessly idealistic in the beginning, however, after receiving divine guidance from Krishna and introspection, he resolves to action and ultimately wins the Mahabharata War.

Krishna

He is the charioteer, the driving force, an external agent or an inner higher conscience that- as a friend and as a guide, shows Arjuna the path towards righteousness. This paper does not validate his historical existence but appreciates the character as the symbol of the higher intellect (*purusha* or the Spirit) that guides the lower self (*prakriti*) towards the path of self-realization. He is the manifested form of the absolute (Brahma) which he reveals in his *Vishwaroop Avatar* (the Universal Form).

The *Vishwaroop Avatar* of God may seem very thrasonical on the surface as He proclaims that He's everything and one must give up every other faith to realize Him. But when a deeper analysis is done, one realizes that the idea of God is not as anthropomorphic and anthropocentric as it seems. It is a higher consciousness that is all encompassing, which facilitates the co-existence of the material and the spiritual in complete harmony. In fact, it will be appropriate to call it 'It' and not 'He' as it is formless, structure-less and indefinite. Rather than godifying a person (which the *Gita* opposes), Krishna personifies the God, in its material *avatar*.

Kauravas

They basically symbolize the dominance of *prakriti* (the lower natural evolutionary self) over the *purusha* (the higher intellect, or the spirit), with their egos and their urges to have material possessions. They are disillusioned by *Maya* (illusory drives), are submissive to their impulsive and egoist selves, mostly driven by their *indriyas* (organs of sense, perception and action). The demonic and divine qualities within us are in constant struggle, one over-powering the other. Every person faces struggles on personal, societal and even universal levels at some point or the other.

Dhritarastra and Sanjaya

Dhritarastra, the blind king and the father of the Kauravas is the ultimate symbol of ignorance (*avidya*). His blindness may symbolize his *avidya*, ego and materialistic desires, without any offense to differently-abled persons. He can be compared to the modern-day ego-centric human in various forms and colors such as a power-thirsty politician, a rapacious industrialist and so on. The blind king receives a live commentary of the events occurring in the Battlefield through Sanjaya (a man who has *divya drishti* or divine vision).

Sanjaya represents stability, awareness and *vidya* (knowledge), as the advisor to Dhritarastra. He was also the latter's charioteer both in a metaphorical and real sense of the word. He, as a typical armchair philosopher, narrates the episode of the Gita and provides his insights (only when asked for) on the same.

The Goal of the Gita and the Means

Individuals, societies, countries and even the global community, often find them in states of dilemma regarding the ends they ought to pursue and regarding making the proper choice out of various means to achieve any such purpose. Sometimes subjects have no idea regarding the right course of action (problems of planning, rationalization, theorizing and legislation), and, at other times, are clueless how to implement those (problems of execution and praxis). Often, they are constrained by their contradictory and inconsistent inner impulses, by conflicting social ethics and for the lack of dedicated will and effort. Thinkers like Albert Camus, Jean-Paul Sartre, Fyodor Dostoyevsky and so on consider life and any action implemented in its pursuit as being absolutely absurd and in lacking any purpose. The *Gita*, however, offers a philosophical as well as a practical beacon, seeking to bridge the theory-praxis gap, that may be applicable to all (in different ages, at various times, and in different circumstances) to find the right way and to tread it the right manner.

The *Gita* attempts to educate the readers, or make them capable of self-realizing- the absolute wisdom or the absolute truth, that is- *Brahmavidya*, or the metaphysical knowledge of the *Brahma*- the all-encompassing and all-transcending Absolute. It includes the scientific knowledge of the *Brahmanda*- the Cosmic Egg. It assumes that all matter, energy, phenomenal egos, and all other ontological elements of the *Brahmanda* are imperfect parts of the absolute *Brahma,* and the *Brahma* manifests Itself in and as everything through the immanent and transcendental spirit- *Atma.* It, therefore, upholds the principle of holism over atomism, that is, the idea that every component in a given system is a part of the larger whole that is irreducible to the sum of its atomistic parts (Melsen, 2019). However, it does not rule out the bounded free will of certain parts, which belongs to the ambit of entities comprising consciousness and intellect.

The *Vedas*, the most ancient surviving texts of wisdom in Indian philosophy, had identified the *Rita,* as the cosmic and natural law, that all entities- from the atoms to the galaxies and beyond, from deterministic automata to free willed individuals, to even the *Iswaras* or the personal and conceptualized Gods (or forces of nature and of societies), all being part of the *Brahma,* obey or are subjected to the constraints of. *Dharma* (or *Dhamma*) is the subjective and contextual law of moral righteousness and ethical conduct, following which every entity can reach its higher self, attain inner peace and freedom, and contribute to universal harmony, in the quest for attaining oneness with the Absolute Reality.

He who does not, in this world, help to turn the wheel thus set in motion, is evil in his nature, sensual in his delight, and he...lives in vain. III, 16 (Radhakrishnan, 2014, p. 157)

Conscious agents, it implies, possessing free will, if choose to act in consonance with the *Rita* (the universal law), identifying their individual duty (*swadharma*) and collective righteousness (*sadharana dharma*) consequently, tethering the codes of their moral, ethical, legal, social and international behavior accordingly, would go on to create institutions, societies, polities and international order, that are orderly (or appropriately disorderly), just and good for everything (that deserves a place). It therefore advocates the virtues of enlightened communitarianism, cosmopolitanism, ecologism and progressively transcendental universalism.

Sages see with an equal eye, a learned and humble Brahmin, a cow, an elephant or even a dog or an outcaste (Radhakrishnan, 2014, p. 210).

These principles are in vehement opposition to egoism, which is at the root of anthropocentrism- the meta-ideology of privileged human exceptionalism and of the instrumentalism of the underprivileged, which again forms the ideational basis of most human actions, something that will be explained later. The *Gita* goes on to identify the various ways to achieve the Absolute Knowledge by making one's actions compatible with the *Rita* and relevant *Dharma,* in the pursuit of the Absolute *Brahma.*

It espouses the practical virtues of the *Yoga* philosophy that holds that conscious subjects must liberate them from their natural and egoistic bodily and mental constraints that are based on materialistic desires and ignorance, in order to find enduring individual bliss and universal cohesion. *Yoga* is a very broad philosophical school that involves the action or deliberate inaction of various mental and physical processes to achieve the said ends. *Yoga*, here, should not be restricted to the contemporary narrower idea of a set of physical exercises and meditation techniques, but, must be understood in the context of its broader objectives- to help conscious beings achieve enlightenment through the employment of physical as well as spiritual methods, recognizing the unity of the embodied mind and the transcendental soul, of matter and of spirit, of *prakriti* and of *purusha.*

Yoga shares some of its fundamental assumptions with the *Sankhya* school of Indian philosophy that is based on the synthetic dualism between *prakriti* and *purusha,* that is, between deterministic nature and free spirit, which is united into a whole scheme of things by the addition of the Universal Spirit that permeates everything, material and spiritual (Radhakrishnan, 2014, p. 45).

Thus far I have declared to you the analytical knowledge of sankhya philosophy. Now listen to the knowledge of yoga whereby one works without fruitive result … when you act by such intelligence, you can free yourself from the bondage of works. II, 39 (Prabhupada, 1972)

On the path of self-realization, the major obstacles are the all-consuming desires (*kama*), ego (*ahankara*) and ignorance (*avidhya*). Ego generates various identities which leads to identity- based distinctions and discriminations like those based on race, caste, class, nationality, religion, species and so on. This is the manifestation of anthropocentrism.

Bhagavad Gita identifies three major types of *yogas* or *margas* (paths) to achieve the ultimate end. They are that of- *Gyaan, Karma,* and *Bhakti. Gyaan yoga* refers to the path of realizing one's ultimate self in relation to and as a part of the ultimate *Brahma.* This broadly entails acquiring all the knowledge that is required to achieve the expressed goal of Gita. Epistemologically, it is similar to the *Sankhya* doctrine as is expressed above. Second is the *Karma yoga* or the path of informed righteous action that is considered to be the most practically effective way of achieving real knowledge, leading a blissful life and achieving cosmic harmony. Finally, *Bhakti Yoga,* or, the path of absolute devotion and renunciation is necessary to put into effect one's ideals and corresponding duties with a sense of hope and faith.

Gyaan Yoga is necessary to identify the purpose, content, methods and so on of performing one's *karma*, in accordance with the cosmic laws and the ethics of righteousness and in the immediate direction of societal (or ecological) welfare (*Loksamgraha*). It requires one to identify one's talents (inherent and acquired), availability of appropriate opportunities and resources, one's limitations (as the outcome of one's natural and social conditions). Once one's *Dharma* is theorized, practice should naturally follow while still adhering to the spiritually detached transcendental idealism of *Gyaan Yoga.*

The Gita considers the performance of *Nishkam Karma* or selfless action as the best possible path to achieve its ends, considering the assumption that human beings are material bodies endowed with a transcendental spirit, thus advocating a synthesis of spiritual knowledge, material action, and emotive devotion. It recognizes that altruistic and purposive action may be impossible to be achieved by quasi-rational-quasi-whimsical humans if sought to be done just for the sake of it. Humans can be philosophically and scientifically rational (for which there is a need of *Gyaan Yoga*) as well as sometimes controlled by matters of theism and dogmatism (for which there is *Bhakti Yoga*). The synthesis of the need of the human agency for scientific rationalism and spiritual devotion for the effective performance of one's duties results in the doctrine of rationalistic theism, that remain the ideological basis and the compass for the performance of *Nishkam Karma*.

Nishkam Karma involves a synthesis of materialistic determinism and spiritual free will, or transcendence (without complete renunciation) of the former by the latter. It involves utilizing the bodily and sensory organs for the ultimate realization of *Brahma* and *Moksha. Moksha,* in a literal sense means salvation from the bondage of recurring life and death. However, in a metaphorical sense, it may also mean redemption from the travails of pleasure and pain, from wants and disappointments, and from desires and agony, not only of one's own but also of all other sentient beings. *Loksamgraha* or enabling the redemption of other elements of society, especially by people of eminence (like Arjuna was) is one of the most immediate practicable prescriptions in the *Gita.*

One who is beyond duality and doubt, whose mind is engaged within, who is always busy working for the welfare of all sentient beings (and not just any class of humans), and who is free from all sins, achieves liberation in the Supreme. V, 25 (Prabhupada, 1972)

From a narrower perspective, the *Bhakti Marga* (path of devotion) advocated in the *Gita,* along with the prescribed sacrifices and renunciations (including of all other faiths), may, *prima facie*, appear (and even be misused by religious perverts) as blind ego-centric submission to an anthropomorphic God, who is calling for universal proselytization. However, if granted an enlightened and scientific interpretation, it would make much more sense even to an atheist. The Enlightened Charioteer, ultimately resorts to revealing his *Vishwaroop Avatar* (The Universal Form of God), in which the Absolute Reality is described to compose all that is known and knowable, all that is transcendentally being and ontologically becoming, all the matter, anti-matter, energy, spirit and imagination, everything that is tangible and otherwise, the culmination of the Ultimate Right and Ultimate Good, the end point of all spiritualism or idealism and materialism.

To an idealist, like Plato (and Socrates) and Hegel, the God in *the Gita* may be the Universal Spirit or the Ultimate Truth, of which all other ideas and matter are parts and transitional manifestations. To a materialist, like Democritus and Hobbes and even a modern scientist, It may be the sum total of all matter, energy, and all that is scientifically established. It would point towards organic unity of all material entities in the universe, and to adopt a holistic attitude about everything in a given system. At a global-contextual level, it promotes the idea of material sameness of all ecological entities-living and non-living (ecologism), the organismic similarity of all living entities– human and non-human (biocentrism), the communitarian unity of all human beings (cosmopolitanism), *inter alia*. As a matter of fact, all living matter (including plants and animals) has evolved from and composed of similar chemical compounds, sharing genetic characteristics with one another. For instance, a human shares 100 percent genes with another human (in different sequences), 98 percent with chimpanzees, 92 percent with mice, 26 percent with yeast, and, around 18 percent with thale cress (a weed, a plant) (Koshland Science Museum, 2019).

It may be of special interest to the thinkers like Karen Barad, Elizabeth Grosz, Rosi Braidotti, Jane Bennett, Vicki Kirby, and Manuel DeLanda, associated with the emerging discipline of New Materialism, which is an "interdisciplinary, theoretical, and politically committed field of inquiry, emerging roughly at the millennium as part of what may be termed the post-constructionist, ontological, or material turn" having been inspired from the insights from philosophy, feminism, cultural theory and science studies (Sencindiver, 2017).

IDEALISM, MATERIALISM, MIND, CONSCIOUSNESS AND INTELLECT

The materialism-idealism debate is an enduring one throughout the dialogue of the *Gita*. Idealism holds that the idea, soul, or spirit is the essence of the universe (possibly being part of some cosmic spirit) and the driving force of history, being more real than the so called real itself, the latter of which may merely be the projection of the mental rationality and sensual perception of a conscious subject, being in some transitional stage in the realization of the ideal or absolute spirit or God. The idealistic conception of the all-immanence of the Universal Spirit is fused together with the non-rejection of material reality. This may be attributed to the combined influence of dualistic Sankhya and the monism of the Upanishads. It holds that matter, including the human body (with the nervous system as the seat of consciousness and the sense organs as the media), is the transitional but nevertheless real manifestation of the *Brahma* in its evolution towards the spiritual through the material.

Consciousness is an oft-underrated concept that may be highlighted here, keeping in mind its relevance at all times, and especially as this is, when the outcomes of privileged brains are shaping forces of history, while the consciousness of other sentient creatures is blatantly neglected as of tertiary importance. Consciousness is the seat of the so-called mind that includes the organs of senses and the information conveying-cum-processing nervous system with the brain at the centre. One can rightly argue that all philosophy or science would be practically irrelevant and even impossible to conceive of if there was no consciousness. Therefore, it would be valid to contend that the ambit of the practical relevance of the *Gita* extends till the extent of one's consciousness. The spiritual insights offered in the *Gita* are to make conscious existence more sublime and in consonance with macro-level processes to attain universal harmony. Consciousness is a very complex and challenging subject to comprehend and to conceptualize. It is the centre of any free will, and of the abilities of thinking and of perception, that is, of rationality and of empiricism, however bounded by naturalistic elements of determinism. Therefore, it is the source of any free-willed action. Different entities have consciousness of different levels and of different types.

The *Taittiriya Upanishad* recognizes five stages of matter – *anna* (abiotic matter), *prana* (biotic matter), *manas* (conscious mind), *vijnana* (enlightened intelligence), and *ananda* (transcendental bliss), with every subsequent one being the manifestation of a greater level of spiritual existence, getting closer to *Brahma* (Radhakrishnan, 2014, p. 92). The *Gita* holds-

The working senses are superior to dull matter; mind is higher than the senses; intelligence is still higher than the mind; and he [the Soul] is even higher than the intelligence. III, 42 (Prabhupada, 1972)

The *Gita* upholds the realization of spiritual consciousness as more liberating and as involving a positive-sum game (vis-à-vis other humans) than merely bodily or material consciousness that may require ten Earths for its satisfaction. However, it also is tolerant to those (including other animals) at various intermediate stages of such a realization, retaining deterministic natural processes, by virtue of their inherited genetic predispositions. It, however, is not tolerant to intolerants who cause harms to other conscious entities and afflict global sustainability and larger ideals.

Bewildered by the modes of material nature, the ignorant fully engage themselves in material activities and become attached. But the wise should not unsettle them, although these duties are inferior due to the performers' lack of knowledge. III, 29 (Prabhupada, 1972).

It advocates finding ways to overcome the limitations of the ordinary human body in realizing one's spiritual potential. It contends that Godliness is latent in all, realizing which every conscious being can realize bliss, but, are obstructed by the limitations of egoism, purposeless hedonism and bounded rationality. True wisdom can only be achieved when one conquers over his organs of perception (*Gyana indriyas*) and puts into action his organs of action (*Karma indriyas*) in order to perform selfless duty (*Niskam Karma*) for the welfare of all (*Loksamgraha*), that is simply having a control of the mind over the body. One has to gain control over one's latent subconscious tendencies (*vasanas*) or inherited genetic liabilities (which are mainly based on Hobbesian instincts of survival and maximization of power). A person who is guided by her Ignorance (*avidhya* or *agyan*) is dominated with *vasanas* which prevent her from understanding the Ultimate Truth. *Avidya* is the outcome of the veil of ignorance (*Maya*) which in turn arises from the three *Gunas* (temperaments) of animalistic human nature (*prakriti*) - *Sattva* (goodness), *Rajas* (passion), *Tamas* (darkness or destruction). *Yoga* helps people get over the bondage of material existence and attain a more spiritual disposition. It must be accompanied by the right and enlightened knowledge (*Gyan* and *Vijnyan*).

DETERMINISM VERSUS FREE WILL

The *Gita,* very interestingly synthesizes the doctrine of absolute devotion to the supreme spirit without granting the latter deterministic agency, while championing the cause of genuine freedom of intellectually conscious individuals, through the use of free will (which although is naturally-, socially- and circumstantially- bounded) to overcome ignorance, desires and purposeless ego that cause the alienation of the individual spirit from the Absolute. In other words, it says that the Absolute Reality exists as a source of true knowledge and freedom, as the end point of all material and spiritual existence, having immanent as well as transcendental qualities in all existence. It, however, is not interested in running the affairs of mortals, as it is not the kind of anthropomorphic Gods that humans like to imagine. Humans must make the conscious effort to realize their immanent Godliness, by transcending their ego, desires, and ignorance. It identifies the survivability- and power- maximizing natural human nature, that is- *prakriti*, being dominated by self-alienating instincts of *animus dominandi* and hedonistic egoism. It identifies the divine duty of humans to overcome such natural deterministic impulses by exercising the free will of the higher self- *purusha*. It also identifies most of the societal, legal, cultural, and religious paraphernalia (including the personalized, anthropomorphic Gods or *Ishwaras*) as being regressive institutions, invented by anthropocentric humans that hold individuals back from realizing their real spiritual potential.

Such an idea that a similar *purusha* (or higher spiritual self) or *atma* inhabits *in and as* us all, taking similar inspiration from the absolute *Brahma,* is based on the assumption that all material objects (including the human body and brain), at similar levels of consciousness, *ceteris paribus,* would behave similarly, if divested of their individual egos, desires, illusions, and incognizance. It can be compared to the social idea of the "General Will", which is broadly composed of the collective will of the aggregate of higher particular egos, which, having transcended their lower selves, return similar outputs on questions of general welfare, as advocated by philosophers like Nicolas Malebranche, Denis Diderot, and especially- Jean-Jacques Rousseau (Bertram, 2017; Munro, 2019).

Therefore, real free will, in a state of inner-liberation and bliss, on condition of absolute merger with the *Brahma,* would, in fact, be under the deterministic automation of the Universal Spirit. Thus, a society or organization composed of a large proportion of enlightened beings or being run on such principles of enlightened duty, or at least on lesser anthropocentric ideals would do better work, be more efficient in its processes and outcomes, and would not harm similar chances of others, while upholding the virtues of horizontal, vertical and inter-generational sustainability. It would possibly imply that whatever global actions or processes are based on the evolutionarily deformed Hobbessian human nature, in the form of realist or liberal politics, growth-oriented libertarian (or even Marxist) economics, machiavellian work-ethics, identity-based social organizations and so on, may be successful in achieving limited material possessions (like the Kauravas did), but, containing the seeds of their own decay, would ultimately be doomed out of their inner contradictions.

ANTHROPOCENTRISM, SPECIESISM, AND ANIMAL AGRICULTURE

This is the age of the Anthropocene- the name of the geologic age, which is named for the first time after a single species, the collective actions of which have substantial and far-reaching consequences, to the extent of shaping history and altering ecological processes (Rafferty, 2019). It is fuelled by the ideology of anthropocentrism. Note that *anthropos* is the Greek word for human.

Anthropocentrism stands for belief in human exceptionalism and tendency to treat non-human entities as objects of instrumental benefit. At a subtler level, this exceptionalism does not apply to all the humans equally but only those in power and who treat other humans (who form the numerical majority of Homo sapiens) as sub-humans or non-humans. Arguably, anthropocentrism is the root cause of most of the major problems that the world faces today including international conflicts, uneven distribution of 'resources' (and conflicts over the same), climate change, over-population among humans, extinction of species, and miserable living conditions of the surviving species. Anthropocentrism is the root cause of nationalism (and imperialism), class and caste-based exploitation, racism, sex- and gender-based exploitation (including homophobia), ableism (physical, psychological and intellectual), social Darwinism, majoritarianism, differences on the basis of ethnicity and culture, elitism, and so on. However, the most underrated, neglected, most widespread, and acute basis of discrimination and exploitation is Speciesism.

Speciesism is the differential treatment and often exploitation accorded on the basis of difference in species. For instance, a human child, at a similar level of intellectual development as another mature animal (with intellect being defined in human terms) is viewed as a societal asset and nurtured with special care, while, the latter is often not even entitled to the basic right to a dignified life and death (Singer, Animal Liberation, 1975, pp. 6-23).

From the aforementioned assertions, it can be deduced that speciesism (which has anthropocentric roots) is, in fact, the ideological basis for animal agriculture. Animal agriculture is the present-day globalized industry of producing animal products- meat, dairy, leather, and so on, often by the use of augmenting technologies and 'resources'. Mushrooming human population with its burgeoning material (including nutritional and gustatory) demands has turned this industry into the greatest inter-species crime in known history. It has been established that the said industry is being responsible for a wide range of global problems, few of which are described below. The list is non-exhaustive and lacks details.

MAJOR CHALLENGES IN THE ANTHROPOCENE CAUSED BY ANIMAL AGRICULTURE

Environmental Insecurity

Environmental insecurity is inclusive of insecurities caused by climate change, resource insecurity, water insecurity, food insecurity, and considering the assumption of universal environmental holism, all of these are inter-related. As far as environmental pollution is concerned, animal agriculture has a substantial role to play. The aforementioned industry is responsible for 18% of greenhouse gas emissions which is far more than that generated by transportation (FAO, 2006). Animal agriculture leads to extinction of species, creates dead zones in oceans, causes water pollution and destroys the natural habitat at an alarming rate (ibid.). The need to maintain sustainability of agricultural assistance without compromising environmental integrity is indispensable (Tilman, Cassman, & Polasky, 2002).

Resource Insecurity

Due to the ever-increasing human population and the subsequent scarcity in resources, the world is in a pretty vulnerable position with 'resources' being consumed at a higher rate than they can be replenished (Dimick, 2014). The emphasis on the word 'resource', whether biotic or abiotic, is to underscore its anthropocentric roots. Rampant deforestation to clear the land to be used as pastures and for growing feed crops has led to an imbalance in the environment which has its own demerits, for instance, animal agriculture results in 91% of the destruction of the Amazon rainforests (Oppenlander, 2013). The water consumed for the production of 1 kilo of rice is around 3500 litres but at the same time, the production of 1 kilo of beef requires around 15000 litres of water and therefore it is necessary in this age of water scarcity to reflect upon our dietary plans (UNDESA, 2014). One can refer to the documentary *Cowspiracy-The Sustainability Secret* or read Food and Agriculture Organization's comprehensive report titled- *Livestock's Long Shadow* to find a large collection of other facts associated with the unsustainability caused by animal agriculture.

Food Insecurity

Apart from the most common and major causes of food insecurity being droughts and social instabilities (also contributed by animal agriculture), animal agriculture (and its subsequent ill-effects caused by unsustainable land use practices, deforestation to create pastures, desertification of land, and so on) has become one of the most crucial problems to reflect upon (UN, 2015). Around 821 million people are hunger-stricken in a world that produces enough food to feed around 10 billion people (Holt-Gimenez, 2012). While 37,000 pounds of plant-based food can be produced using 1.5 acres of land, the same area can only produce 375 pounds of beef (Oppenlander, 2013). Highlighting another point, for instance, soya bean, which is rich in high-grade protein, and, can be used to feed millions of hungry stomachs, is, instead, used largely (around 85% of the total world production) to feed animals, leaving less than ten percent for human consumption (MacDonald & Iyer, 2011). Almost one-third of the harvest of grains in the world is fed to livestock. To produce 28 metric tons of animal protein, 157 million metric tons of plant protein is required (Robbins, 1999, p. 221). The scintilla of energy that we receive (after wasting so much of plant protein) from meat, could have been gained by directly eating a much less amount of plant-based products.

Social and Political Problems Arising From the Above Causes

The significant problems of the world on a deeper level have ecological roots, although on the surface they, on the trunk of the society, have political, economic, religious and ethnic branches. The ever-growing population of the world has resulted in people jockeying over limited resources which in turn leads to large scale antagonisms (Scientist, 2008).

Let us take for instance the Darfur crisis, a series of violent conflicts caused by ecological (including climatic) changes, in Sudan. The conflict started at the local level (aggravated by the famine in the mid-1980s) and eventually gave way to religious, political, and economic tensions at the national level (UNEP, 2007). Scarcity of resources was among the major driving forces (ibid).

The Fulani tribe (inhabiting Sahel and West Africa), the largest nomadic pastoral community of the world, is turning violent against the already settled agriculturists in order to save its own herds and eventually its way of living (Patience, 2016). With the already scanty land and water resources slowly diminishing, the Fulanis are turning to agricultural lands for cattle ranching and thereby destroying crops, while, every rebellion on the part of the farmers is being suppressed with a more violent reaction from the Fulani herdspeople (Mcgregor, 2017).

Migration, based on environmental catastrophes and their impacts, along with the ensuing refugee crisis, is an escalating phenomenon, which the international community will have a hard time responding to.

The resource-based and climate-change-induced-conflicts and related personal, political, social, food-insecurities among humans, *inter alia*, are therefore ecological in origin in which the industry of animal agriculture is one of the greatest causal factors.

Sentience, Moral Degradation and Speciesism

Animal sentience is the capability on the part of animals of subjective perception, feeling, and experience, considering them corporeally, intellectually, and emotionally conscious beings (Allen & Zalta, 2010). According to Jeremy Bentham, the great utilitarian thinker, animals should not be subjected to suffering because of the fact that they are biologically or intellectually different from humans (Crimmins, 2019). In this anthropocentric world, the sufferings of humans are treated with much more gravity than the sufferings of animals, which is the outcome of speciesism. Speciesism, the term popularized by Peter Singer (the author of *Animal Liberation*, 1975), refers to the mass-scale discrimination and abuse on the basis of difference in species (Singer & Yancy, 2015).

A Case for Veganism as a Possible Response to Some of Those Challenges

The industry of animal agriculture has sustained for ages for it has been feeding fat to the anthropocentric human's greed, regardless of the threats it poses to the environment. Apart from its contributions to the clothing industry, the fertilizer industry, and so on, its major contribution is to the food industry.

The plant kingdom can easily stand as a replacement and provide us with all the basic necessities that we otherwise get from the aforementioned industry. Animals (including humans) are highly energy-inefficient creatures- they consume a lot and utilize only a negligible amount of energy for the same. In the food chain, when energy is transferred from one trophic level to another, only at most ten percent of the transferred energy is utilized and the rest is lost. So, when a person consumes an animal that is at a higher trophic level (heterotrophs) than plant products (autotrophs), she tends to waste at least ten times more energy than a person with a vegetarian diet would (Brennan, 2017).

The fact needs to be realized that meat is not a necessity and its ever-rising demands to satisfy human gluttony needs to be put to an end by shifting to plant-based or vegan diets and to other similar choices. Another alternative would be to enhance their physiological systems and change the way human body processes and digests food. Till this transhuman (or technologically enhanced) approach is actualized, the least we could do is spare the (mostly artificial) lives of those billions of animals who are bred to only lose their lives in the cruelest way possible only to fill our huge platters. The best and easiest way to do that would be adopting veganism.

DOES GITA PROMOTE VEGANISM?

No and yes! The *Bhagwad Gita* does not give any specific and particular prescription about anything. Whatever instruction Krishna furnished to Arjuna in the battlefield of Kurukshetra was of a very local and temporal nature. What of eternal and universal significance it offers are broad principles of how to arrive at virtuous principles of actions. It therefore is a text offering meta-principles, to be referred to while diagnosing problems of a contextual nature, in their special circumstances. It therefore can be deduced with maximum certainty, as will be reasoned subsequently, that the *Gita* would oppose tooth-and-nail the anthropocentric and exploitative industry of animal agriculture, one of the antidotes to which is changing individual dietary habits to more plant-based ones, towards absolute veganism.

It is an established fact that the industry of animal agriculture is a key factor in global affairs that is responsible for a great deal of global problems and even greater level of individual sufferings among sentient beings. It is appropriate, therefore, to assume that it is being run on wrong, unsustainable, and immoral principles, and has adopted dreadful means to achieve egoistic ends.

Any so called 'problem' or 'suffering' as is mentioned above, being value-laden, according to what conscious subjects may understand and evaluate, by its very nature, is a problem associated with and dependent upon the use of or appeal to consciousness. It is only because human subjects have consciousness, that they distinguish between good and bad, right and wrong, with such an evaluation being dependent upon the previous assumptions of some value-based principles or some naturally acquired instincts, based on some limited context. Therefore, so long as we do not understand all the mysteries of nature, the reason and purpose (if any) behind the expansion of the galaxies, and the strange quantum-level behavior of subatomic particles, it would be most desirable and pragmatic to focus on the issues of this world, all of which are issue associated with consciousness, something the *Gita* is most concerned with, and, most of the macro-level ones are the result of anthropocentrism, something the *Gita* is dia-metrically opposed to.

The industry of animal agriculture, as has been established, is not only preposterously harmful for the major stakeholders- the billions of conscious animals exploitatively involved, and, also the majority of humans (as is argued earlier), but also has wide-ranging direct and indirect impacts on the personal, economic, and moral wellbeing of humans, as well as causes purposeless and extensive harms of a systemic (global) nature. Therefore, the said industry even does not stand the test of the anthropocentric ethics (that humans have invented for interactions among them, based on human-consciousness) by far. Various studies have conclusively proven that animal-based foods, in fact, are harmful for human health and wellbeing, and afflict humans through a number of different ways which may not be highlighted in this paper.

That happiness which is derived from contact of the senses with their objects and which appears like nectar at first but poison at the end is said to be of the nature of passion. XVIII, 38 (Prabhupada, 1972)

Talking about today's *Dharma*, utilitarianism arguably is the leading theory behind most of human legal, ethical, and moral considerations. It holds that conscious subjects are predisposed to maximize pleasure, and more importantly, to minimize sufferings, and so- all legal, ethical and moral considerations should be designed to achieve or further such ends. In its original form, as enunciated by the likes of Jeremy Bentham (whose ideas have revolutionized the modern legal and ethical systems), it considers all sentient subjects, irrespective of their species, as worthy of equitable moral considerations, only on the basis of their ability to feel pain and the tendency to avoid it, and on no other basis as rationality, intelligence, power, and so on. Such an idea is also consistent in its essence with an enlightened interpretation of Kantian doctrine of Categorical Imperatives that may hold, among other things, that every conscious entity (and not merely humans as in the original doctrine) must be treated as an end in itself and never a means to further another's ends.

Associated as well as rival theories to utilitarianism, as the theories of Kantian Ethics (and other Deontological theories), Theological Ethics, Epicureanism, Stoicism, Buddhist Ethics, Ethical (or Moral) Intuitionism, theories related to Virtue Ethics, and so on, arguably, are concerned with achieving similar ends associated with subjects' consciousness, although may differ in their approaches.

Animal agriculture, if put to test, based on the broader principles of these ethical theories of the day (if taken to their logical conclusion and after removing the egocentric inconsistencies), is bound to fail by a steep margin, exposing the massive deep-rooted contradictions and organized hypocrisies inherent in anthropocentric practices of a systemic nature.

The Mahabharata War was fought over issues and principles. One of the major ones was the alleged outraging the modesty of Draupadi (the wife to the Pandava princes), by the Kauravas. Krishna reasons it as a crime of a social nature, of an enormous magnitude, and not just a personal wrong. Today, the world witnesses speciesism as arguably the greatest ethical scourge in the known history of inter-species relations. The globalized industry of animal agriculture is arguably the greatest organized crime in the history of earth, inflicted by the members of one species over others. Even extinction would be preferred over such undignified survival- undergoing harrowing experiences, just to ultimately end up on a plate.

The God in the *Gita,* being devoid of any attributes, is disposed to treat every entity, at a similar level of material and conscious existence, equitably and similarly, without entertaining unreasonably discriminating ideologies like racism, nationalism, communalism, sexism, and also- speciesism.

Speciesism, today (and since known times), is debatably the greatest threat to *Dharma,* responsible for the agonizing slaying of approximately three billion conscious beings daily, at an age when more environmentally sustainable alternatives are widely available and physical sufferings among privileged humans are at an all-time low. Such a paradox is the outcome of anthropocentrism, which is becoming a liability upon it, responsible for all the macro-level problems one can conceive, and something the *Gita* strongly opposes, considering any egoistic ideology as sinful.

Therefore, animal agriculture, fails the test of the *Dharma* of the age, and arguably is not in tune with the *Riti,* as far as the writer understands it. It would, therefore, be the *dharmic karma* (righteous duty) of the enlightened subject to rescue the global system of its massive ethical cleavage, being based on unreasonable and purposeless anthropocentrism that are taking it away from order and towards anarchical chaos. Anarchy and chaos, just like any other localized destruction is not altogether ruled out in the *Gita*. However, any such destruction must be constructive in its purpose and intent, in the broader scheme of things, leading to strengthening of the global *dharma,* without involving unwarranted sufferings upon conscious subjects (such as hapless animals). Even while exhorting Arjuna to kill the Kauravas in battle, for the sake of essentialist *dharma,* Krishna advised Arjuna to cleanse his heart of any evil purpose and of hatred, and to treat his enemies with fundamental respect, love, and empathy. Mahatma Gandhi had once said- "The greatness of a nation and its moral progress can be judged by the way its animals are treated", was also influenced by this doctrine of avoiding unnecessary violence and sufferings (both in action and in intent) in the pursuance of one's duty. The *Gita* considers it the moral duty of persons of eminence to adopt *Dharmic* principles in the direction of *loksamgraha* or general welfare.

Kings such as Janaka and others attained the perfectional stage by performance of prescribed duties. Therefore, just for the sake of educating the people in general, you should perform your work. III, 20 (Prabhupada, 1972)

Today's celebrities, intellectuals, leaders, *inter alios,* and have a special responsibility of spreading awareness and leading by example. Antonio Gramsci, in his theory on intellectuals, considers it to be a much larger category of individuals than is commonly understood, who may not even realize their roles in legitimizing or delegitimizing ideologies, therefore, there is a role of every social being in the creation and propagation of norms and upholding *Dharma*.

The *Gyan Marga* or the path of knowledge would possibly lead a rational human subject to arrive at this conclusion regarding the wastefulness, unsustainability, and immorality associated with the said industry. It neither helps humans attain their spiritual bliss and of course- nor the other animals. Rather, it is the manifestation of the unquenchable human ego, in the pursuit of gustatory pleasure that makes any spiritual transcendence impossible. Moreover, it also prevents such a large number of animals from realizing their subjective peace, by overwhelming their consciousness with harrowing sensory sufferings. Transcendence of both hedonistic pleasure (in case of privileged humans) and of physical and psychological agony (as in exploited animals and underprivileged humans) is the *sine qua non* for realizing their relative spiritual experience.

Other animals, lack free will, as compared to and in nature of that in humans, and, therefore are under the greater deterministic influence of their natural impulses, which makes them lead more agitated and tormented lives, at least physically (if not psychologically), making the attainment of peace an impulsively determined phenomena. It would, therefore, be befitting upon conscious human subjects to show greater empathy and care to other animals, with respect to the treatment appropriate at their level of consciousness, at least of a sensorial and physical nature. The *Gita,* as emphasized earlier, promotes the adoption of the principle of *laissez-faire* and of tolerance, with respect to those entities that may not be able to achieve the expected level of consciousness, or have it of a different kind.

He who has no ill will to any being, who is friendly and compassionate, free from egoism, and self-sense, ever-minded in pain and pleasure and patient... XII, 13 (Radhakrishnan, 2014, pp. 350-351)

The egoistic and exploitative *anthropos* in anthropocentrism is the one who, in nature, is not much different from another animal, being slavish to her natural impulses, and even adding fuel to those by employing the capacities of an advanced and more rational brain towards irrational ends. Advocates of voluntarism like Leibniz, Augustine, Nietzsche, Kant, Pascal, *inter alios*, maintain that- humans are anything but truly intellectually rational agents, who tend to use their reasons towards securing practical, rather than pure or Godly ends. Therefore, any solution must require the transcendence from anthropocentrism. The *Gita* also recognizes that even conscious subjects, even after having attained spiritual knowledge, are constrained by their impulsive natures (*prakriti*), and, show a tendency of reverting to their original impulsive states.

Even a man of knowledge acts according to his own nature, for everyone follows his nature. III, 33 (Prabhupada, 1972)

The *Gita*, nevertheless, has some direct references with respect to the food one may eat:

Foods in the mode of goodness increase the duration of life, purify one's existence and give strength, health, happiness and satisfaction. Such nourishing foods are sweet, juicy, fatty and palatable. Foods that are too bitter, too sour, salty, pungent, dry and hot, are liked by people in the mode of passion. Such foods cause pain, distress, and disease. Food cooked... (that takes relatively longer to prepare)... which is tasteless, stale, putrid, decomposed and unclean, is food liked by people in the mode of ignorance. XVII, 8, 9, 10 (Prabhupada, 1972)

Analyzing the above stanza just with respect to plant-based and animal-based foods, one can scientifically conclude that the prescribed foods broadly can be associated with plant-based ones. It is scientifically proven that a vegan diet is good for digestion; tastes decent; causes less inflammation, diseases, obesity, and other bodily problems; is easier to prepare (and to grow, store, transport, and dispose); causes infinitely lesser pain (including to the eaten); is cleaner (containing less of bad fat, puss, biomagnified pollutants, parasites, microorganisms, and so on, and causes much less defiling of local surroundings and damage to the environment); keeping arguments of moral purity aside.

Moreover, the *Gita* considers the restrains put on consumption of different kinds foods, and intake of 'sacred food' as ways of performing *yajnya* or sacrifice, in the process of expressing devotion to the absolute, noting that restraint is the essence of all sacrifices and means to spiritual growth (Radhakrishnan, 2014, p. 195).

The *Gita* considers those who prevent others from realizing their spiritual or even material truths as sinners, and thus advocates as much individual freedom from external constraints as possible, bearing in mind the 'harm principle' and other truly 'reasonable restrictions', of an individual (*svadharmic*) and of a systemic (*sadharan-dharmic*) nature. The *Gita* is genuinely concerned with maximizing individual freedom, which is quite distinct, more universally inclusive, and much more sustainable than the liberal notion of economic liberty or Marxian notion of material freedom, being in consonance with social and ecological harmony.

It may be argued that killing other animals in it may be justified in some contexts, as in maintaining the natural ecological balance. However, the present day industry of animal agriculture is doing anything but that, by trying to respond to the unquenchable and egoistic wants (and not needs) of an ever-expanding population (with its exponentially magnifying material demands), by taking any means possible, including of artificially reproducing animals in large quantities, expanding production with the input of latest technologies, with least respect to the quality of their conscious existence.

CONCLUSION

Therefore, considering the essence of the *Gita;* the nature of the God described; the contextual understanding of *Dharma* in the 21ˢᵗ Century; the capabilities of conscious humans and the options available to them; the bane of anthropocentrism and of speciesism and the mega-level harms they lead to; the scourge of the industry of animal agriculture over global sustainability and over individual sentient beings; the practical far-reaching and comprehensive benefits of moving towards plant-based diets; it could be contended with conviction that the *Gita* would vigorously promote veganism!

The *Gita* adopts the universal (or the global) as the level of analysis, with the all-encompassing (spiritual and material) *Brahma* as the whole, to evaluate the principles of righteousness and of ethical conduct, to respond to individuals (especially conscious ones) as the units of analysis. It attempts to rationalize and synthesize individual wellbeing with universal sustainability. It does not discriminate on the basis of any imaginary grounds, and is dedicated to enhance the genuine freedom and happiness of all in the most sustainable way possible. The only distinction it makes is on the basis of material existence (including the level of consciousness) and spiritual transcendence, while adhering to equitability and tolerance in individual treatment, including prescribing more empathetic treatment to entities at a lower level of consciousness.

On the eve of the battle, Arjuna requests Krishna to take the chariot to the center of the field so that he could do a better analysis of the situation at hand. This shows the significance of taking into consideration all the possible perspectives available before arriving at any action or conclusion. The warrior gets an equidistant view of the entire scenario which helps him to take an informed decision through the guidance of Krishna. This symbolically means being reflective and going beyond the confines of one's senses, biases, pre-occupations, while at the same time trying to analyze the situation of the antithesis from a closer perspective. Coming to the non-fictional world, the case for veganism demands a similar retrospection. A macro level analysis would show us the gruesome impacts of the industry of animal agriculture on our environment, not to mention the suffering of the animals and the unnecessary exhaustion of various kinds of resources. Further, we need to introspect over our reaction to the entire problem, going beyond our inherent biases. The idea of turning vegan, although challenging, would be the best way to handle some of the major problems of the world today.

Veganism remains one of the most revolutionary ideas, more relevant than ever in the Anthropocene, and the *Gita* remains one of the most effective ways for any individual to attain philosophical guidance, practical direction, spiritual contentment, and lasting peace, while contributing to universal harmony, while not renouncing one's worldly roles, without the need of turning nuns and monks. India has witnessed the all-incorporating and non-violent doctrines of Jainism, Buddhism, and Sanatan Dharma, has witnessed philosophers and leaders who have espoused vegetarian and even vegan ethics, which are part of the faith of the large section of its population. The recent surge of veganism, in the Western

Hemisphere, is associated with the contextual and rationalistic realization of *Dharma* or *Gyan* relevant to this age. A synthesis of associated ideas regarding the right *Gyan*, appropriate *Karma* and effective *Bhakti* would go a long distance to make the world a more livable place for all!

REFERENCES

Allen, C., & Zalta, E. N. (2010, 10 13). *Animal Consciousness*. Retrieved 02 13, 2019, from Stanford Encyclopedia of Philosophy (Summer 2011 Edition): https://plato.stanford.edu/archives/sum2011/entries/consciousness-animal/

Aronson, R. (2017, 04 10). *Albert Camus*. Retrieved 02 18, 2019, from The Stanford Encyclopedia of Philosophy: https://plato.stanford.edu/entries/camus/

Bertram, C. (2017). *Jean Jacques Rousseau*. Retrieved 02 13, 2019, from The Stanford Encyclopedia of Philosophy: https://plato.stanford.edu/entries/rousseau/#IdeaGeneWill

Brennan, J. (2017, 04 25). *How Does Being a Vegetarian Conserve Overall Energy in Trophic Levels*. Retrieved 02 14, 2019, from Sciencing: https://sciencing.com/being-vegetarian-conserve-overall-energy-trophic-levels-3342.html

Chatterjee, S., & Datta, D. (2018). *An Introduction to Indian Philosophy*. New Delhi: Rupa Publications.

Crimmins, J. E. (2019, 01 28). *Jeremy Bentham*. Retrieved 02 13, 2019, from The Stanford Encyclopedia of Philosophy: https://plato.stanford.edu/entries/bentham/

Dimick, D. (2014, 08 21). *As World's Population Booms, Will Its Resources Be Enough for Us?* Retrieved 02 13, 2019, from National Geographic: https://news.nationalgeographic.com/news/2014/09/140920-population-11billion-demographics-anthropocene/

Duignan, B. (2018, 09 27). *Democritus*. Retrieved 02 18, 2019, from Encyclopædia Britannica: https://www.britannica.com/biography/Democritus

FAO. (2006). *Livestock's Long Shadow - Environmental Issues and Options*. LEAD - FAO.

Flynn, T. (2011, 11 05). *Jean-Paul Sartre*. Retrieved 02 18, 2019, from The Stanford Encyclopedia of Philosophy: https://plato.stanford.edu/entries/sartre/

Holt-Gimenez, E. (2012). *We Already Grow Enough For 10 Billion People... and Still Can't End Hunger*. Common Dreams.

Khan, D. (2012, 12 13). *Energy Consumption of The Human Body*. Retrieved 02 14, 2019, from Stanford University: http://large.stanford.edu/courses/2012/ph240/khan1/

Koshland Science Museum. (2019). *Tracing Similarities and Differences in Our DNA*. Retrieved 02 18, 2019, from Putting DNA to work: https://www.koshland-science-museum.org/sites/all/exhibits/exhibitdna/intro03.jsp

MacDonald, M., & Iyer, S. (2011). Skillful Means - The Challenges for China's Encounter with Factory Farming - [New York: Brighter Green.]. *Policy Brief*, 1.

Mcgregor, A. (2017, February). *The Fulani Crisis: Violence and Radicalization in the Sahel*. Retrieved February 12, 2019, from Combating Terrorism Center: https://ctc.usma.edu

Melsen, A. G. (2019). *Atomism*. Retrieved 02 11, 2019, from Encyclopædia Britannica: https://www.britannica.com/topic/atomism#ref561364

Morson, G. S. (2019, 02 14). *Fyodor Dostoyevsky*. Retrieved 02 18, 2019, from Encyclopædia Britannica: https://www.britannica.com/biography/Fyodor-Dostoyevsky

Munro, A. (2019). *General Will - Philosophy of Rousseau*. Retrieved 02 13, 2019, from Encyclopædia Britannica: https://www.britannica.com/topic/general-will

Oppenlander, R. A. (2013). *Food Choice and Sustainability: Why Buying Local, Eating Less Meat, and Taking Baby Steps Won't Work*. Minneapolis: Publish Green.

Patience, M. (2016, 07 10). *Nigeria's deadly battle for land: Herdsmen v farmers*. Retrieved 02 13, 2019, from BBC News: https://www.bbc.com/news/world-africa-37021044

Philosophy Index. (2019). *Absurdism*. Retrieved 02 18, 2019, from Philosophy Index: http://www.philosophy-index.com/existentialism/absurd.php

Prabhupada, A. B. (1972). *Bhagavad-gita As It Is*. Los Angeles: www.Krishna.com

Prabhupada, B. S. (1998). *Bhagavad-Gita As It Is*. Los Angeles: Bhaktivedanta Book Trust International.

Radhakrishnan, S. (1948). *Indian Philosophy* (Vol. I). London: George Allen & Unwin Ltd.

Radhakrishnan, S. (1948). *Indian Philosophy* (Vol. II). London: George Allen & Unwin Ltd.

Radhakrishnan, S. (2014). *The Bhagavadgita*. Noida: Harper Element.

Radhakrishnan, S., & Moore, A. C. (1957). *A Source Book in Indian Philosophy*. Princeton: Princeton University Press. doi:10.1515/9781400865062

Rafferty, J. P. (2019). *Anthropocene Epoch*. Retrieved 02 16, 2019, from Encyclopædia Britannica: https://www.britannica.com/science/Anthropocene-Epoch

Redding, P. (2015, 08 04). *Georg Wilhelm Friedrich Hegel*. Retrieved 02 18, 2019, from The Stanford Encyclopedia of Philosophy: https://plato.stanford.edu/entries/hegel/

Robbins, R. (1999). *Global Problems and the Culture of Capitalism*. Allyn and Bacon.

Ruzsa, F. (2019). *Sankhya*. Retrieved 02 18, 2019, from Internet Encyclopedia of Philosophy: https://www.iep.utm.edu/sankhya/

Scientist, N. (2008, 12 10). *New Scientist*. Retrieved 02 13, 2019, from Darfur crisis is stripping the environment: https://www.newscientist.com/article/dn16248-darfur-crisis-is-stripping-the-environment/

Sencindiver, S. Y. (2017, 07 26). *New Materialism*. Retrieved 02 15, 2019, from Oxford Bibliographies Online: http://www.oxfordbibliographies.com/view/document/obo-9780190221911/obo-9780190221911-0016.xml

Singer, P. (1975). *Animal Liberation*. Harper Collins.

Singer, P., & Yancy, G. (2015, May 27). *Peter Singer: On Racism, Animal Rights and Human Rights.* Retrieved 02 14, 2019, from The New York Times: https://opinionator.blogs.nytimes.com/2015/05/27/peter-singer-on-speciesism-and-racism/

Sorell, T. (2018, 11 30). *Thomas Hobbes.* Retrieved 02 18, 2019, from Encyclopædia Britannica: https://www.britannica.com/biography/Thomas-Hobbes

Tilman, D., Cassman, K. G., & Polasky, S. (2002). Agricultural sustainability and intensive production practices. *Nature, 418*(6898), 671–677. doi:10.1038/nature01014 PMID:12167873

UNDESA. (2014). *International Decade for Action 'Water for Life' 2005-2015.* Retrieved 02 13, 2019, from Water for Life Decade: http://www.un.org/waterforlifedecade/food_security.shtml

UNEP. (2007). *Sudan- Post-Conflict Environmental Assessment.* Nairobi: UNEP.

This research was previously published in Science and Spirituality for a Sustainable World edited by Deepanjali Mishra; pages 125-152, copyright year 2019 by Information Science Reference (an imprint of IGI Global).

Index

B

C

D

F

M

T

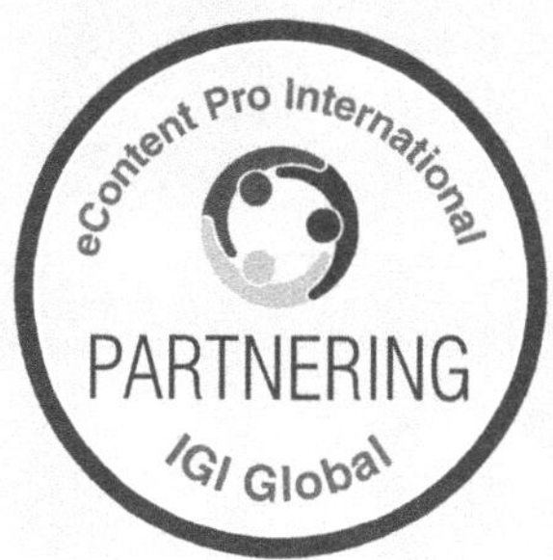

IGI Global Proudly Partners With eContent Pro International

Receive a 25% Discount on all Editorial Services

Editorial Services

IGI Global expects all final manuscripts submitted for publication to be in their final form. This means they must be reviewed, revised, and professionally copy edited prior to their final submission. Not only does this support with accelerating the publication process, but it also ensures that the highest quality scholarly work can be disseminated.

English Language Copy Editing

Let eContent Pro International's expert copy editors perform edits on your manuscript to resolve spelling, punctuaion, grammar, syntax, flow, formatting issues and more.

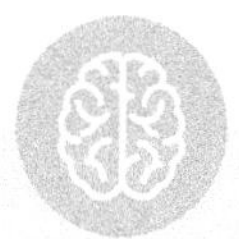

Scientific and Scholarly Editing

Allow colleagues in your research area to examine the content of your manuscript and provide you with valuable feedback and suggestions before submission.

Figure, Table, Chart & Equation Conversions

Do you have poor quality figures? Do you need visual elements in your manuscript created or converted? A design expert can help!

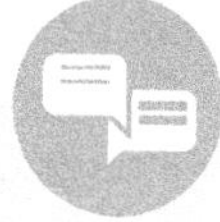

Translation

Need your documjent translated into English? eContent Pro International's expert translators are fluent in English and more than 40 different languages.

Email: customerservice@econtentpro.com　　　　**www.igi-global.com/editorial-service-partners**